TUREK'S ORTHOPAEDICS

Principles and Their Application

FIFTH EDITION

Editors

Stuart L. Weinstein, MD

Ignacio V. Ponseti Professor of Orthopaedic Surgery
University of Iowa College of Medicine
Iowa City, Iowa

Joseph A. Buckwalter, MD

Professor of Orthopaedic Surgery
University of Iowa College of Medicine
Iowa City, Iowa

27 Contributors

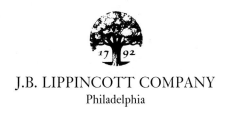

J.B. LIPPINCOTT COMPANY
Philadelphia

Acquisitions Editor: James D. Ryan
Sponsoring Editor: Delois Patterson
Associate Managing Editor: Grace R. Caputo
Designer: Doug Smock
Cover Designer: Tom Jackson
Production Manager: Caren Erlichman
Senior Production Coordinator: Kevin P. Johnson
Indexer: Alexandra Nickerson
Compositor: Tapsco, Inc.
Prepress: Jay's Publishers Services, Inc.
Printer/Binder: Arcata Graphics/Kingsport
Color Insert Printer: Princeton Polychrome Press

5th Edition

Copyright © 1994 by J.B. Lippincott Company.
Copyright © 1984, 1977, 1967, 1959 by J.B. Lippincott Company. All rights reserved. No part of this book may be used or reproduced in any manner whatsoever without written permission except for brief quotations embodied in critical articles and reviews. Printed in the United States of America. For information write J.B. Lippincott Company, 227 East Washington Square, Philadelphia, PA 19106.
This book printed on acid-free paper.

6   5   4   3   2

Library of Congress Cataloging-in-Publication Data

Turek's Orthopaedics, principles and their application.—5th ed./
    editors, Stuart L. Weinstein, Joseph A. Buckwalter; 27 contributors.
        p.   cm.
    Rev. ed. of: Orthopaedics, principles and their application/Samuel L. Turek. 4th ed. ©1984.
    Includes bibliographical references and index.
    ISBN 0-397-50692-9
    1. Orthopaedics.   I. Turek, Samuel L. Orthopaedics.
II. Weinstein, Stuart L.   III. Buckwalter, Joseph A.   IV. Title:
Orthopáedics, principles and their application.
    [DNLM: 1. Orthopedics.   WE   168   T9342   1994]
RD731.T8   1994
617.3—dc20
DNLM/DLC
for Library of Congress   93-39198
                                                                    CIP

Every effort has been made to ensure drug selections and dosages are in accordance with current recommendations and practice. Because of ongoing research, changes in government regulations, and the constant flow of information on drug therapy, reactions, and interactions, the reader is cautioned to check the package insert for each drug for indications, dosages, warnings, and precautions, particularly if the drug is new or infrequently used.

Contributors

Robert F. Ashman, MD
Professor and Director
Rheumatology Division
University of Iowa College of Medicine
Iowa City, Iowa

George S. Bassett, MD
Associate Professor of Orthopaedic Surgery
University of Southern California School of Medicine
Los Angeles, California

Joseph A. Buckwalter, MD
Professor of Orthopaedic Surgery
University of Iowa College of Medicine
Iowa City, Iowa

John S. Cowdery, MD
Associate Professor of Medicine
University of Iowa College of Medicine
Iowa City, Iowa

Edward V. Craig, MD
Associate Professor
University of Minnesota Medical School—
  Minneapolis
Attending Physician
University of Minnesota Hospital
Minneapolis, Minnesota

Alan D. Croock, MD
Assistant Professor of Medicine
Rheumatology Division
Baylor College of Medicine
Houston, Texas

Frederick R. Dietz, MD
Professor of Orthopaedic Surgery
University of Iowa College of Medicine
Iowa City, Iowa

Georges Y. El-Khoury, MD
Professor of Radiology and Orthopaedic Surgery
University of Iowa College of Medicine
Iowa City, Iowa

Elizabeth H. Field, MD
Associate Professor of Medicine
University of Iowa College of Medicine
Department of Veterans Affairs Medical Center
Iowa City, Iowa

Neil E. Green, MD
Professor and Vice Chairman
Orthopaedics and Rehabilitation
Vanderbilt University School of Medicine
Nashville, Tennessee

Eric T. Jones, MD
Clinical Professor of Orthopaedic Surgery
West Virginia University School of Medicine
Morgantown, West Virginia

Mary M. Jones, MD
Assistant Professor of Pediatrics
University of Iowa College of Medicine
Iowa City, Iowa

Robert W. Karr, MD
Division of Rheumatology
University of Iowa College of Medicine
Iowa City, Iowa

Roger A. Mann, MD
Associate Clinical Professor of Orthopaedic Surgery
Director, Foot Fellowship Program
University of California, San Francisco, Medical
  School
Oakland, California

Philip Mayer, MD
Associate Professor of Clinical Orthopaedics
Wayne State University School of Medicine
Detroit Medical Center
Detroit, Michigan

Roy A. Meals, MD
Associate Professor of Orthopaedic Surgery
University of California, Los Angeles, UCLA School
  of Medicine
Chief, Combined Orthopaedic–Plastic Hand Surgery
  Service
UCLA Medical Center
Wadsworth VA Medical Center
Los Angeles, California

Mark A. Mehlhoff, MD
Private Practice
Iowa Medical Clinic
Mercy Medical Center
Cedar Rapids, Iowa

Timothy E. Moore, MB, ChB, FRACP
Associate Professor of Radiology
University of Nebraska Medical Center
Omaha, Nebraska

Stanley J. Naides, MD
Associate Professor of Medicine
Division of Rheumatology
University of Iowa College of Medicine
Clinical Investigator
Department of Veterans Affairs Medical Center
Iowa City, Iowa

Richard R. Olson, MD
Assistant Professor of Medicine
University of Iowa College of Medicine
Iowa City, Iowa

Peter D. Pizzutillo, MD
Professor of Orthopaedic Surgery and Pediatrics
Jefferson Medical College of Thomas Jefferson
  University
Attending Orthopaedic Surgeon
Thomas Jefferson University Hospital
Philadelphia, Pennsylvania

John W. Rachow, PhD, MD
Assistant Professor of Medicine
University of Iowa College of Medicine
Iowa City, Iowa

Karim Rezai, MD
Associate Professor of Radiology
University of Iowa College of Medicine
Iowa City, Iowa

Louise H. Sparks, MD
Mercy Hospital
Iowa City, Iowa

M. Paul Strottmann, MD
Associate Professor of Internal Medicine
Division of Rheumatology
University of Iowa College of Medicine
Iowa City, Iowa

Stuart L. Weinstein, MD
Ignacio V. Ponseti Professor of Orthopaedic Surgery
University of Iowa College of Medicine
Iowa City, Iowa

Russell E. Windsor, MD
Associate Professor of Surgery (Orthopaedics)
Cornell University Medical College
Associate Chief, The Knee Service
Hospital for Special Surgery
New York, New York

Preface

Since the first edition of Samuel Turek's *Orthopaedics: Principles and Their Application*, no specialty has grown more rapidly or developed the ability to provide medical, surgical, and orthotic care to a more diverse group of patients than has orthopaedics. This rapid progress has dramatically improved the quality of life for children and adults with painful and disabling conditions of the musculoskeletal system. As the specialty has grown and diversified, so have the methods of providing orthopaedic education. The past several decades have seen the appearance of many new orthopaedic journals, textbooks, monographs, courses, video tapes and computer-based programs that meet the needs of orthopaedic subspecialties. These changes in the specialty of orthopaedics and in orthopaedic education require significant revision of Dr. Turek's classic textbook to provide a concise, current presentation of pediatric and adult musculoskeletal disorders.

The fifth edition of *Turek's Orthopaedics* retains the broad approach to adult and pediatric orthopaedics, but musculoskeletal trauma and the details of surgical techniques have been eliminated. The book has been shortened to one volume and reorganized to reflect current orthopaedic knowledge and practice. It now includes a detailed section on imaging of the musculoskeletal system. The eight basic science chapters have been updated and condensed, and the chapters on peripheral vascular disease, skin grafting, and amputation have been deleted. Each section includes concise annotated bibliographies selected by the authors.

Reading *Turek's Orthopaedics* cover to cover will provide orthopaedic residents, residents in other specialties, and medical students with a strong interest in orthopaedics a broad presentation of the specialty of orthopaedics and current adult and pediatric orthopaedics. It consists of three sections: Orthopaedics and the Musculoskeletal System, General Disorders of the Musculoskeletal System, and Regional Disorders of the Musculoskeletal System. Section I provides the reader with an overview of the specialty of orthopaedics and its relation to the musculoskeletal system, covering the current organization and scope of the clinical specialty, the tissues of the musculoskeletal system, and the imaging of these tissues. Readers familiar with the specialty of orthopaedics may want to skip the first chapter. Section II covers the generalized disorders of the musculoskeletal system, including infection, rheumatic diseases, neuromuscular diseases, hereditary and idiopathic diseases, and neoplasms. The final section covers the specific regional disorders of the musculoskeletal system, including the neck, the spine, and the upper and lower extremities.

Although this fifth edition of *Orthopaedics* differs considerably from the first, it has the same purpose—to transmit a fund of knowledge that stimulates enthusiasm for the practice of orthopaedics and creates interest and curiosity that lead to further investigations that advance the specialty.

Stuart L. Weinstein, MD
Joseph A. Buckwalter, MD

Contents

TUREK'S
ORTHOPAEDICS
Principles and Their Application

I

Orthopaedics and the Musculoskeletal System

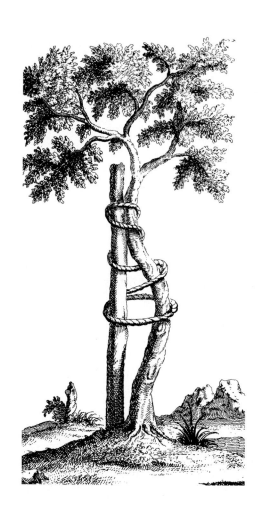

1

Turek's Orthopaedics: Principles and Their Application, Fifth Edition, edited by Stuart L. Weinstein and Joseph A. Buckwalter. J.B. Lippincott Company, Philadelphia, © 1994.

Joseph A. Buckwalter

The Specialty of Orthopaedics

Orthopaedics is the broad-based medical and surgical specialty dedicated to the prevention, diagnosis, and treatment of diseases and injuries of the musculoskeletal system. The frequency and impact of these diseases and injuries combined with recent advances in diagnosis and treatment of musculoskeletal disorders make orthopaedics a critical part of health care. Most medical students learn that orthopaedists treat fractures, repair athlete's knee injuries, and replace arthritic hips and knees, but only a few receive a broader education in orthopaedics. As a result, many physicians, including some orthopaedic residents in the early years of their orthopaedic education, have limited understanding of the specialty of orthopaedics.

This chapter introduces the specialty of orthopaedics. It reviews the importance of musculoskeletal disorders, the development of the specialty of orthopaedics, the evaluation of orthopaedic patients, the spectrum of current orthopaedic treatments, the subspecialties of orthopaedics, and the role of orthopaedic research in improving care for patients with musculoskeletal disorders.

MUSCULOSKELETAL DISORDERS

Diseases and injuries of the musculoskeletal system cause pain, deformity, and loss of function. They limit activity and cause disability for more people than disorders of any other organ system. Musculoskeletal problems rank second in frequency as the reason that patients seek medical attention, and about 10% of US citizens have musculoskeletal problems severe enough to restrict their activity. Congenital malformations of the musculoskeletal system—such as spina bifida, congenital dislocation of the hip, and congenital scoliosis—occur more frequently than malformations of any other organ system. Diseases and injuries of the musculoskeletal system rarely threaten life, but they adversely affect the quality of life, and they rank second only to diseases of the circulatory system in economic cost.

Physicians usually classify musculoskeletal disorders by the functional units of the musculoskeletal system—for example, disorders of the hip, knee, cervical spine, or hand. The tissues that form these functional units include bone, cartilage, dense fibrous tissues (tendon, ligament, fascia, and joint capsule), muscle, peripheral nerves, and peripheral blood vessels. These tissues and the specific structures formed from them change with development, growth, aging, and changes in use. With skeletal maturation, bones change not only in size and shape but also in density and material properties. With aging, bone shape, density, and strength continue to change. A persistent decrease in repetitive loading of bone (eg, immobilization of the leg in a cast) decreases bone density and strength. A persistent increase in repetitive loading of bone (eg, training for athletic competition) increases bone density and strength. Failure to use a joint for a prolonged time decreases the extensibility of the periarticular tissues including tendons, ligaments, and muscles, and may cause loss of articular cartilage and accumulation of fibrous and fatty tissue in the joint; as a result, joint motion decreases. In contrast, repetitive use of a joint, accompanied by attempts to stretch the periarticular tissues, can increase the joint range of motion. The other musculoskeletal tissues show similar changes with development, growth, aging, and persistent changes in use and repetitive loading. Thus, successful treatment of disorders like a clubfoot deformity requires methods of correcting the initial deformity and of maintaining the correction that accommodate for the age-related changes and adaptability of the musculoskeletal system.

Musculoskeletal disorders vary in extent, chronicity, and the tissues affected. They may be localized like an idiopathic clubfoot deformity or degenerative joint disease of the thumb carpometacarpal joint, or generalized like Marfan's syndrome and rheumatoid arthritis. Acute problems, like a septic hip joint, require emergency medical and surgical treatment. Chronic problems, like degenerative disease of the hip, may be treated symptomatically for many years in most patients. Although many problems treated by orthopaedists involve bony abnormalities, musculoskeletal disorders frequently involve multiple tissues in addition to bone, and some have minimal or no affect on bone. An idiopathic congenital clubfoot deformity may appear to result from disturbances of bone formation and development, but the deformity also includes abnormalities of tendons, ligaments, peripheral nerves, skeletal muscle, and other soft tissues.

The causes of musculoskeletal disorders include trauma and immunologic, inflammatory, degenerative, neoplastic, psychological, endocrinologic, neuromuscular, hereditary, and developmental diseases. Acute trauma causes readily apparent damage to the tissues, but repetitive minor trauma or overuse also causes tissue damage, pain, and loss of function. Rheumatoid arthritis, systemic lupus erythematosus, ankylosing spondylitis, and other rheumatic and inflammatory diseases cause pain and alter the function of all of the musculoskeletal tissues. Bacterial, microbacterial, viral, and fungal infections involve bone, joints, tendons, and muscles. Degenerative diseases, like osteoarthritis, and degenerative disease of the intervertebral disks cause pain and significant functional limitation. Neoplasms of the musculoskeletal system include primary benign or malignant tumors originating in bone or soft tissues, or metastatic tumors. Tumors can cause pain, loss of function, and death. Joint contractures, weakness and paralysis, paresthesias, anesthesia, and pain may result from psychiatric and psychological disorders. Endocrinologic and metabolic disorders, such as hyperparathyroidism and osteoporosis, weaken the musculoskeletal system and cause progressive disability. Arthrogryposis, cerebral palsy, and other neuromuscular diseases cause weakness, loss of joint motion, and deformity. Hereditary and developmental diseases—including achondroplasia, neurofibromatosis, and idiopathic scoliosis—affect multiple musculoskeletal tissues and cause crippling deformities.

DEVELOPMENT OF ORTHOPAEDICS

The specialty of orthopaedics has grown and diversified far beyond the original definition of the term *orthopaedic*. Nicolas Andry (1658 to 1742), a professor of medicine in the Royal College in Paris, derived *orthopaedic* from the Greek words *orthon* (straight, free from deformity) and *paidion* (child). He distinguished orthopaedics from other medical and surgical specialties with his book *L'Orthopedie*, published in 1741. In 1743 an English translation appeared with the title *Orthopaedia: or, The Art of Correcting and Preventing Deformities in Children*. Belgian and German editions helped spread Andry's approach to deformities in children and use of the term *orthopaedic*.

Andry did not practice surgery and did not advocate surgical treatment of musculoskeletal problems or discuss treatment of traumatic injuries of the musculoskeletal system. He emphasized the value of moderate exercise for health, the role of body mechanics in the function and form of the musculoskeletal system, and the importance of muscle strengthening to improve musculoskeletal function. He understood how the musculoskeletal system could change with growth and changes in loading and use; he advised manipulation, splinting, and active exercise to prevent and treat deformities. To treat a "crooked" leg in a child he recommended fastening an iron plate to the "hollow" side of the leg and then tightening the plate against the leg daily until the leg became straight. He noted that the same method could straighten "the crooked trunk of a young tree" and illustrated the method with a drawing of a young tree tied to a stake. This illustration became the symbol for the specialty of orthopaedics.

In the 19th century, the introduction of anesthesia and methods of preventing infection made it possible to correct musculoskeletal deformities surgically. The discovery and clinical application of radiographs let orthopaedists see the bony abnormalities responsible for a deformity before surgery and revealed fractures and joint dislocations. Orthopaedists found that osteotomies could correct angulatory and rotatory deformities of the long bones or restore motion for patients with stiff hips by creating a pseudarthrosis. Arthrodesis could correct joint deformity or stabilize a flail joint; excision of a diseased or deformed joint could provide motion, restore alignment, and sometimes decrease pain. In the latter part of the 19th century and early part of the 20th century, orthopaedists found that they could transplant the tendons of healthy muscles to restore the function of paralyzed muscles and could transplant bone from one part of the body to another to stimulate bone healing or replace lost segments of the skeleton.

Because many of the conditions that were correctable by these procedures affected skeletally mature patients as well as children, orthopaedists extended the scope of the specialty to include adults with musculoskeletal disorders. Surgeons with experience in the surgical and nonsurgical treatment of skeletal deformities began to treat patients with acute traumatic injuries including fractures and joint dislocations. Successful treatment of people injured in World War I stimulated further development of the specialty, and by the early part of the 20th century trauma had become a well-recognized primary area of orthopaedic practice along with pediatric orthopaedics and adult orthopaedics.

Since then, advances in surgical and nonsurgical orthopaedic treatments including internal and external stabilization of fractures and osteotomies, arthroscopy, and microsurgery have stimulated further diversification of orthopaedics. Although many orthopedists continue to work exclusively with children, and the prevention and nonsurgical treatment of deformities in children forms an important part of the specialty, orthopaedics now includes the diagnosis and surgical and nonsurgical treatment of musculoskeletal diseases and injuries affecting bone, cartilage, tendon, ligament, meniscus, nerve, and vessel in patients of all ages. The regions of the body included in orthopaedic care are the limbs, shoulder, and pelvic girdles and the spine. Orthopaedic treatment uses medical, surgical, orthotic, prosthetic, and physical methods, including braces, splints, exercises, and manipulation. Musculoskeletal problems treated by orthopaedists range from congenital deformities such as clubfeet in newborns to degenerative diseases such as osteoarthritis of the hip in elderly patients.

EVALUATION OF ORTHOPAEDIC PATIENTS

The diagnosis of some orthopaedic disorders, like a bunion or a syndactyly of the index and long fingers, may seem readily apparent by inspection of the involved part. The diagnosis of other disorders, such as shoulder pain and weakness caused by throwing a ball or painless diffuse enlargement of the calf, may remain obscure even after extensive study. For any musculoskeletal disorder, a precise diagnosis that forms the basis for educating patients about their problem and for selecting the most appropriate treatment requires a careful, complete evaluation that includes a detailed history of the problem, a musculoskeletal examination, appropriate laboratory studies, and often imaging studies.

This section provides a brief overview of the evaluation of orthopaedic patients. Subsequent chapters explain the details of the orthopaedic evaluation, including the use of imaging studies and the history, physical findings, and imaging findings in specific orthopaedic disorders.

History

Most patients who seek orthopaedic care complain of (1) symptoms that include pain, numbness, tenderness, weakness, or crepitus (often the patients can identify a specific movement or activity that produces or exacerbates their symptoms); (2) deformities that include angulatory or rotational abnormalities as well as discrete masses or diffuse swelling; (3) disturbances of musculoskeletal function, including instability, weakness, loss of function, restricted motion, or stiffness; or (4) combinations of musculoskeletal symptoms, deformities, and loss of function.

Occasionally, an orthopaedic problem is discovered incidentally during the course of evaluation for other reasons. A radiograph taken to evaluate an acute knee injury may reveal a destructive lesion in the proximal tibia. A routine physical examination may reveal a mass in the thigh or restricted motion of the knee. Musculoskeletal deformities can progress unnoticed for a prolonged period. Large soft tissue and bone masses or curvature of the spine may develop for months or even years without patients or family members noticing the deformity.

Once the physician has defined the symptoms, location, and functional effects of the patient's musculoskeletal disorder, he or she must establish its detailed history. Important questions include the circumstances surrounding the onset of the problem (eg, did the problem develop suddenly or gradually, or in association with traumatic injury or systemic illness?); the course of the disorder (whether it has improved or has been progressive, stable, or episodic); and factors that exacerbate or alleviate the problem (in particular, movements or specific activities associated with the exacerbation or alleviation of the problem).

Equally important, the physician should determine the patient's perception of their musculoskeletal problem and the effects of the problem on the patient. This determination often includes assessing the effects of the musculoskeletal disorder on a patient's family, close friends, and work and recreational activities. Patients with similar musculoskeletal disorders often view the problem differently, and the effects of similar problems on daily activities differ among patients. For example, degenerative disease of the knee may severely disrupt the life and cause

emotional distress for a socially and physically active 62-year-old woman. Indefinite use of a cane and medications may not give this patient an acceptable result, but she may find that a total knee replacement substantially improves the quality of her life. A similar patient with comparable disease of her knee may find that nonsurgical treatment provides adequate function and relief of symptoms.

Examination

The physician may find it difficult to resist the temptation to examine immediately a painful region or deformity identified by the patient and then to order imaging studies. Observing the patient before an examination, however, often provides essential information. The physician should assess general muscular development, posture, gait, resting position of joints, the joint contours, and the appearance of the skin and should compare the symmetry of contralateral parts. The patient's demonstration of a deformity or disturbance of musculoskeletal function often suggests the correct diagnosis and may be more helpful than palpation or imaging studies. For example, a tentative diagnosis may be possible from observation of a patient's gait or attempt to use the upper extremity.

For many localized musculoskeletal disorders, the physician can compare the injured or diseased part of the musculoskeletal system with the contralateral normal part; comparison of the normal and abnormal sides and examination of the normal side first often make the type and degree of the disorder clearer. For example, unilateral muscular atrophy can confirm disuse, whereas symmetrically well-developed muscles argue against a chronic disability.

Palpation of the affected region will demonstrate tenderness, increased temperature, or crepitus. The examiner should compare the sensation and deep tendon reflexes of the affected and unaffected areas. The vascular examination includes inspection and palpation of the skin to assess skin temperature, color, the presence or absence of ulcers, and the pulses or major arteries. Palpation of joints will document the presence or absence of effusions, and gentle stress applied to a joint will allow the examiner to assess joint stability. Measuring the circumference of the affected and contralateral unaffected part will reveal the presence of swelling or atrophy.

Asking patients to demonstrate the active range of motion of the affected region and then comparing active motion of the affected and contralateral unaffected regions will show limitations of active motion. Assessment of active motion includes evaluation for possible muscle spasm and joint or tendon crepitus. Joint motion should be described in terms of the type of motion relative to the anatomic position of the body (flexion, extension, internal rotation, external rotation, adduction, abduction) and the range of motion in degrees.

The physician can help clarify the reason for a limitation of the active range of motion by assessing the passive range of motion. This must be done carefully to avoid causing patients unnecessary discomfort. Equal limitations of active and passive motion suggest a mechanical block to joint or muscle tendon unit motion. Common causes of mechanical blocks to motion include scarring of joint capsules and tendons, and interposition of cartilage or meniscal fragments between joint surfaces. When passive motion exceeds active motion, it suggests muscle weakness, tissue disruption (eg, a tendon or muscle rupture), paralysis, or inhibition of muscle contraction. Inhibition of muscle contraction may result from pain, or the patient may intentionally fail to demonstrate his or her full active range of motion.

Evaluation of many musculoskeletal problems requires assessment of muscle strength. If possible, the examiner should evaluate the specific actions of individual muscles, but such isolation is impossible in some regions and the physician can assess only the strength of a muscle group. The generally accepted method for describing muscle strength based on physical examination has five grades:

Grade 0—no visible or palpable muscle contraction
Grade 1—a trace of palpable or visible muscle contraction, but no associated joint motion
Grade 2—muscle contraction that produces a joint motion with gravity eliminated
Grade 3—muscle contraction that produces joint range of motion against gravity
Grade 4—muscle contraction that produces a range of motion against gravity plus some resistance
Grade 5—normal muscle contraction that produces a full range of motion against full resistance

The inability of this grading scheme to distinguish differences in muscle strength within a grade limits its value for the evaluation of some orthopaedic problems or sequential evaluation of changes in muscle strength. When more precise quantitative measures of muscle strength are needed, devices that measure the force and speed of muscle contraction can provide quantitative measures of muscle performance. These devices augment the physical examination, particularly for complex musculoskeletal problems and during rehabilitation of patients with muscle weakness or restricted range of motion.

Laboratory Studies

Most benign neoplasms and localized congenital, developmental, and degenerative diseases of the musculoskeletal system do not cause serum and urine abnormalities. Localized infections of the musculoskeletal system may elevate the white blood cell count and erythrocyte sedimentation rate, but these studies occasionally remain normal or near normal in patients with chronic infections. Localized primary musculoskeletal malignant neoplasms may cause abnormalities in the complete blood count, erythrocyte sedimentation rate, serum calcium, and phosphorous and serum alkaline phosphatase. Metastatic neoplasms and metabolic diseases involving bone often cause abnormalities in serum calcium and phosphorous and alkaline phosphatase. Serum studies—including latex fixation and antinuclear antibodies, immunoglobulins, erythrocyte sedimentation rate, and complete blood count—may be helpful in making the diagnosis of rheumatologic disorders including rheumatoid arthritis, systemic lupus erythematosus, and ankylosing spondylitis. Analysis of synovial fluid for white cell count, Gram stain, culture, and crystals may identify the cause of joint, tendon sheath, and bursal inflammation.

Imaging Studies

Imaging studies have become an essential part of the diagnosis of many musculoskeletal disorders. They also have a critical role in planning surgical and orthotic treatment and in assessing the results of treatment.

Complete evaluation of many musculoskeletal disorders requires plain radiographs, including at least two views of the affected region. Not only do plain radiographs show most focal bone abnormalities including fracture, bone formation, or bone destruction, they also provide information about bone shape and density, the relations between adjacent bones, the presence of air or foreign bodies in the tissues, and the shape and density of the soft tissues. In children, examination of plain radiographs allows the examiner to estimate skeletal maturity. When inspection of the plain radiographs suggests but does not establish the presence of an abnormality, comparison of the suspicious radiographs with similar studies of the contralateral normal side may help the physician make a diagnosis or determine whether other diagnostic studies are needed. Even when plain roentgenograms show only normal tissues, they may help eliminate some causes of pain, deformity, or loss of function. Depending on the results of plain anteroposterior and lateral roentgenograms, the physician may find that oblique roentgenograms, fluoroscopic studies, or tomograms will help clarify an abnormality demonstrated by plain films or reveal an abnormality not visible on the plain roentgenograms.

Computed tomography (CT) has become a critical part of the evaluation of many bone and some soft tissue lesions. Three-dimensional reconstructions using CT have proved helpful in designing surgical procedures and assessing the extent of disease. CT combined with injection of contrast media or air can provide clear three-dimensional outlines of joint cavities and the spinal subarachnoid space.

Scanning after injection of radioactive isotopes, especially technetium, can identify regions of increased activity within the musculoskeletal system, especially within bone. These scans may help the physician evaluate musculoskeletal pain of unknown etiology or may demonstrate the presence and extent of multiple skeletal lesions. Gallium scanning may reveal lesions not demonstrated by technetium scanning and, combined with technetium scanning, may help identify the cause of some skeletal lesions.

Magnetic resonance imaging (MRI) can show the precise anatomic location, size, and shape of musculoskeletal soft tissue lesions as well as bone marrow involvement by inflammatory and neoplastic processes. MRI also provides excellent visualization of spinal lesions and intraarticular abnormalities, including meniscal and ligament tears.

Ultrasonography can image soft tissue masses and has proved useful in evaluation of conditions such as congenital dislocation of the hip and tears of the rotator cuff. The lack of radiation exposure and relatively low cost of ultrasonography give it important advantages over other imaging methods for initial evaluations of some of these conditions.

CURRENT ORTHOPAEDIC TREATMENT METHODS

Current treatment of orthopaedic conditions includes use of medications, physical treatments, orthotics, prosthetics, and surgery. Although physicians frequently separate the treatment choices for musculoskeletal disorders into surgical and nonsurgical categories, optimal treatment of many orthopaedic problems includes surgical and nonsurgical therapy.

Medical, Physical, Orthotic, and Prosthetic Treatments

Arthritis, infections, and musculoskeletal pain often require treatment with medications. For this reason, orthopaedists commonly use nonsteroidal antiinflammatory agents, antibiotics, and analgesics. Exercises to improve range of motion of musculoskeletal tissues, strengthen muscles, and improve flexibility form part of the physical treatment of many musculoskeletal conditions. Orthotics can help straighten or stabilize the limbs or spine, and can decrease pain resulting from some musculoskeletal conditions. They are used in the treatment of scoliosis, low-back pain, foot pain, and some foot deformities. Although orthotics generally do not correct fixed skeletal deformities, especially in adults, serial casts can progressively correct some foot deformities and other selected musculoskeletal deformities in children. Many patients with congenital or acquired amputations can benefit from prosthetic devices. These artificial limbs or parts of limbs often significantly improve musculoskeletal function and the patient's quality of life.

Surgical Treatments

Operative orthopaedic treatment consists of manipulation, arthroscopic surgical procedures, and open surgical procedures. Closed manipulations can reduce dislocations or fractures and can increase joint motion by stretching contractures. Orthopaedists use arthroscopy to identify the cause of joint pain or dysfunction, remove or repair torn menisci, remove cartilage fragments, and replace or repair cruciate ligaments. Common open surgical procedures include open reduction and internal fixation of fractures, repair of damaged tendons and ligaments, joint replacements, correction of spine and foot deformities in children, removal of herniated intervertebral disks, and arthrodesis of painful joints.

Recent advances in orthopaedic treatment include improvements in surgery and anesthesia, new synthetic materials and surgical instruments, and better methods of rehabilitation of the musculoskeletal system. Improvements in anesthesia and surgical techniques have made it possible to perform procedures that correct major skeletal deformities, including those of the spine, hip, and pelvis. Development of new synthetic materials and better understanding of musculoskeletal system biomechanics have improved prosthetic joints, methods of stabilizing injured tissues, and methods of correcting skeletal deformity. Invention of instruments for arthroscopic procedures has stimulated rapid growth of arthroscopic surgery for diagnosis and treatment of intraarticular injuries and diseases. Refinements in operating microscopes and instruments have made reattachment of severed limbs and transplantation of vascularized tissue for reconstruction of musculoskeletal deformity standard treatments. Physical therapy programs based on understanding of the effects of loading and motion on the musculoskeletal tissues have helped patients regain strength and motion after surgery or injury.

ORTHOPAEDIC SUBSPECIALTIES

Orthopaedic subspecialties have developed that reflect the diversity of clinical problems and treatment methods. These subspecialties include children's (pediatric) orthopaedics, musculoskeletal trauma, adult hip and knee reconstructive surgery, hand surgery, adult spine surgery, sports medicine, foot and ankle surgery, orthopaedic oncology, microvascular surgery, shoulder and elbow surgery, and orthopaedic rehabilitation. Many of these special areas overlap, and all are changing rapidly. Some focus on a particular anatomic area, such as the hand or foot; others define themselves by the age group of the patients, such as children's orthopaedics; and others center on the cause of the musculoskeletal problem, such as trauma, sports medicine, or oncology. A few areas focus on methods of treating musculoskeletal disorders, such as rehabilitation, microvascular surgery, and arthroscopy.

Pediatric Orthopaedics

Pediatric orthopaedists diagnose and treat musculoskeletal disorders in skeletally immature patients. Disorders frequently treated by pediatric orthopaedists include clubfoot deformities, congenital dislocations of the hip, infections of bones and joints, and scoliosis. Some children's orthopaedists also care for patients with traumatic injuries and neoplasms.

Trauma

Musculoskeletal trauma includes not only fractures but also injuries to cartilages, tendons, ligaments, muscles, peripheral nerves, and peripheral blood vessels. Orthopaedists have special expertise in reduction and stabilization of fractures and joint injuries including use of external skeletal fixation devices, and surgical reduction and internal fixation. Musculoskeletal injuries may occur in association with other injuries; therefore, orthopaedists often form part of multidisciplinary trauma teams to provide care for patients with trauma to multiple organ systems.

Adult Reconstructive Surgery

Generally, orthopaedic adult reconstructive surgery refers to the diagnosis and treatment of degenerative and rheumatic joint disease, most commonly involving the hip and knee. Common nonsurgical treatments of these problems include antiinflammatory and analgesic medications, physical therapy, orthoses, canes, and crutches. Surgical treatments include arthrodeses, osteotomies, and arthroplasties. Total joint arthroplasties of the hip and knee are among the most successful group of surgical procedures in any specialty. Current total hip and total knee replacements can restore near-normal function to patients with severe pain and markedly limited function. Although orthopaedists replace other synovial joints less frequently, improved elbow and shoulder arthroplasties have made it possible to relieve pain and improve function for patients with advanced disease of these joints.

Adult Spine

Orthopaedists with a special interest in adult spine problems treat patients with back and neck pain, spinal deformity, tumors of the spine, and traumatic injuries. Development of improved imaging techniques has made it possible to better define the causes of adult spine problems, including chronic back pain. As a result, orthopaedists have devised new treatments for spine problems including surgical stabilization of the spine, surgical correction of structural deformities, and improved methods of rehabilitation.

Sports Medicine

Orthopaedic sports medicine specialists provide care for recreational and competitive athletes injured during athletic training and competition. Rapid advances in arthroscopic surgery have improved the ability of orthopaedists to diagnose and treat injuries to major synovial joints, including the knee, shoulder, and ankle. Sports medicine specialists also develop methods of preventing injury including improved training techniques, rule changes, and protective orthoses and other protective equipment.

Oncology

Orthopaedists with special interest and experience in oncology treat patients with primary neoplasms and lesions that resemble neoplasms of the bone and musculoskeletal soft tissues. Orthopaedists also diagnose and treat patients with metastatic disease of the skeleton. Improved imaging methods and surgical techniques have made possible limb-sparing operations for many primary malignant tumors of the musculoskeletal system and improved treatment of benign aggressive tumors. Advances in methods of skeletal stabilization have made possible treatment of many patients with painful disabling metastatic diseases of the skeleton including pathologic fractures or impending pathologic fractures.

Hand Surgery

Hand surgeons treat patients with disorders of the hand and the upper extremity. These conditions include infections, congenital deformities, neoplasms, traumatic injuries, and degenerative and rheumatologic diseases. Many orthopaedists with special interest and experience in hand and upper extremity surgery use microvascular surgery to reattach traumatically amputated digits and hands and to transplant tissues to reconstruct damaged or lost parts of the musculoskeletal system.

Microvascular Surgery

Orthopaedists with special interest and expertise in microvascular surgery reattach amputated parts, transplant vascularized tissues to repair skeletal defects, or replace lost or damaged tissue. Microvascular transplantation of vascularized tissue has proved especially beneficial in treatment of large, open wounds with extensive full-thickness soft tissue loss.

Foot and Ankle Surgery

Orthopaedists with special interest and expertise in foot and ankle surgery treat patients with localized and systemic conditions affecting the foot and ankle.

Common problems include degenerative and rheumatologic problems of the joints of the foot, bunions, foot deformities, and traumatic injuries.

Rehabilitation

All orthopaedists participate in the rehabilitation of their patients, that is, in the restoration of the patient to maximum musculoskeletal function after disease or injury. Rehabilitation includes physical therapy, such as range of motion and muscle strengthening, and use of orthotics, prosthetics, or other devices to restore maximum musculoskeletal function. More complex musculoskeletal problems may require specialized vocational and occupational counseling or therapy. Specialized rehabilitation programs help patients with sports injuries, upper extremity impairment, and intractable chronic low-back pain achieve the maximum level of musculoskeletal function. Patients with spinal cord injuries, including patients with hemiplegia and paraplegia, require highly specialized long-term rehabilitation programs. Their rehabilitation must be integrated with other orthopaedic treatment of their musculoskeletal dysfunction, including orthotics and surgical correction of deformity.

ORTHOPAEDIC RESEARCH

In addition to the diagnosis and treatment of diseases and injuries of the musculoskeletal system, the specialty of orthopaedics includes scientific investigations of the musculoskeletal system that help improve the prevention, diagnosis, and treatment of musculoskeletal diseases and injuries. The types of investigations vary from epidemiologic studies of musculoskeletal disorders to basic investigations of the control of cell and tissue function.

During the last third of the century, great progress has been made in defining the composition, structure, and function of the musculoskeletal tissues. Work in biomechanics and biomaterials has led to development and use of prosthetic joint replacements and devices for stabilization of fractures and correction and stabilization of skeletal deformity. Other work has provided improved understanding of the ability of musculoskeletal tissues to repair injuries and of the processes of aging and degeneration in the musculoskeletal system. Study of musculoskeletal injury mechanisms and patterns of occurrence have provided the information necessary to prevent injuries. Preservation and transplantation of bone, tendon, ligament, and cartilage allografts have become part of orthopaedic clinical practice.

Current work with control of mesenchymal cell function through use of growth factors, electrical fields, and mechanical loading shows great promise for further improvement in orthopaedic treatment. Progress in use of mesenchymal cell culture and transplantation offers potential for replacement of lost, damaged, or diseased musculoskeletal tissues. Better understanding of the effects of mechanical loads on musculoskeletal tissues and the optimal methods of applying these loads will improve treatment of deformities and injuries. As these scientific and technical advances continue to increase the ability of orthopaedists to improve the function of patients suffering from musculoskeletal injuries and diseases, they expand the specialty of orthopaedics and broaden the meaning of the term *orthopaedic.*

Annotated Bibliography

Andry N. Orthopaedia: or, the art of correcting and preventing deformities in children. London, A Millar, 1743.
This two-volume English translation of Andry's book describes his recommendations for maintaining health and preventing and correcting deformities in children. He stated that he compounded the word orthopaedia *from the Greek words* orthon *(straight, free from deformity) and* paidion *(child) to express in one term his intent to teach methods of preventing and correcting the deformities of children. Andry did not advocate surgical treatment but rather stressed the value of exercise and advised manipulation and splinting to treat deformities.*

Bick EM. Source book of orthopaedics. New York, Hafner, 1968.
Bick reviews the history of orthopaedics beginning with the pre-historic use of splints to treat fractures. His review shows how advances in the basic sciences have influenced the practice of orthopaedics and how certain methods of treating musculoskeletal injuries and diseases have been discovered, abandoned, and then rediscovered.

Keith A. Menders of the maimed: the anatomical and physiological principles underlying the treatment of injuries to muscles, nerves, bones, and joints. London, Oxford University Press, 1919.
The discovery of anesthesia, antisepsis, and asepsis in the 19th century made possible effective surgical treatment of many acute traumatic injuries and restoration of musculoskeletal function for patients with impairments resulting from injuries. At the time Keith published his book, British orthopaedic surgeons were treating thousands of men injured in World War I. Keith stressed that "effective and rational treatment must be based on our knowledge of the structure and mechanism of the human body." To aid orthopaedic surgeons in their efforts to restore musculoskeletal function, he summarized the principles underlying orthopaedic surgery and the lives of the individuals who helped to define those principles—the "menders of the maimed."

Praemer A, Furner S, Rice DP. Musculoskeletal conditions in the United States. Park Ridge, IL, American Academy of Orthopaedic Surgeons, 1992.
This book describes the breadth and scope of the problems imposed by musculoskeletal disorders on the United States. It shows that most musculoskeletal problems do not directly cause mortality, but they can cause diminution of the quality of life, morbidity, disability, and economic loss.

Turek's Orthopaedics: Principles and Their Application, Fifth Edition,
edited by Stuart L. Weinstein and Joseph A. Buckwalter.
J.B. Lippincott Company, Philadelphia, © 1994.

2

Joseph A. Buckwalter

Musculoskeletal Tissues and the Musculoskeletal System

The stability and mobility of the body depend on the tissues that form the musculoskeletal system—bone, cartilage, dense fibrous tissue, and muscle. These tissues differ in vascularity, innervation, mechanical and biologic properties, and composition, but they share a common origin from undifferentiated mesenchymal cells. Understanding of diseases and injuries of the musculoskeletal system and their treatment necessarily depends on knowledge of these tissues. Failure to consider the biologic and mechanical properties of the tissues, tissue changes caused by disease or injury, or the responses of the tissues to persistent changes in use can lead to misinterpretation of diagnostic information, suboptimal treatment decisions, and undesirable results of treatment. Furthermore, future advances in the diagnosis and treatment of musculoskeletal problems will depend on increased knowledge of the cell and matrix biology of the musculoskeletal tissues.

To provide the basis for understanding orthopaedic diseases, this chapter reviews the structure and composition of the musculoskeletal tissues. The first section summarizes the distinctive general characteristics of connective tissues, including mesenchymal cells and the matrices they synthesize. The next sections review the structure, composition, and properties of bone, periosteum, the dense fibrous tissues (tendon, ligament, and joint capsule), tendon, ligament, joint capsule insertions into bone, articular cartilage, growth cartilage, meniscus, synovium, muscle tendon junction, and intervertebral disk. Although skeletal muscle is not a connective tissue, because it forms a critical part of the musculoskeletal system it is included in this chapter.

CONNECTIVE TISSUE

The gross and microscopic studies of 19th-century histologists and pathologists led them to view connective tissue as a continuous basic tissue, or connecting substance, that extended throughout the body and assumed specialized forms—including cartilage, periosteum, bone, tendon, fibrous septa, and fascia—in different locations without altering the basic character of the tissue. The definition of basic connective tissue structure proposed by Virchow, "the greater part of the tissue is composed of intercellular substance, in which, at certain intervals cells are embedded," remains unchanged.

The role of connective tissue is most apparent in the musculoskeletal system, but all tissues and organ systems of multicellular organisms depend on connective tissue for mechanical support. The parenchymal cells of liver, kidney, and brain could not maintain the organization of these tissues or the tissue functions without their structural connective tissue framework. Normal function of the respiratory and cardiovascular systems depends on the repetitive mechanical performance of the connective tissues that form the airways and the blood vessels.

The group of specialized connective tissues that form the supporting structure and joints of the musculoskeletal system (bone, cartilage, dense fibrous

tissue ligaments, tendons, and joint capsules) have primarily mechanical functions. Because of their obvious mechanical roles, and the prominence of their matrix component relative to their cellular component, these tissues are often regarded as homogeneous and inert. Yet, even in the mature skeleton, they remain metabolically active; the cells and matrices are degraded and replaced, and the tissues respond to hormonal, metabolic, and mechanical stimuli.

Mesenchymal Tissues Versus Epithelial Tissues

During embryonic development two morphologic and functional classes of tissues appear—epithelium and mesenchyme. The skeletal connective tissues originate from a subdivision of the mesenchyme. Mesenchyme (from the Greek *mesos,* or middle, and *enchyma,* or infusion) refers to the location of mesenchyme between the epithelial layers of endoderm and ectoderm. Epithelial tissues may develop from endoderm, ectoderm, and mesoderm but mesenchyme appears to develop from only mesoderm.

The relation of the cells to each other and the relation of the cells to the matrix distinguish epithelia from mesenchyme (Fig. 2-1). Epithelial cells form sheets or layers of cells. They establish close relations with adjacent cells, frequently binding their membranes together with specialized cell junctions and devoting a large portion of their membranes to contact with other cells. Epithelial tissues generally have a sparse extracellular matrix, and a specialized form of matrix, the basement membrane, frequently serves as the bed for epithelial cells and separates them from mesenchymal tissue. Mesenchymal cells do not generally form sheets or layers. In the mesenchyme that forms the skeletal connective tissues, cells rarely establish extensive contact with other cells, and they surround themselves with an abundant extracellular matrix consisting of a macromolecular framework synthesized by the cells and water that fills the macromolecular framework. The cell membranes bind to specific macromolecules within the matrix, and although the cells may appear fixed in place by the surrounding matrix, they can migrate through the matrix.

Mesenchymal Cells

Undifferentiated mesenchymal cells not only can move through the tissue but also have the potential to divide rapidly and differentiate into specialized

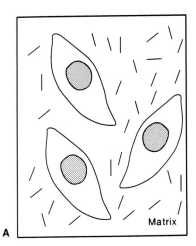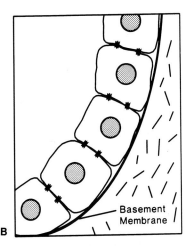

FIGURE 2-1. Diagramatic representation of the differences between mesenchymal and epithelial tissues. (A) Mesenchymal cells have little or no contact with other cells, and surround themselves with an extracellular matrix. (B) Epithelial cells establish and maintain close cell-to-cell contact and often rest on a basement membrane that separates them from mesenchymal tissue. (Buckwalter JA, Cooper RR. The cells and matrices of skeletal connective tissues. In: Albright JA, Brand RA, eds. The scientific basis of orthopaedics. Norwalk, CT, Appleton & Lange, 1987:3)

musculoskeletal tissue cells, including the cells of cartilage, bone, dense fibrous tissues, and muscle (Fig. 2-2). Systemic factors (including nutrition and hormonal balance) combined with local factors in the cell environment (including the composition of the matrix, concentrations of oxygen, cytokines and nutrients, and pH and mechanical forces) influence mesenchymal cell proliferation and differentiation. These systemic and local factors interact with the genomic potential of the cell to determine the progression from undifferentiated stem cells to highly differentiated cells like chondrocytes and osteocytes.

The progressive differentiation proceeds through a series of stages with transition from one stage to the next dependent on signals from the local environment. The variety of forms these mesenchymal cells can assume include blood, fat, and muscle cells as well as the specialized connective tissue cells, fibroblasts, chondrocytes, osteoblasts, and osteocytes. Cell differentiation creates persistent but not necessarily permanent changes in the cells. In general, the differentiated cell form persists through many generations of the cell. Some cells, like chondrocytes, rarely divide but maintain their differentiated form for their entire life. During cell differentiation the cells change not only their form but also the types

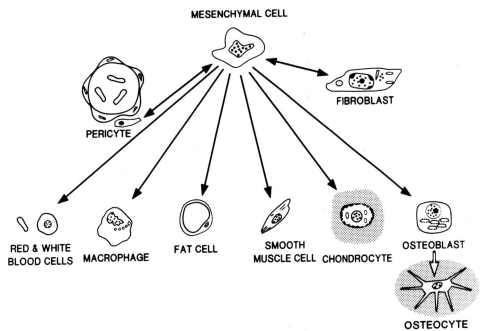

FIGURE 2-2. Diagramatic representation of the differentiation of specialized connective tissue cells from undifferentiated mesenchymal cells. (Buckwalter JA, Cooper RR. The cells and matrices of skeletal connective tissues. In: Albright JA, Brand RA, eds. The scientific basis of orthopaedics. Norwalk, CT, Appleton & Lange, 1987:3)

of molecules they synthesize and thus the composition and organization of the matrix that surrounds them.

Even in the skeletally mature individual, undifferentiated mesencyhmal cells persist. With increasing age they may lose some of their capacity for proliferation and differentiation, but they can still respond to appropriate signals by migrating, proliferating, and differentiating into the mature cells of bone, cartilage, and dense fibrous tissue, including osteoblasts, osteocytes, chondrocytes, and fibroblasts.

Mesenchymal Matrices

The matrices of the musculoskeletal tissues consist of elaborate, highly organized frameworks of organic macromolecules filled with water. Light microscopic

examination of these matrices shows fibrils embedded in an amorphous ground substance. Biochemical examination shows that the fibrils consist of multiple types of collagen and elastin, the ground substance consists primarily of water and proteoglycans, and the matrix contains another class of macromolecules called noncollagenous proteins. In addition to an organic matrix, bone has an inorganic matrix that consists primarily of calcium phosphate. Figure 2-3 shows the differences in matrix composition among the general types of musculoskeletal connective tissue.

Organic Matrix Macromolecules

COLLAGENS.   Collagens give all connective tissues their basic form and tensile strength; however,

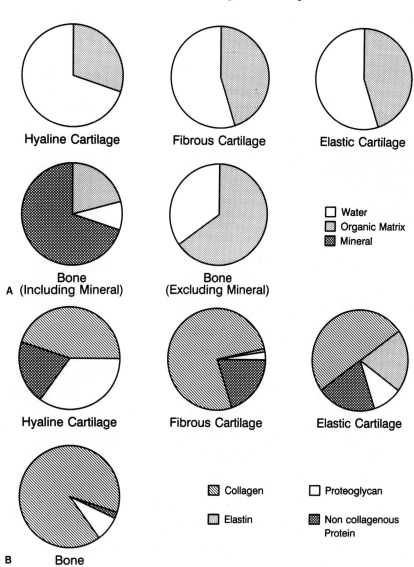

FIGURE 2-3. Pie charts showing the matrix composition of the general types of musculoskeletal connective tissue. (**A**) Hyaline cartilage has the highest concentration of water, and bone has the lowest. (**B**) Hyaline cartilage has the highest concentration of proteoglycans, and bone has the lowest. Dense fibrous tissues like tendon and ligament have a matrix composition similar to that of fibrocartilage. (Buckwalter JA. Cartilage. In: Dulbecco R, ed. Encyclopedia of human biology. New York, Academic Press, 1991)

the tissues vary in collagen concentration and organization and in the types of collagens that form part of their organic matrix. All collagens function as structural proteins in the extracellular matrix and a significant portion of each collagen molecule consists of a triple helix formed from three amino acid chains. This helical structure gives the molecules stiffness and strength.

More than 20 genes direct the synthesis of at least 13 different types of collagen. Differences in molecular topology and polymeric form divide the 13 known collagen types into three classes—fibrillar collagens (class I), basement membrane collagens (class II), and short-chain collagens (class III). A specific type of collagen may vary slightly among tissues. For example, bone type I collagen, which normally mineralizes, appears to differ in structure and composition from tendon type I collagen, which does not mineralize under normal conditions.

Class I Collagens (Fibrillar Collagens). Class I collagens form the cross-banded fibrils seen by electron microscopy in all connective tissues. The five collagens in this group—types I, II, III, V, and XI—have triple helical domains consisting of about 1000 amino acid residues in each of three polypeptide chains. Type I collagen forms the principal matrix macromolecule of skin, bone, meniscus, annulus fibrosis, tendon, ligament, joint capsule, and all other dense fibrous tissues. Figure 2-4 shows the assembly of type I collagen microfibrils. Type II collagen forms the banded fibrils found in hyaline cartilage, the nucleus pulposus of the intervertebral disk, and the vitreous humor of the eye. The "minor" fibrillar collagens, types V and XI, also contribute to the matrices of the connective tissues. Type V forms part of the matrix in tissues containing type I collagen, usually about 3% of the amount of type I. Type XI forms part of the type II collagen fibrils. Type III collagen occurs

FIGURE 2-4. Type I collagen. (A) A stained microfibril of collagen exhibiting characteristic cross-striations with a regular repeat period (D) of approximately 680 Å. (B) A two-dimensional representation of the packing arrangement of tropocollagen macromolecules in the microfibril. (C) Each tropocollagen molecule has large numbers of darkly staining bands, and five of these that are separated by a regular distance of 680 Å account for the repeat period (D) in the microfibril. The H₂N terminal and probably the HOOC terminal ends of the molecule are atypical and nonhelical in structure, and are called *telopeptides*. (D) Each tropocollagen molecule consists of three polypeptides, two with identical amino acid sequences (α_1 chains) and one with a slightly different amino acid sequence (α_2 chain). Each α chain is coiled in a tight left-handed helix with a pitch of 9.5 Å, and the three chains are coiled around each other in a right-handed "superhelix" with a pitch of about 104 Å. (E) Gly occurs in every third position throughout most of the polypeptide chains, and there are large amounts of Pro and Hypro in the other two positions. X and Y represent any amino acid other than Gly, Pro, Hypro, Lys, or Hys. (Grant ME, Prockop DJ. The biosynthesis of collagen. N Engl J Med 1972;286: 194, 242, 291)

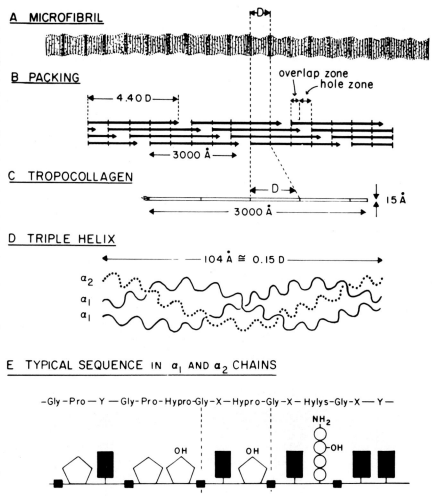

in association with type I collagen in most tissues other than bone and appears in repair tissue.

Class II Collagens (Basement Membrane Collagens). The class II collagens—types IV, VII, and VIII—form critical parts of basement membranes. Type IV contributes the major structural component of basement membranes. Type VII acts as an anchoring filament in epithelial basement membranes, and type VIII forms part of endothelial basement membranes.

Class III Collagens (Short-Chain Collagens). The forms and functions of class III collagens—types VI, IX, and X—remain less well understood than the forms and functions of the other classes of collagens. Type VI collagen appears in small amounts in many tissues. When examined by electron microscopy, it appears as filamentous banded aggregates. These aggregates often appear in the matrix immediately surrounding cells. Type IX collagen forms covalent bonds with type II collagen molecules and thus contributes to the extracellular matrix of hyaline cartilage. It may influence type II collagen fibril diameter and the organization of the hyaline cartilage matrix. Type X collagen occurs in the calcified cartilage region of the physis, articular cartilage, and bone fracture callus. Although its limited distribution suggests that it may have an important role in chondrocyte enlargement or cartilage mineralization, its functions remain unknown. The forms and functions of type XII and XIII collagens likewise remain unknown.

ELASTIN. Elastin, like collagen, forms protein fibrils, but elastin fibrils lack the cross-banding pattern seen in electron microscopic studies of fibrillar collagens (Fig. 2-5) and differ from collagens in amino acid composition, confirmation of the amino acid chains, and mechanical properties. In addition, elastin also forms lamellae or sheet-like structures. Unlike collagen, elastin can undergo some deformation without rupturing or tearing. Following deformation it returns to its original size and shape. Amino acid chains of elastin contain two amino acids not found in collagens (desmosine and isodesmosine), and the elastin amino acid chains form random coils, unlike the highly ordered triple helices of collagens. The random coil confirmation of the amino acid chains makes it possible for elastin fibers and sheets to undergo some deformation without molecular damage and then resume their original shape and size.

Elastin does not form part of the matrices of hyaline cartilage or bone, and it contributes only a small amount to the extracellular matrices of most other connective tissues. Trace amounts appear in the intervertebral disk and meniscus. Many ligaments also have some elastin, usually less than 5%. A few ligaments, however, such as the nuchal ligament and the ligamentum flavum, have high elastin concentrations, up to 75%.

PROTEOGLYCANS. Proteoglycans form the major nonfibrillar macromolecule of the cartilage, intervertebral disk, dense fibrous tissue, and bone and muscle matrices. These musculoskeletal tissues vary considerably in the concentration and possibly the function of proteoglycans. The highest concentrations of proteoglycans occur in hyaline cartilages and nu-

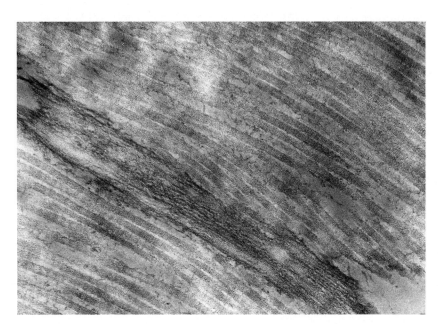

FIGURE 2-5. Electron micrograph showing cross-banded collagen fibrils lying parallel to an elastic fiber consisting of multiple dark microfibrils and regions of amorphous elastin.

cleus pulposus. In these tissues the concentration of proteoglycans may approach 30% to 40% of the tissue dry weight, and these molecules significantly influence fluid flow through the matrix and help give the tissues stiffness to compression and resilience. They may have similar space filling and mechanical roles in the other tissues, but their much lower concentrations in these tissues (in the dense fibrous tissues and bone, they contribute at most a few percent of the dry weight) make their effect on the tissue mechanical properties proportionately less. Muscle also contains specific types of proteoglycans, but they form only a small fraction of the tissue.

Proteoglycan monomers, the basic units of proteoglycan molecules, consist of polysaccharide chains covalently bound to protein. Most types of proteoglycans contain relatively little protein, about 5% or less. Glycosaminoglycans, a special class of polysaccharide consisting of repeating disaccharide units containing a derivative of either glucosamine or galactosamine and carrying one or two negative charges, form the principal part of proteoglycan molecules (Fig. 2-6). Connective tissue glycosaminoglycans include hyaluronic acid, chondroitin 4 sulfate, chondroitin 6 sulfate, dermatan sulfate, and keratan sulfate. Proteoglycan monomers assume multiple forms, including large aggregating proteoglycans, large nonaggregating proteoglycans, and small nonaggregating proteoglycans.

Large Aggregating Proteoglycans. Aggregating proteoglycan monomers consist of protein core filaments with multiple covalently bound oligosaccharides and longer chondroitin and keratan sulfate chains. Each glycosaminoglycan chain creates a string of negative

charges that bind water and cations in solution. Because of this property, proteoglycans can expand to fill a large domain in solution. In most musculoskeletal tissues, an intact collagen fibril network limits the swelling of the proteoglycans, but loss or degradation of the collagen fibril network will allow a tissue that contains a high concentration of large proteoglycans to swell, increasing the water concentration and the permeability of the tissue.

Aggregating proteoglycan monomers may exist as free monomers or as aggregates formed by the noncovalent association of multiple monomers with hyaluronic acid filaments and small proteins called link proteins. Aggregates, consisting of a central hyaluronic acid filament with multiple attached monomers and link proteins, may reach a length of more than 10,000 nm with more than 300 monomers (Fig. 2-7). Link proteins stabilize the association between monomers and hyaluronic acid and may have a role in directing the assembly of aggregates in the matrix. Aggregates appear to help anchor monomers within the matrix, preventing their displacement and thereby organizing and stabilizing the macromolecular framework. They also help determine the permeability of the matrix, and thus the flow of water through the matrix.

Large Nonaggregating Proteoglycans. Large nonaggregating proteoglycans may result from the breakdown of aggregating proteoglycans, or they may represent a distinct population of molecules that have a composition similar to that of aggregating proteoglycans. Their function remains uncertain, although it appears likely that they have a role in providing tissue stiffness to compression and binding water.

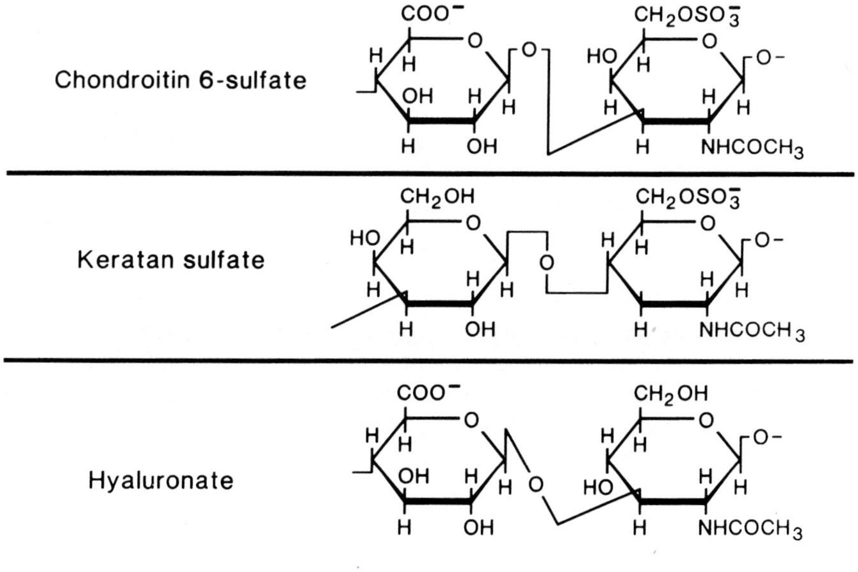

FIGURE 2-6. Diagramatic representation of the structures of the glycosaminoglycans, chondroitin sulfate, keratan sulfate, and hyaluronate. Chondroitin sulfate has two negative charges per disaccharide, and the others have one. (Buckwalter JA, Cooper RR. The cells and matrices of skeletal connective tissues. In: Albright JA, Brand RA, eds. The scientific basis of orthopaedics. Norwalk, CT, Appleton & Lange, 1987:23)

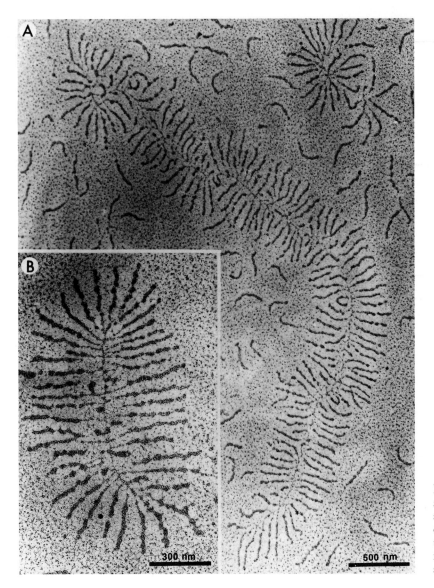

FIGURE 2-7. Electron micrographs showing the structure of proteoglycan aggregates. (A) A large aggregate. The central filament is hyaluronic acid, and the projecting side arms are proteoglycan monomers. (B) A smaller proteoglycan aggregate.

Small Nonaggregating Proteoglycans. Small nonaggregating proteoglycans may contain chondroitin sulfate and dermatan sulfate. They form specific associations with collagen fibrils and may influence matrix organization and the ability of cells to bind to the matrix collagen fibrils, but their specific functions remain unknown.

NONCOLLAGENOUS PROTEINS. Less is known about noncollagenous proteins and glycoproteins than about the collagens, elastin, or proteoglycans. Although they form part of the macromolecular framework of musculoskeletal tissues, few noncollagenous proteins have been identified, and their functions have not been well defined. Most of them consist primarily of protein with small numbers of attached monosaccharides and oliosaccharides. They

appear to have roles in the organization and maintenance of the macromolecular structure of the matrix and in establishing and maintaining the relations between the cells and the other matrix macromolecules.

Examples of noncollagenous proteins found within the musculoskeletal tissue matrices include link protein, chondronectin, anchorin CII, fibronectin, osteonectin, and tenascin. Link protein helps organize and stabilize the extracellular matrix through its effect on proteoglycan aggregation. Chondronectin appears to mediate the adhesion of chondrocytes to the matrix and may help stabilize the phenotype of hyaline cartilage chondrocytes. Anchorin CII may have similar functions. Fibronectin exists in soluble and insoluble forms. Soluble fibronectin occurs in many body fluids, including plasma, urine, amniotic fluid, and cerebral spinal fluid. Insoluble or cellular fibronectin appears in most musculoskeletal tissue matrices except for normal mature cartilage. Fibronectins examined by electron microscopy appear as fine filaments or granules. They may coat the surface of fibrillar collagens and associate with cell membranes. Osteonectin, a bone associated glycoprotein, binds to type I collagen and hydroxyapatite. The ability of osteonectin to bind hydroxyapatite to the organic matrix suggests that it may have a role in initiating mineralization. Tenascin, another matrix glycoprotein, occurs in perichondrium, periosteum, tendon, and muscle tendon junction. Its function remains unclear.

Inorganic Matrix

Normal function of the musculoskeletal tissues depends on rapid, controlled mineralization (deposition of relatively insoluble mineral within the organic matrix) of some organic matrices and prevention of mineralization in others; yet the conditions that control and promote normal and pathologic mineralization of musculoskeletal tissues remain poorly understood. Bone, the growth plate cartilage longitudinal septa, and a thin zone of articular cartilage organic matrices mineralize normally. The organic matrices of other cartilage regions and dense fibrous tissues mineralize in association with certain diseases, including chondrocalcinosis, and muscle and some dense fibrous tissues mineralize following some injuries. The deposition of mineral in the organic matrix radically changes the properties of the tissue. It increases stiffness and compressive strength of bone, but pathologic mineralization of cartilage and dense fibrous tissue may accelerate or be associated with degenerative changes in these tissues.

BONE

The strength and stiffness of bone combined with its light weight gives vertebrates their mobility, dexterity, and strength. Bone has an elaborate vascular supply and several specific types of bone cells that from and resorb the bone matrix. Like the other musculoskeletal tissues, bone consists of mesenchymal cells and an extracellular matrix, but unlike the other tissues bone matrix mineralizes.

Structure

Gross Structure

SHAPES. Bones assume a remarkable variety of shapes and sizes. They vary in size from the ear ossicles to the long bones of the limb. The variety of shapes allows bones to be classified into three groups—long, short, and flat. Long bones like the femur, tibia, or humerus have an expanded metaphysis and epiphysis at either end with thick-walled tubular diaphysis. The thick cortical walls of the diaphysis become thinner and increase in diameter as they form the metaphysis, and articular cartilage covers the epiphyses where they form synovial joints. The metacarpals, metatarsals, and phalanges, like the larger limb bones, have the form of long bones. Short bones, like the tarsals, carpals, and centra of the vertebrae, have about the same length in all directions. Flat or tabular bones have one dimension that is much shorter than the other two, like the scapula or wing of the ilium.

CORTICAL AND CANCELLOUS BONE. Examination of the cut surface of a bone shows that the tissue assumes two forms—the outer cortical or compact bone, and the inner cancellous or trabecular bone (Fig. 2-8). Cortical bone forms about 80% of the skeleton and surrounds the thin bars or plates of cancellous bone with compact lamellae. In long bones, dense cortical bone forms the cylindric diaphysis that surrounds a marrow cavity containing little or no trabecular bone. In the metaphyses of long bones, the cortical bone thins, and trabecular bone fills the medullary cavity. Short and flat bones usually have thinner cortices than the diaphyses of long bones and contain cancellous bone. Cancellous and cortical bone modify their structure in response to persistent changes in loading, hormonal influences, and other factors.

Because of their differences in density and organization, equal size blocks of cortical and cancellous bone have different mechanical properties. The two types of bone have the same composition, but

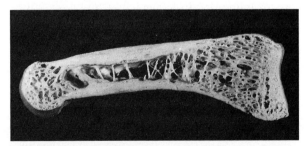

FIGURE 2-8. Longitudinal section of a human phalanx. Outer lamellae of cortical bone surround the inner cancellous bone. The metaphyses contain more cancellous bone than the diaphysis, and the thick cortical bone of the diaphysis becomes thinner in the metaphysis. Larger bones like the femur follow the same structural pattern. (Buckwalter JA, Cooper RR. Bone structure and function. AAOS Instruct Course Lect 1987;36: 27–48)

cortical bone has much greater density. Because the compression strength of bone is proportional to the square of the density, cortical bone has compressive strength that may be in order of magnitude greater than that of cancellous bone. Differences in the organization and orientation of cortical and cancellous bone matrices may also make a difference in their mechanical properties.

Microscopic Structure

MINERALIZED AND UNMINERALIZED BONE MATRIX. During skeletal growth and bone remodeling, osteoblasts form seams of unmineralized bone organic matrix, osteoid, on the surface of mineralized bone matrix. Normally, osteoid mineralizes soon after it appears. Therefore, normal bone contains only small amounts of unmineralized matrix.

Osteoid lacks the stiffness of mineralized bone matrix. For this reason, failure to mineralize bone matrix during growth or during normal turnover of bone matrix in skeletally mature individuals produces weaker bone. Individuals with impaired mineralization of bone matrix may develop skeletal deformities or fractures. In children, the clinical condition associated with impaired mineralization, rickets, predisposes the patient to skeletal deformity. In adults, the clinical condition associated with impaired mineralization, osteomalacia, predisposes the patient to fractures.

WOVEN AND LAMELLAR BONE. Mineralized bone exists in two forms—woven (immature, fiber, or primary) and lamellar (mature, secondary). Woven bone forms the embryonic skeleton and the new bone formed in the metaphyseal parts of growth plates. Mature bone replaces this woven bone as the skeleton develops and during skeletal growth. Small amounts of woven bone may persist after skeletal maturity as part of tendon and ligament insertions, the suture margins of cranial bones, and the ear ossicles. With these exceptions, woven bone rarely appears in the normal human skeleton after 4 or 5 years of age, although it is the first bone formed in many healing fractures at any age, and it also appears during the rapid turnover and formation of bone associated with metabolic, neoplastic, and infectious or inflammatory diseases.

Woven and mature bone differ in mechanical properties and the rate of bone formation. Cells rapidly form the irregular, almost random, collagen fibril matrix of woven bone. The appearance of the irregular arrangement of collagen fibrils gives woven bone its name. It contains about four times as many os-teocytes per unit volume of lamellar bone, and they vary in size, orientation, and distribution. The mineralization of the woven bone matrix also follows an irregular pattern with mineral deposits varying in size and their relation to collagen fibrils. In contrast, cells form lamellar bone more slowly, and the cell density is less. The collagen fibrils of lamellar bone vary less in diameter and lie in tightly aligned parallel sheets forming distinct lamellae 4 to 12 μm thick with an almost uniform distribution of mineral throughout the matrix.

Because of the lack of collagen fibril orientation, the high cell and water content, and the irregular mineralization, the mechanical properties of woven bone differ from those of lamellar bone. It is more flexible, more easily deformed, and weaker than mature lamellar bone. For this reason, the immature skeleton and healing fractures have less stiffness and strength than the mature skeleton or a fracture remodeled with lamellar bone.

Composition

Cells

The formation and maintenance of bone depends on the coordinated actions of different types of bone cells. The morphology, function, and characteristics of bone cells separates them into four groups—undifferentiated or osteoprogenitor cells, osteoblasts, osteocytes, and osteoclasts.

UNDIFFERENTIATED OR OSTEOPROGENITOR CELLS. Undifferentiated or osteoprogenitor cells, small cells with a single nucleus, few organelles, and irregular form, remain in an undifferentiated state until stimulated to proliferate or differentiate into osteoblasts. They usually reside in the canals of bone, the endosteum and the periosteum, although cells that can differentiate into osteoblasts also exist in tissues other than bone.

OSTEOBLASTS. Osteoblasts, cuboidal cells with a single usually eccentric nucleus, contain large volumes of synthetic organelles—endoplasmic reticulum and Golgi membranes (Fig. 2-9). They lie on bone surfaces where, when stimulated, they form new bone organic matrix and participate in controlling matrix mineralization. When active, they assume a round to oval or polyhedral form, and a seam of new osteoid separates them from mineralized matrix. Their cytoplasmic processes extend through the osteoid to contact osteocytes within mineralized matrix.

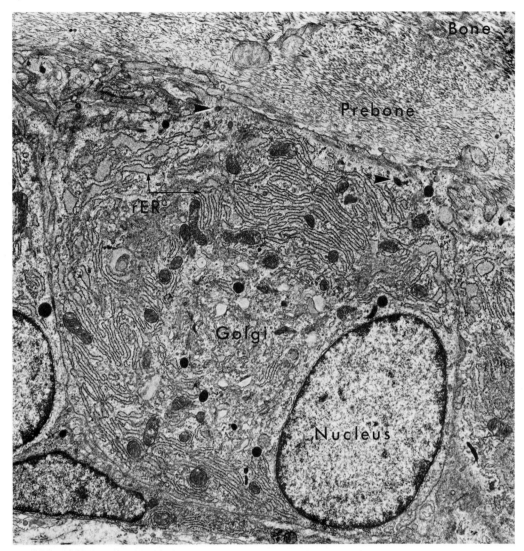

FIGURE 2-9. Electron micrograph of an osteoblast from demineralized rat alveolar bone showing the arrangement of the organelles. Numerous collagen fibrils, which these cells secrete, are present in the adjacent prebone, or osteon and bone (*upper right*). The procollagen, which is the precursor of the collagen fibrils, is carried within secretory granules (*arrowheads*) originating from the Golgi saccules. Procollagen is released into the prebone by fusion of the secretory granule with the apical plasma membrane of the cell (× 12,000). (Courtesy of Melvyn Weinstock; Ham AW, Cormack DH. Histology, ed 8. Philadelphia, JB Lippincott, 1979)

Once actively engaged in synthesizing new matrix, they can follow one of two courses. They can decrease their synthetic activity, remain on the bone surface, and assume the flatter form of a bone surface lining cell, or they can surround themselves with matrix and become osteocytes.

OSTEOCYTES. Osteocytes contribute over 90% of the cells of the mature skeleton. Combined with the periosteal and endosteal cells, they cover the bone matrix surfaces. Their long cytoplasmic processes extend from their oval or lens-shaped bodies to contact other osteocytes within the bone matrix or the cell processes of osteoblasts forming a network of cells that extends from the bone surfaces throughout the bone matrix (Figs. 2-10 and 2-11). The cell membranes of the osteocytes and their cell processes cover over 90% of the total surface area of mature bone matrix. This arrangement gives them access to almost all the mineralized matrix surface area and may be critical in the cell- mediated exchange of mineral that occurs between bone fluid and the blood. In partic-

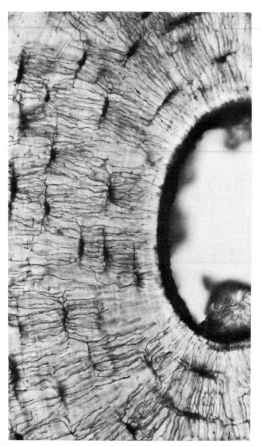

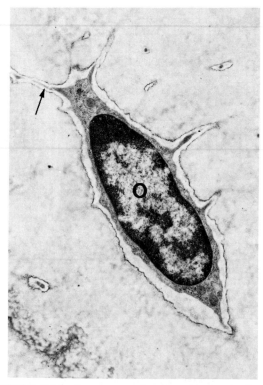

FIGURE 2-11. Low-power electron micrograph of an osteocyte and its processes in a section of decalcified bone. The nucleus (O) and an arrow point to a process in a canaliculus. Two processes in canaliculi cut in cross section can be seen, one near the upper right corner and the other toward the lower left corner. (Courtesy of S.C. Luk and G.T. Simon; Ham AW, Cormack DH. Histology, ed 8. Philadelphia, JB Lippincott, 1979)

FIGURE 2-10. A photomicrograph of a ground bone section. The lacunae in which the osteocytes reside are dark, flattened oval structures. The fine lines connecting these are canaliculi. The canaliculi extend to the empty canal on the right. In life, this canal contained blood vessels that supplied tissue fluid to the canaliculi. (Preparation by H. Whittaker; Ham AW, Cormack DH. Histology, ed 8. Philadelphia, JB Lippincott, 1979)

ular, they may help maintain the composition of bone fluid and the body's mineral balance.

OSTEOCLASTS. Osteoclasts, large irregular cells with multiple nuclei, fill much of their cytoplasm with mitochondria to supply the energy required for these cells to resorb bone. They usually lie directly against the bone matrix on endosteal, periosteal, and haversian system bone surfaces (Fig. 2-12), but unlike osteocytes, and presumably osteoblasts, they can move from one site of bone resorption to another. Osteoclasts appear to form by fusion of multiple bone marrow–derived mononuclear cells. When they have finished their bone resorbing activity, they may divide to reform multiple mononuclear cells.

One of the most distinctive features of osteoclasts is the complex folding of their cytoplasmic membrane where it lies against the bone matrix at sites of bone resorption (Fig. 2-13). This ruffled or brushed border appears to play a critical role in bone resorption, possibly by increasing the surface area of the cell relative to the bone and creating a sharply localized environment that rapidly degrades bone matrix. The fluid between the brush boarder and the bone matrix probably has a high concentration of hydrogen ions and proteolytic enzymes. The acidic environment could demineralize bone matrix, and the enzymes could degrade the organic bone matrix. In cancellous bone, osteoclasts resorbing the bone surface create a characteristic depression called a Howship lacuna. In cortical bone, several osteoclasts lead the osteonal cutting cones that remodel dense cortical bone.

Bone Matrix

Bone matrix consists of the organic macromolecules, the inorganic mineral, and the matrix fluid. The inorganic matrix component contributes about

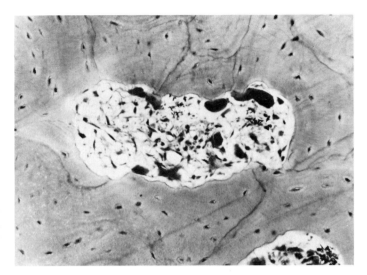

FIGURE 2-12. Photomicrograph of a cross section of the shaft of a bone showing a resorption cavity in cross or somewhat oblique section. The large dark cells are osteoclasts; their activity explains the etched-out borders of the cavity. (Ham AW, Cormack DH. Histology, ed 8. Philadelphia, JB Lippincott, 1979)

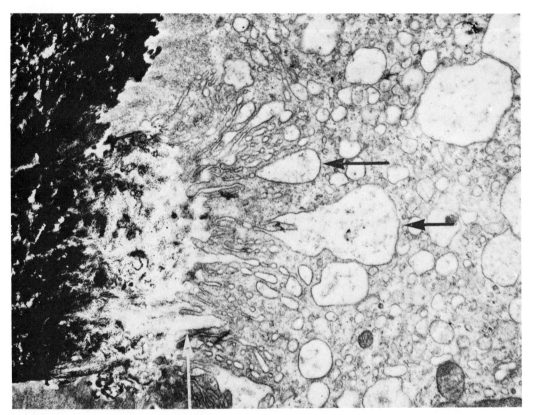

FIGURE 2-13. Electron micrograph of a section of a bone surface undergoing resorption. Calcified bone appears black (*left*). The main part of the picture is occupied by the cytoplasm of an osteoclast. Extending from the top to the bottom, in the middle of the picture, is the ruffled border of the osteoclast; this consists of complex folds and projections that abut on the bone at the left. Between the ruffled border of the osteoclast and the heavily calcified bone is an area where the calcium content is much less, which suggests that the osteoclast is dissolving or otherwise removing mineral from this area. Black granules of mineral can be seen in some of the large vesicles (*horizontal arrows*), which probably form because of the bottom of crypts being pinched off. In the original print a collagenic microfibril showing typical periodicity could be seen at this site indicated by the vertical arrow ($\times$ 20,000). (Courtesy of B. Boothroyd and N.M. Hancox; Ham AW, Cormack DH. Histology, ed 8. Philadelphia, JB Lippincott, 1979)

70% of wet bone weight, although it may contribute up to 80%. The organic macromolecules contribute about 20% of the wet bone weight, and water contributes 8% to 10% (see Fig. 2-3). The organic matrix gives bone its form and provides its tensile strength; the mineral component gives bone strength in compression.

Removal of the bone mineral or digestion of the organic matrix shows the contributions of the inorganic and organic matrix components to the mechanical properties of bone. Removal of either component leaves bone with its original form and shape, but demineralized bone, like a tendon or ligament, has great flexibility. A demineralized long bone, such as the fibula, can be twisted or bent without fracture. In contrast, removal of the organic matrix makes bone brittle. Only a slight deformation will crack the inorganic matrix, and a sharp blow will shatter it.

ORGANIC MATRIX. The organic matrix of bone resembles that of dense fibrous tissues like tendon, ligament, annulus fibrosis, meniscus, and joint capsule. Type I collagen contributes over 90% of the organic matrix. The other 10% includes small proteoglycans, many of noncollagenous proteins including osteonectin, and small amounts of type V collagen and possibly other collagens.

Mineralization changes and stabilizes the composition of the bone organic matrix. Compared with bone organic matrix, osteoid contains more noncollagenous macromolecules and water. Once mineralization occurs, the organic matrix remains stable until resorbed. Abnormalities of the organic matrix can weaken bone. For example, many patients with osteogenesis imperfecta have disturbances of synthesis, secretion, or assembly of the collagen component of the bone organic matrix that increase bone fragility.

INORGANIC MATRIX. The mechanisms that initiate and control the transformation of osteoid into mineralized bone matrix remain unclear. However, morphologic studies show that soon after osteoblasts produce osteoid, mineral appears within the bone type I collagen fibrils and then extends through the matrix without altering the organization of the collagen fibrils (Fig. 2-14) or affecting osteocytes within the mineralized matrix. Mineralization of the bone matrix not only increases the stiffness and strength of bone but also provides a reservoir for minerals

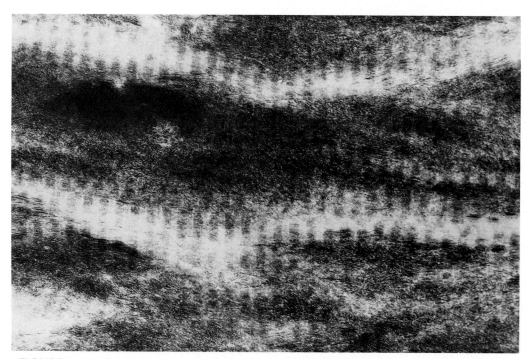

FIGURE 2-14. Electron micrograph of an undecalcified, unstained section of embryonic chick bone. The ordered disposition of the dense mineral phase along the axial direction of the collagen fibrils is evident. The mineral phase is in lateral register as well ($\times$ 110,000). (Glimber MJ. A basic architectural principle in the organization of mineralized tissues. Clin Orthop 1961;61:16)

needed for normal function of other tissues and organ systems. The bone matrix contains about 99% of the body's calcium, 80% of the phosphate, and large proportions of the sodium, magnesium, and carbonate.

Newly mineralized bone matrix contains a variety of calcium phosphate species that range from relatively soluble complexes to insoluble crystalline hydroxyapatite. As bone matures, the inorganic matrix becomes primarily crystalline hydroxyapatite, although sodium, magnesium, citrate, and fluoride may also be present. Because the degree of mineralization increases with maturation, the material properties of bone change as well. In particular, with increasing mineralization, bone stiffness increases. This helps explain why children's and adult's bones may differ in their patterns of fracture. When subjected to excessive load, normal adult bone usually breaks rather than deforming permanently. In contrast, children's bones may bow or buckle rather than break.

Control of Bone Cell Activity

Throughout life, osteoclasts remove bone matrix, and osteoblasts replace it. The reason for this physiologic turnover of bone tissue not been established, but it may have a role in maintaining the structural integrity of the bone tissue. To preserve normal bone mass and mechanical properties, osteoblastic bone formation must balance osteoclastic bone resorption. A variety of stimuli can alter this balance. For example, repetitive loading of the skeleton can increase bone formation relative to bone resorption and thereby increase bone mass and strength. Immobilization decreases bone formation relative to bone resorption, thereby decreasing bone mass and strength.

Bone mass normally changes with age. It increases to a maximum value about 10 years after completion of skeletal growth, remains stable for a variable period, and then begins to decrease, progressively weakening the skeleton. The reasons for the age-related loss of bone mass and the mechanisms that normally coordinate and control bone cell function remain poorly understood, but investigations of bone turnover show that both systemic and local factors help control osteoclast and osteoblast function.

Systemic Factors

Systemic factors that influence the balance between bone resorption and bone formation include nutrition, exercise, and hormonal activity, especially parathyroid hormone, vitamin D and its metabolites, thyroid hormone, growth hormone, insulin, estrogens, testosterone, and calcitonin. Dietary abnormalities, lack of physical activity, and some disturbances of hormone balance are the most commonly known causes of clinically significant systemic increases in bone resorption relative to bone formation. Protein malnutrition impairs bone formation during bone growth and remodeling. Prolonged lack of exercise decreases bone mass. Vitamin D deficiency and abnormalities of vitamin D metabolism produce rickets or osteomalacia. Excessive parathyroid hormone increases bone turnover and decreases bone mass; excessive thyroid hormones can have similar effects. Exogenous corticosteroids decrease the synthetic activity of osteoblasts and may interfere with the ability of undifferentiated cells to assume the form of osteoblasts and adversely affect calcium balance. As a result, patients receiving corticosteroids for prolonged periods may develop severe osteopenia and multiple pathologic fractures. Estrogen also influences bone cell function. In many women, bone mass begins to decrease rapidly after menopause and then continues to decrease rapidly for 5 to 10 years. Estrogen replacement can slow or reverse this rapid loss.

Local Factors

In addition to systemic factors, local factors—including oxygen tension, pH, local ion concentrations, interactions between cells, local concentrations of nutrients and metabolites, mechanical and electrical signals, and interaction between cells and matrix molecules—can influence the balance between bone loss and bone formation. Localized mechanical loading of bone has particular significance. Immobilization or decreased loading of a limb causes a relatively rapid loss of bone mass, whereas repetitive increased loading can increase bone density.

Recent work suggests that cytokines, small protein molecules that influence multiple cell functions, can influence bone cell function and may help couple bone resorption and formation. Cytokines produced by neoplasms may increase bone formation or, more frequently, increase bone resorption. Interleukin-1, a cytokine produced by monocytes, stimulates osteoclast formation and osteoclastic bone resorption. It may contribute to the loss of bone in conditions like rheumatoid arthritis. Transforming growth factor β (TGF-β), a cytokine present in bone matrix, may be one of the factors that balances bone resorption and bone formation. Osteoclastic resorption of bone matrix may release or activate TGF-β. Activated TGF-β then may inhibit osteoclastic activity and stimulate osteoblasts to form bone.

Blood Supply

An elaborate system of vessels extends throughout bone, penetrating even the most dense cortical bone (Fig. 2-15). No cell lies more than 300 μm from a blood vessel.

Long-bone diaphyses and metaphyses have three sources of blood supply—nutrient arteries, epiphyseal and metaphyseal penetrating arteries, and periosteal arteries (Fig. 2-16). The nutrient arteries pass through the diaphyseal cortex and branch proximally and distally forming the medullary arterial system

that supplies the diaphysis. The proximal and distal branches of the nutrient arteries join multiple fine branches of periosteal and metaphyseal arteries that contribute to the medullary vascular system. Under normal circumstances, this medullary vascular system supplies most periosteum-covered bone; therefore, the primary direction of blood flow through the cortex is centrifugal. In regions of dense fascial insertions into bone, such as muscle insertions or interosseous membrane insertions, periosteal or insertion site vessels usually supply the outer third of the bone cortex.

Before closure of the physis, medullary vessels rarely cross the growth plate, and epiphyses depend on penetrating epiphyseal vessels for their blood supply. With closure of the physis, interosseous anastomoses develop between the penetrating epiphyseal arteries and the medullary arteries, but these anastomoses rarely provide sufficient blood

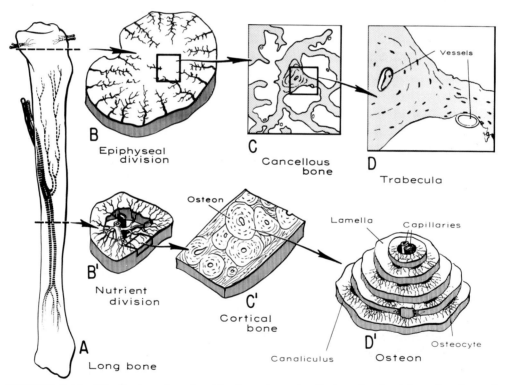

FIGURE 2-15. Distribution of nutrient blood supply to the diaphyseal and epiphyseal regions of a long bone. (**A**) Basic pattern of nutrient circulation to a long bone (human tibia). (**B**) Pattern of circulation in epiphyseal–metaphyseal region. Arteries perforate thin cortical shell to enter cancellous bone. (**C**) Structure of cancellous bone. (**D**) A trabeculae of bone. Capillaries abut against thin trabecula. In thicker trabecula, an osteon can be seen. (**B'**) Cross section of middiaphysis. Here there is a single nutrient artery and vein. Lateral branches arise from the artery to supply the cortical bone. (**C'**) Cortical bone. Osteons and interstitial bone between osteons. (**D'**) Diagramatic concept of a single osteon. Canaliculi of the osteocytes are canals in which the processes of the osteocytes are located. It is by way of these canaliculi that nutrition is derived from the vessels in the haversian canal. (Kelly PJ, Peterson LFA. The blood supply of bone. Heart Bull 1963;12:96)

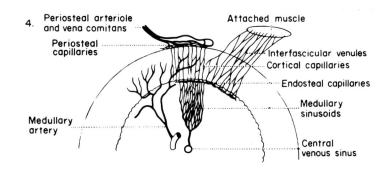

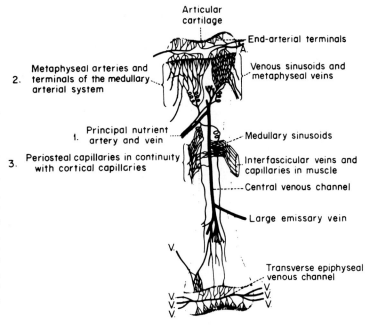

FIGURE 2-16. Blood supply of a long bone. Three basic blood supplies are shown: (1) nutrient; (2) metaphyseal, which anastomoses with epiphyseal after epiphyseal closure; and (3) periosteal. The numerous metaphyseal arteries arise from periarticular networks and anastomose with terminal branches of ascending and descending medullary arteries. Periosteal capillaries emerge from the cortex (efferent blood flow). (4) A periosteal arteriole feeds capillaries that provide afferent blood flow to a limited outer layer of cortex (Rhinelander FW. Circulation of bone. In: Bourne GH, ed. Biochemistry and physiology of bone, ed 2. New York, Academic Press, 1972:2)

flow to support the epiphyseal bone cells without the contribution of the epiphyseal vessels. For this reason, even after closure of the physis the blood supply to many epiphyses is vulnerable to interruption. This is a particular problem in the region of the femoral head where a dislocation of the hip or damage to the epiphyseal penetrating vessels can cause necrosis and eventually collapse of the femoral head.

Nerve Supply

Nerve fibers have been identified within the medullary canals of bone and particularly in association with blood vessels. Presumably, these nerves have the primary function of controlling bone blood flow. Specialized complex nerve endings have not been described within bone tissue.

PERIOSTEUM

Except for the articular cartilage surfaces and the insertions of tendons, ligaments joint capsules, and interosseous membranes, a tough thin membranous fibrous tissue, the periosteum, covers the external surface of bone. It allows for attachment of some ligaments, tendons, and joint capsules to bone and provides a source of cells that can form new bone or cartilage.

Structure

Two tissue layers form the periosteum—an outer fibrous layer and an inner, more cellular and vascular layer (Fig. 2-17). The outer layer consists of a dense fibrous tissue matrix and fibroblast-like cells. Tendon,

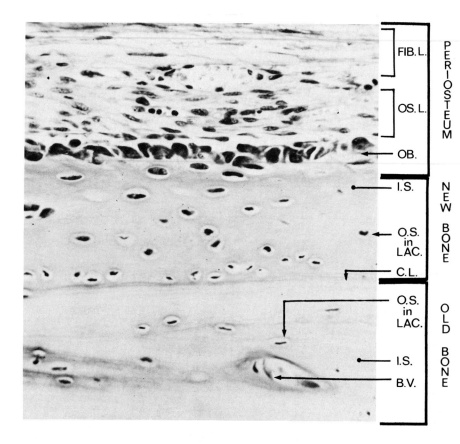

FIGURE 2-17. A longitudinal section of a rabbit's rib close to a fracture that had been healing for a short time. During this time the osteogenic cells of the periosteum have proliferated, and some have differentiated into osteoblasts that have laid down a layer of new bone on the original bone that was fractured. Three layers are labeled at the right: periosteum, new bone, and old bone. Periosteum: FIB. L., fibrous layer; OS.L., osteogenic layer; OB., layer of osteoblasts. New bone: I.S., intercellular substance; O.S. in LAC., osteocyte in a lacuna; C.L., cementing line between the new bone and the old. Old bone: I.S., intercellular substance; O.S. in LAC., osteocyte in a lacuna; B.V., blood vessel in a canal. (Ham AW, Cormack DH. Histology, ed 8. Philadelphia, JB Lippincott, 1979)

ligament, and joint capsule insertions that do not penetrate directly into bone attach to this layer. In some regions, the dense fibrous tissue insertions form a continuous sheet or membrane of tissue with the periosteum. The inner, osteogenic or cambium layer contains cells capable of forming cartilage and bone.

Periosteum changes with age. The thick cellular vascular periosteum of infants and children readily forms new bone. It shows this capacity when osteomyelitis or trauma destroys the diaphysis of a young individual's bone, and the periosteum regenerates a new diaphysis. With increasing age, periosteum becomes thinner and less vascular, and its ability to form new bone declines. The cells of the deeper layer become flattened and quiescent, but they continue to form new bone that increases bone diameter, and they still have the potential to form bone or cartilage in response to injury.

Blood Supply

In many areas, a plexus of small vessels lies on the outer fibrous layer of the periosteum. At intervals these periosteal blood vessels anastomose with the vessels of the overlying muscle. Branches of the vessels on the surface of the periosteum penetrate the fibrous layer and contribute to the vascular system of the deeper layer of the periosteum and to the blood vessels that penetrate bone to join the medullary vascular system.

Nerve Supply

Nerve cell processes lie on the external periosteal surface and often accompany periosteal blood vessels. Presumably, they help regulate periosteal blood flow.

TENDON, LIGAMENT, AND JOINT CAPSULE

The specialized musculoskeletal dense fibrous tissues—tendon, ligament, and joint capsule—have a major role in providing the stability and mobility of the musculoskeletal system. These tissues differ in shape and location and vary slightly in structure, composition, and function. However, they have in common their insertion into bone and their ability to resist large tensile loads with minimal deformation. Tendons transmit the muscle forces to bone that produce joint movement; ligaments and joint capsules stabilize joints and the relations between adjacent bones while allowing and guiding joint movement. Diseases or injuries that affect these tissues can destabilize joints or lead to loss of muscle function. Contractures of these tissues limit muscle and joint motion and contribute to skeletal deformity.

Structure

Tendons, ligaments, and joint capsules take the form of tough yet flexible and pliant fibrous sheets, bands, and cords that consist of highly oriented dense fibrous tissue. The high degree of matrix organization and density of the matrix, reflecting a high concentration of collagen (Fig. 2-18), distinguish these tissues from irregular dense fibrous tissues and loose fibrous tissues.

Tendon

Tendons vary in shape and size from the small fibrous strings that form the tendons of the lumbrical muscles to the large fibrous cords that form the Achilles tendons. In any shape or size, however, they unite muscle with bone and transmit the force of muscle contraction to bone. They consist of three parts—the substance of the tendon itself, the muscle tendon junction, and the bone insertion (Fig. 2-19). Connective tissues surrounding tendons allow low

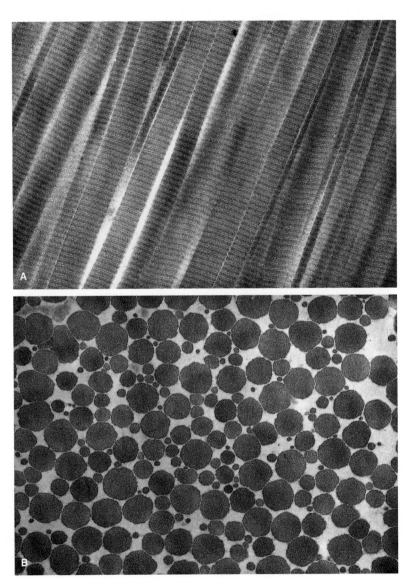

FIGURE 2-18. Electron micrographs of the type I collagen fibrils of ligament. (**A**) A longitudinal section shows the densely packed highly oriented collagen microfibrils. (**B**) A transverse section also shows the densely packed collagen microfibrils.

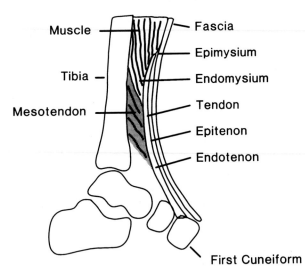

FIGURE 2-19. Diagramatic representation of the tibialis anterior tendon showing the muscle tendon junction, the tendon substance, and the bone insertion. The epimysium and endomysium of muscle, and the epitenon and endotenon of tendon form continuous structures. The epimysium consists of a fibrous envelope that surrounds the muscle, and the endomysium consists of the fine sheaths that surround individual muscle fibers. Perimysium refers to the fibrous sheath enveloping primary bundles of muscle fibers. Loose connective tissue surrounds the tendon proximally where it pursues a straight course, but a sheath forms distally where it changes direction. (Buckwalter JA, Maynard JA, Vailis AC. Skeletal fibrous tissues: Tendon, joint capsule, and ligament. In: Albright JA, Brand RA, eds. The scientific basis of orthopaedics. Norwalk, CT, Appleton & Lange, 1987:388)

friction gliding and access for blood vessels to the tendon substance. Many tendons have a well-developed mesotendon, a structure that attaches the tendon to the surrounding connective tissue and consists of loose elastic connective tissue that can stretch and recoil with the tendon and provide a blood supply to the tendon substance. In certain locations, the surrounding connective tissue forms sheaths that enclose the tendon and specialized pulleys of dense fibrous tissue that influence the line of tendon action.

TENDON SUBSTANCE. Multiple fascicles or bundles, consisting of fibroblasts and dense linear arrays of collagen fibrils, form the tendon substance and give tendons their fibrous appearance. The endotendon, a less dense connective tissue containing fibroblasts, blood vessels, nerves, and lymphatics, surrounds individual tendon fascicles. The separation of tendon fascicles by endotendon may allow small gliding movements between adjacent tendon bundles. The endotendon tissue continues to form the

epitenon, a thin layer of connective tissue that covers the surface of the tendon. Where the tendon joins the muscle, the fibrous tissue of the epitenon continues as the thin fibrous covering of the attached muscle called the epimysium.

MUSCLE TENDON JUNCTIONS. Muscle tendon junctions must efficiently transmit the force of muscle contraction to the tendon. The attachment of muscle to tendon occurs through continuation of the collagen fibrils of the fibrous tissue layers of muscle (epimysium, perimysium, and endomysium) into the collagen fibrils of the tendon and through elaborate interdigitation of the muscle cell membrane with the collagen fibrils of the tendon. This interdigitation of muscle cell and tendon has the appearance of interlocking fingers when examined by electron microscopy, and provides a strong bond between the muscle cell and the tendon collagen. Collagen fibrils do not enter the muscle cells but lie next to their basement membranes. The muscle cell plasma membrane thickens at the muscle tendon junction, and muscle myofilaments extend directly to it.

PERITENDINOUS STRUCTURES. Normal tendon gliding, efficient transmission of muscle forces to move joints, and tendon nutrition depend on the peritendinous connective tissue structures sometimes called peritenon. These structures range from loose connective tissue to elaborate well-defined mesotendons, sheaths, and pulleys.

Where tendons follow a straight course, the surrounding tissue usually consists of loose areolar tissue. In some locations, this tissue must stretch several centimeters and then recoil without tearing or disrupting the tendon blood supply. It consists of an interlacing meshwork of thin collagen fibrils and elastic fibers filled with abundant soft, almost fluid, ground substance.

Where tendons change course between their muscle attachment and their bone insertion, often as they cross or near a joint, the surrounding connective tissue may form a bursa or a discrete tendon sheath. These structures allow low-friction movement between the tendon and adjacent bone, joint capsule, tendon, ligament, fibrous tissue retinacula, or fibrous tissue pulleys. Tendon bursae and sheaths consist of flattened synovial lined sacks that usually cover only a portion of the tendon circumference. Tendon sheaths and bursae resemble synovial joints in that they consist of cavities lined with synovial-like cells, they contain synovial-like fluid, and they facilitate low-friction gliding between two surfaces. Mesotenons generally attach to one surface of a tendon within a tendon sheath and provide the blood supply to this portion of the tendon.

Distinct dense fibrous tissue retinacula, pulleys, or fascial slings lie over the outer surface of some regions of tendon sheaths. These firm fibrous structures direct the line of tendon movement and prevent displacement or bowstringing of the tendon that would decrease the efficiency of the muscle tendon unit. For example, the dense fibrous tissue extensor tendon retinacula of the wrist keeps the wrist and digital extensor tendons from displacing dorsally when they extend the fingers and dorsiflex the wrist. The flexor tendons of the fingers and thumb pass through a more elaborate series of pulleys and sheaths that make possible efficient finger flexion.

Joint Capsule and Ligament

Joint capsules and ligaments have similar structures and functions, and in some regions ligament and capsule form a continuous structure. Like tendon, both of them consist primarily of highly oriented, densely packed collagen fibrils. Unlike tendons, they more often assume the form of layered sheets or lamellae. Both ligament and capsule attach to adjacent bones and cross synovial joints, yet allow at least some motion between the bones. Ligaments have the primary function of restraining abnormal motion between adjacent bones. Joint capsules also restrain abnormal joint motion or displacement of articular surfaces, but usually to a lesser extent. Both capsule and ligament consist of a proximal bone insertion, ligament or capsular substance, and a distal bone insertion, and both contain nerves that may sense joint motion and displacement.

JOINT CAPSULE. Joint capsules form fibrous tissue cuffs around synovial joints. A synovial membrane lines the interior of the joint capsule, and loose areolar connective tissue covers the exterior. This loose tissue often contains networks of small blood vessels that supply the capsule. Nerves and blood vessels from this loose connective tissue penetrate the fibrous capsule to supply the capsule and outer later of synovium. Each end of the capsule attaches in a continuous line around the articular surface of the bones forming the joint, usually near the periphery of the articular cartilage surface. Tendons and ligaments reinforce some regions of joint capsules. For example, the glenohumeral ligaments form part of the glenohumeral joint capsule, and the expansion of the semimembranosus tendon contributes to the posterior oblique ligament of the knee and part of the knee joint capsule.

LIGAMENT. Surgeons and anatomists have named ligaments by their location and bony attachments (eg, the anterior glenohumeral ligament or the anterior talofibular ligament) or by their relation to other ligaments (eg, the medial collateral ligament of the knee or the posterior cruciate ligament of the knee). Unlike joint capsules, ligaments vary in their anatomic relation to synovial joints. This variability separates ligaments into three types—intraarticular or intracapsular, articular or capsular, and extraarticular or extracapsular. Intraarticular ligaments, including the cruciate ligaments of the knee, have the form of distinct separate structures. In contrast, capsular ligaments, like the glenohumeral ligaments, appear as thickenings of joint capsules. Extraarticular ligaments, like the coracoacromial ligament, lie at a distance from a synovial joint. Despite these differences in relation to joints, the function of the three ligament types remains that of stabilizing adjacent bones or restraining abnormal joint motion.

Composition

Individual tendons, ligaments, and capsules differ slightly in cell and matrix composition. However, they all contain the same basic cell types, share similar patterns of vascular supply and innervation, and have the same primary matrix macromolecule, type I collagen.

Cells

Fibroblasts form the predominant cell of tendon, ligament, and joint capsule. The endothelial cells of blood vessels, and in some locations nerve cell processes, exist within tendon, ligament, and joint capsule, but they form only a small part of the tissue. The fibroblasts surround themselves with a dense fibrous tissue matrix and throughout life continue to maintain the matrix. They vary in shape, activity, and density among ligaments, tendons, and joint capsules and among regions of the same structure. Most dense fibrous tissue fibroblasts have long small diameter cell processes that extend between collagen fibrils throughout the matrix. Generally, younger tissues have a higher cell density and cells with a larger cytoplasmic volume and intracellular density of endoplasmic reticulum. With increasing age, the cell density usually decreases, and the cells appear to become less active.

Matrix

Tissue fluid contributes 60% or more of the wet weight of most dense fibrous tissues, and the matrix macromolecules contribute the other 40%. Because most dense fibrous tissue cells lie at some distance from blood vessels, these cells must depend on diffusion of nutrients and metabolites through the tissue fluid. In addition, the interaction of the tissue fluid and the matrix macromolecules influences the mechanical properties of the tissue.

Collagens, elastin, proteoglycans, and noncollagenous proteins combine to form the macromolecular framework of the dense fibrous tissues. Collagens, the major component of the dense fibrous tissue molecular framework, contribute 70% to 80% of the dry weight of many dense fibrous tissues. Type I collagen commonly forms over 90% of the tissue collagen. Type III collagen also occurs within the dense fibrous tissues; in some tissues it forms about 10% of the total collagen, and other collagen types may also be present in small amounts. Most dense fibrous tissues have some elastin, less than 5% of their dry weight. Some ligaments, in particular the nuchal ligament and ligamentum flavum, have much higher elastin concentrations, up to 75% of the tissue dry weight. Proteoglycans usually contribute less than 1% of the dry weight of dense fibrous tissues but may have important roles in organizing the extracellular matrix and interacting with the tissue fluid. Most dense fibrous tissues appear to contain both large aggregating proteoglycans and small nonaggregating proteoglycans. The large proteoglycans presumably occupy the interfibrillar regions of the matrix, and the small proteoglycans lie directly on or near the surface of collagen fibrils. Noncollagenous proteins also form a critical part of the dense fibrous tissue matrix even though they contribute only a few percent to the dry weight of most of the tissues. Fibronectin occurs in all dense fibrous tissues; other noncollagenous proteins also contribute to the structure of these tissues, but their composition, structure, and function have not been well defined.

Insertions Into Bone

The bony insertions of tendons, ligaments, and joint capsules attach the flexible dense fibrous tissue securely to rigid bone, yet they allow motion between the bone and the dense fibrous tissue without damage to the dense fibrous tissue. Despite their small size, insertions have a more complex and variable structure than the substance of the tissue, and they have different mechanical properties. They vary in size, strength, and the angle of their collagen fiber bundles relative to the bone and in the proportion of their collagen fibers that penetrate directly into bone. Based on differences in the angle between the collagen fibers of the dense fibrous tissue structure and the bone and on the proportion of collagen fibrils that penetrate directly into bone, dense fibrous tissue insertions can be separated into two types—direct insertions (insertions in which many collagen fibrils pass directly into bone) and indirect or periosteal insertion (insertions in which only a few collagen fibrils pass directly into bone; Fig. 2-20).

Direct Insertions

Direct insertions, like the insertion of the medial collateral ligament of the knee into the femur, consist of sharply defined regions where the ligament joins

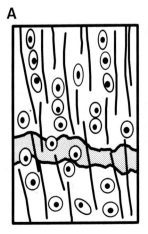
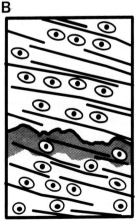

Ligament

Fibrocartilage

Mineralized Fibrocartilage

Bone

FIGURE 2-20. Diagramatic representations of direct and indirect dense fibrous tissue insertions into bone. (**A**) In direct insertions a high proportion of the collagen fibers pass directly into bone, and the fibrocartilage and mineralized fibrocartilage zones are well developed. (**B**) In direct insertions a high proportion of the collagen fibers pass into the periosteum, and the fibrocartilage and mineralized fibrocartilage zones often are not well developed. (Buckwalter JA, Maynard JA, Vailis AC. Skeletal fibrous tissues: Tendon, joint capsule, and ligament. In: Albright JA, Brand RA, eds. The scientific basis of orthopaedics. Norwalk, CT, Appleton & Lange, 1987:391)

the bone; only a thin layer of the substance of the ligament, tendon, or capsule joins the fibrous layer of the periosteum. Most of the collagen fibrils at the insertion pass directly from the substance of the tendon, ligament, or joint capsule into the bone cortex, usually entering at a right angle to the bone surface. These fibrils then mingle with the collagen fibrils of the organic matrix of bone creating a strong bond between the tendon, ligament, or capsule and the bone matrix. Where dense fibrous tissue structures approach the bone surface at oblique angles, the collagen fibrils may make a sharp turn to enter the bone at a right angle.

The deeper collagen fibers that enter the bone pass through four zones of increasing stiffness—the substance of the dense fibrous tissue structure, fibrocartilage, mineralized fibrocartilage and bone. In the fibrocartilage zone, the cells are larger and more spherical than the fibroblasts of the tendon, joint capsule, or ligament. A sharp border of unmineralized matrix separates the zone of fibrocartilage from the mineralized fibrocartilage zone.

Indirect Insertions

The less common indirect insertions, like the insertion of the medial collateral ligament of the knee into the tibia, usually cover more bone surface area than direct insertions because a larger proportion of their collagen fibrils join the periosteum. Like direct insertions, indirect insertions have superficial and deep collagen fibrils, but most collagen fibrils form the superficial layer that joins the fibrous layer of the periosteum. The deep collagen fibrils enter the bone cortex, but they generally do not pass through sharply defined zones of mineralized and unmineralized fibrocartilage.

Blood Supply

Most dense fibrous tissues have well-developed networks of blood vessels extending throughout their substance. Generally, these vascular systems follow the longitudinal pattern of the collagenous matrix, but they may have multiple anastomoses between parallel vessels. Some blood vessels in tendon, ligament, and joint capsule insertions enter the bone.

Nerve Supply

In addition to nerve cell processes next to blood vessels, like those found in periosteum and bone, dense fibrous tissues have specialized nerve endings that lie on the surface or within the substance of the tissue. Presumably, the nerve fibers in the dense fibrous tissues function as pain receptors, vasomotor efferents, and mechanoreceptors sensitive to stretch or distortion. The mechanoreceptors presumably sense joint position, muscle tension, and loads applied to ligaments, capsules, and tendons. In tendon they can adjust muscle tension. In ligament and capsule they may have a role in initiating protective reflexes that oppose potentially damaging joint movements.

MENISCI

Like articular cartilages, menisci perform important mechanical functions in synovial joints, including load bearing, shock absorption, and participation in joint lubrication. They may also contribute to joint stability. Menisci and meniscus-like structures consist of dense fibrous tissue or fibrocartilage and project from the margins of synovial joints to interpose themselves between articular cartilage surfaces. They include the knee menisci (two C-shaped menisci that lie on the tibial plateaus and form part of the knee joint), the articular disks of the sternoclavicular and acromioclavicular joints, the triangular fibrocartilage that binds the distal ends of the ulna and radius together and forms part of the wrist joint, and the labra found in some joints like the hip and shoulder. Because the structures other than the knee menisci have not been extensively studied, this section refers only to the knee menisci.

Structure

Within the knee menisci, collagen fibril diameter and orientation and cell morphology vary from the surface to the deeper central regions. The superficial regions that lie against articular cartilage usually consist of a mesh of fine fibrils. Immediately deep to these fine fibrils, small diameter collagen fibrils with a radial orientation relative to the body of the meniscus form a thicker subsurface layer. The flattened ellipsoid-shaped cells of this layer orient their maximum diameter roughly parallel to the articular surface. In the deeper central or middle region, making up the bulk of the meniscus, large diameter collagen fibril bundles surround larger cells with a more spheric shape. The deeper collagen fibril bundles follow the curve of the menisci, and smaller radially oriented fibril bundles weave among the circumferential fibril bundles. The circumferential arrangement of the large collagen bundles gives the menisci great tensile strength for loads applied parallel to the orientation of the fibers. The radial fibers may resist the development and propagation longitudinal tears between the larger circumferential collagen fiber bundles.

Composition

Cells

Meniscal cells, like many other types of mesenchymal cells, lack cell–cell contacts and attach their membranes to specific matrix macromolecules. They have the primary function of maintaining the meniscal matrix. Most of them lie at a distance from blood vessels, so like chondrocytes they rely on diffusion through the matrix for transport of nutrients and metabolites.

Matrix

Water contributes 60% to 75% of the total wet weight of meniscus. As in the other musculoskeletal tissues, the interactions between the matrix fluid and the macromolecular framework significantly influence the mechanical properties of menisci.

The macromolecular framework of meniscus contributes 25% to 40% of the meniscus wet weight and consists of collagens, noncollagenous proteins, proteoglycans, and elastin. The collagens give menisci their form and tensile strength and contribute about 75% of the dry weight of the tissue. Type I collagen makes up over 90% of the total tissue collagen. Types II, V, and VI collagen each contribute 1% to 2% of the total tissue collagen. Noncollagenous proteins, including link protein, fibronectin, and other noncollagenous proteins, contribute 8% to 13% of the dry weight. Large aggregating proteoglycans and smaller nonaggregating proteoglycans together contribute about 2% of meniscal dry weight. Presumably they have functions like the proteoglycans found in other dense fibrous tissues. Elastin forms less than 1% of the tissue dry weight. This small amount of elastin probably does not significantly influence the organization of the matrix or the mechanical properties.

Blood Supply

Most menisci and meniscal-like structures have some blood supply, at least in their more peripheral regions. Branches from the geniculate arteries form a capillary plexus along the peripheral borders of the knee menisci. Small radial branches project from the circumferential parameniscal vessels into the meniscal substance. These vessels penetrate into 10% to 30% of the width of the medial meniscus and 10% to 25% of the width of the lateral meniscus, leaving the cells of the inner portions of the menisci dependent on diffusion of nutrients and metabolites.

Nerve Supply

Nerves lie on the peripheral surface of the knee menisci and other meniscal-like structures. Although these nerves enter the more superficial regions of some parts of the tissue, they generally do not penetrate into the central regions. The functions of these nerve endings have not been clearly defined, but they may contribute to joint proprioception.

SYNOVIUM

Synovium lines the nonarticular regions of synovial joints and the bursae and sheaths of tendons. In synovial joints, synovium attaches directly around the margins of the articular cartilage. It covers the inner surfaces of the joint capsule, bone surfaces, and intraarticular ligaments and tendons. Normally, it does not extend over articular cartilage, intraarticular disks, or menisci. When examined from inside a joint, most of the synovial membrane has a smooth, even surface. However, some regions may have small projections or villi, and in others the synovium may form folds or fringes that project into the joint cavity. Fat lying outside the synovial membrane contributes to the ability of synovium to fill potential spaces in the joint cavity.

Structure

Synovial membranes consist of two layers—an inner intimal layer and a peripheral subintimal layer that lies on joint capsule or periarticular fat. Both layers vary in thickness among joints and among different regions of the same joint.

Intima

In most areas the intima consists of one or more layers of synovial cells in an amorphous matrix. The cells vary considerably in shape from flattened ellipsoids to elongated cells and polyhedral or spherical cells, and they may have cell processes. The synovial cells do not form a continuous layer; in some regions they leave gaps between cell membranes that fill with extracellular matrix. Unlike epithelial cells, the superficial synovial cells do not lie on a basement membrane.

Two types of synovial cells (A and B cells) have been identified. Type A cells have surface filopodia, plasma membrane invaginations, and vesicles. They contain mitochondria, lysosomes, cytoplasmic filaments, and Golgi membranes. B cells lack most of these characteristics, but contain a high concentration of endoplasmic reticulum. Some investigators have proposed that A and B cells have different primary functions. They suggest that A cells produce the hyaluronic acid that serves as part of the synovial fluid and have phagocytic capability and that B cells synthesize proteins, including enzymes. Cells with features of both A and B cells appear commonly; the two cell types may not represent distinct phenotypes but morphologic variants of the same cell.

Subintima

The subintimal layer separates the initmal synovial cell layer from the joint capsule or the other synovial covered tissues, including bone, tendon, and ligament. The cells of the subintima include blood vessel endothelial cells, fibroblasts, macrophages, mast cells, and fat cells. The subintimal matrix may have a loose areolar form or a denser matrix with a higher concentration of collagen and elastin.

Blood Supply

The subintimal layer of synovium commonly has an extensive network of small blood vessels. The network forms from vessels that pass through the joint capsule. Where synovium covers bone, tendon, or ligament, the subintimal blood vessels form anastomoses with blood vessels from the underlying tissue.

HYALINE CARTILAGE

Like bone and dense fibrous tissues, cartilage consists of a sparse population of mesenchymal cells embedded within an abundant extracellular matrix. The cells contribute about 5% of the total tissue volume, and the matrix contributes about 95%. The roughly spheric shape of most cartilage cells, or chondrocytes; the unique composition of the matrix they synthesize, assemble, and maintain; and the lack of blood vessels and nerves distinguish cartilage from dense fibrous tissues and bone.

Differences in matrix composition, distribution within the body, mechanical properties, and gross and microscopic appearance differentiate three types of adult human cartilage—hyaline, fibrous, and elastic cartilage. Elastic cartilage forms the auricle of the external ear, a portion of the epiglottis, and some of the laryngeal or bronchiolar cartilages; it does not form part of the musculoskeletal system. Fibrous cartilage (also considered a form of dense fibrous tissue) forms part of the intervertebral disks, pubic symphysis and tendon, ligament, and joint capsule insertions. Menisci consist of a specialized form of fibrous cartilage. The most widespread form of cartilage, hyaline cartilage, forms most of the skeleton before it is removed and replaced by bone through the process of endochondral ossification. It also forms the physeal cartilages that produce longitudinal bone growth until skeletal growth ceases; in adults it persists as the nasal, laryngeal, bronchiolar, articular, and costal cartilages. This section discusses the structure of two specialized forms of hyaline cartilage that have important roles in the musculoskeletal system—articular cartilage and growth cartilage.

Structure

Articular Cartilage

Function of synovial joints (eg, the hip or the knee) depends on the unique mechanical properties of the articular cartilage that forms their bearing surfaces. It distributes loads, thereby minimizing stresses on subchondral bone. When loaded it deforms, and when unloaded it regains it original shape. It provides a surface with almost unequaled gliding properties and has remarkable durability.

Although only a few millimeters thick at most, articular cartilage has an elaborate internal organization. This organization can be described by dividing articular cartilage into four successive zones beginning at the joint surface—the superficial or gliding zone; the intermediate, middle, or transitional zone; the deep or radial zone; and the calcified cartilage zone (Fig. 2-21 and Color Fig. 2-1). Within zones, differences in matrix composition and organization distinguish three regions or compartments—pericellular, territorial, and interterritorial.

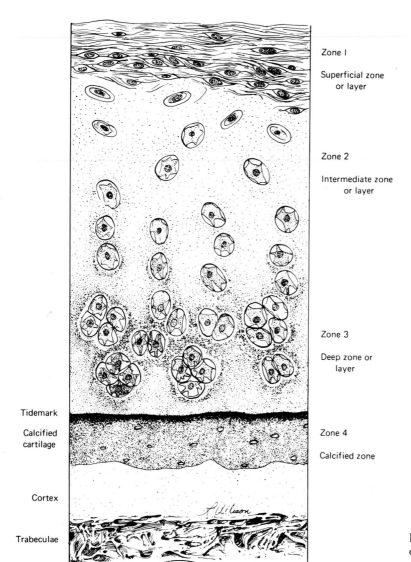

Zone 1

Superficial zone
or layer

Zone 2

Intermediate zone
or layer

Zone 3

Deep zone or
layer

Tidemark

Calcified
cartilage

Zone 4

Calcified zone

Cortex

Trabeculae

FIGURE 2-21. Diagramatic representation of the organization of articular cartilage into zones.

CARTILAGE ZONES. Cartilage zones differ in matrix composition, water concentration, collagen fibril orientation, and cell alignment and morphology.

Superficial Zone. The superficial or gliding zone, the smallest cartilage zone, forms the joint surface. A thin cell-free layer of matrix, containing primarily fine fibrils, lies directly next to the synovial cavity. Deep to this layer, elongated flattened chondrocytes surrounded by a larger volume of matrix per cell align their major axes parallel to the articular surface. The collagen fibrils of this zone lie roughly parallel to the articular surface.

Middle Zone. The middle or transition zone has several times the volume of the superficial zone. Its more spheric cells contain greater volumes of en-doplasmic reticulum, Golgi membranes, mitochondria, and glycogen. The larger interterritorial matrix collagen fibrils of the transitional zone have a more random orientation than those of the gliding zone.

Deep Zone. The cells of the deep or radial zone resemble the spheric cells of the transitional zone but tend to align themselves in columns. This zone has the largest collagen fibrils, the highest proteoglycan content, and lowest water content.

Calcified Cartilage Zone. The thin calcified cartilage zone separates the hyaline cartilage from the stiffer subchondral bone. Collagen fibrils penetrate from the deep zone of cartilage directly through calcified cartilage into bone, thereby anchoring articular cartilage to subchondral bone.

MATRIX REGIONS. Matrix regions differ in their proximity to chondrocytes, collagen content, collagen fibril diameter, collagen fibril orientation, and proteoglycan and noncollagenous protein content and organization.

Pericellular Matrix. The smallest matrix compartment, the pericellular matrix, consists of a thin layer of matrix containing little or no fibrillar collagen. It appears to attach directly to the chondrocyte cell membranes and probably contains noncollagenous proteins that help chondrocytes bind themselves to the matrix.

Territorial Matrix. An envelope of territorial matrix surrounds the pericellular matrix and sometimes pairs or clusters of chondrocytes and their pericellular matrices. Thin collagen fibrils in the territorial matrix near the cells appear to bind to the pericellular matrix. At a distance from the cell they spread and intersect at various angles, forming a basket-like structure around the cells.

Interterritorial Matrix. The interterritorial matrix, the largest matrix compartment, has collagen fibrils of greater diameter than the territorial matrix. The organization and orientation of these interterritorial collagen matrix fibrils changes as they pass from the articular surface to the deep region of the cartilage. In the most superficial zone, they lie primarily parallel to the joint surface; in the transition zone, they assume a more random orientation; and in the deep zone, they tend to lie perpendicular to the joint surface.

Growth Cartilage

Bones elongate by growth of the cartilage, forming the physes or growth plates (Fig. 2-22). The complex structure of the physes (Fig. 2-23) makes it possible for them to produce precisely directed longitudinal bone growth. The growth cartilages increase their volume and therefore bone length by synthesizing new matrix and by cell swelling. The organization of the growth cartilage matrix and the

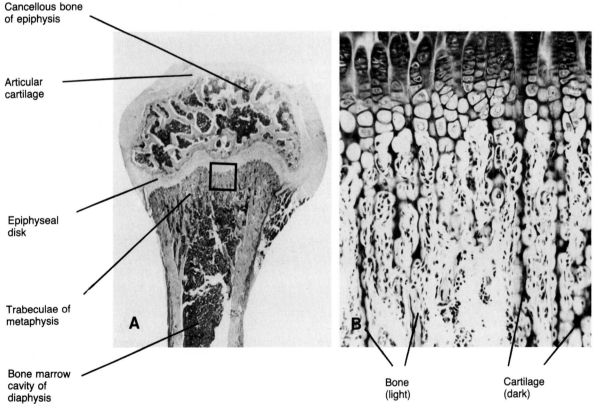

Cancellous bone of epiphysis

Articular cartilage

Epiphyseal disk

Trabeculae of metaphysis

A

Bone marrow cavity of diaphysis

B

Bone (light)

Cartilage (dark)

FIGURE 2-22. Micrographs showing the structure of a long bone physis. (**A**) Low-power photomicrograph of a longitudinal section cut through the end of a long bone of a growing rat. At this stage of development, osteogenesis has spread out from the epiphyseal center of ossification so that only the articular cartilage above and the epiphyseal plate below remain cartilaginous. (**B**) On the diaphyseal side of the epiphyseal plate are the metaphyseal trabeculae, which consist of cartilage cores on which bone has been deposited. (Ham AW, Cormack DH. Histology, ed 8. Philadelphia, JB Lippincott, 1979)

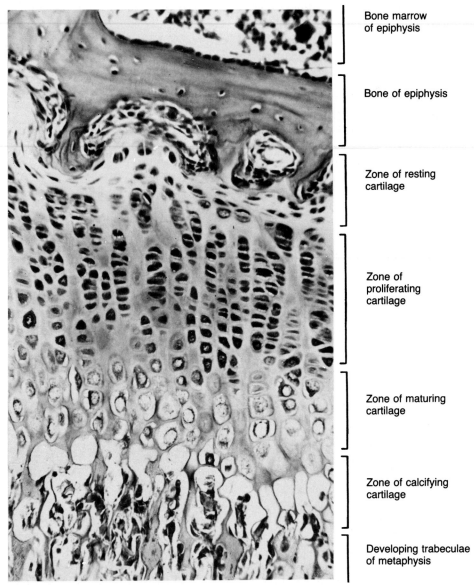

Bone marrow
of epiphysis

Bone of epiphysis

Zone of resting
cartilage

Zone of
proliferating
cartilage

Zone of maturing
cartilage

Zone of calcifying
cartilage

Developing trabeculae
of metaphysis

FIGURE 2-23. High-power photomicrograph of longitudinal section cut through upper end of tibia of a guinea pig. Different zones of cells are visible in the epiphyseal plate. (Ham AW, Cormack DH. Histology, ed 8. Philadelphia, JB Lippincott, 1979)

surrounding fibrous tissue directs the increasing volume of cells and matrix so that it produces longitudinal bone growth. In the region of the growth cartilage nearest to the metaphysis, the longitudinal cartilage septae of the growth cartilage mineralize, and in the metaphysis, osteoblasts cover the mineralized cartilage bars with new woven bone. Osteoclasts then resorb the woven bone, and calcified cartilage and osteoblasts form lamellar bone to complete the replacement of cartilage by mature bone.

ORGANIZATION. Growth cartilages have a layered or zonal organization and a regional organization similar to that found in articular cartilage. The matrix regions, like those of articular cartilage, consist of the pericellular, territorial, and interterritorial compartments. The layered or zonal organization differs considerably from that of articular cartilage. The identified growth cartilage layers or zones consist of reserve or resting, proliferative, and hypertrophic or maturing zones.

Reserve or Resting Zone. Reserve zone cells, located in a thin layer at the epiphyseal pole of the growth plate, show relatively little evidence of metabolic activity. The functions of these small cells have not been clearly established, but they may serve as stem cells for the proliferative zone.

Proliferative Zone. In the proliferative zone, chondrocytes rapidly divide, synthesize new matrix, and assume a highly oriented flattened disk-like shape. In rapidly growing bones, they create long columns of highly ordered cells that resemble stacks of plates.

Hypertrophic or Maturing Zone. Toward the bottom of the proliferative zone, the proliferative cells begin to enlarge, creating the hypertrophic zone. From the proliferative zone to the last part of the hypertrophic zone, they increase their volume 5 to 10 fold, contributing significantly to bone growth, and assume a spheric or polygonal shape. As the cells enlarge their matrix changes. The territorial matrix volume per cell increases significantly as its collagen concentration decreases and mineral appears in the interterritorial matrix.

The orientation of the interterritorial matrix collagen fibrils of the growth cartilage changes among zones. In the reserve zone and upper region of the proliferative zone, the fibrils have little apparent orientation. In the middle and lower regions of the proliferative zone and throughout the hypertrophic zone, however, these interterritorial matrix collagen fibrils lie parallel to the long axis of the bone, forming longitudinal columns or septae that surround the chondrocyte columns and their territorial and pericellular matrices.

In the last part of the hypertrophic zone, the zone of provisional calcification, the longitudinal septae mineralize. The enlarged chondrocytes condense, and metaphyseal capillary sprouts penetrate the territorial matrix and cell lacunae bringing osteoblasts that begin to form new bone on the calcified cartilage septae.

Composition

Chondrocytes

Unlike the other musculoskeletal tissues, cartilage contains only one cell type, the chondrocyte (Figs. 2-24 and 2-25), and no nerve cell processes or blood vessels. Like many other mesenchymal cells, chondrocytes surround themselves with the matrix they synthesize, attach themselves to the matrix macromolecules, and do not form contacts with other cells.

The relation between chondrocytes and their matrix does not end with the synthesis and assembly of the matrix. The normal degradation of matrix macromolecules, especially proteoglycans, forces the cells to synthesize new matrix components to preserve the tissue. In addition, the matrix acts as a mechanical signal transducer for the chondrocytes. Deformation of the matrix generates signals, transmitted through the matrix, that cause the cells to alter their synthetic activity. For example, absence of joint loading and motion causes deterioration of the articular cartilage matrix, possibly because of the lack of mechanical signals to stimulate normal chondrocyte function.

Matrix

Tissue fluid forms the largest component of cartilage (see Fig. 2-3). Depending on the type of cartilage and its age, water contributes 60% to 80% of the wet weight of cartilage. The volume concentration, organization, and behavior of the tissue fluid depend on its interaction with the structural macromolecules. These molecules contribute 20% to 40% of the wet weight of cartilage and include collagens, proteoglycans, and noncollagenous proteins. Hyaline cartilage does not contain elastin. In most hyaline cartilages, collagens contribute about 50% of the tissue dry weight, proteoglycans contribute 30% to 35%, and noncollagenous proteins contribute about 15% to 20%. The collagens form the fibrillar meshwork that gives cartilage its tensile strength and form. The proteoglycans and noncollagenous proteins bind to the collagen network or become mechanically entrapped within it, and the chondrocytes attach themselves to the matrix macromolecules.

Type II collagen fibrils form the cross-banded fibrils identified by electron microscopy and account for 90% to 95% of total hyaline cartilage collagen. Hyaline cartilage also contains at least two other collagens, types IX and XI, and may contain trace amounts of other collagens. The mineralizing regions of articular cartilage and growth plate cartilage also contain small amounts of type X collagen.

Proteoglycans form a much larger portion of the matrix structure in hyaline cartilage than in any other musculoskeletal tissue except for the nucleus pulposus. Hyaline cartilage has a high concentration of large aggregating proteoglycans that give the tissue

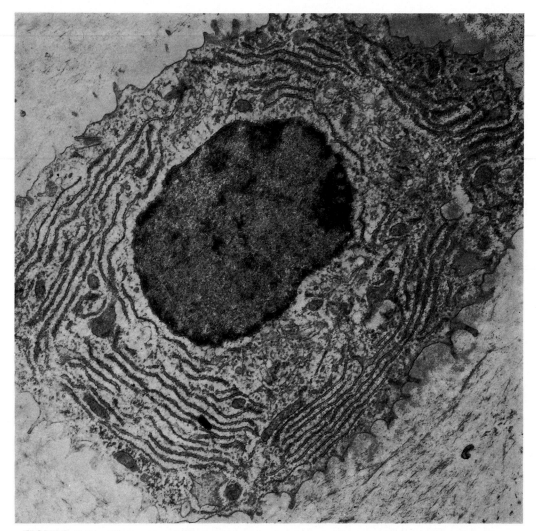

FIGURE 2-24. Ultrastructural characteristics of a chondrocyte. The cytoplasm reveals well-developed rough-surfaced vesicles of endoplasmic reticulum and a well-developed Golgi apparatus. The cytoplasmic processes extend off into the intercellular substance (cytoplasmic footlets). As the chondrocyte becomes older and synthesis of protein is less, the rough-surfaced vesicles and Golgi apparatus become less prominent, and glycogen and lipid material accumulate in the cytoplasm. (Ham AW. Histology, ed 7. Philadelphia, JB Lippincott, 1974)

its unique material properties in compression. It also contains smaller nonaggregating proteoglycans like those found in dense fibrous tissues. The large aggregates help control the fluid flow through the matrix.

Noncollagenous proteins also have an important role in hyaline cartilage. Link proteins stabilize and increase the size of proteoglycan aggregates. Chondronectin and anchorin CII may have a role in matrix organization and in establishing and maintaining the relations between the chondrocytes and the matrix macromolecules.

INTERVERTEBRAL DISK

Normal function of the spine depends greatly on the mechanical properties of the intervertebral disks. These 23 specialized connective tissue structures unite adjacent vertebral bodies from the second and third cervical vertebrae to the fifth lumbar vertebrae and sacrum. They vary in size from the small diameter, thin disks in the cervical region to the large diameter, thick disks of the lower lumbar region. Throughout the spine they contribute to stability while allowing movement between vertebrae and

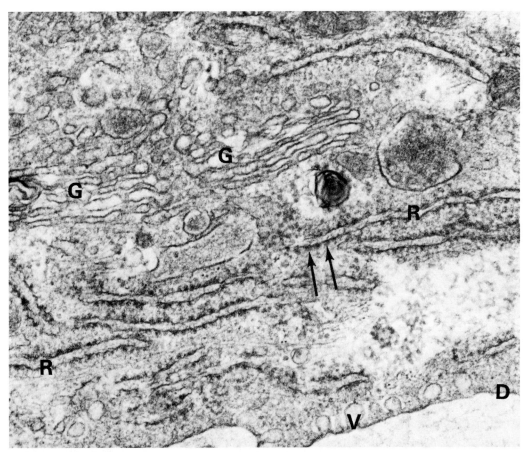

FIGURE 2-25. Transmission electron micrograph of (glutaraldehyde; × 37,500) of part of a chondrocyte showing paired membranes of rough endoplasmic reticulum (R) with ribosome granules (*arrows*). The rough endoplasmic reticulum contrasts with the smooth membranes of the Golgi apparatus (G). Micropinocytotic vesicles (V). Limiting cell membrane (D). (Meachim G. The matrix. In: Freeman MA, ed. Adult articular cartilage, ed 2. London, Pitman, 1973:1)

absorbing compressive loads. With age, the gross and microscopic appearance, cell content, and matrix composition of disk tissues change more than any other tissues.

Structure

Human intervertebral disks consist of four tissues—hyaline cartilage end-plate, annulus fibrosis, transition zone, and nucleus pulposus. These tissues vary in structure, composition, cell populations, and mechanical properties.

Cartilage End-Plate

Hyaline cartilage end-plates cover the superior and inferior surfaces of each disk and separate the other disk tissues from the vertebral bone. Grossly and microscopically, they closely resemble other hyaline cartilages. The dense collagen fibers of the annulus fibrosis pass through the outer edges of the end-plates into the vertebral bodies. With age, the cartilage plates mineralize and eventually cannot be identified as distinct structures.

Annulus Fibrosis

Annulus fibrosis consists primarily of densely packed collagen fibers formed into two components—the outer circumferential rings of collagen lamellae or layers (Fig. 2-26) and an inner, larger fibrocartilaginous component. The collagen lamellae that form the outer concentric rings of the annulus have a high degree of orientation: collagen fibrils within a layer lie parallel to each other, and those within adjacent layers lie at 40- to 70-degree angles to the collagen fibers within layers on either side. In

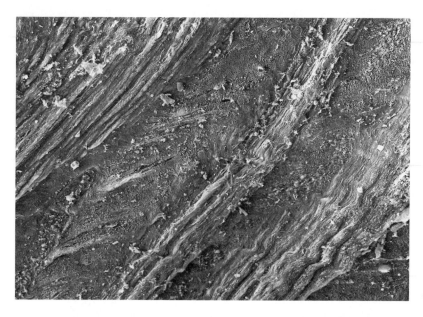

FIGURE 2-26. Electron micrograph of the cut surface of a human annulus fibrosus. Notice the dense layers of collagen fibers.

the fibrocartilaginous component of the annulus, collagen fibrils run concentrically and vertically but lack the high degree of orientation found in the outer concentric rings.

Transition Zone

When the intervertebral disk first forms, the nucleus pulposus and annulus fibrosus have a sharp boundary where the gelatinous nucleus pulposus lies directly against the fibrous annulus. With growth, a transition zone appears that lies between the fibro-

cartilaginous component of the annulus fibrosis and the nucleus pulposus.

Nucleus Pulposus

In newborns and young individuals the soft gelatinous nucleus pulposus tissue has a translucent appearance. It contains relatively few collagen fibers, and they lack any apparent orientation (Fig. 2-27). With age, the nucleus pulposus becomes more fibrous, making it increasingly difficult to separate the

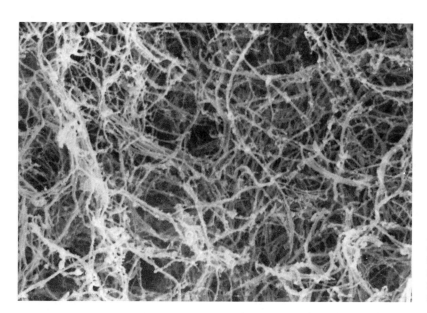

FIGURE 2-27. Electron micrograph showing the collagen fibers of a human nucleus pulposus. Notice loose arrangement of the fibers compared with the annulus fibrosus.

nucleus pulposus from the transition zone and the fibrocartilaginous part of the annulus fibrosus.

Composition

Intervertebral disk tissues consist of water, cells, and matrix macromolecules. The composition of the hyaline cartilage plates has not been extensively studied, but it appears to resemble other hyaline cartilages. The annulus, like other dense fibrous tissues, has water concentration of 60% to 70% throughout life. In contrast, the water concentration of the nucleus pulposus declines from about 80% to 90% at birth to about 70% in adults.

Cells

Intervertebral disks contain two principal cell types—notochordal cells and connective tissue cells. Notochordal cells form the nucleus pulposus in the fetus. With growth, development, and aging, they gradually disappear, and the cells found in the nucleus of older individuals have the appearance of connective tissue cells, often resembling chondrocytes. The connective tissue cells of the outer annulus have the appearance of fibroblasts, like those found in other dense fibrous tissues. The connective tissue cells of the inner regions of the annulus and other disk components have a more spheric form, like chondrocytes. The cells of the cartilage end-plate tissue have the shape and organelles of hyaline cartilage chondrocytes.

NOTOCHORDAL CELLS. Clusters and cords of large, irregular notochordal cells populate the nucleus pulposus of the newborn human intervertebral disk (Fig. 2-28). These cells contain endoplasmic reticulum, Golgi membranes, mitochondria, glycogen, and bundles of microfilaments. Unlike mesenchymal cells, notochordal cells form multiple specialized junctions with other cells, and their membranes form elaborate interdigitations with those of other cells. During skeletal growth, the notochordal cell clusters or cords disappear, and the glycogen content of the cells declines. In some regions they retain cell–cell contact by elongated cell processes. With aging, the density of notochordal cells declines further, and definite notochordal cells have not been identified in the human nucleus pulposus after age 32.

CONNECTIVE TISSUE CELLS. In the outer annulus the fibroblasts lie with their long axes parallel to the collagen fibrils. In the inner fibrocartilaginous region of the annulus, more of the cells assume a spheric form like those seen in other fibrocartilages (Fig. 2-29). In the nucleus pulposus, connective tissue cells have oval nuclei and slightly elongated form, but most have a more spheric shape. The proportion of viable nucleus pulposus cells declines with age, but even in disks from elderly people some viable connective tissue cells survive.

Matrix

The matrix macromolecular framework of the human intervertebral disk forms from collagens,

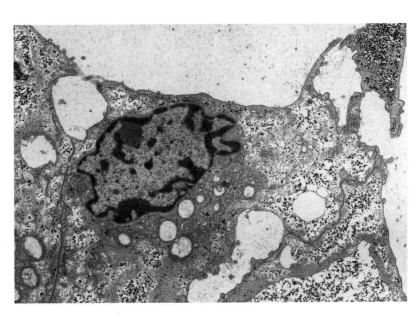

FIGURE 2-28. Electron micrograph of human nucleus pulposus notochordal cells. Unlike connective tissue cells, the membranes of notochordal cells bind to the membranes of adjacent cells.

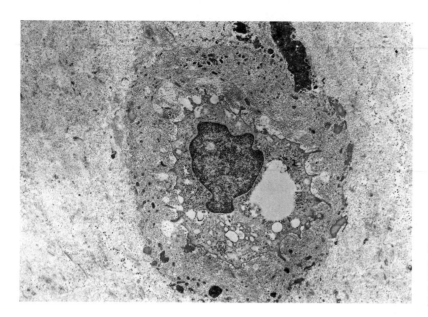

FIGURE 2-29. Electron micrograph of a human connective tissue cell from the inner region of the annulus fibrosus. This cell lacks any contact with other cells and has formed a distinct pericellular matrix.

elastin, proteoglycans, and noncollagenous proteins. The concentrations and specific types of these molecules vary among the disk tissues.

The collagens, including fibrillar and short-chain collagens, give the disk its form and tensile strength. The concentration of collagen decreases progressively from the outer annulus to the most central portion of the nucleus. In the adult disk the contribution of collagen to the tissue dry weight declines from 60% to 70% in the outer rim of the annulus to 10% to 20% in the most central part of the nucleus.

The annulus fibrosus contains fibrillar and short-chain collagens. The fibrillar collagens found in the annulus fibrosis include types I, II, III, and V. The concentration of type I collagen declines from about 80% of the total collagen in the outer rim of the annulus to zero in the transition zone and nucleus. The concentration of type II collagen follows the opposite pattern. It increases from zero to 80% of the total collagen from the outer rim of the annulus to the transition zone and nucleus. Type III collagen occurs in trace amounts, and type V collagen contributes about 3% of the total collagen of the annulus fibrosus. The short-chain collagens found in annulus fibrosus include types VI and IX. Type IX collagen forms only about 1% of annulus fibrosus collagen, but type VI occurs in unusually high concentrations and forms about 10% of total annulus fibrosis collagen.

Fibrillar and short-chain collagens also form part of the matrix of the nucleus pulposus. It contains at least three fibril-forming collagens—types II, III, and XI. Type II is the predominant collagen contributing

about 80% of the total nucleus pulposus collagen. Type III occurs in trace amounts, and type XI contributes about 3% of the total collagen of the nucleus. Nucleus pulposus short-chain collagens include types VI and IX. As in the annulus fibrosis, type IX forms only about 1% of the total collagen, but type VI contributes even more to the nucleus than to the annulus, forming about 14% to 20% of the total collagen. The reason for the unusually high concentration of type VI collagen in the annulus and nucleus remains unknown. This short-chain collagen forms banded fibrillar aggregates of longitudinal fibrils about 5 nm in diameter with alternating transverse bands consisting of two 15-nm-wide dark bands separated by a 15-nm-wide lucent strip. These fibrillar aggregates occur most frequently in the matrix immediately surrounding cells. They may have a role in resisting tensile loads on the matrix or may provide a loose fibrillar network that helps organize other matrix molecules.

Aggregating and nonaggregating proteoglycans form a significant part of the disk macromolecular framework and help give disk stiffness to compression and resiliency. Their concentration increases from the periphery of the disk to the center. They contribute about 10% to 20% of the dry weight of the outer annulus and as much as 50% of the dry weight of the central nucleus.

Annulus fibrosus and nucleus pulposus proteoglycans differ from those found in hyaline cartilages like the disk cartilage end-plates, articular cartilage, or epiphyseal or growth plate cartilage. The proteoglycan populations found in annulus fibrosus and nucleus pulposus include fewer aggregates, smaller aggregates, and smaller more variable monomers. Many disk proteoglycan aggregates consist of star-shaped clusters of monomers rather than long aggregates. Aggregated and nonaggregated disk proteoglycan monomers have shorter protein core filaments, vary more in size, and have less chondroitin sulfate and more keratan sulfate than those found in hyaline cartilages. The high concentration of these small variable monomers in the nucleus pulposus suggests that fragments of degraded proteoglycans accumulate in the central regions of the disk.

Elastin occurs in trace amounts in annulus fibrosis and nucleus pulposus. In the annulus, elastin appears as fusiform or cylindric fibers lying parallel to the collagen fibrils. In the nucleus, elastin assumes irregular lobular shapes without apparent relation to collagen fibrils. The contribution of elastin to disk mechanical properties remains unclear.

As in other musculoskeletal tissues, noncollagenous proteins appear to help organize and stabilize the extracellular matrix of intervertebral disk and may facilitate adhesion of cell membranes to other matrix macromolecules. The concentration of disk noncollagenous proteins increases with age. In the annulus, the proportion of tissue dry weight contributed by noncollagenous proteins increases from 5% to 25% with increasing age, and in the nucleus it increases from 20% of the dry weight to 45% of the dry weight. Some of the increasing concentration of noncollagenous proteins may be due to accumulation of degraded molecules. Electron microscopic studies have identified dense granular sheaths around disk collagen fibers. These sheaths increase in volume with increasing age, suggesting that they represent collections of noncollagenous proteins.

Blood Supply

Small blood vessels and networks of vessels lie on the surface on the annulus fibrosis, and occasional small vessels penetrate a short distance into the outer layers of the annulus. The intraosseous blood vessels of the vertebrae contact but do not penetrate the cartilage end-plates. This arrangement of blood vessels leaves the central disk as the largest avascular structure in the body. The cells must rely on diffusion of nutrients and metabolites through a large volume of matrix. Mineralization of the end-plates with increasing age may further compromise diffusion of nutrients to the central regions of the disk.

Nerve Supply

Perivascular and free nerve endings lie on the outer surface of the annulus, and some of these nerve cell processes penetrate the outer most collagen lamellae. Despite multiple investigations of disk innervation, no nerves have been identified deep to the outer annular layers. The cartilage plates also have perivascular nerves.

Age-Related Changes in Disk Tissues

Growth, maturation, and aging dramatically alter disk tissues, especially the nucleus pulposus. The four tissue components of the disk are easily identified in the newborn. A clear gelatinous nucleus fills almost half the disk and consists almost entirely of notochordal tissue. A narrow transition zone and larger ring of annulus fibrocartilage surround the nucleus. The outermost layers of the annulus encircle the annular fibrocartilage. As the disk grows and matures during childhood, the nucleus gradually becomes opaque. The decreasing water concentration makes it dense, firm, and difficult to separate from the fibrocartilage and transition zones. The annular fibrocartilage ring increases in size as the proportion of the disk occupied by the nucleus decreases. In the elderly, the components of the disk inside the outer annular layers consist almost entirely of fibrocartilage, and clefts and fissures appear in the central parts of the disk.

The disk cells also change with age. Viable notochordal cells fill most of the fetal nucleus pulposus. With growth and maturation their numeric density progressively decreases, and cells with the morphologic features of connective tissue cells appear in the nucleus pulposus. In adults, few if any notochordal cells remain, and the percentage of necrotic cells in the nucleus increases from about 2% in the fetus to about 50% in adults. In adults and elderly persons, a dense pericellular matrix forms around most cells in the nucleus pulposus and the inner annulus fibrosus, possibly because of accumulation of cell products and metabolites. In the elderly less than 20% of the nucleus cells remain viable. The causes of these age changes remain unclear. They may result from decreased nutrition of central disk cells because of increased disk volume, decreased diffusion of nutrients into the disk following mineralization of the cartilage end-plates, and accumulation of cell products and metabolites in the matrix.

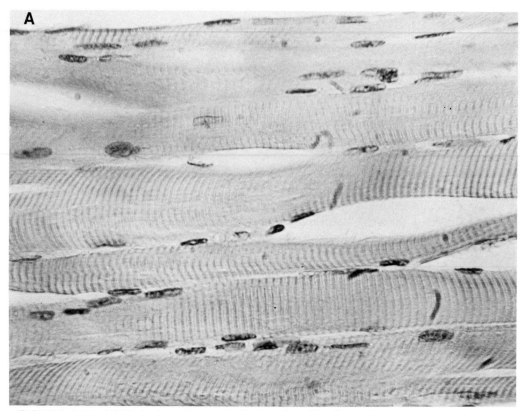

FIGURE 2-30. (A) Skeletal muscle, longitudinal section. The fibers do not branch or anastomose. Each fiber has many flattened, slender sarcolemmal nuclei lying peripherally beneath the membrane and oriented parallel with the long axis of the fiber. In muscle disease, these nuclei come to occupy a central position. Large numbers of axially disposed myofibrils are contained within the fiber ($\times$ 670). (B) Striated muscle, cross section. An enlargement of a muscle fiber is depicted. The myofibrils are separated by sarcoplasm. The matrix consists of the endomysium, perimysium, and epimysium.

MUSCLE

The ability of muscle cell contraction to produce joint motion or stabilize joints against resistance depends not only on the composition and structure of the muscle cells but also on the muscle nerves and blood vessels, the organization of the tissue, and the attachment of muscle cells to tendons. Unlike the musculoskeletal connective tissues, muscle consists primarily of cells contained within a small volume of highly organized matrix (Fig. 2-30). The matrix contains collagens, elastin, proteoglycans, and noncollagenous proteins that maintain the structure of the tissue, including the muscle nerves and blood vessels.

Structure

Muscle cells (myofibers or muscle fibers) cluster into bundles called fascicles. Aggregates of fascicles combined with their extracellular matrix form named muscles. Although the extracellular matrix makes up only a small fraction of muscle volume (see Fig. 2-30), it is critical for normal muscle function, maintenance of muscle structure, and healing. A basal lamina containing collagens, noncollagenous proteins, and muscle-specific proteoglycans surrounds each myofiber. The basal lamina together with the surrounding irregularly arranged fine collagen fibers form the endomysium. A thicker matrix sheath composed primarily of collagen fibers and elastic fibers (the perimysium) covers muscle fasciculi. The epimysium, a denser peripheral sheath of connective tissue, covers the entire muscle and usually joins with the fascia overlying the muscle and with the muscle tendon junction.

Composition

Cells

Muscles contain connective tissue cells, endothelial cells of blood vessels, and nerve cell processes, but most of the tissue consists of large, highly dif-

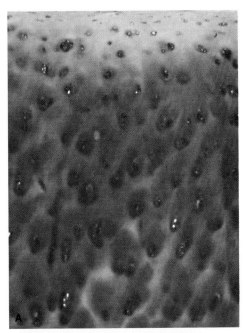

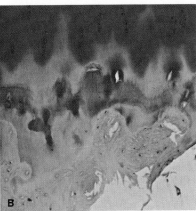

COLOR FIGURE 2-1. Normal adult (70-year-old patient) human cartilage stained with safranin-O)
to demonstrate specifically, by the intensity of the stain, the concentration of glycosaminoglycans;
counterstained with hematoxylin. (**A**) Superficial zone: elongated cells are arranged with the long axis
parallel to articular surface. The acellular bright line at the articular surface is the lamina splendens.
The matrix does not stain with safranin-O. Transitional zone: rounded cells are in random arrangement;
some cells are in pairs. This zone stains with safranin-O. Radial zone: rounded cells are in short
columns arranged perpendicular to the articular surface. The zone stains with safranin-O. (**B**) Basilar
portion. The cell columns of the radial zone are surrounded by an intensely stained matrix indicating
an increased concentration of glycosaminoglycans at this level. The "tidemark" separates the radial
from the calcified zone. Calcified zone: rests on the subchondral bony end plate (× 100). (Courtesy of
Dr. Charles Weiss)

B

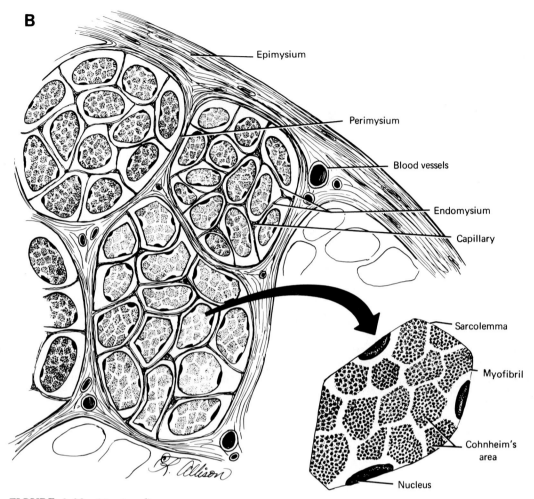

Epimysium

Perimysium

Blood vessels

Endomysium

Capillary

Sarcolemma

Myofibril

Cohnheim's area

Nucleus

FIGURE 2-30. (*Continued*)

ferentiated muscle cells. Each muscle cell, or myofiber, contains multiple nuclei, a unique form of endoplasmic reticulum called the sacroplasmic reticulum and contractile protein filaments (actin and myosin) organized into cylindric organelles called myofibrils (Fig. 2-31). When viewed by the electron microscope, actin filaments appear as thin filaments, and myosin filaments appear as thick filaments (Figs. 2-32 and 2-33). Each myofibril consists of regular repeating units, consisting primarily of actin and myosin, called sarcomeres. These myofibrils often extend through the entire length of the cell and fill most of the cell volume. Flattened vesicles of sarcoplasmic reticulum surround the myofibrils and a series of invaginations of the cell membrane, called transverse tubules, extend from the cell surface to lie next to each myofibril and the membranes of the sarcoplasmic reticulum (Fig. 2-34). The interfibrillar sarcoplasm contains mitochondria, lysosomes, and ribosomes.

Myofibers form by fusion of multiple small mesenchymal cells called myoblasts. Myofibers cannot proliferate; therefore, increase in muscle mass occurs through cell growth. The myofibers can grow in length by fusion with myoblasts, thereby increasing the number of nuclei. They can grow in diameter by increasing the size and number of myofibers. In mature individuals, some myoblasts survive. They remain next to mature myofibers, and following muscle injury, they can proliferate and fuse to form new muscle cells.

Matrix

Because of difficulties in extracting, purifying, and studying the small volume of matrix found in muscle, the composition and organization of the muscle matrix remains poorly understood. The muscle basal lamina contain laminin (a noncollagenous protein that forms part of basement membranes),

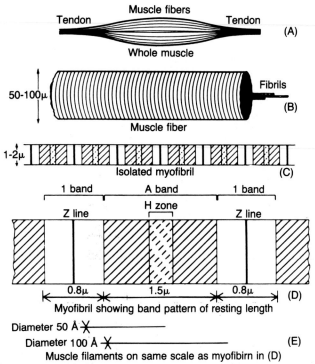

FIGURE 2-31. The dimensions and arrangement of the myofibrils in a muscle. The whole muscle (**A**) is made up of fibers (**B**) that contain cross-striated myofibrils (**C** and **D**). Myofibrils consist primarily of actin and mysin filaments (**E**) that overlap and interdigitate in a stereospecific manner. (Huxley HE. The molecular basis of contraction. In: Bourne GH, ed. The structure and function of muscle. New York, Academic Press, 1972)

types IV and V collagen, and heparin sulfate proteoglycan. The outer connective tissue envelopes of muscle consist primarily of type I collagen fibrils.

Blood Supply

Many blood vessels penetrate the epimysium, passing between muscle fasciculi within the muscle tissue matrix. They then enter the muscle fascicles to form rich capillary networks around individual myofibrils.

Innervation

Initiation, coordination, and control of muscle contraction require elaborate innervation. Nerves that sense muscle tension terminate on intrafusal fibers and Golgi tendon organs. Three types of motor neurons that supply myofibers follow: (1) α motor neurons innervating extrafusal myofibers, (2) β motor neurons innervating both extrafusal and intrafusal myofibers, and (3) γ motor neurons innervating intrafusal myofibers.

One motor neuron innervates each myofiber, but each motor neuron generally innervates more than one myofiber. A motor unit consists of the motor neuron and the muscle fibers it innervates. Motor nerves attach to myofibers through a neuromuscular

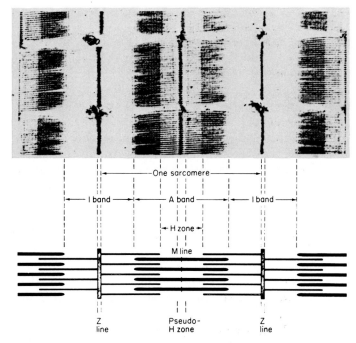

FIGURE 2-32. Longitudinal section of frog sartorius muscle (*top*) together with a diagram showing the overlap of filaments that gives rise to the band pattern. The A band is most dense in its lateral zones, where the thick and thin filaments overlap. The central zone of the A band (the H zone) is less dense, because it contains thick filaments only. The I bands are less dense still because they contain only thin filaments. The sarcomere length here is about 2.5 μm. (Huxley HE. The molecular basis of contraction. In: Bourne GH, ed. The structure and function of muscle. New York, Academic Press, 1972)

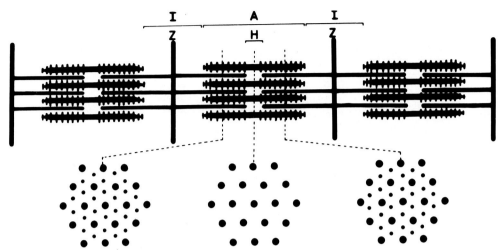

FIGURE 2-33. Structure of striated muscle, showing overlapping arrays of actin- and myosin-containing filaments, the latter with projecting cross-bridges on them. To facilitate showing the relations, the diagram is drawn with considerable longitudinal foreshortening, with filament diameters and side spacings as shown. The filament lengths should be about five times the lengths shown. (Huxley HE. The molecular basis of contraction. In: Bourne GH, ed. The structure and function of muscle. New York, Academic Press, 1971)

junction that transmits signals from the motor nerve terminas to limited regions of the myofibers. Neuromuscular junctions consist of five principal parts: (1) the nerve terminal filled with thousands of vesicles containing neurotransmitters, (2) a Schwann cell overlying the nerve terminal, (3) a synaptic space lined with basement membrane, (4) the postsynaptic membrane containing receptors for the neurotransmitters, and (5) postjunctional sarcoplasm necessary for the structural and metabolic support of the postsynaptic membrane. Release of neurotransmitters from the motor nerve terminal into the synaptic space creates an action potential in the muscle cell membrane. The action potential in the muscle cell membrane extends into folds in the cell membrane to the sarcoplasmic reticulum. The sarcoplasmic reticulum releases calcium ions, and the rapid increase in intracellular calcium triggers simultaneous contraction of myofibers throughout the cell.

FORMATION AND DEVELOPMENT OF THE MUSCULOSKELETAL SYSTEM

Normal structure and function of the musculoskeletal system depend on the formation and growth of the specific skeletal connective tissues and muscle, and the integration of these tissues into the system that provides the stability and mobility of the body. Car-

tilage, muscle, bone, and dense fibrous tissue form, grow, and become organized into the musculoskeletal system during early prenatal life so that by 6 months the final form of the musculoskeletal system is easily recognized (Fig. 2-35). Disturbances of these processes cause congenital abnormalities, including failure of segmentation of vertebrae, congenital dislocations of the hip, clubfeet, and absence of part or all of a limb. Following birth, the musculoskeletal system continues to grow and modify its form until the physes close.

Cartilage, Muscle, and Bone

Within the first few weeks of intrauterine life, the embryo takes shape, developing the head, trunk, and protrusions called limb buds. Between the ectoderm and the entoderm lies the diffuse, loose, cellular mesenchyme, which differentiates into the musculoskeletal connective tissues and skeletal muscle. The first recognizable musculoskeletal structures appear as dense concentrations of mesenchymal cells that take the shape of the bones. Figure 2-36 shows the development of cartilage and skeletal muscle from mesenchyme.

As early as the fifth embryonic week, mesenchymal cells enlarge, become more compact, and differentiate into a sheet of cells recognized as precar-

(text continues on page 55)

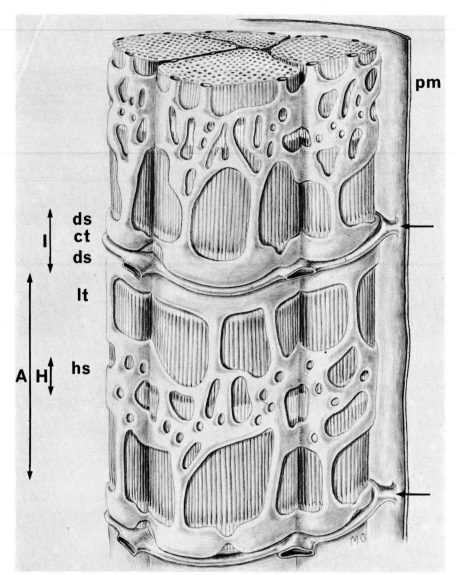

FIGURE 2-34. Three-dimensional drawing of parts of four myofibrils to illustrate (1) the sarcolemma (labeled pm on the right); (2) the transverse tubules that extend into the substance of the fiber from the sarcolemma (from points indicated by arrows on the right); and (3) the sarcoplasmic reticulum, which is interposed and so lies between myofibrils over their I, A, and H portions (labels for the latter on left). The transverse tubules are delicate tubules that are invaginations of the sarcolemma; hence their walls are composed of cell membrane, and their lumens open onto the outer surface of the sarcolemma. Transverse tubules (in the frog) enter the fiber at the level of Z line (indicated by arrows on right side), and each one branches as it extends across the fiber so as to surround myofibrils whose Z lines are in register with the site where it entered, as is shown by following the two tubules in this illustration, from right to left. The sarcoplasmic reticulum consists of cisternae and channels of smooth-surfaced endoplasmic reticulum that lie between and so surround myofibrils. In the region of the I band, the extent of which is indicated at the left of the illustration, the cisternae, known as terminal cisternae, are large and flattened, but they may be more or less distended (ds); they lie to either side of the transverse tubule (ct). The cisternae, by means of channels that run longitudinally (lt) over the A band to the region of the H zone, connect with a network of more or less flattened sacs called the H sacs (hs). The site of the H zone in the A band is indicated at the left of the illustration. (Courtesy of C.P. Leblond; Ham AW. Histology, ed 7. Philadelphia, JB Lippincott, 1974)

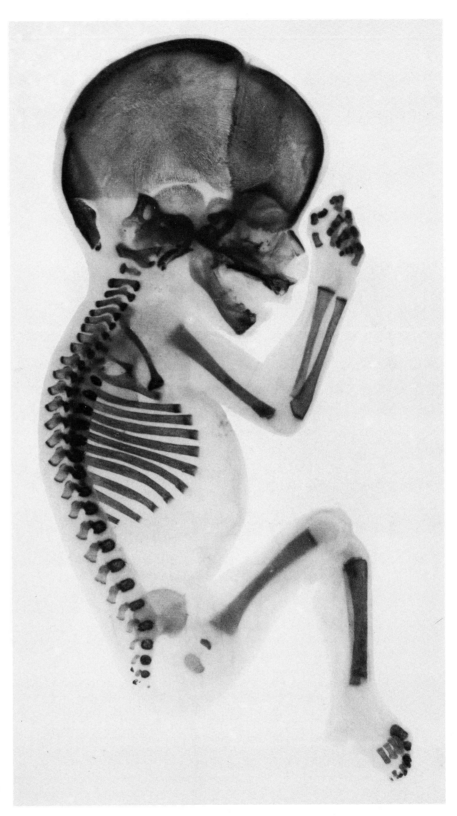

FIGURE 2-35. Skeletal development of a 6-month-old fetus.

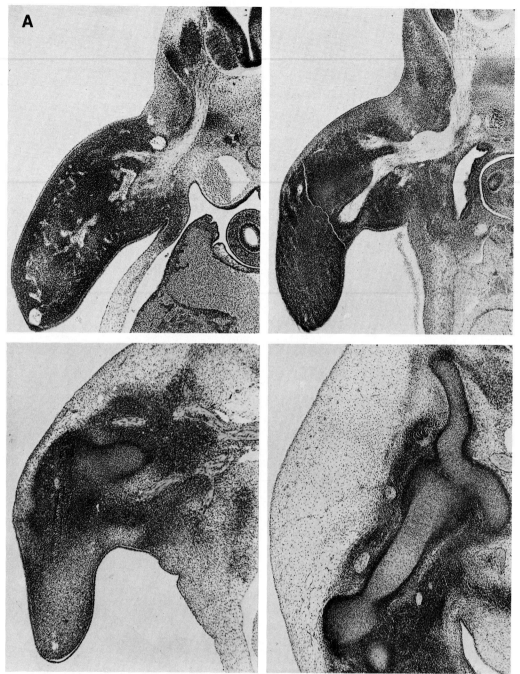

FIGURE 2-36. (A) Origin of a limb bud. Development of the upper limb bud and histogenesis of the humerus are shown. The limb bud originates as a small elevation of the body wall and at first consists of a condensed mass of proliferating mesoblastic cells. Within a few days, a central condensation of mesoblasts occurs. This is the skeletomuscle condensation, so called because separate muscle and skeleton cannot be identified. At the same time, a broad sheet of branching nerve trunks from the cord and the spinal ganglia stream into the base of the arm bud (*top left*). A few days later, muscular and skeletal condensations become distinct, and massive nerve trunks enter the center of the muscle condensations (*top right*). Next section: definite muscle groups can be identified (*bottom left*) containing conspicuous nerve trunks, and major branches of the brachial plexus are obvious. At the same time, the central part of the skeletal condensation is being transformed into cartilage (this tissue appears lighter in color). The cartilage of different bones is deposited separately in the last section (*bottom right*) so that these central cartilaginous cores within the skeletal bed acquire the shape of the bones of which they are forerunners. These sections represent developmental periods of about 2 days each. (B) These diagram drawings correspond to these sections in **A**. (Streeter GL. Developmental horizons in human embryos. Contrib Embryol 1949;33:149. Publication 583 from the Carnegie Institution of Washington)

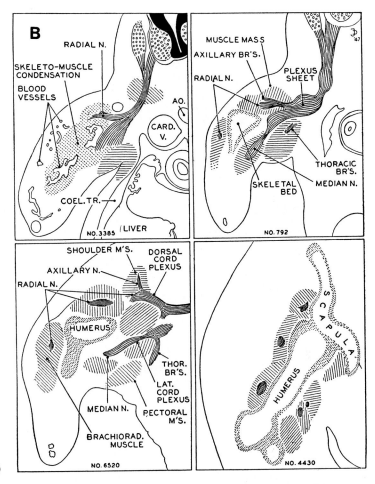

FIGURE 2-36. (*Continued*)

tilage. Then matrix is laid down between the cells (Fig. 2-37). Cartilage increases in thickness by growth, both internally and externally (Fig. 2-38). Internal growth occurs by multiplication of cartilage cells and production of new matrix. Peripheral growth occurs from the investing sheath (the perichondrium), whose inner cells are transformed into chondrocytes.

Bone first appears after the seventh embryonic week. It forms either from mesenchymal membranes (eg, facial and cranial bones) or from cartilage (eg, the long bones of the limbs). Although the bone is identical in each instance, in the latter type the cartilage must first be removed before bone can be laid down.

Intramembranous Bone Formation

The mesenchymal or connective tissue membrane first forms the original model of the facial and the cranial bones. At one or more central points of the

membrane, intramembranous ossification begins (Fig. 2-39). These ossification centers are characterized by the appearance of osteoblasts that lay down a meshwork of bony trabeculae spread radially in all directions. The mesenchyme at the periphery differentiates into a fibrous sheath (the periosteum), the undersurface of which differentiates into osteoblasts, which in turn deposit parallel plates of compact bone (the lamellae). This is periosteal ossification, by which the inner and the outer tables of the skull are form. Trabeculae are arranged mainly along lines of greatest stress.

Enchondral Bone Formation

A cartilaginous model of the structure precedes destruction of cartilage and its replacement by bone. Two processes are involved—ossification centrally within the cartilage, or endochondral ossification; and ossification peripherally beneath the perichondrium

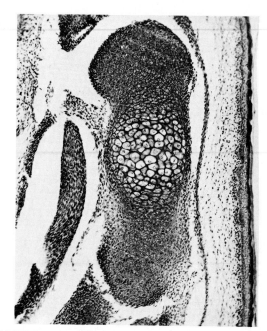

FIGURE 2-37. Early fetal anlage of a long bone. It is composed of mesenchyme at the center of which the cells become rounded and assume the appearance of chondrocytes. Later, the peripheral mesenchyme will give rise to vascular tissue that will invade the calcified cartilage and replace the latter with bone.

(or periosteum), or perichondrial or periosteal ossification.

In the center of the cartilaginous precursor, the cells enlarge and become arranged radially as the matrix mineralizes. Invading from blood vessels the perichondrium (Figs. 2-40 and 2-41) bring osteoblasts that deposit new bone that replaces the cartilage.

As the central bone formation occurs, the cells of the inner layer of perichondrium (now more appropriately name the periosteum), lay down parallel layers of compact bone. The cartilaginous physes form at the end of each long bone and produce endochondral bone throughout skeletal growth. Periosteal ossification contributes to growth thickness of the structure.

Joints

Two types of joints develop between bones—synarthroses, which allow little movement, and diarthroses, which allow low-friction movement. The synarthroses form by the differentiation of mesenchyme into a uniting layer of connective tissue (the suture or syndesmosis), cartilage (the synchondrosis),

or bone (the synostosis). Diarthroses have joint cavities that arise from a cleft in the mesenchyme. The joint capsule and ligaments form from the dense external tissue, which is continuous with the periosteum. The cells on the inner surface of the capsule flatten into the synovial membrane. Menisci and meniscus-like structures form from mesenchyme that projects into the joint cavity.

The Axial Skeleton

The notochord is the primitive axial support for the body. Mesenchymal tissue (designated as sclerotomes) migrate toward the notochord and come to lie in paired segmental masses alongside the notochord. Intersegmental arteries separate each sclerotomic mesenchymal mass from similar masses before and behind. Each sclerotome then differentiates into a caudal compact portion and a cranial less-dense half. The denser caudal half then unites with the looser cranial half of the succeeding sclerotome to form the substance of the vertebra (Fig. 2-42). Both the condensed and the looser portions grow about the notochord to form the body of the vertebra. From the denser (now cranial) half, dorsal extensions pass around the neural tube to form the vertebral arch, and paired ventrolateral outgrowths form the costal processes or forerunners of the ribs. The mesenchymal tissue in the intervertebral fissure gives rise to the intervertebral disk. The nucleus pulposus in the disk constitutes the remnant of the notochord. The two parts of sclerotomes, in joining, enclose the intersegmental artery, which, therefore, passes through the center of the vertebral body. In the seventh embryonic week, centers of chondrification appear— two in the vertebral body and one in each half of the vertebral arch. These four centers enlarge and fuse into a complete cartilaginous vertebra. Vertebral ossification starts in the tenth week. A single center in the body and one in each half of the arch appears, but union is not completed until several years after birth (Fig. 2-43).

Continued growth in length of the body occurs by endochondral ossification at the cephalad and the caudad epiphyseal plates. About the rim of the superior and the inferior surfaces, a prominent ring of cartilage exists to which is attached the fibers of the longitudinal ligament of the spine (Fig. 2-44). It does not participate in growth. Gradually, it develops secondary ossification centers that are triangular in cross section but actually skirt the rim of the body. Even-

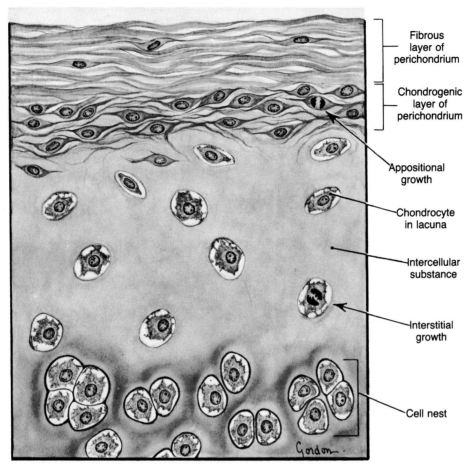

Fibrous layer of perichondrium

Chondrogenic layer of perichondrium

Appositional growth

Chondrocyte in lacuna

Intercellular substance

Interstitial growth

Cell nest

FIGURE 2-38. Appositional and interstitial cartilage growth. Cartilage grows from the perichondrium when fibroblast-like cells enlarge into chondroblasts and become encapsulated. They multiply, form groups, and synthesize new matrix-producing appositional growth. Cells within the tissue also proliferate and synthesize matrix-producing interstitial growth. (Ham AW. Histology, ed 7. Philadelphia, JB Lippincott, 1974)

tually, this center appears as a line parallel with the upper and lower surfaces of the body and resembles a plate (Fig. 2-45). The term *plate* is reserved for the growth cartilage that intervenes between the ring and the main body of bone. The secondary centers fuse with the main body by age 17. The central artery can be seen up to age 6, after which it is obliterated (Fig. 2-46). It may persist beyond this time in certain conditions (eg, Scheuermann disease).

An exception in the development of the vertebra occurs in the atlas. The body differentiates typically but soon is taken over by the axis serving as a peg-like extension (dens) of the latter, about which the atlas rotates. The atlas is left as a ring. The sacral and the coccygeal vertebrae represent vertebra with reduced vertebral arches. The sacral vertebrae eventually fuse into a single mass. The coccygeal vertebrae

exist as rudimentary structures. The entire spine at birth displays one continuous curve convex posteriorly. As the erect posture is assumed after the first year, secondary forward curves develop the cervical and the lumbar regions. Finally, the lordosis in the cervical and the dorsal regions is balanced by the kyphosis in the thoracic and the sacral regions.

The original union of the costal process with the vertebra is replaced by a joint for the head of the rib. The center of ossification appears at the tangle of the rib. The distal ends of the long ribs, however, always remain cartilaginous. In the neck, the ribs are represented by their tubercles, which are fused with the transverse processes and their heads fused with the bodies; between these processes is an interval, the transverse foramen, through which the vertebral arteries course. When the costal processes are over-

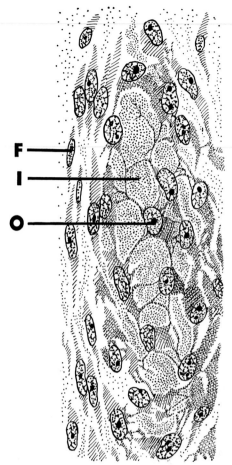

FIGURE 2-39. Intramembranous bone formation. Collagenous fibrils are no longer visible. Connective tissue cells (O) have developed processes to become osteoblasts and later osteocytes. F, fibroblast; I, homogeneous interstitial bone substance.

developed in the cervical region, a supernumerary rib is formed, which may lead to compression of nerve structures.

The sternum originates from the junction of two bars of ventrolaterally placed mesenchyme, which initially have no connection with the ribs or each other.

At birth, the posterior bony arch is separated from the anterior bony centrum by cartilaginous bridges. The bony arch is completed by the second year. Junction between arch and body occurs between the third and sixth years.

The Appendicular Skeleton

The appendicular skeleton is derived directly from the unsegmented somatic mesenchyme. Definite

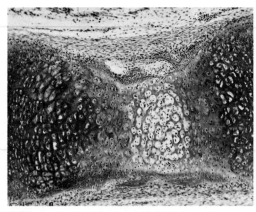

FIGURE 2-40. Ossification of a fetal cartilaginous long bone. The cartilage cells at the center of the calcified cartilage have become enlarged, and the matrix is sparse. A bone collar has formed about this level and is gradually replacing the cartilage.

masses are formed at the sites of the future pectoral and pelvic girdles and limb buds. This is followed by the sequence of bone development through cartilaginous and osseous stages.

The clavicle is the first bone of the skeleton to ossify. Before ossification, a peculiar tissue resembling both membranous and cartilaginous tissue makes it difficult to classify the origin. Two primary centers of ossification appear.

The scapula is a single plate with two chief centers of ossification and several epiphyseal centers that appear later. An early primary center forms the body and the spine. The other, after birth, gives rise to the coracoid process.

The humerus, the radius, and the ulna all ossify from a single primary center in the diaphysis and an epiphyseal center at each end. Additional epiphyseal centers are constant at the lower end of the humerus. Each carpal bone ossifies from a single center. The metacarpals ossify from a single primary center and an epiphyseal center (Figs. 2-47 and 2-48).

At first, the cartilaginous plate of the pelvis lies perpendicular to the vertebral column. Later, it rotates to a position parallel with the vertebral column and in relation to the first three sacral vertebrae. Three main centers of ossification appear for the ilium, ischium, and pubis. The three elements join at a cup-shaped depression, the acetabulum, which is the articulation for the head of the femur.

The development of the femur, the tibia, the fibula, the tarsus, the metatarsals, and the phalanges corresponds to that of the bones of the upper extremity (Figs. 2-49 and 2-50).

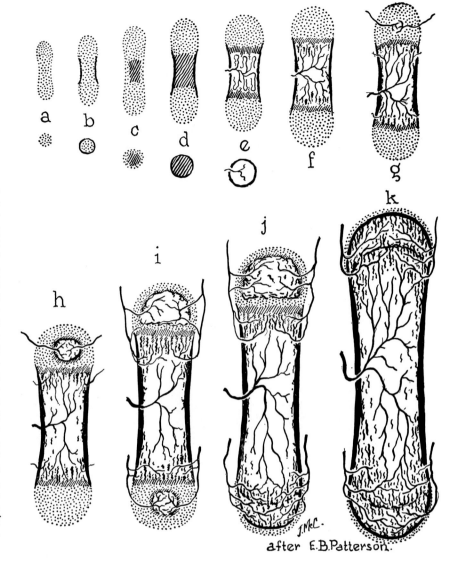

FIGURE 2-41. Development of a typical long bone. (a) Cartilage model. (b) Periosteal bone collar appears. (c) Center of calcifying cartilage. (d) Further development of calcified cartilage. (e) Vascular mesenchyme enters, resorbs calcified cartilage, and new bone is laid down toward either extremity of the model. (f) Endochondral ossification is further advanced and bone increased in length. (g) Blood vessels and mesenchyme enter upper epiphyseal cartilage. (h) Development of epiphyseal ossification center. (i) Ossification center develops in lower epiphysis. (j and k) The lower and then the upper epiphyseal cartilage plates disappear, bone ceases to grow in length, a continuous bone marrow cavity traverses the entire length of the bone, and blood vessels of diaphysis, metaphysis, and epiphysis intercommunicate. (Adapted from Maximow AA, Bloom W. Textbook of histology. Philadelphia, WB Saunders, 1968)

after E.B.Patterson

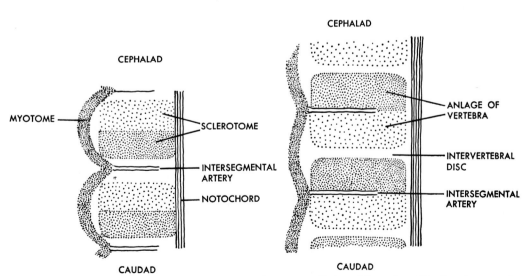

FIGURE 2-42. Early stages of differentiation of vertebrae. (Adapted from Arey LB. Developmental anatomy. Philadelphia, WB Saunders, 1974)

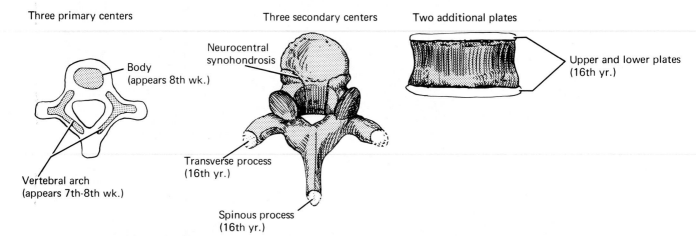

FIGURE 2-43. Development of vertebra. Three primary ossification centers develop in utero; three secondary centers appear during the growth period and, with epiphyseal plates, become completely ossified as growth is completed. (Adapted from Goss CM. Gray's anatomy, ed 28. Philadelphia, Lea & Febiger, 1966)

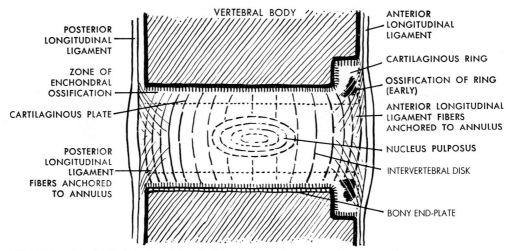

FIGURE 2-44. Sagittal section through adjacent vertebral bodies during ossification of the cartilaginous ring. (Adapted from Schmid P. Zur Entstehung der Adolezentenkyphose. Dtsch Med Wochenschr 1949;74:798)

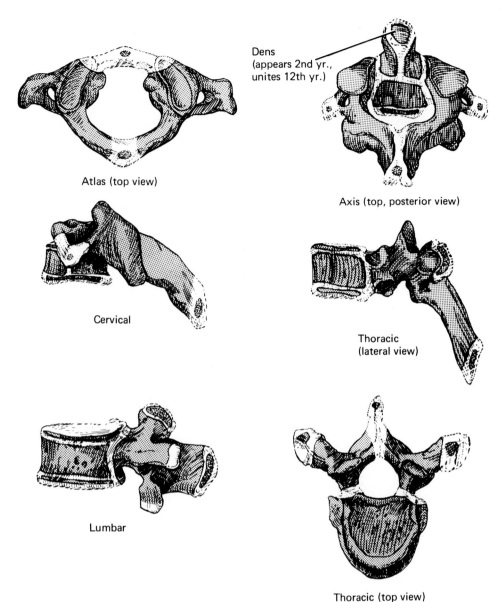

Dens
(appears 2nd yr.,
unites 12th yr.)

Atlas (top view)

Axis (top, posterior view)

Cervical

Thoracic
(lateral view)

Lumbar

Thoracic (top view)

FIGURE 2-45. Ossification of the vertebrae.

SUMMARY

The musculoskeletal system consists of skeletal connective tissues (bone, cartilage, and dense fibrous tissues) and muscle formed into functional units that make possible movements that vary from the finely controlled motions of the upper limbs necessary to play musical instruments, to the powerful motions of all four extremities and the spine necessary to lift a heavy weight from the ground, to the rapid coordinated repetitive motions required for success in many sports. Mesenchymal cells form all musculoskeletal tissues, but specific tissues differ in structure, composition, mechanical properties, innervation, and blood supply. The skeletal connective tissues (bone, cartilage, and dense fibrous tissue) consist of sparsely distributed cells surrounded by a large volume of extracellular organic matrix synthesized by the cells. Their matrix molecular frameworks consist of collagens, proteoglycans, and noncollagenous proteins. Each tissue has a unique combination of these three classes of macromolecules, and in some tissues (eg,

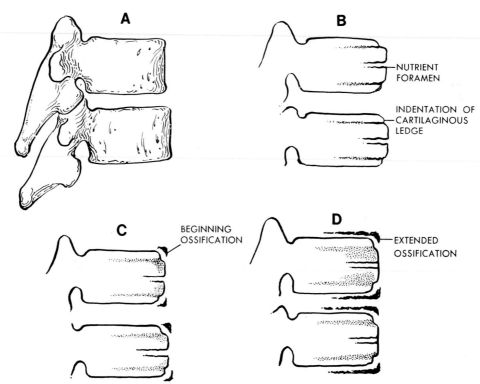

FIGURE 2-46. The appearance of normal thoracic vertebrae in children at various ages. (**A**) Normal thoracic vertebrae, fully developed, lateral view. (**B**) Lateral roentgenographic view of vertebral bodies in children under 6 years of age. (**C**) Lateral view in children, 6 to 9 years of age. Ossification starting in the cartilaginous ring is most visible anteriorly. (**D**) At 9 to 15 years of age. Ossification is more extensive in the ring and progresses posteriorly. The nutrient foramen normally is obliterated after 6 years of age.

meniscus, intervertebral disk, and ligament), elastin also forms part of the organic matrix. In addition to their organic matrix, bone and some cartilage regions have an inorganic matrix consisting of relatively insoluble mineral deposited within the organic matrix. These differences in matrix composition give the skeletal connective tissues different mechanical properties. Hyaline cartilage has the stiffness in compression, the ability to distribute loads, and the durability to form the low-friction gliding surfaces of synovial joints. The dense fibrous tissues have the tensile strength and flexibility to serve as tendons and ligaments, and bone has the stiffness and strength to provide the rigid support necessary for normal function of the other tissues. Hyaline cartilage lacks nerves. Bone contains perivascular nerves, and some regions of the dense fibrous tissues have nerves that may sense tissue deformation as well as perivascular nerves; however, none of the connective tissue cells has direct innervation. Hyaline cartilage,

the intervertebral disk (except for the outermost layers of the annulus fibrosus), and some regions of dense fibrous tissue lack blood vessels. Unlike the skeletal connective tissues, skeletal muscle consists primarily of cells with only a small volume of extracellular matrix, the tissue has a network of blood vessels that reaches every cell, a motor nerve innervates each muscle cell, and the cells generate the force necessary to produce movement.

Although knowledge of the tissues provides the basis for understanding orthopaedic diseases, musculoskeletal function and dysfunction cannot be understood in terms of individual tissues alone. The mobility, strength, and stability of the body depend on the organization and integration of these tissues into functional units. Voluntary movement requires skeletal muscle contraction, but the mechanisms by which muscle contraction produces joint motion, or the failure of muscle contraction to produce joint motion, cannot be understood by considering muscle

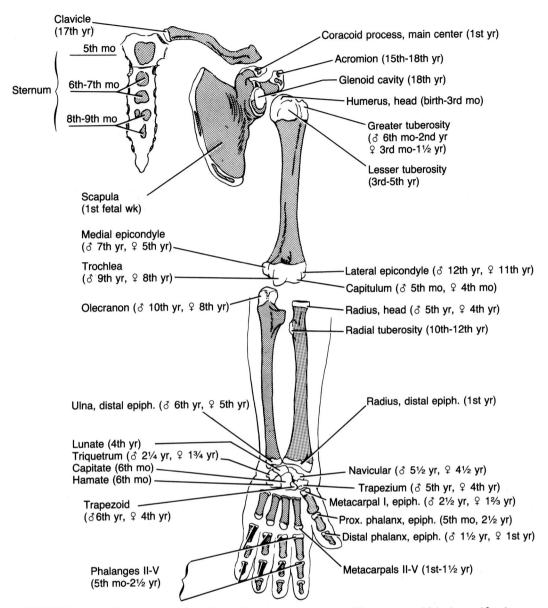

Clavicle (17th yr)

5th mo

Sternum

6th-7th mo

8th-9th mo

Coracoid process, main center (1st yr)

Acromion (15th-18th yr)

Glenoid cavity (18th yr)

Humerus, head (birth-3rd mo)

Greater tuberosity (♂ 6th mo-2nd yr ♀ 3rd mo-1½ yr)

Lesser tuberosity (3rd-5th yr)

Scapula (1st fetal wk)

Medial epicondyle (♂ 7th yr, ♀ 5th yr)

Trochlea (♂ 9th yr, ♀ 8th yr)

Olecranon (♂ 10th yr, ♀ 8th yr)

Lateral epicondyle (♂ 12th yr, ♀ 11th yr)

Capitulum (♂ 5th mo, ♀ 4th mo)

Radius, head (♂ 5th yr, ♀ 4th yr)

Radial tuberosity (10th-12th yr)

Ulna, distal epiph. (♂ 6th yr, ♀ 5th yr)

Radius, distal epiph. (1st yr)

Lunate (4th yr)
Triquetrum (♂ 2¼ yr, ♀ 1¾ yr)
Capitate (6th mo)
Hamate (6th mo)

Trapezoid (♂6th yr, ♀ 4th yr)

Navicular (♂ 5½ yr, ♀ 4½ yr)

Trapezium (♂ 5th yr, ♀ 4th yr)

Metacarpal I, epiph. (♂ 2½ yr, ♀ 1⅔ yr)

Prox. phalanx, epiph. (5th mo, 2½ yr)

Distal phalanx, epiph. (♂ 1½ yr, ♀ 1st yr)

Phalanges II-V (5th mo-2½ yr)

Metacarpals II-V (1st-1½ yr)

FIGURE 2-47. The appearance at birth of the upper extremity. The ages at which the ossification of the epiphyses appear are shown with the differentiation between male and female indicated.

cells alone. Muscles move or stabilize synovial joints and the spine by transmitting the force generated by individual muscle cells to tendons through elaborate muscle tendon junctions. Many tendons pass through sheaths and retinacula that make it possible to effectively transmit the force generated by muscle to bone through distinct insertions into bone or periosteum. The force then acts on synovial joints consisting of articular cartilage, menisci, bone, joint capsule, synovium, and ligaments or the spine. The spine includes these tissues with the addition of the intervertebral disk. Ultimately, muscle contraction causes joint motion or stabilizes joints against resistance. However, synovial joint or spine function can be understood only by considering how the multiple musculoskeletal tissues perform simultaneously as parts of a functional unit. Likewise, understanding orthopaedic diseases depends on considering how disturbances in the structure or function of one or more

(*text continues on page 67*)

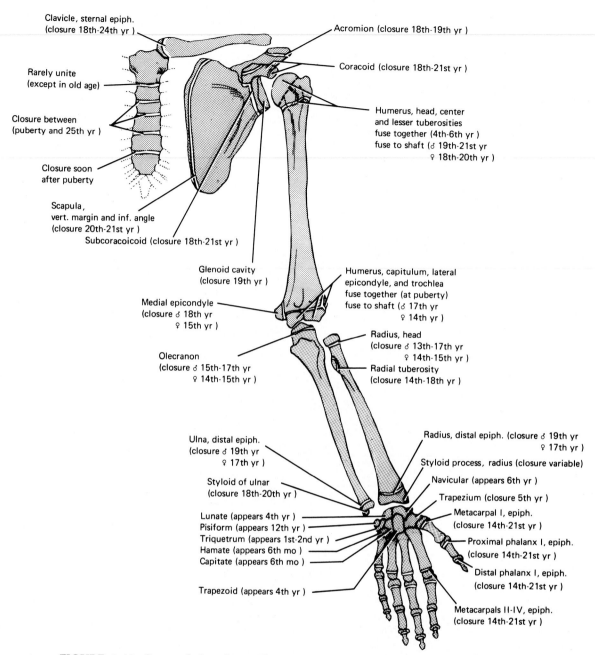

FIGURE 2-48. Stages of advancing ossification and epiphyseal closure of the upper extremity.

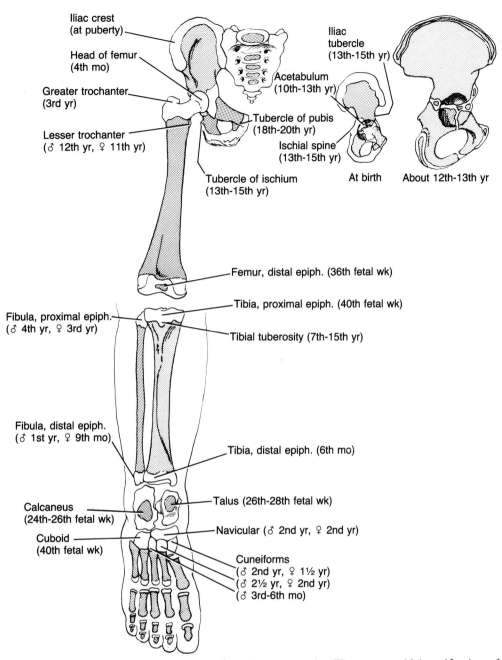

Iliac crest
(at puberty)

Head of femur
(4th mo)

Greater trochanter
(3rd yr)

Lesser trochanter
(♂ 12th yr, ♀ 11th yr)

Tubercle of ischium
(13th-15th yr)

Iliac tubercle
(13th-15th yr)

Acetabulum
(10th-13th yr)

Tubercle of pubis
(18th-20th yr)

Ischial spine
(13th-15th yr)

At birth

About 12th-13th yr

Femur, distal epiph. (36th fetal wk)

Tibia, proximal epiph. (40th fetal wk)

Fibula, proximal epiph.
(♂ 4th yr, ♀ 3rd yr)

Tibial tuberosity (7th-15th yr)

Fibula, distal epiph.
(♂ 1st yr, ♀ 9th mo)

Tibia, distal epiph. (6th mo)

Talus (26th-28th fetal wk)

Calcaneus
(24th-26th fetal wk)

Navicular (♂ 2nd yr, ♀ 2nd yr)

Cuboid
(40th fetal wk)

Cuneiforms
(♂ 2nd yr, ♀ 1½ yr)
(♂ 2½ yr, ♀ 2nd yr)
(♂ 3rd-6th mo)

FIGURE 2-49. The appearance at birth of the lower extremity. The ages at which ossification of the epiphyses appear are shown with the differentiation between male and female indicated.

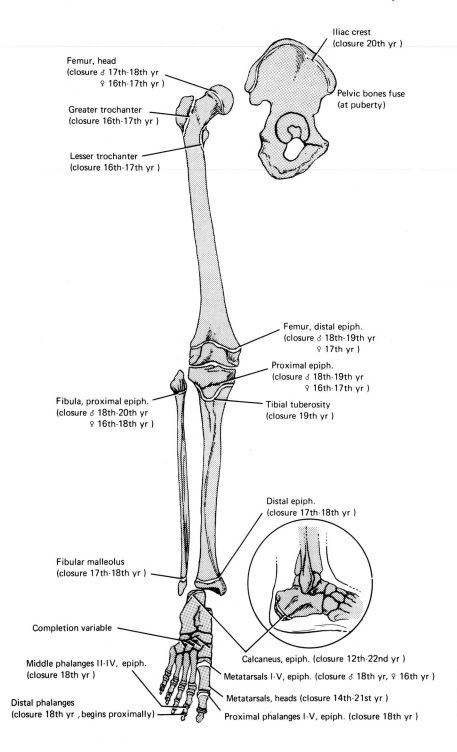

Iliac crest
(closure 20th yr)

Femur, head
(closure ♂ 17th-18th yr
♀ 16th-17th yr)

Greater trochanter
(closure 16th-17th yr)

Pelvic bones fuse
(at puberty)

Lesser trochanter
(closure 16th-17th yr)

Femur, distal epiph.
(closure ♂ 18th-19th yr
♀ 17th yr)

Proximal epiph.
(closure ♂ 18th-19th yr
♀ 16th-17th yr)

Fibula, proximal epiph.
(closure ♂ 18th-20th yr
♀ 16th-18th yr)

Tibial tuberosity
(closure 19th yr)

Distal epiph.
(closure 17th-18th yr)

Fibular malleolus
(closure 17th-18th yr)

Completion variable

Middle phalanges II-IV, epiph.
(closure 18th yr)

Calcaneus, epiph. (closure 12th-22nd yr)

Metatarsals I-V, epiph. (closure ♂ 18th yr, ♀ 16th yr)

Metatarsals, heads (closure 14th-21st yr)

Distal phalanges
(closure 18th yr , begins proximally)

Proximal phalanges I-V, epiph. (closure 18th yr)

FIGURE 2-50. The stage of advancing ossification and epiphyseal closure of the lower extremity.

tissues alters musculoskeletal function measured in terms of motion, strength, and stability.

Annotated Bibliography

Albright JA, Brand RA, eds. The scientific basis of orthopaedics. Norwalk, CT, Appleton & Lange, 1987.
The chapters of this book discuss the cells and matrices of the skeletal connective tissues, genetics, the development of the musculoskeletal system, bone structure, function, physiology and healing, articular cartilage structure and function, joint lubrication, the skeletal fibrous tissues, skeletal muscle, nerve, blood vessels, inflammation, and immunology.

Buckwalter JA. Fine structural studies of human intervertebral disk. In: White AA, Gordon SL, eds. Proceedings of the Workshop on Idiopathic Low Back Pain. St Louis, CV Mosby, 1982:108–143.
This chapter summarizes the structure, composition, and age-related changes of the human intervertebral disk.

Buckwalter JA, Cooper RR. Bone structure and function. AAOS Instruct Course Lect 1987;36:27–48.
This article reviews the structure and function of bone.

Orthopaedic science: a resource and self-study guide for the practitioner. Park Ridge, IL, American Academy of Orthopaedic Surgeons, 1986.
This book and slide set provides illustrations and descriptions of the structure composition and mechanics of the musculoskeletal tissues.

Woo SL, Buckwalter JA, eds. Injury and repair of the musculoskeletal soft tissues. Park Ridge, IL, American Academy of Orthopaedic Surgeons, 1988.
This book reviews the structure, composition, function, and response to injury of the musculoskeletal soft tissues—tendon, ligament, and tendon and ligament insertions into bone, muscle tendon junctions, skeletal muscle, peripheral nerve, peripheral blood vessel, articular cartilage, and meniscus.

Turek's Orthopaedics: Principles and Their Application, Fifth Edition,
edited by Stuart L. Weinstein and Joseph A. Buckwalter.
J.B. Lippincott Company, Philadelphia, © 1994.

Georges Y. El-Khoury
Karim Rezai
Timothy E. Moore

3

Imaging of the Musculoskeletal System

PLAIN RADIOGRAPHY
PLAIN OR CONVENTIONAL
TOMOGRAPHY
COMPUTED TOMOGRAPHY
MAGNETIC RESONANCE
IMAGING
Physical Principles
Definitions
Safety and Contraindications
Application in the
Musculoskeletal System

RADIONUCLIDE BONE
SCANNING
Technique and Instrumentation
Metastatic Disease of the
Skeleton
Primary Bone Lesions
Trauma
Infection
Osteonecrosis and Bone
Infarction
Reflex Sympathetic Dystrophy
Miscellaneous Bone Disorders

PLAIN RADIOGRAPHY

Despite the rapid advances in technology, conventional radiography continues to be the mainstay of the orthopaedic examination. Proper selection of equipment and radiographic technique are crucial in obtaining diagnostic examinations and protecting patients from excessive irradiation.

The following are considered standard equipment:

- Four-way floating top table with a Bucky grid (12:1 ratio) focused at 80 to 90 cm (36 to 40 inches)
- 500-mA three-phase generator
- X-ray tube with relatively small focal spot (0.6 mm)
- Chest board with a stationary grid
- Rare earth screens

Special setups are needed to perform scoliosis surveys, upright lateral flexion and extension lumbar spine examinations, upright views of the knees (Fig. 3-1) and feet, and magnification views. Fluoroscopy with spot filming or video taping is needed for arthrography, joint aspirations, needle biopsies, and dynamic studies.

Although orthpaedists employ radiographs extensively in their work, few are formally trained in radiation protection. Some simple rules apply to all personnel working with ionizing radiation:

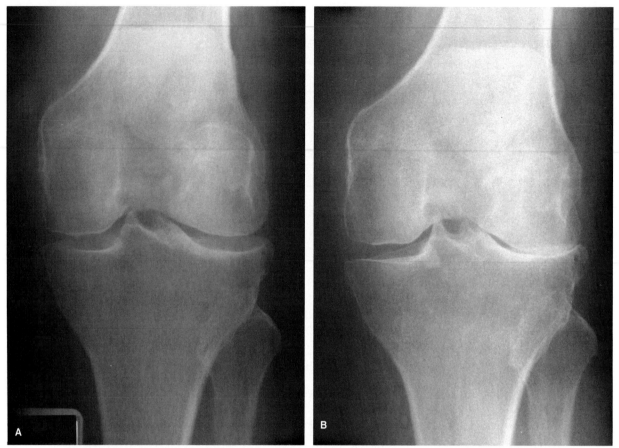

FIGURE 3-1. Standing view of the knee in osteoarthritis. (A) AP view of the left knee taken supine shows degenerative changes, but the joint space appears to be well preserved. (B) Examination repeated with patient standing demonstrates total obliteration of the joint space laterally; moderate valgus is present.

1. Wearing a radiation monitoring badge at all times is mandatory.
2. Use protective lead apron, lead gloves, and thyroid shield when performing fluorscopy and positioning or stressing an extremity for plain radiography.
3. In all diagnostic procedures the fastest appropriate film-screen combination should be used.
4. Never expose your hands or other parts of your body to the direct x-ray beam even when protected by lead gloves and apron. Protective devices are designed to shield from scattered radiation only.
5. Avoid using fluoroscopy when you can use radiography.
6. Limit your fluoroscopy time to short bursts of exposure.
7. Protect patients with gonadal shields whenever possible.
8. Consult with a radiologist when it is necessary to perform a radiographic examination on a pregnant patient.

PLAIN OR CONVENTIONAL TOMOGRAPHY

Plain or conventional tomography is still useful in orthopaedic radiology and is well suited for the evaluation of organs with inherent tissue contrast such as bone. Selection of tube motion and the interval between sections is determined by the anatomy of the structure studied and the clinical problem under investigation. In evaluating nonunion in the scaphoid, for example, 36-degree circular or hypocycloidal motion at 2-mm intervals is usually required, whereas for large parts, like the spine sections, 5- to 10-mm intervals would be adequate. Plain tomography is the technique of choice for evaluation of nonunion in spine fusions (Fig. 3-2). To assess the hips through a thick plaster cast in a child with congenital dislocation of the hip, an 8-degree tomographic section using circular motion at the appropriate level is sufficient to blur out the cast and visualize the relation

(text continues on page 75)

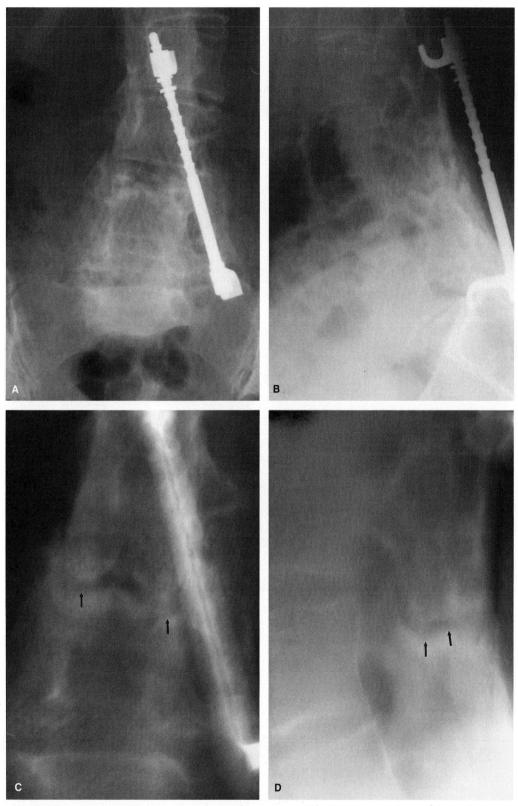

FIGURE 3-2. Nonunion at the site of spine fusion. (**A** and **B**) AP and lateral views of the lumbosacral spine demonstrate the posterior fusion mass. Motion is suspected at the L3-L4 level. (**C** and **D**) AP and lateral tomographic sections clearly show the break and nonunion in the fusion mass (*arrows*).

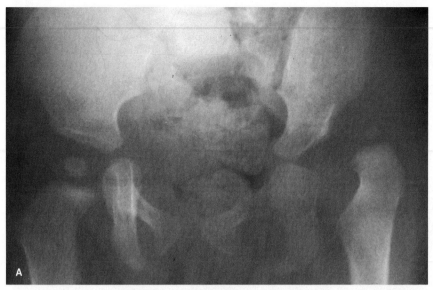

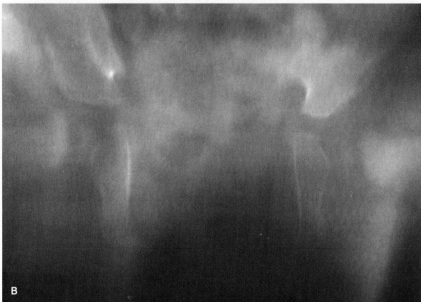

FIGURE 3-3. Illustration of the usefulness of thick-section tomography in evaluating bony structures not visualized by plain radiography. This technique keeps the radiation dose to a minimum. **(A)** AP film of the pelvis demonstrates congenital dislocation of left hip discovered at the age of 10 months. The patient underwent open reduction and was placed in a thick plaster cast. Plain radiography through the cast failed to show the left femoral head and its relation to the acetabulum. **(B)** An 8-degree tomographic section using circular motion demonstrates the proper position of the left femoral head within the dysplastic acetabulum.

FIGURE 3-4. C4 facet fracture-dislocation with locking. **(A)** Lateral view of the cervical spine showing malalignment with anterior displacement of C4 or C5. **(B)** On lateral tomography there is fracture (*arrow*) of the inferior articular facet of C4 with anterior dislocation of the inferior facet of C4 (*asterisk*) on the superior facet of C5. The dislocated facet is locked in the dislocated position.

FIGURE 3-5. A 15-month-old boy with congenital scoliosis resulting from a hemivertebra in the lower thoracic spine. **(A)** Plain AP view of the spine demonstrates the hemivertebra. **(B)** Tomography shows the abnormality in more detail. The hemivertebra is demonstrated to have a pedicle, a lamina, and superior and inferior articular facets.

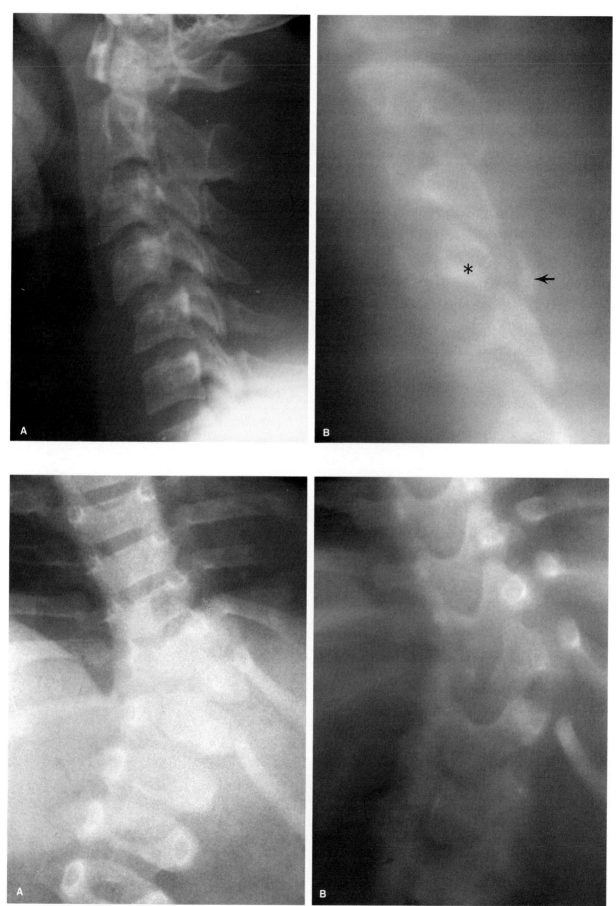

FIGURE 3-5.

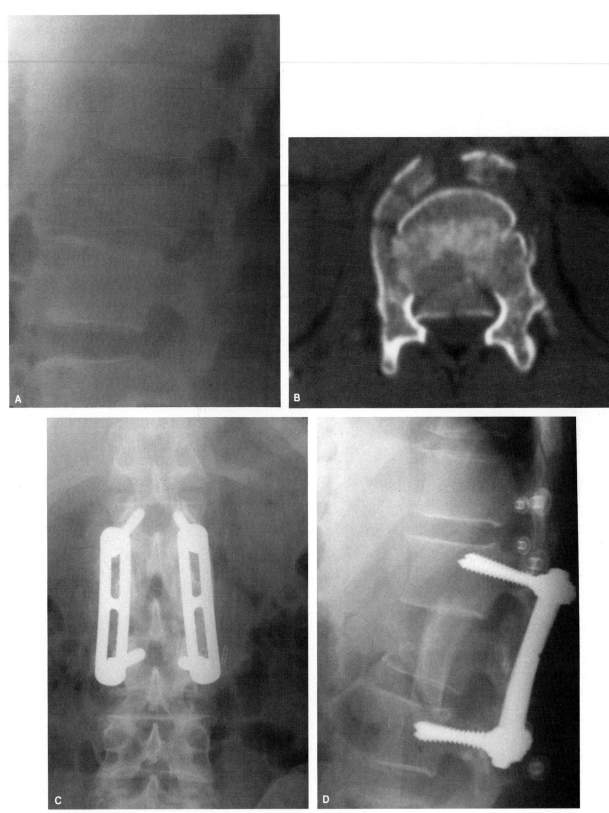

FIGURE 3-6. Diagnostic CT examinations are obtainable in the presence of metallic hardware. (**A**) Lateral view of the lumbar spine shows at least a two-column fracture of L2 with retropulsion of the fractured body into the spinal canal. (**B**) CT shows a comminuted fracture of L2 with the retropulsed fragments obliterating the spinal canal. (**C** and **D**) Postoperative AP and lateral views demonstrate resection of the retropulsed fragments and placement of a bone graft bridging the end-plates of L1 to L3. Fixation with Stephie plates and screws was performed. (**E**) CT demonstrates restoration of the spinal canal postsurgically. The metal artifacts did not significantly interfere with visualization of the spinal canal and graft (*arrow*).

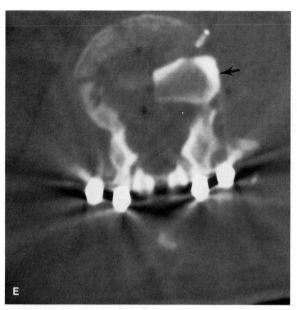

FIGURE 3-6. *(Continued)*

of the femoral heads to the acetabula (Fig. 3-3). Plain tomography is useful in studying cervical spine fractures and segmentation anomalies of the spine (Figs. 3-4 and 3-5). It is also used in the evaluation of occult wrist fractures, infections, tarsal coalitions, benign and malignant bone tumors, and bone erosions at the craniovertebral junction in patients with rheumatoid arthritis. Much of the diagnostic work previously performed with conventional tomography is currently being done with computed tomography (CT) and magnetic resonance imaging (MRI); however, when these modalities are not available, conventional tomography is still a useful diagnostic tool.

COMPUTED TOMOGRAPHY

Computed tomography, like plain radiography and tomography, uses ionizing radiation to obtain images. The scanning gantry contains an x-ray tube, a series of detectors, and a couch with a precision positioning system. The x-ray beam is highly collimated, and the x-ray tube typically moves 360 degrees during a single CT slice. The detectors capture the attenuated beam, and the resulting data are processed by a computer that displays the image on a matrix of 512 × 512 small squares called pixels. Each pixel is given a CT number related to data obtained by the detectors. On CT images, the numbers are displayed as various shades of gray where the lowest numbers appear black (eg, air), and the highest numbers appear white

(eg, cortical bone). The operator at the console can manipulate the window width (range of CT numbers in the gray scale) and window level (center of the gray scale) to study either bone or soft tissue detail.

Planning an examination for CT requires a good deal of expertise needed to select thickness of slices, couch index or interval of slices, gantry angulation, filming at the proper window width and level, and reconstruction of appropriate sagittal and coronal images. For three-dimensional (3D) reconstructions, slices should not exceed 3 mm in thickness and should usually be contiguous or overlap by 1 mm. As with all radiographic procedures, the clinical problem should be communicated clearly to the radiologist on the radiologic requisition, or better still, discussed with the radiologist directly. The CT examination should always be tailored to the needs of the patient and designed to answer a specific clinical problem, using the least amount of radiation.

Some diagnostic problems that were, until recently, studied by CT, are now better addressed by MRI. Most notable in this category are intervertebral disk herniations, metastatic disease to the spine with cord compression, bone and soft tissue tumors, and avascular necrosis. CT, however, continues to be useful in the evaluation of complex fractures of the spine, pelvis, acetabulum, knee, ankle, calcaneus, wrist, and shoulder. Detection and evaluation of burst fractures with retropulsion of bony fragments into the spinal canal are adequately demonstrated by CT. If, however, cord contusion or hematoma are suspected, then MRI would be the examination of choice. CT is the method of choice in studying burst fractures of C1 (Jefferson's fracture) and C1-C2 rotary dislocations. CT is also useful following reduction of spine fractures internally fixed with metal rods or plates, where demonstration of the size and contour of the spinal canal can be achieved by using a wide window, hence reducing metal streak artifacts caused by beam hardening (Fig. 3-6). Some manufacturers have produced special computer software to remedy the problem of metal streaking, thereby greatly improving the capabilities of CT in scanning areas where metal devices are present.

Complex fractures of the acetabulum, knee, ankle, calcaneus, and wrist are commonly evaluated by 3D CT (Fig. 3-7). Thorough knowledge of the fracture components before surgery gives the surgeon an added advantage and often results in reduction of the operating time.

CT is effective in the evaluation of some bone

(text continues on page 78)

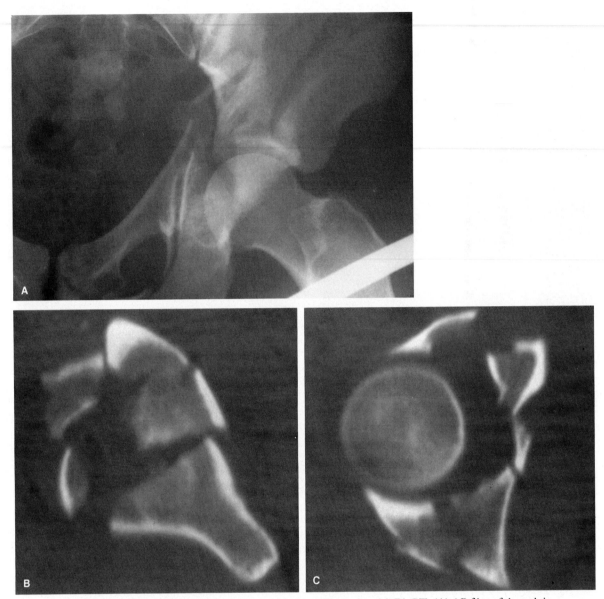

FIGURE 3-7. Acetabular fracture studied with three-dimensional (3D) CT. (**A**) AP film of the pelvis reveals a comminuted fracture of the right acetabulum with extension into the ilium. There is also a comminuted fracture of the right symphysis pubis. (**B** and **C**) Axial CT sections through the acetabulum show the fracture with involvement of the anterior column, posterior column, and acetabular roof. The next five images are 3D CT images using the surface rendering technique, whereby structures close to the person viewing the image appear bright (in all these images, the femoral head has been edited out): looking at the acetabulum from the front (**D**), from the side (**E**), from the back (**F**), from inside the pelvis (**G**), and from below, primarily to inspect the acetabular roof (**H**). Asterisk, anteroinferior iliac spine; P, superior pubic ramus; I, ischium; IS, ischial spine; G, greater sciatic notch.

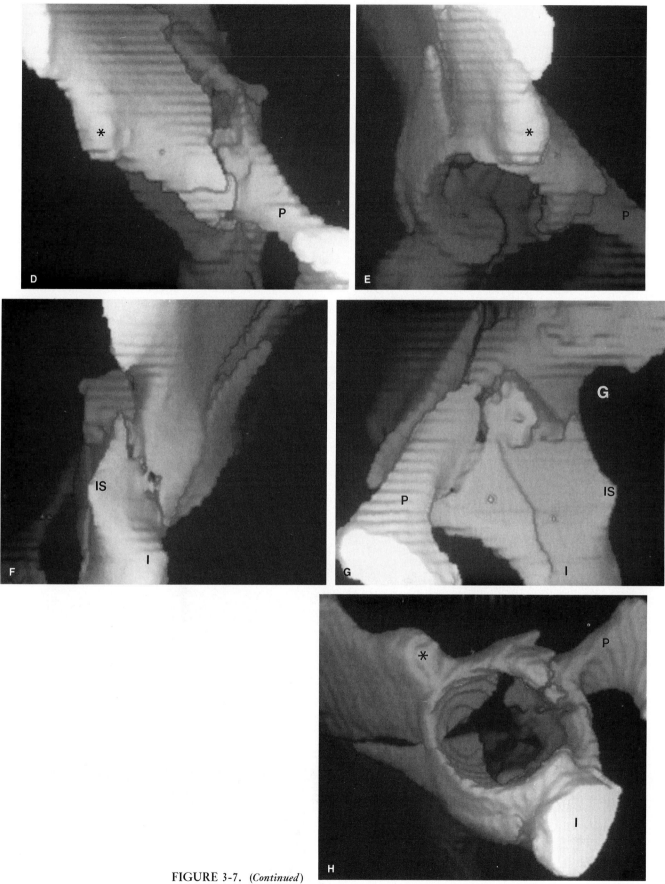

FIGURE 3-7. (*Continued*)

and soft tissue tumors. Tumors are considered to be malignant if they have poor margination, areas of diminished density, blurring of adjacent fat, multiple muscle group involvement, and bony invasion. Sharp margins alone, however, do not guarantee that a lesion is benign.

Focal metastatic disease detected by radionuclide scans but not visualized on plain films can be accurately mapped by CT (Fig. 3-8). Because of enhanced tissue contrast, CT can detect fine calcifications not seen by plain radiography or MRI. Tumors such as osteoid osteoma or osteoblastoma can be elegantly demonstrated by CT. The nidus in osteoid osteoma is usually difficult to demonstrate on plain films but is easily depicted on thin-section CT images filmed with a wide window (Figs. 3-9 and 3-10).

Double-contrast arthrotomography with CT is the technique of choice for the evaluation of labral tears in the shoulder (Fig. 3-11). The technique is also used to detect uncalcified intraarticular loose bodies and osteochondral fractures.

Tarsal coalitions are clearly demonstrated by CT (Fig. 3-12). Disk space infections with associated paraspinal abscesses, and muscle abscesses are routinely investigated with CT.

Early spondylolysis is best studied by CT (Fig. 3-13). Healing can be achieved in early stages of the disease and can also be followed by CT. On axial CT images pars interarticularis defects are commonly overlooked because they resemble normal facet joints. Thorough knowledge of sectional anatomy is essential to avoid such mistakes.

MAGNETIC RESONANCE IMAGING

Magnetic resonance imaging is a new technology that produces sectional images in any desirable plain revealing excellent anatomic detail with high-contrast resolution. The demand for musculoskeletal MRI examinations is rapidly increasing, and because of this unprecedented expansion, well-controlled studies of its diagnostic efficacy were initially slow in coming. Excellent retrospective and prospective studies have shown the efficacy of MRI in diagnosing and staging a variety of musculoskeletal diseases. The full po-

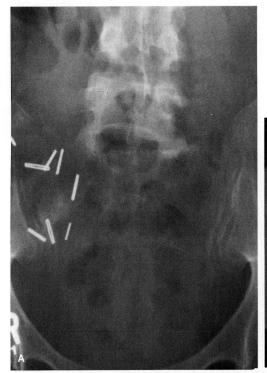 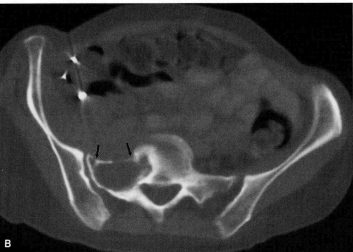

FIGURE 3-8. Metastasis to the sacral ala. (A) Plain AP radiograph of the pelvis performed on a 45-year-old woman with a pelvic mass. The right scaral ala appeared lucent, but the observers were not sure whether this was due to metastasis or overlying gas. (B) CT section through the upper sacrum shows definite destruction of the right sacral ala (*arrows*).

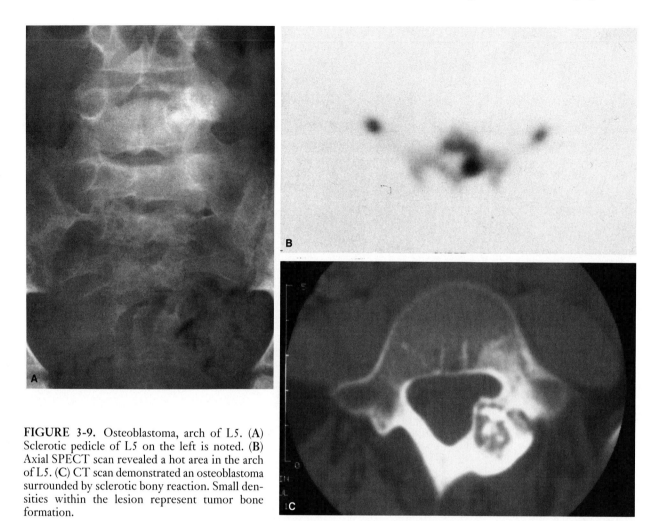

FIGURE 3-9. Osteoblastoma, arch of L5. (**A**) Sclerotic pedicle of L5 on the left is noted. (**B**) Axial SPECT scan revealed a hot area in the arch of L5. (**C**) CT scan demonstrated an osteoblastoma surrounded by sclerotic bony reaction. Small densities within the lesion represent tumor bone formation.

tential of MRI has not been reached; nevertheless, its impact on orthopaedics has altered our approach to many diagnostic problems. Already MRI is the primary imaging technique for disk disease, internal derangement of the knee, muscle and tendon injuries, early avascular necrosis, soft tissue tumors, and malignant bone tumors.

MRI is different from other diagnostic modalities, and a basic understanding of its physical principles, terminology, applications, health hazards, contraindications, and future directions is essential for practicing state-of-the-art orthopaedic surgery.

Physical Principles

Nuclei with an odd number of protons or neutrons (^{1}H, ^{31}P, ^{23}Na) exhibit a spin. Because these nuclei are charged particles in motion, they create a mag-

netic field, thus behaving like small magnets. The nucleus most commonly used for medical imaging is hydrogen because of its abundance in biologic tissues and its favorable magnetic characteristics. Normally these small magnets (nuclei) are randomly oriented, but when placed in a strong magnetic field they orient themselves in the direction of the external magnetic field and therefore are considered to be in a state of equilibrium. In this state, the nuclei, in addition to spinning, also precess around the axis of the external field, in a manner similar to the wobble of a spinning top (Fig. 3-14). The frequency of precession is directly proportional to the strength of the external field. If a specific radiofrequency (RF) pulse, resonant with (frequency equal to) the precessing frequency, is applied to these nuclei, they are deflected from their alignment with the external magnet. When the strength of the RF pulse is chosen to cause a 90-

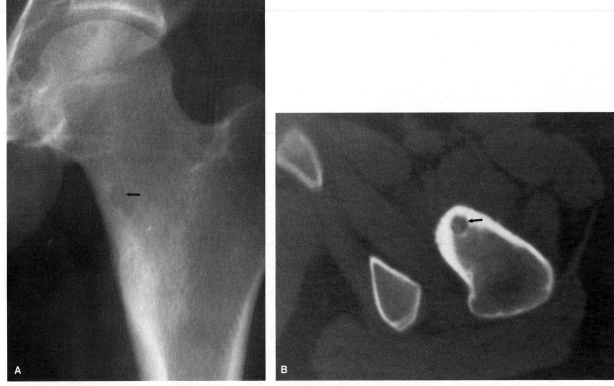

FIGURE 3-10. Osteoid osteoma in the femoral neck. (**A**) AP view of the left hip shows a lucency in the femoral neck medially (*arrow*). (**B**) CT scan through the femoral neck demonstrates a nidus (*arrow*) and a small calcification within it. The nidus is surrounded with reactive sclerotic bone.

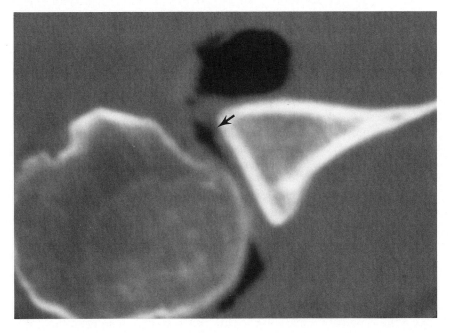

FIGURE 3-11. Labral tear. Double-contrast arthrogram of the shoulder followed by CT shows a small cleft between the articular cartilage of the glenoid and the labrum anteriorly (*arrow*). This is diagnostic of a labral tear.

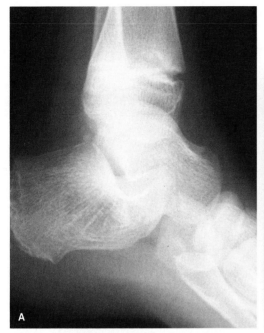
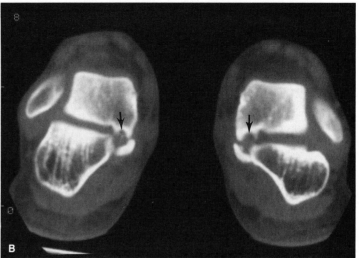

FIGURE 3-12. A 9-year-old boy presented with pain in the subtalar joint bilaterally. (A) Special plain views of the subtalar joint failed to show any abnormalities. (B) CT of the subtalar joint reveals a coalition (*arrows*) at the middle subtalar joint bilaterally.

degree deflection, the nuclei tip 90 degrees and precess perpendicular to the external magnetic field. Magnetic moments perpendicular to the external field are capable of producing an alternating current in a receiver coil placed adjacent to the part being examined. When the RF pulse stops, the nuclei gradually return to their equilibrium state (alignment with the external field), and the emitted signals diminish. The signals are captured by the receiver coil and eventually transformed into clinically useful images or spectra.

Definitions

RESONANCE. As mentioned previously, the frequency of precession is directly proportional to the strength of the external magnet. The external magnetic field is set at a gradient where field strength gradually decreases across the scanned part, so that each slice or position is encoded with a known frequency of precession. Resonance is the synchronizing of the RF pulse emitted by the transmitter with the precessing frequency of the nuclei in the sample for energy transfer to occur.

T1 RELAXATION TIME. Also called longitudinal relaxation or spin lattice relaxation time, this is a tissue-specific time constant. It is the time required for 63% of the deflected nuclei to realign with the external magnetic field or return to equilibrium state, after the termination of a 90-degree RF pulse.

T2 RELAXATION TIME. Also called transverse relaxation time or spin-spin relaxation time, this is a tissue-specific time constant describing the rate at which nuclei get out of phase or out of precessing as one unit and start to precess as individual nuclei. After the 90-degree RF pulse, all the deflected nuclei lying in the tranverse plain precess in phase. In a matter of milliseconds, they slip out of phase because of interactions with neighboring nuclei. As a result, transverse magnetization ceases, and the signal emitted from the scanned tissue diminishes. Maximum transverse magnetization is achieved immediately after the 90-degree RF pulse followed by an exponential decay at a time constant T2. To put the nuclei back in phase, a 180-degree RF pulse is used.

T1 and T2 relaxation following the 90-degree RF pulse occur simultaneously. The T2 decay, however, takes a shorter time than T1 relaxation. For most soft

(text continues on page 84)

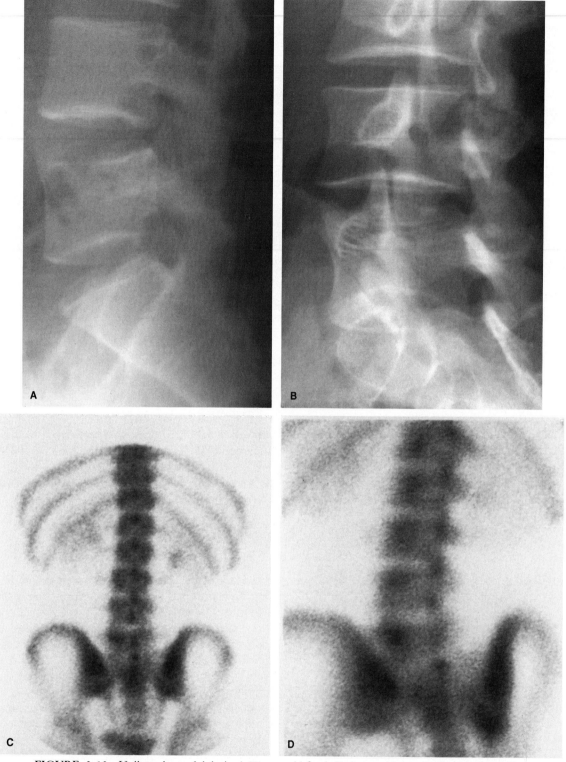

FIGURE 3-13. Unilateral spondylolysis. A 20-year-old football player with low-back pain of 3 weeks' duration. (**A** and **B**) Lateral and oblique views of the lumbar spine failed to show any abnormalities. (**C** and **D**) Posterior and oblique bone scans of the lumbar spine show increased radionuclide uptake in the region of L5 on the left. (**E**) Thin section CT scan demonstrates a pars defect in L5 on the left (*arrowheads*). (**F**) Sagittal reconstruction through the pars interarticularis on the left clearly shows the defect (*arrow*). (**G**) The pars interarticularis on the right is normal.

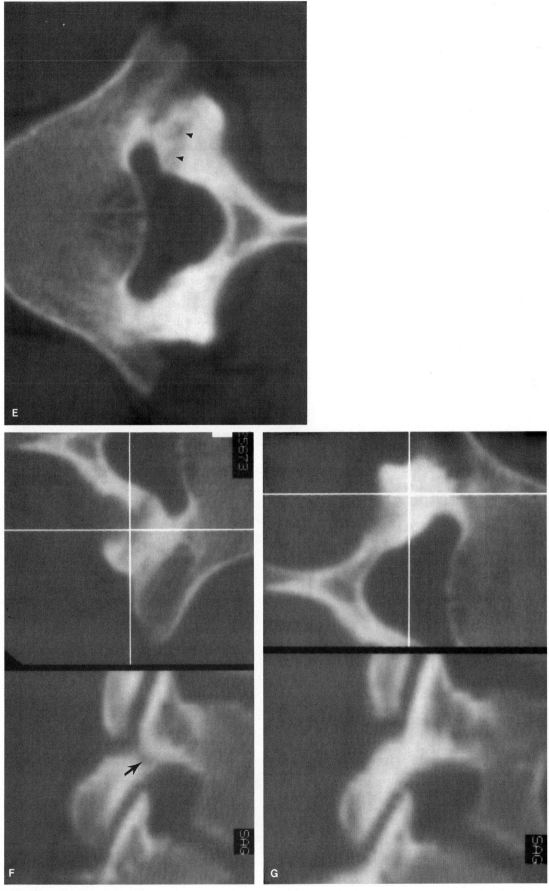

FIGURE 3-13. (*Continued*)

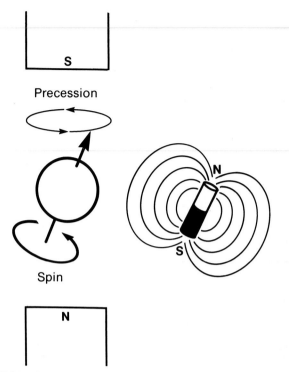

FIGURE 3-14. Each hydrogen atom behaves like a small magnet. When placed in an external magnetic field, these small magnets align with the external field. Each hydrogen atom has an intrinsic spin; it also precesses around the long axis of the external magnet at a rate determined by the strength of the magnet.

tissues, the range of T1 is 220 to 3000 ms; T2 varies from 55 to 200 ms.

TISSUE CONTRAST. Why do certain tissues appear bright or black with particular pulse sequences? Tissue contrast is dependent on the following inherent tissue properties: free hydrogen in the tissue (also known as proton density), T1 and T2 relaxation times, and flow. Tissues with a higher density of free protons emit greater signal and therefore appear brighter than tissues with lower proton density. Most soft tissues in the body, however, have almost similar proton densities; therefore, proton density alone is not

TABLE 3-1.
Relative Relaxation Times of Practical Value in the Musculoskeletal System

Normal Tissue	T1	T2
Water	Long (dark)	Long (bright)
Cerebrospinal fluid	Long (dark)	Long (bright)
Fat	Short (bright)	Medium (gray, bright)
Fibrous connective tissue	Long (dark)	Very short (dark)
Tendons and ligaments	Very long (dark)	Very short (dark)
Bone	Very long (dark)	Very short (dark)
Muscle	Medium (gray)	Medium (gray)
Cartilage		
Hyaline cartilage	Medium (gray)	Medium (gray)
Fibrocartilage	Long (dark)	Very short (dark)

a major contributor to tissue contrast. Flowing tissue such as blood within arteries does not persist in a fixed place for scanning and therefore appears black on both T1- and T2-weighted images. This is explained as being due to the migration of the excited (stimulated by RF pulses sequence) cylinder of blood from the scanning field and replacement by unexcited blood before the receiver coil is ready to detect the emitted signals. This leaves T1 and T2 relaxation times of tissues as the most important factors in determining tissue contrast in images. Exploiting these tissue properties by selecting the proper pulse sequences is the key to obtaining diagnostic quality images (Table 3-1).

A pulse sequence is a precisely defined pattern of RF pulses and listening times. The most commonly used pulse sequence in the study of the musculoskeletal system is the spin echo sequence. It consists of a 90-degree pulse followed by a pause, after which a 180-degree pulse is applied. Then after an additional pause, the receiver coil is set to listen to a signal (echo) emitted from the tissues; after a longer pause, the cycle is repeated (Fig. 3-15). The spin echo sequence can be T1 weighted, accentuating the T1

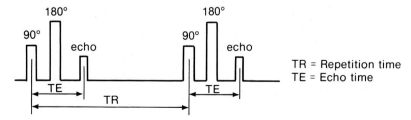

TR = Repetition time
TE = Echo time

FIGURE 3-15. A diagram of a spin echo pulsing sequence.

properties of tissue, or T2 weighted, accentuating the T2 properties of the tissue. T1-weighted sequences, sometimes called partial saturation sequences, have an echo time (TE) less than or equal to 40 ms and repetition time (TR) less than or equal to 800 ms (see Fig. 3-15). T2-weighted sequences have a TE greater than or equal to 80 ms and TR greater than or equal to 1500 ms. In general, T1-weighted images depict anatomy better, and T2-weighted images show pathology better.

On T1-Weighted Sequences
- Tissues with short T1 have high signal intensity (bright)—for example, fat.
- Tissues with long T1 have low signal intensity (dark)—for example, cerebrospinal fluid (CSF).

On T2-Weighted Sequences
- Tissues with short T2 have low signal intensity (dark)—for example, tendon or ligament.
- Tissues with long T2 have high signal intensity (bright)—for example, CSF.

Inflamed tissue appears dark on T1-weighted images and bright on T2-weighted images when compared with the healthy neighboring tissue, because of prolongation of T1 and T2 relaxation times. The increased water in the form of edema is offered as an explanation. Neoplasm generally increases the T1 and T2 relaxation times relative to the host tissue; therefore, it appears dark or isointense on T1-weighted sequences and bright on T2-weighted sequences. This is also thought to be due to an increase in the free water content (Table 3-2).

SURFACE COILS. Surface coils are sophisticated antennae designed to transmit or receive radio waves generated by the precessing nuclei. In a receiver coil, these radio waves impinge on the coil and generate an alternating current. The efficiency of this process is dependent on how closely the wires in the coils are applied to the body part being examined. The design of the surface coil is dependent on the anatomic region; therefore, a surface coil for the shoulder is different in design from a lumbar spine coil or a knee coil. Surface coils greatly improve the quality of the image by increasing the signal-to-noise ratio.

CONTRAST AGENTS. The contrast agent approved by the Food and Drug Administration for clinical use is gadolinium–diethylenetriaminepentaacetic acid (Gd-DTPA), which is a paramagnetic agent. Paramagnetic atoms possess unpaired electrons in their outer shells, thus creating their own small local magnetic field. Paramagnetic agents act in enhancing (shortening) the T1 and T2 relaxation times of surrounding hydrogen nuclei under evaluation. T1 shortening produces higher (brighter) signals on T1-weighted images. Gd-DTPA displays pharmacokinetics similar to those of iodinated contrast media in that it penetrates highly vascularized areas and produces an increase in signal intensity in these areas on T1-weighted images. The paramagnetic properties of Gd-DTPA reduce the T1 relaxation time of penetrated tissues. In the musculoskeletal system, there is preliminary evidence that it is useful in differentiating edema, cyst formation, and necrosis from the actual tumor and, therefore, helps in delineating the extent of a neoplastic process. It has also been used extensively in differentiating epidural scarring from recurrent disk herniation following surgery.

Nonionic Gd compounds with lower osmolality than Gd-DTPA are being developed. These newer compounds can be safely injected in larger quantities than permitted with Gd-DTPA.

Safety and Contraindications

With the current clinical level of exposures, MRI is generally a safe technique. Recent studies indicate no interference with cardiac function or nerve conduction at 2 to 7 Tesla. Forceful attraction of ferromagnetic objects to the magnet is a definite risk. Caution must be exercised when there are ferromagnetic objects embedded in the patient such as shrapnels, foreign bodies lodged within the eye, or aneurysm clips on the brain. As a rule, MRI should not be performed on patients with cardiac pacemakers, aneurysm clips, or cochlear implants. Metallic ortho-

TABLE 3-2.
Relative T1 and T2 Relaxation Times of Some Pathologic Processes

Abnormal Process	T1	T2
Infection/inflammation	Long (dark)	Long (bright)
Neoplasm	Long (dark) or medium (isointense)	Long (bright)
Fibrosis	Long (dark)	Very short (dark)
Fatty infiltration	Short (bright)	Medium (bright)
Hemorrhage (acute)	Long (dark)	Long (bright)

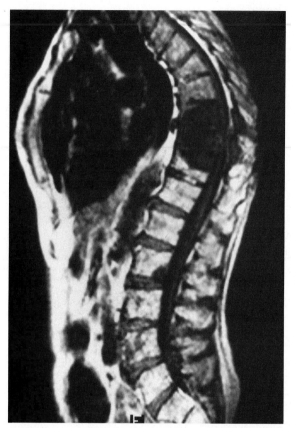

FIGURE 3-16. Metastasis to the spine. Eighty-one-year-old man with prostatic cancer, presenting with weakness in both lower extremities. T1-weighted sagittal image of the spine shows metastasis to the lower thoracic spine and to L3. The mass in the thoracic region has invaded the epidural space and compressed the cord.

paedic appliances are generally not ferromagnetic, but they do create significant local artifact that precludes scanning in the immediate vicinity of the appliance. In pregnancy, MRI should be avoided during the first trimester.

Application in the Musculoskeletal System

Spine

With the use of surface coils and other technical advances, MRI is becoming the most important imaging study of the spine. The demand for myelography in most institutions is decreasing, and some authorities predict that myelography will soon become obsolete. MRI has the advantage of direct visualization of the cord, conus, cauda equina, intervertebral disks, ligaments, vertebrae, and bone

marrow. From an orthopaedic standpoint, MRI has been useful in the evaluation of neoplastic disease of the spine, degenerative disk disease, trauma, infection, and congenital anomalies.

MRI is currently the technique of choice to evaluate spine metastases with cord compression (Fig. 3-16). The entire spine and its content are evaluated without any discomfort to the patient. Typically these patients have weakness in the lower extremities or paraplegia and are unable to withstand the rigors of a complete myelogram. MRI also shows promise in the typically vexing problem of vertebral body compression without obvious evidence of malignancy in the elderly patient. The question is frequently raised as to whether the compression fracture is due to neoplastic infiltration or osteoporosis.

Congenital cord abnormalities associated with spinal dysraphism are most advantageously studied

(text continues on page 90)

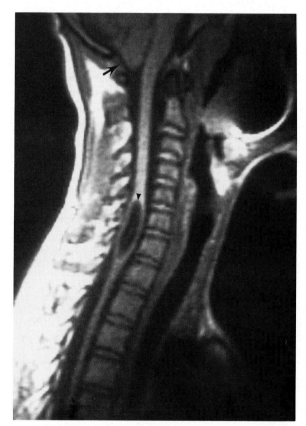

FIGURE 3-17. A 15-year-old boy with atypical scoliosis. The entire spine was screened with MRI to look for cord abnormalities. Sagittal midline image of the cervical spine shows Arnold-Chiari malformation with the cerebellar tonsils (*arrow*) extending below the foromen magnum; there is also hydromyelia in the lower cervical cord (*arrowhead*).

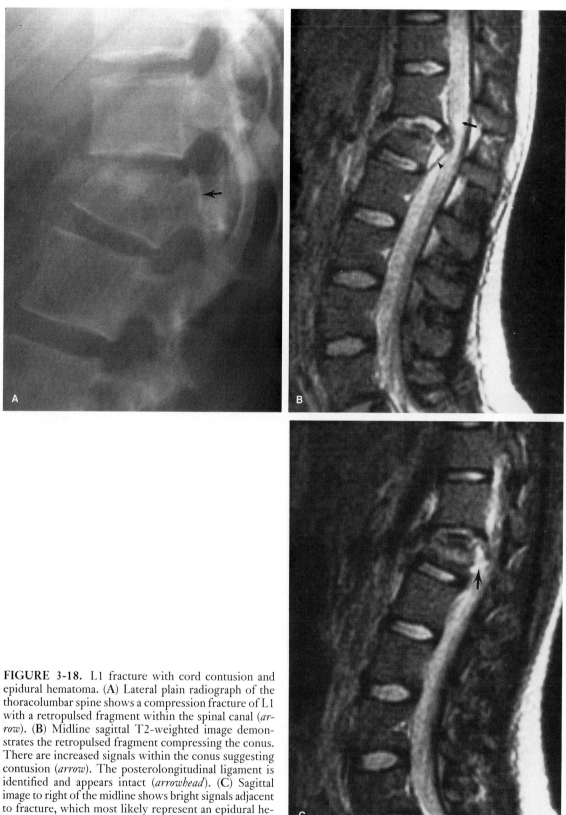

FIGURE 3-18. L1 fracture with cord contusion and epidural hematoma. (**A**) Lateral plain radiograph of the thoracolumbar spine shows a compression fracture of L1 with a retropulsed fragment within the spinal canal (*arrow*). (**B**) Midline sagittal T2-weighted image demonstrates the retropulsed fragment compressing the conus. There are increased signals within the conus suggesting contusion (*arrow*). The posterolongitudinal ligament is identified and appears intact (*arrowhead*). (**C**) Sagittal image to right of the midline shows bright signals adjacent to fracture, which most likely represent an epidural hematoma (*arrow*).

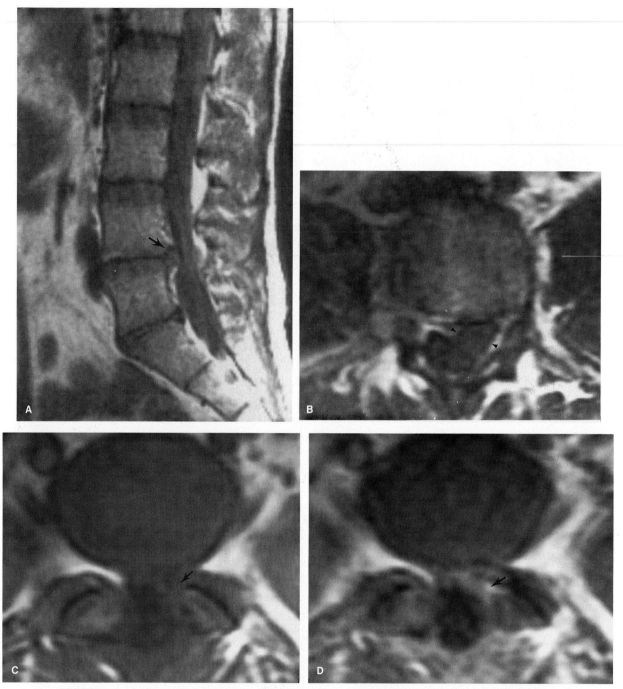

FIGURE 3-19. Acute disk herniation. (**A**) Sagittal T1-weighted image showing disk herniation at the L4-L5 level (*arrow*). (**B**) Axial T1-weighted image. The herniated disk is seen as a mass (*arrowheads*) compressing the thecal sac. (**C**) Epidural postsurgical scarring. A 32-year-old man who had diskectomy at the L5-S1 level 7 months before this exam. T1-weighted axial image at the L5-S1 level shows a low signal intensity mass interposed between the disk and the thecal sac (*arrow*). It is uncertain from this image whether this represents a recurrent disk herniation, residual disk material, or scarring from the previous surgery. (**D**) The same image is retaken after the patient has been injected with Gd-DTPA. The mass now appears bright (*arrow*); this highly suggests scarring rather than recurrent or residual disk herniation.

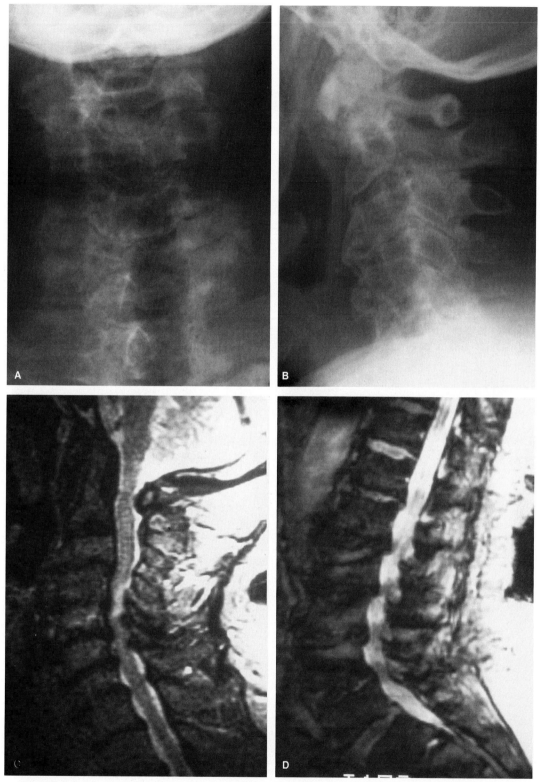

FIGURE 3-20. Multilevel cervical and lumbar spinal stenosis. (A and B) Plain radiographs of the cervical spine show severe degenerative disk and facet disease. (C) Sagittal T2-weighted image of the cervical spine shows multiple levels of stenosis and cord compression. (D) Midline sagittal image of the lumbar spine in the same patient also shows multilevel spinal stenosis.

by MRI. Screening the entire spine and its contents for anomalies before scoliosis surgery is effectively accomplished with MRI (Fig. 3-17).

In trauma to the spine, bony detail is better delineated by CT. Associated soft tissue injuries, including epidural hematoma, disk herniation, and cord compression or contusion, however, are all clearly visualized by MRI (Fig. 3-18).

For disk disease, MRI has capabilities that combine the advantages of myelography, CT myelography, and diskography without being invasive (Fig. 3-19A and B). Healthy disks have high water content and, therefore, appear bright on T2-weighted images. Degenerated and herniated disks have diminished water content and show decreased signal intensity on T2-weighted sequences. Postoperative epidural fibrosis can be reliably distinguished from recurrent disk herniation with the use of Gd-DTPA; fibrosis enhances, showing increased signal intensity, whereas recurrent disk herniation does not enhance on T1-weighted sequences (see Fig. 3-19C and D). Spinal stenosis is believed to be better evaluated by

CT; however, MRI continues to gain some ground (Fig. 3-20).

Disk space infections exhibit a characteristic appearance on MRI, and there is the added advantage of showing soft tissue extension or abscess formation in muscle and epidural space.

Neoplasms

In dealing with malignant bone tumors, plain films continue to be the most effective modality in determining tissue characterization, biologic activity of the tumor, and evaluation of associated periosteal reaction. For staging of musculoskeletal tumors, MRI has an advantage over other imaging modalities, including CT, because of its superior tissue contrast and, therefore, better assessment of soft tissue extension, and bone marrow and neurovascular bundle involvement. MRI has the capability of imaging directly in multiple planes and without the use of ionizing radiation. Images in the coronal and sagittal planes are particularly useful in surgical planning

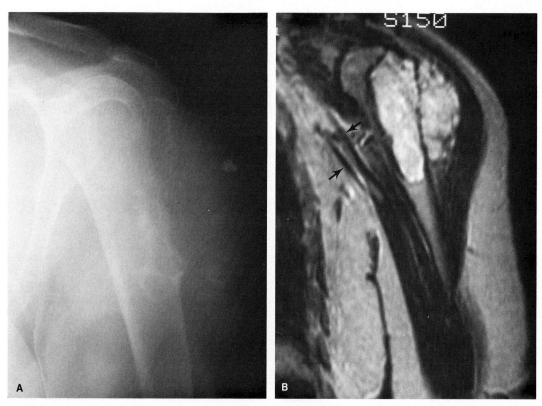

FIGURE 3-21. Chondrosarcoma arising from an exostosis. **(A)** AP view of the left shoulder shows a surface lesion destroying the lateral cortex. The lesion is exophytic and has a chondroid matrix. The diagnosis of chondrosarcoma was made at the basis of the radiographic appearance. **(B)** Coronal T2-weighted image demonstrates the soft tissue and marrow extension of the lesion. Tissue characterization is not possible from the MRI appearance. The neurovascular bundle (*arrows*) is not involved.

(Fig. 3-21). The fact that neurovascular bundles can be traced by MRI has reduced the need for preoperative angiography, which is both invasive and expensive. There is excellent correlation of intramedullary tumor extent as determined by MRI and pathologic examination.

MRI, with few exceptions, has no tissue specificity, and calculation of T1 and T2 relaxation times of tumors has failed to yield any tissue characterization (Fig. 3-22). MRI is incapable of reliably distinguishing between benign and malignant soft tissue tumors. Increased signal intensity on T2-weighted images in the skeletal muscles adjacent to a neoplasm indicates that the neoplasm is malignant. This sign is not helpful, however, when the masses are in-

flamed or caused by an abscess. MRI is inferior to CT in the detection of air bubbles and soft tissue calcifications.

MRI has proved to be highly sensitive to bone marrow changes and is the only modality that allows direct imaging of bone marrow without the use of contrast agents or radioisotopes. Although bone marrow aspirate and biopsy are the gold standards in the diagnosis of marrow packing diseases, such as leukemia, MRI offers important information as to the extent of the disease because of the large volume of marrow that can be scanned (Figs. 3-23 and 3-24). Measurements of the T1 value of bone marrow in patients with marrow packing disorders showed significant prolongation of T1 when compared with

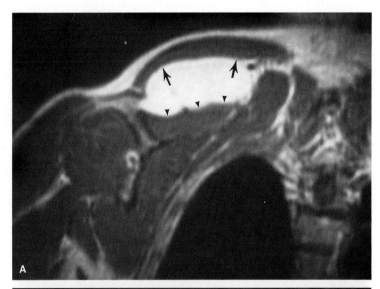

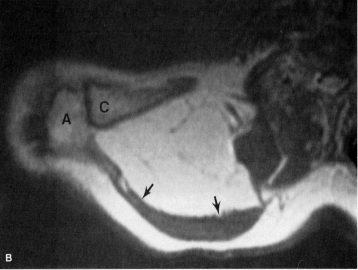

FIGURE 3-22. Lipoma of the right shoulder. (A) T1-weighted coronal image of the right shoulder shows a lipoma (*bright mass*) situated between the trapezius (*arrows*) muscle and supraspinatus muscle (*arrowheads*). Lipomas and hemangiomas have a characteristic appearance on MRI. (B) In the axial plain the lipoma (*bright mass*) is seen displacing the trapezius muscle (*arrows*) posteriorly. C, clavicle; A, acromion.

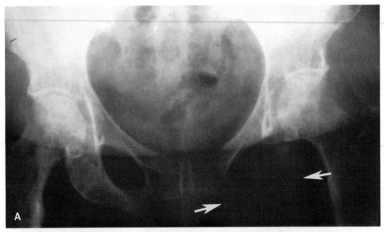

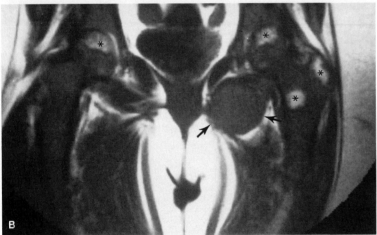

FIGURE 3-23. Multiple myeloma. **(A)** A 44-year-old woman presenting with a large lytic lesion (*arrows*) in the left ischium that proved to be a myeloma. **(B)** T1-weighted image was performed to study the extent of the disease and to determine if this lytic lesion (*arrows*) represents a solitary myeloma or disseminated disease. All the dark-appearing marrow is infiltrated with myeloma. Only the small bright areas (*asterisks*) in the femoral heads, left greater trochanter, and left interrochanteric region are spared.

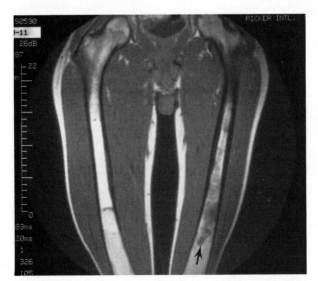

FIGURE 3-24. Lymphoma. Twelve-year-old boy with stage IV lymphoma. Coronal T1-weighted image through the femurs shows areas of low signal intensity (*dark*) within the marrow of the left femur. This represents marrow infiltration with lymphoma (*arrow*). Lymphoma and hairy cell leukemia tend to have patchy marrow infiltration. Leukemias in general show diffuse marrow involvement.

normal controls. Aplastic anemia can be distinguished from normals by the significant shortening of the T1 value.

A significant contribution of MRI to the management of musculoskeletal neoplasm has been in the follow-up of treated lesions. Lesions with low-signal intensity on T2-weighted images, in patients who have undergone radiation therapy or surgery, indicates absence of residual or recurrent tumor. Conversely, high-signal intensity lesions after surgery alone indicate recurrence. In patients who have had radiation alone, high-signal intensity lesions on T2-weighted images indicate that the patient either has active tumor or radiation-induced inflammation. Differentiation of these two processes is not possible without a biopsy. Early attempts at studying bone and soft tissue tumors with phosphorus-31 MRI spectroscopy have been published.

Trauma

The fact that MRI can scan in the sagittal and coronal planes helps in studying muscle injuries.

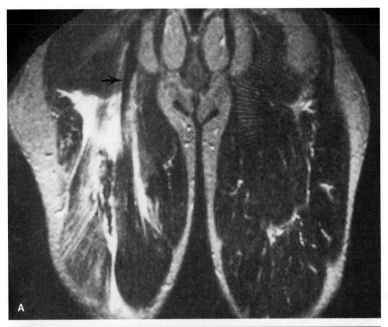

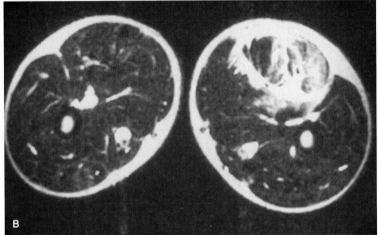

FIGURE 3-25. Musculotendinous sprain of the right hamstring group. (A) T2-weighted coronal section through the posterior thighs reveals the hamstring tendons (*arrow*) to be intact bilaterally; however, there is extensive bleeding (*bright areas*) within the fascial plains in the posterior compartment of the right thigh. (B) T2-weighted axial section through the proximal thigh demonstrates the bleeding (*bright areas*) around the hamstring group on the right and some bleeding within the belly of the biceps femoris.

Muscle hematomas, tears, and avulsions are easily demonstrated by MRI; tendon rupture and attenuation can also be seen (Figs. 3-25 and 3-26). Acute hematomas show low signal intensity on T1-weighted images and high signal intensity on T2-weighted images. This pattern, however, changes as the hematoma becomes subacute or chronic. There are reports of subtle fractures, not detected by plain radiography, that are detected by MRI (Fig. 3-27).

MRI is used extensively in the evaluation of internal derangement of the knee. MRI, in contradistinction to arthrography and arthroscopy, is capable of demonstrating intracapsular and extracapsular abnormalities. The anatomic detail in and around the knee with MRI images is exquisite, and in many institutions knee arthrography has become a rarity. The menisci in the sagittal and coronal sections appear as black triangles, whereas the articular hyaline cartilage appears somewhat brighter on T1-weighted images (Fig. 3-28). The posterior cruciate is consistently visualized in the sagittal plain and is seen as a thick, dark band on both T1- and T2-weighted images (Fig. 3-29). The anterior cruciate is more difficult to show with consistency because it is smaller in size than the posterior cruciate and has more internal signals; it appears as a dark gray ribbon-like or striated structure on T1-weighted sagittal images (Fig. 3-30).

The medial collateral ligament is visualized on the coronal plane as a dark linear band originating from the medial femoral condyle and inserting on the medial tibia distal to the tibial condyle (Fig. 3-31). The lateral collateral ligament can be seen both

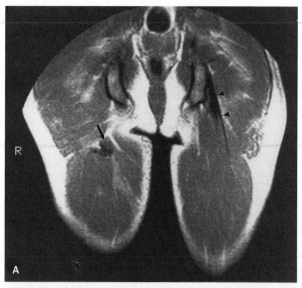

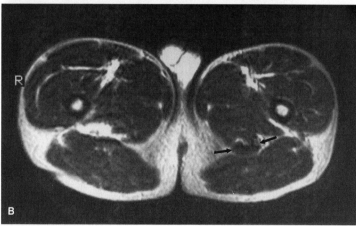

FIGURE 3-26. Avulsion of the right hamstring tendon off the ischial tuberosity. **(A)** T1-weighted coronal image through the posterior thigh shows avulsion of right hamstring tendon. The tendon is seen retracted and curled in the midthigh (*arrow*). The tendons on the left side are normal (*arrowheads*). **(B)** T2-weighted axial image through the proximal thigh shows normal hamstring tendons (*arrows*) on the left and absent tendon on the right.

on the coronal and sagittal plane; it appears as a dark cord arising from the lateral femoral condyle and extending inferiorly and posteriorly to insert along with the biceps femoris tendon on the head of the fibula (Fig. 3-32).

Meniscal tears are diagnosed when bright signals within the menisci on T1-weight images are detected (see Figs. 3-28 and 3-32). For these signals to be significant, they should reach the surface of the meniscus. When a meniscus is deformed or amputated, this also represents a tear (see Fig. 3-28C). In most series where findings on MRI are compared with arthroscopy and arthrotomy, the accuracy of diagnosing meniscus tears approaches 90%.

Diagnosis of ligamentous injury is made when increased signal intensity is seen within the normally dark ligamentous structure on both T1- and T2-weighted images. The reliability for assessment of ligamentous tears is not yet adequately tested. Di-

agnosing posterior cruciate tears by MRI is reliable with an accuracy of 90% and 84% for the anterior cruciate (see Figs. 3-29B and 3-30B). Medial collateral ligament disruptions are easier to diagnose in the acute phase than later (see Fig. 3-31B).

In the shoulder, the presence of the rotator cuff tears as well as the extent of the tear can be demonstrated on MRI (Fig. 3-33). Labral tears are still studied by double-contrast arthrography followed by thin-section CT, but early attempts with MRI at showing labral abnormalities are promising (see Figs. 3-11 and 3-33B).

Avascular Necrosis

Avascular necrosis (AVN) is a major medical problem leading to severe joint dysfunction with the

(text continues on page 98)

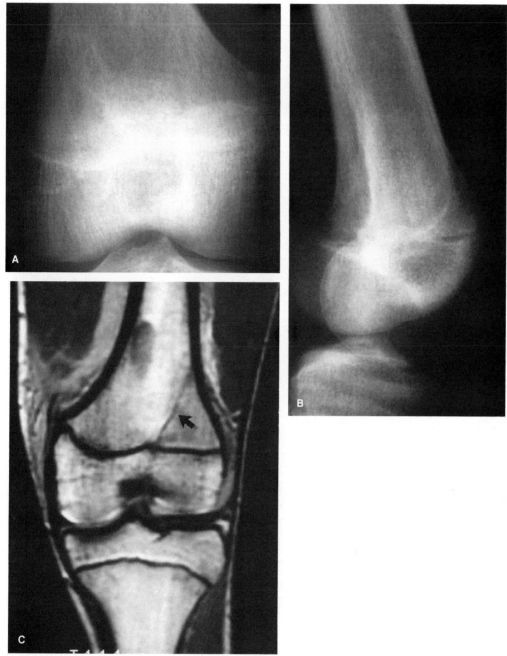

FIGURE 3-27. Occult Salter II fracture of the distal femur detected by MRI. (**A** and **B**) AP and lateral radiographs of the left knee in a 16-year-old boy injured during a football game appear normal. The patient continued to have pain and was unable to bear weight; MRI was performed to evaluate internal derangement. (**C**) Coronal image of the knee shows an unsuspected Salter II fracture of the distal femur without displacement.

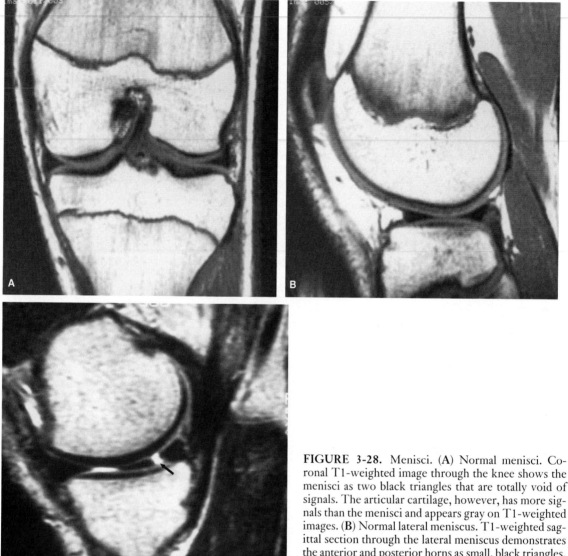

FIGURE 3-28. Menisci. **(A)** Normal menisci. Coronal T1-weighted image through the knee shows the menisci as two black triangles that are totally void of signals. The articular cartilage, however, has more signals than the menisci and appears gray on T1-weighted images. **(B)** Normal lateral meniscus. T1-weighted sagittal section through the lateral meniscus demonstrates the anterior and posterior horns as small, black triangles. **(C)** T2-weighted sagittal image of the medial meniscus shows a tear in the posterior horn. Fluid is present within the tear (*bright signals; arrow*). A joint effusion is present.

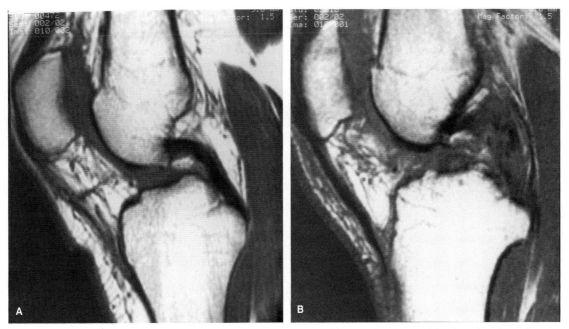

FIGURE 3-29. Posterior cruciate. **(A)** Normal posterior cruciate. Sagittal T1-weighted section through the posterior cruciate shows a thick and moderately curved posterior cruciate. **(B)** Torn posterior cruciate. Sagittal T1-weighted image demonstrates the fragmented posterior cruciate ligament.

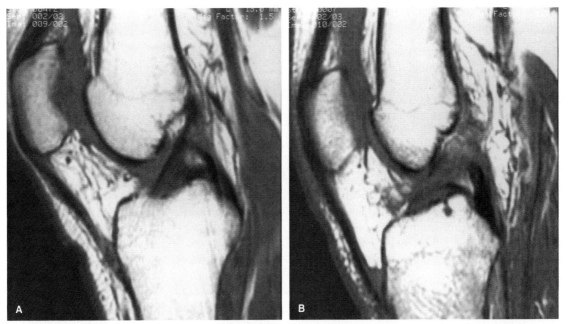

FIGURE 3-30. Anterior cruciate. **(A)** Normal anterior cruciate seen on T1-weighted image. It always appears straight and has more signals than the posterior cruciate. It is also smaller in diameter than the posterior cruciate. **(B)** Torn anterior cruciate ligament seen on a sagittal T1-weighted image.

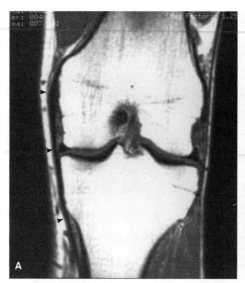
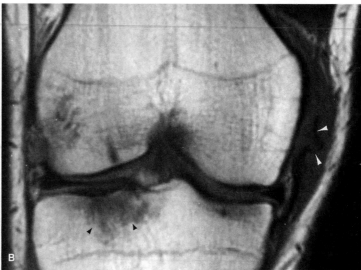

FIGURE 3-31. Medial collateral ligament. (**A**) Normal medial collateral ligament demonstrated on a coronal T1-weighted image (*black arrowheads*). The medial collateral ligament originates on the medial femoral condyle and inserts on the tibia distal to the medial tibial condyle. (**B**) Coronal T1-weighted image of the knee shows the disrupted fibers of the medial collateral ligament close to the medial femoral condyle (*white arrowheads*). Note also the marrow contusion in the lateral tibial plateau (*black arrowheads*).

hips being the most commonly affected joint. The number of patients at risk for AVN is large, and some authorities believe that early diagnosis and treatment is important for a favorable outcome; however, there is no convincing evidence to support this contention.

MRI is superior to radionuclide imaging and CT for the detection of early AVN. It should be emphasized, however, that MRI is not necessary when plain films are diagnostic because the cost of the examination is high.

Bone marrow in the peripheral skeleton in adults is fatty and, therefore, appears bright on T1-weighted images. Avascular necrosis reveals well-defined areas with irregular margins of low-signal intensity on T1-weighted images adjacent to bright marrow signals (Fig. 3-34); a low-cost 5-minute T1-weighted sequence is all that is needed to make the diagnosis, and anything more than this is considered a diagnostic overkill.

Differentiating between acute bone infarction and infection in patients with sickle cell anemia is still a diagnostic problem. Both acute bone infarction and infection would show decreased signal intensity on T1-weighted images and high signals on T2-weighted images.

In Legg-Calvé-Perthes disease, involved areas in the femoral capital epiphysis show diminished or absent signal intensity. MRI is at least as sensitive as

a radionuclide scan, but MRI has better spacial resolution; therefore, it shows better delineation of the lesion.

Infection

Radionuclide bone scans are highly sensitive for the diagnosis of osteomyelitis; however, radionuclide uptake associated with cellulitis may simulate osteomyelitis, and this problem limits the specificity and accuracy of bone scans. MRI promises to be helpful in the diagnosis of musculoskeletal infections because of its sensitivity in detecting free water within tissues. The diagnosis of osteomyelitis is made when the bone marrow appears dark on T1-weighted images and bright on T2-weighted images (Fig. 3-35). Decreased signals of the soft tissues on T1-weighted images and increased signals on T2-weighted images, along with ill-defined margins, are considered to represent cellulitis. Well-defined collections that are dark on T1-weighted images and bright on T2-weighted images typically represent soft tissue abscesses (Fig. 3-36). Detection of fluid in deep joints such as the hip, shoulder, and in tendon sheaths is also easily achieved with MRI and is often employed in the search for a source for sepsis (Fig. 3-37).

(text continues on page 101)

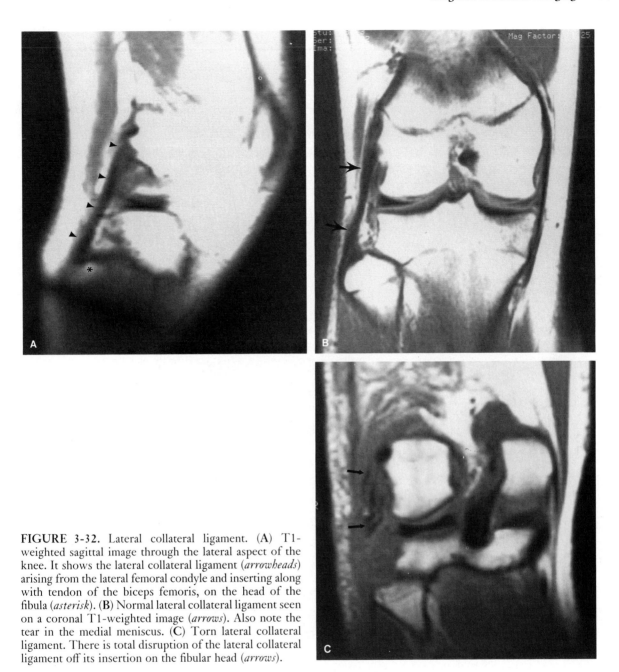

FIGURE 3-32. Lateral collateral ligament. (**A**) T1-weighted sagittal image through the lateral aspect of the knee. It shows the lateral collateral ligament (*arrowheads*) arising from the lateral femoral condyle and inserting along with tendon of the biceps femoris, on the head of the fibula (*asterisk*). (**B**) Normal lateral collateral ligament seen on a coronal T1-weighted image (*arrows*). Also note the tear in the medial meniscus. (**C**) Torn lateral collateral ligament. There is total disruption of the lateral collateral ligament off its insertion on the fibular head (*arrows*).

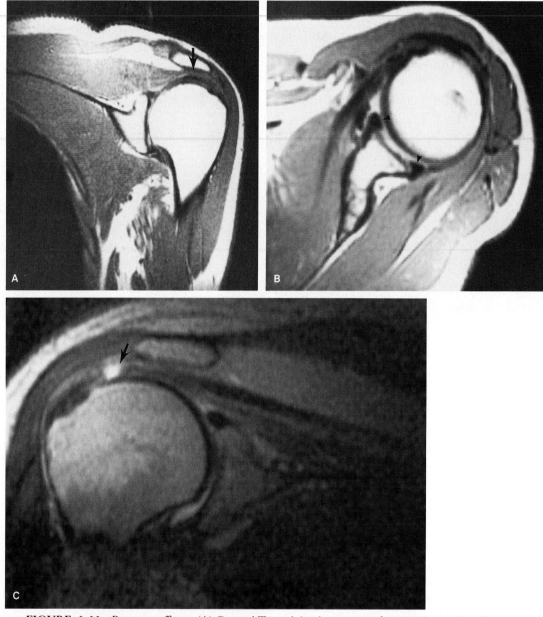

FIGURE 3-33. Rotator cuff tear. **(A)** Coronal T1-weighted sequence of a normal shoulder. Note the supraspinatus tendon and its insertion on the greater tuberosity (*arrow*). **(B)** Axial section of the shoulder revealing normal labrum, seen as small black triangles on the edges of the glenoid (*arrowheads*). **(C)** T2-weighted oblique coronal section of the shoulder showing a tear in the supraspinatus tendon (*arrow*). The size of the tear can also be delineated on MRI.

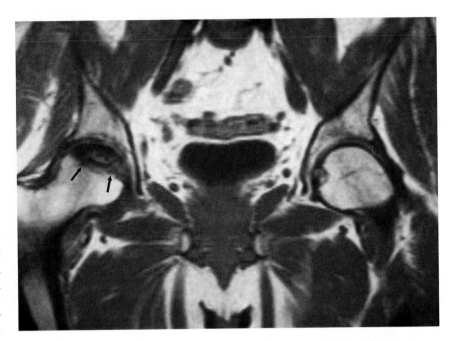

FIGURE 3-34. Avascular necrosis of the right femoral head. Coronal T1-weighted image through the hips demonstrates avascular necrosis involving the weight-bearing area of the right femoral head (*arrows*). Note the normal bright signals in the left femoral head due to the presence of normal marrow fat.

It should be cautioned that on MRI the bone marrow changes in acute osteomyelitis are nonspecific, and a healing fracture or metastasis may have similar changes.

Synovial Diseases

Most centers now perform MRI to study patients with rheumatoid arthritis complicated with atlantoaxial subluxation or cranial settling. Massive pannus formation with impingement on the cord or brain stem can be easily detected with MRI (Fig. 3-38). Multiple subaxial subluxations in the cervical spine resulting in multilevel spinal stenosis can also be well demonstrated by MRI.

In joints with effusions, T2-weighted images have an arthrographic effect whereby abnormalities of the synovial lining can be detected. Pigmented villonodular synovitis is particularly suited for initial evaluation and follow-up by MRI (Fig. 3-39).

RADIONUCLIDE BONE SCANNING

The introduction of radioisotopes into medical imaging has significantly enhanced the armamentarium for diagnostic bone imaging. The strengths of this approach are in the ease of surveying the entire skeleton, and its high sensitivity for detection of neoplastic, inflammatory, and traumatic bone abnormalities. The technique involves intravenous administration of radiopharmaceuticals that localize in bone according to specific physiologic or pathologic processes. A scintigraphic image, also referred to as a scan, is then generated by a γ-camera that captures and records the photon emissions of the radioactive tracer. These images primarily depict a function rather than morphology and, therefore, should be supplemented by the available clinical information and the findings of other imaging modalities to formulate a diagnosis.

The standard bone scan uses a photon-emitting radionuclide, technetium-99m (^{99m}Tc), which, coupled to a phosphate or phosphonate ligand, localizes in the bone at a rate commensurate with the regional blood flow and osteoblastic activity. The technique is useful in the assessment of osteomyelitis, osteonecrosis, and bone injuries, but its major application is currently in the evaluation of skeletal neoplasm. Other scintigraphic techniques are also available that permit specific investigation of bone infection, bone marrow distribution, and measurement of bone mineral density.

Technique and Instrumentation

The radioisotopes of the natural constituents of bone are not suitable for in vivo imaging. Phosphorus-32

(text continues on page 105)

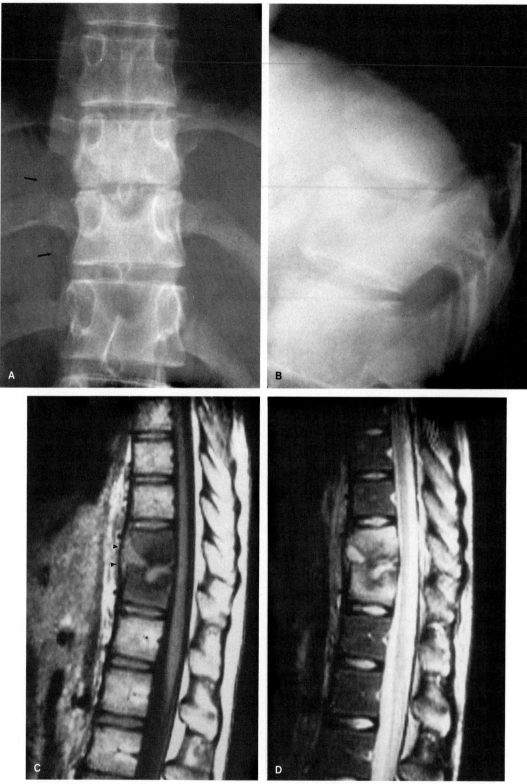

FIGURE 3-35. Disk space infection. (**A** and **B**) AP and lateral radiographs of the thoracic spine reveal narrowing T10-T11 disk space with erosions at the end-plates. The paraspinal stripe on the right is elevated because of fluid collection (*arrows*). (**C** and **D**) Sagittal T1- and T2-weighted midline sections, T10 and T11 weighted, show the end-plate destruction and abscess formation elevating the anterior longitudinal ligament (*arrowheads*). The thecal sac and epidural space are intact. Note the appearance of the marrow in T10 and T11; black on T1-weighted image and bright on T2-weighted image are due to infiltration of the marrow with pus and edema fluid. (**E**) Axial T1 section through the T10-T11 disk delineated a fluid collection on the left side between the crus of the diaphragm and the vertebra (*arrows*). CT-guided needle aspiration yielded pus that grew *Staphylococcus aureus*.

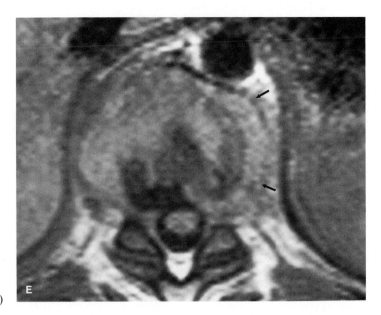

FIGURE 3-35. (*Continued*)

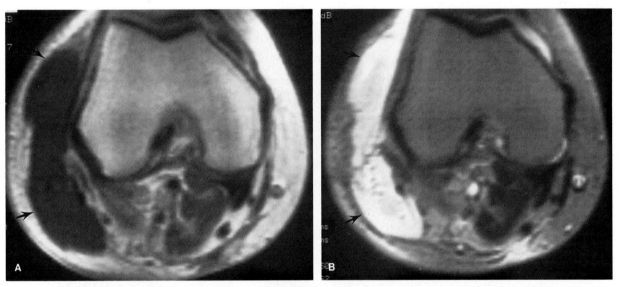

FIGURE 3-36. Subcutaneous abscess. This is a 45-year-old diabetic who presented with fever, swelling, redness, and hotness over the lateral aspect of the right knee. Clinically, the question was whether the patient had cellulitis or an abscess that has organized enough to be drained. Axial T1- and T2-weighted images through the knee demonstrated a well-defined fluid collection in the subcutaneous tissues of the knee representing an abscess (*arrows*).

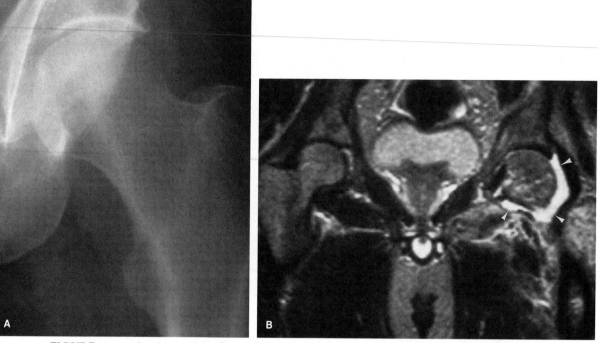

FIGURE 3-37. Septic arthritis of the left hip. A 39-year-old diabetic with left hip pain and fever. **(A)** AP film of the left hip shows no abnormalities. **(B)** T2-weighted MRI of the hips in the cornonal plane revealed a large joint effusion on the left side. Bright signals are seen around the left femoral head and neck (*arrowheads*). Hip aspiration yielded pus, and culture of the aspirate grew *Staphylococcus aureus*.

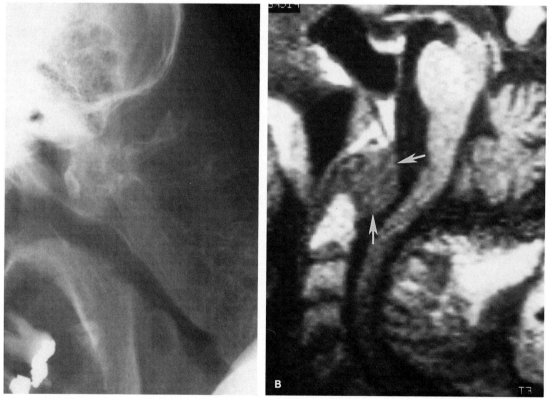

FIGURE 3-38. Rheumatoid arthritis of the cervical spine. **(A)** Plain lateral film of the cervical spine taken in flexion shows erosion of the dens and C1-C2 anterior subluxation. **(B)** Midline sagittal image of the craniovertebral junction reveals a large pannus engulfing the entire dens and encroaching on the spinal canal (*arrows*).

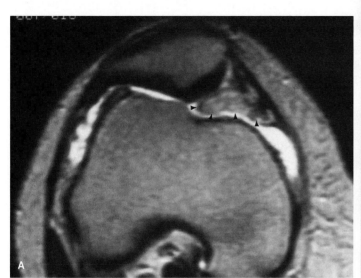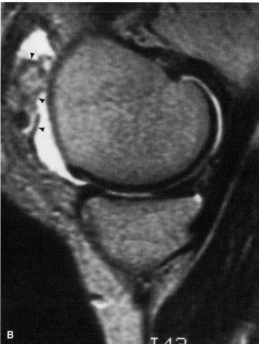

FIGURE 3-39. Pigmented villonodular synovitis. Axial and sagittal T2-weighted images of the knee reveal a large mass arising from the synovium (*arrowheads*). A joint effusion is also present.

is a pure β-emitter and is used therapeutically in the management of polycytemia vera and intractable bone pain secondary to osseous metastases. Strontium-85, strontium-87m, and fluorine-18 were used in the early days of bone scanning with great difficulty, but were supplanted in 1972 by the introduction of ^{99m}Tc phosphonate compounds.

^{99m}Tc emits pure γ-photons at an energy of 140 keV, which is optimal for imaging. The relatively short half-life of 6 hours is advantageous for reducing the radiation burden to the patient, and yet poses no logistic problems because the nuclide is available from a molybdenum-99 generator with a much longer half-life of 67 hours. ^{99m}Tc has no particular affinity for osseous tissue and relies on the presence of a phosphonate ligand for bone localization. Methylene diphosphonate and hydroxymethylene diphosphonate are the two ligands most commonly used. The exact mechanism for localization of these compounds in bone is not clear. It is known that the diphosphonates adsorb to the surface of the newly formed bone crystals at the interface between the uncalcified and calcified bone matrix. Because less mature bone contains smaller crystals and thus presents a larger surface area for deposition of the radionuclide, ^{99m}Tc-diphosphonate scans tend to represent a spatial map of the osteoblastic activity throughout the body. Bony abnormalities in general give rise to a focal or segmental increase in tracer uptake, but a small fraction of the lesions may exhibit reduced tracer uptake. This is especially true for cases in which the blood supply is compromised.

Only about 30% to 45% of injected ^{99m}Tc-diphosphonate localizes in the bones. The remainder distributes throughout the body in the vascular and interstitial fluid spaces and is subject to excretion by the kidneys in about 3 to 4 hours. The radiation dose to the bladder wall approaches 3 to 6 rad from a typical 20 mCi dose of radiopharmaceutical but can be substantially reduced if patients drink extra fluids and void frequently. Imaging is performed 3 to 4 hours after the injection of the tracer to allow for adequate clearance from the soft tissues.

γ-Cameras cover a field of view measuring 35 to 40 cm in diameter. Thus, multiple images are obtained to cover the entire skeleton. Alternatively, a "moving table" can be used to scan the entire length of the patient's body (Fig. 3-40). The spatial resolution of the γ-cameras is primarily governed by the aperture size of their collimator holes. A standard collimator can typically resolve 15- to 20-mm lesions, whereas a so-called high-resolution collimator may

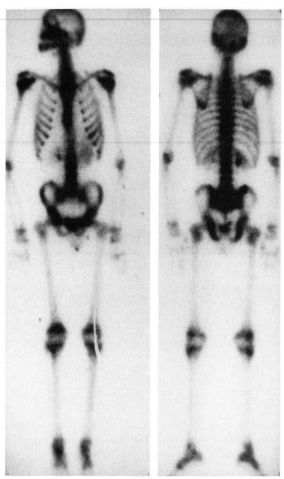

FIGURE 3-40. Normal bone scan. AP views of a technetium-99m diphosphonate study obtained 4 hours after the injection of radionuclide.

body. A computer can then reconstruct tomographic slices from this set of data in axial, sagittal, or coronal planes. Tomography does not improve the image resolution but provides a significant gain in contrast by eliminating the superimposed activity from overlying structures. Image acquisition and reconstruction for SPECT takes about 1 hour for each region of the body and, therefore, is not suitable for whole body imaging.

The diagnostic yield of a ^{99m}Tc-diphosphonate study can be enhanced by obtaining a radionuclide angiogram and blood-pool images at the time of tracer injection. This is done by recording a rapid sequence of images (1 to 3 seconds each) while injecting the radiopharmaceutical, followed by one or more images obtained after the equilibration of the radionuclide in the body. The "three-phase" bone study so obtained provides information about the blood flow changes in the area of interest and differentiates inflammation or malignant neoplasm from other bony disorders.

Other radiopharmaceuticals used in bone scintigraphy include ^{99m}Tc-colloidal preparations for bone marrow imaging, and gallium-67 (^{67}Ga)– and indium-111 (^{111}In)–labeled leukocytes for detection of bone or soft tissue infection. These radiopharmaceuticals are generally employed in combination with a standard bone scan. Because ^{67}Ga and ^{111}In emit higher energy photons than ^{99m}Tc, it is possible to inject either radionuclide simultaneously with ^{99m}Tc-diphosphonate and perform dual photon imaging. This ensures perfect alignment of the bone scans with the ^{67}Ga or ^{111}In white blood cell (WBC) images and facilitates the localization of bony abnormalities.

achieve a resolution on the order of 12 to 15 mm. A considerable degree of magnification and some improvement in image resolution can be obtained by using a pin hole collimator. This is especially advantageous for examining small bony structures. Hot lesions are defined as those with greater radiotracer activity than the surrounding areas and are generally detected with greater ease than the cold lesions that contain lesser radionuclide concentrations. Single-photon emission computed tomography (SPECT) refers to the technique of tomographic scanning that is useful for examining complex bony structures, such as the facial bones, the hip joints, or the posterior elements of the vertebrae (see Fig. 3-9B). The technique involves acquisition of multiple scintigraphic images while a γ-camera rotates around the patient's

Metastatic Disease of the Skeleton

Assessment of neoplastic disease in the skeleton constitutes the most frequent indication for radioisotopic bone imaging. Bone scanning is the primary imaging modality in the detection of bony metastases and plays a lesser but nevertheless significant role in the management of primary bone tumors.

Bone scintigraphy provides a convenient means of surveying the entire skeleton with a single injection of radiopharmaceutical and a moderate radiation burden to the patient. Although most osseous metastases occur in the axial skeleton, about 10% will be found in the appendicular skeleton, and another

10% will occur in the skull. The sensitivity of the bone scan for detecting osseous lesions is unmatched by any other imaging modality. Comparative studies from large series of patients have shown that, on the average, 22% of patients with extraosseous malignancies will have bone metastases visible on scintigrams but not on radiographs. Conversely, a positive radiograph accompanied by a negative scintigram will only occur in less than 3% of the cases. A 10% increase in radiotracer localization associated with a bony metastasis would be readily visible on bone scintigrams, but as much as a 50% reduction in bone mineral content is needed before a lytic lesion can be identified on conventional radiography.

Bone scanning is also used in the follow-up of patients to assess response to treatment. A definitive sign of deterioration is either an increase in the number of lesions or an expansion of the existing lesions. A mere increase in the intensity of radiopharmaceutical uptake is not a sign of worsening prognosis and may herald a favorable response to therapy. This flare phenomenon is typically observed 2 to 3 months after initiation of successful chemotherapy in patients with breast cancer and is followed by general quiescence of the lesions in 6 months. It is not unusual for some lesions to disappear totally. The presumed mechanism for the flare phenomenon is the intensification of osteoblastic activity to reestablish normal bone matrix following tumor regression. A similar response is not observed after radiation therapy. Irradiation of osseous tissue at levels above 3000 rad results in near-complete suppression of ^{99m}Tc-diphosphonate uptake in the bone. The scan will show a photon-deficient "cold" area whose margins correspond to the port of the radiation therapy. The effect is long-lived, and recovery is never complete.

Bone scintigraphy permits accurate localization of osseous lesions for resection, biopsy, or local irradiation. Special markers can be affixed to the skin or inserted directly into the lesion under γ-camera monitoring. Biopsy is indicated when the primary site is unknown. It is common for patients with primary cancer of the lung, breast, or prostate to present with skeletal pain as their initial complaint. If radiographs of the painful area are negative, a bone scan should be obtained and would typically show numerous sites of bony metastasis.

Bone scans should be routinely obtained in the initial staging of the common malignancies mentioned earlier but also in certain less common tumors that tend to metastasize to the skeleton with great frequency. These include renal cell carcinoma, thyroid carcinoma, lymphoma, and neuroblastoma. Neoplasms that rarely metastasize to the bone include gynecologic tumors, gastrointestinal malignancies, bladder cancer, and carcinomas of the head and neck. Routine bone imaging in these cases is not indicated unless specific symptoms suggest bone involvement.

The characteristic pattern of diffuse bony metastases consists of numerous foci of increased radiotracer uptake predominantly in the axial skeleton and distributed in an asymmetric manner (Fig. 3-41). The pattern is rarely mimicked by other polyostotic bone lesions, such as fibrous dysplasia, Paget disease, or multiple enchondromatosis. Difficulty arises when only few lesions of moderate or low intensity are seen that are localized to the vertebral column, ribs,

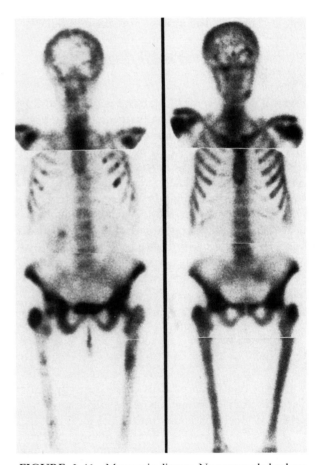

FIGURE 3-41. Metastatic disease. Numerous skeletal metastases from breast carcinoma are seen on the study dated February 1985. The follow-up scan obtained 5 months later shows proliferation of the metastases giving rise to a "super scan" appearance. Individual lesions are no longer identified because of the coalescence of many metastases.

or joint areas. Patients undergoing metastatic screening are typically old and have arthritic changes in their spines and weight-bearing joints; the rib cage is notorious for showing focal increased uptake as a result of minor trauma. The uncertainty is even greater for single lesions. According to literature, the likelihood of a unifocal scintigraphic abnormality representing a bony metastasis in a patient with known extraosseous malignancy ranges from 10%, if found in a rib, to about 50%, if found in a long extremity bone. In such cases, if demonstration of a bony metastasis will radically change the patient's clinical management, verification should be obtained by plain films, CT, or MRI, and if negative, by biopsy of the lesion. If, conversely, such a finding is not likely to alter the patient's treatment plan, one may elect to follow the patient with radiography or bone scanning alone. Scintigraphy will generally demonstrate a change in the intensity or size of uptake or the number of lesions in patients with metastases, whereas the benign lesions will remain stable or regress entirely.

Focal increase in radiotracer uptake is not the universal pattern for metastatic disease. About 2% of bony metastases, especially those arising from breast or renal cell carcinoma, may appear as cold defects (Fig. 3-42) at the time of initial evaluation or convert to such an appearance after 1 to 2 years of follow-up. This is generally coincident with the appearance of a predominantly lytic lesion on radiographs. In patients with bronchogenic carcinoma, a linear pattern of abnormal uptake along the periosteum of the long bones indicates the onset of hypertrophic pulmonary osteoarthropathy. The finding could present without any evidence of concomitant metastases to the appendicular skeleton and commonly precedes the appearance of periosteal reaction on conventional radiography.

Finally, a peculiar, normal-appearing scan may occasionally be obtained in patients with extensive involvement of the skeleton by metastases from prostate or breast cancer. This superscan represents the coalescence of numerous metastatic lesions that makes it difficult to identify individual focal lesions. A superscan shows uniform intense activity throughout the skeleton with relative paucity of counts in the kidneys that are regularly seen on bone scans. The pattern should be differentiated from metabolic bone disorders, such as hyperparathyroidism, renal osteodystrophy, and hypervitaminosis-D, which may also produce a superscan. Radiographic

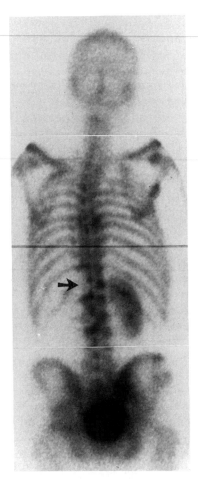

FIGURE 3-42. Photopenic osseous metastasis. Multiple bony metastases are present in the right scapula, the vertebral column, and the pelvis 6 months after left nephrectomy for renal cell carcinoma. Lesion with reduced uptake of radionuclide (photopenic) may occur in a small fraction of metastases from breast or renal cell carcinoma (*arrow*).

correlation would obviate the diagnosis in cases of diffuse metastases.

Primary Bone Lesions

Bone scintigraphy plays a complementary role to conventional radiography, CT, and MRI in the evaluation of primary bone lesions. It assists in delineation of the primary site, but, more important, it facilitates surveying the skeleton with high sensitivity for detection of remote sites of involvement. This is useful both in the initial evaluation and the follow-up of such bone disorders as Paget disease, fibrous dysplasia, and osteochondromas that tend to be polyostotic, and also in the management of such bone malignancies as osteosarcoma and Ewing sarcoma that tend to metastasize to bone.

A notable exception to the foregoing is the primary benign tumor, osteoid osteoma, which can be detected with greater ease using scintigraphy than conventional radiography. Osteoid osteoma occurs relatively commonly, accounting for about 10% of benign bone tumors. Radiographic examination should be attempted first and if negative, a scintigram of the symptomatic area with a wide margin around it should be obtained. A hot focus corresponding to the nidus of the osteoid osteoma will be demonstrated. The sensitivity of bone scan for osteoid osteoma exceeds that of the plain radiologic studies. Radiographic detection is most difficult when the tumor occurs in the pelvis or vertebrae. The bone scan guides the radiographic or tomographic examination for verification. Scintigraphy is also helpful in the operating room to localize the tumor and verify that the nidus has been removed.

Osteosarcoma and Ewing sarcoma represent the bony malignancies in which ^{99m}Tc-diphosphonate bone scintigraphy is helpful in detecting the sites of osseous metastases (Fig. 3-43). At the time of initial evaluation, secondary tumor foci are more prevalent with Ewing sarcoma than with osteosarcoma. Skeletal metastases, however, occur with considerable frequency as a late sequel in both tumors and warrant serial bone scintigraphy. In the past, bone scanning was not recommended after the resection of osteosarcoma because of the much higher incidence of pulmonary metastasis than bony metastasis. With the advent of adjuvant chemotherapy, bone metastases are seen with increasing frequency without any concomitant pulmonary metastases.

Bone scan is also helpful in detecting recurrence of the tumor at the bony stump following amputation. Although scans remain hot in the terminal portion of the stump for as long as 6 months because of bone remodeling, persistence of abnormal activity beyond this period is suggestive of tumor recurrence, infection, or fracture. Scintigraphic studies are less reliable for evaluation of the primary tumor at the time of initial presentation. Intense uptake would be present in the primary lesion and may extend a variable distance proximally, but this does not correlate with tumor involvement and therefore should not be relied on for determining the level of bone resection. Lack of abnormal radiotracer uptake in regions proximal to the primary lesion, however, is a reliable sign of normal bone. This is in contrast to soft tissue sarcomas for which bone scintigraphy is a reliable indicator both for demonstration and exclusion of tumor extension into the adjacent bone (Fig. 3-44).

Benign bone lesions such as osteochondroma, enchondroma, and various cystic lesions generally present with moderate or minimal uptake on bone scintigraphy (Fig. 3-45), and large cystic lesions may appear as cold areas. The degree of uptake in osteochondromas is only slightly greater than the adjacent normal bone and increases considerably with malignant transformation (Fig. 3-46). Bone scan, however, is of little value in predicting such an outcome. Multiple myeloma has a variable appearance on bone

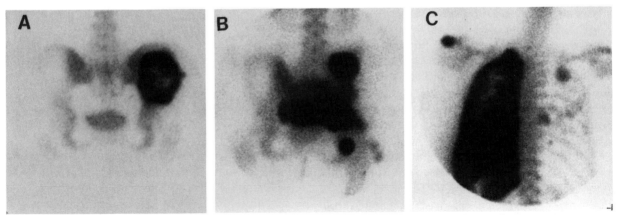

FIGURE 3-43. Osteosarcoma. (**A**) The primary tumor in the right iliac crest. (**B** and **C**) Recurrence in the pelvis, lungs, ribs, and the left shoulder 8 months after the resection of the primary tumor. The intense activity in the left hemithorax is due to presence of malignant pleural effusion.

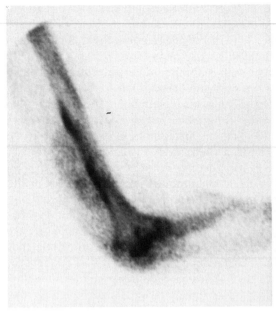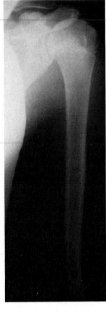

FIGURE 3-44. Fibrosarcoma of the left arm. The soft tissue tumor is faintly outlined on a technetium-99m bone scan. The intense activity in the adjacent humerus, however, denotes bone involvement by the tumor. Radiograph of the arm is unremarkable for bone involvement.

scanning, and about one half of the lesions appear as either cold or indistinguishable from normal bone. Thus, isotopic bone imaging is not indicated in this disorder.

Paget disease is another entity characterized by intense uptake of radiotracer on bone scans (Fig. 3-47). The uptake pattern is usually extensive and involves the greater portion of the affected bone. In long bones, the involvement usually starts at the articular end and extends toward the shaft. In flat bones, a contiguous area of intense, uniform radiotracer activity is the characteristic presentation. Osteoporosis circumscripta of the skull typically presents with a hot rim corresponding to the margins of the lytic area demonstrated on radiographs.

The application of bone scintigraphy in Paget disease is primarily for mapping the sites of skeletal involvement. Several series in the literature have convincingly shown that this can be accomplished more effectively with bone scanning than with radiographic examination. The lesions most difficult to detect on radiographs were those in scapula, ribs, and sternum. The reported distribution of Paget disease in the skeleton, based on scintigraphic studies, has differed little from that reported from radiographic examinations. The highest incidence is usually in the pelvis (15%), followed by spine (13%), skull (9%), femur (9%), scapula (7%), tibia, and other long bones (3% to 4% each) and less than 1% in the remaining bones. The appearance of the bone scan changes with the occurrence of such complications as fracture or sarcomatous changes. A fracture line can usually be distinguished by its pattern of intense

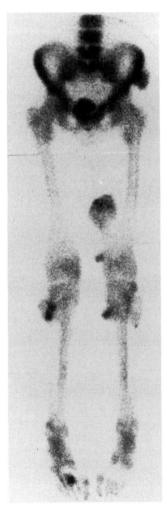

FIGURE 3-45. Familial exostoses. Multiple lesions are shown in the lower extremity bones and the left hemipelvis.

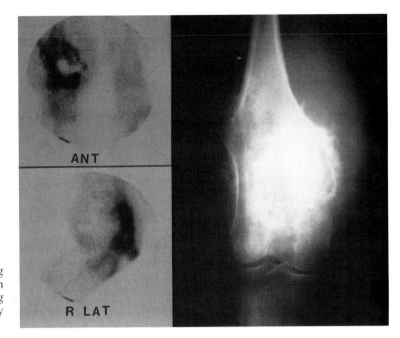

FIGURE 3-46. Chondrosarcoma arising from an osteochondroma. In patients with multiple bony exostoses, serial bone scanning may be used to survey the skeleton for early signs of malignant transformation.

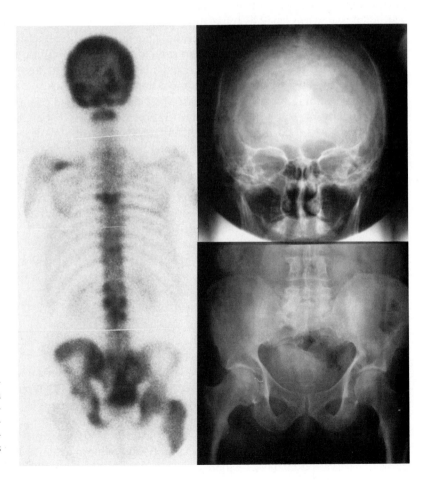

FIGURE 3-47. Paget disease. The intense uniform uptake of technetium-99m diphosphonate shown in the skull, vertebrae, pelvis, and the right femur is characteristic of Paget disease. Bone scan provides a useful tool for mapping the sites of skeletal involvement.

linear uptake traversing the diseased bone. Sarcomatous degeneration cannot be reliably studied with bone scintigraphy. Radiographic signs of rapid destruction in a stable lesion with CT or MRI evidence of a mass lesion are definitive signs of sarcomatous degeneration.

Trauma

As a mechanical apparatus, the bony skeleton is exposed to a wide range of disruptive forces, but as a living tissue, it can cope with them by continually repairing itself. This process, however, fails when the structural elements of the bone are depleted, as in osteoporotic fractures, when the rate of destruction exceeds the repair capacity of the bone as in stress fractures and when the bone receives violent trauma overwhelming its structural strength, as in acute fractures. Bone scintigraphy plays a different role in the evaluation of each of these conditions.

The time-course of scintigraphic changes following bone injury has been extensively studied. Within 24 hours, there will be hyperemia and intense radiotracer localization at a fracture site. The lag phase may be prolonged to 72 hours in the elderly population. Thereafter, the bone scan remains hot for 3 to 6 months and gradually returns to a normal appearance by 1 year in 63% of the cases and by 2 years in nearly all cases. If the fracture fragments unite without adequate alignment, there will be continued activity at the fracture site for many years as a result of bone remodeling. This chronology can help estimate the age of collapsed vertebrae that are frequently encountered on spinal radiographs. In most cases this is the sequel of profound osteoporosis, but the question becomes more critical if the patient has had recent onset of back pain, if there is an extraosseous malignancy with likelihood of metastasis to the bone, or in medicolegal cases. A negative bone scan (ie, uptake equal to the rest of the vertebrae) would indicate that the vertebral collapse occurred at least 1 year before the examination and would effectively eliminate association with any recent event. A positive scan, conversely, does not establish a causal relation and should be evaluated in the light of other available information.

Patients presenting with unexplained bone pain are also candidates for a radioisotopic bone study. Two entities—namely, pain related to sports injury and pain secondary to spondylolysis or spondylolisthesis—deserve special mention in this context. Stress fractures, once thought to occur in soldiers on marching exercises, are now diagnosed with increasing frequency in athletes and nonathletes. Joggers typically present with pain in the legs and feet. Following a negative radiographic examination, bone scintigraphy should be obtained. Bone scan may reveal a spectrum of findings in this condition ranging from a totally normal study to one showing only mild or moderate periosteal reaction as linear uptake along the cortex, or a grossly abnormal study demonstrating intense focal activity at the point of bony tenderness. A normal scan effectively eliminates any bony etiology for the pain, whereas a focal pattern of uptake is highly suggestive of a stress fracture (Fig. 3-48). Orthogonal views should be obtained to ascertain cortical extension. Several series have now verified that these patients go on to develop overt fractures visible on subsequent radiographic examinations if the limb is not put to rest. With proper curtailment of the activities, however, the scintigraphic findings revert back to normal usually within 1 to 2 months. The significance of the linear uptake confined to the periosteum is presently less clear. Available evidence indicates that this pattern can be seen in a variety of nonspecific conditions, including the clinical entity of shin splints and probably calls for a moderate reduction in physical activity.

The low-back pain syndrome is another area of diagnostic difficulty for which bone scintigraphy has shown promising results. A great deal of clinical research has been carried out in recent years on this subject, spawned by the introduction of SPECT imaging. The tomographic approach permits detailed visualization of the various components of a vertebra such as the end-plates, the body, the neural arch, and the pars interarticularis, previously not attainable with planar scintigraphy. Preliminary data indicate that SPECT imaging may evolve into a significant diagnostic tool in the management of patients with back pain resulting from inflammation, tumor, or traumatic injuries (Fig. 3-49).

Infection

Diagnosis of osteomyelitis continues to be a perplexing clinical problem. Acute hematogenous osteomyelitis typically occurs in the pediatric age group and requires prompt detection. Bone radiographs may take as long as 10 to 12 days before the characteristic changes of bone resorption and periosteal reaction are evident. The standard ^{99m}Tc-diphosphonate bone scan can be employed in this setting to diagnose the disease as early as 24 to 48 hours after onset of

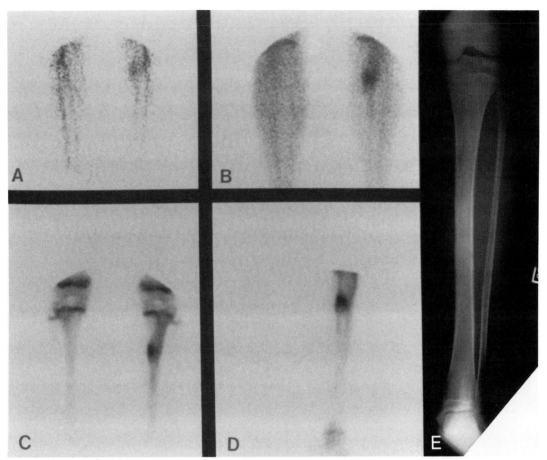

FIGURE 3-48. Stress fracture. A three-phase bone scan in a 16-year-old runner who has been experiencing leg pain for the last 2 weeks. (**A** and **B**) Radionuclide angiogram and blood-pool images show hyperemia in the proximal part of the left tibia. (**C** and **D**) Anterior and lateral bone scans show intense focal uptake involving the cortex of the bone. (**E**) A radiograph of the left tibia is negative for stress fracture at this stage.

symptoms. Using a three-phase study, one can also assess blood flow changes in the symptomatic area and thereby improve the specificity of the test. Presence of hyperemia effectively excludes other diagnoses such as leukemia and bone infarction, which are also considered in this setting.

The orthopaedic surgeon may face an even more perplexing problem, namely, diagnosing osteomyelitis in the presence of fractures, surgical implants, prostheses, or diabetic changes in the foot. In these situations all imaging modalities are hampered to variable degrees, and a combined approach frequently becomes necessary. Two additional radiopharmaceuticals, ^{111}In leukocytes and ^{67}Ga, can be used in conjunction with the standard bone scan to facilitate the detection of bone or soft tissue infection.

^{67}Ga is a trivalent cation that localizes in a variety of tumors and in sites of soft tissue or bone infection.

The mechanism of localization for this radionuclide is poorly understood and is probably multifactorial. It binds to specific plasma and tissue proteins such as transferrin and lactoferrin, which abound in inflammatory sites, and it also directly labels leukocytes and certain bacteria. The result is a considerable concentration of the radionuclide in infected areas. ^{67}Ga is used in a standard dose of 5 mCi, and images are obtained at 6 to 24 hours postinjection of radionuclide. Colonic excretion may render the interpretation of pelvic and abdominal regions difficult and, therefore, require bowel preparation with laxatives or cleansing enemas.

For the ^{111}In WBC imaging, a 50-mL sample of the patient's blood is drawn from which leukocytes are harvested by sedimentation and centrifugation. The radioactive tracer is introduced into the cells by the aid of lipophilic chelating agents, such as oxine

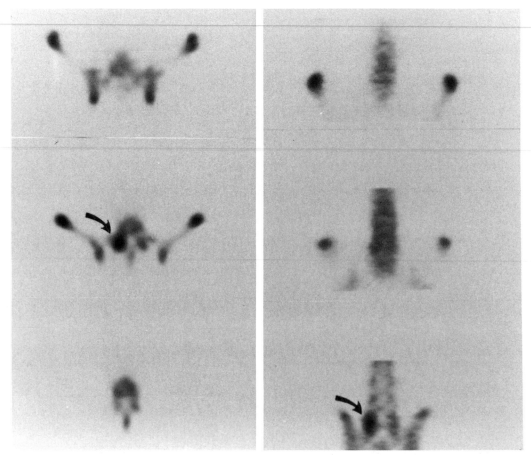

FIGURE 3-49. SPECT imaging of the spine. Tomographic bone scanning helps visualize complex bony structures such as the posterior elements of vertebrae. Axial (*left*) and coronal (*right*) sections of a bone scan are shown in a patient with spondylolysis of the L5 vertebra (*arrow*).

or tropolone, and the final preparation is injected intravenously. Many centers currently perform ^{111}In WBC imaging in preference to ^{67}Ga for its superior image quality, lack of colonic excretion, and greater overall sensitivity and specificity for detection of infection. Ga, however, is considered to be more effective for chronic osteomyelitis, probably because ^{111}In WBC preparations lack a sufficient number of functioning lymphocytes and mononuclear cells.

Evaluation of osteomyelitis should begin with standard radiography, and if negative, a bone scan would suffice in most cases. The typical presentation on three-phase bone scintigraphy consists of increased blood flow and hyperemia demonstrated on the early phases coupled with diffusely increased radiotracer localization on the delayed images. In cellulitis alone, there will be diffuse hyperemia but no significant enhancement of the radiotracer uptake in the bone on delayed images. With septic arthritis, there will be hyperemia and increased tracer uptake over the joint area; however, the bony uptake would be limited to the periarticular regions and would be present on both sides of the joint. Patients with leukemic infiltrates or those with advanced osteonecrosis also exhibit abnormal bone uptake on scintigraphy, however, without the characteristic hyperemic pattern. In the pediatric age group, osteomyelitis occurring adjacent to the growth plate of the bones may be obscured by the intense radiotracer uptake normally present in this region. High-resolution scintigrams would be helpful and should include the contralateral bone for comparison.

Controversy surrounds the use of bone scanning in osteomyelitis of the neonatal age group. ^{99m}Tc-diphosphonate scans have been reported to be normal or show only cold defects in a small fraction of neonates with proven acute osteomyelitis. The presumed mechanism is disruption of the blood supply secondary to elevated intramedullary pressure, subperiosteal abscess formation, or septic embolism to the vessels near the growth plate that result in impaired delivery of the radiopharmaceutical to the infected bone. ^{67}Ga scan has been suggested as a more sensitive alternative. Recent reports using improved instrumentation, however, have found the ^{99m}Tc scan to be as effective in the neonates as in other age groups.

The sensitivity and specificity of ^{99m}Tc-diphosphonate bone scan for detection of acute osteomyelitis affecting an intact bone exceeds 90%. Addition of blood flow and blood-pool images (three-phase study) does not improve the sensitivity appreciably but enhances the specificity. The specificity can be further improved by addition of ^{67}Ga or ^{111}In WBC imaging; however, considering the extra time, cost, and the radiation burden to the patient, neither of these procedures is indicated in detection of osteomyelitis in an intact bone. Their use, however, is imperative for diagnosing infection in the presence of orthopaedic appliances, fractures, or other confounding factors.

Chronic osteomyelitis cannot be reliably assessed by technetium bone imaging alone. In most cases, bone scans show enhancement of the radiotracer uptake, generally without any appreciable hyperemia, but this pattern can also be found even after successful treatment of acute osteomyelitis, presumably because of continued remodeling of the bone. ^{67}Ga is the preferred mode of scintigraphy in chronic osteomyelitis with an overall sensitivity of 80% to 90%. The role of ^{111}In WBC in chronic osteomyelitis has not been clearly defined, but available evidence indicates that it is inferior to ^{67}Ga for this application.

Detection of infection associated with fractures and surgically implanted devices unequivocally calls for combining the Tc bone scan with either ^{67}Ga or ^{111}In WBC imaging. Despite the longer experience available with ^{67}Ga, there is a growing tendency to use ^{111}In WBC preferentially for this application (Figs. 3-50 and 3-51). ^{67}Ga localizes to a variable extent in the normal bone, and as such, infection is only suggested when the gallium uptake exceeds the intensity of ^{99m}Tc-diphosphonate activity on comparable bone scans (incongruent pattern). Studies, therefore, will be nondiagnostic if this requirement is not met. Such encumbrance, however, does not apply to leukocyte imaging. Leukocyte imaging, however, is not reliable within the first 2 months after an acute fracture. Hematoma formation acutely, and normal bony repair and callus formation in later stages, have been shown

to cause ^{111}In WBC localization in the fracture area in the absence of infection. Leukocyte imaging also provides valuable information about the presence of infection in soft tissues adjacent to the target bony area or elsewhere in the body.

The question of prosthesis infection arises when the patients complain of continued pain in an operated joint. A bone scan may be obtained and will be diagnostic if it shows no significant abnormal uptake around the prosthetic device. The evolution of scintigraphic findings after placement of a prosthetic device has been best described for hip joint prostheses. Intense radionuclide uptake is generally present in the bones surrounding the prosthesis up to 6 months following the operation. Thereafter, only a minimal uptake is detected in the acetabulum, the greater trochanter, and the tip of the stem. A diffuse pattern of uptake outlining the contour of the prosthesis strongly suggests loosening (Fig. 3-52), and intense focal activity anywhere along the bone–metal interface suggests osteomyelitis. A leukocyte scan should be obtained for maximum diagnostic accuracy. Infection will be characterized by abnormal ^{111}In WBC localization, whereas a negative study would effectively rule out such a diagnosis.

Detection of osteomyelitis in the diabetic foot is difficult by any imaging modality. The typical patient presents with Charcot joint, extensive bone destruction, and infected soft tissue ulcers. Bone scan and ^{111}In WBC scan are helpful in demonstrating bone infection (Figs. 3-53 and 3-54). A clear distinction between bone versus soft tissue involvement, however, is not always possible because of the limited resolution of these imaging modalities. Recently, MRI has shown promising results.

Osteonecrosis and Bone Infarction

Radiopharmaceuticals used in bone scintigraphy are injected intravenously and reach their target area through the blood vessels. With reduction of blood supply there will be a corresponding decrease in the intensity of tracer uptake in the affected bone on scintigraphic images. A partial reduction in blood supply would affect the delivery of the radiotracer to the involved area, whereas a more complete cessation of blood flow would also result in death of the cellular elements and total absence of scintigraphic activity. An example of the former is the irradiated bone in which a permanent reduction in radiotracer uptake is observed following exposure to 3000 rad during a 3-week period because of injury to the mi-

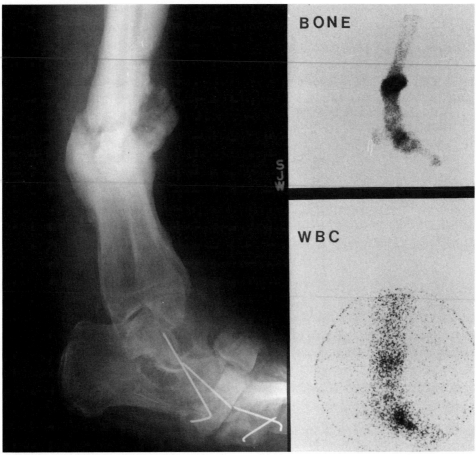

FIGURE 3-50. Fracture nonunion with osteomyelitis. This patient suffered multiple fractures in a motor vehicle accident. Scintigraphy performed 11 months later for evaluation of fracture nonunion shows abnormal uptake on bone scan in distal tibia and the tarsal bones. Findings may represent bone remodeling or superimposed infection. Indium-111 leukocyte imaging clearly shows localization in both sites and indicates osteomyelitis. Bone infection in the tarsal bones was not suspected clinically, but was verified on bone biopsy and culture.

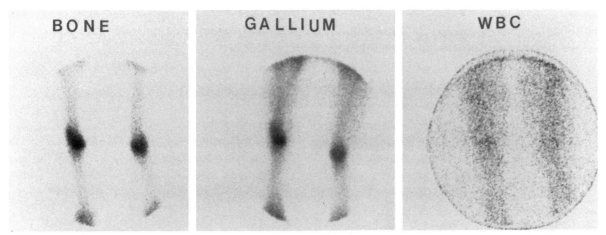

FIGURE 3-51. Fracture nonunion without infection. Delayed healing of the bilateral tibial fractures prompted this combined scintigraphy with technetium-99m diphosphonate, gallium-67, and indium-111 white blood count. The bone scan and the gallium scan both show increased radiotracer localization at the fracture site, which may be construed to indicate osteomyelitis. The gallium uptake, however, is not significantly greater than that of the bone scan and therefore is equivocal. Leukocyte imaging shows no appreciable radiotracer localization in the fracture sites and, therefore, rules out infection. No infection was found on bone biopsy and cultures.

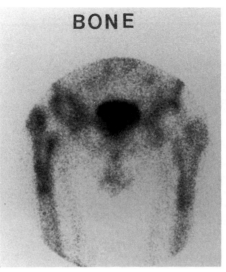 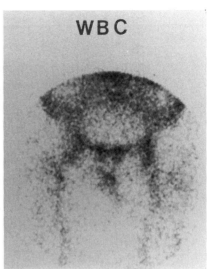

FIGURE 3-52. Prosthesis loosening. Bilateral hip prostheses are depicted in this scintigram from a 64-year-old patient with right hip pain. Abnormal uptake of radiotracer technetium-99m MDP around the right hip prostheses is characteristic of loosening. Asymptomatic prostheses (*left*) generally elicit no significant uptake on bone scan, or may only show slight enhancement in the acetabulum, the greater trochanter, and around the tip of the prosthesis. WBC, white blood count.

crovasculature of the bone. Examples of the latter kind of ischemic injury include the well-known clinical entities of osteonecrosis that affect the femoral capital epiphysis most frequently.

Necrosis of the femoral head can follow a variety of causes, including fracture, dislocation, slipped femoral capital epiphysis, treatment with steroids, or systemic disorders like lupus erythematosus, hemoglobinopathies, and alcoholism. In about 25% of the cases, no definite cause can be found. The greatest utility of the bone scan is in the detection of disease shortly after the onset of ischemia when radiographic signs have not yet developed. At this stage, the radionuclide angiogram, the blood-pool images, and the standard bone scintigrams would show reduced or totally absent radiotracer activity in the region of the femoral head (Fig. 3-55). If a fracture precedes the osteonecrosis, it will be evident as a line of in-

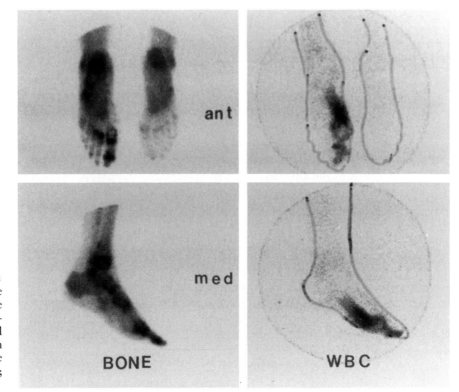

FIGURE 3-53. Osteomyelitis in the foot. Osteomyelitis of the first metatarsal and the great toe is demonstrated in this 52-year-old diabetic man by the abnormal uptake present on the bone scan and the indium-111 leukocyte scan. Ant, anterior; med, medial; WBC, white blood count.

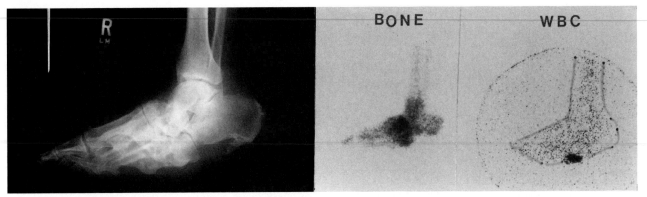

FIGURE 3-54. Foot infection. This diabetic patient with a known infected foot ulcer was studied for osteomyelitis. The radiograph shows Charcot changes in the midfoot, which make evaluation of osteomyelitis difficult. The bone scan is also equivocal, since it shows diffuse uptake, which may be ascribed to degenerative changes or bone infection. Leukocyte imaging, however, only shows abnormal uptake in the region of the infected soft tissue ulcer and clearly rules out bone infection.

creased activity adjacent to the cold femoral head. Radiographs typically disclose no evidence of avascular necrosis at this time. Several reports in literature have indicated that SPECT imaging may be superior to planar scintigraphy for detection of the cold defects secondary to osteonecrosis. Both planar and SPECT imaging will eventually show a transition from the initial cold appearance to one of increasing activity in the femoral head within several weeks after the onset of aseptic necrosis.

Reflex Sympathetic Dystrophy

Radioisotopic imaging has been used in the detection of reflex sympathetic dystrophy with the aggregate evidence indicating that scintigraphy is more useful in diagnosing this condition than conventional radiography. The pathophysiology is thought to be vasomotor instability in the affected limb and typically follows such insults as trauma, neoplasia, stroke, myocardial infarction, or disk disease. A three-phase ^{99m}Tc-diphosphonate study exhibits hyperemia in the painful region on the initial set of images followed by demonstration of intense radiotracer uptake in the juxtaarticular regions and occasionally in the shaft of the bones involved. These findings are present in about 80% to 90% of the cases and generally predate the appearance of osteoporosis on radiographs. Furthermore, those with positive scintigrams have been shown to respond more favorably to steroid therapy than those who have negative scans.

Miscellaneous Bone Disorders

Scintigraphic techniques in general have played a limited role in the management of inflammatory joint diseases. Both blood-pool agents and bone-seeking radiopharmaceuticals as well as inflammation-specific tracers such as ^{67}Ga or ^{111}In WBC have been employed in patients with rheumatoid arthritis. All three classes of radiopharmaceuticals tend to show enhanced activity over the involved joints with a sensitivity comparable with or somewhat superior to that achieved by radiography. These findings, however, are nonspecific and do not add significantly to the information available from clinical and radiographic examinations alone. The high sensitivity of bone imaging with ^{99m}Tc- diphosphonate, however, has proved useful in detection of inflammation in the sacroiliac and hip joints. In patients with sacroiliitis and ankylosing spondylitis, bone scintigraphy will reveal enhanced radiotracer uptake in the inflamed joints and facilitate the diagnosis of this condition in a patient with unexplained low-back pain. A successful clinical treatment with antiinflammatory drugs will usually result in subsidence of the abnormal findings on bone scintigraphy. Low-grade inflammation of the joint, however, may not be detected with this approach.

Transient (toxic) synovitis of the hip occurs with some frequency in children under age 10 and presents a diagnostic challenge. Bone scanning will be abnormal in most of these cases but will have a variable pattern of abnormal findings. A few children will show hyperemia and increased tracer localization,

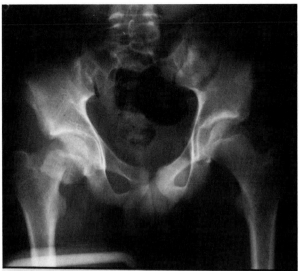

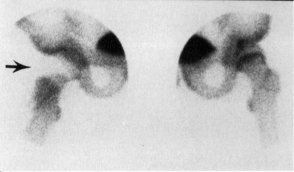

FIGURE 3-55. Avascular necrosis following bone fracture. Lack of tracer localization on bone scintigraphy is characteristic of avascular necrosis in the early stages of the disease. At this time, radiographs are usually nondiagnostic.

but most children will exhibit a pattern of decreased blood-pool activity and decreased bone tracer localization. This photon-deficient appearance is believed to represent the accumulation of fluid within the joint capsule and has been shown to disappear following arthrocentesis.

Metabolic diseases affecting the bony skeleton generally do not yield specific patterns of abnormality on bone scintigraphy. In hyperparathyroidism, the bone scan may be normal, but frequently will show a generalized pattern of enhanced uptake in the skeleton, most pronounced at the costochondral junction of the ribs, the sternum, and the skull. Typically, the kidneys fail to visualize on these superscans when the film exposure is adjusted for the high intensity of uptake in the skeleton. A dramatically abnormal scintigram, demonstrating intense radiotracer uptake in the lungs, stomach, and other soft tissues,

may occasionally be found in patients with primary hyperparathyroidism or renal osteodystrophy.

Assessment of patients with involutional osteoporosis is currently possible with one of three different approaches. Most nuclear medicine centers perform measurements of bone mineral density with dual photon absorptiometry. In this technique, an external source of ^{153}Gd is used, whose dual photon emissions of 44- and 100-keV energy, penetrate the body and are recorded with a scintillation device. The differential attenuation of the two photons as they traverse the soft tissues and the bony structures permits the calculation of the bone mineral density in units of g/cm^2. Measurements are typically obtained from the lumbar spine with a precision of 2% to 3% and from the hip area with a precision of 3% to 5%. Normal values have been defined for both regions. The other two methods include the use of CT and the more recent technique of absorptiometry with an x-ray generator rather than an isotopic source. With the CT approach, attenuation numbers are compared with a set of known references included in the scanning field. A major problem presently encountered with all three methods is the considerable degree of overlap found between data obtained from normal subjects and from patients known to be at risk for osteopenic fractures.

Annotated Bibliography

Aisen AM, Martel W, Ellis JH, McCune WJ. Cervical spine involvement in rheumatoid arthritis: MRI imaging. Radiology 1987;165:159.
This study of 18 patients with rheumatoid arthritis and suspected cervical involvement found that MRI provided valuable information regarding the status of the spinal cord and dura.

Angtuaco EJC, McConnell JR, Chadduck WM, Flanigan S. MRI imaging of spinal epidural sepsis. AJR 1987;149:1249.
A study of MRI and CT studies on four patients with spinal infection showed that MRI was more definitive in the early demonstration of epidural abscesses.

Beckly DE, Anderson PW, Pedegana LR. The radiology of the subtalar joint with special reference to talo-calcaneal coalition. Clin Radiol 1975;26:333.
The authors discuss normal anatomy and radiography of the subtalar joint. They also describe the secondary signs of subtalar coalition, namely, talar beaking, narrowing of the posterior talocalcaneal joint, rounding of the lateral process of the talus, and failure to visualize the middle subtalar joint on lateral views.

Beltran J, Noto AM, Herman LJ, Lubbers LM. Tendons: high-field-strength surface coil MRI imaging. Radiology 1987;162:735.
Normal anatomic appearances of tendons are described and illustrated in addition to experimentally produced tears of the domestic swine Achilles tendons.

Beltran J, Noto AM, Mosure JC, Weiss KL, Zuelzer W, Christofordis AJ. The knee: surface-coil MRI imaging at 1.5 T. Radiology 1986;159:747.

This article on the early use of surface coil MRI imaging of the knee correctly predicted its rapidly increasing replacement of the more invasive arthrography.

Beltran J, Simon DC, Katz W, Weis LD. Increased MRI signal intensity in skeletal muscle adjacent to malignant tumors: pathologic correlation and clinical relevance. Radiology 1987;162: 251.
This study of MRIs of 50 patients with musculoskeletal disorders found that increased signal in T2-weighted images adjacent to neoplasms was usually caused by edema and was suggestive of malignancy. Edema was also observed adjacent to infection, myositis, and hematoma.

Berquist TH. Imaging of adult cervical spine trauma. Radiographics 1988;8:667.
This is an excellent review of trauma to the cervical spine. The text is succinct, and the article is well illustrated with examples from different types of injuries.

Berquist TH, ed. Imaging of orthopedic trauma and surgery. Philadelphia, WB Saunders, 1986.
The first chapter in this book describes the physical principles and applications of the different diagnostic techniques, including plain radiography, conventional tomography, CT, nuclear medicine, and MRI. This chapter is a concise introduction to the topic.

Bloem JL, Taminiam AHM, Eulderink F, Hermans J, Pauwels EKJ. Radiologic staging of primary bone sarcoma: MRI imaging scintigraphy, angiography, and CT correlated with pathologic examination. Radiology 1988;169:805.
This prospective study of 56 patients with primary bone sarcomas concluded that MRI is the modality of choice for local staging. They found it equal or superior to CT, ^{99m}Tc bone scanning, and angiography in defining the extent of tumors and the relation to major neurovascular bundles.

Bluemm RG, Falke THM, Ziedses des Plantes BGZ Jr, Steiner RM. Early Legg-Perthes disease (ischemic necrosis of the femoral head) demonstrated by MRI. Skeletal Radiol 1985;14:95.
This is a case report of early Legg-Perthes disease demonstrated by MRI. The MRI appearances and comparison with normal appearances are discussed.

Brant-Zawadzki M, Jeffrey RB Jr, Minagi H, Pitts LH. High resolution CT of thoracolumbar fractures. AJR 1982;138:699.
The authors stress the usefulness of CT is the evaluation of thoracolumbar fractures. Vertebral body and posterior element fractures can be missed on plain films. CT also detects unsuspected spinal canal compromise. CT with intrathecal contrast can show dural tears.

Bundschuh C, Modic MT, Kearney F, Morris R, Deal C. Rheumatoid arthritis of the cervical spine: surface-coil MRI imaging. AJR 1988;151:181.
This study of 15 patients with cervical involvement with rheumatoid arthritis compared the findings in plain films, pluridirectional tomography, and MRI. The authors found that MRI was an excellent imaging procedure that demonstrated the most clinically important parameters better than the other imaging modalities.

Collier BD, Carrera GF, Johnson RP, et al. Detection of femoral head avascular necrosis in adults by SPECT. J Nucl Med 1985;25:979.
Twenty-one patients with avascular necrosis of the femoral head were studied. Radionuclide tomographic imaging had a sensitivity of 85% versus 55% for planar scintigraphy.

Collier BD Jr, Hellman RS, Krasnow AZ. Bone SPECT. Semin Nucl Med 1987;17:247.
An excellent review on the subject of tomographic bone imaging with special consideration of the technical aspects.

Collier BD, Johnson RP, Carrera GF, et al. Painful spondylolysis or spondylolisthesis studied by radiology and single-photon emission computed tomography. Radiology 1985;154:207.

This article describes a broad range of applications for bone scintigraphy in the work-up of patients with skeletal pain.

Crues JV III, Mink J, Levy TL, Lotysch M, Stoller DW. Meniscal tears of the knee: accuracy of MRI imaging. Radiology 1987;164: 445.
This comparison of surgical and MRI findings concluded that MRI can separate surgically significant from nonsignificant meniscal lesions based on a grading system of MRI appearances.

Daffner RH, Lupetin AR, Dash N, Deeb ZL, Sefczek RJ, Schapiro RL. MRI in the detection of malignant infiltration of bone marrow. AJR 1986;146:353.
Thirty patients with myeloma were studied with MRI and radionuclide bone scans. Most had normal bone scans, but all 30 had abnormal MRI studies. Metastatic disease was also studied, and MRI was found to be a sensitive method of detecting malignancy within bone marrow.

Ehara S, Khurama JS, Kattapuram SV. Pyogenic vertebral osteomyelitis of the posterior elements. Skeletal Radiol 1989;18:175.
The authors describe three patients with pyogenic vertebral osteomyelitis involving only the posterior elements. Two of the patients had diabetes mellitus. In all three patients the facets were involved, which makes this condition difficult to differentiate from an erosive arthritis if a biopsy is not performed.

El-Khoury GY, Kathol MH, Chandler JB, Albright JP. Shoulder instability: impact of glenohumeral arthrotomography on treatment. Radiology 1986;160:669.
This study showed strong correlation between labral pathology and anatomic instability. Labral tears were seen in 86% of patients with anatomic instability and in only 40% of patients with functional instability.

Evancho AM, Stiles RG, Fajman WA, et al. MRI imaging diagnosis of rotator cuff tears. AJR 1988;151:751.
A study of MRI, arthroscopy, and arthrography of the shoulder suggested that MRI is an accurate procedure for the diagnosis of complete rotator cuff tears.

Feldman F, Singson RD, Rosenberg ZS, Berdon WE, Amdio J, Abramson SJ. Distal tibial triplane fractures: diagnosis with CT. Radiology 1987;164:429.
The authors stress that CT is the method of choice for preoperative and postoperative evaluation of triplane fractures. This is due to the special geometry of these fractures, which have important transverse components involving the tibial plafond.

Fleckenstein JL, Weatheral PT, Parkey RW, Payne JA, Peshock RM. Sports-related muscle injuries: evaluation with MRI imaging. Radiology 1989;172:793.
This study found that pain associated with muscle strain and occurring several days after exercise were both associated with prolongation of muscle T1 and T2.

Fogelman I, ed. Bone scanning in clinical practice. London, Springer-Verlag, 1987.
This book comprehensively reviews the clinical and technical aspects of radioisotopic bone imaging.

Fogelman I, Collier BD. An atlas of planar and SPECT bone scans. St Louis, CV Mosby, 1989.
This book comprehensively reviews the clinical and technical aspects of radioisotopic bone imaging.

Ghelman B, Thompson FM, Arnold WD. Intraoperative radioactive localization of an osteoid-osteoma: case report. J Bone Joint Surg 1981;63A:826–827.
The authors describe their experience with presurgical and intraoperative localization of osteoid ostemoas.

Gill K, Bucholz RW. The role of computerized tomographic scanning in the evaluation of major pelvic fractures. J Bone and Joint Surg 1984;66A:34.
The authors studied 25 patients with double vertical fractures of the pelvic ring using plain radiography and CT. In one third of

the patients, CT added additional anatomic information. CT is recommended for evaluation of major pelvic fractures.

Gilula LA. Carpal injuries: analytic approach and case exercises. AJR 1979;133:503.
A classic article in which the author describes the three arcs of the wrist and how they assist in the diagnosis of a variety of carpal dislocations and fracture dislocations.

Gilula LA, Weeks PM. Post-traumatic ligamentous instabilities of the wrist. Radiology 1978;129:641.
The authors discussed the patterns of instability and the different angles drawn on the lateral radiograph to arrive at a diagnosis. They also stress the usefulness of the "instability series."

Golimbu C, Firooznia H, Rafii M. CT of osteomyelitis of the spine. AJR 1984;142:159.
CT studies of 17 adult patients with spine osteomyelitis are presented. The principal features were paravertebral soft tissue swelling, abscess formation, bone erosion, and disk involvement. CT guided needle biopsy was helpful in establishing a specific diagnosis.

Harbert JC. Nuclear medicine therapy. New York, Thieme Medical Publishers, 1987:169.
This textbook is an excellent reference for the therapeutic applications of radionuclides and includes a comprehensive description of the treatment procedures for osseous metastatic disease and radiation synovectomy.

Harley JD, Mack LA, Winquist RA. CT of acetabular fractures: comparison with conventional radiography. AJR 1982;138:413.
Plain radiography and CT were compared in 26 adult patients with acetabular fractures. CT was more sensitive than plain radiography in detecting fractures of the acetabular roof, posterior acetabular lip, and quadrilateral surface. Entrapped bony fragments were also better detected by CT.

Harms SE, Morgan TJ, Yamanashi WS, Harle TS, Dodd GD. Principles of nuclear magnetic resonance imaging. Radiographics 1984;4:26.
This is a basic review of the physical principles of MRI. The article also discusses the commonly used scanning sequences and why certain tissues appear the way they do on certain sequences.

Hartzman S, Reicher MA, Bassett LW, Duckwiler GR, Mandelbaum B, Gold RH. MRI imaging of the knee. II. Chronic disorders. Radiology 1987;162:553.
Sixty patients with chronic knee symptoms were evaluated with MRI. A wide variety of disorders was encountered, and the MRI appearances are described. The authors conclude that MRI imaging can provide information that may otherwise require multiple, sometimes invasive, diagnostic procedures.

Herman LJ, Beltran J. Pitfalls in MRI imaging of the knee. Radiology 1988;167:775.
Discrepancies between the findings of MRI and those of arthroscopy were reviewed retrospectively in 52 knee examinations. Some of these discrepancies were caused by misinterpreting normal structures, which mimicked meniscal tears. These are discussed.

Hudson TM, Schabel M II, Springfield DS. Limitation of computed tomography following excisional biopsy of soft tissue sarcomas. Skeletal Radiol 1985;13:49.
The authors demonstrate convincingly that CT is not an effective method to follow patients after complete or incomplete excisional biopsy of soft tissue sarcomas. In about half the patients, CT failed to detect residual tumor.

Hueftle MG, Modic MT, Ross JS, et al. Lumbar spine: postoperative MRI imaging with Gd-DTPA. Radiology 1988;167:817.
This study of 30 patients with failed back surgery found that MRI studies with Gd-DTPA could, in most cases, differentiate between epidural scar and extruded disk material.

Hughes J. Techniques of bone imaging. In: Silberstein EB, ed. Bone scintigraphy. Mount Kisco, NY, Futura, 1984:39.
A good reference for patient positioning in bone scintigraphy.

Jelinek JS, Kransdorf MJ, Utz JA, et al. Imaging of pigmented villonodular synovitis with emphasis on MRI imaging. AJR 1989;152:337.
The authors describe the MRI appearances of pigmented villonodular synovitis with emphasis on the differential diagnosis and the tendency for hemosiderin deposition to result in a decrease.

Kathol MH, Moore TE, El-Khoury GY, Yuh WTC, Montgomery WJ. Magnetic resonance imaging of athletic soft tissue injuries. Iowa Orthop 1989;9:44.
This review of 54 cases of sports-related soft tissue injuries concluded that MRI is well suited for detecting these injuries and is usually superior to other imaging modalities.

Kirchner PT, Simon MA. The clinical value of bone and gallium scintigraphy for soft-tissue sarcomas of the extremities. J Bone Joint Surg 1984;66A:319.
A rare source of information on the outcome of bone scanning in soft tissue tumors.

Kowalski HM, Cohen WA, Cooper P, Wisoff JH. Pitfalls in the CT diagnosis of atlantoaxial rotary subluxation. AJR 1987;149:595.
Functional CT scanning through C1 and C2 is proposed as the best technique to differentiate atlantoaxial rotary fixation from other forms of torticollis. Patient with rotary fixation demonstrate no motion at C1-C2 during this maneuver, whereas patients with transient torticollis show reduction or reversal of the C1-C2 rotation.

Kransdorf MJ, Jelinek JS, Moser RP, et al. Soft-tissue masses: diagnosis using MRI imaging. AJR 1989;153:541.
MRI images of 112 soft tissue masses were reviewed retrospectively. The authors found that in most cases a preoperative diagnosis could not be made, although some types of lesions did show specific features (lipomas, hemangiomas, hematomas, and pigmented villonodular synovitis). MRI could not reliably distinguish between benign and malignant lesions.

Kulkarni MV, Bondurant FJ, Rose SL, Narayana PA. 1.5 Tesla magnetic resonance imaging of acute spinal trauma. Radiographics 1988;8:1059.
The MRI appearances of hemorrhage and edema in the injured spinal cord are described. The correlation between MRI patterns of cord injury and neurologic recovery was excellent in this series of 50 patients.

Levenson RM, Sauerbrunn BJL, Bates HR, Eddy JL, Ihde DC. Comparative value of bone scintigraphy and radiography in monitoring tumor response in systemically treated prostatic carcinoma. Radiology 1983;146:513.
This article describes the flare phenomenon seen on bone scans after initiation of chemotherapy.

Manaster BJ, Osborn AG. CT patterns of facet fracture dislocations in the thoracolumbar region. AJR 1987;148:335.
Thoracolumbar facet dislocations are less common than cervical spine facet dislocations; however, the injury is unstable, and early diagnosis is essential. The authors present three patterns of thoracolumber facet fracture dislocation, which are diagnosable by CT.

Matin P. Appearance of bone scans following fractures: including immediate and long-term studies. J Nucl Med 1979;20:1227.
This article describes the appearance of bone scan in various types of osseous injury. In particular, the second article elaborates on the value of bone scanning in sports-related injuries in 238 patients.

McKillop JH, McKay I, Cuthbert GF, Fogelman I, Gray HW, Storrock RD. Scintigraphic evaluation of the painful prosthetic joint: a comparison of gallium-67 citrate and indium-111 to labeled leukocyte imaging. Clin Radiol 1984;35:239.
This article defines the outcome of ^{67}Ga citrate scanning in chronic osteomyelitis. The authors found ^{67}Ga to be superior to leukocyte imaging in 15 patients.

McKinstry CS, Steiner RE, Young AT, Jones L, Swirsky D, Aber V. Bone marrow in leukemia and aplastic anemia: MRI imaging before, during and after treatment. Radiology 1987;162:701.

Serial MRI studies of cervical bone marrow were performed in patients undergoing bone marrow transplant for aplastic anemia and chronic granulocytic leukemia. MRI was felt likely to be useful in the assessment and treatment of hematologic disorders.

McNeil BJ. Value of bone scanning in neoplastic disease. Semin Nucl Med 1984;14:277.
This publication provides an excellent review of the role of bone scintigraphy in the management of skeletal metastases.

Merkel KD, Fitzgerald RH, Brown ML. Scintigraphic evaluation in musculoskeletal sepsis. Orthop Clin North Am 1984;15:401.
This is a good general review of the radionuclide procedures available for work-up of osteomyelitis.

Mettler FA Jr, ed. Radionuclide bone imaging and densitometry. New York, Churchill Livingstone, 1988.
This book comprehensively reviews the clinical and technical aspects of radioisotopic bone imaging.

Mink JH, Deutsch AL. Occult cartilage and bone injuries of the knee: detection, classification, and assessment with MRI imaging. Radiology 1989;170:823.
This article describes four types of bone and cartilage knee injuries, which may be seen in MRI studies but not in plain films.

Mitchell DG, Rao VM, Dalinka MK, et al. Femoral head avascular necrosis: correlation of MRI imaging, radiographic staging, radionuclide imaging, and clincial findings. Radiology 1987;162:709.
This article describes the MRI appearances of avascular necrosis of the femoral heads and describes a chronologic pattern of MRI signal features, which may allow staging by MRI imaging.

Mitchell MD, Kundel HL, Steinberg ME, Kressel HY, Alavi A, Axel L. Avascular necrosis of the hip: comparison of MRI, CT and scintigraphy. AJR 1986;147:67.
In a comparison of CT, radionuclide scanning, and MRI, MRI was found to be the most sensitive imaging technique for the early diagnosis of avascular necrosis of the hip.

Modic MT, Feiglin DH, Piraino DW, et al. Vertebral osteomyelitis: assessment using MRI. Radiology 1985;157:157.
Thirty-seven patients, clinically suspected of having vertebral osteomyelitis, were prospectively evaluated with MRI, radiography, and radionuclide studies. The MRI appearances of vertebral osteomyelitis were characteristic, and MRI was found to be as accurate and sensitive as radionuclide scanning in the detection of osteomyelitis.

Modic MT, Masaryk TJ, Ross JS, Cartor JR. Imaging of degenerative disk disease. Radiology 1988;168:177.
This is a comprehensive article that reviews current opinions on the pathophysiology of degenerative disk disease and the effect imaging has had on the study of this disorder.

Nair N. Bone scanning in Ewing's sarcoma. J Nucl Med 1985;26:349.
Seventy-two patients with Ewing sarcoma are described. Bony metastases were found in 51% of the patients, with no clinical signs being present in 76% of them.

Papanicolaou N. Osteoid osteoma: operative confirmation of complete removal by bone scintigraphy. Radiology 1985;154:821.
The author describes his experience with presurgical and intraoperative localization of osteoid osteomas.

Paulson DF, Uro-Oncology Research Group. The impact of current staging procedures in assessing disease extent of prostatic adenocarcinoma. J Urol 1979;121:300.
This publication provides an excellent review of the role of bone scintigraphy in the management of skeletal metastases.

Pettersson H, Gillespy T III, Hamlin DJ, et al. Primary musculoskeletal tumors: examination with MRI imaging compared with conventional modalities. Radiology 1987;164:237.
A study of 176 cases of musculoskeletal tumors found that MRI was excellent in the determination of intraosseous extent, although

not proven to be better than CT or scintigraphy. MRI was found to be inferior to plain films and CT in assessment of periosteal reaction, calcification, and bone destruction. It was found superior to other modalities in assessment of soft tissue tumors and the soft tissue extension of bone tumors.

Rafii M, Firooznia H, Golimbu C, Bonamo J. Computed tomography of tibial plateau fractures. AJR 1984;142:1181.
Twenty patients with tibial plateau fractures were studied by conventional tomography and CT. CT proved more accurate in assessing depressed and split fractures when they involved the anterior and posterior border of the plateau and in demonstrating the extent of fracture comminution.

Raghavam N, Barkovich AJ, Edwards M, Norman D. MRI imaging of the tethered spinal cord syndrome. AJR 1989;152:843.
In a study of 25 patients with a clinical diagnosis of tethered spinal cord, MRI imaging was found to be extremely useful. The authors were able to visualize the conus medullaris, assess the thickness of the filum terminale, identify traction lesions, and evaluate associated bony dysraphisms.

Rao S, Solomon N, Miller S, Dunn E. Scintigraphic differentiation of bone infarction from osteomyelitis in children with sickle cell disease. J Pediatr 1985;107:685.
This article describes the complementary roles of bone and bone marrow scanning in evaluation of bone infarction in 40 children with sickle cell disease.

Redmond OM, Stack JR, Dervan PA, Hurson BJ, Garney DN, Ennis JT. Osteosarcoma: use of MRI and MRI spectroscopy in clinical decision making. Radiology 1989;172:811.
This study of 14 patients with osteosarcoma compared the pathologic findings with those of the MRI images. There was an excellent correlation of intramedullary tumor extent. They found the T2-weighted images were optimal in demonstrating soft-tissue bulk and breach of cortex.

Reicher MA, Hartzman S, Bassett LW, Mandelbaum B, Duckwiler G, Gold RH. MRI imaging of the knee. I. Traumatic disorders. Radiology 1987;162:547.
One hundred thirty patients with knee injuries were evaluated with MRI. The authors report on the accuracy of MRI when compared with surgical findings in a wide variety of traumatic lesions.

Rossleigh MA, Lovegrove FT, Reynolds PM, Byrne MJ, Whitney BP. The assessment of response to therapy of bone metastases in breast cancer. Aust NZ J Med 1984;14:19.
This article describes the flare phenomenon seen on bone scans after initiation of chemotherapy.

Rupani HD, Holder LE, Espinola DA, Engin SI. Three-phase radionuclide bone imaging in sports medicine. Radiology 1985;156:187.
This article describes the appearance of bone scan in various types of osseous injury. In particular, the second article elaborates on the value of bone scanning in sports-related injuries in 238 patients.

Rush BH, Bramson RT, Ogden JA. Legg-Calvé-Perthes disease: detection of cartilaginous and synovial changes with MRI imaging. Radiology 1988;167:473.
This study of 20 patients with Legg-Calvé-Perthes disease concluded that MRI provides a means of evaluating the acetabular and epiphyseal cartilage, allowing assessment of femoral head containment, congruity of the acetabular and femoral articular surfaces, and intracapsular soft tissue irregularities.

Saks BJ. Normal acetabular anatomy for acetabular fracture assessment: CT and plain film correlation. Radiology 1986;159:139.
This article discusses in detail the radiographic anatomy of the acetabulum both on plain radiographs and by CT. It is helpful for interpretation of acetabular fractures as described by Judet and Letournel.

Schaffer DL, Pendergrass HP. Comparison of enzyme, clinical, radiographic, and radionuclide methods of detecting bone me-

tastases from carcinoma of the prostate. Radiology 1976;121:431.
This publication provides an excellent review of the role of bone scintigraphy in the management of skeletal metastases.

Schauwecker DS, Park H-M, Mock BH, et al. Evaluation of complicating osteomyelitis with 99mTc MDP, In-111 granulocytes, and Ga-67 citrate. J Nucl Med 1984;25:849–853.
The authors compare the usefulness of ^{67}Ga and ^{11}In leukocyte imaging in the evaluation of chronic osteomyelitis. They conclude that leukocyte imaging is superior to gallium, as the latter was found to be either insensitive or equivocal in a substantial number of cases.

Schutte HE, Park WM. The diagnostic value of bone scintigraphy in patients with low back pain. Skeletal Radiol 1983;10:1.
This article describes a broad range of applications for bone scintigraphy in the work-up of patients with skeletal pain.

Seabold JE, Nepola JV, Conrad GR, et al. Detection of osteomyelitis at fracture nonunion sites: comparison of two scintigraphic methods. Am J Radiol 1989;152:1021.
The authors compare the usefulness of ^{67}Ga and ^{111}In leukocyte imaging in the evaluation of chronic osteomyelitis. The authors concluded that leukocyte imaging was superior to Ga, as the latter was found to be either insensitive or equivocal in a substantial number of cases.

Smith SR, Williams CE, Davies JM, Edwards RHT. Bone marrow disorders: characterization with quantitative MRI imaging. Radiology 1989;172:805.
Quantitative MRI of the lumbar spine was performed on 15 healthy control subjects and 30 patients with hematologic disorders. Infiltrative bone marrow disorders showed significantly more prolonged T1 times, and aplastic anemia showed significantly shortened T1 when compared with normal individuals.

Smoker WRK, Godersky JC, Knutzon RK, Keyes WD, Norman D, Bergman W. The role of MRI imaging in evaluating metastatic spinal disease. AJR 1987;149:1241.
The authors stress the usefulness of MRI over myelography in the evaluation of metastatic disease to the spine with cord compression, especially when there are multiple sites of myelographic blocks.

Subramanian G, McAfee JG, Blair RJ, Mehter A, Connor T. ^{99m}Tc-EHDP: a potential radiopharmaceutical for skeletal imaging. J Nucl Med 1972;13:947.
A landmark publication that spawned the widespread use of diphosphonates in bone scanning.

Sundaram M, McGuire MH. Computed tomography or magnetic resonance for evaluating the solitary tumor or tumor-like lesion of bone. Skeletal Radiol 1988;17:393.
In a study of 89 cases, the authors conclude that for long-bone tumors MRI should be used instead of CT as a staging procedure. In flat bones, they recommend CT with MRI being reserved for depiction of lesion extent.

Tang JSH, Gold RH, Bassett LW, Seeger LL. Musculoskeletal infection of the extremities: evaluation with MRI imaging. Radiology 1988;166:205.
In this series of 17 patients referred for possible osteomyelitis, MRI was found particularly useful for seeking foci of active infection in areas of chronic osteomyelitis complicated by surgical intervention or fracture.

terMeulen DC, Majd M. Bone scintigraphy in the evaluation of children with obscure skeletal pain. Pediatrics 1987;79:587.
This article describes a broad range of applications for bone scintigraphy in the work-up of patients with skeletal pain.

Totty WG, Murphy WA, Lee JKT. Soft-tissue tumors: MRI imaging. Radiology 1986;160:135.
CT and MRI studies of 32 soft tissue masses were compared. The authors found MRI to be superior or equal to CT in 92 possible comparisons in four categories.

Tumeh SS, Aliabadi P, Weissman BN, McNeil BJ. Chronic osteomyelitis: bone and gallium scan patterns associated with active disease. Radiology 1986;158:685.
This article defines the outcome of ^{67}Ga citrate scanning in chronic osteomyelitis. The authors found ^{67}Ga scan to be specific only when the uptake of ^{67}Ga was greater than ^{99m}Tc MDP uptake on standard bone scan.

Utz JA, Lull RJ, Galvin EG. Asymptomatic total hip prosthesis: natural history determined using ^{99m}Tc MDP bone scans. Radiology 1986;161:509.
The evolution of bone scan findings in patients with asymptomatic hip prostheses are described.

Van Lom KJ, Kellerhouse LE, Pathria MN, et al. Infection versus tumor in the spine: criteria for distinction with CT. Radiology 1988;166:855.
CT criteria to diagnose spinal infection include prevertebral soft tissue involvement, diffuse osteolytic destruction, gas within both bone and soft tissue, and a process centering within an intervertebral disk. Neoplastic disease is characterized by posterior element involvement, partial or absent prevertebral soft tissue swelling, and osteoblastic and osteolytic lesions.

Wahner HW. Assessment of metabolic bone diseases: review of new nuclear medicine procedures. Mayo Clin Proc 1985;60:827.
This article provides a good review of the applications of ^{99m}Tc bone scintigraphy in various metabolic bone diseases.

Wahner HW, Dunn WL, Riggs BL. Assessment of bone mineral. J Nucl Med 1984;25:1134–1141, 1241.
This is a two-part article broadly covering the techniques and applications of bone mineral density determinations.

Weekes RG, McLeod RA, Reiman HM, Pritchard D. CT of soft-tissue neoplasms. AJR 1985;144:355.
The authors developed criteria to differentiate malignant from benign lesions, and these criteria were helpful in 88% of their cases. Different malignant tumors did not have characteristics that are specific enough to differentiate them from each other.

Wilson AJ, Totty WG, Murphy WA, Hardy DC. Shoulder joint: arthrographic CT and long-term follow-up, with surgical correlation. Radiology 1989;173:329.
This is an excellent study of shoulder arthrotomography both normal and abnormal. The article discusses the variations in the shape of the labrum and the variations in the insertion of the capsule to the glenoid. The authors conclude that a limited number of plain radiographs combined with contiguous CT sections should be sufficient to answer most diagnostic questions.

Yao L, Lee JK. Occult intraosseous fracture: detection with MRI imaging. Radiology 1988;167:749.
Eight patients with recent symptomatic knee injuries and normal radiographs were found on MRI to have intraosseous regions of decreased signal intensity on T1-weighted and proton density imaging and increased signal intensity on T2-weighted imaging. The authors speculate that the MRI findings represent microscopic compression fractures of trabecular bone.

Yuh WTC, Corson JD, Baraniewski HM, et al. Osteomyelitis of the foot in diabetic patients: evaluation with plain film, ^{99m}Tc-MDP bone scintigraphy, and magnetic resonance imaging. AJR 1989;152:795.
This study compared the findings of MRI, plain films, and bone scans with the histologic findings in suspected osteomyelitis in the feet of diabetic patients. MRI was found to have much higher sensitivity and specificity than the other imaging modalities. The authors found MRI to be useful and slightly superior to both radionuclide bone scanning and plain radiography for detection of foot osteomyelitis in diabetic patients.

II

General Disorders of the Musculoskeletal System

Turek's Orthopaedics: Principles and Their Application, Fifth Edition,
edited by Stuart L. Weinstein and Joseph A. Buckwalter.
J.B. Lippincott Company, Philadelphia, © 1994.

4

Neil E. Green

Bone and Joint Infections in Children

DIAGNOSIS AND TREATMENT OF OSTEOMYELITIS AND SEPTIC ARTHRITIS

The treatment of bone and joint infections in children has continued to evolve since the development of antibiotics in the early 1940s. We have witnessed the development of penicillin resistance by staphylococci and the subsequent development of the semisynthetic penicillins and cephalosporins, which eradicate these penicillin-resistant staphylococci. Because of the risk of chronic bone infection, acute hematogenous osteomyelitis was traditionally treated with 6 weeks of intravenous (IV) antibiotics in the hospital. Recently, however, a short course (5 to 10 days) of IV antibiotics in the hospital followed by a longer course of oral therapy has been shown to be effective in eradicating these infections.

ACUTE HEMATOGENOUS OSTEOMYELITIS

Classification

Osteomyelitis in the child may be classified in various ways. The age of the child at the onset of the infection determines the type of infection that develops. Acute hematogenous osteomyelitis behaves differently in neonates from the way it does in children. Because of the existence of blood vessels that cross the growth plate in the neonate and infant younger than age 18 months, the bone infection that develops in that age group will likely cross the physis; however, in the child older than this age, acute infections rarely cross the growth plate (Fig. 4-1).

Osteomyelitis may also be classified according to the severity of the infection and the rapidity with which it develops. Acute hematogenous osteomyelitis has a rapid onset, and children with this illness are usually seen within 1 to several days from the onset of the infection. Another form of bone infection is subacute hematogenous osteomyelitis, which resembles the acute form; however, the children are less

ill, and the infection causes fewer systemic findings (Table 4-1). Chronic osteomyelitis is usually present for months before either detection or treatment. It may also result from inadequate treatment of an acute bone infection. It more commonly is the result of an infection that is secondary to an open fracture of a long bone.

Osteomyelitis may result from hematogenous spread of the infecting organism. This is the most common means of production of osteomyelitis in the child. Bone may also become infected secondarily from the spread of a contiguous area of infection, although this is an uncommon means of development of a bone infection. A bone infection may also result from direct inoculation of bacteria. If this occurs, it is usually the result of an open fracture of a long bone or penetration of a bone such as is seen after nail punctures of the foot. Lastly, bone infections may be classified according to the type of infectious agent. Both pyogenic and granulomatous organisms may infect bone. We discuss only pyogenic infections in this chapter.

Pathogenesis

The metaphyses of long bones is where acute hematogenous osteomyelitis begins. The nutrient artery of the long bone divides within the medullary canal

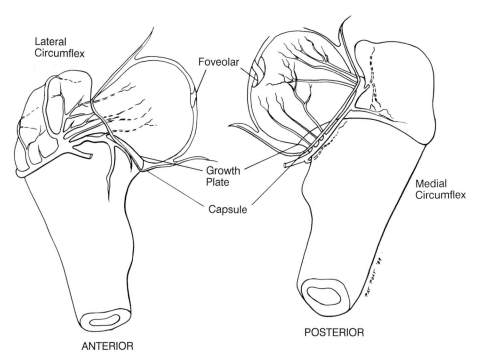

FIGURE 4-1. Views of the hip in a neonate. The intraosseous circulation in the femoral head of a neonate is different from that in a child older than 12 to 18 months. Blood vessels are seen crossing the growth plate in the femoral neck and head of a neonate.

TABLE 4-1.
Comparison of Acute and Subacute Hematogenous Osteomyelitis

	Subacute	Acute
White blood cell count	Frequently normal	Frequently elevated
Erythrocyte sedimentation rate	Frequently elevated	Frequently elevated
Blood cultures	Rarely positive	50% positive
Bone cultures	60% positive	90% positive
Localization	Diaphysis, metaphysis, epiphysis, cross physis	Metaphysis
Pain	Mild to moderate	Severe
Systemic illness	No	Fever, malaise
Loss of function	No or minimal	Marked
Prior antibiotics	30%–40%	Occasional
Initial radiograph	Frequently abnormal	Bone normal

of the bone, ending in small arterioles that ascend toward the physis. Just beneath the physis, these arterioles bend away from the physis and empty into venous lakes that drain into the medullary cavity. It is here, in the bend of these arterioles, that the infection begins. Bacteria injected into the osseous circulation are phagocytosed in the medullary cavity of the bone; phagocytosis, however, seems to be less active in the metaphysis. This differential in phagocytosis may explain the predilection of the metaphysis for the development of acute hematogenous osteomyelitis. A lack of reticuloendothelial cells in the metaphysis often exists, so bacteria that lodge there are more likely to multiply and establish an infection. The bacteria may also lodge in the metaphysis because of a decrease in the rate of circulation at the bend of the terminal arterioles before they empty into the venous lakes.

Trauma may be associated with the establishment of a bone infection in a certain location. Children with acute hematogenous osteomyelitis frequently complain of trauma as an inciting incident. It is well known that the trauma may simply bring the child's attention to a preexisting lesion. It has been shown, however, that rabbits in whom a bone is traumatized develop an infection more frequently in the traumatized bone than in nontraumatized areas after the production of a bacteremia.

Once established, the infection produces an exudate, and if the infection remains untreated, pus is produced. The fluid formed seeks the path of least resistance for egress from the metaphysis. The fluid can spread in one of three ways. It can spread from the metaphysis into the diaphysis; it can spread into the epiphysis across the physis; or it can exit the cortex of the bone, producing a collection of subperiosteal pus. Although an infection that commences in

the metaphysis of a long bone may occasionally spread into the diaphysis, it rarely does so. Instead, the infection generally spreads through the cortex of the metaphysis of the bone of a child. It is important to this discussion to understand the anatomy of the bone of a human at different ages to appreciate how the same infection behaves differently in patients of different ages. For example, the presence of transphyseal vessels in the neonate allows an infection that begins in the metaphysis of a long bone to easily spread into the epiphysis through these vessels (see Fig. 4-1).

In the child older than 1 year to 18 months, an osteomyelitis that begins in the metaphysis of a long bone usually spreads through the cortex of the metaphysis. The metaphyseal cortex of the infant is porous, thereby providing easy access for the egress of an exudate or pus. As the fluid exits the bone cortex, it elevates the periosteum, which in the child is loosely adherent to the cortex of the bone. The periosteum is, however, thick and therefore not easily penetrated, so the pus remains subperiosteal until there is enough periosteal destruction to allow the development of a soft tissue abscess. The periosteum of the adult is more thickly adherent to the bone cortex, but it is also much thinner and easily torn.

If an osteomyelitis progresses in a child, the infection that begins in the metaphysis produces loss of the endosteal blood supply of the involved bone because of thrombosis of the venous and arterial blood supply. Once pus escapes through the metaphyseal cortex, it elevates the periosteum, thereby depriving the bone of its remaining vascular supply. The portion of the bone that has become avascular is termed a *sequestrum*. The elevated periosteum remains viable because its blood supply, which is derived from the overlying muscle, is undisturbed. The cambium layer of the periosteum continues to produce bone; however, this bone is produced at a distance from the bone cortex because the periosteum has been elevated. This new periosteal bone is termed the *involucrum.*

Acute hematogenous osteomyelitis begins with a "cellulitis" phase in which no obvious pus has been produced. The patient will exhibit at the signs of a bone infection, but there will be no obvious pus formation. If this infection is left unchecked, however, an abscess will form. The pus then escapes through the cortex of the metaphysis of the long bone, producing a subperiosteal abscess. This concept of an initial cellulitis of bone is important because it is during this stage that medical treatment alone usually results in cure of the infection.

Staphylococcus aureus coagulase positive is the organism that causes the most cases of acute hematogenous osteomyelitis, being responsible for more than 90% of cases in otherwise normal children. Other organisms may rarely produce acute hematogenous osteomyelitis, such as bacteroides, pneumococcus, *Kingella kingae*, and *Haemophilus influenzae*. In neonates, *Staphylococcus* is still common, as are group B *Streptococcus* and gram-negative organisms. In patients with sickle cell disease, both *Staphylococcus* and *Salmonella* are known to cause acute hematogenous osteomyelitis.

Diagnosis

The diagnosis of acute hematogenous osteomyelitis depends on a high index of suspicion. Children with acute bone pain and systemic signs of sepsis should be considered to have acute hematogenous osteomyelitis until proved otherwise. Unfortunately, not all children with osteomyelitis have the characteristic findings that one typically associates with this disease, so the diagnosis is not always easily made. It is important, however, to make the diagnosis of acute hematogenous osteomyelitis early in the course of the disease, because both the course of the disease and its ultimate prognosis depend on the rapidity and adequacy of treatment.

For those instances in which an absolute diagnosis has not been established, the diagnosis of acute hematogenous osteomyelitis may be established if a patient fulfills two of the following criteria: (1) bone aspiration yielded pus; (2) bacterial culture of bone or blood was positive; (3) presence of the classical signs and symptoms of acute osteomyelitis exists; and (4) radiographic changes typical for osteomyelitis occur. It is important to have diagnostic criteria for acute

hematogenous osteomyelitis; these criteria should include the typical patient history and physical findings, because occasionally the cultures of bone may be negative; however, even with negative cultures one may make the presumptive diagnosis of acute hematogenous osteomyelitis if other criteria have been established. Most of the time, however, one makes the diagnosis of acute hematogenous osteomyelitis as a result of the typical history and physical findings combined with positive bone cultures.

History and Physical Examination

Children with acute hematogenous osteomyelitis usually present with a history of bone pain of one to several days' duration. The pain may be well localized if the child is old enough to cooperate. The pain may be poorly localized if the child is young or if the area of involvement produces confusing findings such as might be seen in patients with osteomyelitis of the pelvis. The pain usually is severe enough to seriously limit or completely restrict the use of the involved extremity. The child usually is febrile and relates a history of generalized malaise consistent with the generalized sepsis. Some children, however, present without generalized sepsis and therefore do not exhibit all of these complaints. Thus, one must not exclude the diagnosis of acute hematogenous osteomyelitis simply on the basis of a lack of sepsis, because this disease may be more or less virulent depending on the organism involved and the host resistance.

The physical examination of these children is extremely important for the establishment of the correct diagnosis. The examination may be difficult to perform, because these children are frightened and experience considerable pain. One must approach the child slowly and carefully, gaining the child's confidence before beginning the examination. This usually takes a few extra minutes, but the time is well spent. One should first attempt to establish the limb involved before the examination begins and also have an idea where in the limb the pain is localized. The examiner begins by palpating the uninvolved areas of the extremity after the rest of the child has been examined. The final portion of the examination focuses on the area of involvement.

Children with acute hematogenous osteomyelitis usually have swelling of the involved extremity. The swelling is localized to the area of the infection unless the infection has spread to involve much of the soft tissues of the extremity. Early in the course of the disease, the swelling is localized to the metaphysis of the involved long bone, which is warm. The overlying skin, however, is not red unless the bone involved is subcutaneous or unless the infection has spread and a subcutaneous abscess has developed.

Laboratory Data

It is important to obtain laboratory studies in every child suspected of having osteomyelitis; however, it must be emphasized that acute bone and joint infections are diagnosed by clinical means, and laboratory studies are used only as confirmatory evidence and never to make a diagnosis.

A complete blood count and an erythrocyte sedimentation rate should be obtained, both of which are usually elevated. In addition, there is frequently a left shift of the differential count of the white blood cells. Although these blood studies are usually abnormal in children with acute hematogenous osteomyelitis, one must never dismiss the diagnosis of acute hematogenous osteomyelitis simply because the white blood cell (WBC) count or the sedimentation rate is normal. Neonates frequently have no signs of infection, which makes the diagnosis of osteomyelitis more difficult in them.

Radiographic Findings

Radiographs of the involved extremity should be obtained; however, the bone changes that are characteristic of osteomyelitis are not seen for at least 10 to 14 days after the onset of the infection. Soft tissue swelling with loss of the normal soft tissue planes is seen before bone changes become apparent. The radiographic finding of soft tissue swelling, however, simply confirms the findings of a good physical exam that has established the existence of the swelling and determined its location (Fig. 4-2). Magnetic resonance imaging (MRI) has not been shown to be of greater benefit for the evaluation of suspected osteomyelitis than have other more conventional modalities.

Bone Scan

Bone scanning has become a popular method for the evaluation of children with suspected osteomyelitis. With the advent of technetium-99m (^{99m}Tc) bone scanning, the evaluation of the abnormal bone in the child became possible. The low radiation dose of this radioisotope and its affinity for bone make it ideal for the evaluation of the skeleton. ^{99m}Tc is taken up in areas of rapid bone formation or in areas of increased blood flow. Thus, one would expect that there would be increased uptake of ^{99m}Tc in areas of acute hematogenous osteomyelitis, but this is not always the case. The bone scan has been shown to have an accuracy rate as low as 80% in patients with acute hematogenous osteomyelitis. In some children, especially those in whom the infection is fulminant, the involved bone may have become avascular by the time of the scan, producing a cold scan. The reason for the cold scan is the loss of the endosteal circulation as a result of occlusion of the nutrient artery along with the loss of the periosteal circulation resulting from the elevation of the periosteum by a subperiosteal abscess. This cold scan should alert one that the infection of the bone demands immediate drainage.

The bone scan may be used to help confirm the diagnosis of osteomyelitis much as one would use the sedimentation rate or the WBC count; however, treatment must never be delayed while awaiting the results of a bone scan. It is important to note that needle aspiration of a bone does not alter the bone scan. Thus, bone aspiration itself will not cause a bone scan to be positive.

Bone scanning may be helpful when the exact localization of an acute infection is in doubt, such as in infections of the spine or the pelvis. Bone scanning may be of use in neonates, in whom multiple sites of infection are common, and it may also be helpful in the case of bone pain in children with sickle cell disease, for whom the differential diagnosis of acute hematogenous osteomyelitis from acute bone infarction is difficult.

Gallium scanning has been advocated by some authors, because radioactive gallium localizes in white blood cells and therefore would seem to be more specific for osteomyelitis than is ^{99m}Tc. Gallium scanning may be more specific than technetium scanning, but it is not more sensitive. If a ^{99m}Tc scan is negative, a gallium scan is likely to be negative also. In addition, the gallium scan requires at least 24 to 36 hours for an adequate study. Some authors have advocated the use of gallium scanning for the differentiation of bone infarction from osteomyelitis in patients with sickle cell disease.

Bone Aspiration

Once a clinical diagnosis of acute hematogenous osteomyelitis is established, a bacteriologic diagnosis is made by culturing the involved bone. Bone aspiration is mandatory not only to establish an accurate bac-

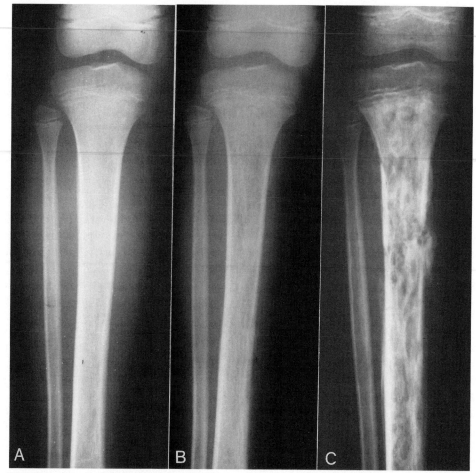

FIGURE 4-2. Radiographs of a child with progressive radiographic changes as the result of acute hematogenous osteomyelitis of the tibia. (**A**) AP radiographs of the tibia that demonstrate soft tissue swelling with loss of the normal tissue planes. (**B**) Radiographs of the same leg taken 2 weeks after the one in **A**. Here one can note the early mottled appearance of the tibia with a small amount of periosteal new bone seen on the medial cortex of the tibia. (**C**) Five weeks after presentation this AP radiograph of the tibia shows progressive destruction of the entire diaphysis and proximal metaphysis of the tibia. (Courtesy of Dr. R.H. Hensinger)

teriologic diagnosis but also to determine whether an abscess is present. Aspiration of the bone should be performed immediately after completion of the physical evaluation so that treatment may be started without delay.

The bone should be aspirated at the point of maximum swelling and pain, which is usually at the metaphyseal end of a long bone. One should use a large bore needle such as a 16- or 18-gauge spinal needle with an inner stylet. The stylet is necessary to prevent plugging of the end of the needle with bone. The needle is inserted just to the outer cortex of the bone, and the subperiosteal space is aspirated. If an abscess is encountered, the pus is cultured and a Gram stain is performed. In this instance, the di-

agnosis has been firmly established, and the need for drainage of the abscess has been determined. If no abscess is encountered, the needle is advanced into the bone through the cortex, which can be accomplished with ease in the metaphysis. The needle is gently twisted as it is advanced into the bone. Once the needle is through the cortex and is in the medullary cavity of the bone, the marrow is aspirated. Usually one obtains only marrow, but this must be cultured because almost invariably the cultures are positive. If no pus is found, the infection is in an early cellulitis stage (ie, before an abscess has developed). If an abscess is encountered, it should be cultured and surgically drained.

In addition to obtaining cultures of the involved

bone, one should obtain cultures of any and all lesions that could potentially have been the source of a bacteremia. Blood cultures should also be obtained, but they should not be relied on to make a bacterial diagnosis because only 50% of patients with acute hematogenous osteomyelitis have positive blood cultures. Ten percent of patients with acute hematogenous osteomyelitis have negative bone cultures, and in these instances, one may enhance the likelihood of obtaining a bacteriologic diagnosis if cultures of all possible sources plus the blood have been obtained.

Treatment

To effectively treat acute hematogenous osteomyelitis, sufficient antibiotic must be delivered to the site of the infection for an adequate period to sterilize the bone and eradicate the infection. Controversy occasionally arises between pediatrician and orthopaedist concerning the appropriate form of treatment. The pediatrician may recommend only parenteral antibiotic therapy, whereas the orthopaedic surgeon may recommend both surgical drainage and antibiotic treatment. This controversy will not arise if acute hematogenous osteomyelitis is considered an infectious disease rather than either a surgical or a medical disease. Principles of the treatment of infection then become evident. It is well established that sequestered abscesses require surgical drainage, but areas of simple inflammation without abscess formation respond to antibiotics alone. Bone aspiration is therefore important in determining the future course of therapy of the child with an osteomyelitis. If an abscess is encountered either under the periosteum or within the bone itself, surgical drainage of the abscess is required. If no abscess is found, antibiotics alone should suffice in eradicating the infection, because treatment begins during the cellulitis stage of the infection, before the formation of an abscess.

Surgical drainage should also be considered when the patient does not respond to appropriate antibiotic therapy after a negative bone aspiration. In that instance, an abscess may have developed that requires drainage. If a child with acute hematogenous osteomyelitis does not show symptomatic improvement with decrease in swelling and tenderness after 36 to 48 hours of appropriate antibiotic treatment, the bone should be aspirated again and consideration given to surgical drainage. The fever should also begin to decline, although it may remain elevated for several more days.

If surgical treatment is necessary, the bone involved should be approached directly over the area of involvement. A subperiosteal abscess should be thoroughly drained and débrided. Whether or not the bone should be opened is subject to debate. Some authors think that if a subperiosteal abscess is found, an intraosseous abscess is not likely because it would have spontaneously drained itself into the subperiosteal space through the porous metaphyseal cortex. Conversely, if no abscess is found under the periosteum, the intraosseous abscess will not have drained itself into the subperiosteal space, and the bone must be opened. Although we and others have not found pus under pressure within the bone cortex at the time of drainage of a subperiosteal abscess, it is probably wise to drill the metaphyseal cortex to be certain that no abscess is sequestered within the bone. It is probably not necessary to widely open the bone to curette it unless pus is discovered at the time of drilling of the bone cortex.

Surgical treatment, if needed, should not create more tissue damage than has already been created by the infection itself. If pus escapes through the metaphyseal cortex, the periosteum is elevated and the periosteal blood supply is compromised, leaving the bone cortex avascular. When draining an abscess, one should not elevate the periosteum more than it has already been elevated, so as to avoid creating further sequestration of the bone.

Once the abscess is adequately débrided, the wound may be closed over a drain. It is not necessary nor recommended to leave the wound open, unless one is dealing with a chronic, long-standing osteomyelitis. A suction drain or a Penrose drain may be used and removed in 2 to 4 days. Closed suction-irrigation is not necessary and introduces a significant risk of superinfection with gram-negative organisms.

Antibiotics

Antibiotics are begun immediately after all cultures are obtained, whether or not surgical drainage is necessary. The initial choice of antibiotic is made on a best-guess basis. At least 90% of the cases of acute hematogenous osteomyelitis in otherwise normal children are caused by coagulase-positive staphylococci. Thus, the antibiotic chosen should be one that effectively treats this organism. For patients who are not allergic to penicillin, a semisynthetic penicillin that is β-lactamase resistant should be chosen. The antibiotic of choice is either oxacillin or nafcillin. Methicillin is also effective, but this antibiotic carries a higher risk of interstitial nephritis than do the others. If one choses nafcillin, one must be careful with peripheral needle sites for the administration of the drug IV, because nafcillin may cause significant sloughing of the skin and subcutaneous tissues if infiltration of the IV solution occurs.

The recommended dosage of these antibiotics is 150 to 200 mg/kg administered in divided doses over 24 hours. The appropriate length of therapy has been a subject of debate for many years. In the past, children with acute hematogenous osteomyelitis were treated for 6 weeks with IV antibiotics in the hospital. It became apparent that this was excessive, and a regimen of 3 weeks of IV antibiotics followed by 3 weeks of oral therapy was adopted. Because it has been shown more recently that adequate blood levels of antibiotic may be achieved with oral administration, the current mode of therapy involves a shorter period of initial IV therapy, given a good response by the patient, followed by oral therapy.

Combined IV and oral antibiotic therapy has now become accepted as the standard treatment for acute hematogenous osteomyelitis. This mode of therapy is more complicated than the simple treatment of the child with IV antibiotics for the entire course, because it requires the complete cooperation of the family and the child. In addition, one must be certain that the antibiotic is adequately absorbed from the gastrointestinal tract, providing sufficient blood levels of the drug.

The current regimen is to begin treatment of the patient with IV antibiotics. If the patient responds quickly to this form of therapy, one may consider switching the child to oral antibiotics (Table 4-2). To be able to do this, one must meet certain requirements (Table 4-3).

Antistaphylococcal antibiotic therapy is started while awaiting the culture results. Once the organism

TABLE 4-2.
Contraindications to Oral Antibiotic Therapy

Inability to swallow or retain medicine

Etiologic agent not established

Inability of the laboratory to perform analysis of serum bactericidal activity

Infection with agent for which no effective oral therapy exists (eg, *Pseudomonas*)

Failure of patient to demonstrate clinical response to parenteral antibiotics

(Jackson MA, Nelson JD. Etiology and medical management of acute suppurative bone and joint infections in pediatric patients. J Pediatr Orthop 1982;2:320)

TABLE 4-3.
Requirements for Oral Therapy of Osteomyelitis

Adequate response to intravenous therapy needed

Compliance must be ensured

Organism must be obtained and sensitivity to proposed antibiotics must be good

Serum concentration of the antibiotic must be determined

Serum bactericidal concentrations of at least 1:8 must be obtained

Laboratory must be capable of performing these studies

is identified, the antibiotic is adjusted if necessary. It is important to retain the bacteria so that the laboratory may be able to test it against the antibiotic being used to be certain that adequate blood levels can be obtained. If the child responds quickly to the initial therapy with IV antibiotics, consideration is given to beginning oral therapy. The IV antibiotics are continued for at least 5 days, although some physicians prefer to treat with IV antibiotics for a longer period before beginning oral therapy. Oral therapy is begun 5 to 7 days after the initiation of IV therapy if there has been a good clinical response to the initial treatment.

Oral therapy is begun in the hospital to be certain of compliance and patient tolerance of the drug. Peak serum levels of the antibiotic are determined by obtaining a blood sample 1 hour after the oral dosage of the drug. The bactericidal level of the drug in the blood should be 1:8 or greater. If the patient is reliable, he or she may be discharged from the hospital and followed as an outpatient once all studies have been completed. If compliance is not assured, the child should be followed in the hospital. If the child is discharged, he or she should be seen weekly and blood levels of the antibiotic determined at that time to be certain that the drug is being taken and that it is being absorbed. Treatment should continue for a total of 6 weeks, which includes the time of IV and oral therapy combined.

If there is adequate response to the IV therapy, oral dicloxacillin may be started at a dosage of 50 mg/kg/24 h. As an alternative, cephalexin may be administered at a dosage of 150 mg/kg/24 h. The oral suspension form of dicloxacillin is not palatable, and parents may find it difficult to persuade young children to swallow it. For that reason, cephalexin may be preferred, as the oral suspension of this antibiotic is more palatable. Cephalexin may also be used as the IV drug, at a dosage of 150 mg/kg/24 h, in place of the semisynthetic penicillin. Other authors favor the use of clindamycin for both IV and oral therapy. The dosage of clindamycin is 30 mg/kg/24 h IV, followed by 50 mg/kg/24 h by mouth. This is particularly attractive in patients who are allergic to penicillin. Methicillin-resistant staphylococcal organisms are rare but have been reported, and for these one should use vancomycin, 50 mg/kg/24 h IV, combined with rifampin, 15 mg/kg/24 h orally. Although in vitro sensitivity tests of methicillin-resistant staphylococci may show sensitivity to cephalosporins, in vivo these organisms have not responded to this class of antibiotics.

Neonatal Osteomyelitis

Osteomyelitis in the neonate is a different disease from that seen in children because of the variety of organisms involved, the frequency of multiple sites of infection, and the presence of transphyseal vessels until age 12 to 18 months, which leads to infection on both sides of the physis. As a result, this will likely result in destruction of the center of ossification of the epiphysis and the physis itself, producing complete growth arrest (Fig. 4-3). This is most likely to occur in the proximal femur, where the result is destruction of the head of the femur. The infection frequently spreads out of the involved epiphysis into the joint, producing a septic arthritis.

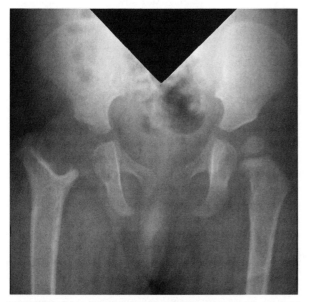

FIGURE 4-3. AP radiograph of the pelvis of a 1-year-old girl who had an osteomyelitis of the proximal femur and a septic arthritis of the hip as a neonate. This resulted in destruction of the physis and the epiphysis.

Osteomyelitis in the neonate frequently produces fewer clinical and laboratory signs than in the child. Although *Staphylococcus* may be the etiologic agent of the osteomyelitis, gram-negative organisms and group B *Streptococcus* are also common; therefore, antibiotics that cover all of the organisms must be given while awaiting the results of cultures. Neonates with acute hematogenous osteomyelitis frequently have multiple sites of involvement—as often as 40% of the time. Infants with multiple sites of osteomyelitis are usually sick before the onset of the infection, and most have an umbilical catheter. Infants with single sites of osteomyelitis have a milder disease and are generally less ill than those with multiple sites of infection.

Special Sites of Infection

Acute hematogenous osteomyelitis of the pelvis may be difficult to diagnose, requiring a high index of suspicion for establishment of the correct diagnosis. Children with acute infection of the pelvis often are initially thought to have infection of the hip joint because the pain is frequently intense and often limits motion of the hip joint. The correct diagnosis can be established by performing a careful examination. Carefully moving the hip joint usually demonstrates a free, painless range of movement, whereas palpation of the pelvis establishes the area of maximum tenderness. Septic arthritis of the sacroiliac joint is also frequently confused with osteomyelitis of the pelvis. In this disease, tests specific for pain in the sacroiliac joint—such as the figure 4 test (one leg is placed across on top of the other leg with the knee bent to 90 degrees, as in the number 4, and the pelvis is then rocked using the crossed leg as a lever arm) and pelvic compression—are positive. Plain radiographs of the pelvis are normal in the early stages of osteomyelitis of the pelvis and in septic arthritis of the sacroiliac joint. Bone scintigraphy usually is positive. As in acute osteomyelitis of other bones, however, a certain percentage of these infections have false-negative bone scans. Bacterial confirmation of the diagnosis is established by bone aspiration.

An abscess may develop in patients with acute hematogenous osteomyelitis of the pelvis. If this occurs, surgical drainage of the abscess is necessary. A child with acute hematogenous osteomyelitis of the pelvis should be evaluated in the same manner as the child with an infection of a long bone, with an appropriate history and physical examination. In addition, laboratory data should be obtained. Bone aspiration should also be performed, and antibiotics should be started once all cultures have been obtained. Because of the possibility of developing an intrapelvic abscess that is not detectable either on physical examination or through needle aspiration, CT scanning of the pelvis should be performed. If an abscess is seen, it should be drained through an appropriate surgical approach and the child treated with antibiotics to sterilize the bone (Fig. 4-4).

Osteomyelitis of the spine in children and infants is rare. A much more common presentation of infection of the spinal column is the disk space infection, which is discussed in the subacute osteomyelitis section. True osteomyelitis of the spine produces significant bone destruction. Neonates with osteomyelitis of the spine develop abnormalities of the spine that resemble congenital defects.

Sickle Cell Disease

Acute hematogenous osteomyelitis in patients with sickle cell disease differs from osteomyelitis in otherwise normal patients. The two major differences in the two forms of osteomyelitis are that the infection in patients with sickle cell disease is usually located in the diaphysis of long bones rather than in the metaphysis. In addition, the organism responsible for the infection is frequently salmonella, although *Staphylococcus* is also common in patients with sickle cell disease. The salmonella bacteria enter the blood stream through microinfarcts in the gut lining, producing a bacteremia. The bacteria may then produce bone infection at the site of an acute bone infarction.

Patients with sickle cell disease and acute bone pain present a difficult diagnostic problem, because acute bone infarcts are painful and produce clinical findings often identical to those of patients with osteomyelitis. Thus, it is frequently difficult to differentiate between an area of acute bone infarction and one of acute osteomyelitis. The infarction and the infection are usually located in the diaphysis of a long bone, and both are associated with severe pain and restricted use of the involved extremity. Patients with acute osteomyelitis usually have a higher and more persistent fever than those with infarction. The sedimentation rate and peripheral WBC count may be elevated in both but are usually higher in patients with infection.

The diagnosis of acute osteomyelitis in these children is therefore difficult. As mentioned earlier, children with infection exhibit somewhat severer clinical findings. Bone scanning maybe helpful in

these patients. A cold bone scan usually indicates a bone infarct, whereas normal uptake or increased uptake on the bone scan usually indicates infection. Cultures of the patient's stool should be performed, as should bone aspiration.

SUBACUTE HEMATOGENOUS OSTEOMYELITIS

Subacute hematogenous osteomyelitis differs from acute osteomyelitis in the severity of the clinical signs. The systemic signs seen in patients with subacute forms of the disease are either absent or much less severe than those seen in patients with the acute form of the disease. In addition, the location of the subacute form of the disease may differ from that seen with acute osteomyelitis (see Table 4-1).

Classification

Some authors have classified subacute osteomyelitis according to the location and radiographic appearance of the lesion. This, however, does not consider the differences in clinical presentation of these different forms of subacute osteomyelitis. The classification based on radiographic appearance was first described by Gledhill and subsequently modified by others. In this classification, the type 1 lesion is a central metaphyseal lesion. The type 2 lesion is also metaphyseal, but it is eccentrically placed with cortical erosion present. The type 3 lesion is an abscess in the cortex of the diaphysis, and the type 4 lesion is a medullary abscess in the diaphysis without cortical destruction but with periosteal reaction present. The type 5 lesion is primary epiphyseal osteomyelitis. The type 6 lesion is a subacute infection that crosses the physis (Fig. 4-5).

This classification system excludes the subacute osteomyelitis that begins in the metaphysis and crosses the physis to involve the epiphysis. Acute hematogenous osteomyelitis in the child older than age 18 months rarely crosses the physis; however, subacute osteomyelitis frequently does. The lesion may be primarily metaphyseal with only a small portion of the physis and epiphysis involved (Fig. 4-6). Conversely, much of the physis may be involved (Fig. 4-7). In the neonate with acute hematogenous osteomyelitis that crosses the physis to involve the epiphysis, the physis is frequently destroyed as is the growth center of the epiphysis (see Fig. 4-3). Con-

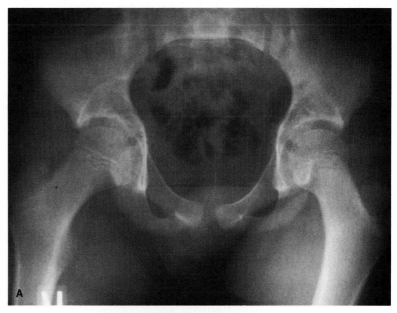

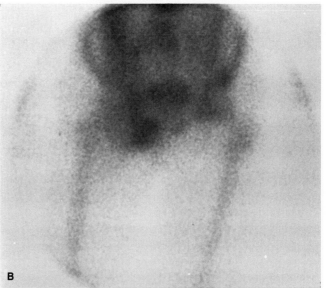

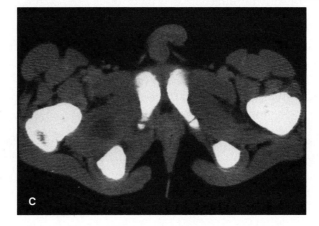

FIGURE 4-4. Eight-year-old boy with osteomyelitis of the pubis and a pelvic abscess. (**A**) AP radiograph of the pelvis of this child demonstrating no bony abnormalities. (**B**) Technetium-99m bone scan demonstrating increased uptake of the isotope in the region of the right pubis. (**C**) CT scan through the obturator region of the pelvis demonstrating an abscess in the obturator region of the right hemipelvis.

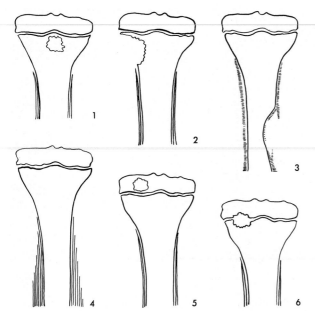

FIGURE 4-5. Classification of subacute osteomyelitis. Type 1 is a central metaphyseal lesion. Type 2 is an eccentric metaphyseal lesion with erosion of cortex. Type 3 is a lesion of cortex of diaphysis. The type 4 lesion of the diaphysis demonstrates periosteal new bone formation but without a definite bone lesion. Type 5 is primary subacute epiphyseal osteomyelitis, and type 6 represents subacute osteomyelitis that crosses physis involving both the metaphysis and epiphysis.

versely, the subacute infection that crosses the physis rarely causes permanent damage to the growth plate.

One may also subclassify subacute hematogenous osteomyelitis into two types according to the rapidity of onset and severity of presenting symptoms. One type has a fairly acute presentation, and children with this type of infection usually present within a week or two of the onset of symptoms. Radiographic changes may be present at the time of presentation; however, the infection is usually diaphyseal. This type of infection thus encompasses types 3 and 4 of the Gledhill classification system. This diaphyseal infection could easily be confused with Ewing sarcoma, and a biopsy may be necessary to exclude this diagnosis. Frequently, however, the clinical and radiographic picture is characteristic enough to make a presumptive diagnosis of infection. Children with this type of subacute infection may have a fever, although it will not be as elevated as one would see in acute hematogenous osteomyelitis. In addition, children with this type of infection usually continue to walk even if the femur, the most commonly involved bone, is infected. They will, however, limp and complain of pain. The peripheral WBC count and the sedimentation rate may be ele-

vated, although the sedimentation rate is more commonly elevated (Fig. 4-8). The second type of subacute infection encompasses types 1, 2, 5, and 6. Children with this type of infection have minimal symptoms, but the complaints are frequently of longer duration. There are no systemic signs, and the peripheral WBC count and the sedimentation rate usually are normal. Radiographic changes are present at the time of presentation and may be described as a lucency located anywhere within a bone.

Diagnosis and Treatment

The diagnosis in patients with subacute infection of the diaphysis of a long bone is confirmed by bone aspiration for bacterial culture. The cultures usually are positive for *S aureus* and are coagulase-positive. The treatment of this lesion depends on several fac-

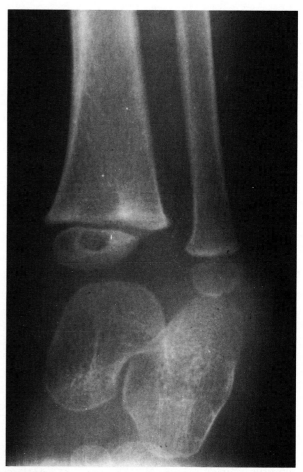

FIGURE 4-6. AP radiograph of the distal tibia demonstrating an area of subacute osteomyelitis that involves the metaphysis, physis, and the epiphysis.

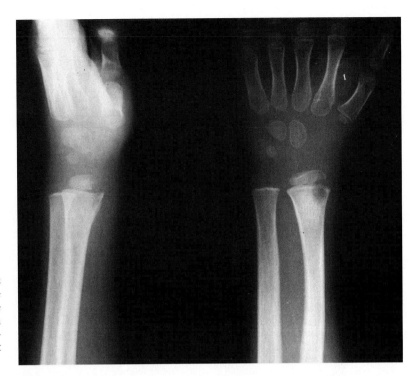

FIGURE 4-7. AP and lateral radiographs of a distal radius of a child with subacute osteomyelitis that crosses the physis. The AP radiograph demonstrates that the lesion involves both the metaphysis and the epiphysis. On the lateral radiograph, significant erosion of the epiphysis is seen.

tors. If the diagnosis is in question, open biopsy may be required, at which time débridement is carried out if infection is established at the time. If a sequestrum is present, sequestrectomy is required for eradication of the infection. Most commonly, however, the patient presents with minimal radiographic bone changes, and simple antibiotic therapy alone usually results in eradication of the infection, because there is no abscess present.

Lesions of subacute osteomyelitis can usually be diagnosed as subacute osteomyelitis radiographically; however, there are instances in which the diagnosis is in question. Open biopsy is therefore frequently required in making the diagnosis (Fig. 4-9). In addition, because there is a radiographic lesion, an abscess has formed and débridement is usually required, although some authors have reported healing without débridement. Frequently no pus is evident at exploration; however, one may find granulation tissue within the cavity that should be débrided. Cultures may be sterile, but *S aureus* and *S epidermidis* are the most common organisms.

The treatment of subacute osteomyelitis should be similar to that of acute osteomyelitis. One begins with IV antibiotics and may then switch to oral antibiotics if there are no contraindications. As mentioned earlier, débridement is usually necessary for subacute osteomyelitis with a radiographic lesion or if a sequestrum has formed or if the patient has not responded adequately to antibiotics.

CHRONIC MULTIFOCAL OSTEOMYELITIS

Chronic osteomyelitis may be defined as osteomyelitis presenting with symptoms that have been present for months or longer. Also included in the diagnosis of chronic osteomyelitis is any recurrent osteomyelitis. This chapter does not deal with the chronic osteomyelitis that results from a recurrence of a previously treated infection or from an open wound such as an open fracture. The only exception is the special circumstance of nail puncture wound infections of the foot, which are covered in the next section.

The etiology of chronic multifocal osteomyelitis is unknown at the present time, but it is presumed to be due to an infectious agent. The disease produces vague bone pain in multiple sites. Frequently the symptoms seem to be unilateral, despite the fact that lesions occur bilaterally. Children with this disease usually do not exhibit systemic signs of infection such as an elevated temperature. Although the peripheral WBC count is normal, the sedimentation rate is frequently elevated.

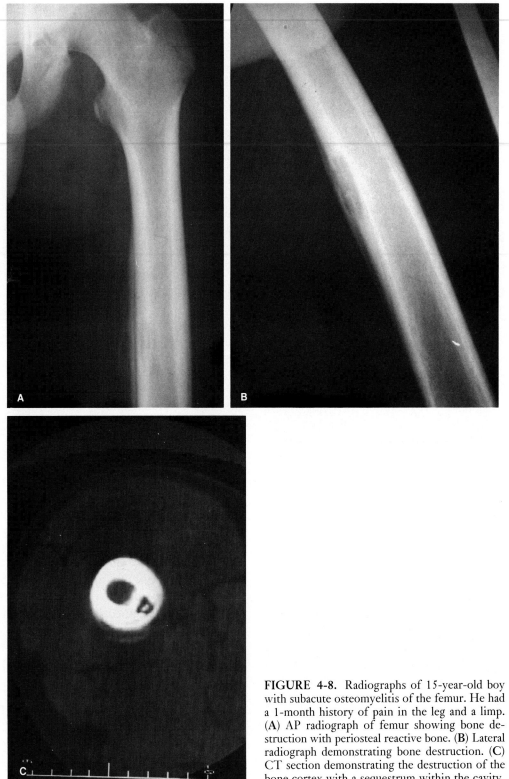

FIGURE 4-8. Radiographs of 15-year-old boy with subacute osteomyelitis of the femur. He had a 1-month history of pain in the leg and a limp. (A) AP radiograph of femur showing bone destruction with periosteal reactive bone. (B) Lateral radiograph demonstrating bone destruction. (C) CT section demonstrating the destruction of the bone cortex with a sequestrum within the cavity.

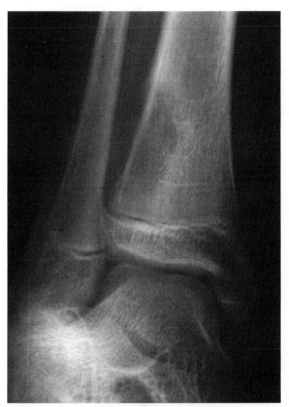

FIGURE 4-9. Oblique radiograph of the distal tibia of an 11-year-old girl with a 1-month history of pain, swelling, and redness of ankle. There is a metaphyseal lesion of the distal tibia that resembles subacute osteomyelitis; however, the biopsy revealed that the lesion was an osteogenic sarcoma.

Multiple lytic lesions that have little surrounding bone reaction and are generally located in the metaphyses of the long bones are seen radiographically (Fig. 4-10). The medial end of the clavicle seems to be the bone that is most frequently involved, followed by the distal tibia and then the distal femur.

Based on clinical and radiographic findings, these lesions are thought to be caused by an infectious agent. The histology of these lesions is typical of osteomyelitis; however, the agent responsible has not as yet been identified with certainty. The treatment is symptomatic. The natural history of this disease usually involves spontaneous resolution of the lesions and the clinical signs and symptoms, which may take anywhere from 1 to 15 years.

DISK SPACE INFECTION

Etiology

Controversy has arisen as to the etiology of disk space infections, resulting in the term *diskitis*. This disease is usually regarded, however, as an osteomyelitis of the vertebral end-plates that secondarily invades the disk without producing an acute osteomyelitis of the vertebral body. The organism that produces the infection in children is usually *S aureus*, although other organisms are common in older patients, especially drug abusers, and in debilitated patients.

Clinical Findings

Although disk space infection may occur at any age, it is most common in the younger child, who may present with an inability to walk as the primary presenting feature, although the most common complaint is back pain. Unfortunately, in the infant and toddler the diagnosis of back pain may be difficult. Some children present with abdominal pain as the primary complaint. Frequently, the infant is irritable without other definite complaints.

The physical findings in these patients are characteristic, and the diagnosis can usually be established on the basis of the physical examination alone. Because the disk space infection usually occurs in the lumbar spine, the child splints the spine, refusing to flex it. Although the child may be able to bend at the waist, no flexion occurs in the spine itself. Some children are adept at compensating for the pain and may function relatively normally. They will, however, exhibit complete restriction of motion of the spine on examination.

This disease entity differs from osteomyelitis of the spine in that there are usually few, if any, systemic signs in patients with disk space infection. The patient's body temperature is usually normal as is the peripheral WBC count. The sedimentation rate is frequently, although not invariably, elevated.

Radiographic Findings

The radiographic findings depend on the delay in diagnosis. The disease characteristically produces narrowing of the disk space with irregularity of the adjacent vertebral end-plates. This may be difficult to see radiographically, especially in a young child early in the course of the disease. Lateral tomography of the involved area of the spine is helpful in demonstrating the disk space and bone abnormality. These radiographs help eliminate the overlying gas that frequently obscures the spine in the lumbar region.

Bone scanning has been a popular method of diagnosing disk space infections. The bone scan usually demonstrates an area of increased uptake in the infected disk space, but some scans will be false-

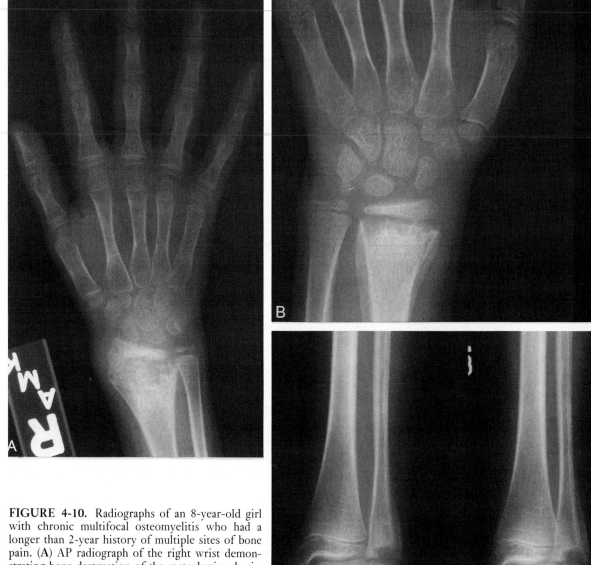

FIGURE 4-10. Radiographs of an 8-year-old girl with chronic multifocal osteomyelitis who had a longer than 2-year history of multiple sites of bone pain. (**A**) AP radiograph of the right wrist demonstrating bone destruction of the metaphysis, physis, and epiphysis. (**B**) AP radiograph of the left wrist demonstrating bone destruction in the metaphysis with periosteal reactive bone. (**C**) Radiographs of the left ankle demonstrating metaphyseal and physeal destruction of the distal fibula with periosteal reactive bone.

negative. Therefore, the diagnosis of disk space infection should not be excluded because of a normal bone scan. MRI has been shown to be able to accurately demonstrate an abnormal disk space, and the authors have recently demonstrated that the MRI is abnormal before the bone scan is positive and before radiographic changes are evident (Fig. 4-11).

Diagnosis

The diagnosis of disk space infection is usually made on clinical grounds because of the characteristic physical findings. The clinical diagnosis is confirmed with radiographs that show the characteristic disk space narrowing and erosion of the vertebral endplates. Normally with a bone infection, a tissue or bacteriologic confirmation of the diagnosis would be necessary; however, because of the morbidity of needle aspiration of the spine, this procedure is usually not justified for the child exhibiting the characteristic findings of a disk space infection. The infecting

organism is usually *S aureus*. Aspiration biopsy of the spine should be reserved for the child who does not respond to initial treatment with antistaphylococcal antibiotics. One should also perform a biopsy of the disk space when the disease is unusual in any respect. If the infection involves an older child such as a teenager, or if drug abuse is suspected, a biopsy should be performed because of the possibility of a gram-negative organism being the etiologic agent.

Treatment

Some authors have advocated the use of spinal immobilization for children with disk space infection. They have shown that many patients respond to immobilization alone and consequently reserve antibiotics for the child who does not respond to immobilization alone. Most authors, however, favor the use of antibiotics as one would for any other bone infection. These children should, therefore, be started on oxacillin or cephalosporin in doses that would be

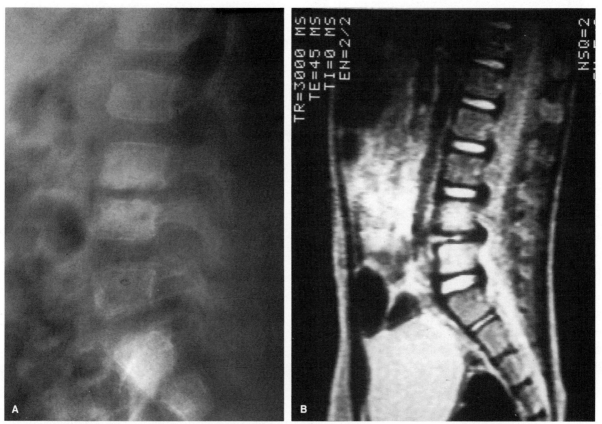

FIGURE 4-11. MRI of the spine demonstrating an abnormal L4-L5 disk. Note the loss of height and the change in the density of the disk. The bone scan, the plain radiographs, and the lateral tomograms of this patient were normal. The lateral radiograph of the spine subsequently demonstrated the typical changes seen in disk space infections.

used for osteomyelitis. Treatment should be continued for 1 to 2 weeks with IV antibiotics, followed by oral antibiotics for another 4 weeks.

Immobilization of the spine has been a mainstay of the treatment of disk space infection. However, most children with disk space infection usually respond quickly to IV antibiotics. Therefore, immobilization is used only in those patients who do not exhibit a rapid and dramatic response to the IV antibiotic treatment.

PSEUDOMONAS INFECTIONS OF THE FOOT FOLLOWING PUNCTURE WOUNDS

Clinical Presentation

Puncture wounds of the foot are relatively common injuries. The exact number of complications of these injuries is not known, although a 10% rate has been reported.

The presentation of the infectious complications of nail punctures is characteristic. Typically, the patient is a child with tennis shoes who steps on a nail, sustaining a puncture of the foot that invariably either enters a bone or joint or punctures the plantar fascia. These children experience pain from the initial puncture wound, but this pain usually diminishes quickly. Children who develop a pseudomonal infection experience increasing pain in the foot 2 to 4 days after the initial trauma. These symptoms worsen so that within a day or so the children is not able to bear weight.

At presentation there is pain and swelling about the area of the puncture wound and throughout the area of the bone or joint infection, with signs of inflammation, including redness of the skin. Careful examination of the foot reveals pain and tenderness on the dorsum of the foot over the involved bone or joint.

Despite the fact that this is an infection of the foot, there frequently are no or few systemic signs of infection. The child's temperature usually is normal, as is the WBC count. Unfortunately, these findings have prompted many to underestimate the seriousness of this infection.

Treatment

The infection of the foot following puncture wounds is almost always caused by *Pseudomonas aeruginosa*, which has been grown from cultures taken from within the sole of tennis shoes. This infection requires thorough surgical débridement and prolonged antibiotic treatment. Antibiotic coverage alone does not eradicate the infection and only allows the infection to destroy more tissue. Once the diagnosis of bone or joint infection of the foot following puncture wound is made, a thorough débridement is performed. Prior aspiration of the area of infection may be performed, but this is not always necessary because the signs and symptoms of this infection are so typical that culture of the tissues at the time of débridement is sufficient. It is important, however, that no antibiotics be given until adequate cultures of the area of infection are obtained. Superficial cultures from the area of the puncture wound are not sufficient; it is necessary to obtain cultures from the bone or joint involved. *Pseudomonas* rarely produces the thick pus typical of other infections. Rather, one finds a thin, watery, serosanguineous fluid typical of early *Pseudomonas* infections.

The surgical approach to the area of infection depends on the area of involvement. If one is dealing with a septic arthritis of the metacarpophalangeal joint, the joint may be drained through a dorsal incision rather than through the puncture wound itself. If infection exists only within the sole of the foot under the plantar fascia, a plantar incision is necessary. If there is extensive infection of one of the bones of the foot, débridement may be required, using both dorsal and plantar incisions.

After thorough débridement and culture, IV antibiotics are required. Because the involved organism is usually *Pseudomonas*, no oral antibiotics are able to treat this organism. Generally, aminoglycoside antibiotics are used. Either gentamicin or tobramycin is administered in a dosage of 5 mg/kg/24 h in three divided doses. The length of treatment depends on the patient's response, the extent of the infection, and the thoroughness of the débridement. In general, the more thorough the débridement, the shorter the length of antibiotic treatment necessary. Some authors have recommended a minimum of 3 weeks of antibiotics to a maximum of 6 weeks. The sedimentation rate may be used as a guide to the length of therapy, with the recommendation that antibiotics be discontinued when the sedimentation rate falls to normal.

The sequelae of this infection depend on the interval between the puncture wound and the onset of appropriate treatment. The longer the delay before débridement of the foot and the commencement of aminoglycoside therapy, the worse the sequelae. To minimize sequelae, it is important to quickly establish the correct diagnosis and to perform the surgical débridement.

SEPTIC ARTHRITIS

Pathogenesis

Acute septic arthritis is a relatively uncommon disease. It may be associated with acute osteomyelitis, especially in the proximal femur, where bacteria escape the cortex of the metaphysis and invade the adjacent joint, producing a joint infection. In other cases, the joint infection is simply the result of hematogenous infection of the synovium or synovial fluid without prior bone infection. This isolated joint infection may be treated differently from the bone infection, which requires longer antibiotic therapy, because of the possible presence of necrotic bone within the area of the infection. With a pure septic arthritis, bone sequestration does not occur. In addition, antibiotics are delivered across the synovium into the joint in high concentrations.

Organisms

Different organisms prevail as the most common infecting organisms depending on the age of the patient. *S aureus* is the most common organism over all age groups. In the neonate, as we have seen in bone infections, group B *Streptococcus* is common, as are gram-negative organisms. In the child between the age of 6 months to 5 years, type B *H influenzae* is common, and in some series the most common agent in septic arthritis in this age group. In the older child *S aureus* becomes the most common organism. In the teenager, however, *Neisseria gonorrhoeae* is common and may be the most common cause of septic arthritis. It is certainly the most common cause of polyarthritis in that age group.

Diagnosis

Children with septic arthritis usually exhibit all the clinical signs of sepsis, with elevated temperature, malaise, and local signs of inflammation. The onset of septic arthritis is frequently more acute than is the onset of osteomyelitis. The child, especially the neonate, may present with pseudoparalysis of the extremity. The older child will protect the extremity, and if a joint of the lower extremity is involved, the child will usually refuse to walk.

The physical examination reveals an irritable child with a painful joint. Few other diseases produce such exquisite joint pain. The differential diagnosis includes acute rheumatic fever or acute juvenile arthritis, both of which may produce acute joint inflammation that is as painful as that produced by septic arthritis. In both of these diseases, the joint effusion also is significant, and the WBC count in the synovial fluid may occasionally be as high as 100,000 cells. The diagnosis usually can be made by other laboratory means, although the diagnosis occasionally is made retrospectively after treating a child for an infection.

Inspection of the child reveals a warm and painful joint with an effusion. The child will resist movement, splinting the joint in the position of greatest comfort. Laboratory data may be helpful. The peripheral WBC count is usually elevated, as is the sedimentation rate, although the diagnosis of septic arthritis should not be excluded simply on the basis of normal values for these two studies. Radiographs may demonstrate the joint swelling, although they are of little benefit early in the course of the disease except to exclude other problems.

Joint aspiration is mandatory for fluid analysis and culture of the synovial fluid. The joint fluid should be inspected visually. The fluid in patients with an infection of the joint varies in color from cloudy yellow to creamy white or gray, especially if the infection has been present for a period or if the organism is particularly virulent. Thus, the earlier the infection is diagnosed and the joint aspirated, the clearer the fluid. The fluid should be analyzed for cell count with a differential count of the WBCs. In most septic joints, the WBC count is greater than 50,000, and usually greater than 100,000. The one exception is in gonococcal arthritis, in which the WBC count is frequently lower than 50,000 cells. The differential count of polymorphonuclear leukocytes demonstrates that they constitute over 90%, and usually over 95%, of the total WBCs in the fluid.

A Gram stain and culture of the synovial fluid is obviously important and provides the basis for the definitive diagnosis of septic arthritis. The fluid should be transported immediately to the laboratory and plated on the appropriate medium. Laboratory personnel must be informed that the fluid is from a joint and should also know what the physician suspects, which enables the technician to perform the appropriate cultures. There are some special circumstances that require special techniques for organism retrieval. *H influenzae* is difficult to culture, and the plates must be incubated under a carbon dioxide environment. Despite meticulous culture techniques, a percentage of septic joints yield negative cultures. In some series, the percentage of organism retrieval was only 70%. Therefore, blood cultures should also be performed. Despite this, the diagnosis of septic arthritis may have to be made on clinical grounds in some patients because of negative bacterial cultures.

Because of the possibility of negative joint fluid cultures, one should also perform glucose determination on the joint fluid. In addition, lactic acid determination of the joint fluid and counterimmunoelectrophoresis may be helpful for the detection of *H influenzae*.

Treatment

The principles of treatment of septic arthritis do not differ from those of the treatment of infections in other areas of the body. The infection should be considered an abscess that requires drainage for eradication of the infection. In addition, the infection requires appropriate antibiotic therapy to sterilize the joint. The joint infection differs from other infections, in that it occurs in a closed space with easy access for needle aspiration and irrigation. In addition, antibiotics readily cross the synovial barrier and are concentrated in the synovial fluid.

Thorough débridement of the joint is required to completely eradicate the infection of the joint. In some instances, this may be accomplished with aspiration and irrigation of the joint without surgical débridement. Most reports of aspiration and irrigation technique of joint débridement of infection have reported good results. The requirements for this technique are specific. The major contraindication to aspiration irrigation technique for the treatment of joint infections is the hip joint being the site of infection. This joint must always be surgically drained in the face of an acute infection, because the vascular supply of the hip joint is intracapsular, and therefore these vessels are easily obliterated if the pressure within the hip joint is elevated. In the case of acute septic arthritis of the hip joint, the joint must be surgically drained as an emergency.

The technique of aspiration irrigation of infected joints requires that the joint be easily accessible for aspiration. Because of its accessibility, the knee joint is the joint most frequently treated with this technique. The ankle joint is also relatively accessible. The other joints of the body are less accessible and therefore more difficult to adequately débride through a needle.

Joint aspiration must be performed sterilely with the use of a large-bore needle. The fluid is fully drained from the joint and sent for appropriate studies. Without removing the needle, the joint is irrigated with sterile IV saline until the fluid that is returned is clear. The joint should be splinted and the patient started on antibiotics while awaiting the culture results. If the WBC count of the fluid is low (ie, below 80,000 to 100,000), and there is no particulate matter in the aspirate, this aspiration-irrigation may be the only mechanical treatment needed. The joint should be inspected the following day, and if the fluid has reaccumulated, a second aspiration-irrigation should be performed. If the reaccumulation of fluid is significant, and if the patient is still febrile, consideration should be given to performing surgical drainage. If in addition the WBC count of the aspirated fluid is not significantly lower on the second day than that seen in the initial aspirate, surgical débridement should be strongly considered. If a second aspiration is performed and the fluid reaccumulates significantly on the third day, surgical drainage should be performed. Parenteral antibiotics enter the inflamed joint so readily that there is no need for direct joint instillation of antibiotics.

Initial arthrotomy of the joint should be performed when the fluid is thick (ie, with a WBC count over 100,000), and when particulate matter is seen in the aspirate. This particulate matter is precipitated fibrin that must be removed to eradicate the infection. The arthrotomy of the knee joint should be performed through a small lateral parapatellar incision that allows inspection of the joint. A medial parapatellar incision is not performed because release of the medial retinaculum might lead to patellar subluxation. The joint may be closed over a small drain such as a Penrose drain. Suction drainage may be used; however, a suction irrigation system should not be employed because of the possibility of superinfection with gram-negative organisms. Arthroscopy has become a popular tool for the inspection of the joint and has been proposed for the débridement of the infected joint. Proponents state that one can effectively débride the joint and that the fibrinous material may be removed with the débridement tools available to the arthroscopist.

IV antibiotics should be started immediately after the joint fluid has been cultured and the other studies such as Gram staining and WBC count have been performed. The diagnosis may have to be confirmed on a presumptive basis; however, it is important to begin treatment as long as the criteria for making the diagnosis of septic arthritis have been met. In the child older than 5 years, most acute septic arthritis is caused by *S aureus*. In children 6 months to 5 years, *H influenzae* is a common cause. In the neonate, group B *Streptococcus* and gram-negative organisms are common etiologic organisms. While awaiting the culture results, appropriate antibiotics should be started to cover the most likely organisms. Because

Staphylococcus is ubiquitous, all acute septic joints are treated initially with an anti-*Staphylococcus* drug. Another drug may be added in the appropriate-aged patients. For example, in a 3-year-old child with a septic arthritis of the knee, one would treat initially for *Staphylococcus* and for *Haemophilus* flu while awaiting the culture results. The antibiotics are then modified when the culture and sensitivity results are known.

The treatment of a suspected *H influenzae* septic arthritis is begun with an antibiotic that is effective against β-lactamase–producing *H influenzae*, because 20% of *Haemophilus* flu strains are resistant to ampicillin. Therefore, one may begin the child on either chloramphenicol or cefuroxime while awaiting cultures, as both are effective against β-lactamase–producing *Haemophilus*. Cefuroxime has the advantage of also effectively eradicating *S aureus*, and thus does not require the addition of oxacillin. It also does not produce bone marrow suppression. Cefamandole should not be used because it does not cross the blood–brain barrier, and children with a septic arthritis caused by *H influenza* may have a concurrent meningitis.

The dosages of the antibiotics are the same as given for the patient with acute hematogenous osteomyelitis. The duration of antibiotic treatment, however, is not as long as in osteomyelitis, because antibiotics reach the infected joint readily and in high concentration. In addition, one does not have to deal with necrotic bone in a septic arthritis as one would in a patient with osteomyelitis. Treatment of the septic joint should be started with IV antibiotics for 5 to 7 days. The patient may then be switched to oral antibiotics if there has been a good response to the treatment. The total length of treatment is generally 2 to 4 weeks.

Hip Joint

An infection of the hip joint must be treated as an emergency because of the potential for the development of avascular necrosis of the femoral head. The initial evaluation of the hip joint is performed in the same manner used for any other joint. However, because the hip joint is deep and may be difficult to aspirate accurately, it must be aspirated using fluoroscopy. The needle may be directed from the anterior or medial approach. The anterior approach is used if the child is able to extend the hip. If because of pain the hip is in a position of abduction, flexion, and external rotation, a medial approach to the hip is easier. The exact needle entry point through the

skin is easily determined by placing the needle on the skin and positioning the needle point using fluoroscopy. After skin penetration, the needle is directed toward the femoral neck at about the level of the junction of the head and the neck. If no fluid is collected from the joint, contrast medium is injected into the joint and an arthrogram obtained, which will reveal whether the hip joint has been entered.

Once the diagnosis of septic arthritis of the hip joint has been confirmed, the joint must be surgically drained as mentioned earlier. One need not await culture reports before draining the infected hip. Strong presumptive evidence is sufficient. Therefore, a positive Gram stain or WBC count of the joint fluid of more than 90,000 to 100,000 cells is sufficient evidence if seen in combination with the characteristic history and physical findings.

The hip joint should never be treated with aspiration and irrigation because of the danger of avascular necrosis developing as a result of increased joint fluid pressure from the infection. The hip may be drained from either an anterior or a posterior approach. Each approach has its proponents. The posterior approach is generally easier and less damaging to the muscles of the hip. In addition, it allows for dependent drainage. If the femoral neck must be opened because of an intraosseous abscess, this cannot be performed posteriorly because the blood supply to the femoral head would be damaged. Thus, if one thinks that the femoral neck should be windowed, the hip should be approached anteriorly. This allows one to drill the femoral neck in every patient (Fig. 4-12). The decision as to whether this is required may be made on clinical grounds. Regardless of the approach to the joint, the joint should be closed over a drain in the same manner as for any other joint.

The joint should be immobilized for several days to allow for a decrease in the acute inflammation. The hip may be placed in split Russell traction and the other joints splinted. Once the acute inflammation has subsided, motion should be instituted. Continuous passive motion has been advocated, and it may be used in children of adequate size. Joint motion helps prevent fibrosis and assists in cartilage nutrition.

Sacroiliac Joint

Septic arthritis of the sacroiliac joint is somewhat unusual because of its symptomatology and treatment, and therefore deserves separate discussion. Sacroiliac (SI) joint infection may be difficult to diagnose unless one is familiar with its signs and symptoms and con-

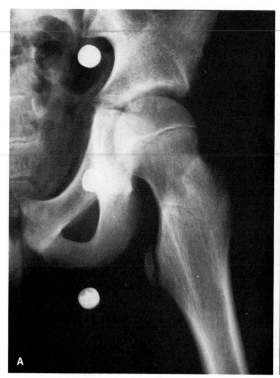
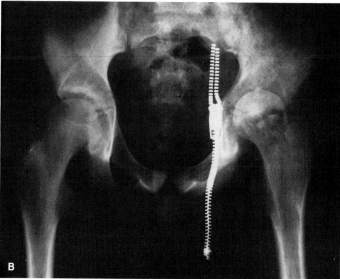

FIGURE 4-12. A 14-year-old boy with septic arthritis of his left hip. (A) AP radiograph of the left hip at the time of presentation. The hip was drained posteriorly, but the femoral neck was not drained. (B) AP radiograph of the left hip taken 6 weeks later demonstrating chondrolysis, avascular necrosis of the femoral head, and chronic osteomyelitis of the femoral neck with sequestrum within the femoral neck.

siders it in patients with pain about the pelvis and hip. Frequently, children with this disease are referred with abdominal or hip pain. Occasionally, they may be thought to have back pain. A careful history and examination, however, reveal that the pain is localized to the posterior pelvis. Pelvic compression is positive and usually produces exquisite pain in the region of the SI joint. The figure 4 test or Fabre test produces exquisite pain in the region of the SI joint.

The child usually is febrile, with signs of a systemic infection. The initial radiographs of the pelvis are usually normal, although tomograms of the SI joint may show some erosion of the margins of the joint if the infection has remained untreated for a sufficiently long period. Usually, however, all radiographs are normal. ^{99m}Tc bone scanning may be positive; however, false-negative bone scans are seen in 25% or more of patients with acute infections. The diagnosis, therefore, depends on a careful history and examination, combined with confirmatory laboratory studies.

As in any other infection, joint aspiration is necessary to determine the bacteriologic cause of the infection; however, the SI joint is difficult to aspirate. Several descriptions of SI joint aspiration technique have been published, but even with this assistance the technique is demanding. Children with SI joint infection experience considerable pain and are usually distraught, making aspiration even more difficult. The SI joint may be aspirated directly by approaching the joint through the ilium. This is easily accomplished by directing the aspiration needle perpendicular to the ilium at the level of the SI joint using fluoroscopic control. The large-bore needle with a stylet is carefully drilled through the ilium and into the SI joint. To be certain that the SI joint has been entered, the needle is drilled into the sacrum and as the needle is withdrawn slowly, aspiration is performed. Both the marrow contents and the contents of the SI joint are aspirated. This material is then submitted for Gram stain and culture. Appropriate antibiotics are immediately begun while awaiting culture results. The infecting organism seen most commonly in non–drug-abusing children is *Staphylococcus*. Surgical drainage is not required unless the infection does not respond to IV antibiotics.

Gonococcal Arthritis

Septic arthritis secondary to infection with *N gonorrhoeae* is probably the most common form of septic arthritis in the sexually active population. The typical syndrome of disseminated gonococcal infection frequently consists of three stages, although all patients with gonococcal septic arthritis do not go through all of these stages. The first stage is a septic stage that is similar to a septicemia caused by any other bacteria. The second stage is a transition stage, and the final stage is the septic joint stage. Eighty percent of patients with gonococcal arthritis complain of a migratory polyarthralgia, which is most commonly seen on the dorsum of the hands, wrists, ankles, and feet. This history is so characteristic that the diagnosis of gonococcal arthritis may be made on the basis of the history of migratory polyarthralgia combined with the typical joint findings.

About 60% of patients with gonococcal arthritis have more than one involved joint. The joints of the upper extremity, especially those of the fingers and wrist, are more commonly involved than are the joints of the lower extremity.

Joint aspiration is mandatory for culture and fluid analysis. Typically, the WBC count of the fluid is much lower than one would see in the fluid of a joint infected with another organism. In a series of teenagers with gonococcal arthritis, the average WBC of the synovial fluid was 48,000, with a range of 3800 to 152,000. The organism is difficult to culture in the laboratory, and joint fluid cultures of septic joints are positive only half of the time. Therefore, it is necessary to culture all orifices in patients suspected of having gonococcal arthritis.

Surgical drainage of the infected joints is usually not required, because the organism is so easily eradicated with appropriate antibiotic therapy. In addition, the organism usually does not destroy the involved joint until late in the course of an infection; therefore, if an infection is treated promptly, no joint destruction should be expected. Penicillin is the drug of choice for the treatment of this infection. In treating patients with gonococcal arthritis, one should follow the Centers for Disease Control and Prevention recommendations, which are to treat with 10 million units of penicillin IV for 3 days followed by ampicillin or amoxicillin, 0.5 g orally four times a day for 4 days. One may also treat this disease with oral therapy alone; however, patient compliance must be assured. A loading dose of 3.5 g of ampicillin or amoxicillin plus 1 g of probenecid is given orally, followed by either ampicillin or amoxicillin, 0.5 g orally four times a day for a total of 7 days. Tetracycline should be used for penicillin-sensitive patients. Spectinomycin is used if the organism is resistant to penicillin.

Annotated Bibliography

Canale ST, Harkness RM, Thomas PA, Massie JD. Does aspiration of bones and joints affect results of later bone scanning? J Pediatr Orthop 1985;5:23.
The authors demonstrate that bone aspiration with a needle does not alter the bone scan. They emphasize that if bone scanning is to be done in acute hematogenous osteomyelitis, it should not delay a bone aspiration and treatment. Treatment should be carried out immediately, and if a bone scan is necessary, it may be done without fear of altering the results after needle aspiration.

Cole WG, Dalziel RE, Leitl S. Treatment of acute osteomyelitis in childhood. J Bone Joint Surg 1982;64B:218.
The authors present a review of 55 children with acute hematogenous osteomyelitis. Ninety-two percent were cured if diagnosed early, and their cure was effected with a single course of antibiotics without operation. The patients were kept in the hospital for less than 1 week. The authors quickly switched to oral antibiotics as soon as the patient had responded to the IV antibiotics with excellent results.

Crosby LA, Powell DA. The potential value of the sedimentation rate in monitoring treatment outcome in puncture wound-related *Pseudomonas* osteomyelitis. Clin Orthop 1984;188:168.
The authors used the sedimentation rate for determining the course of antibiotic treatment for pseudomonal osteomyelitis of the foot after puncture wounds. They found that once the sedimentation rate had returned to normal, the antibiotic therapy could be stopped.

Curtiss PH Jr, Klein L. Destruction of articular cartilage in septic arthritis. J Bone Joint Surg 1963;45A:797.
The authors demonstrate the effect of staphylococcal pus and various proteolytic enzymes on the structural integrity of articular cartilage. They show that collagenase did produce proteolytic destruction of cartilage. They also thought that a mechanical process was necessary for cartilage destruction.

Gillespie WJ, Mayo KM. The management of acute hematogenous osteomyelitis in the antibiotic era. J Bone Joint Surg 1981;63B:126.
The authors review the treatment of acute hematogenous osteomyelitis seen in children between 1947 and 1976. They had a high failure rate of 20% and found that failure was more common in surgically treated patients. Their results are worse than one would expect today. The organism recovered was S aureus in more than 90%, but they isolated the organism in only 55% of patients who were treated successfully.

Green N. *Pseudomonas* infections of the foot following puncture wounds. AAOS Instruct Course Lect 1983;32:43.
The author identifies the cause of pseudomonal infections of the foot after puncture wounds. These require débridement in all cases and prolonged antibiotic therapy.

Green N, Beauchamp R, Griffin P. Primary subacute epiphyseal osteomyelitis. J Bone Joint Surg 1981;63A:107.
The authors identify lesions of the epiphysis as representing primary subacute epiphyseal osteomyelitis. The lesions are characteristic with well-circumscribed borders. The treatment is débridement and antibiotic therapy.

Griffin PP, Green WT Jr. Hip joint infections in infants and children. Orthop Clin North Am 1978;9:123.
The authors outline the appropriate treatment for acute septic arthritis. They emphasize that early treatment of the infection is

mandatory and that poor results are more likely to be seen in infants and young children than in older children and that poor results are more common in children with a delay in the diagnosis and treatment. They also point out that associated osteomyelitis of the femoral neck is more likely to result in a poor outcome.

Gutman L. Acute, subacute, and chronic osteomyelitis and pyogenic arthritis in children. Curr Probl Pediatr 1985;15:1.
This is a good review of the diagnosis and treatment of osteomyelitis in children. All forms of osteomyelitis are discussed, and the means of diagnosis and treatment are outlined.

Jackson MA, Nelson JD. Etiology and medical management of acute suppurative bone and joint infections in pediatric patients. J Pediatr Orthop 1982;2:313.
The authors review the etiology and management of acute bone and joint infections and outline oral therapy of acute hematogenous osteomyelitis.

Johanson PH. *Pseudomonas* infection in the foot following puncture wounds. JAMA 1968;204:262.
The author was the first to identify Pseudmonas as the primary etiology for infections of the bones of the foot after nail puncture wounds. These should be treated aggressively.

Meller Y, Yugupsky P, Elitsur Y, Inbar-Ianay I, Bar-Ziv J. Chronic multifocal symmetrical osteomyelitis. Am J Dis Child 1984;138:349.
The authors identify the syndrome of chronic multifocal osteomyelitis. This is an unusual disease with no known etiology as of yet. It seems to run a self-contained course that may last as long as 15 years.

Morrissy RT. Bone and joint sepsis in children. AAOS Instruct Course Lect 1982;31:49.
The author presents a good review of the etiology, diagnosis, and treatment of bone and joint infections in children. He emphasizes the need for aspiration of the bone and joint for diagnosis and treatment.

Nelson JD, Bucholz RW, Kusmiesz H, Shelton S. Benefits and risks of sequential parenteral–oral cepalosporin therapy for suppurative bone and joint infections. J Pediatr Orthop 1982;2:255.
The authors outline the sequential IV-oral treatment of acute bone and joint infections in children. They emphasize the need for high-dose antibiotics both in the IV and oral route. They stress that the oral antibiotics should not be given unless the child has had an excellent response to the IV antibiotics.

Roberts JM, Drummond DS, Breed AL, Chesney J. Subacute hematogenous osteomyelitis in children: a retrospective study. J Pediatr Orthop 1982;2:249.
The authors outline the diagnosis of subacute hematogenous osteomyelitis in children. This disease does not produce systemic symptoms but does produce local findings. Treatment is débridement and antibiotic therapy.

Rotbart HA, Glode MP. *Haemophilus influenzae* type b septic arthritis in children: report of 23 cases. Pediatrics 1985;75:254.
The H influenzae type B is shown to be a common causative organism in children under age 6 with acute septic arthritis.

Scoles P, Quinn T. Intervertebral discitis in children and adolescents. Clin Orthop 1982;162:31.
The authors identify the syndrome of intervertebral diskitis in children. This is an infection of the disk space that should be treated aggressively.

Sullivan JA, Vasileff T, Leonard JC. An evaluation of nuclear scanning in orthopaedic infections. J Pediatr Orthop 1981;1:73.
The authors demonstrate that bone scanning is less than 100% accurate in patients with acute hematogenous osteomyelitis. As a matter of fact, they find in their series only 80% of the children with acute hematogenous osteomyelitis had a positive bone scan. Therefore, the diagnosis of acute hematogenous osteomyelitis should not depend on bone scanning.

Szalay E, Green N, Heller R, Horev G, Kirchner SG. MRI disc space infection. J Pediatr Orthop 1987;7:164.
The authors believe that MRI is the most sensitive means of early diagnosis of disk space infection in children.

Trueta J. The three types of acute hematogenous osteomyelitis: a clinical and vascular study. J Bone Joint Surg 1959;41B:671.
The author describes the three types of osteomyelitis—namely, neonatal, childhood, and adult—and demonstrates the difference in blood supply that forms the basis for this classification system.

Wenger DR, Bobechko WP, Gilday DL. The spectrum of intervertebral disc-space infection in children. J Bone Joint Surg 1978;60A:100.
The authors elucidate the etiology, diagnosis, and treatment of disk space infection in children. They emphasize the infectious nature of this disease.

Turek's Orthopaedics: Principles and Their Application, Fifth Edition,
edited by Stuart L. Weinstein and Joseph A. Buckwalter.
J.B. Lippincott Company, Philadelphia, © 1994.

5

Stanley J. Naides
Robert F. Ashman
Elizabeth H. Field
M. Paul Strottmann
John S. Cowdery
Robert W. Karr

Richard R. Olson
Mary M. Jones
John W. Rachow
Louise H. Sparks
Alan D. Croock

Rheumatic Diseases: Diagnosis and Management

(continued)

The Normal Synovium

Robert F. Ashman

The *synovium*, or *synovial membrane*, is a thin, delicate tissue that, with the hyaline cartilage, completely encloses the synovial cavity of diarthrodial joints. On its inner surface is a layer of lining cells that is one or two cells thick and consists of a mixture of phagocytic cells (type A) and secretory cells (type B). Under this surface layer, a delicate connective tissue stroma encloses a few capillaries and some adipose tissue. In places, it is wrinkled into folds. At its base, it merges with the joint capsule or periosteum.

Synovial fluid is a plasma transudate from synovial capillaries, modified by the secretory activities of the type B synovial lining cells. They secrete the hyaluronic acid–protein complex (mucin) that gives synovial fluid its viscosity and lubricating properties. Glucose and electrolytes are in equilibrium between synovial fluid and serum. The nutrition of hyaline cartilage depends on synovial fluid exchanged by diffusion plus compression and decompression of the cartilage during motion and weight bearing.

CHARACTERISTICS OF NORMAL SYNOVIAL FLUID

Normal fluid is clear, pale yellow, and sufficiently viscous that droplets expelled from a needle tip fall in a long string. When a drop is pressed between the thumb and forefinger, the sticky viscous consistency is apparent. Normal synovial fluid does not clot because it lacks fibrinogen. The normal volume of fluid in the largest synovial cavity, the knee, is 0.2 to 4 mL. Thus, aspiration of the normal joint may yield only enough fluid to wet the needle.

Laboratory analysis of normal fluid shows (1) sterile culture; (2) less than 100 leukocytes per cubic millimeter, mostly lymphocytes and monocytes; (3) specific gravity of 1.008 to 1.015; (4) protein content of 20 to 200 mg/mL, with an albumin/globulin ratio of 1.5:1; (5) mucin content that varies widely and is the main determinant of the high viscosity; (6) glucose that is normally more than 75% of the concentration in serum; and (7) no crystals.

EXAMINATION OF SYNOVIAL FLUID

Aspiration of synovial fluid is a helpful diagnostic maneuver whenever the cause of arthritis is in doubt, but especially when the inflammation is concentrated in a single joint or has an acute onset. Ruling out infection or crystal deposition as a cause of arthritis is the strongest indication for synovial fluid analysis, because the treatment of these disorders is substantially different from that of other causes of joint inflammation. In the case of bacterial infection, the results of misdiagnosis can be catastrophic.

Routine analysis of synovial fluid includes (1) inspection for color, transparency, and viscosity; (2) cell count; (3) crystal examination; (4) bacterial culture; and, if bacterial infection is suspected clinically, (5) Gram stain. Samples for both cell count and crystals can be collected in sodium heparin (green-top) tubes. All these tests are most reliable when performed on fresh specimens, but culture of the fastidious gonococcus requires plating of fluid on chocolate agar and culture in a high carbon dioxide incubator within a few minutes of collection.

Additional tests sometimes performed include the following:

> *Mucin clot test:* Add 1 mL of synovial fluid to 4 mL of 2% acetic acid, and mix with glass rod. Normal fluid forms a single tight clump. If inflammatory cells are present, they degrade the mucin so that the clump is easily fragmented.
> *Glucose:* Any condition that causes a high neutrophil count in the fluid reduces the glucose because neutrophils metabolize it. A glucose level that is less than half the serum level supports the diagnosis of infection or inflammation but adds little to the information already provided by cell count, crystal examination, and culture.
> *Protein level:* Protein levels rise in inflammation but add no important information.
> *Complement component levels:* C_3 and C_4 levels normally bear the same relation to protein levels as in the serum, unless complement is being activated in the joint cavity. Joint fluid complement levels rarely contribute to decisions regarding diagnosis or therapy.

CRYSTAL EXAMINATION

Crystal examination is the only known means of making the diagnoses of gout, pseudogout, and basic calcium phosphate (BCP) crystal disease. Examination of fresh synovial fluid on a polarizing microscope with a first-order red compensating filter permits the recognition of the sign of birefringence in addition to crystal morphology. *Sodium urate* crystals are thin, pointed, and strongly negatively birefringent (yellow if their axis is parallel to that of the compensator). *Calcium pyrophosphate dihydrate* (CPPD) crystals are short, thick, and weakly positively birefringent. *BCP* (including hydroxyapatite) crystals may be identified

under ordinary light microscopy as small, chunky Alizarin red–staining crystals in clumps. Diagnosis is more certain if crystals are seen within phagocytes.

Crystal artifacts occasionally encountered include steroid crystals (flat parallelograms occurring in joints recently injected with depot steroid preparations), glass fragments, and lithium heparin or oxalate crystals (hence the recommendation of sodium heparin as anticoagulant).

Table 5-1 summarizes the results of synovial fluid analysis, with usual diagnostic implications. Typical cell counts and fluid characteristics overlap among the classifications, and only in the case of a positive crystal examination or culture can a definitive diagnosis be made from fluid alone. Since septic joints (especially if partially treated) may have low leukocyte counts, culture should be performed regardless of the fluid's appearance. Furthermore, more than one diagnosis may be present, as in the gout or rheumatoid arthritis (RA) patient with a septic joint.

A frankly bloody fluid may mean tumor, trauma, or hemophilia. A dark brown fluid full of hemosiderin is seen in hemophilia and pigmented villonodular synovitis. Fat floating on a bloody fluid indicates fracture or tumor exposing the marrow cavity to the synovial space. Floating fragments resembling ground pepper represent pigmented cartilage fragments in ochronosis. Small white clots ("rice bodies") represent fibrin bits seen in some inflammatory fluids. Phagocytic mononuclear cells with vacuoles may appear in RA and in Reiter syndrome.

SYNOVIAL BIOPSY

The indications for synovial biopsy are rare, since fluid analysis, direct visualization by arthroscopy, or arthrography usually provides most of the information required for diagnosis. The suspicion of tumor, pigmented villonodular synovitis, tuberculous or fungal arthritis, sarcoidosis, amyloidosis, or synovial chondromatosis may be confirmed by synovial biopsy.

Biopsy is most commonly obtained by arthroscopy but may also be obtained by an open procedure or with a biopsy needle. In the latter case, a hollow guide needle is inserted into the synovial space. The hooked core needle can then be inserted multiple times through the guide needle, manipulated until it impales synovial tissue, then withdrawn to provide the specimen. Biopsy tissue is usually formalin fixed for hematoxylin and eosin staining, but preservation

TABLE 5-1.
Results of Synovial Fluid Analysis

Group	Appearance	Mucin Clot	Cell Count/μL	Neutrophils (%)	Glucose (% of Serum)	Culture	Typical Diagnosis
Normal	Clear, colorless to straw colored, good string, low volume	Firm	< 100	< 25	75–100	—	None
I (Noninflammatory)	Clear, straw colored, good string	Firm	200–2000	< 25	75–100	—	Degenerative arthritis, internal derangement, trauma, aseptic necrosis
IIA (Mild inflammatory)	Faintly cloudy, moderate string	Friable if shaken	1000–10,000	25–50	75–100	—	Systemic lupus erythematosus and other immune complex arthritides, mild rheumatoid arthritis, spondyloarthropathies
IIB (Severe inflammatory)	Translucent but cloudy, yellow, drops like water	Friable	2000–75,000	50–75	50–100	Rarely positive for tuberculosis	Moderate to severe rheumatoid arthritis, gout, pseudogout, tuberculosis
III (Septic)	Creamy, opaque, poor string	Friable to none	> 50,000	> 80	< 50	Often positive for bacteria	Acute gout, bacterial infection

of urate crystals requires absolute ethanol, and cultures require unfixed sterile samples. The yield of positive cultures from synovium in tuberculous and fungal arthritis is superior to that of fluid cultures. Other special staining procedures include iron stains for hemosiderin in pigmented villonodular synovitis or hemochromatosis and Congo red stains for amyloid.

Histologic findings of diagnostic import include the cartilage metaplasia of synovial chondromatosis, malignant synovial sarcoma or chondrosarcoma, metastatic tumors or leukemias, caseating granulomas (tuberculosis), noncaseating granulomas (sarcoidosis), the histiocytes and giant cells of multicentric reticulohistiocytosis, and the periodic acid Schiff–positive macrophages of Whipple disease. Of course, inflam-

mation is a far more common finding, but unfortunately, the histology of inflamed synovium is similar in the major rheumatic diseases. Early in inflammatory arthritis, the synovial lining cells accumulate, capillaries proliferate, and then mononuclear cells (mostly monocytes and T lymphocytes) infiltrate the tissue. Finally, in the chronic phase, complete germinal centers resembling those of lymph nodes may appear. The exuberant thickening of this hypercellular synovium resembles granulation tissue, forms long villous fronds, begins to erode cartilage at the joint margins, and may even enter bone along the haversian canals. These latter changes (called *marginal erosions* by the radiologist) are most typical of RA but can occur in any severely and chronically inflamed joint.

Degenerative Joint Disease
Elizabeth H. Field

RADIOLOGIC FEATURES

In addition to the history and physical examination, radiographic studies are extremely valuable in establishing a diagnosis of degenerative arthritis and assessing its progression. The characteristic radio-

graphic features of degenerative arthritis are osteophyte formation, asymmetric joint space narrowing, bony sclerosis, and subchondral cysts. The radiographic abnormalities of degenerative joint disease (DJD) can be scored as to severity based on these four common features (Table 5-2).

TABLE 5-2.
Radiographic Classification of Degenerative Joint Disease

Grade	Description
KNEES	
0	Normal
1	Doubtful narrowing of joint space and possible osteophytic lipping
2	Definite osteophytes and possible narrowing of joint space
3	Moderate multiple osteophytes, definite narrowing of joint space, some sclerosis, and possible deformity of bone ends
4	Large osteophytes, marked narrowing of joint space, severe sclerosis, and definite deformity of bone ends. Subchondral cysts may be present.
HIPS	
0	Normal
1	Possible narrowing of joint space medially and possible osteophytes around the femoral head
2	Definite narrowing of joint space inferiorly, definite osteophytes, and slight sclerosis
3	Marked narrowing of joint space, slight osteophytes, some sclerosis and cyst formation, and deformity of femoral head and acetabulum
4	Gross loss of joint space with sclerosis and cysts, marked deformity of femoral head and acetabulum, and large osteophytes

(Adapted from the Council for International Organization of Medical Sciences, 1963)

General

The osteophyte, or bone spur, is the single most common feature of osteoarthritis. An *osteophyte* is an osseous outgrowth that most commonly arises at the joint margin. There are two areas where diagnosing osteophytes may be difficult—the axial skeleton and the distal interphalangeal (DIP) and proximal interphalangeal (PIP) joints of the fingers and toes. In the axial skeleton, osteophytes may be confused with *syndesmophytes* (another type of new bone formation), which are oriented vertically, as if flowing from one vertebral body to the next. Syndesmophytes indicate an underlying inflammatory spondyloarthropathy. Osteophytes from degenerative arthritis are oriented more horizontal to their point of origin (Fig. 5-1). In the DIP and PIP joints, osteophytes of degenerative arthritis need to be distinguished from the proliferative new bone formation seen in psoriatic arthritis (Fig. 5-2). Osteophytes in DJD have been described as seagull wings, because the combination of irregular joint space narrowing and marginal osteophytes resembles a seagull flying. In psoriatic arthritis, the proliferative changes at the DIP and PIP joints may resemble mouse ears, resulting from a combination of new bone formation at the enthesis of the joint and erosions that begin at the margins and progress centrally.

Joint space narrowing, also a characteristic of DJD,

results from loss of hyaline cartilage and should be present to some degree in all joints that exhibit osteophytes. Because joint space loss is greatest where the stress on the joint is greatest, joint space narrowing in DJD is asymmetric, in contrast to the uniform narrowing seen in inflammatory arthritis.

Subchondral bony sclerosis and *cyst formation* occur in the most stressed areas of the joint, where the joint space is narrowed. In this area, the bony surfaces often rub and polish each other, a process termed *eburnation*. Cysts form in the subchondral bone beneath eburnated or sclerotic surfaces late in the degenerative process and signify severe disease.

Other, less common features of DJD include detached pieces of bone or cartilage (*joint mice*) within the joint space. The significant soft tissue swelling and the osteopenia characteristic of inflammatory arthritis do not occur.

Knees

Knee joints of suspected DJD patients should have a radiograph taken in the weight-bearing position. Joint spaces that look normal on supine films may have significant joint space narrowing with weight bearing. Frequently, the knee shows angulation, *valgus deformity*, as a result of greater joint space narrowing in the medial compartment (Fig. 5-3). Bony

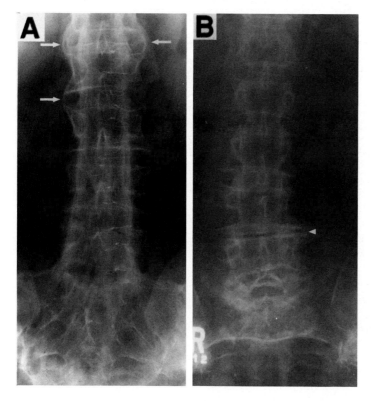

FIGURE 5-1. Osteophytes versus syndesmophytes. Osteophytes can be distinguished from syndesmophytes by their orientation. Syndesmophytes of spondylarthropathy project vertically and seem to flow from one vertebral body to the next (*arrows in* **A**), whereas osteophytes of degenerative arthritis project laterally (*arrowheads in* **B**).

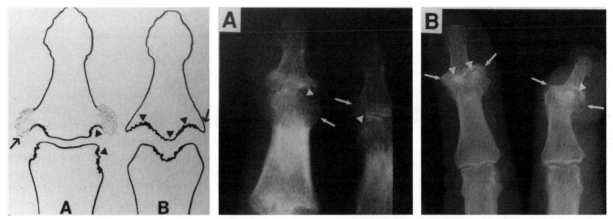

FIGURE 5-2. Mouse ears versus seagull wings. (A) In psoriasis, because new bone formation at the enthesis (*arrow*) is accompanied by erosions that begin at the margins and progress centrally (*arrowhead*), the joint resembles a mouse ear. (B) In osteoarthritis, the combination of osteophytes at the margin (*arrow*) and irregular joint space narrowing (*arrowhead*) resembles a seagull flying.

sclerosis with or without subchondral bone cysts may be seen. Osteophytes occasionally arise from the tibial spines or intercondylar notch as well as from the patella and joint margins of the tibia and femur. Tricompartmental (medial, patellar, and lateral) uniform involvement is extremely rare in simple DJD and suggests a previous inflammatory process. For example, RA produces uniform cartilage damage, but when the inflammation is controlled, degenerative changes of DJD may follow.

Hips

The DJD changes in the hip are concentrated in the superolateral aspect of the joint, which is the area under most mechanical stress. Joint space narrowing is followed by osteophyte formation, sclerosis, and cyst formation. Remodeling of the medial and lateral femoral head occurs and can lead to its collapse and flattening. The medial acetabulum space fills in with osteophytes, resulting in the gradual superolateral migration of the femoral head (Fig. 5-4). There can be thickening of the cortex with new bone formation along the medial aspect of the femoral neck (*buttressing*). In contrast, diffuse loss of joint space and medial migration along the axis of the femoral head, *protrusio acetabuli,* suggest an inflammatory arthritis, such as RA.

Spine

Degenerative arthritis most frequently involves the lumbar and lower cervical spine, although any level of the spine may be affected. The spine is made up of a series of synovial lined joints, *apophyseal joints;* cartilaginous joints, *nucleus pulposus of the intervertebral disks;* and fibrous articulation, *annulus fibrosus of the intervertebral disk.* Disease can arise from any

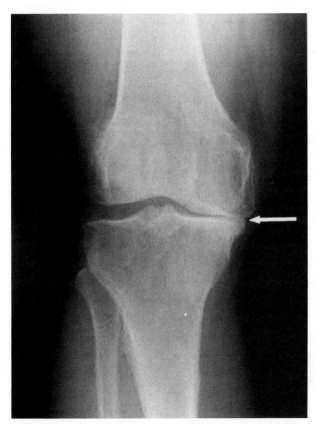

FIGURE 5-3. Degenerative joint disease of the knee is manifested by asymmetric joint space narrowing. The medial compartment (*arrow*) is affected primarily over the lateral compartment.

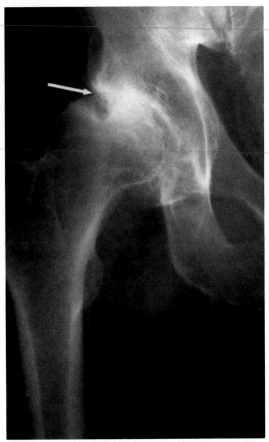

FIGURE 5-4. Degenerative joint disease of the hip. An AP view of the hip joint illustrates superolateral migration of the femoral head (*arrow*) with asymmetric joint space narrowing.

of these structures and produce distinct radiographic findings (Fig. 5-5). These features may be found in the same place in the same patient, since the pathologic process that leads to the degeneration of cartilage or fibrous tissue also leads to reactive new bone formation. But for clarity, each pathologic process is described separately.

Osteoarthritis of the apophyseal joints and uncovertebral joints (neurocentral joints of Luschka) involves joint space narrowing, marginal osteophytes, and sclerosis. *Spondylolisthesis*, or the forward movement of one vertebral body over another, may result from osteoarthritis of the facet joints and is diagnosed by lateral radiographs.

Intervertebral osteochondritis begins with the degeneration of the nucleus pulposus of the intervertebral disk. Radiographically, there is progressive uniform or nonuniform narrowing of the disk space and reactive subchondral sclerosis at the end plate. Progressive desiccation or rupture of the disk can lead to a release of gas into the disk substance, appearing as a thin linear lucency within the disk (*vacuum sign*) on extension, which disappears on flexion. A vacuum sign on a radiograph excludes infection. Progressive degeneration of the disk may lead to herniation into the adjacent vertebral body, producing a *Schmorl node* (Fig. 5-6).

Spondylosis deformans refers to degenerative disease of the annulus fibrosus of the intervertebral disk. Disk space narrowing occurs with osteophyte for-

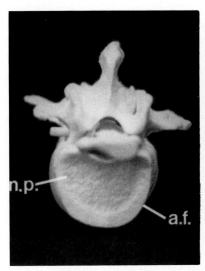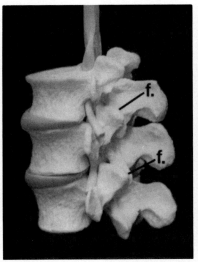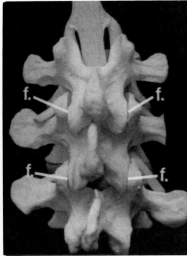

FIGURE 5-5. The vertebral bodies and intervertebral disc contain three structures that can be affected by degenerative joint disease. Involvement of the facet joint (f) is termed *osteoarthritis*. The intervertebral disc is composed of the central nucleus pulposus (n.p.) surrounded by the anulus fibrosis (a.f.). Disease of the nucleus pulposus is termed *intervertebral osteochondritis* and disease of the anulus fibrosis is *spondylosis deformans*.

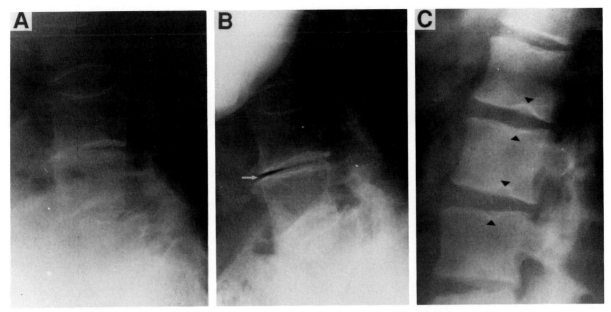

FIGURE 5-6. Lateral views of the lumbosacral spine in flexion (**A**) and extension (**B**) sometimes yield the vacuum sign (*arrow*), a horizontal linear lucency in the intervertebral disc space created when gas forms in the disc as a result of negative pressure. The vacuum sign rules out infection and indicates intervertebral osteochondritis. (**C**) A Schmorl node (*arrowhead*) forms when the nucleus pulposus herniates into an adjacent vertebral body.

mation along the anterior or lateral aspect of the spine.

To adequately evaluate DJD in the spine, anteroposterior (AP) and lateral views in both extension and flexion are required. The oblique views of the lumbar spine to show the facet joints are probably unnecessary. More sophisticated radiographic studies, such as computed axial tomography or magnetic resonance imaging (MRI), are helpful in diagnosing herniated intervertebral disk disease and lumbar spinal stenosis that can occur secondary to osteoarthritis. In suspected cases, the physician should establish a specific diagnosis of disk disease or lumbar spinal stenosis, since physical therapy designed to benefit one of these disorders may aggravate the other.

Hands and Wrists

About 30% of the US population has DJD changes of the hand, and 8% are symptomatic. Degenerative arthritis of the hands and wrist frequently involves the DIP and PIP joints along with the first carpometacarpal (trapeziometacarpal) joints. There is uniform or nonuniform loss of joint space, marginal osteophytes, bony sclerosis, and subchondral cyst formation. In extreme cases, angular deformity, dislocation, or ankylosis may occur. Occasionally, the metacarpophalangeal (MCP) joints are involved, but never without concomitant involvement of the DIP or PIP joints. Osteophytes of the DIP joints lead to *Heberden nodes*, and osteophytes of the PIP joints lead to *Bouchard nodes* (Fig. 5-7).

Erosive osteoarthritis, a disease of primarily middle-aged and older women, is characterized by degenerative changes plus bone erosions in a bilateral polyarticular pattern involving mainly the DIP and PIP joints. The erosions occur centrally but can extend laterally along the joint margin. Coupled with marginal osteophytes, these erosions give a scalloped appearance to the joint on plain radiographs. Erosive osteoarthritis should be distinguished from RA and psoriatic arthritis because these three diseases warrant different management. In RA, DIP involvement and central erosions are rare. In psoriatic arthritis, the DIP and PIP joints may be involved in a unilateral, bilateral, uniarticular, oligoarticular, or polyarticular fashion, and psoriatic skin lesions and nail bed changes frequently overlie the affected joint. Swelling of psoriasis may involve the whole finger in a sausage-like pattern, called *dactylitis*. The psoriatic joint is characterized by progressive expansion of the distal margin of the interphalangeal joint from fluffy periosteal new bone formation and erosion of the lateral aspects of the proximal margin, resulting in a "pencil-in-cup" appearance.

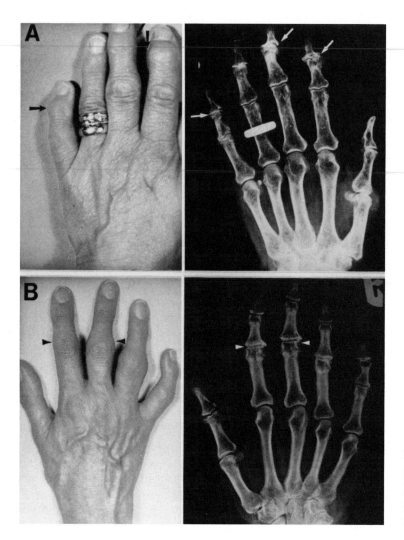

FIGURE 5-7. Heberden and Bouchard nodes. (**A**) Enlargement of the distal interphalangeal joint (*arrow*) is termed a *Heberden node* when caused by osteophytes. (**B**) A similar deformity at the proximal interphalangeal joint is called a *Bouchard node* (*arrowhead*).

Other

The sacroiliac joint frequently exhibits degenerative arthritis in older age groups. Asymmetric joint space narrowing, osteophytes at the inferior aspect of the joint, and distinct sclerotic joint margins are radiographic features. The presence of either pseudo-widened joint spaces, indistinct joint margins, erosions, or fusion of the joint should suggest inflammatory sacroiliitis.

Degenerative disease of the first metatarsophalangeal joint of the foot is characterized by joint space narrowing, osteophyte formation, sclerosis, and subchondral cysts. Osteoarthritis of this joint can lead to *hallux rigidus*, limitation of dorsiflexion or plantar flexion of the metatarsophalangeal (MTP) joint, or *hallus valgus*, abduction of the great toe with lateral angulation of the joint. Frequently, an inflamed bursa, *bunion*, may form, overlying the hyperostosis of the MTP joint with hallus valgus deformity.

LABORATORY FEATURES

No laboratory studies are specific for degenerative arthritis, but studies are often performed to rule out diseases that can be associated with or mimic DJD. Synovial fluid analysis reveals normal viscosity, good mucin clot, and less than 1000 cells/μL. Frequently, the cell count is less than 100 cells/μL, but elevations as high as 2000 cells/μL may occur early in the disease. The synovial fluid should be carefully examined for crystals, since the incidence of both CPPD and apatite crystals is increased in degenerative arthritis.

In clearcut cases of primary DJD with classic radiographic findings and noninflammatory synovial fluid, additional laboratory studies are not needed. In less clearcut cases, where an underlying metabolic disease or other form of arthritis is suspected, determination of complete blood count, erythrocyte sedimentation rate (ESR), calcium, magnesium, liver enzymes, serum iron and iron saturation, thyroid functions, glucose, rheumatoid factor (RF), and antinuclear antibodies (ANA) may be useful. In the elderly male patient with back pain, metastatic disease from prostatic malignancy with an acid phosphatase should be ruled out. The ESR is usually normal in DJD, except in severe cases of erosive osteoarthritis.

MEDICAL MANAGEMENT

Medical management of the patient with degenerative arthritis requires a team approach targeted toward educating the patient and family, evaluating and sometimes altering the patient's lifestyle, offering assistive devices, and prescribing physical therapy and pharmacotherapy.

Education is the first step in patient management. The term *arthritis* conjures up visions of deformity and wheelchairs for most patients, and the word *degenerative* is equally pejorative. Frequently, an explanation of the distinctions between degenerative arthritis and inflammatory arthritis reassures patients. Patients need to know that significant disability is unusual in degenerative arthritis, and continued activity of everyday living will not accelerate the degenerative process. Patients need to understand the benefits and limitations of their medicines; medications are prescribed to alleviate pain and any inflammation that may occur and may not alter the disease process.

Obese patients should be evaluated by dietitians and given dietary instructions on weight reduction because even small amounts of weight reduction can reduce the amount of stress on weight-bearing joints. The beneficial effects of weight reduction on non–weight-bearing joints has not been explained.

Occupational and physical therapy are integral parts of management of degenerative arthritis. Patients should be encouraged to rest the degenerative joint periodically to relieve pain, particularly if significant loss of cartilage is present. Splints used on the wrists and thumbs and other adaptive devices are helpful in bracing and protecting the joint. Insoles, braces, and orthopaedic shoes can benefit DJD of the feet and ankles. Walking aids, such as a cane, are useful in decreasing weight-bearing stress on knees and hips. A cane should always be held in the contralateral hand. Cervical collars and cervical traction are of benefit in selected patients with DJD of the cervical spine. Prolonged use of cervical collars, however, should be avoided or coupled with an isometric exercise program to keep the neck muscles from atrophying. A transcutaneous electrical nerve stimulation (TENS) unit may be extremely useful in controlling severe pain of specific areas and should be tried instead of narcotics. Paraffin baths are particularly useful in erosive osteoarthritis.

Specific exercise programs are extremely beneficial in the management of back pain from degenerative arthritis. The exact diagnosis must be made, however, since these programs are tailored for specific conditions. The pain from DJD of the intervertebral disk responds to a program of back extension exercises, because extension removes pressure from the anterior aspect of the disk and from the disk itself. Patients with disk disease need to be instructed on the body mechanics of lifting, sitting, standing, and walking to prevent unnecessary flexion of the spine, which aggravates disk pain. In contrast, patients who exhibit mainly facet joint degeneration or spinal ste-

TABLE 5-3.
Nonsteroidal Antiinflammatory Agents

Drug	Total Daily Dose	Dosage Schedule
Acetylsalicylic acid (ASA)	2–4 g	qid, check levels
Antrhranilic acids		
Meclofenamate	200–400 mg	tid or qid
Arylacetic acids		
Diclofenac	100–150 mg	bid or tid
Fenoprofen	900–3200 mg	tid or qid
Nabumetone*	1000–2000 mg	bid or qd
Naproxen	500–1500 mg	bid or tid
Carboxylic acids		
Diflunisal	500–1500 mg	bid or tid
Heterocarboxyindole acetic acids		
Etodolac	600–1200 mg	bid, tid, or qid
Indomethacin	75–200 mg	bid or tid†
Sulindac	300–400 mg	bid
Tolmetin	600–1600 mg	tid
Nonacetylated ASA		
Salsalate	1.5–3 g	bid or tid
Choline magnesium trisalicylate	2–3 g	qd, bid, or tid
Oxicams		
Piroxicam	10–20 mg	qd
Phenylproprionic acids		
Flurbiprofen	200–300 mg	bid, tid, or qid
Ketoprofen	150–300 mg	tid or qid
Ibuprofen	1200–3200 mg	tid or qd
Oxaprozin	600–1200 mg	qd

* Active metabolite is a phenylacetic acid.
† Sustained release tablets are available for all day delivery.

nosis benefit from exercises that emphasize flexion of the spine, thus reducing pressure on the facet joints. These patients need to be instructed on protection of their lower back from hyperextension.

Pharmacotherapy is traditionally given to relieve pain, since the course of degenerative arthritis is usually benign and no therapy is thought to alter the course of the disease. This view, however, was recently challenged because some scientific evidence suggests that DJD may be reversible. Sometimes, the use of analgesics, such as acetaminophen, low-dose aspirin, or propoxyphene, is sufficient to control pain. Because of growing evidence that nonsteroidal anti-inflammatory drugs (NSAIDs) and acetylsalicylic acid affect bone metabolism and may impact on the course of DJD, NSAIDs and aspirin are usually the first drugs of choice. Table 5-3 outlines the available NSAIDs and their starting doses. Treatment is empiric, since no one NSAID is more efficient than another for all patients, and striking individual differences in response occur. It is best to try three or four different NSAIDs, each for 10 to 14 days, before deciding which drug is most effective. Frequently, as many as six or more NSAIDs must be tried before failure of treatment can be declared for a given patient. Starting doses need to be adjusted to individual patients. Elderly patients do not tolerate higher doses of NSAIDs because of lower metabolism and glomerular filtration rate and thus should be started on lower doses.

The most common side effects of the NSAIDs are gastritis and gastrointestinal bleeding. Renal effects include fluid and sodium retention, hyperkalemia, decreased renal perfusion, hypertension, and tubulointerstitial nephropathy. Elderly patients in particular should be monitored within 2 to 3 weeks of beginning NSAIDs to determine whether deleterious effects on the kidney are present. The liver functions should be checked within 2 to 3 months of starting an NSAID. Patients on chronic NSAID therapy need to be monitored for side effects with complete blood count, creatinine, blood urea nitrogen, and liver function studies one to three times a year.

Systemic steroids are never indicated in degenerative arthritis. Localized injections of steroids into joints may be of benefit, particularly in patients who have a significant inflammatory component to their disease, such as large joint effusion and warm joint. Repeated intraarticular injections of steroids can lead to steroid arthropathy, tendon rupture, postinjection flare, and infection in rare instances and should be avoided. Benefit from steroid injection lasts for 2 to 3 weeks but may be considerably longer in some patients.

SURGICAL MANAGEMENT

Surgical intervention is considered for intractable pain or deformity that limits function and is discussed separately elsewhere. It does not obviate the need for continued medical treatment.

Rheumatoid Arthritis
M. Paul Strottman

Rheumatoid arthritis is a disease in which chronic inflammation is largely responsible for the familiar clinical features and frequently for impairment of function. The nature of the inflammatory process and its interaction with the immune response in patients with classic RA are important in understanding this disease.

RA occurs in 1% to 3% of white adults, depending on the rigor of the classification criteria used. The ratio of women to men with RA (about 3:2) also varies somewhat with the criteria used and declines with increasing age. RA is seen in all races and occurs worldwide.

Products of the D region or class II genes of the major histocompatibility complex were demonstrated to control both immune responses and the susceptibility to several autoimmune diseases, including RA. People with HLA-DR4 and certain subtypes of DR1 are at greater risk for developing RF-positive (seropositive) erosive RA than are those without these genes. Even so, most with the HLA-DR4 gene do not develop RA. Other genetic factors and environmental influences important to RA susceptibility have not been fully clarified.

Extensive investigation into the cause of RA has been carried out for more than 40 years. The types of leukocytes and cell products involved in normal immune and inflammatory responses to bacteria and viruses carry on their activities in the RA joint, but the initiating and sustaining factors remain a mystery.

Bacterial and viral causes continue to be the most heavily studied, but as yet no conclusive evidence has been developed pointing to any particular responsible agent.

RHEUMATOID FACTORS

Rheumatoid factors are antibodies that react specifically with the Fc region of human immunoglobulin G (IgG) and have cross-reactivity with IgG of other species. The most readily measured RFs are of the IgM class, but RF activity is often demonstrable by special methods in IgG, IgA, and IgE. RF is detectable in normal sera but is elevated in the sera of most patients with RA and in patients with a variety of other diseases. In most conditions associated with elevated RF, including RA, individual sera contain a variety of RFs with differing reactivity, indicating their polyclonal nature.

The standard tests for RF determine essentially only IgM RF and include the latex fixation test and nephelometric assays. Results obtained by the various methods are qualitatively similar, but their sensitivity and quantitative results differ. Screening tests that indicate the presence or absence of RF at a predetermined concentration and quantitative methods are both readily available.

Elevated RF is seen in a large and heterogeneous group of diseases, including the following:

- RA
- Systemic lupus erythematosus (SLE)
- Sjögren syndrome
- Systemic sclerosis (scleroderma)
- Polymyositis and dermatomyositis
- Sarcoidosis
- Bacterial endocarditis (chronic)
- Tuberculosis
- Chronic hepatitis

The upper limit of normal is set so that about 5% of the normal population demonstrate low-titer positive RF in their sera, but the frequency and concentration increases modestly with advancing age.

PATHOLOGY

The earliest pathologic events in the joints of patients with RA are seen in the synovium: edema, microvascular proliferation, and perivascular T-lymphocyte infiltration in the subsynovial tissue. Subsequently, there are synovial lining cell proliferation and an increasing mononuclear cell infiltra-

tion consisting of additional T lymphocytes, macrophages, and fibroblasts. B cells and plasma cells also appear in chronic lesions, where germinal centers may resemble those of lymph nodes. Although T cells outnumber B cells at all stages, plasma cells increasingly secrete immunoglobulin, including RF, giving rise to complement-activating immune complexes. With continuation of the process, fibrin deposits on the surface of the synovium and granulation tissue develop, with further proliferation of fibroblasts, synovial lining cells, and additional new vessel formation to the point at which the redundant synovium forms folds and villi and is easily palpable as a spongy mass. All these features are those of a chronic inflammatory process. Granulocytes are relatively sparse in the synovial tissue.

In chronic RA, the layer of proliferating granulation tissue (*pannus*) gradually advances across the joint surface, destroying the margin of the articular cartilage as it progresses. Frequently, the pannus invades vascular foramina and destroys the supporting subchondral bone as well as the cartilage. This inflammatory process often involves joint capsules, ligaments, and tendons, resulting in extensive damage to these tissues. Fibrotic adhesions may develop within joints or may involve joint capsules and ligaments. Adhesion between tendons and tendon sheaths is also a frequent finding. These changes produce the contractures that cause permanent limitation of motion of joints and impaired joint function. The cellular biochemical processes underlying these clinical changes are outlined next.

An intense inflammatory process occurs in the synovial fluid simultaneous with that in the synovial tissue. It is largely an acute process, and granulocytes are prominent in the effusion. These granulocytes are derived from the blood and migrate through the capillary walls and synovial tissues into the joint space, attracted by chemotactic factors generated in part by complement activation. Once in the joint space, these cells remain and are destroyed there. Lysosomal enzymes from disintegrating granulocytes are a final means of tissue destruction in RA. They are released in quantities too great to be cleared from the joint by diffusion into the circulation. Thus, hydrolases, DNAases, proteinases (including elastase and collagenase), and other enzymes with capacity for damage to joint tissue accumulate within the synovial fluid and destroy the proteoglycan responsible for the viscosity of synovial fluid. They diffuse into the synovium, articular cartilage, and exposed bone in amounts that may overwhelm the inhibitors of these enzymes that are normally present, such as α_2-

macroglobulin and α_1-antitrypsin. In this way, granulocytes in synovial fluid, with the chronic inflammatory cells and fibroblasts in the synovium, release substances responsible for the progressively destructive nature of RA.

No consistent changes are seen in the numbers or ratio of types of lymphocytes in the peripheral blood of RA patients, in contrast to the characteristic composition of the various types and subsets of lymphocytes within the rheumatoid synovium. Evidence that an active immunologic process occurs within the joints in RA includes the presence of a high proportion of T cells bearing surface markers characteristic of activated T cells, such as class II major histocompatibility complex. Furthermore, synovial T cells are enriched for T cells bearing certain antigen receptors, whereas these same populations are depleted in the peripheral blood.

Soluble substances produced by active lymphocytes, monocytes, and macrophages (cytokines, lymphokines, E series prostaglandins, leukotriene B$_4$) are generated in the rheumatoid joint. These cell products have a variety of effects, including granulocyte, lymphocyte, and mononuclear cell activation, regulation, and chemotaxis; increase in vascular permeability; and activation of synovial cells, osteoclasts, mononuclear cells, and fibroblasts. Injection of these lymphokines into the joints of animals results in development of synovial inflammation. Thus, the soluble mediators liberated in RA may be important in augmentation and perpetuation of the inflammatory response, attracting more inflammatory cells to the synovium, which in turn produce more soluble mediators. Active inflammation is accompanied by attempted repair as the fibroblasts respond to the cytokines produced by local inflammatory cells by proliferating and secreting not only collagenases, which destroy cartilage and connective tissue, but also collagen itself. As inflammation wanes, collagen production may become dominant, leading to fibrosis and contractures.

The role of RF in the pathogenesis of RA is unclear. Patients with agammaglobulinemia, having extremely low serum levels of IgG and undetectable RF, may develop arthritis that closely resembles RA. Yet, patients who are seropositive for RF generally have more severe disease than those who are RF negative. IgM RF is actively produced in the rheumatoid joint, especially during flares of the disease. The resulting complexes activate complement, producing neutrophil chemotactic factors and agents that increase vascular permeability, providing a mecha-

nism for augmenting the inflammatory process. Thus, RF may intensify and perpetuate the inflammatory process, but there is no evidence that it is causative or even necessary.

CLINICAL FEATURES

Rheumatoid arthritis is a systemic disease that is variable in all its clinical features. Joint pain, stiffness, and fatigue are the most common symptoms. Patients may also have myalgia, malaise, mild fever, and weight loss of modest degree. These constitutional symptoms are more common in patients with severely active joint disease and in those with involvement of other organs. RA usually begins gradually, but occasionally the onset is more abrupt and rarely is precipitous, developing in the course of a day. Joint involvement is usually persistent, with inflammation continuing in affected joints for weeks to years, rather than being intermittent or migratory. There is a clear tendency for RA to be progressive, with involvement of increasing numbers of joints as the disease evolves. A definite predilection for small joints in the hands, feet, and wrists, usually in a fairly symmetric pattern is another common characteristic. There is relative sparing, however, of the DIP joints of the fingers and toes. Involvement of the large joints of the extremities in a relatively symmetric manner also occurs frequently. Inflammation of tendons and tendon sheaths resulting in tenosynovitis is common in RA and is an important cause of impaired function, especially of the hand.

Examination of the musculoskeletal system in RA patients who have active disease reveals signs of inflammation in the affected joints, with compression tenderness or pain on motion being the most frequent finding. Because the pathologic process in RA results in a major increase in synovial tissue and fluid volume, swelling of joints or tendon sheaths is common and is a major diagnostic feature. Increased warmth of the skin overlying joints is also common, but the magnitude of increase is intermediate between normal and that of a gouty joint. Similarly, although erythema of the skin overlying the joints may occur, it is not invariable.

Tenderness, swelling, and heat are clinical evidence of active inflammation. In RA, however, the chronic inflammatory process commonly results in varying degrees of damage to tissues, especially the articular cartilage, joint capsules, tendons, ligaments, and subchondral bone. Much of this damage is permanent, and it contributes greatly to the overall impairment of function of individual joints and collectively to impairment of the function of the patient.

The features of RA to be described next are examples of damage to tissues that may result from persistent inflammation. They illustrate another aspect of the natural history of RA, the frequently progressive nature of the disease. Many of these abnormalities are common in patients with established RA and are important clinically because they cause impairment of function.

Damage to the capsule and ligaments at the radiocarpal joint allows rotation of the carpometacarpal complex on the radius (counterclockwise when viewed from the dorsum) in response to the more dominant radially deviating forces that operate at the wrist. Volar subluxation of the carpus on the radius may occur because of capsular damage, often in combination with erosion of articular cartilage at the radiocarpal joint. The functional result of these deformities or of contracture of the joint may be pain on motion, a weak grip, or impaired ability to position the hand in performance of tasks.

The distal radioulnar joint is frequently affected in RA. There may be painful or restricted rotation of the forearm due to contracture, due to malalignment of the joint resulting from ligament laxity and dorsal subluxation of the distal ulna, or due to erosions within the joint. Wrist pain and inability to properly position the hand cause decreased hand function.

At the MCP joints, damage to the joint capsule and collateral ligaments results in weakness and laxity of these structures. When combined with the rotational deformity of the carpometacarpal complex, MCP joint laxity leads to ulnar deviation of the fingers at the MCP joints, one of the most common deformities seen with RA. It is often accompanied by volar or ulnar subluxation of the proximal phalanx at the MCP joint and by erosion of articular cartilage, resulting in compromise of hand function for strength of grip, for tasks requiring opposition of the thumb and index finger, or for positioning of the fingers for skilled tasks.

Inflammation may involve the intrinsic muscles of the hand, resulting in spasm. When prolonged and severe, it may lead to fibrosis and contracture of these muscles. Because the tendons of these muscles attach to the extensor tendons of the fingers, intrinsic muscle contracture often causes impairment of hand closure. In the late far-advanced stage, it may result in *swan-neck deformities* of the fingers, in which there is fixed hyperextension of the PIP joint and accompanying flexion of the DIP joint.

Boutonniere deformity of a finger is present when there is a flexion contracture of the PIP joint in association with hyperextension of the DIP joint. This occurs as a result of damage to the central portion of the extensor tendon overlying the PIP joint, resulting in loss of active PIP joint extension. In addition, damage to the ligaments that support and maintain the position of the lateral bands of the extensor tendon along their course to the point of attachment at the base of the distal phalanx leads to volar displacement of the lateral bands to a level below the axis of rotation of the PIP joint. As a result, their extension force is converted to a flexion force at the PIP joint. The combined result of these lesions is loss of active extension with unopposed flexion forces at the PIP joint, leading to contracture of this joint while active extension of the DIP joint is maintained.

Baker cysts often develop in the popliteal space when inflammation in the knee results in persistent effusion of moderate or greater size. There is marked increase in intraarticular pressure; and gradually a portion of the posterior capsule weakens, and the synovial membrane is forced outward through the defect. Because the pressure within the knee is intermittently greater than in the cyst, the cyst may gradually enlarge and dissect along fascial planes downward into the calf. The cyst does not have a normal supporting fibrous capsule, and therefore, it is prone to rupture with leakage of the inflammatory synovial fluid into the tissues of the calf of the leg. When this occurs, there is often abrupt pain, swelling, and heat in the calf, frequently mimicking deep venous thrombosis or cellulitis. In the absence of rupture, the popliteal cyst may cause chronic pain or partial venous compression, resulting in edema of the calf and foot. The diagnosis of a popliteal cyst may be accurately made by arthrography of the knee, which demonstrates a communication with the cyst and outlines the extent of its dissection. Ultrasonography is also helpful in diagnosis and is a noninvasive procedure. A period of rest and conservative treatment is indicated for acute rupture. Cysts that are large and symptomatic or that rupture repeatedly are treated by synovectomy of the knee to reduce the rate of formation of synovial fluid, rather than by excision of the cyst.

RA frequently involves the cervical spine and may affect any of its articulations or ligaments, resulting in pain, laxity, or restricted motion. Of particular importance is damage to the ligaments that attach to the odontoid process of C2 and to the lateral masses of C1. When these ligaments become lax during flexion of the neck, anterior subluxation of C1 relative to C2 and the odontoid process may occur, with simultaneous decrease of the AP diameter of the spinal canal, a condition called *atlantoaxial subluxation.* With progression of the subluxation, compression of the spinal cord may occur and cause severe neurologic damage. Subluxation may also occur at any of the lower levels of the cervical spine (*subaxial subluxation*), with similar potential for neurologic damage.

Less frequently occurring than atlantoaxial subluxation, but with even greater potential for serious neurologic injury, is the condition of cranial settling in which erosion of the occipital condyles or the lateral masses of C1 results in a gradual caudal movement or settling of the skull relative to the odontoid process. With progression of the lesion, the odontoid process may gradually protrude into the foramen magnum. There it may compress the medulla or pons, resulting in a variety of neurologic complications, including sensory or motor impairment in the extremities, cranial nerve dysfunction, and impairment of rectal and urinary bladder sphincter function. The course and severity of cervical spine subluxation correlates with the severity of peripheral joint erosion.

The forefoot is commonly involved in RA, and a number of problems frequently occur as a result. These include widening or splaying of the forefoot, hallux valgus, hallux rigidus, and cock-up deformities of the small toes. Atrophy or anterior migration of the soft tissue pad on the plantar surface of the MTP joints may occur in later stages of the disease, resulting in prominence of the metatarsal heads, pain when bearing weight and, at times, ulceration. These forefoot deformities often occur in combination and result in difficulty in proper fitting of shoes, painful feet, or both. They are a common cause of severe impairment of ambulation.

The hindfoot is also frequently involved in patients with RA. The results are variable and include contracture, especially of the subtalar joints or, alternatively, excessive laxity of these joints with development of a valgus deformity, often associated with laxity of other tarsal joints, and abduction and pronation of the midfoot and forefoot.

COURSE AND PROGNOSIS

The course of RA is extremely variable, from active disease of several months duration followed by prolonged spontaneous remission without residual evidence of joint disease to persistently and severely active arthritis that progressively damages joints over several years, producing multiple deformities and incapacitating impairment of function, even for the necessary activities of personal care and daily living. The number of patients who have early and complete remission is not accurately known, and estimates vary from 10% to 30%. Most patients with RA who seek ongoing care have chronic disease that continues for many years, with varying degrees of disease activity. Periods of severe joint inflammation may be interspersed with periods of milder disease during which symptoms and signs are less prominent. Damage to joints and other musculoskeletal tissues increases progressively in RA, correlating reasonably well with the degree and duration of inflammation.

EXTRAARTICULAR RHEUMATOID DISEASE

Lesions outside the musculoskeletal system occur frequently in patients with RA. They are essentially restricted to those who have RF in their serum and ultimately are seen in about 25% of all patients with RA. Like the joint disease, the extraarticular lesions are characterized by chronic inflammation, usually classified as rheumatoid nodules, serositis, or vasculitis. If persistent, this chronic inflammation can result in fibrosis or destruction of tissue.

Rheumatoid nodules are the most common extraarticular lesion and are seen in about 25% of all patients. They usually do not appear early in the course of RA, most often occurring sometime after the first year of disease. Pathologically, rheumatoid nodules reveal a central area of fibrinoid necrosis surrounded by histiocytes and chronic inflammatory cells. They are most frequently found in the subcutaneous tissue or in tendons. The most common locations are on the extensor surfaces of the forearm just distal to the elbow and around the hands, wrists, feet, and ankles. The location of nodules is often at sites of repeated application of pressure, such as the forearm and posterior aspect of the heel. Less frequent locations of rheumatoid nodules include the ischial tuberosities in patients who are infirm and who sit a good deal, and over the occiput in patients who are bedridden. Rarely, nodules occur in viscera or in the pleura. Excision of nodules is generally not recommended because they tend to recur.

Other extraarticular manifestations of RA are less common than rheumatoid nodules and usually do not appear until after the arthritis has been present for several years. Their appearance may not be synchronous with the activity of disease in the joints. Not uncommonly, clinical manifestations of extraarticular disease become severe and may overshadow the joint disease in their impact on the patient's life.

Sjögren syndrome occurs in about 10% of RA patients. It is caused by chronic inflammation that involves various exocrine glands, most often the lacrimal and salivary glands, resulting in impaired secretory function and drying of the cornea or mucous membranes. Often, complications arise as a result of the loss of secretion, such as infection, accelerated dental caries, or desiccation and loss of corneal epithelium.

Felty syndrome is characterized by the occurrence of splenomegaly and peripheral blood cytopenia, most often granulocytopenia. It may result in increased susceptibility to bacterial infections, which may be persistent and life-threatening. Interestingly, the increased risk of infection does not correlate well with the absolute granulocyte count in the peripheral blood, indicating that additional factors operate to impair the response to infection.

Leg ulcers due at times to cutaneous vasculitis and at other times to pyoderma gangrenosum occur in patients with RA. They are seen with increased frequency in patients with Felty syndrome.

Evidence of previous serositis, either pleuritis or pericarditis, is found at autopsy in about 40% of patients with erosive RA, but clinically it is much less common because it is so often painless. The most frequent manifestation is moderate or large pleural effusion with a recurrent or persistent course. Although constrictive pericarditis is known to occur in these patients, it is uncommon for the process to progress to significant impairment of hemodynamic function.

Rheumatoid disease affecting the parenchyma of the lung may take the form of single or multiple rheumatoid nodules. The nodules may cavitate and become secondarily infected, creating a lung abscess. Because the nodules are frequently subpleural, bronchopleural fistulas may occur, at times leading to empyema. Noninfectious pneumonic infiltrates may occur.

More common than pulmonary rheumatoid nodules or pneumonic infiltrates is the development of diffuse interstitial pulmonary fibrosis. Pulmonary fibrosis in RA patients has the same pathologic and clinical features as the fibrosis seen in idiopathic pulmonary fibrosis or in patients with scleroderma. It is bilateral and diffuse, and it affects the lower portions of the lungs to a somewhat greater degree than the upper portions. The process varies in severity but often progresses to moderate or severe degrees of impairment of pulmonary function and hypoxemia.

Secondary pulmonary hypertension with resulting cor pulmonale may occur.

Sjögren syndrome may also affect the bronchial exocrine glands. This may result in impairment of mucociliary function with development of recurrent or chronic bronchitis. At times, this may lead to severe obstructive pulmonary disease, bronchiectasis, or both.

Inflammation in the eye, unrelated to Sjögren syndrome, may occur, most often in the form of episcleritis or scleritis. *Episcleritis* is a clinically mild condition in which there is inflammation of the superficial episcleral coat of the eye, resulting in injection, which is often asymptomatic. *Scleritis*, however, may cause extensive damage of the scleral coat of the eye. This may result in perforation of the sclera, herniation of ocular tissue, and loss of the eye.

Systemic necrotizing vasculitis occurs rarely in patients with RA and is considered to be the most severe expression of this disease. It is most often characterized by focal inflammatory or ischemic lesions of the skin, presenting as papules, purpura, ulcers, or gangrene, most often appearing in the distal portions of the extremities, especially fingers and toes. Vasculitis of the vasa nervorum can lead to ischemic damage of nerve trunks with resultant sensory and motor nerve deficits. Often, several nerve trunks are involved, leading to the designation of mononeuritis multiplex. Nerve involvement is often asymmetric, in contrast to the more symmetric involvement seen in diabetic peripheral neuropathy. Similarly, vasculitis may involve arterioles or venules in skeletal muscle, leading to muscle pain or tenderness. Weakness may occur as the result of vasculitis of muscle but is more frequently the result of peripheral nerve involvement. Rarely, the vasculitis may become more widespread and involve viscera. Patients who develop vasculitis are seriously ill, with extreme morbidity and increased mortality.

In patients with relatively more severe seropositive RA, small, 1- to 2-mm hemorrhagic cutaneous infarcts may occur, usually in the periungual regions of the digits, on the dorsum of the PIP or MCP joints, or on the extensor surface of the elbow. These are the result of obliterative vasculopathy and do not indicate that systemic necrotizing vasculitis is present.

LABORATORY FEATURES

Laboratory test abnormalities commonly seen in patients with RA reflect the systemic inflammatory nature of the disease. Mild normocytic normochromic anemia (hemoglobin concentration, 10 g/dL or greater) is present in most patients with active RA. Mild leukocytosis without obvious abnormality of the differential count is also common. Leukopenia is rare in the absence of Felty syndrome. Thrombocytosis is common in RA, the degree of increase in the platelet count correlating well with disease activity. Both the ESR and C-reactive protein (CRP) tests are commonly elevated, and the results correlate well with disease activity.

RF is elevated in the serum of about 80% of patients diagnosed as having RA, so it is not a sensitive test for RA. Neither is RF a specific test for RA, since it is found in the sera of patients with a wide variety of other inflammatory or infectious diseases.

Synovial fluid analysis in patients with RA gives evidence of the chronic inflammatory process occurring in joints. The fluid is mildly to moderately turbid on direct visual inspection, the turbidity correlating with the concentration of cells in the fluid. The mucin clot test, a measure of the integrity of the joint fluid proteoglycan, is abnormal, indicating depolymerization of the hyaluronate–protein complex. Viscosity is decreased because of the abnormal proteoglycan, as can be easily demonstrated by observing the length of the "strings" of synovial fluid drops as they are slowly ejected from a syringe.

The leukocyte count in synovial fluid in RA is increased, commonly in the range of 5000 to 50,000 cells/μL. Polymorphonuclear neutrophils are present in increased numbers, commonly in the range of 30% to 60%. No findings specific for RA are present in the synovial fluid, since the results only confirm the presence of chronic inflammation. The main value of synovial fluid analysis is in helping to rule out other causes of joint inflammation, for example, crystal-induced arthritis (by polarization microscopy) or bacterial infection (by culture).

DIAGNOSIS OF RHEUMATOID ARTHRITIS

Rheumatoid arthritis is a clinical syndrome, and the diagnosis is made by careful evaluation of the history, physical findings, laboratory tests, and radiographs. No specific physical finding or laboratory test result proves the diagnosis. As detailed earlier, clinical features most useful in supporting the diagnosis of RA include morning stiffness, progression to involve multiple joints, symmetric distribution, and a tendency to involve MCP, PIP, MTP, and wrist joints, sparing the DIP joints. Involvement of a single joint

or recurrences in a migratory pattern argue against RA. Arthritis in any MCP, MTP, or PIP joint on both sides meets the definition of symmetry. Involvement of the temporomandibular joints (TMJs) and the cervical spine is also frequent but is not of great diagnostic value.

Physical examination of the joints of patients with RA reveals signs of inflammation that reflect the pathologic nature of the disease. Inflamed synovium and joint effusion produce the typical soft, boggy swelling of the joint. The temperature of inflamed joints is increased to a mild or moderate degree, which is easily overlooked. Erythema of joints is slight or absent, in contrast to the greater inflammation seen in septic or gouty joints.

In patients with disease of longer duration, several deformities may occur that are characteristic of RA, but these rarely occur in the first few months when diagnosis is most often uncertain. Deformities such as ulnar deviation of the fingers, laxity, and subluxation of other joints are frequent but are also seen in other forms of chronic inflammatory arthritis.

In early RA, there is rarely evidence of inflammatory disease in other organs. Although extraarticular rheumatoid disease (such as Sjögren syndrome or Felty syndrome) occurs in 20% or more of RA patients, these features rarely appear at the time of onset of the arthritis. This is an important point in the differential diagnosis because if at onset there is evidence of active disease in other organs, such as rash or pleurisy, along with the arthritis, one must seriously investigate the possibility that the patient has a different disorder, such as SLE, vasculitis, or an infectious disease that may cause arthritis, such as hepatitis B.

As already discussed, the presence of RF is helpful but is not essential to the diagnosis and is often absent in the first 6 months of symptoms, when it would be most useful diagnostically. Radiographic examination of the joints often gives normal results if done early in the course of the disease. Typical changes consisting of demineralization of bone, uniform narrowing of joint spaces, and erosion of bone are commonly seen after 6 months or later.

In an effort to standardize the diagnosis of RA for purposes of clinical or epidemiologic investigations, the American Rheumatism Association (now the American College of Rheumatology) developed criteria for the classification of RA to facilitate accuracy of diagnosis. These criteria are clearly useful for their intended purposes and are also helpful as guides to diagnosis in individual cases. Because these criteria for definite or classic RA are stringent, however, clinical judgment must be used when patients present with inflammatory arthritis of recent onset that cannot yet be classified as definite or classic disease. Among the diseases that resemble early RA, the most common is RA itself.

MANAGEMENT OF PATIENTS WITH RHEUMATOID ARTHRITIS

Rheumatoid arthritis varies greatly in the manner and degree to which it may affect a patient's general health, ability to perform common daily tasks, capacity for work, and quality of life. Many patients have slowly progressive gradual decrease in functional capacity with increasing duration of disease. This gradual loss of function is largely due to progressive damage to joints and tendons. During the course of disease, however, there are frequently variations in the severity of the inflammatory process in joints, with resulting changes in the degree to which pain, stiffness, and fatigue affect the patient. Thus, skillful evaluation of patients to determine their treatment needs is essential for effective management. Periodic reassessment is necessary to ensure that changes in therapy are made when indicated.

Goal of Therapy

We cannot arrest the course of RA or induce a true remission with the treatment that is available. It is essential that we establish a goal of treatment toward which we can work as we care for patients with RA, so that our approach is orderly and focused. I believe that the appropriate goal is to improve and maintain a patient's functional capacity and quality of life. We will have varying degrees of success, and our results in those patients with more severe disease will be less favorable than in the others. Even though functional capacity will decline somewhat for many patients despite of our best efforts, in most instances, we can make substantial progress toward this goal.

Assessment of the Patient

The therapeutic needs of a patient can be determined by the history, physical examination, and readily available laboratory tests along with radiographs of selected joints when indicated. The first step in assessment of the patient is to learn whether the ar-

thritis is interfering to an important degree with the patient's ability to work, with personal and family life, or with sleep. If so, the approximate degree and rate of change of functional impairment of the patient's activities should next be determined.

If the patient has functional impairment, the relative contributions of inflammation and of structural damage to this impairment are assessed. Increased inflammation in joints commonly results in a decrease in functional capacity. With increased disease activity, the patient usually has increase in severity of pain, more prolonged morning stiffness, increased fatigue, and symptoms appearing in joints not previously symptomatic. Thus, a few questions can help the physician to ascertain whether a patient has had a recent flare of disease. On the other hand, damage to joints, ligaments, and tendons also occurs to some degree in most patients with RA, causing impaired function and even disabling restriction of activity, as, for example, when advanced hip joint destruction hampers walking.

It is important in the management of RA patients to assess and record the severity of joint inflammation and the spread of inflammation among joints, the two essential elements in the assessment of disease activity. Several methods were developed and shown to give results reproducible and accurate enough for clinical use. Commonly used measures include the patient's estimate of the *duration of morning stiffness*, that is, the time elapsed from arising in the morning until the stiffness maximally improves. This period may vary from no time for a patient whose arthritis is inactive, to 5 or 6 hours for those with moderately active disease, to the entire day for those with severe disease. The patient then estimates the time of day when *fatigue* generally appears, recording the number of hours that elapse from the time of arising. With increase in disease activity, there is regularly a decrease in muscle strength. Although the mechanism for this is not known, it occurs frequently and is one basis for a standard measure of disease activity in studies of patients with RA, namely grip strength.

Additional information is then obtained from examination of the extremity joints. First, the presence or absence of *tenderness* is determined for each joint. (For the hips, pain on motion is substituted for tenderness.) The degree of tenderness may be graded for additional information. Similar observations are made for *swelling* and *heat* for each joint. Usually, tenderness is the earliest and most sensitive sign of inflammation, followed by swelling; the presence of heat usually is noted only in the more actively inflamed joints. The number of joints that show each of these signs is recorded. *Erythema* of joints occurs relatively infrequently and thus is not of great help in the day-to-day evaluation of patients with RA.

The ESR or CRP concentration may be added as an additional measure of inflammation. With modest experience, these data can be interpreted to give a useful estimate of disease activity. The degree to which active disease contributes to impaired function influences the aggressiveness of therapy. The recording of comparable information at successive evaluations is also helpful in determining the effectiveness of treatment, especially with drugs that are slow acting, requiring several months for an adequate trial. The determination of disease activity eliminates an otherwise purely subjective approach to assessing the role of joint inflammation in a patient's problems and is essential to good management of patients with RA.

Just as important as the evaluation of the contribution of inflammation to decreased function in patients with RA is the assessment of the degree to which previous damage to joints, ligaments, and tendons impairs functional capacity. These manifestations of rheumatoid disease are the consequence of previous active inflammation but do not imply current inflammation, and so they do not justify treatment. Commonly encountered abnormalities include contracture of joints, laxity of joints with subluxation or instability, joint surface destruction, tendon rupture, and weakness and atrophy of muscle. Contracture results from adhesions developing within joints, from fibrosis of capsules or ligaments, or from fibrosis of muscle. Laxity of joints occurs as a result of damage to capsules or ligaments, with resulting loss of the joint-stabilizing function. Joint laxity may also occur because of articular cartilage destruction by the inflammatory process, which shortens the distance between the attachment points of ligaments. A commonly occurring example of laxity of ligaments and joint capsules, often accompanied by articular cartilage destruction, is ulnar deviation of the fingers at the MCP joints. Tendon rupture may occur because of destruction of tendons by the rheumatoid inflammatory process or by mechanical damage, which may occur when repetitive movement of a tendon over the irregular surface of an eroded bone results in tendon damage and ultimate rupture. Muscle weakness and atrophy may result from any of several factors and are often caused by several in combination. With contracture of a joint, the permanent loss of motion usually is accompanied by atrophy and weakness of muscle. Persistent pain is the most frequent cause of weakness because it

commonly prevents the normal application of muscle force necessary for maintenance of strength. Malaise, chronic fatigue, general debilitation, loss of interest, or depression may contribute to muscle weakness as well.

The latter group of problems ascribed to structural damage (contracture, joint laxity, joint surface destruction, tendon rupture, and muscle weakness) share common features that allow easy identification and evaluation. Although any may be present in more than one location, at each site, the problem presents with localized symptoms (eg, decrease in grip strength in the case of MCP joint contracture). In addition, the symptoms generally occur only when the abnormal structure is used or subjected to stress. In contrast, pain due to inflammation of a joint usually is more persistent, and there is usually accompanying prominent morning stiffness of that joint and constitutional symptoms. For all these conditions except joint surface destruction, physical examination reveals the anatomic abnormality. In the case of articular cartilage destruction, the problem is inferred from the history of pain with use of the joint (eg, pain on weight bearing in the case of knee joint surface damage), and radiograph confirms the finding.

Thus, physical examination and radiograph of appropriate joints can lead to accurate determination of the degree of anatomic abnormalities in patients with RA. Careful history taking usually enables the physician to estimate accurately the contribution of a particular abnormality to the impairment of function. Evaluation of the patient with RA requires only a modest investment of time. For therapeutic decisions, no battery of laboratory tests or radiographs of numerous joints can substitute for an accurate clinical evaluation. The most important aspect of the evaluation is the first step: careful assessment of the degree and nature of impairment of function because all treatment decisions should be based on this. For example, if a patient has clearly had a decrement of function that interferes with important activities, and evaluation reveals a moderately severe flare of the arthritis, more intensive antiinflammatory treatment is clearly indicated. In contrast, if a patient reports no recent change in functional status, and pain and stiffness are reasonably well controlled, it would not be appropriate to intensify therapy even though several joints may have tenderness or swelling. Finally, if pain or functional impairment appears to be due to structural damage in the absence of current inflammation, treatment should center on analgesia, physical therapy, or surgery, rather than antiinflammatory treatment.

Systemic Lupus Erythematosus and Immune Complex Disease

John S. Cowdery

Systemic lupus erythematosus is an autoimmune inflammatory disease of uncertain etiology that may affect multiple organ systems. Patients with SLE frequently exhibit serum antibodies that react with self antigens; additionally, these patients often have antigen–antibody complexes present in both serum and tissue. Thus, the arthritis of SLE and immune complex disease are discussed together.

Inflammatory arthritis or noninflammatory arthralgias are seen in most patients with SLE, with up to 100% of patients experiencing joint problems at some point in the course of their disease. Abnormal formation of immune complexes may occur in association with a variety of diseases distinct from SLE, including hepatitis B virus infection and other systemic infections, such as endocarditis. These diseases are characterized by a high level of circulating foreign antigen, which can, in combination with host antibody, form an immune complex. Additionally, serum sickness is seen with increasing frequency because of the clinical use of monoclonal antibodies derived from nonhuman sources. It is not clear whether the pathogenesis of the arthritis of SLE and that of immune complex arthritis are due to the same etiologic mechanism.

CLINICAL FEATURES

The diagnosis of SLE arthritis rests primarily on making the diagnosis of SLE. In SLE, the female/male ratio is about 9:1, with onset most common during the childbearing years. Common clinical features of SLE include an erythematous rash (frequently in sun-exposed areas); oral ulcers; pleuritis or pericarditis; nephritis; anemia, leukopenia, or thrombocytopenia; central nervous system manifestations; the presence of a number of autoantibodies; and arthritis. The arthritis of SLE may be polyarticular and, on occasion, difficult to distinguish from the polyarthritis associated with other rheumatic diseases. In SLE, the joints most commonly affected by arthritis are the knees and the small joints of the hands. Wrists, elbows, shoulders, ankles, and hips are less commonly involved. The axial skeleton is almost always spared. The symptoms of SLE arthritis are not strikingly different from those experienced by any patient with inflammatory arthritis. Prominent symptoms include pain (on motion and at rest) accompanied by tenderness to palpation and morning stiffness. Patients with SLE arthritis may experience pain of similar intensity to that experienced by patients with RA; however, the swelling and erythema that accompany SLE arthritis are frequently less striking than in RA. The clinical signs of SLE arthritis *may* distinguish it from other forms of inflammatory arthritides in that the arthritis of SLE is rarely destructive of bone, and the observed changes such as swan-neck deformity or marked ligamentous laxity are generally reducible. In contrast, RA is destructive of bone and results in permanent deformity.

An arthropathy commonly seen in SLE, especially in patients taking corticosteroids, is avascular necrosis of bone. Although this entity may affect virtually any joint, the hip, knee, and shoulder are most commonly affected. The abrupt onset of arthritis in a single large joint of an SLE patient should alert the clinician to the possibility of avascular necrosis. MRI scanning, which can reveal decreases in blood flow in avascular necrosis, is useful in determining whether a patient's symptoms arise from arthritis or from avascular necrosis.

The clinical features of immune complex arthritis not associated with SLE are much more difficult to categorize because the clinical symptoms may be more evanescent. The chief clinical feature identifying this entity is a clinical setting that could give rise to circulating immune complexes. The large joints—elbows, shoulders, knees, and hips—are the most commonly involved. The onset may be relatively abrupt, and the patient may experience severe pain in one or more affected joints accompanied by low-grade fever and, occasionally, a macular skin rash. The joint pain may be accompanied by objective signs of inflammation, such as redness, warmth, or an effusion. The severity of symptoms may appear out of proportion to the objective physical findings.

PATHOLOGIC AND RADIOLOGIC FEATURES

In SLE arthritis, radiographic abnormalities are usually absent. Sometimes, soft tissue swelling or joint subluxation are seen. Erosions are seen far less commonly than in RA. Since the subluxation in the small joints of the hand may be reducible (as occurs from placing them on a flat radiographic plate), a patient with clinically obvious subluxations may have a hand radiograph that shows normal bone alignment. Histopathologic studies of synovium in SLE have failed to demonstrate consistent pathologic features, and thus synovial biopsy is not useful in diagnosis. Documented findings include synovial fibrin deposition, hypercellularity, and perivascular inflammation.

LABORATORY FEATURES

As mentioned previously, the arthritis of SLE is most often seen in the setting of active disease in other organs. Laboratory features that document lupus activity therefore are useful in supporting the diagnosis of SLE arthritis. Specifically, arthritis may be accompanied by an elevated ESR, anemia, leukopenia, thrombocytopenia, a positive ANA test, and, in some patients, antibodies to double-stranded DNA. SLE is a clinical diagnosis that is based on symptoms, physical findings, and laboratory tests. The clinician cannot rely on a battery of laboratory tests to make the diagnosis of SLE. RF is usually negative. Synovial fluid findings are most consistent with an inflammatory arthritis with modest elevations in both the total number of leukocytes and the proportion of granulocytes. Leukocyte counts above 50,000 are unusual, however, and should increase suspicion of infection.

The arthritis seen in connection with other immune complex diseases is frequently not accompanied by diagnostic, or even strongly suggestive, laboratory tests. The ESR is variably elevated, and other laboratory tests may be normal. Synovial fluid is frequently scant, making aspiration difficult. When synovial fluid is analyzed, it shows less inflammatory characteristics than joint fluid from patients with SLE arthritis. Specifically, the leukocyte count is frequently below 10,000, with relative preservation of both viscosity and mucin clot formation.

MEDICAL MANAGEMENT

Since the articular manifestations of SLE frequently occur in the setting of disease affecting other organ systems, medical management is usually directed toward treating disease activity in major organs, such as kidney, bone marrow, or central nervous system.

Traditionally, a cornerstone of lupus therapy has been corticosteroids. These potent antiinflammatory medications can greatly diminish the patient's symptoms of fatigue, fever, rash, and arthritis. Unfortunately, corticosteroids have little impact on the long-term natural history of the disease, and these compounds have predictable toxicity that occurs with chronic use. In addition to obesity, glucose intolerance, osteoporosis, hypertension, and cataracts, which are experienced by most patients chronically taking steroids, patients with SLE who take steroids have an increased risk of infection and avascular necrosis of bone. Infectious complications and avascular necrosis can occur in lupus patients not taking steroids; however, steroid therapy significantly increases the risk of both these well-documented complications. The adverse effects of corticosteroids become most prominent at doses exceeding 20 mg daily. Cytotoxic agents such as azathioprine and cyclophosphamide are used to treat major organ involvement in SLE. Their use carries considerable risk, and they are of unproved benefit in SLE arthritis. Antimalarial agents, such as hydroxychloroquine, are used with some success in treating the cutaneous manifestations of disease but are of unproved benefit in SLE arthritis.

Management of SLE arthritis requires that the physician weigh the risk of therapy against the severity of the patient's symptoms. In many cases, symptoms can be effectively managed with NSAIDs. Some patients, however, continue to have disabling symptoms despite an adequate trial of these agents. These patients may benefit from a low dose of supplemental corticosteroid given as either a stable daily dose (5 to 15 mg) or as alternate day therapy (15 to 25 mg alternating with 5 to 10 mg daily). In general, it is best to avoid using a "burst-and-taper" regimen. Patients with SLE arthritis have a chronic condition that responds to the initial high doses but frequently flares with the attendant rapid taper. Thus, it may be advisable to identify the lowest dose that acceptably controls the patient's symptoms and, after maintaining the patient for several weeks, to attempt a slow taper to test whether a lower dose will suffice.

The arthritis seen in patients with SLE usually responds to the previously outlined medical regimen. Because this arthritis is rarely destructive of bone, joint replacement is rarely indicated. On occasion, ligamentous laxity (which accounts for the reducible deformities seen in SLE arthritis) may be of sufficient severity to warrant surgical reconstruction, particularly in the MCP joints of the hand. This surgical intervention is almost always intended to restore function (hand closure) and is rarely helpful in managing painful symptoms of SLE arthritis. In the case of immune complex arthritis, management consists of addressing the underlying condition that causes circulating immune complexes and treating the accompanying arthritis conservatively with analgesics, rest, and NSAIDs. Because the duration of this arthritis is defined by the presence of circulating or tissue immune complexes, this condition does not behave as a chronic arthritis. Because of the limited duration of the symptoms and the possible presence of an underlying infectious disease (eg, hepatitis, endocarditis), corticosteroids should be avoided.

Enthesopathies
Robert W. Karr

Several distinct forms of arthritis share the clinical features referred to as enthesopathy and spondyloarthropathy. Enthesopathy is an inflammatory process that involves an enthesis, the anatomic site of insertion of a ligament into bone. *Spondyloarthropathy* refers to a type of arthritis that involves the sacroiliac joints and the vertebrae. These shared features are the basis for classifying ankylosing spondylitis (AS), reactive arthritis, and psoriatic arthritis as enthesopathies and often as spondyloarthropathies as well.

ANKYLOSING SPONDYLITIS

Clinical Features

Ankylosing spondylitis is a form of arthritis that always involves the sacroiliac joints, often involves the spine, and may also involve peripheral joints. The cardinal symptom of AS is back pain. Because back pain is a common symptom, however, the physician must differentiate the back pain of AS from the more common mechanical back pain. Several characteristic features of the back pain of AS have been defined. The back pain of AS usually begins insidiously in the third or fourth decades. In contrast to mechanical back pain, however, the back pain of AS persists for longer than 3 months and tends to be relieved by exercise. Back stiffness in the morning is another common feature of AS. Peripheral joint involvement, which occurs in about 20% of AS patients, is typically an asymmetric oligoarthritis that involves the large joints of the lower extremities. The inflammatory synovitis of peripheral joints may cause pain, erythema, warmth, swelling, and effusion. These findings in an involved peripheral joint are indistinguishable from RA, although the pattern of involvement is different. Extraarticular manifestations of AS include weight loss, fatigue, fever, chronic prostatitis, conjunctivitis, and uveitis. Enthesopathic symptoms may include heel pain at the insertion of the Achilles tendon or the plantar fascia.

In early disease, the examination often reveals a mildly abnormal erect posture with slightly flexed hips and decreased motion of the lower spine. In more advanced disease, there may be loss of the normal lumbar lordosis, decreased motion of the cervical and lumbar spine, decreased chest expansion, and increased hip flexion when standing. There is a typical manner of body movement in AS that is characterized by movement of the torso as one block because of spinal stiffening. Evidence of enthesopathy on examination may include heel tenderness due to Achilles tendonitis or plantar fasciitis or soft tissue swelling over the Achilles tendon.

The prevalence of AS is about 1%. Among the 7% of the population who are HLA-B27–positive, however, about 20% develop AS. Recent evidence indicates that AS occurs with equal frequency in men and women, although the patterns of disease differ. Women tend to have generally milder disease with more severe cervical spine involvement and early peripheral joint involvement. Symptoms of sacroiliac and lumbar disease are much more common in men.

Pathologic Features

The distinctive pathologic feature of AS is involvement of the enthesis, the site of insertion of ligaments and joint capsules into bone. Enthesopathy may cause bony erosions at the enthesis. The reparative process that follows the initial inflammatory phase is characterized by ossification at these sites. This enthesopathic process is the basis for many of the findings in AS: for example, heel pain and spurs, syndesmophyte formation, and squaring of the vertebral bodies. The synovitis that may also occur in AS is pathologically indistinguishable from the synovitis of RA.

Radiologic Features

Sacroiliitis is essential for the diagnosis of AS. Radiographic involvement of the sacroiliac joints, which may be adequately assessed on a routine AP radiograph of the pelvis, range from minimal blurring of the joint margins in early disease to complete ankylosis of the joints in advanced disease. In intermediate stages, erosions, narrowing of the joint space, and sclerosis along the joint margins may be seen. Other radiographic manifestations of AS include squaring of normally concave anterior surfaces of vertebral bodies due to enthesopathic erosions of the upper and lower corners of the vertebrae and syndesmophyte formation. Syndesmophytes, which appear radiographically as fine lines of ossification that bridge the outer aspects of the intervertebral disks between vertebral bodies, result from ossification of the outer fibers of the annulus fibrosis. Radiographic manifestations of extraspinal disease include bony erosions in involved peripheral joints and erosions and new bone formation at sites of enthesopathy. For example, erosions, periostitis, or bone spurs may be seen in the calcaneus at the insertion of the Achilles tendon or the plantar fascia. Asymmetric involvement is more common in the periphery than in the spine.

Laboratory Features

No laboratory tests are diagnostic for AS. The ESR rate may be elevated, but in general, it does not correlate well with disease activity. The histocompatibility antigen HLA-B27, which occurs in only 7% of normal people, is present in over 90% of white patients with AS. Similar associations also exist in other racial groups. This strong association of B27 and AS is thought to be an important clue to the etiopathogenesis of the disease; however, B27 testing, which is expensive, adds little to the evaluation of an individual patient with symptoms suggestive of AS. The history and physical examination and radiographic findings should remain the basis for the diagnosis of AS.

Medical Management

The goals of medical management of AS are pain relief and preservation of function. When the disease is recognized early, before significant changes in posture occur, a motivated patient, who will faithfully conduct a prescribed daily spinal range-of-motion exercise program, may be able to minimize the development of spinal deformities. Although no therapeutic measures are known to halt the underlying process of ossification and fusion, careful attention to posture and exercises may lead to the maintenance of a functional, erect posture as the spine mobility decreases. Therefore, patient education and the involvement of a physical therapist are essential to management of the disease. Because fusion of the costochondral and costovertebral joints may decrease chest expansion, patients should be encouraged to cease smoking.

Many of the NSAIDs may be used in the treatment of AS. Indomethacin is often the first medication used because of its potency and acceptable toxicity; it may be given in doses of 25 to 50 mg three times per day. Sulindac, naproxen, and tolmetin are often effective, and aspirin is less so. Because of its potential toxicity, phenylbutazone should be reserved for those cases in which the pain of AS is unresponsive to indomethacin and other NSAIDS.

REACTIVE ARTHRITIS

Clinical Features

The clinical syndrome of reactive arthritis consists of postinfectious inflammatory oligoarthritis that may occur in association with involvement of the eyes, skin, and mucus membranes. The preceding infection occurs in either the genitourinary or the gastrointestinal tract. Nongonococcal urethritis, in some cases due to *Chlamydia trachomatis,* may be the preceding illness; whereas dysenteric illnesses with *Campylobacter, Yersinia, Shigella,* or *Salmonella* sp may also precede the development of the clinical syndrome. The arthritis usually begins acutely 1 to 3 weeks after the infection and typically presents as an asymmetric inflammatory arthritis involving primarily the large joints (knees and ankles) of the lower extremities. Involvement of a toe may result in a typical "sausage toe" appearance. Enthesopathic symptoms such as heel pain may also occur. Back pain is common during the initial episode, and spine involvement with sacroiliitis may eventually develop in 20% of patients with reactive arthritis. Conjunctivitis or uveitis may also occur with reactive arthritis. Cutaneous lesions include inflammation of the glans penis (circinate balanitis) and hyperkeratotic lesions that occur primarily on the soles of the feet (keratodermia blennorrhagicum).

Reiter syndrome describes a specific clinical presentation of reactive arthritis that includes the classic triad of arthritis, conjunctivitis, and urethritis. The concept of *reactive arthritis* is preferred to the previous terminology of *complete* or *incomplete Reiter syndrome* to describe the variable symptom complex that may be associated with postinfectious inflammatory arthritis. Organisms implicated include *Klebsiella, Yersinia, Chlamydia,* and other pathogens of the gastrointestinal tract; yet the arthritis occurs long after the infection and has not been shown to be altered by antibiotic treatment. The clinical course of reactive arthritis is variable; patients may have only the initial episode or a pattern of recurrent episodes of arthritis, but at least half of patients have chronic joint symptoms. Therefore, a significant percentage of patients with reactive arthritis may have chronic disability associated with the disease.

Reactive arthritis occurs in both men and women, with women constituting 10% to 20% of the cases. Some patients with an inflammatory oligoarthritis that involves primarily large joints of the lower extremities suggestive of reactive arthritis may not have had an identifiable antecedent infection. It is reasonable to categorize patients who maintain this pattern of joint involvement as having reactive arthritis.

Pathologic Features

The synovial changes in reactive arthritis are nonspecific and are similar to those found in RA.

Radiologic Features

Generally, no radiographic abnormalities are present at the time of the initial presentation of reactive arthritis. Chronic arthritis of a knee or ankle may result in joint space narrowing, erosions, and juxtaarticular osteoporosis, changes that are indistinguishable from those found in RA. At the site of enthesopathic involvement, such as the insertion of the Achilles tendon or plantar fascia, erosions or periostitis may be visible. Sacroiliitis occurs in about 20% of patients with reactive arthritis. In contrast to the symmetric sacroiliitis of AS, the sacroiliitis of reactive arthritis may be asymmetric. Spinal involvement is characterized by asymmetric, nonmarginal syndesmophytes that may skip some vertebrae.

Laboratory Features

No laboratory test is diagnostic of reactive arthritis. The ESR does not correlate well with disease activity, so a normal value does not exclude active reactive arthritis. The synovial fluid analysis is typical of an inflammatory arthritis, with a high leukocyte count (up to 75,000 cells/μL, although there is a wide range). In those patients who present with inflammatory oligoarthritis, septic arthritis should be included in the differential diagnosis, and the fluid should be cultured. By definition, however, the joint fluid is sterile in reactive arthritis. HLA-B27 is found in 80% to 90% of white patients with reactive arthritis, compared with about 7% of normal controls. B27 testing, however, is of minimal usefulness in the evaluation of individual patients. Reactive arthritis remains a clinical diagnosis based on the history, pattern of joint involvement, and presence of associated ocular or mucocutaneous manifestations.

Medical Management

Nonsteroidal antiinflammatory drugs are used in the treatment of the joint and enthesopathic symptoms of reactive arthritis. Indomethacin, 50 mg three times per day, is often beneficial and is usually the first drug prescribed. The minority of patients with progressive disease unresponsive to NSAIDs may require therapy with methotrexate.

PSORIATIC ARTHRITIS

Psoriatic arthritis is a form of inflammatory arthropathy that occurs in association with psoriasis. About 10% of patients with psoriasis develop an inflammatory arthritis. There is an association between psoriatic nail involvement and psoriatic arthritis; nail involvement occurs in 80% of patients with psoriatic arthritis and in 30% of patients without arthritis. Several different patterns of joint involvement occur in psoriatic arthritis. The most common pattern is an asymmetric oligoarthritis. Other patterns of joint involvement include a symmetric polyarthritis that is similar to RA, an arthritis with predominant involvement of the DIP joints, a severe deforming arthritis characterized by osteolysis and ankylosis, and a pattern resembling AS in 5%. "Sausage digits" may occur in psoriatic arthritis as well as in reactive arthritis. Enthesopathic symptoms, such as heel pain, may also occur in psoriatic arthritis. In most patients, the skin lesions of psoriasis develop before the arthritis. In about 15% of patients, however, the arthritis precedes the skin disease.

The pathologic features of the synovium in psoriatic arthritis are indistinguishable from those found in RA. Likewise, many of the radiologic features of psoriatic arthritis, such as joint space narrowing, erosions, and juxtaarticular osteoporosis, do not differ from those of RA. The DIP joint involvement with erosions and osteolysis of the terminal phalanx are,

however, different from changes found in RA or osteoarthritis. Spinal involvement in psoriatic arthritis includes sacroiliitis and syndesmophytes, which are often asymmetric. Most patients with psoriatic arthritis may be treated adequately with an NSAID. In patients with the symmetric polyarthritis pattern of disease, therapy with gold may be effective. The treatment of the skin and joints should be approached individually; in general, the arthritis does not improve significantly as the skin improves in response to therapy.

Juvenile Rheumatoid Arthritis

Richard R. Olson
Mary M. Jones

Juvenile rheumatoid arthritis (JRA) is a group of chronic inflammatory diseases that occur before the age of 16 years. Important to our understanding of JRA has been the identification of three distinct modes of onset of disease: *pauciarticular, polyarticular,* and *systemic.* The pertinent differential diagnoses, the prognoses, and the complications vary with the mode of JRA onset (Table 5-4). Common to all forms of JRA are the challenges involved in ther-

apy of a chronic inflammatory condition occurring in growing, developing individuals. A multidisciplinary approach, including physical therapist, occupational therapist, medical social worker, orthopaedist, ophthalmologist, and rheumatologist, is necessary to ensure the best possible outcome.

The etiology and pathogenesis of JRA remain unknown. As with adult RA, genetic susceptibility related to HLA may play an important role. *Juvenile*

TABLE 5-4.
Juvenile Rheumatoid Arthritis Subgroup Types

Onset Type	Gender Ratio	Clinical Features	Outcome
Pauciarticular (50% of cases)	F > M	Involves four or fewer joints	Generally good for joint disease
		High frequency of ANA-positive and uveitis	Risk of vision damage
		Subgroup may develop ankylosing spondylitis, especially HLA-B27–positive patients	
Polyarticular (40% of cases)	F > M	Usually older age at onset	Severe arthritis in about half of RF-positive and one fourth of RF-negative patients
		Symmetric involvement of many joints	
		Subgroup has positive serum rheumatoid factor and nodules	
Systemic (10% of cases)	F = M	Fever, rheumatoid rash, serositis, leukocytosis, negative RF and ANA	Severe arthritis in one fourth of patients
		Systemic symptoms may predate onset of chronic arthritis by months	

ANA, antinuclear antibody; HLA, histocompatibility antigen; RF, rheumatoid factor.

rheumatoid arthritis is the most commonly used diagnostic term for children with chronic arthritis of unknown etiology and is the term designated by the American College of Rheumatology in its classification criteria. In some other countries, the term *rheumatoid* is reserved for those children with circulating serum RF and an inflammatory arthritis similar to adult RA; and other forms of idiopathic arthritis are called *juvenile arthritis* or *juvenile chronic arthritis*.

DIFFERENTIAL DIAGNOSIS

Chronic arthritis in children and many other conditions that present with arthralgias or apparent arthritis have multiple etiologies. Essential to the diagnosis of JRA is the presence of *chronic* arthritis (longer than 6 weeks' duration) and the exclusion of other conditions by history, physical examination, and appropriate laboratory testing. Laboratory criteria are not used in the diagnosis of JRA, except those that exclude alternative diagnoses. The possibility of malignancy or infection must always be considered in the evaluation of a child with joint pain (Fig. 5-8). Synovial fluid aspiration and analysis is often helpful when fluid is detectable clinically and is mandatory in cases in which infection is a diagnostic possibility. "Growing pains," or benign limb pains, are common in school-aged children. These poorly localized pains usually occur in the lower extremities in the evening or at night and normally last a few days to weeks. Severe pain, altered gait, morning stiffness, and abnormalities on physical examination such as joint swelling suggest consideration of alternative diagnoses, including JRA.

CLINICAL CHARACTERISTICS

Several features distinguish JRA from adult RA. Inflammatory arthritis in children (particularly younger children) is much less likely to present with complaints of pain, even when there is easily demonstrable inflammatory arthritis on examination. Like adults, children with chronic arthritis may develop destructive bony changes and soft tissue flexion contractures. Children, however, are much more prone to develop ankylosis of peripheral joints and particularly the cervical spine. Growth disturbances can result from suppression of linear growth by inflammatory disease and premature epiphyseal closure. Only a minority of JRA patients are RF positive (10% to 20%); all of these have polyarticular onset.

Pauciarticular Onset

Pauciarticular (oligoarticular) disease is the most common form of JRA, constituting over half of cases. Up to four joints are affected, most commonly large

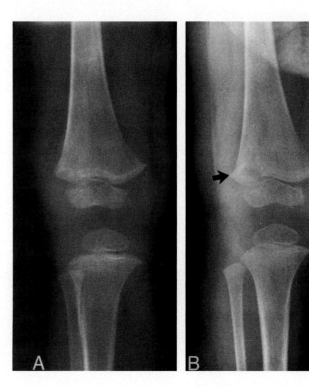

FIGURE 5-8. Osteomyelitis. An 18-month-old girl with persistent right knee swelling. **(A)** The first radiograph was taken 3 days into her illness and was read as normal. **(B)** A radiograph obtained 17 days later shows a subtle lucency in the lateral distal femoral metaphysis.

joints in an asymmetric fashion. In about half of pauciarticular patients, disease is limited to a single joint, most often the knee. Elbows and ankles are also commonly involved. In distinction from polyarticular JRA and adult RA, small joints of the hands and feet are less frequently involved. This presentation often afflicts young girls, with a peak age of onset at about 2 years of age. These girls have a high incidence of concomitant inflammatory eye disease (uveitis) as well as ANA in sera. A smaller peak of disease onset occurs in the 10- to 15-year-old age group. These patients are generally boys, who in many cases ultimately develop AS. Indeed, 75% of patients with pauciarticular JRA who are HLA-B27–positive develop spondylitis.

Joint symptoms in pauciarticular disease are often mild and of insidious onset. The patient may present to the pediatrician for evaluation of abnormal gait or a reluctance to walk or play. These patients do not appear systemically ill. Undiagnosed or untreated disease may result in (and present with) muscular atrophy and joint contractures, particularly of the knee. As with other subtypes of JRA, growth distur-

bances of variable degree occur depending on severity of disease, age of affliction, and duration of joint inflammation. Localized growth disturbances are particularly common in the pauciarticular form (Fig. 5-9).

Polyarticular Onset

Thirty to 40% of patients present with disease involving more than four joints. Girls are most commonly affected, and both large and small joint involvement may be seen. Patients with serum RF often have a persistent destructive arthropathy and associated subcutaneous rheumatoid nodules. This small group of patients represents the onset in childhood of classic adult RA. RF-negative patients generally have less aggressive disease without rheumatoid nodules but a striking tendency for ankylosis, particularly in the cervical spine (Fig. 5-10).

Patients often present with a gradual onset of symptoms: decreased activity, morning stiffness, joint swelling, and occasionally joint pain. Systemic

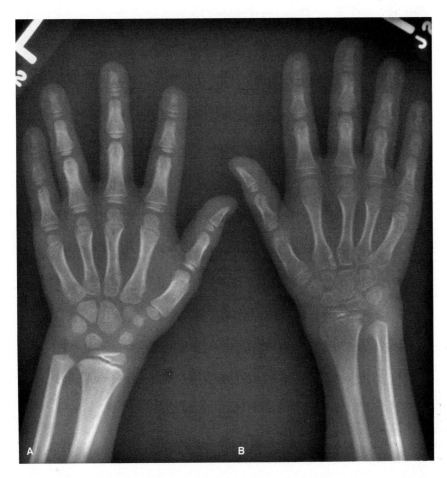

FIGURE 5-9. Pauciarticular juvenile rheumatoid arthritis with discrepancy in bone age. Radiographs of a 7-year-old girl with right wrist arthritis of 3 years' duration. Soft tissues of the right hand and forearm are underdeveloped compared with the left. Radiographs demonstrate osteopenia as well as enlargement of carpal bones, distal radius, and ulnae.

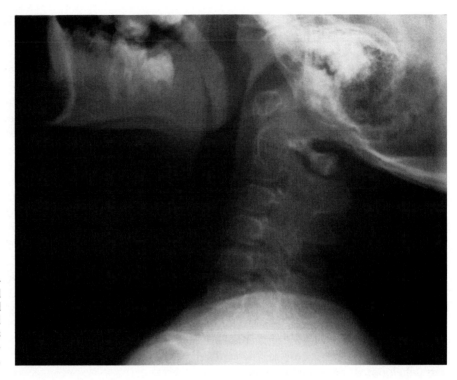

FIGURE 5-10. Juvenile rheumatoid arthritis (JRA) of cervical spine. Radiograph of 12-year-old with long-standing JRA. Lateral radiograph of cervical spine shows C2–C4 and occipital–atlantal fusion as well as diffuse osteopenia.

symptoms occur but are generally mild. Low-grade fever, fatigue, and poor appetite may occur for weeks or months before diagnosis. Examination reveals proliferative synovitis and effusions and often loss of joint motion. Mild adenopathy or hepatosplenomegaly is sometimes present. Chronic uveitis occurs less frequently than in pauciarticular JRA.

The differential diagnosis of polyarticular onset disease is extensive. Acute rheumatic fever, viral arthritis, prodromal hepatitis, and metabolic bone diseases warrant consideration. Neuroblastoma and lymphoid malignancies are the most common neoplasms that present as polyarthritis in children.

Systemic Onset

Systemic onset of JRA (Still disease) occurs in 10% to 20% of cases. Inflammatory arthritis is not always present on initial evaluation, but when present, it is an important clue to the diagnosis. These children present with high fever, malaise, and rash. The fever pattern in Still disease is classically hectic, with one or more daily spikes to the 38.8°C to 40.5°C (102°F to 105°F) range, followed by a return to normal or occasionally subnormal temperatures. The rash is often present only during fever spikes or after a hot bath, when it transiently appears as a fine, salmon-colored, macular eruption of the trunk, proximal ex-

tremities, and skin overlying affected joints. Most patients have adenopathy and hepatosplenomegaly and are found to have moderate to severe anemia and a striking neutrophilic leukocytosis. Other manifestations of systemic onset disease may include pericarditis, myocarditis, pleural effusion, and interstitial lung disease. Renal disease is rare during the presentation of Still disease and suggests consideration of alternative diagnoses such as SLE or systemic vasculitis. Other important considerations in the differential diagnosis include infections (particularly osteomyelitis and abdominal abscesses), inflammatory bowel disease, and malignancy. RF and ANA are usually absent, and diagnosis is made on clinical findings.

COURSE, COMPLICATIONS, AND PROGNOSIS

Considerable variability is found in the severity and the responsiveness to therapy of JRA. Patients with pauciarticular disease generally have milder synovitis and a better prognosis. However, 10% to 15% of patients with pauciarticular onset later progress to polyarticular disease. Patients with pauciarticular disease may develop significant disability due to joint contractures and muscular atrophy, even with control of inflammatory arthritis activity. One cannot overemphasize the importance of physical therapy in the management of these patients.

Polyarticular disease has a variable prognosis. Patients with RF often develop progressive disease extending into the adult years and disability in the absence of effective therapy. Patients with systemic onset generally recover from the acute systemic illness without major sequelae, but synovitis with either an oligoarticular or polyarticular pattern may then persist.

Ocular Complications

Eye involvement occurs in about 25% of pauciarticular JRA patients, in 5% of polyarticular patients, and rarely in systemic-onset patients. A chronic anterior uveitis occurs most commonly in young girls who are ANA positive. Insidiously progressive disease may result in posterior synechiae with resultant pupillary abnormalities, and occasionally band keratopathy may be seen. Loss of vision results from the development of secondary glaucoma, cataracts, and keratopathy. Early detection and treatment are essential to improving the outcome of JRA-associated uveitis. The eye disease is usually asymptomatic at onset, and patients with pauciarticular disease should be seen by an ophthalmologist at least every 3 months during the first 2 to 3 years of disease and then every 6 months for several more years. There is no correlation between the severity of arthritis and risk for development of uveitis.

Growth Disturbances

Children with chronic inflammatory disease of any type may have generalized inhibition of growth and subsequent short stature. Occasionally, periarticular hyperemia results in premature epiphyseal fusion with resultant shortening of the affected extremity. Prolonged hyperemia may at times cause accelerated bone growth (see Fig. 5-9). Leg length discrepancies are the most common orthopaedic sequelae of JRA and can be severe. TMJ involvement may result in a shortened mandible and micrognathia. This may result in disturbances of speech and chewing in addition to the cosmetic alteration. Surgery may be complicated by difficulties with endotracheal intubation, particularly in patients with associated cervical spine fusion.

Hip disease is unusual at onset of JRA but is commonly seen in patients with polyarticular disease.

Muscle spasm and disuse results in flexion contracture. Hip involvement in early childhood may contribute to valgus deformity of the femoral neck, persistent femoral anteversion, and dysplasia of both femoral head and acetabulum. Postoperative ectopic bone formation occasionally complicates surgical management of severe disease. Nonetheless, joint replacement can be successful in patients with disabling, end-stage disease. Knee involvement typically results in flexion contracture. Associated leg length discrepancy and hip disease may also contribute to development of contracture as well as genu valgus. Secondary scoliosis may occur. In the hand and wrist, deformities similar to adult rheumatoid disease are seen, although ulnar deviation at the wrist and *radial* deviation at the MCP joints is common. Additionally, some patients develop extensive fusion of carpal bones (Fig. 5-11). Ankles and feet are similarly prone to fusion, particularly at the subtalar joint. Complex foot deformities may be seen as a result of soft tissue damage and growth disturbances.

MANAGEMENT

Essential to optimal outcome in JRA is the early diagnosis and prompt institution of physical therapy measures. The greatest challenges in treatment, however, may be in the maintenance of psychosocial growth and development. Both the parents and the patient need education and emotional support. Integration of the patient into usual childhood activities should be attempted whenever possible. The effects of chronic illness and deformity on self-image must be kept in mind.

NSAIDs are the most commonly used drugs in the treatment of JRA. They control pain, swelling, and stiffness but have no effect on the long-term outcome. NSAIDs approved by the US Food and Drug Administration for use in childhood arthritis include aspirin, ibuprofen, naproxen, and tolmetin sodium. Other NSAIDs are used for patients who cannot tolerate the FDA approved NSAIDs. Ibuprofen, naproxen, and several salicylate preparations are available in liquid form. Aspirin has a long historical record of use in JRA but has more gastrointestinal side effects and can induce elevation of serum transaminases, particularly in systemic JRA patients. Because of the slight risk of Reye syndrome, salicylates are temporarily discontinued in JRA patients with concomitant influenza or varicella infections. In the newly diagnosed JRA patient, an NSAID is tried for

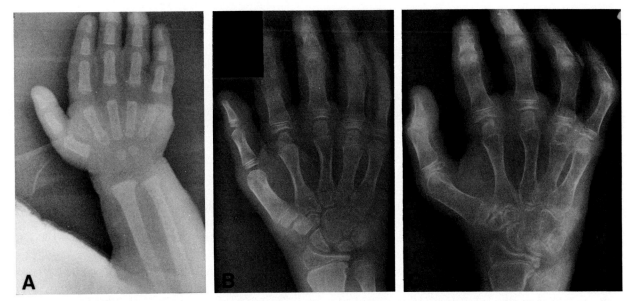

FIGURE 5-11. Juvenile rheumatoid arthritis (JRA) with progressive joint destruction. Radiographs of a 15-year-old boy with severe polyarticular JRA, who is negative for rheumatoid factor and antinuclear antibodies. The patient presented at age 2 years with arthritis. (A) The right hand at age 2 years is normal except for decreased bone age. (B) By age 12 years, extensive changes are noted, including soft tissue swelling, diffuse osteopenia, and bony erosions. (C) At age 15 years, films demonstrate fusion of the carpal bones, progressive joint irregularity, and worsening osteopenia.

several weeks, then additional agents are added if the clinical response is not adequate. Specific agents include hydroxychloroquine, gold salts, sulfasalazine, and methotrexate.

Systemic corticosteroids are reserved for refractory cases of JRA and are particularly useful in the treatment of severe systemic JRA. The lowest possible dose should be used. Intraarticular injections of corticosteroids are safe in children, and the indications for use are similar to those for adults. Local anesthesia is sufficient for the older child, but a younger child may need sedation before intraarticular injection.

About 10% of children with JRA seen in a pediatric rheumatology center require surgical intervention, and the specific procedures used are reviewed more extensively in the references. Children with severe JRA have significant osteoporosis and can experience spontaneous fractures. JRA patients require surgical intervention when medical and physical therapy (eg, splinting, casting) are not sufficient to control pain, improve contracture, or correct deformity. The most common procedure in JRA pa-

tients is soft tissue release, particularly of the knee or hip. Occasionally, synovial biopsy may be necessary for diagnostic reasons. Synovectomy can be helpful for the child with severe pain or loss of function and is most commonly required for the knee in pauciarticular patients. Arthroscopy can be performed, but the presence of severe pericapsular contracture may decrease distensibility and visibility of the joint. Severe bone ankylosis may require a corrective osteotomy to improve joint position. Joint replacement is a well-established treatment of end-stage JRA. Children with severe polyarticular or systemic JRA are often smaller and lighter than other children of the same age, and the joint prosthesis may need to be custom made.

Careful preoperative medical and anesthetic evaluation is necessary in all children. Children on systemic corticosteroid therapy need intravenous stress corticosteroid coverage and are at greater risk of infection. Involvement of the cervical spine, TMJs, and cricoarytenoid joints can make airway management difficult.

Infectious Arthritis
Stanley J. Naides

Infectious agents have been demonstrated to play an etiologic role in the initiation and propagation of certain chronic arthritides. Still other clinical syndromes, such as RA, lack a defined etiology; but an array of infectious agents have been hypothesized to contribute to pathogenesis. The recent discovery of the spirochete *Borrelia burgdorferi* as the cause of chronic Lyme arthritis has spurred efforts to identify other arthritogenic infectious agents. Although these efforts promise to provide new insights into the role of microbial agents in chronic arthritis, several clinical entities have already been defined that confront the practitioner regularly. Infectious arthritis is usually a medical emergency, since failure to recognize and treat appropriately may result in otherwise avoidable catastrophic joint destruction.

ACUTE SEPTIC ARTHRITIS

Direct invasion of the joint by pyogenic bacteria causes acute septic arthritis. Invasion may occur by hematogenous spread or contiguous spread from soft tissue infection or osteomyelitis. Patients with altered joint anatomy from old injury, chronic inflammatory arthritis, or joint prosthesis are at greater risk of joint infection, as are those with compromised immunity, for example, those with diabetes melitis, alcoholism, anemia, sickle cell anemia, malignancy, allogeneic transplants, RA, intravenous drug abuse, or human immunodeficiency virus (HIV) coinfection or those on steroid or cytotoxic drugs. Immunocompromise may stunt or abort the usual signs and symptoms of infection, making the clinical diagnosis of septic arthritis difficult. Recurrent infection in an apparently healthy person raises the possibility of inherited or acquired immunodeficiency.

Acute septic arthritis is a medical emergency. Delay in initiating therapy may lead to joint destruction. Acute septic arthritis usually presents with joint swelling, heat, pain, erythema, and loss of function. Usually, a single joint is affected. In some cases, especially in the immunocompromised, multiple joints may be infected. Sudden onset of monarticular arthritis should be considered septic until proved otherwise. Any joint may be involved, although the large weight-bearing joints, especially the knees, are most often involved. The ankle, shoulders, elbows, and wrists are other commonly affected sites. In the patient with known inflammatory polyarthritis, such as RA, the sudden worsening of a single joint or the worsening of a single joint out of proportion to the disease activity in the other joints should suggest the possibility of intervening septic arthritis. Nonarticular infection, such as cellulitis, pneumonia, dental, or urinary tract infections, are often the distant source for bacterial seeding of joints. Constitutional signs and symptoms, when present, are helpful in suggesting an infection but in themselves are nonspecific, as are general laboratory studies. An elevated ESR is common. Leukocytosis occurs in up to two thirds of patients.

The diagnosis of acute septic arthritis is confirmed by arthrocentesis with synovial fluid analysis and culture. Arthrocentesis provides bacteriologic diagnosis as well. Synovial fluid is usually purulent, with greater than 50,000 cells/μL and over 80% polymorphonuclear leukocytes. Initial leukocyte counts, however, may be only minimally elevated. In immunocompromised hosts, leukocyte counts in synovial fluid may remain low or even normal. In cases with low or normal leukocyte counts, repeat arthrocentesis in 12 to 24 hours may demonstrate rising counts. A high leukocyte count in itself is not pathognomonic, since high counts may be seen in nonseptic inflammatory arthritis, especially crystal-induced arthritis or Reiter syndrome. Identification of crystals, however, does not rule out septic arthritis, since both entities may occur simultaneously. Synovial glucose may be less than one third of serum levels, but depressed synovial glucose may also be seen in RA. Poor mucin clot is a nonspecific finding. The definitive diagnosis requires demonstration of the causative bacteria on Gram stain, by culture, or using both. Aerobic and anaerobic cultures of synovial fluid should be obtained.

Plain radiographs are usually normal early in infectious arthritis, except perhaps for evidence of soft tissue swelling or joint effusion. Nevertheless, joints with suspected infection should be radiographed at presentation, since a baseline study is useful in interpretation of subsequent examinations. Periarticular osteopenia may be seen but is nonspecific. Gas-producing organisms such as *Escherichia coli* or anaerobes may generate articular gas. In joints with limited joint capsule volume and distensibility, subluxation may occur, for example, in the hips in children and the shoulders in adults. Joint space narrowing due to cartilage destruction may occur in several days to a week without appropriate treatment. Subchondral bone destruction is a late finding. Contiguous osteomyelitis is a late but grave complication. Radionuclide imaging techniques, such as technetium, gallium, or indium-leukocyte scans, may aid diagnosis of septic arthritis in joints difficult to aspirate, such as intervertebral, sacroiliac, or hip joints.

Treatment must be initiated even before availability of culture results. Initial choice of antibiotics is made based on the clinical setting and Gram stain, and they should be given parenterally in the hospital. Suspected primary sites of infection, as well as synovial fluid, should be cultured and, when appropriate, examined by Gram stain. Blood cultures should be performed routinely. The most common nongonococcal bacterium causing arthritis in adults is *Staphylococcus aureus*, followed by *Streptococcus* sp. Gram-negative bacteria are commonly the offending agent in geriatric patients, intravenous drug abusers, and the seriously ill. *E coli, Proteus* sp, and *Serratia* sp are common. Sickle cell anemia patients are at increased risk for *Salmonella* sp infection. Anaerobic bacterial arthritis is most often seen in the setting of gastrointestinal pathology, open fractures, joint prosthesis, or RA. Mixed aerobic and anaerobic infection is becoming more frequent. Therefore, anaerobic cultures should be performed routinely on all synovial fluid samples sent for culture.

Daily needle aspiration of the joint is required for drainage and monitoring efficacy of therapy. Serial synovial fluid leukocyte counts fall in response to appropriate therapy. Open drainage should be considered only if the loculation of synovial fluid prevents adequate needle drainage or if the infection fails to respond to appropriate antibiotic therapy within an appropriate time. The time required before considering opened drainage depends on the site, organism, and antibiotic sensitivity. Culture and sensitivity results may suggest a change in the antibiotic regimen. Joint rest should be enforced until inflammation subsides, at which time physical therapy with passive range of motion may be started cautiously. Parenteral antibiotics should be continued long enough to prevent relapse. The duration of parenteral therapy depends on the clinical response and the offending organisms, ranging from 10 days to 6 weeks. Parenteral antibiotics penetrate the synovium to attain adequate intraarticular drug levels. Injection of intraarticular antibiotics is contraindicated owing to the risk of inducing chemical synovitis and superinfection.

GONOCOCCAL ARTHRITIS

Infectious arthritis due to *Neisseria gonorrhoeae* follows dissemination from a primary site, such as urethra, cervix, rectum, or pharynx. The clinical course is classically biphasic. The first stage, characterized by migratory polyarthralgias, polyarthritis, or tenosynovitis, is associated with pathogenic circulating immune complexes. Multiple vesiculopustular skin lesions that develop necrotic centers may be seen. Cultures from these skin lesions and from blood are often positive for *N gonorrhoeae* during this stage. Untreated, the patient may develop the second stage, in which infection settles into one or a few joints, which become purulent. Cultures from purulent joints are positive only one quarter of the time because *N gonorrhoeae* is a fastidious organism and difficult to grow. Patients with suspected gonococcal infection should have all possible sites examined and cultured, including pharynx, rectum, blood, cervix in women, and urethra in men. Special transport media should be used if samples will be delayed in reaching the microbiology laboratory. The gonococcus is usually sensitive to most parenteral antibiotic therapy, especially penicillin. Penicillinase-producing *N gonorrhoeae* strains, however, are encountered frequently in the Far East, West Africa, New York, California, and Florida, and penicillin is no longer the drug of first choice in such cases. Failure to respond to or relapse on penicillin therapy should alert the physician to the possibility of infection with a penicillinase-producing strain. A history of recurrent episodes of gonococcal or meningococcal infection requires investigation for deficiency of a terminal complement component (ie, C_5 through C_9).

BACTERIAL ENDOCARDITIS

Bacterial endocarditis may be associated with immune complex–mediated polyarthritis. Rarely, septic arthritis or diskitis results from septic emboli. Myalgias and hypertrophic osteoarthropathy may also be associated with bacterial endocarditis.

BRUCELLA ARTHRITIS

Brucellosis (Mediterranean Fever, Malta Fever, undulant fever) is usually acquired from contact with animals or animal products. Human infection is carried by one of four species of gram-negative coccobacilli: *Brucella abortus* (cattle), *B suis* (hogs), *B mel-*

itensis (goats), and in a few cases, *B canis* (dog). Human infection is acquired through abraded skin or ingestion of infected tissue or milk. Veterinarians and slaughterhouse workers are at special risk. Iowa, California, Texas, and Virginia have most of the cases reported in the United States. In areas of the world where ingestion of fresh milk or cheese is common, brucellosis is not limited to those in an occupation at risk.

In the acute form of the disease associated with bacteremia, fever, which may be high, is accompanied by diaphoresis, polyarthralgia, myalgias, headache, and general malaise. In the subacute form that occurs more than 8 weeks but less than 1 year after infection, fever is less prominent. Constitutional symptoms of diaphoresis and weight loss may be undulant. Ocular and urologic damage may occur. Hepatosplenomegaly is common. Leukopenia may be noted in acute and subacute forms of brucellosis. Patients with disease for more than 1 year are considered chronic. They have frequent arthralgias and often low-grade fever. Uveal lesions, hepatic dysfunction, and anemia are common.

Peripheral arthritis is the most common articular manifestation of brucellosis. Most cases are monarticular, involving the large weight-bearing joints of the lower extremity (ie, knee, hip, or ankle). Rarely, the arthritis may have a symmetric rheumatoid-like distribution. Failure to isolate organisms in some instances suggests that peripheral arthritis may be reactive in some cases. Sacroiliitis is the second most common articular manifestation. Usually unilateral, sacroiliitis is most commonly seen in the chronic form of brucellosis. The articular surfaces of the sacroiliac joint are usually blurred on radiographs, but erosions are infrequent. Spondylitis occurs in about one tenth of patients and is most common in the lumbar spine. The characteristic changes are erosions at the anterosuperior margin of the vertebral body with disk narrowing. Unlike Pott disease (tuberculous spondylitis), however, brucella spondylitis is characterized by early repair with sclerosis and formation of "parrot-beak" osteophytes. The concurrence of erosion and osteoblastic repair suggests the diagnosis of brucella spondylitis. Brucella osteomyelitis is rare. Tendonitis, bursitis, and epicondylitis have been reported in brucellosis.

Diagnosis of brucellosis is based on a positive culture or rising or high-titer brucella serology. Culture of bone marrow may be helpful. About half of synovial fluid cultures are positive in peripheral arthritis. Special medium is required for optimal culture results. Synovial biopsy typically shows cellular infiltrates and granuloma formation.

Treatment of acute and subacute forms of brucellosis relies on oral tetracyclines given for 1 month initially, but 5 months may be required in difficult cases. Some authors suggest adding rifampin to decrease the incidence of relapse. Both diagnosis and treatment of chronic brucellosis are difficult.

TUBERCULOUS ARTHRITIS

Tuberculous arthritis should be considered in the differential diagnosis of monarticular and pauciarticular arthritis at any age. The arthritis is frequently insidious in onset. It tends to appear "cold," lacking the usual signs of active inflammation, especially erythema and heat. Pott disease, tuberculous involvement of the spine, classically involves the thoracolumbar junction. Anterior destruction of vertebral bodies and disks eventually leads to angulation of the spine and kyphosis (gibbous deformity). Although constitutional signs of tuberculosis (eg, fever, malaise, or weight loss) may be present, active pulmonary tuberculosis is rare. A history of past infection may be absent. A positive skin test for tuberculosis is helpful, although a negative test in the presence of anergy does not rule out the diagnosis. Diagnosis is based on finding acid-fast bacilli in synovium or synovial fluid or caseating granulomas in biopsied synovium. Synovial fluid or tissue cultures are positive 90% of the time. Tuberculosis and its complications should be considered in patients with acquired immunodeficiency syndrome (AIDS) or a history of immigration from an endemic area. Atypical mycobacterial infection should be considered in the setting of immune compromise, especially AIDS.

LEPROSY

Leprosy may be acquired in the United States in Texas or Louisiana. Additional patients may come from endemic areas abroad, such as Mexico. Leprosy may present in several ways. Lepromatous leprosy may present with polyarthralgia or polyarthritis. Erythema nodosa leprosum is an associated finding and consists of nodose lesions of the legs, arms, or trunk. Malaise and fever may occur. Swollen hands syndrome is another presentation of leprosy. Thickening of peripheral nerves and typical skin changes suggest the diagnosis. Diagnosis is made by identifying *Myco-bacterium leprae* in aspirates of skin lesions or in scrapings of the nasal septum. *M leprae* may be found in synovial and periarticular tissues.

SYPHILIS

Syphilis is a rare cause of arthritis but should not be overlooked, since the incidence of syphilis is increasing. "Saber shins" are a classic manifestation of congenital syphilis. Bony abnormalities include osteochondritis, osteomyelitis, osteitis, and periostitis. Gummas have rarely been reported in tubular or flat bones. In older children, painless effusions, especially of the knees (Clutton joints), may occur.

In acquired primary syphilis, transient bone pain of a boring nature may be prominent. The tibia, humerus, and cranium are most frequently involved, but radiographs are normal. In secondary syphilis, pain and tenderness with overlying soft tissue swelling may be seen in superficial bones, such as anterior tibia, sternum, ribs, and frontal calvarium. Symptoms and signs are variable but characteristically worse at night. Proliferative periostitis is the most common radiographic change. It is associated with new bone formation that may be extensive, resulting in marked cortical thickening. The tibia, sternum, ribs, and calvarium are most significantly involved, but changes may also been seen in the femur, fibula, clavicle, hands, and feet. Of interest, periostitis in the adult that involves both clavicles or tibiae is frequently syphilitic. Destructive bony lesions suggest syphilitic osteomyelitis or osteitis, but these are less common than periostitis. Areas of lysis may be seen in the skull, although any bone may be effected. Skull involvement may present as headache with localized swellings. In the long bones, lytic foci, periostitis, and epiphyseal separation may be seen. Syphilitic arthritis, especially of the sternoclavicular joints, may complicate the picture.

Tertiary syphilis may be complicated by gummatous osseous lesions. The lesion pathologically resembles a tubercle with necrosis of adjacent bone. Lytic and sclerotic areas of bone may reach large size and may be associated with pathologic fracture. Periostitis adjacent to gummatous lesions is frequent. Nongummatous osseous lesions that consist of periostitis, osteitis, or osteomyelitis may occur in conjunction with or in the absence of gummatous bony lesions.

Charcot joints, characteristically of the knees, results from loss of proprioception due to tabes dorsalis in tertiary syphilis. Hip, ankle, shoulder, elbow, spine, and other joints may be affected as well in tabes dorsalis. The frequency of direct syphilitic involvement of the joint is low. It may result from contiguous spread from a bony lesion or direct involvement of synovial or parasynovial tissues.

Diagnosis is based on serology. Parenteral penicillin is the drug of choice for treatment of syphilis.

LYME DISEASE

Originally described as Lyme arthritis, Lyme disease is a multisystemic disease caused by the tick-borne spirochete, *B burgdorferi.* At least 42 states have reported Lyme disease, but most cases in the United States are found in the endemic areas of the Northeast, upper Midwest, and West. The white-tailed deer tick, *Ixodes dammini,* is the principle vector from Massachusetts to Maryland and in Wisconsin and Minnesota. *I pacificus* carries the spirochete in California and Oregon. Lyme disease is endemic in eastern and western Europe, where it is carried by the sheep tick, *I ricinus. Ixodes* ticks are small, measuring only a few millimeters in the unengorged state. Many patients do not recall a tick bite. A characteristic lesion, erythema chronicum migrans (ECM), occurs at the bite site after 3 to 32 days. ECM begins as a red macule or papule but expands to form an annular, or target, lesion with a bright red, frequently indurated border and central clearing. Within several days, additional ECM lesions may appear due to hematogenous dissemination of spirochetes. The initial ECM lesion frequently occurs in the thigh, groin, or axilla, where the tick prefers feeding. Constitutional signs and symptoms during this initial phase of disease may be intermittent and include fever, malaise, fatigue, chills, nonproductive cough, sore throat, myalgias, arthralgias, headache, neck stiffness, generalized lymphadenopathy, hepatitis, conjunctivitis, iritis, or panophthalmitis. As many as one fourth of patients lack the characteristic ECM lesion, making the diagnosis less obvious. Symptoms usually improve or resolve in several weeks.

After several weeks or months, a second stage of disease occurs. Significant neurologic manifestations occur in 15% of infected patients, including cranial neuritis, Bell palsy, opthalmic nerve atrophy, meningitis, encephalitis, motor and sensory radiculopathy, mononeuritis multiplex, plexopathy, myelitis, or chorea. Deficits may wax and wane. Although neurologic manifestations frequently improve over several months, deficits may become fixed in some patients. Chronic infection can lead to cognitive deficits, dementia, or multiple sclerosis–like illness.

Less than 10% of infected patients develop cardiac involvement within several weeks of illness, including atrioventricular conduction blocks, myocarditis, pericarditis, ventricular dysfunction, and cardiomegaly. Although cardiac involvement is usually self-limited, it may prove fatal in a few cases.

Rheumatologic manifestations during the second stage of disease include migratory arthralgia, myalgia, and tendon and bone pain. Joint swelling is uncommon. A third stage of disease, however, occurs in about 60% of those infected and is characterized by intermittent monarticular or oligoarticular arthritis of large joints. The knee is most commonly effected. Symmetric arthritis of large or small joints is much less common. Attacks may last for months and recur over years. About 10% of patients develop chronic erosive arthritis of large joints.

Diagnosis is usually made by specific IgM serology in stage 1 disease or by rising specific IgG titers. Specific IgM peaks at 3 to 6 weeks after disease onset. Specific IgG titers rise slowly and are highest during arthritis. Early in disease, a significant proportion of serologies are negative and therefore should be repeated in several weeks if the index of suspicion remains high. Unfortunately, serologic diagnosis is complicated by the lack of laboratory standardization of serologies and the presence of regulatory T lymphocytes that suppress anti-*Borrelia*–antibody response early in disease. Occasionally, antibody responses are absent despite vigorous T-lymphocyte proliferative responses that indicate infection. The clinical significance of low IgG titers in patients living in endemic areas may be difficult to assess; about half of infections may be asymptomatic. Synovial fluid findings are nonspecific. Spirochetes are rarely identified in synovial fluid or synovium. The diagnosis of Lyme disease remains clinical; the laboratory has a confirmatory role.

Tetracycline is the treatment of choice for early disease; penicillin and erythromycin are alternatives in children and tetracycline-allergic patients. Recently, doxycycline was recommended as the drug of choice, with amoxicillin the choice for children. Late neurologic or cardiac disease requires parenteral antibiotics. Lyme arthritis requires parenteral high-dose penicillin. Ceftriaxone was used in recent trials, with fewer apparent treatment failures. A repeat antibiotic course with the same or a different drug usu-ally treats initial therapeutic failures effectively. Occasionally, synovectomy may be useful in patients who fail antibiotic therapy.

FUNGAL ARTHRITIS

Fungal arthritis usually presents as an indolent monarthritis, much like tuberculous arthritis. Coccidioidomycosis occurs in the southwestern United States. It may present with erythema nodosum, periarthritis, and bihilar lymphadenopathy. This triad is also seen in sarcoidosis (where it is known as Lofgren syndrome), and therefore, the two entities must be differentiated. In coccidioidomycosis, the triad is a hypersensitivity reaction to primary infection and resolves spontaneously within weeks. Persistent arthritis is uncommon, resulting from hematogenous spread or extension from contiguous osteomyelitis. The most commonly involved joints are knees, wrist and hand, ankle, elbow, and foot, in order of decreasing frequency. Arthritis progression is slow and indolent. Diagnosis is by synovial biopsy and culture.

Blastomycosis occurs as a primary pulmonary infection in central and southern United States. Hematogenous spread to skin and bone may occur. Monarthritis may occur uncommonly and typically involves a knee, ankle, or elbow in a middle-aged man. Constitutional signs and symptoms may accompany pulmonary and skin disease. The organism may be isolated from sputum, skin, and synovial fluid.

Sporotrichosis typically occurs in agricultural or mine workers or in gardeners after minor skin trauma. Indolent arthritis occurs rarely and involves the knee, hand, wrist, or ankle, in order of decreasing frequency. More than one joint is involved in about half the patients. Alcoholism or myeloproliferative disease predisposes to infection. Diagnosis is by synovial histology and culture.

Candida arthritis is rare. It is usually seen in the setting of immune compromise. Some infections may be indolent. The knee is typically involved; polyarticular involvement occurs in 40% of infections. Osteomyelitis may occur in up to 65% of patients. Mortality is high.

Treatment of fungal arthritis is limited to amphotericin B. Surgery is reserved for debridement of involved bone or synovium in those patients with coccidioidomycosis or sporotrichosis who fail to respond to amphotericin B alone.

VIRAL ARTHRITIS

The occurrence of inflammatory arthritis acutely in some viral infections has long been recognized. The development of chronic arthralgias or arthritis after an acute infection in some patients has spurred investigators to search for virally induced alterations in the immune system or persistent viral infection to explain chronic sequelae of acute viral infection. The number of patients in the rheumatologic population with postviral arthralgia or arthritis may be significant, but diagnosis of the acute infection is rarely confirmed by acute-phase serology or viral isolation because patients often present late in their course. As improvements in biotechnology provide simpler and more sensitive tests for viral diagnosis, it will become incumbent on the clinician to consider specific viruses in the differential diagnosis of arthritis.

Hepatitis B infection is associated with a significant viremia early in its course. As anti–hepatitis B surface antigen (HB$_s$Ag) antibodies are produced, they form soluble immune complexes with circulating HB$_s$Ag, leading to an immune complex–mediated arthritis. The period of circulating immune complexes, and therefore arthritis, usually precedes onset of jaundice. Urticaria may be associated with the arthritis prodrome. Onset of arthritis is usually sudden and often severe. The joints of the hand and knee are most often affected, but wrists, ankles, elbows, shoulders, and other large joints may be involved as well. Joint involvement is usually symmetric and migratory or additive, but simultaneous involvement of several joints at onset does occur. Arthritis may precede jaundice by days to weeks and may persist for several weeks. Although arthritis is usually limited to the preicteric prodrome, those patients who develop chronic active hepatitis or chronic hepatitis B viremia may have recurrent arthralgias or arthritis. Polyarteritis nodosa and mixed essential cryoglobulinemia are two entities frequently associated with chronic hepatitis B viremia. As many as 40% of polyarteritis nodosa patients may have immune complexes involving hepatitis B virus in their cryoglobulins.

Rubella infection leads to a high incidence of joint complaints in adults, especially in women. Joint symptoms may occur 1 week before or after onset of the characteristic rash. Arthralgias are more common than frank arthritis, although stiffness is prominent; and periarthritis, tenosynovitis, and carpal tunnel syndrome are known complications. Joint involvement is usually symmetric and may be migratory,

resolving over a few days to 2 weeks. The PIP and MCP joints of the hands, knees, wrists, ankles, and elbows are most frequently involved. In some patients, symptoms may persist for a few months. In a few patients, arthralgias may occur for up to 1 year.

Live, attenuated vaccines have been employed in rubella vaccination. A high frequency of postvaccination arthralgia, myalgia, arthritis, and paresthesias have been associated with some vaccine preparations. The HPV77/DK12 strain is the most arthritogenic of the three vaccine strains available in the United States. The pattern of joint involvement is similar to natural infection. Arthritis usually occurs 2 weeks after inoculation and usually lasts less than 1 week, but symptoms may persist in some patients for more than a year. In children, two syndromes of rheumatologic interest may occur. In the *arm syndrome*, a brachial radiculoneuritis causes arm and hand pain and dysesthesias that are worse at night. The *catcher's crouch syndrome* is characterized by popliteal fossa pain on arising in the morning. Those affected assume a baseball catcher's crouching position. The pain gradually decreases through the day. This lumbar radiculoneuropathy is associated with delayed nerve conduction times. Both syndromes occur 1 to 2 months after vaccination. The initial episode may last up to 2 months, but recurrences usually are shorter. Episodes of catcher's crouch syndrome may recur for up to 1 year, but there is no permanent damage.

Infection with human parvovirus, designated B19, may be responsible for as many as 15% of patients presenting with recent-onset polyarthralgia or polyarthritis. B19 is common and widespread, causing the common childhood exanthem erythema infectiosum, or fifth disease, characterized by "slapped cheeks" and a lacy or blotchy rash of the torso and extremities. Up to 60% of adults have serologic evidence of past infection. About 10% of children with fifth disease have arthralgias, and 5% have arthritis, usually short lived. Up to 78% of infected adults develop joint symptoms.

The illness is usually mild in children, but an influenza-like illness tends to be more severe in adults. Adults lack the "slapped-cheek" rash, and the reticular rash on the torso or extremities may be subtle or absent. Arthralgia is more common than frank arthritis. The distribution of involved joints is rheumatoid-like. Symmetric involvement of MCP, PIP, knee, wrist, and ankle joints is prominent. Patients usually experience sudden onset followed in 2 weeks by improvement. Joint symptoms in infected adults are usually self-limited, but a minority of adults may have symptoms for up to 5 years (the longest follow-up to date). The course in those with chronic symptoms is that of intermittent flares. Only one third of patients are symptom-free between flares. Morning stiffness is prominent. Patients usually meet at least four of the seven American College of Rheumatology 1987 criteria for a diagnosis of RA. RF is usually absent in parvovirus B19 arthropathy but is reported occasionally. Joint erosions and rheumatoid nodules have not been reported. Specific serologic diagnosis is possible; however, there is a brief window of opportunity to make the diagnosis based on the presence of anti-B19 IgM antibodies, which may be elevated for only 2 months after an acute infection. Joint symptoms occur 1 to 3 weeks after initial infection; anti-B19 IgM antibodies are usually present at the time of onset of rash or joint symptoms. The high prevalence of anti-B19 IgG antibodies in the adult population limits their diagnostic usefulness. Treatment is with NSAIDs. Parvovirus B19 also was shown to cause most cases of transient aplastic crisis in patients with chronic hemolytic anemias, some cases of hydrops fetalis with fetal loss, and, in immunocompromised patients, chronic bone marrow suppression.

The alphavirus genus of the Togaviridae family includes a number of arthritogenic viruses responsible for major epidemics of febrile polyarthritis in Africa, Australia, Europe, and Latin America. All are mosquito-borne, with the specific species depending on the virus and the locale. The known viral pathogens in this genus include Chikungunya fever virus, O'nyong-nyong virus, Ross River virus, Sindbis virus, and Mayaro virus.

Apart from specific viral infections noted previously in which arthralgia, arthritis, or both are typically a prominent feature, there is a host of commonly encountered viral syndromes in which joint involvement is occasionally seen. Children with varicella are reported rarely to develop brief monarticular or pauciarticular arthritis that is thought to be viral in origin. This is to be differentiated from the occasional bacterial arthritis due to contiguous spread

from an infected vesicle. Adults who develop mumps occasionally develop small or large joint synovitis that lasts up to several weeks. Arthritis may precede or follow parotitis by up to 4 weeks.

Infection with coxsackieviruses A9, B2, B3, B4, and B6 and adenovirus is associated with recurrent episodes of polyarthritis, pleuritis, myalgia, rash, pharyngitis, myocarditis, and leukocytosis. Epstein-Barr virus–associated mononucleosis is frequently accompanied by polyarthralgia, but frank arthritis is rare. Polyarthritis, fever, and myalgia due to echovirus infection were reported in only a few cases. Arthritis associated with herpes simplex virus or cytomegalovirus infections are likewise rare. Vaccinia virus was associated with postvaccination knee arthritis in two reported cases. In one case of monarticular knee arthritis, vaccinia virus was recovered from synovial fluid. In the other case, both knees and a single PIP joint were involved.

Organisms such as *Salmonella, Shigella, Campylobacter, Yersinia, Mycoplasma, Ureaplasma,* and *Chlamydia* that have been associated with reactive spondyloarthropathies are discussed elsewhere in this chapter. Infection with HIV is associated with an increased incidence of such reactive arthritides, probably owing to associated gastrointestinal and urinary tract infections. Most patients with AIDS have musculoskeletal signs and symptoms. About a third of patients have arthralgias, about 10% have Reiter syndrome, and few have psoriatic arthritis, myositis, or vasculitis. Another 10% of patients have a unique syndrome of severe intermittent pain that involves three or fewer joints without evidence of synovitis. Episodes last 2 to 24 hours and require therapy with NSAIDs or narcotics for pain control. Another 10% have arthritis that involves the lower extremities for 1 week to 6 months. The arthritis in this syndrome may be monarticular, oligoarticular, or polyarticular. There is some concern that HIV infection may be capable of causing synovitis. As the worldwide AIDS epidemic continues to grow, clinicians will be confronted with an expanding spectrum of clinical presentation of HIV infection. The differential diagnosis of many arthritides, especially Reiter syndrome, needs to be expanded to include HIV infection.

Crystal-Induced Arthritis

John W. Rachow

DEFINITION

Few clinical presentations are as distinct and dramatic as an acute gout attack. With its clinical description rooted in antiquity, gout can be considered the prototype acute monarthritis. Gout, which is due to the presence of monosodium urate (MSU) crystals in articular tissues, is also the prototype crystal-induced arthritis. But other crystals in articular tissues also directly cause clinical manifestations of arthritis. These other crystals include CPPD, BCP, and calcium oxalate. (BCP is composed mostly of carbonate-substituted hydroxyapatite but may include varying amounts of octacalcium phosphate and tricalcium phosphate.) For MSU and CPPD crystals, criteria reminiscent of Koch postulates have been fulfilled: either synthetic crystals or crystals recovered from inflamed joints induce acute monarthritis when injected into normal human or animal joints.

In acute clinical situations, the essential information needed to diagnose crystal-induced arthritis can be readily obtained from microscopic examination of fresh synovial fluid. Joint radiographs provide supportive evidence. These tools, combined with synovial fluid Gram stain and culture, enable the clinician efficiently to work through the differential diagnosis of acute monarthritis and apply specific therapy.

CLINICAL FEATURES

Symptoms

Hallmarks of the acute crystal-induced attack of arthritis include rapid onset over a few hours, extreme pain and tenderness, swelling, and redness. The earliest attacks of gout tend to occur in the first MTP joint (podagra), the midfoot, or ankle joints. With long-standing disease, similar attacks can occur in knees, wrists, and elbows. Only rarely are the central joints involved. The axial joints are spared. In 1977, a subcommittee of the American Rheumatism Association published preliminary criteria for the classification of gout (Table 5-5), forming a concise description of the most important clinical features of gout.

With CPPD crystal-induced acute attacks (often termed *pseudogout*), the first attack most commonly

occurs in the knee; however, wrist, MCP, and shoulder joints are often involved. Although acute inflammation due to BCP (mostly composed of hydroxyapatite) is more likely to be a periarthritis such as shoulder bursitis or tendinitis, acute monarthritis also has been documented with this crystal. Calcium oxalate crystal-induced acute arthritis is uncommon, occurring in the setting of chronic renal failure and dialysis.

Acute crystal-induced attacks are usually self-limited and resolve in less than 2 weeks without treatment. Later in the disease course, recurrent acute attacks tend to become less intense, to resolve more slowly, and to involve more than one joint at a time. Eventually, a picture of chronic polyarthritis may emerge, which can be easily confused with either RA or osteoarthritis.

With gout, in which tophi often develop along the proximal ulna resembling rheumatoid nodules, confusion with RA is possible. This is an important distinction to make, since gout and RA are managed differently. Also, they tend to be mutually exclusive; simultaneous occurrence in the same patient is extremely rare. With calcium phosphate crystal-induced arthritis, incidence of concurrent RA is probably the

TABLE 5-5.
Preliminary Criteria for the Classification of Acute Gout*

Suspected tophus (not examined microscopically for crystals)
More than one acute attack
Maximal inflammation developed in 1 day
Acute monarthritis
Redness
First metatarsophalangeal joint involved
Unilateral first metatarsophalangeal joint attack
Unilateral tarsal joint attack
Hyperuricemia
Asymmetric joint swelling on radiograph
Subcortical cysts without erosion on radiograph
Negative synovial fluid culture during attack

* These criteria are not intended to replace polarized light microscopy of synovial fluid in the diagnosis of gout or other crystal-induced arthropathies. The presence of six of these criteria alone identifies only 88% of gout patients; but when combined with microscopic examination of synovial fluid, 98% are correctly identified.

(Wallace SL, Robinson H, Masi AT, et al. Preliminary criteria for the classification of the acute arthritis of primary gout. Arthritis Rheum 1977;20:895)

same as in the general age-matched population, so the finding of intraarticular calcium-containing crystals does not rule out RA. CPPD crystal deposition arthropathy, which typically occurs in older age groups, is more likely to be confused with osteoarthritis.

Signs

Examination of the patient who presents with acute musculoskeletal complaints suggestive of monarthritis should determine whether a true joint is involved. Cellulitis, bursitis, and tendinitis can all result in warmth, redness, and swelling around the joints. Demonstration of a joint effusion or pain on slight movement of the affected joint helps to confirm true joint involvement. Swelling or tenderness directly over a joint or joint line is a helpful but less specific sign of true joint involvement.

Redness over a joint with exquisite tenderness is seen almost exclusively in infection, acute crystal-induced arthritis, or occasionally acute trauma. Because joint infection is so serious, the finding of redness in the setting of acute arthritis requires immediate vigorous investigation, including arthrocentesis.

In gout, several joints in the foot may be involved simultaneously, resulting in diffuse redness, swelling, and tenderness over much of the foot. Especially in foot or ankle involvement, widespread proximal edema and redness of the affected extremity may be noted. This, combined with sympathetic effusions in joints proximal to the presenting joint, may lead the examiner to conclude falsely that polyarticular arthritis is present.

The finding of tophi (subcutaneous or bursal deposits of MSU) suggests that the presenting attack is due to gout. Tophi occur in the helix of the external ear, along extensor and dorsal surfaces of the extremities, and in any area subjected to repeated pressure or trauma. Tophi may drain spontaneously and may be confused with draining cutaneous, joint, or bursal abscesses. The drainage from tophi usually includes prominent particles of white, chalky material and may even have an appearance suggestive of toothpaste.

In CPPD crystal-induced acute monarthritis, the joint findings are similar to those in acute gout except for patterns of joint involvement. Since CPPD deposition can occur simultaneously with gout, RA, and osteoarthritis, the finding of tophi, rheumatoid nodules, or Heberden and Bouchard nodes does not rule out superimposed CPPD crystal disease.

BCP crystal deposition is less likely to be associated with acute inflammatory arthritis and more likely to be found in settings of advanced osteoarthritis of the knee or shoulder. There is little on the physical examination to suggest specifically calcium oxalate crystal-induced acute arthritis.

Epidemiology

Gout implies preceding prolonged periods of sustained hyperuricemia; therefore, the epidemiology of gout closely parallels the epidemiology of hyperuricemia. Since lower levels of serum uric acid are found in the normal population of prepubertal men and premenopausal women, gout develops mostly in postpubertal men or postmenopausal women. Any other factors that result in sustained elevations of serum uric acid above the solubility product of MSU can lead to increased total-body urate and predispose to gout. Such factors can be divided into those that involve either uric acid underexcretion or overproduction (Table 5-6).

TABLE 5-6.
Classification of Hyperuricemia

OVERPRODUCTION OF URIC ACID
Complete deficiency of HGPRT (Lesch-Nyhan syndrome)
Partially deficient or mutant HGPRT
Overactive PRPP synthetase
Glucose-6-phosphatase deficiency
Diseases involving increased tissue turnover
    Myeloproliferative and lymphoproliferative disorders
    Malignancies
    Hemolytic anemia
    Psoriasis
Idiopathic

UNDEREXCRETION OF URIC ACID
Chronic diseases leading to renal underexcretion
    Renal failure
    Hypertension
    Lead nephropathy
    Obesity
Drugs that might be used chronically
    Diuretics
    Low-dose salicylates
    Pyrazinamide
    Ethambutol
    L-dopa
Ethanol

HGPRT, hypoxanthine-guanine phosphoribosyltransferase; PRPP, phosphoribosylpyrophosphate.

A classification of CPPD crystal deposition arthropathy follows:

- Familial
- Posttraumatic
- Metabolic and endocrine disease associated
  - Hypothyroidism
  - Hemochromatosis
  - Hyperparathyroidism
  - Hypomagnesemia
  - Hypophosphatasia
  - Gout
  - Amyloidosis
- Idiopathic (age associated)

CPPD crystal deposition occurs only in adults; and unless associated with familial chondrocalcinosis or prior joint trauma, CPPD crystal-induced arthritis rarely occurs before the sixth decade. Incidence of chondrocalcinosis on radiographs steadily rises and may exceed 30% of the asymptomatic population over 85 years old. CPPD deposition also occurs more frequently in certain metabolic diseases: hypothyroidism, hyperparathyroidism, hemochromatosis, hypomagnesemic states, and hypophosphatasia. Although these metabolic disease associations give helpful clues in pondering the pathogenesis of CPPD crystal formation, they account for a small minority of cases of CPPD crystal deposition. CPPD crystal deposition occurs more commonly in patients with urate gout than in normal people for unknown reasons. The presence of amyloid in articular tissues also appears to increase the likelihood of developing CPPD deposition. Chondrocalcinosis due to either CPPD or BCP crystals is a frequent finding in ochronosis (alkaptonuria), especially in the vertebral disks.

BCP crystal arthropathy tends to occur in the same population as osteoarthritis but may be present in any joint with advanced degenerative disease. Calcium oxalate crystal-induced arthritis occurs in the setting of chronic renal failure, dialysis, and vitamin C administration.

PATHOGENESIS

In gout, prolonged hyperuricemia at concentrations yielding supersaturation with respect to sodium and uric acid leads to precipitation of MSU crystals in soft tissues. When sufficient MSU accumulates within joints, several factors, such as trauma, abrupt dietary changes, acute illness, dehydration, and administration of serum urate–lowering medications, probably induce acute MSU crystal precipitation within joints or shedding of crystals from deposits in synovium into synovial fluid. MSU crystals recovered from

joints are coated with a variety of serum proteins, notably immunoglobulins, which attract and enhance phagocytosis by polymorphonuclear leukocytes. Crystal contact with leukocytes results in generation of mediators of inflammation and chemoattractants, including interleukin-1 and a specific polymorphonuclear leukocyte–derived, crystal-induced chemotactic factor. A massive influx of polymorphonuclear leukocytes into the joints ensues. Partially due to the membranolytic properties of the MSU crystals, polymorphonuclear leukocyte lysis occurs, releasing lysosomal contents that further intensify the inflammatory response. Simultaneous influx of serum factors into the joint, including lipoproteins and proteolytic enzyme inhibitors, help make gout attacks self-limited.

Metabolic abnormalities that allow CPPD crystals to form intraarticular deposits are not well understood. There does not appear to be an increased whole-body load of inorganic pyrophosphate (PPi), as exists for urate in gout. Plasma, serum, and urinary levels of PPi are no different in most patients with CPPD crystal deposition than normal, except in hypophosphatasia. Synovial fluid PPi concentrations are higher than plasma in many arthropathies but are highest in patients with CPPD crystal deposition. Accumulated evidence suggests that elevated intraarticular PPi concentrations are more likely due to excess production of PPi by cartilage than to impaired PPi clearance mechanisms.

Analysis of the metabolic diseases associated with CPPD crystal deposition suggests that impaired PPi hydrolysis may be an important factor in some cases. Breakdown of PPi in vitro by inorganic pyrophosphatases, which are widely distributed in human tissue, is inhibited by high calcium and low magnesium. This may partially explain the association of CPPD deposition with hyperparathyroidism and hypomagnesemia. Adult hypophosphatasia is a rare, inherited partial deficiency of alkaline phosphatase, an enzyme for which PPi is a natural substrate. These patients, who are prone to CPPD crystal deposition, excrete increased amounts of PPi in the urine.

RADIOLOGIC FEATURES

Radiographs of a joint undergoing an acute gout attack may only show nonspecific soft tissue swelling. With long-standing disease and a history of several attacks, asymmetric periarticular swelling suggestive of a soft tissue mass may indicate the existence of a tophus. This finding typically is found over the first MTP joint, the olecranon, or extensor surfaces of the finger joints. Tophi may also develop inside juxtaarticular bone and appear on radiographs as subchondral cystic lucencies. Still later in the gout disease course, nonmarginal bone erosions may be seen proximal to the point of confluence of synovium, cartilage, and subchondral bone (joint margin). These erosions may exhibit a characteristic blown-out appearance in which overhanging lips of the disrupted bone cortex are displaced outward. There is often overlying soft tissue swelling, which may contain small calcified fragments, contributing to the overall impression that a subcortical explosion has taken place. In the most advanced stages, total joint destruction suggestive of a Charcot joint may be seen.

The radiographic hallmark of CPPD deposition is the relatively specific finding of chondrocalcinosis (uncommonly, chondrocalcinosis may be due to deposition of other calcium-containing crystals). CPPD crystal deposits in cartilage have a finely stippled appearance on joint radiographs. The stippled deposits may merge, continuously involving the articular cartilage in a manner that suggests the presence of a double subchondral bone cortex. Within fibrocartilage, the stippling may be partially arranged in streaks, giving a multilaminar appearance.

CPPD crystal deposits are found only in cartilage. Although hyaline articular cartilage is often involved, there tends to be a predisposition for deposition in fibrocartilage, especially the knee menisci and triangular cartilage of the wrist. Other fibrocartilage occasionally involved includes the sternoclavicular joint, symphysis pubis, and intervertebral disks.

No radiographic findings are specific for intra-articular BCP or calcium oxalate crystal deposition. Ligament, tendon, and cutaneous calcific deposits seen on radiographs are due to BCP crystals.

LABORATORY FEATURES

The essential laboratory finding in crystal-induced arthritis is demonstration of crystals in synovial fluid drawn from the affected joint. In the cases of gout, CPPD crystal deposition, and calcium oxalate deposition, this is accomplished with compensated polarized light microscopy of the synovial fluid sample. Occasionally, crystals may also be seen in tiny droplets of fluid drawn from periarticular inflamed soft tissue. In the case of gout, MSU crystals appear as strongly negatively birefringent needle-shaped crystals. CPPD crystals usually appear as smaller weakly positively birefringent rhomboids. Calcium oxalate crystals are positively birefringent bipyramids. The observation of any of these crystals within polymorphonuclear leukocytes is proof of phagocytosis and further verifies that the arthritis is crystal induced.

BCP crystals are uncommonly seen on light microscopy but can be detected in fluid samples by several techniques that are not widely available in clinical settings: radiographic diffraction, electron microscopy, or the ethane-1,1-hydroxy diphosphonate binding assay. Alizarin red staining detects any calcium-containing particulate and therefore is not specific for BCP. This technique can have some clinical utility if CPPD crystals are ruled out by polarized light microscopy and weaker grades of staining ignored.

Other tests on synovial fluid are of limited use in diagnosing acute crystal-induced arthritis. Synovial fluid leukocyte count should be clearly in the inflammatory range, usually greater than 10,000 cells/μL, and often in the 20,000 to 100,000 cells/μL range. In acute gout and pseudogout attacks, synovial fluid leukocyte counts are as high as those seen in septic arthritis, or higher. Acute crystal-induced and septic arthritis can rarely occur simultaneously. Therefore, if clinical suspicion persists even after crystals are identified, synovial fluid Gram stain and culture should be obtained. Failure to detect crystals on polarized light microscopy of synovial fluid in the setting of acute monarthritis should greatly increase the suspicion that septic arthritis is present.

Serum uric acid levels are often misused in evaluating patients with suspected acute gout. Although a gout attack is preceded by many months of sustained hyperuricemia, at the time of an acute attack, serum uric acid concentration may be low, normal, or elevated. Serum uric acid levels are not helpful in diagnosing acute gout; however, levels are useful in guiding uric acid–lowering therapy later.

When the acute gout attack resolves, further laboratory investigation may be indicated to determine the cause of total-body urate accumulation. Hyperuricemia is usually due to renal uric acid underexcretion. This is either an idiopathic condition in middle-aged men who are otherwise normal or occurs in patients who have a readily identifiable reason for renal underexcretion: medication, renal insufficiency, or alcohol abuse. If the onset of gout occurs in a man before the age of 20 years, in a menstruating woman, or in a patient without an obvious reason for renal underexcretion, it is appropriate to determine whether urate accumulation is a result of overproduction or underexcretion. This is accomplished by measuring 24-hour urine uric acid excretion. An excretion of greater than 800 mg of uric acid, on an unrestricted diet and in the absence of uricosuric drug ingestion, is clear evidence of uric acid overproduction. In the presence of normal renal function, a 24-hour urinary uric acid of less than 800 mg in a hyperuricemic patient indicates underexcretion. Once this basic classification step is made, investigation for the specific conditions indicated in Table 5-6 can be pursued.

In the case of CPPD crystal-induced arthritis, no laboratory tests other than examination of joint fluid establish the diagnosis. If CPPD crystal deposition is established, it is appropriate to rule out the metabolic conditions occasionally associated with CPPD crystal deposition. This can be accomplished by determining levels of serum thyroxine, calcium, iron, transferrin saturation, magnesium, and alkaline phosphatase activity.

No laboratory evaluation has been established for BCP or calcium oxalate deposition.

MEDICAL MANAGEMENT

The primary diagnostic maneuver in acute crystal-induced monarthritis, joint aspiration, is also therapeutic. Since the crystals induce and probably promote the acute attack, their removal alone sometimes gives noticeable relief. Oral colchicine, 0.6 mg given hourly until improvement in the attack, until the onset of diarrhea, or until 10 doses have been taken, traditionally is used in the treatment of acute gout. Response to this regimen has been touted to be diagnostic for gout as well. In fact, however, oral colchicine used in this manner for acute gout frequently results in onset of severe diarrhea at unpredictable intervals after the last colchicine dose and tends to work poorly in attacks that have been established for a day or more. Response to colchicine is not specific to gout but occurs with CPPD crystal-induced arthritis as well.

The treatment of choice for acute crystal-induced arthritis, which works equally well with gout and pseudogout, is oral administration of one of the NSAIDs. Indomethacin, 50 mg taken every 6 hours until marked improvement is noted, followed by tapering to an every-8-hour schedule for an additional 10 days, is effective even in established attacks.

In patients who have a history of peptic ulcer disease, tolmetin, naproxen, sulindac, or ibuprofen may be substituted, since these agents are associated with less gastric irritation than indomethacin. Renal insufficiency, congestive heart failure, and diabetes are encountered often in older patients with gout. These patients are therefore more likely to develop acutely worsening renal function from suppression of renal prostaglandin synthesis by any of the NSAIDs. In these patients, pretherapy serum creatinine and potassium levels are obtained, and lower doses of NSAIDs should be used. Creatinine and potassium levels are then repeated 3 to 5 days after therapy is started in case further adjustment is needed. Sulindac may spare renal prostaglandins relative to other NSAIDs, a theoretic advantage in this setting.

Aspirin and the other salicylates should be avoided in gout, since they are likely to acutely perturb serum uric acid levels and lead to prolongation of the attack. Allopurinol and the uricosuric medications are not used in the management of acute gout for the same reason.

Administered intravenously, colchicine pharmacology is much different than given orally: absorption is complete, gastrointestinal side effects are rare, a *single* 2 mg dose is effective in both gout and pseudogout, but if given in *repeated* doses, bone marrow toxicity can be severe. This may be the treatment of choice in the hospitalized postsurgical patient with unstable cardiovascular hemodynamics, who cannot take oral medication and who is suffering an acute gout or pseudogout attack. Care must be taken to avoid extravasation during infusion, since severe skin sloughing and ulceration can occur, similar to that encountered with vincristine. Extreme care must be taken in administering intravenous colchicine to patients with renal or hepatic insufficiency, and it should not be administered to patients with combined renal and hepatic failure. Intravenous colchicine should not be given to patients who are already receiving it orally. After an intravenous dose, colchicine should not be given by any route for 1 month.

If the preceding therapies are contraindicated or ineffective in 1 to 2 days, injection of the affected joint with a long-acting microcrystalline steroid ester, such as triamcinolone hexacetonide, is usually effective.

Treatment of BCP or calcium oxalate crystal-induced arthritis should begin with joint aspiration (also diagnostic) and NSAID administration. Little is known about the use of colchicine in acute arthritis due to these crystals. Steroid injection is likely to be effective.

The long-term management plan for gout must be individualized. In principle, it is desirable to treat the underlying condition of long-standing hyperuricemia. Some patients, however, may only suffer a small number of gout attacks in their lifetime and never develop detectable tophi or joint damage. Therefore, urate-lowering therapy should be applied only when there is reason to believe the patient will continue to experience increasingly frequent attacks or progressive joint or renal damage. Such certainty can come from an elicited history of many past attacks, the finding of tophi on physical examination, or the radiographic findings of bone tophi, nonmarginal erosions, or other joint destruction.

The preferred hypouricemic agent is allopurinol. Allopurinol is a synthetic hypoxanthine analog that acts as a false substrate and binds irreversibly to liver xanthine oxidase, thereby preventing the conversion of hypoxanthine to xanthine and xanthine to uric acid. Because of the long half-life of allopurinol, only one dose per day is required. The allopurinol dose can be adjusted upward from 300 mg/d in 100-mg increments every 2 weeks until serum uric acid falls to about 5 mg/dL (soft tissue urate deposits begin dissolving when uric acid concentration falls below 6 mg/mL). Initiation of allopurinol therapy is associated with increased frequency of acute gout attacks; therefore, prophylaxis against acute attacks is usually administered along with allopurinol for the first 6 to 12 months in the form of colchicine 0.6 mg orally twice daily.

Uricosuric drugs, which can lower serum uric acid and also mobilize tophi, seem a rational choice in patients with uric acid underexcretion. There are some limitations to this approach:

1. Normal renal function is required for the uricosuric drugs to be effective.
2. Increased concentration of urine uric acid can result in acute stone formation, so uricosuric drugs should not be used in patients with a history of stones.
3. Serum uric acid reductions are likely to be modest compared with reductions achievable with allopurinol.
4. Uricosurics have a short half-life and must be given 4 times a day.

Probenecid and sulfinpyrazone are both uricosuric drugs used in the long-term management of gout. Probenecid is usually begun at 500 mg/d and increased up to 3000 mg/d in four divided doses as needed to lower the serum uric acid. Sulfinpyrazone can be initiated at 100 mg/d and increased as needed to 800 mg/d in four divided doses. Increased fluid intake is recommended to lessen the risk of acute urinary stone formation. Just as with allopurinol, acute lowering of uric acid with the uricosuric agents can precipitate acute gout attacks, and colchicine prophylaxis should be used.

Synovial Chondromatosis
Louise H. Sparks

DEFINITION

Synovial chondromatosis or osteochondromatosis is the development of cartilaginous or osteocartilaginous bodies within the synovial membrane of joints, bursa, or tendon sheaths as a result of metaplasia of synovial fibroblasts. The evolution is characterized by three stages: the *active stage*, characterized by the formation or presence of nodules confined within the synovial lining; the *intermediate stage*, characterized by the presence of both loose and synovial cartilage nodules; and the *final stage*, characterized by loose bodies only.

CLINICAL FEATURES

The clinical features of synovial chondromatosis relate to its presence in joints, bursa, and tendon sheaths (with up to 21% extraarticular). Earlier re-

ports suggested a male predominance of 2:1, but more recent studies suggest a female predominance of 1.4:1. Presentation is in young to middle-aged adults, with a mean age of 48 years and a range from 17 to 79 years. Isolated TMJ disease is more dominant in middle-aged women, with hand and foot involvement more common in elderly women. Synovial chondromatosis is not thought to be hereditary.

Large diarthrodial joints are most commonly affected, and 10% of patients have bilateral involvement. The knee is affected in a monarticular fashion half of the time, and hip, elbow, shoulder, and ankle involvement are common. When multiple joints are simultaneously involved, the hands and feet are typically affected, and the metacarpal and metatarsal joints or the tendon sheath are the most frequent sites. Distal radioulnar and TMJ involvement also were described.

Typical symptoms are local pain and swelling with active (stage 1) synovial involvement and mechanical symptoms (transient locking, grating, or crepitus) with intermediate or late disease. TMJ disease is characterized more often by pain. Average duration of symptoms before diagnosis is 4.5 years, with a range from 3 to 8 years. Associations with non–insulin-dependent diabetes mellitus and simultaneous pigmented villonodular synovitis have been suggested.

Physical examination reveals joint tenderness, soft tissue swelling, synovial thickening, or discrete masses and, depending on symptoms, marked audible or palpable crepitus.

PATHOLOGIC FEATURES

Gross pathologic examination reveals a thickened synovial lining with multiple shiny blue-white glistening cartilage nodules either embedded in the cartilage or attached by pedicles along the surface like cobblestones. The synovium is moist, folded, and often hyperemic. Loose bodies may be present and average 1 to 2 cm in diameter (Fig. 5-12). The nodules of metaplastic cartilage formed within the synovial tissue are initially attached by a synovial pedicle deriving nutritional support, which allows hypertrophy and endochondral ossification (synovial osteochondromatosis). After separation, the synovial fluid provides nutrition for continued hypertrophy, but the osseous portion (if any) dies. Trauma by direct pressure can cause bony erosions.

Histologically, metaplastic synovial fibroblasts produce nodules of hyaline cartilage within the synovial tissue. Attached by a pedicle, these develop vascular ingrowth with subsequent endochondral ossification with woven and lamellar bone. The adjacent unaffected synovium is entirely normal.

Although characterized by focal atypia, binucleate cells, and nuclear enlargement, synovial chondromatosis does not metastasize and is not thought to be sarcomatous. Malignant degeneration to chondrosarcoma and de novo intraarticular chondrosarcoma in association with synovial chondromatosis have been described, but the incidence is too low (less than 1%) to affect management. From these reports, it is difficult to determine whether primary occurrence was in bone or joint, since bone, soft tissue, and joint involvement are present at presentation.

RADIOGRAPHIC FEATURES

Plain radiographs may reveal multiple juxtaarticular radiodense shadows with the discrete stippled appearance of cartilaginous lesions (Fig. 5-13). As chondromas hypertrophy, the opacities become larger, with peripheral linear densities, radiolucent centers, and bony trabeculation. Pressure erosions of adjacent bony surfaces are seen primarily in the femoral neck when the hips are involved and on the anterior aspect of the lower femur when the knees

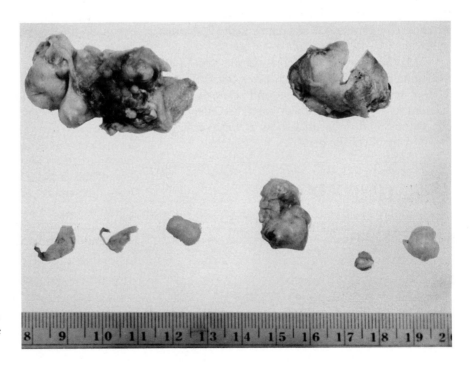

FIGURE 5-12. Osteochondromatosis. These loose bodies were recovered from a knee joint.

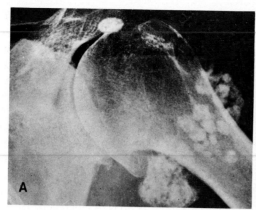
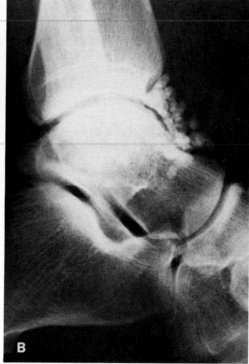

FIGURE 5-13. (A) Osteochondromatosis of the shoulder joint. (B) Osteochondromatosis of the ankle.

are involved. Associated DJD is characterized by patellofemoral disease and osteophytes rather than loss of joint space. Air or double-contrast arthrography has been the standard procedure to demonstrate chondromas; however, reports of MRI used for this purpose are promising. Bone scan of involved joints reveals increased activity in a synovial distribution. Neither MRI nor bone scan can differentiate between synovial chondromatosis and pigmented villonodular synovitis.

TMJ radiography may demonstrate joint space widening and additional features of calcified loose bodies, irregular joint surface, and sclerosis of the glenoid fossa and mandibular condyle. Osteochondromatous tendon sheaths show a linear arrangement of small calcific densities.

LABORATORY FEATURES

No characteristic abnormal laboratory features have been established for synovial chondromatosis.

MANAGEMENT

Surgical management has long been standard, but the type and extent of surgery has become more controversial. Total synovectomy predicated to cure the disease and prevent DJD is thought to be unnecessary, and recent studies support partial synovectomy, simple loose-body removal by arthroscopy, or both. An operation designed to relieve symptoms seems most appropriate (ie, if mechanical symptoms, removal of loose bodies; if pain and swelling, partial synovectomy). Histologic staging of the disease at time of surgery best predicts recurrence: active or intermediate stages are more likely to result in recurrences. When only loose bodies are removed by arthroscopy, however, some studies suggest that the best correlation with functional results is the condition of the cartilage of the tibiofemoral joint, not the histologic grade of the chondroma. Overall, the prognosis is good, and synovial chondromatosis and osteochondromatosis remain uncommon, benign, self-limited conditions.

Villonodular Synovitis
Louise H. Sparks

DEFINITION

Villonodular synovitis is a term that characterizes a spectrum of idiopathic lesions involving exuberant proliferation of the synovial membrane of joints, tendon sheaths, or bursae, which may invade locally without metastasis or malignant histology. Theories of its etiology are diverse. The childhood disease is polyarticular, has sibling involvement, and is associated with congenital anomalies. An autosomal dominant trait has been implicated. Jaffe's original theory, that a nontraumatic irritant causes a reactive type of synovitis characterized by accumulation of histiocytes and fibroblasts, remains the standard. Jaffe proposed three sequential stages based on clinical findings. The first is synovial cell proliferation, causing synovial hypertrophy with villous overgrowth. In the second stage, nodules form from matted confluent fused synovial projections and villi in the presence of fibrin and blood. The third stage is characterized by fibrosis with hyalinization, forming fibrous nodules firmly adherent to synovial structures. The characteristic forms produced include both localized (LPVS) and diffuse pigmented nodular synovitis (DPVS), localized and diffuse nodular tenosynovitis, and (rarely) localized nodular bursitis.

CLINICAL FEATURES

Measured with respect to all forms, the incidence of villonodular synovitis is 1.8 per million. The disease has an equal gender distribution and occurs in young adults between 20 and 40 years of age. Large joint involvement of mixed diffuse and nodular disease occurs at a mean age of 40 years, with a range from 11 to 73 years; whereas localized nodular tenosynovitis occurs more frequently in women aged 20 to 40 years.

Unilateral knee involvement is seen in greater than 80% of cases, with only rare reports of polyarticular disease. Involvement of hip, ankle, elbow, shoulder, calcaneocuboid, TMJ, hand, and sole of foot is seen. Rarely, the posterior elements of the cervical spine are involved. The tendon sheaths of the fingers and toes are the most common sites of tendon involvement, although larger tendon sheath involvement proximal to the ankle and wrist has been de-

scribed. Bursal involvement is rare, usually occurring diffusely in the popliteal, iliopectineal, or anserine bursae or in the common flexor tendon sheaths of the hand.

The gradual onset of mild to moderate intermittent pain associated with repeated swelling is characteristic of the presenting symptoms, with duration ranging from 1 day to 30 years. The mean duration of symptoms before presentation in large joints is 5 years. Mechanical interference is characterized by stiffness, locking, limitation of motion in extension, and a snapping sensation. The form that is restricted to part of the synovium more frequently presents with locking as a predominant complaint and is occasionally associated with acute pain when the nodule's stalk becomes twisted and infarcted.

Physical examination reveals soft tissue swelling, which enlarges the entire joint and is associated with tenderness and pronounced effusion in diffuse synovial involvement. Localized nodular synovial involvement may present with minimal effusion, slight intermittent swelling, and an occasional palpable mass.

Recurrence in large joints is characterized by painful swelling that occurs after a mean interval of 5 years with a range from 31 days to 20 years.

PATHOLOGIC FEATURES

Gross pathology of diffuse disease reveals a markedly papillary synovial lining with innumerable finger-like villous projections and synovial folds. Projections fuse to form soft or hard confluent nodular masses, which may be sessile or pedunculated and range from 0.5 to 2 cm in diameter. Color ranges from red-brown (secondary to hemorrhage) to yellow-orange (secondary to lipid). Pigmentation may extend deep into the subsynovial structure, through the joint capsule, and into bone. Depending on the extent of invasion, tissue may be coated with strands of red-brown tissue or present as a soft to rubbery red-brown mass with foci of hemorrhagic cysts. Involved tendon sheaths present as sausage-shaped masses distended by synovial proliferation.

Histology reveals proliferation of synovial lining cells both on the surface and with subsynovial invasion. There is no difference in the histologic appearances between variants. Cellular infiltrate is characterized by polyhedral histiocytic cells, fibroblasts, giant cells, and hemosiderin- or lipid-laden (foam cells) macrophages (Fig. 5-14). Hemosiderin is also seen between cells, in synovial lining cells, and in histiocytes. Overall histology cannot predict outcome or recurrence, nor can level of proliferative activity predict an outcome differing from that seen in hemochromatosis and hemosiderosis secondary to trauma. Foci of hemorrhage are common, with some surrounding chronic inflammatory infiltrate.

Nodules reveal villi with characteristic cellular infiltrates surrounding hemorrhage, fibrin plugs, and fibrosis. Nodules are usually smaller than 2.5 cm in diameter but have been reported as large as 7 cm. Older nodules have massive collagen deposition with bands of fibroblasts but little additional cellular activity. Although it is a proliferative lesion, there are few mitoses and no signs of malignancy.

When bone erosion is present, the lesion enters the bone through perivascular foramina, ligamentous attachments, or chondroosseous junctions. This is usually seen on both sides of the joint and frequently

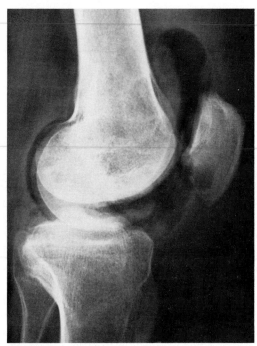

FIGURE 5-15. Pigmented villonodular synovitis. Note the nodular density in the suprapatellar pouch demonstrated by air arthrography.

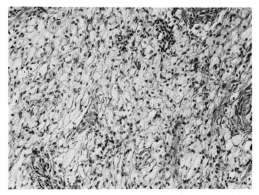

FIGURE 5-14. Xanthoma cells or foam cells. They are large and polyhedral and contain a small, central, usually pyknotic nucleus and transparent, foamy cytoplasm. Lipoid bodies are dissolved out in hematoxylin-eosin stains and are demonstrable by fat stains. Foam cells exist in varying proportion with fibroblasts and collagenous fibrils. When fibrous tissue is abundant, xanthoma cells are enveloped and difficult to demonstrate; this lesion is termed a *fibroxanthoma*. The characteristics of a fibroxanthoma are foam cells; fibrocellular stroma with short, blunt, spindle-shaped cells containing a pale, slightly elongated nucleus; multinucleated giant cells of the epulis type, containing 5 to 40 nuclei; blood pigment, coarse yellow or brown pigment of hemosiderin scattered throughout the groundwork, situated principally intracellularly in macrophages or foam cells; blood vessels, mainly small, abundant capillaries; and, when xanthomatous tumors develop within the synovium of joints (nodular synovitis), synovial villous formation. (DeSanto DA, Wilson PD: Xanthomatous tumors of joints. J Bone Joint Surg 1939;21:531)

close to the reflection of the synovial membrane. Localized nodular tenosynovitis is also associated with bone erosion.

RADIOGRAPHIC FEATURES

Plain radiographs may be normal. Localized disease within the synovial cavity may reveal a nodular soft tissue density (Fig. 5-15). Diffuse disease may show a diffuse bubbly flocculent effect. Localized nodular disease of the lane is usually located in the posterior suprapatellar area or in the junction between the capsule and the meniscus. Diffuse disease has radiographic findings more commonly than localized disease. No osteoporosis, joint space narrowing, or calcification is seen.

Bone erosion and subchondral cyst formation are uncommon but, when present, usually affect both sides of the joint. The cysts are multiple, with well-defined thin sclerotic rims, and can occur on non–weight-bearing surfaces. In the knee, the uncommon bone changes usually involve the intercondylar area. Joints with a higher frequency of bone involvement are the hip (central femoral neck) and the ankle (syndesmotic recesses). Predisposition to erosion in these locations is postulated to be due to higher intracapsular pressures in a smaller synovial volume, where villi have little room to grow. Tenosynovial involvement also causes frequent bone erosions, characterized by a scooped-out excavation rimmed by a sclerotic margin appearing beneath a soft tissue mass following a tendon sheath.

In the past, arthrography was used to provide more detailed information, revealing capsular distension and nodular filling defects. Currently, MRI has the best potential to provide noninvasive diagnosis. Hemosiderin present in villonodular synovitis creates a low-signal intensity on both T_1- and T_2-weighted images, and lipid creates a high-signal intensity. These two substances need to be present in sufficient concentrations to alter signal intensity; and when present, together they can average out owing to their opposing effects. Further experience may improve diagnostic utility, although recent studies diagnosed six of eight cases of pigmented villonodular synovitis by MRI. Until MRI is more firmly established, biopsy, either by closed needle or (more commonly) by arthroscopy, is necessary for diagnosis.

LABORATORY FEATURES

Despite earlier studies suggesting a role for cholesterol in the pathogenesis of villonodular synovitis, there has been no documentation of elevated serum triglycerides or cholesterol. Synovial fluid analysis in villonodular synovitis has been documented to contain numerous birefringent lipid microspherules and foam cells (lipid-laden macrophages). Lipid microspherules are seen as Maltese crosses by polarizing microscopy.

Characteristic synovial fluid in DPVS ranges in color from dark bloody to rusty to thick orange-brown. Cell counts reveal large numbers of red blood cells and less than 2000 leukocytes. In contrast to DPVS, LPVS synovial fluid, when present, is frequently straw-colored without cells.

MANAGEMENT

Total surgical synovectomy is recommended, often requiring multiple incisions (knee, elbow) and joint dislocation (hip) for all DPVS and mixed nodular and diffuse disease. Only well-characterized localized nodules in joint or tendon should be treated with simple excision.

The proposed pathogenesis appears to indicate that prognosis and recurrence rate should be based on stage of disease, with diffuse disease (DPVS) more susceptible to recurrence than localized (LPVS) disease. Recent studies, however, revealed no difference in recurrence rates.

With respect to knee involvement, recurrence was predicted by location, history of previous operative procedures, and incomplete synovectomy, which gives a recurrence free-survival of 65% at 25 years. Recurrences did not correlate with bone involvement. With respect to hip disease, adequate exposure (ie, dislocation during surgery) facilitated a complete synovectomy and was correlated with a lower recurrence rate. Functional outcome in the hip correlated with cartilage preservation. Patients who underwent complete synovectomy and total hip arthroplasty had the best outcomes and the fewest recurrences. No adjuvant therapy, either external beam irradiation or chemotherapy, lowers the recurrence rate. Survival is not altered by recurrence, underscoring the benign nature of villonodular synovitis.

Systemic Sclerosis
Alan D. Croock

Scleroderma literally means tight skin. The characteristic hidebound skin due to fibrosis is of most concern to the patient and provides the only definitive clinical diagnostic criterion. There are many formes frustes of scleroderma (Table 5-7). Perhaps the greatest misconception regarding systemic sclerosis is that the disease always entails progressive internal organ involvement, spelling doom for the patient. On the contrary, optimism is extremely helpful in management and is justified in that not all scleroderma is progressive. Intervention can prolong life despite incipient organ failure (eg, in scleroderma renal crisis [SRC]). Hence, the term *progressive systemic sclerosis* is misleading.

Systemic sclerosis, a multisystem and multistage disorder of unknown etiology with an annual incidence of about 12 per 1 million population, is 4 times more common in women than men. It is characterized

TABLE 5-7.
Classification of Scleroderma

SYSTEMIC SCLEROSIS (GENERALIZED SCLERODERMA)

Diffuse cutaneous

Limited cutaneous (CREST syndrome)

LOCALIZED SCLERODERMA

Morphea

Linear

SCLERODERMA-LIKE SYNDROMES (PSEUDOSCLERODERMA)

Occupational and environmental (eg, vinyl chloride, silicosis)

Eosinophilic fasciitis

Scleredema

Metabolic (eg, porphyria)

Graft-versus-host disease

Drug induced (eg, bleomycin)

Silicone augmentation mammoplasty

SCLERODERMA-ASSOCIATED SYNDROMES

Overlapping or mixed connective tissue syndromes (eg, sclerodermatomyositis, sclerolupus, scleromyxedema)

Tumor-associated (eg, carcinoid syndrome)

Inherited (eg, Werner syndrome)

by proliferative vascular lesions, obliterative microvascular lesions, and consequent atrophy with fibrosis of multiple organs. Mortality from systemic sclerosis depends on the extent of vascular involvement of vital organs. Traditionally, the diffuse cutaneous subtype has been considered to have a worse prognosis and, therefore, potentially earlier and more extensive internal organ involvement than the limited cutaneous variant, which includes calcinosis, Raynaud phenomenon, esophageal hypomotility, sclerodactyly, and telangiectasia (CREST syndrome). CREST syndrome, however, after 10 to 20 years, may become as generalized and life-threatening as diffuse scleroderma is in its first decade, with severe pulmonary hypertension being a particularly feared complication. Fortunately, this severe progression of CREST syndrome is uncommon, occurring in less than 10% of patients. For study purposes, patients with three or more of the five CREST characteristics are considered to have the syndrome.

The clinical diagnostic criteria for scleroderma are outlined in Table 5-8. These criteria, as with diagnostic criteria proposed for other rheumatic diseases, serve mainly as a guideline, particularly for epidemiologic studies. A more recently recognized rare subtype of scleroderma known as *systemic sclerosis sine scleroderma* is characterized by Raynaud phenomenon, nailfold capillary abnormalities, and esophageal dysfunction in the notable absence of skin involvement. Pulmonary and renal disease are unusual, but the extent of other internal organ involvement and the eventual outcome of disease in this subgroup remain to be fully elucidated.

PATHOGENESIS

The etiology of scleroderma remains unknown. The hypothesis is that an immunoinflammatory response to altered endothelium of small arteries and capillaries leads to further endothelial injury, exposure of subendothelium, activation of platelets and the clotting cascade, and migration of smooth muscle cells to the intima with eventual intimal proliferation and narrowing of the vessel lumen. Serum activity toxic to the endothelial cell has been identified in about half of scleroderma patients. This activity may be due to a neutral protease. Factor VIII–von Willebrand factor attachment to subendothelium is an important step in the first phase of platelet interaction with the vessel wall. Increased plasma concentrations of secreted platelet proteins, particularly platelet factor IV and β-thromboglobulin, were documented in scleroderma patients. Increased collagen synthesis and deposition in the skin or internal organs in an unpredictable fashion is viewed as the end result of this

TABLE 5-8.
Preliminary Criteria for Classification of Systemic Sclerosis (Scleroderma)

MAJOR CRITERION

Proximal scleroderma: Symmetric thickening, tightening, and induration of the skin of the fingers and the skin proximal to the metacarpophalangeal or metatarsophalangeal joints. The changes may affect the entire extremity, face, neck, and trunk (thorax and abdomen).

MINOR CRITERIA

Sclerodactyly: Above-indicated skin changes limited to the fingers

Digital pitting, scars, or loss of substance from the finger pad; depressed areas at tips of fingers or loss of digital pad tissue as a result of ischemia

Bibasilar pulmonary fibrosis: Bilateral reticular pattern of linear or lineonodular densities most pronounced in basilar portions of the lungs on standard chest radiograph; may assume appearance of diffuse mottling or "honeycomb lung." These changes should not be attributable to primary lung disease.

cycle of vascular events, but the mechanism of fibrosis is not well understood. Lymphocytes and mast cells are intimately associated in scleroderma lesions, and their interaction may prove to be of great significance in further elucidating the mechanism of fibrosis. Fibroblast activation may result from a lymphokine and monokine stimulus, most likely associated with other growth factor stimuli. Scleroderma fibroblasts behave abnormally in vitro in terms of site and quantity of collagen synthesis. Two hypotheses attempt to explain this difference: one proposes general fibroblast activation and increased collagen synthesis at the cellular level; the second suggests that normal dermal fibroblasts are heterogenous with respect to levels of collagen synthesis and that, in scleroderma, the growth of the fibroblasts that produce the most collagen is selectively favored. These hypotheses are not mutually exclusive. Both cellular and humoral immune mechanisms appear to perpetuate the fibrosis. Anticentromere and antitopoisomerase-1 (topo-1, formerly Scl-70) antibodies are associated with the CREST syndrome and diffuse cutaneous subtype, respectively.

CLINICAL PRESENTATION

At presentation, the typical patient, most often a woman aged 20 to 40 years, has transient pallor or cyanosis of the tips of the fingers or toes on cold exposure and emotional upset for months or years (Raynaud phenomenon). Puffiness of the hands and face is common, usually associated with numbness and tingling of the fingers. Dysphagia or esophageal reflux symptoms may occur early, but other systemic symptomatology is rare until relatively late in the disease. Examination reveals puffy or taut skin, occasionally with pigment changes. There may be scars or tiny atrophic pits of the finger tips (dermal infarcts), and telangiectasia may be found on the face, lips, tongue, palms, fingers, or anterior chest. Nailfold capillary abnormalities on wide-field microscopy are found in 90% of scleroderma patients. These changes include dilated capillary loops, hemorrhages, and in more severe disease, avascular areas. Although highly characteristic of scleroderma, some of these nailfold abnormalities may occur in patients with dermatomyositis or SLE. Less common presenting features of scleroderma include polyarthritis resembling RA, active myositis, and accelerated hypertension.

Progression of skin disease to hidebound, fibrotic skin is unpredictable and may take weeks to months

to develop. The earliest diagnosis can usually be accomplished by a rheumatologist who is familiar with scleroderma. Skin tightening that occurs from the trunk outward rather than from the extremities inward suggests an alternative diagnosis, such as eosinophilic fasciitis or scleredema. The absence of Raynaud phenomenon likewise makes the diagnosis of scleroderma most unlikely.

Raynaud phenomenon, occurring in 95% of scleroderma patients, precedes the onset of skin disease by a variable period (weeks to years). A longer preceding period of Raynaud phenomenon usually suggests a more favorable prognosis in terms of less severe skin disease or internal organ disease. Primary Raynaud phenomenon (Raynaud disease) has a prevalence of 4% to 30% in the general population, depending on age, sex, and occupation, and is not associated with any underlying systemic connective tissue disorder. The skin color changes reported by patients with primary or secondary Raynaud are mostly uniphasic or biphasic rather than the well-known triphasic (white-blue-red) sequence. Clinical studies have documented pulmonary vasoconstriction and altered renal blood flow that occurs during external cold exposure of an extremity.

ORGAN DISEASE

Skin

Cutaneous involvement occurs in 90% to 95% of patients, the remaining 5% to 10% having systemic sclerosis sine scleroderma. Skin involvement proceeds through an early edematous phase of induration and finally an atrophic phase anytime from 3 to 15 years after initial skin changes, indicating the unpredictable natural history of scleroderma. These changes may be stable or progressive. Recurrent, poorly healing ulcers, especially over the knuckles, are extremely debilitating and painful.

Musculoskeletal

Arthralgias, joint stiffness, and swelling are common early. Mild to severe polyarthritis can be confused with early RA, but it rarely progresses. Indeed, in the later stages of the disease, hand stiffness is secondary predominantly to skin fibrosis and flexion contractures rather than destructive joint disease. Tendon sheath involvement contributes to flexion contractures. Nevertheless, radiographic studies occasionally demonstrated erosive arthropathy. Investigators reported marginal or dorsal erosions in 9% to 15% of patients with advanced scleroderma without other evidence of RA or overlap syndromes. Resorption of distal phalangeal tufts of fingers (acroosteolysis) occurs in 40% to 80% of cases of sclerodactyly. In contrast, a transverse band of lysis in the midshaft rather than the terminal tufts of distal phalanges may occur in vinyl chloride–related scleroderma, renal osteodystrophy and, idiopathic or familial types of acroosteolysis. Subcutaneous calcification (dystrophic in type) is characteristic of the CREST syndrome. Muscle involvement is not severe, with secondary (disuse) atrophy being more common than inflammatory myositis.

Gastrointestinal

Esophageal involvement detectable radiologically occurs in up to 80% of patients; however, only 50% suffer symptoms of reflux and dysphagia. Esophageal hypomotility can be documented by barium swallow; esophageal manometry and radionuclide transit studies are even more sensitive. Small bowel abnormalities relate to hypomotility with stasis and varying degrees of malabsorption associated with bacterial overgrowth. Diarrhea and weight loss occur in up to 10% of patients. Colonic disease is usually asymptomatic despite the characteristic wide-mouth sacculation on radiographs.

Pulmonary

Dyspnea is the most frequent symptom (60% of patients have it on exertion, 14% at rest), sometimes with pleuritic pain (17%) and chronic nonproductive cough (10%). Bibasilar rales are found in up to 40% of patients. Autopsy studies revealed lung abnormalities in 70% of patients, interstitial fibrosis being most common. Vascular abnormalities may occur in the absence of interstitial changes and may be associated with more severe symptoms. In fact, severe pulmonary hypertension without interstitial involvement is well documented in 5% to 10% of CREST patients, resulting in a high mortality; it is much rarer in systemic sclerosis patients with parenchymal disease. The incidence and nature of pulmonary disease is similar in CREST and the diffuse cutaneous subgroups.

Restrictive and obstructive abnormalities are found on lung function testing. Reduction of the single breath diffusion capacity is the most common finding, even in the absence of any obvious clinical or radiologic disease. More recently, bronchoalveolar lavage has become a useful tool for early detection of lung inflammation as well as for monitoring progression of disease. Increased numbers of neutrophils, eosinophils, and less commonly, lymphocytes were reported, correlating with a diminished diffusion capacity.

Cardiac

Cardiac involvement can occur in the absence of either systemic or pulmonary hypertension. Manifestations include pericardial disease and disorders of rhythm and conduction. There is a notable discrepancy between the prevalence of clinical myocardial and pericardial disease and that found at autopsy. Clinical pericardial disease (less than 10% of patients) may present as acute pericarditis or as a more chronic, indolent process with a pericardial effusion of variable size. Rarely, frank tamponade or hemodynamically significant constrictive pericarditis are reported. Myocardial fibrosis is present in up to 80% of patients at autopsy, although clinically significant myocardial dysfunction is uncommon. Exercise and radionuclide techniques showed a high frequency of fixed thallium perfusion abnormalities in patients (69% in diffuse scleroderma and 64% in CREST syndrome). In contrast, limited angiographic studies revealed normal coronary arteries in most patients, illustrating the fact that small vessel disease is dominant. About half of CREST and diffuse cutaneous scleroderma patients have an abnormal electrocardiogram, with varying forms of bundle-branch or atrioventricular block, with atrial or ventricular ectopy predominating. These patients rarely require pacemaker insertion. Sudden cardiac death may occur rarely from ventricular tachyarrhythmias or high-grade heart block.

Kidney

Renal involvement in scleroderma may occur with or without SRC. The latter is characterized by a sudden unpredictable rise in arterial blood pressure, severe hypertensive retinopathy (hemorrhages, cotton wool exudates, and papilledema), elevated plasma renin activity, and rapid deterioration of renal function. More recently, a smaller subgroup of normotensive renal failure patients has been recognized, but is not well characterized.

Clinical evidence of renal involvement (without SRC) may be mild (proteinuria, increased blood urea nitrogen, with or without hypertension) or inapparent, with the prevalence varying from 3% to 45% in published studies. In contrast, autopsy studies revealed 58% to 90% renal involvement, with distinctive vascular proliferative lesions, particularly in the cortical interlobular arteries. Fibrinoid necrosis of small arteries and afferent arterioles is commonly observed in patients with SRC. Immune complexes are found uncommonly. Development of SRC is usually sudden and unpredictable, but occasionally, preceding clinical events (weeks to months) include pericardial effusion (rarely tamponade), cardiac failure, and diuretic use.

DIAGNOSTIC EVALUATION

Laboratory screening tests include a complete blood count, electrolytes, creatinine, and urinalysis. Fragmented red cells on peripheral smear indicate ongoing endothelial damage. ANA are commonly found, with one or more of four patterns of immunofluorescence occurring in scleroderma: speckled, homogenous, nucleolar, and centromere. Any combination of the first three patterns may be seen in any one patient. The centromere pattern can only be detected with the use of a mitotic human cell line (eg, Hep-2) as substrate and is found in 60% to 90% of CREST patients. Topo-1 is found in patients with diffuse cutaneous disease (specificity, more than 90%; sensitivity, 10% to 25%). Anticentromere antibody and topo-1 antibodies are considered mutually exclusive, although there are isolated reports of the simultaneous occurrence of both antibodies. The nucleolar pattern is moderately sensitive and specific for scleroderma, occurring in up to 80% of patients and in less than 20% of patients with other rheumatic diseases. The combination of Raynaud phenomenon, anticentromere antibody, and dilated nailfold capillary loop pattern strongly selects (90% relative risk) a subgroup of patients who will insidiously develop the CREST syndrome.

Specialized investigations such as esophageal manometry, bronchoalveolar lavage, Holter monitoring, and thallium perfusion scanning are considered only on an individualized basis or as part of a study protocol. Skin biopsy is of value in the early stages of the disease to obtain fibroblasts for research purposes.

TREATMENT

No single therapeutic modality has been shown to improve all manifestations of scleroderma. Therefore, an approach directed at both the pathophysiologic and the clinical expression of the disease is recommended.

Supportive Measures

Supportive measures are undoubtedly critical in patient management, taking the form of strict avoidance of situations that stimulate vasoconstriction, such as cold exposure (all seasons, outdoor and indoor), smoking (active and passive), and trauma (because of poor healing capacity). Extensive patient and family counseling and the use of physical therapy are of major importance. Continuing emotional support is a pivotal factor that cannot be overemphasized in the overall management. The patient must fully comprehend that meticulous self-care and a positive attitude are imperative, with drug therapy only being of limited benefit. The patient must learn and perform routine active and passive range-of-motion exercises and cold preventive measures. Occupational therapy is essential, particularly in the management of finger and hand contractures. Attempts to avoid contractures must never cease, no matter how rapidly progressive the skin disease. Liberal skin application of lubricants is encouraged, as is swimming in heated pools. Sex and vocational counseling are important; the patient should be encouraged to lead as normal a life as possible within the restraints of the disease.

Drug Therapy

VASODILATORS. These agents are indicated in the more severe cases of Raynaud phenomenon and digital ulceration, particularly in the winter months. A calcium-channel blocker (such as nifedipine 10 to 20 mg, three or four times a day, or as a sustained-release form) is favored. In the setting of hypertension or renal disease, an ACE inhibitor is the drug of choice. Topical nitroglycerin 1% to 2% applied sparingly once or twice daily to affected digits may help to prevent skin breakdown in threatened areas.

ANTIPLATELET THERAPY. The rationale for use of antiplatelet drugs is based on the assumption that platelet activation plays a key role in the initiation and perpetuation of the vascular disease of scleroderma. Although efficacy has not been clearly shown, empirical use of enteric-coated aspirin (325 mg twice weekly or 80 mg daily), together with dipyridamole (200 to 300 mg daily in divided doses) may be used.

D-PENICILLAMINE.   The rationale for using this drug in scleroderma is based on its ability to inhibit cross-linkage of collagen fibers. Uncontrolled retrospective data suggest benefit of this drug in terms of skin softening and reduction of new visceral organ involvement, especially renal disease. These reported benefits may be artifactual, particularly considering the natural history of spontaneously remitting disease in 10% to 15% of untreated patients. In addition, drug toxicity (rash, thrombocytopenia, leukopenia, nephrotic syndrome, myasthenia gravis, and pemphigus) is of major concern. Adverse reactions of this nature were reported in 57% of treated patients, with 29% having to discontinue penicillamine permanently. In view of the potential serious toxicity of the drug, D-penicillamine should only be used in the setting of severe and progressive skin or internal organ disease and with informed consent from the patient. Results of prospective controlled studies are eagerly awaited.

COLCHICINE.   This drug has the ability to prevent extracellular accumulation of collagen by inhibiting the release of procollagen from fibroblasts. Its efficacy in scleroderma is unproved, but its empirical use (0.6 to 1.8 mg/d) may be tried.

CORTICOSTEROIDS.   Oral steroid therapy is generally contraindicated. It may be considered only in the following situations: the very early edematous phase of skin disease; progressive interstitial lung disease in the setting of an abnormal lavage analysis (unproved); and myopathy with biopsy-proven myositis (uncommon in scleroderma). Steroid therapy most recently was observed to be a significant risk factor for development of normotensive renal failure in a subgroup of scleroderma patients. Topical steroid therapy is absolutely contraindicated. Miscellaneous forms of drug therapy, such as vitamin E, potassium-aminobenzoate, and various immunosuppressive agents, are not of proven benefit.

Gastrointestinal Disease

A mucosal barrier agent (sucralfate, 1 g four times a day given orally or in a liquid slurry) is often effective in relieving acid reflux symptoms. Antacids, H_2-blocking agents (cimetidine, ranitidine), and metoclopramide are occasionally of benefit. No synergistic effect of these agents has been demonstrated.

In the unfortunate situation of esophageal stricture formation, dilation procedures become necessary. Malabsorption syndrome is best managed by the use of intermittent courses of broad-spectrum antibiotics (eg, tetracycline or ampicillin 2 weeks per month to reduce bacterial overgrowth). Parenteral hyperalimentation rarely may be required in the extreme case of inanition. Small and large bowel emergencies rarely may necessitate surgical intervention.

Renal Disease

The mortality of SRC was 100% within the first 2 months of onset in the pre-ACE inhibitor era. The introduction of captopril in 1979 dramatically improved the prognosis of SRC patients. Investigators reported a 50% reduction in SRC (14%, 1979 to 1985 versus 27%, 1972 to 1978) and a 1-year cumulative survival rate of 76% (ACE inhibitor-treated) versus 25% before 1979. However, 24 (44%) of 55 patients with SRC treated with ACE inhibitors died early or required permanent dialysis. The serum creatinine value at the time of initiation of ACE-inhibitor therapy appears to be a critical factor, with a level less than 3 mg/dL associated with a good outcome. Experience with newer ACE inhibitors (enalapril, lisinopril) is still limited, and the lower nephrotoxicity hoped for has not been proved. Captopril dosage for SRC is usually 10 mg four times a day, titrating rapidly upward until blood pressure is controlled. The key to management of renal disease without SRC is meticulous monitoring and control of blood pressure, avoidance of vasoconstricting agents, and extreme caution with diuretic therapy.

Pulmonary Disease

The limited role of D-penicillamine and steroid therapy has been discussed. Early eradication of infection, physical therapy, and in more severe cases, readily available oxygen therapy are most important. Abstinence from smoking (active and passive) is critical. Pulmonary hypertension is usually irreversible, with a high mortality rate. Vasodilator therapy is of little or no benefit in this setting.

Cardiac Disease

In the relatively uncommon situation of clinically significant cardiac disease (conduction abnormalities, restrictive cardiomyopathy, or cor pulmonale with right-heart failure), inotropic, vasodilator, or antiarrhythmic agents are used. Diuretics should be used with extreme caution owing to their potential to precipitate hypovolemic renal failure.

Joint Disease

Joint contractures, particularly of the hands, must be vigorously treated with occupational and physical therapy. These measures are aimed at trying to improve range of motion and microcirculation as well as preventing deformities and skin ulcers. Gold, penicillamine, and immunosuppressive drugs do not play a role in the management of scleroderma joint disease.

Surgery

In view of the significant microvascular disease of scleroderma and resultant poor healing of wounds, surgical procedures are relatively contraindicated. Surgery for severe esophageal strictures and rare small and large bowel emergencies are exceptions. The patient should be educated in this respect and in particular that cosmetic surgery is contraindicated. Predisposition to infection in the setting of impaired wound healing must be emphasized.

The role of hand surgery in scleroderma has been documented infrequently. Jones and colleagues published a notable review of 52 surgical hand procedures in 31 patients out of a series of 813 consecutive scleroderma patients seen at one institution over a 9-year period. Raynaud phenomenon (in 96% of patients) and digital tip ulcerations (in 46%) were primarily controlled by conservative means, vasodilators being most effective (nifedipine and prazosin), with meticulous wound care. Digital ulcerations that progressed to frank gangrene in the absence of infection were allowed to autoamputate. Only nine patients required a total of 23 digital amputations owing to infection or extensive gangrene. All the amputation stumps healed normally except for two (in a single patient on steroid therapy). Other procedures in this series included 53 PIP joint arthrodeses (12 patients with flexion contractures of more than 90 degrees and severe dorsal ulcers; postoperative healing of ulcers in every case), 19 MCP capsulotomies, 4 metacarpal head resections (in four patients; results were disappointing), 13 debulking excisions of calcinotic areas (seven patients; subjective improvement in pain and function without healing problems), 5 digital sympathectomies (in five patients symptoms improved, but one later required digital amputation) and 4 successful carpal tunnel releases. In another series of 20 replacement arthroplasties of the PIP joints in six patients over a 9-year period, significant improvement was reported in hand function and appearance in five (one died from diffuse sclerosis), with few complications (no infections, four delayed healing, two prosthesis removals). In a series of 59 patients seen during a 10-year period, Gahhos and colleagues unexpectedly found that conservative fingertip amputations for nonhealing ulcers constituted the treatment of choice to eradicate ulcers, reduce pain, and restore useful hand function. In this series, intraarterial reserpine (12 patients), cervical sympathectomy (8), debridement of ulcers (7), and split-thickness grafts (4) usually resulted in short-term pain relief but failed to promote healing or prevent new ulcer formation. In summary, although these limited studies suggest that scleroderma hand surgery can be successful, the knowledge that severe microvascular disease is central to the pathology should guide the physician toward conservative therapeutic measures, except in extreme situations.

Fibromyalgia
Elizabeth H. Field

DEFINITION

Fibromyalgia is a clinical syndrome characterized by diffuse, vague pain, extreme fatigue, stiffness, painful tender points, and sleep disturbance. The term *fibrositis* should be avoided because there is no evidence of an inflammatory component to this disorder. Fibromyalgia was previously classified as *primary* if there is no associated underlying disease and *secondary* if the fibromyalgia symptoms occur in patients with preexisting rheumatologic or nonrheumatologic disorders. Because the causes of both primary and secondary fibromyalgia are usually the same (ie, a disorder in restorative stage 4 sleep), this distinction between primary and secondary no longer exists for diagnostic purposes. The American College of Rheumatology defined two criteria for diagnosing fibromyalgia in 1990: (1) a history of widespread pain and (2) pain in at least 11 of 18 tender point sites on digital palpation with a force of 4 kg (Fig. 5-16).

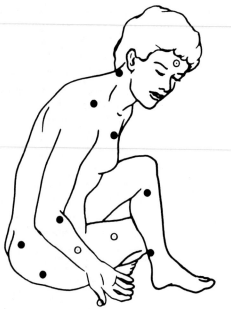

FIGURE 5-16. Eight of the most frequent areas for tender points (*closed circles*) and control areas (*open circles*). Tender points elicit pain directly under the area palpated. The trigger points of myofascial pain syndromes elicit pain away from the area palpated. Pain in 11 of 18 tender-point sites is one of two criteria proposed to diagnose fibromyalgia. *Tender points:* insertion of nuchal muscles into occiput; upper trapezius (midportion); pectoralis muscle just lateral to second costochondral junction; 2 cm below lateral epicondyle; upper gluteal area; 2 cm posterior to greater trochanter; medial knee in area of anserine bursa; junction of gastrocnemius and Achilles tendon. *Control points:* middle of forehead; volar aspect of midforearm; thumbnail; muscles of anterior thigh.

CLINICAL FEATURES

Symptoms

The typical fibromyalgia patient complains of hurting all over or in the shoulder girdle or thighs. Often, patients cannot pinpoint exact locations for their pain, and they describe their pain by rubbing or squeezing whole extremities. The pain can be severe and migratory, affecting both joints and muscles. Numbness and tingling in the extremities may be mistaken for a nerve entrapment syndrome. Patients feel worst in the morning, and fatigue is a major component of the disorder. Frequently, after the interview, the physician is left with a vague history and description of the symptoms but a clear impression that the patient is disabled by the symptoms.

Curiously, patients do not volunteer symptoms of a sleep disorder. Rather, they relate the feeling of chronic tiredness and history of dozing off during the day. On careful questioning, however, patients almost uniformly report frequent waking at night, which may have been their sleep pattern for many years. In patients in whom fibromyalgia is suspected, a detailed history of the sleep pattern is essential in establishing the diagnosis and in helping to educate the patient about this disorder.

Controversy exists about whether patients with fibromyalgia have underlying psychological disorders, but there is consensus that they are perfectionistic and body-aware. Some studies suggest increased depression, hypochondriasis, and neurotic or depressed tendencies in fibromyalgia patients, but others show normal psychological profiles. There is no convincing evidence that fibromyalgia patients as a group are different psychologically from other patients with chronic pain.

Patients commonly feel tense and have difficulty relaxing. They appear hyperirritable because their pain is frequently aggravated by physical and psychological stimuli, such as cold, noise, and stress. An association of fibromyalgia symptoms by occupations that involve prolonged tonic contraction of muscles (orchestra conductors, bus drivers, keyboard operators) is noted. The incidence of migraines and irritable bowel syndrome is increased.

Signs

The most characteristic finding is the presence of tender points. Pressure from the examiner's thumb on these areas elicits exquisite tenderness, with or without palpable "knots" representing local muscle spasm. The patient is usually unaware of these areas and expresses surprise when the physician can so easily find these tender spots. Patients with fibromyalgia have a decreased pain threshold for pressure over these specific areas (see Fig. 5-16). The presence of tender points is diagnostically useful and constitutes one of the criteria to diagnose fibromyalgia if patients have at least 11 painful tender points. Tender points are also found in other disorders, for example, regional pain syndromes (myofascial pain syndromes). In the latter disorder, the tender points are correctly termed *trigger points,* since pressure of a trigger point causes referred pain to a nearby regional area. In contrast, the tender points of fibromyalgia elicit pain in the local area. This distinction is important, since trigger points may respond to local injection with 1% procaine hydrochloride, but tender points usually do not.

Examination of the extremities reveals increased

muscle tone, and the patient has difficulty relaxing the muscles. There may be objective "breakaway" weakness related to pain. Hyperemia of the skin over palpated areas is rarely noted. Patients sometimes exhibit a livedo reticularis rash (lacy superficial purplish discoloration). Notably, there is absence of physical findings to suggest inflammation, such as swollen, red, or warm joints. In fact, palpation of joints rarely elicits pain. The neurologic examination is normal. A useful test is the skinfold roll test. The examiner faces the patient's back and grasps the skin with the thumb and second finger at about the T12 level just lateral to the spine. The skinfold is gradually rolled upward. In normal people, this maneuver does not produce pain. In patients with fibromyalgia, this maneuver causes severe pain on minimal manipulation of the skin.

Incidence

Fibromyalgia commonly affects middle-aged women, but it can affect either gender at any age. The disorder is widespread. As many as 2% of all primary care patients and 15% of all rheumatology clinic patients may present with fibromyalgia, making it the third most common rheumatic disorder, behind osteoarthritis and RA.

PATHOLOGIC FEATURES AND PATHOGENESIS

The most prominent physiologic abnormality identified in fibromyalgia is the abnormal sleep pattern that occurs during stage 4 sleep. The normal electroencephalogram delta waves of stage 4 sleep are interrupted by alpha waves. Similar changes in electroencephalogram patterns can be induced in normal subjects that are deprived of non-REM sleep. These subjects show signs and symptoms of fibromyalgia after such deprivation. This observation has led to the theory that in primary fibromyalgia, there is internal disruption of stage 4 sleep.

Biopsy results in fibromyalgia are controversial, but enough abnormalities were reported to warrant further study. Type II muscle fiber atrophy, motheaten appearance of type I fibers, and ragged red fibers were reported on muscle biopsy, and muscle necrosis was reported on electron microscopy. These changes suggest subclinical injury to muscle, which is thought to be caused by chronic muscle tension or chronic hypoxia. The muscles at the tender points show decreased oxygenation and evidence of abnormal energy metabolism. As yet, none of these findings occurs consistently enough to be useful as a diagnostic test.

RADIOLOGIC AND LABORATORY FEATURES

No radiographic findings of fibromyalgia have been established, and laboratory tests (including the complete blood count and ESR) are characteristically normal. Thyroid function and glucose studies should be performed because hypothyroidism and early diabetes mellitus can mimic fibromyalgia. Once the diagnosis of fibromyalgia is made, extensive workup need not be performed. Other laboratory studies (such as RF and ANA) should be obtained only if the history and physical examination suggest an underlying inflammatory disorder.

In summary, the features that suggest a diagnosis of fibromyalgia are strictly clinical: (1) a history of widespread pain, (2) sleep disturbance, (3) multiple tender points on physical examination, and (4) the absence of clinical or laboratory signs of inflammation. Fibromyalgia does not appear to be a psychosomatic disorder and should be treated with appropriate medical management.

MEDICAL MANAGEMENT

Management of the fibromyalgia patient can be challenging and rewarding. A multifaceted approach must be used because no single modality is effective in long-term use. Education, pharmacotherapy, exercise, relaxation, and patient participation are all important in the treatment of fibromyalgia and need to be equally stressed. The key to successful treatment is to involve the patient in the treatment plan.

Education

Education is the first step. Frequently, patients have seen numerous physicians in the past and have been told their symptoms are psychosomatic. Patients appreciate hearing physicians explain how sleep deprivation can cause and reinforce their symptoms. Describing the sleep deprivation–low pain threshold–more sleep deprivation cycle helps patients understand their condition. The therapeutic goal is then to interrupt these cycles that perpetuate the symptoms. Patients need to set realistic goals for themselves and should be encouraged to focus on small improvements over monthly intervals to avoid treatment dropout. Their fibromyalgia symptoms usually developed over years; therefore, it takes time to reverse the symptoms.

Pharmacotherapy

The importance of reestablishing normal sleep patterns should be stressed as the main focus of therapy. Tricyclics given at bedtime have been shown to benefit fibromyalgia symptoms. Amitriptyline, desipramine, doxepin, and imipramine have all been used at an initial dosage of 10 to 75 mg 1 to 2 hours before bedtime. The dosage can be increased by 25 mg every 3 to 7 days in the absence of significant side effects, such as daytime drowsiness, to a maximal dosage, as tolerated. Amitriptyline is the most commonly used and most extensively studied drug, because it decreases the α-wave intrusion in the δ waves in stage 4 sleep. Patients typically require lower doses than are used to obtain the antidepressant affect and can respond to as little as 10 mg each night, but patients may require up to 100 mg each night. The benefit occurs quickly, before the usual antidepressive effect can take place. Patients should be told that tricyclics are given to improve sleep patterns and not for depression, lest they resent receiving an antidepressant when they are not depressed. Treatment should continue for 6 months or longer. After patients demonstrate improvement, therapy can be gradually withdrawn. Neither steroids nor NSAIDs benefit symptoms of fibromyalgia, but despite increasing evidence against NSAIDs, many physicians still use these agents. Because of the potential toxicity of NSAIDs and lack of benefit, these drugs should *not* be given to treat fibromyalgia. Because of recent evidence that fibromyalgia involves a serotonin deficiency, the new serotonin reuptake inhibitors may benefit patients, and use of these agents is being explored experimentally.

Physical Therapy

Physical therapy should be geared toward a conditioning exercise program, since range-of-motion and stretching exercises do not benefit symptoms. Aerobic exercises, such as swimming, biking, running, or walking, are aimed at increasing cardiovascular work, which improves non-REM stage 4 sleep. Swimming is the exercise of choice because of the added relaxing effect of water on muscles. Exercises should be emphasized as much as pharmacotherapy and performed at least three times a week. TENS may relieve pain when applied to a tender point, but relief is usually transient unless used repeatedly, and use of a TENS unit is impractical for many of the patients with widespread pain. Relaxation exercises are also part of physical therapy. Patients can be taught relaxation techniques and should practice these three times a day. A realistic goal is for the patient to be able to relax muscles on command. Teaching biofeedback may be helpful in patients who have difficulty relaxing. Since much of the success of treatment involves patient participation and high motivation, it is sometimes useful to have patients keep diaries or mark calendars whenever they perform relaxation exercises or physical exercises. This is particularly helpful when the patient is first beginning the treatment protocol, before habits develop or benefits are noted. A follow-up evaluation in 4 to 8 weeks to check the patient's calendar reinforces patient motivation.

Patients with fibromyalgia and other associated rheumatic diseases require a similar treatment program. Since nighttime pain is frequently the cause of the abnormal sleep pattern, adding extra analgesic at night in osteoarthritis or RA patients improves pain control and avoids development of an abnormal sleep cycle, which may precipitate fibromyalgia.

Annotated Bibliography

The Normal Synovium

Schumacher HR. Synovial fluid analysis. In: Kelley WN, Harris ED Jr, Ruddy S, Sledge CB, eds. Textbook of rheumatology, ed 2. Philadelphia, WB Saunders, 1985:561.
This chapter offers a concise but thorough description of diagnostic information to be gained from synovial fluid analysis in rheumatic disease patients.

Steinbrocker O, Neustadt DH. Aspiration and injection therapy in arthritis and musculoskeletal disorders. Hagerstown, MD, Harper & Row, 1972.
This is a brief booklet with informative diagrams and photographs that illustrate the recommended technique for aspiration of joints and tendon sheaths.

Degenerative Joint Disease

Brandt KD. Osteoarthritis. Clin Geriatr Med 1988;4:279.
This article provides a comprehensive discussion of the macromolecular composition and functions of articular cartilage. Brandt compares the biochemical features of articular cartilage in aging versus osteoarthritis and discusses the role of aging in the pathogenesis of osteoarthritis.

Bland JH, Cooper SM. Osteoarthritis: a review of the cell biology involved and evidence for reversibility. Management rationally

related to known genesis and pathophysiology. Semin Arthritis Rheum 1984;14:106.
This is an interesting, albeit controversial, discussion on the pathogenesis and prognosis of osteoarthritis. The authors present experimental data that disputes the concept that osteoarthritis is a result of normal aging and challenges the conventional thinking that osteoarthritis is a nonreversible process. The authors' proposed use of steroids in managing osteoarthritis is not generally accepted.

Docken WP. Clinical features and medical management of osteoarthritis at the hand and wrist. Hand Clin 1987;3:337.
A general review of osteoarthritis of the hands, this article includes comments on the epidemiology, different classifications, and the approach to the differential diagnosis. The review details a practical, nonsurgical approach to patients with hand osteoarthritis, including medical management with nonsteroidal antiinflammatory agents. The treatment approach can be applied to patients with osteoarthritis of other joints as well.

Stefanich RJ. Intraarticular corticosteroids in treatment of osteoarthritis. Orthop Rev 1986;15:65.
This is one of the few reviews of the role that intraarticular steroids play in management of osteoarthritis. This article presents a historical overview of how intraarticular steroid use developed and details past clinical experience. The author concludes that this treatment has a limited place in the management of osteoarthritis. This article also presents an extensive review of potential side effects from intraarticular steroid injection.

Rheumatoid Arthritis

Hastings DE, Evans JA. Rheumatoid wrist deformities and their relationship to ulnar drift. J Bone Joint Surg 1975;57A:930.
This article is an observation of important interrelations among deformities in the wrist and hand.

Pincus T, Callahan LF, Sale WG, Brooks AL, Payne LE, Vaughn WK. Severe functional declines, work disability and increased mortality in 75 RA patients studies over 9 years. Arthritis Rheum 1984;27:864.
The authors present evidence for the progressive and severe nature of rheumatoid disease in many patients.

Stastny P. Association of the B-cell alloantigen DRw4 with rheumatoid arthritis. N Engl J Med 1978;298:869.
In this article, evidence is presented for an association between an HLA-D locus antigen and the development and severity of rheumatoid arthritis.

Winfield J, Young A, Williams P, Corbett M. Prospective study of the radiologic changes in hands, feet and cervical spine in adult rheumatoid disease. Ann Rheum Dis 1983;42:613.
The authors demonstrate correlation severity of cervical spine disease and peripheral joint disease.

Systemic Lupus Erythematosus and Immune Complex Disease

Gladman DD. Prognosis of systemic lupus erythematosus and factors that affect it. Curr Opin Rheumatol 1990;2:694.
SLE is a disease with variable presenting symptoms and varying severity. The natural history of SLE may also be influenced by other factors (such as hormones). This brief review summarizes the clinical manifestations commonly seen in lupus and briefly discusses other factors known to influence disease expression.

Klippel JH, Gerber LH, Pollack L, Decker JL. Avascular necrosis in systemic lupus erythematosus. Am J Med 1979;67:86.
The association of avascular necrosis of bone with SLE is longstanding. This study details the incidence and prevalence of avascular necrosis in lupus patients during a 10-year period. When skeletal surveys were used for diagnoses, over half of the patients exhibited evidence of avascular necrosis during the 10-year period of observation. Not all patients were symptomatic. The patients in this study had more severe lupus and received corticosteroid treatment. The incidence of avascular necrosis may well be lower in patients with less severe disease.

Russel AS, Percy JS, Rigal WM, Wilson GL. Deforming arthropathy in systemic lupus erythematosus. Ann Rheum Dis 1974;33:204.
Patients with SLE frequently have arthralgias and nondeforming arthritis, and certain patients with lupus may have a deforming arthritis (frequently affecting the hands). Unlike RA, the hand deformities in SLE arthritis are usually reducible.

Tan EM, Cohen AJ, Fries J, et al. Revised criteria for the classification of systemic lupus erythematosus. Arthritis Rheum 1982;25:1271.
This paper details the 10 diagnostic criteria used in the classification of patients with system lupus erythematosus. These criteria are used for classification purposes and not for establishing the diagnosis of lupus in a clinical setting. Nonetheless, a patient who presents with four of the criteria is likely to have SLE.

Enthesopathies

Arnett FC. Seronegative spondyloarthropathies. Bull Rheum Dis 1987;37:1.
This review provides a good overview of AS, Reiter's syndrome, and psoriatic arthritis.

Calin A. HLA-B27 in 1982: reappraisal of a clinical test. Ann Intern Med 1982;96:114.
The author reviews the clinical utility of B27 testing.

Fox R, Calin A, Gerber RC, Gibson D. The chronicity of symptoms and disability in Reiter's syndrome: an analysis of 131 consecutive patients. Ann Intern Med 1979;91:190.
A significant percentage of patients with reactive arthritis have chronic disability associated with the disease.

Gladman DD. Psoriatic arthritis: recent advances in pathogenesis and treatment. Rheum Dis Clin North Am 1992;18:247.
This article presents a review of the clinical characteristics of psoriatic arthritis and the current therapeutic options.

Keat A. Reiter's syndrome and reactive arthritis in perspective. N Engl J Med 1983;309:1606.
This review describes the types of infections that may precede arthritis and argues for the utility of the concept of reactive arthritis, which includes Reiter syndrome.

Juvenile Rheumatoid Arthritis

Cassidy JT, Levinson JE, Brewer EJ. The development of classification criteria for children with juvenile rheumatoid arthritis. Bull Rheum Dis 1989;38:1.
The article presents a review of the American College of Rheumatology classification criteria.

Cassidy JT, Petty RE. Textbook of pediatric rheumatology, ed 2. New York, Churchill Livingstone, 1990.
This is an excellent comprehensive general reference.

Swann M. Modern trends in the surgical management of juvenile chronic arthritis. In: Woo P, White PH, Ansell BM, eds. Pediatric rheumatology update. Oxford University Press, 1990.
The authors provide an overview of surgical management of JRA.

Wallace CA, Levinson JE. Juvenile rheumatoid arthritis: outcome and treatment for the 1990s. Rheum Dis Clin North Am 1991;17:971.
The authors present an overview of controversies in the treatment and management of more complex cases of JRA. (This entire volume is devoted to pediatric rheumatology.)

Infectious Arthritis

Benach JL, Bosler EM, eds. Lyme disease and related disorders. Ann NY Acad Sci 1989.
The result of an international conference on Lyme disease and related disorders held by the New York Academy of Sciences and the State of New York Department of Health on September 14–16, 1987, in New York City, this monograph contains papers reviewing the clinical manifestations, pathology, microbiology, antibody response, ecology, veterinary aspects, and treatment of Lyme disease.

Espinoza LR. Infectious arthritis. Rheum Dis Clin North Am 1993.
This timely review of infectious arthritis has chapters on soft tissue infections, nongonococcal bacterial arthritis, gonococcal arthritis, syphilitic arthritis and osteitis, acute rheumatic fever, Chlamydia-induced reactive arthritis, Lyme disease, fungal arthritis, musculoskeletal syndromes of parasitic infection, parvovirus B19 arthritis, HIV-induced arthritis, and rheumatic manifestations of human leukemia virus infection.

Espinoza LR, Goldenberg DL, Arnett FC, Alarcon GS, eds. Infections in the rheumatic diseases. New York, Grune & Stratton, 1988.
This standard text in infectious arthritis contains reviews on the rheumatic manifestations of infection by specific microbial agents. Although some sections may be dated, this remains the standard reference for arthritis caused by specific etiologic agents.

Naides SJ. Parvoviruses. In: Specter s, Lancz G, eds. Clinical virology manual, ed 2. New York, Elsevier, 1992:547.
This chapter presents a comprehensive review of the clinical manifestations of parvovirus B19 infection and a basic review of B19 virology and diagnostic modalities.

Resnick D, Niwayama G. Diagnosis of bone and joint disorders, vol 4. Philadelphia, WB Saunders, 1988.
This standard reference in bone and joint radiology was written by a radiologist and a pathologist. The text is notable for its lucid textual descriptions, extensive radiographic illustrations, and clinicopathologic correlation. This remains an excellent reference for the radiographic manifestation of infectious arthritis.

Schumacher HR, Klippel JH, Koopman W. Primer on the rheumatic diseases, ed 10. Atlanta, Arthritis Foundation, 1993.
This inexpensive text was recently updated and remains a must for the personal library of any physician who cares for patients with rheumatic or orthopaedic disease. The text includes succinct reviews on bacterial, viral, fungal, and reactive arthritides. A separate chapter on Lyme disease is included.

Shope RE. Alphaviruses. In: Fields BN, Knipe DM, Chanock RM, et al. Virology, ed 2. New York, Raven Press, 1990:713.
This chapter in the premier text in virology describes a clinically significant group of arthropod-borne viruses responsible for epidemics of febrile arthritis in Africa, Asia, Europe, and Latin America. Experience in the United States with emerging viruses, previously seen only in developing nations, and the ever-shortening distances in the global village underscore the need for clinicians to be aware of these entities.

Crystal-Induced Arthritis

Antonio J, Reginato MD. Calcium oxalate and other crystals or particles associated with arthritis. In: McCarty DJ, Koopman WJ, eds. Arthritis and allied conditions, ed 12. Philadelphia, Lea & Febiger, 1993:1873.
An exhaustive catalog of the less common particles that cause arthritis.

Daniel G, Baker MD, Schumacher HR Jr. Acute monoarthritis. N Engl J Med 1993;329:1013.
A compact up-to-date review of the clinical paradigm for which crystal-induced arthritis is the prototype.

Lawrence M, Ryan MD, Daniel J, McCarty MD. Calcium pyrophosphate crystal deposition disease: pseudogout, acute chondrocalcinosis. In: McCarty DJ, Koopman WJ, eds. Arthritis and allied conditions, ed 12. Philadelphia, Lea & Febiger, 1993:1835.
This is the definitive discussion of CPPD crystal deposition disease.

Paul B, Halverson MD, Daniel J, McCarty MD. Basic calcium phosphate (apatite, octacalcium phosphate, tricalcium phosphate) crystal deposition diseases. In: McCarty DJ, Koopman WJ, eds. Arthritis and allied conditions, ed 12. Philadelphia, Lea & Febiger, 1993:1857.
This chapter presents a detailed discussion of the many manifestations of calcium phosphate crystal deposition in human tissues.

Kelley WN, Schumacher HR Jr. Gout. In: Kelly WN, Harris ED Jr, Ruddy S, Sledge CB, eds. Textbook of rheumatology, ed 4. Philadelphia, WB Saunders, 1993:1291.
This chapter provides a thorough review of gout and its management.

Synovial Chondromatosis

Dolan EA. Synovial chondromatosis of the TMJ diagnosed by magnetic resonance imaging: report of a case. J Oral Maxillofac Surg 1989;47:411.
This case study is the account of a patient with extracapsular extension diagnosed by MRI.

Dorfman H, et al. Arthroscopic treatment of synovial chondromatosis of the knee. Arthroscopy 1989;5:48.
This article reports on 39 cases with an average follow-up of 3.5 years.

Jaffe HL. Tumor and tumorous conditions of the bones and joints. London, Henry Kimpton, 1958.
This is the classic description within a text.

Maurice H, Crone M, Watt I. Synovial chondromatosis. J Bone Joint Surg 1988:70B:807.
This is a 53-case comparison of radiographic and pathologic features.

Milgram JW. Synovial osteochondromatosis: a histologic study of 30 cases. J Bone Joint Surg 1977;59A:792.
This articles provides a correlation of symptoms, radiographic findings, and histopathology.

Milgram JW. Synovial osteochondromatosis in the subacromial bursa. Clin Orthop 1988;236:154.
This is a case report of true bursal osteochondromatosis.

Murphy EP, et al. Auricular synovial chondromatosis. J Bone Joint Surg 1962;44A:77.
This is a Mayo Clinic review of 32 surgically treated cases with some follow-up.

Perry BE, et al. Synovial chondromatosis with malignant degeneration to chondrosarcoma: report of a case. J Bone Joint Surg 1988;70A:1259.
This is a single case report with histology.

Raibley SO. Villonodular synovitis with synovial chondromatosis. Oral Surg 1977;44:279.
This is a report of a TMJ lesion originally thought to be a malignant parotid tumor.

Schian A. Diabetes and synovial chondromatosis. Diabetes Metab 1976;2:183.
This article explores associations between the two disorders.

Villonodular Synovitis

Byers P, Cotton R, Deacon O. The diagnosis and treatment of pigmented villonodular synovitis. J Bone Joint Surg 1968;50B:290.
This article presents a good historical review of 126 British cases.

Flandry F. Roentgenographic findings in pigmented villonodular synovitis of the knee. Clin Orthop 1989;247:208.
Twenty-nine cases are reviewed, with extensive radiographic correlation to other radiographic studies. Clinical and histopathologic associations are also described.

Gitelis S. The treatment of pigmented villonodular synovitis of the hip. Clin Orthop 1989;239:154.
This article presents a review of 64 cases of pigmented villonodular synovitis of the hip with an example of one case. Some treatment comparison is given.

Goldman, Amy B. Pigmented villonodular synovitis. Radiol Clin North Am 1988;26:1327.
The author presents a radiology-slanted review of diagnosis and differential diagnosis of pigment villonodular synovitis. The article includes good radiographs.

Jaffe HL. Tumors and tumorous conditions of the bones and joints. Philadelphia, Lea & Febiger, 1958:532.
This text provides a classic description of bone and joint tumors.

Jeluneh JS. Imaging of pigmented villonodular synovitis with emphasis on MR imaging. AJR 1989;152:337.
The author describes a seven-patient study of diffuse pigmented villonodular synovitis and provides extensive magnetic resonance images.

Kazuhiro U. Lipid microspherules in synovial fluid of patients with pigmented villonodular synovitis. Arthritis Rheum 1988;31:1442.
This article describes synovial fluid analysis in two cases of pigmented villonodular synovitis.

Kelly J, Rao AS. Pigmented villonodular synovitis (giant cell tumor of tendon sheath and synovial membrane): a review of eighty-one cases. J Bone Joint Surg 1984;66A:76.
A comparison of clinical radiologic and histopathologic features is given, classified by anatomic site. Many good radiographs are included.

Kransdorf MJ. Soft tissue masses: diagnosis using MR imaging. AJR 1939;153:541.
This is a 96-case comparison (6 cases of pigmented villonodular synovitis) of magnetic resonance images with pathologic diagnosis.

Mandelbaum BR. The use of MRI to assist in diagnosis of pigmented villonodular synovitis of the knee joint. Clin Orthop 1988;231:135.
The author describes a single case of MRI diagnosis of pigmented villonodular synovitis.

Myers BW. Pigmented villonodular synovitis and tenosynovitis: a clinical epidemiologic study of 166 cases and literature review. Medicine 1980;59:223.
This is the largest review article that correlates diseases features.

Schwartz HS. Pigmented villonodular synovitis. Clin Orthop 1989;247:243.
This is a retrospective review of 99 patients with an average 13.5-year follow-up. Prognostic indicators were advanced regarding recurrence.

Wendt RG. Polyarticular pigmented villonodular synovitis in children: evidence for a genetic contribution. J Rheumatol 1986;13:921.
The author describes pigmented villonodular synovitis in a single family with multiple lentigines syndrome.

Systemic Sclerosis

Blocka KL, et al. The arthropathy of advanced progressive systemic sclerosis: a radiographic survey. Arthritis Rheum 1981;24:874.
Intrinsic joint disease in scleroderma is generally not well appreciated. In this longitudinal survey of radiographic joint findings, however, significant abnormalities are reported, including marginal erosions and previously undescribed dorsal erosions.

Gahhos F, et al. Management of scleroderma finger ulcers. J Hand Surg 1984;9A:320.
The nonsurgical treatment of scleroderma fingers ulcers is well established, although with variable success. In this retrospective review, the authors surprisingly conclude that conservative finger amputations constitute the treatment of choice for nonhealing ulcers. The extremely limited role of surgery, however, must still clearly be emphasized in this microscopic disorder.

Jones NF, et al. Surgery for scleroderma of the hand. J Hand Surg 1987;12A:391.
With the limited role of hand surgery infrequently documented, this is a noteworthy review. Surprisingly, poor wound healing is not reported in this cohort but must remain of significant potential concern in a disease with pivotal microvascular involvement. Conservative measures for digital gangrene, allowing autoamputation, still remains the treatment of choice in most patients.

Medsger TA. Scleroderma (systemic sclerosis), localized forms of scleroderma and calcinosis. In: McCarty DJ, ed. Arthritis and allied conditions—or a textbook of rheumatology, ed 12. 1993:1253.
This is an excellent, comprehensive, updated text for general reference on all aspects of scleroderma.

Owens GR, Follansbee WP. Cardiopulmonary manifestations of systemic sclerosis. Chest 1987;91:118.
This is an outstanding review of cardiac and pulmonary involvement in scleroderma, including pathogenesis, newer investigative tools, and therapeutic strategies.

Steen VD, et al. Outcome of renal crisis in systemic sclerosis: relation to availability of angiotensin converting enzyme (ACE) inhibitors. Ann Intern Med 1990;113:352.
This notable prospective review clearly highlights the dramatically improved survival of patients with SRC since the introduction of ACE inhibitor therapy in 1979.

Fibromyalgia

Carette S, McCain GA, Bell DA, Fam AG. Evaluation of amitriptyline in primary fibrositis: a double-blind, placebo-controlled study. Arthritis Rheum 1986;29:655.
This article reports the first double-blind, placebo-controlled study of the effectiveness of amitriptyline for treating fibromyalgia. Although patients showed improvement, many of the outcome measures were subjective, and no change was seen in the amount of pain as measured by dolorimeter. Subsequent studies from other groups substantiated the benefit of tricyclics in treating fibromyalgia.

Duna GF, Wilke WS. Diagnosis, etiology, and therapy of fibromyalgia. Comprehens Ther 1993;19:60.
This is a brief, up-to-date review of the new criteria for fibromyalgia. The authors discuss frequent differential diagnostic pitfalls and the two recent pathogenesis theories, serotonin deficiency and a vascular deformity.

Moldofsky H, Scarisbrick P, England R, Smythe H. Musculoskeletal symptoms and non-REM sleep disturbance in patients with "fibrositis syndrome" and healthy subjects. Psychosom Med 1975;37:341.
This classic study describes the stage 4 sleep abnormality in fibromyalgia patients, which is alpha wave intrusion during stage 4 NREM sleep.

Wolfe F, Smythe HA, Yunus MB, et al. The American College of Rheumatology 1990 criteria for the classification of fibromyalgia: report of the Multicenter Criteria Committee. Arthritis Rheum 1990;33:160.
This article reviews different criteria and proposes standard criteria to diagnose fibromyalgia. It underscores the difficulties one encounters in diagnosing these patients.

Turek's Orthopaedics: Principles and Their Application, Fifth Edition,
edited by Stuart L. Weinstein and Joseph A. Buckwalter.
J.B. Lippincott Company, Philadelphia, © 1994.

6

Frederick R. Dietz

Neuromuscular Diseases

CEREBRAL PALSY
  Definition
  Clinical Features
  Natural History
  Evaluation
  Orthopaedic Treatment
  Nonorthopaedic
    Treatment
MYELOMENINGOCELE
  Epidemiology
  Etiology and Diagnosis
  Initial Management
  Orthopaedic
    Management at
    Walking Age and
    After
  Final Comments

ARTHROGRYPOSIS
  MULTIPLEX
  CONGENITA
  Etiology
  Initial Management
  Later Management
MUSCULAR
  DYSTROPHIES
  Definition
  Duchenne and Becker
    Muscular Dystrophy
  Limb-Girdle Muscular
    Dystrophy
  Fascioscapulohumeral
    Dystrophy
  Myotonic Muscular
    Dystrophy
  Spinal Muscular
    Dystrophy

FRIEDREICH ATAXIA
HEREDITARY MOTOR
  SENSORY
  NEUROPATHIES
SYRINGOMYELIA

CEREBRAL PALSY

Definition

Cerebral palsy is a disorder of motion or posture resulting from a fixed, nonprogressive lesion of the immature brain. A movement disorder is the sine qua non of this syndrome that has multiple etiologies (eg, congenital brain malformations, anoxia, and cerebral vascular accident). Many associated disorders occur such as seizures, ocular disturbances, and mental retardation. Variability in severity is found from resolution of motor signs in early life to profound disability requiring total body care.

The movement disorder is characterized by the amount of body involvement and by whether the movement disorder is spastic (Table 6-1). Spasticity of muscle

213

TABLE 6-1.
Cerebral Palsy

GEOGRAPHIC PATTERN

Hemiplegia: Ipsilateral arm and leg involved

Diplegia: Legs involved much more than arms

Quadriplegia: All four limbs involved

MOVEMENT DISORDER

Spasticity: Hyperreflexia, increased muscle tone of
clasp-knife type

Dyskinesia

Athetosis: Slow writhing motions, especially of
wrist and fingers

Chorea: Jerky involuntary movements, more
abrupt than athetosis

Dystonia: Slow rhythmic movements of the trunk and limbs

Hypotonia: Decreased muscle tone

Ataxia: Balance problems and hypotonic muscles

is defined clinically by increased tone of the clasp-knife type, hyperreflexia, sustained clonus, and extensor plantar reflex (Babinski sign). Pathologically, spasticity is caused by injury to the motor cortex or pyramidal tract. Spastic patients are far more prone to fixed muscle contractures than nonspastics. Dyskinetic motions are all increased with voluntary activity, stress, and heightened emotional state. Pathologically, dyskinesias result from injury to extrapyramidal nuclei and tracts, usually those associated with the basal ganglia. Ataxia is present in 1% or less of cerebral palsy patients and is caused by cerebellar injury. Hypotonia is usually a transitory phase in early infancy before a spastic motor pattern becomes apparent. Occasionally, hypotonia may persist as the major motor pattern. Overall, 60% to 70% of cerebral palsy patients have spasticity and 20% to 30% have a mixture of spasticity and dyskinesia, usually athetosis.

Although the brain lesion in cerebral palsy is, by definition, nonprogressive as distinguished from degenerative central nervous system (CNS) disease or CNS tumors, the peripheral manifestation may vary as the child grows and the brain matures. In many mild cases, the motor signs disappear in childhood; hypotonic infants may become spastic; spasticity occasionally evolves into dyskinesia. These changes in movement pattern are attributed to maturation of injured and uninjured brain, or to aberrant maturation of injured areas.

Although cerebral palsy is defined by the presence of a movement disorder, it is important to remember that patients' functional abilities are more determined by intelligence than motor disability.

Epidemiology and Etiology

By age 7 years, 2.3 of 1000 children are found to have cerebral palsy. The major predictors of cerebral palsy are maternal mental retardation, low birthweight, non-CNS fetal malformation, and breech presentation. Several studies have confirmed that neonatal asphyxia accounts for less than 10% of all cerebral palsy. Many children with perinatal hypoxic insults have major organ malformations or other intrinsic defects that predisposed them to such perinatal insults. Although some events and conditions associated with cerebral palsy have been identified, fully two thirds of children with cerebral palsy have no known risk factors. Furthermore, of the 1% of pregnancies at highest risk, only 7% result in a child with cerebral palsy. The implication of these data is that no single preventable cause of cerebral palsy exists; therefore, no specific intervention is likely to significantly reduce the incidence.

Clinical Features

The age and complaints at presentation are variable and depend on the severity of involvement of the child.

Quadriplegia

Children with total body involvement are usually diagnosed neonatally. These babies are apathetic or irritable and often have failure to thrive. Neonatal seizures may occur. Often the children are hypotonic initially but quickly develop signs of spasticity. Over 90% of these children have mental retardation, with most of the retardation being profound. Many children have problems with feeding, aspiration, recurrent pneumonia, and vision. Few of these patients become independent ambulators.

Diplegia

These children usually present neonatally with abnormally low tone and decreased spontaneous movement associated with overactive deep tendon reflexes. Diplegia has been associated with prematurity, but epidemiologic studies have not demonstrated a definite relation between any of the clinical subtypes (quadriplegia versus diplegia versus hemiplegia) and specific predisposing factors. Children with milder degrees of diplegia often present because of delayed motor milestones, especially crawling and walking. Most of these children become ambulators though often dependent on crutches or walker (Fig.

6-1). About 60% of diplegics have normal intelligence (IQ greater than 80). The others have mild to moderate retardation.

Hemiparesis

Children with hemiparesis present in infancy with poor use of one arm and decreased movement of one leg if the hemiplegia is dense (Fig. 6-2). Mild hemiplegics are often not identified until after walking age when a persistent gait asymmetry prompts evaluation. Motor milestones are met at the appropriate time. Seventy percent of hemiplegic children have normal intelligence. The remainder have mild retardation. These children may have seizures and specific learning disabilities. Limb growth asymmetry can result in clinically significant leg length discrepancy.

Dyskinesias

Children with movement disorders are apathetic, hypotonic neonates. During a period of months, the involuntary movements become more obvious. These

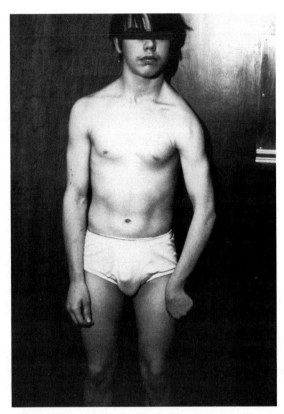

FIGURE 6-2. Fourteen-year-old boy with spastic hemiplegia showing typical arm posture.

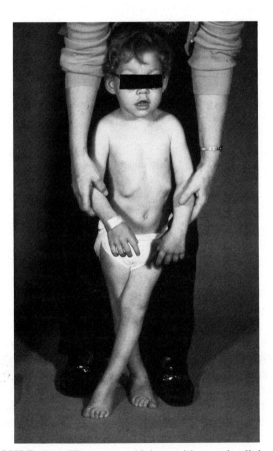

FIGURE 6-1. Three-year-old boy with spastic diplegia. Scissoring and ankle equinus are apparent.

children are severely limited in motor skills and usually need communication aids despite often normal intelligence.

Natural History

Although the syndrome of cerebral palsy is defined and classified by the presence and type of movement disorder, it is intellectual function that most determines level of function, independence, and even survival. Up to half of profoundly retarded children do not survive more than 10 years, whereas children with mild to moderate retardation or normal intelligence can expect normal life-spans regardless of severity of motor involvement.

Resolution of cerebral palsy is common in mild cases diagnosed in infancy. More than two thirds of all children with cerebral palsy classified as mild at 1 year of age resolve their motor deficit by age 7. Even some moderately involved children (especially diplegics) recover their motor function. Many of these children, however, continue to have problems with mental retardation, hyperactivity or visual abnormalities.

Evaluation

The musculoskeletal evaluation of the child with cerebral palsy, regardless of severity, has three major facets: assessment of hip stability, assessment of spinal alignment, and assessment of abnormal muscle activity and contracture that interfere with function.

Assessment of hips and spine is relatively straightforward. The forward-bend test performed standing or sitting, if necessary, suggests the need for spine radiographs. Radiographs should be obtained with the pelvis leveled if possible. Real or apparent (owing to contractures) leg length discrepancy should be compensated for by blocks or sitting radiographs should be taken. Patients who are unable to sit without support may be supported during the radiographs, or supine radiographs may be taken. Such radiographs are inaccurate for determining curve progression and should be interpreted with caution. Radiographs to assess curve progression are generally taken every 6 to 12 months.

Limited abduction of the hip suggests the need for hip radiographs. If hip abduction is more than 45 degrees with the hips in extension, the hips are probably well located. This empirically derived guideline, however, is not true in all cases; therefore an anteroposterior (AP) pelvis radiograph of all children with cerebral palsy in early childhood is prudent. The treatments for early hip subluxation are sufficiently less complex and risky than treatments for severely subluxated and dislocated hips that screening radiographs are warranted. The frequency of radiographs is determined by age of child (less often in older children) and severity of motor involvement (less often in less involved children). In general, radiographs are warranted every 6 months to 2 years in the first 8 to 10 years of life except in children with mild motor involvement.

Assessment of abnormal muscle activity and muscle contractures that interfere with function is difficult. The limitations of this assessment are largely responsible for the historically unpredictable results of orthopaedic surgery in this condition. Assessment of joint range of motion actively and passively on the examining table is not nearly as accurate in spastic or dyskinetic patients as in patients with flaccid paralysis or those with normal neuromuscular function for several reasons. First, selective control (a pyramidal tract function) is often lacking, and extrapyramidal patterned responses must be stimulated to elicit muscle function. The classic response is the "confusion reflex" in which flexion of the hip against resistance causes ankle dorsiflexion in a child with no active dorsiflexion. Ambulatory children often

have a combination of patterned and voluntary control. A muscle that can be controlled voluntarily on the examination table may be overwhelmed by a patterned response during gait. Second, spasticity is dependent on the position of the head and trunk in space. Muscle tone is less in the supine than sitting position and less in the sitting than standing position. Third, range of motion obtained using slow stretch often does not reflect the functional range of motion of a joint when quick stretch is applied as in walking. Finally, there are several tests that purport to determine which muscle is overactive or contracted when the choice is between a muscle crossing one joint and a muscle crossing two joints. The Silverskiöld test attempts to distinguish gastrocnemius from soleus as the cause of ankle equinus by testing dorsiflexion with the knee flexed (gastrocnemius relaxed) and with the knee extended (gastrocneumius stretched). The Ely test attempts to distinguish between iliopsoas and rectus femoris tightness by assessing hip flexion contracture with the knee flexed and extended. The Phelps tests attempts to distinguish gracilis from hamstring contracture by extending the flexed knees with the hips in maximal abduction. Hip adduction during this maneuver suggests gracilis tightness. All of these tests have been shown to be inaccurate in the awake patients by fine-wire electromyograms (EMGs), which showed activity in the supposedly relaxed muscle during the passive maneuver.

These caveats do not mean that conventional physical examination consisting of passive and active range of motion, strength, and assessment of voluntary versus patterned muscle activity should not be done; however, the results should be interpreted in the light of known limitations.

Evaluation of children who function as sitters is relatively straightforward despite the limitations of conventional examination. The main muscle contractures and imbalances interfering with function are equinus or equinovarus of the feet, flexion of the knees, "windswept" hips, and, rarely, extension at the hips. Severe equinus or equinovarus can result in difficult shoeing and pressure areas from a nonplantigrade position on wheelchair foot rests. Severe hamstring contractures can interfere with sitting posture by rotating the pelvis forward when the knees are placed at 90 degrees for sitting. This results in sacral sitting and sliding forward of the pelvis. Hip extension contractures may be primary but are more often due to surgical overweakening of the hip flexors. This contracture or spasticity results in difficulty in maintaining the pelvis posteriorly in the wheelchair. Windswept hips (one hip abducted and the other adducted) may be due to primary muscle imbalance, asymmetric surgical weakening of adductors, or unilateral dislocation. Windswept hips result in difficulty in seating as the windswept hips cause pelvic and trunk rotation making it difficult to seat the child straight and posteriorly in the chair. All these problems can be reasonably assessed by evaluating the sitting child. For example, if the child is constantly sliding forward in his wheelchair and requiring repositioning, the child should be placed with the pelvis in good position at the back of the seat, allowing free knee flexion. The legs are then gradually extended to 90 degrees. If the pelvis rotates forward during this maneuver, overtight hamstrings are part of the problem.

A gray area in children who function as sitters concerns those who will bear weight to transfer. As children grow older and heavier, the ability to transfer independently or aid in transfer can make the difference between living at home or in an institution. The difficulty arises in deciding how much surgery and bracing is appropriate in full-time sitters to attempt to maintain a stable foot and the legs in a sufficiently straight posture to allow weight bearing for transfer. This is a highly individualized decision.

The evaluation of muscle contractures and imbalances in ambulatory children is much more difficult. In addition to the static examination previously described, careful observation of gait must be done. This requires viewing the patient from the front, back, and sides while separately assessing motion of the trunk, pelvis, hip, knee, ankle, and foot. To view and integrate all these elements with their combinations of deviations from normal requires practice and experience. Movies or video tapes of gait make this assessment easier.

More sophisticated assessment of ambulatory patients with cerebral palsy and other neuromuscular disorders can be done by use of gait analysis in centers where the necessary equipment and personnel are available. Gait analysis consists of several or all of the following elements: motion analysis, dynamic electromyograms, force plate, foot switches, and determination of energy consumption. The goals of gait analysis are (1) to improve the clinician's ability to identify pathologic gait abnormalities and their cause, and thereby to improve treatment outcomes; and (2) to accurately document the results of treatment to allow comparison of different therapeutic modalities (Table 6-2).

Gait analysis techniques provide much useful information. Proponents believe that complete and accurate correction of gait abnormalities in complex patients (especially spastic diplegics) can be done safely in a single operative procedure using gait analysis. This promises to decrease the number of operations many patients undergo with an attendant decrease in morbidity, rehabilitation time, and social costs from being away from home and school. However, the information obtained from gait analysis has limitations and does not replace clinical assessment and judgment but rather complements it.

Orthopaedic Treatment

The orthopaedic treatment of all children with cerebral palsy can be broadly broken down into three categories: the treatment of spinal deformity, the treatment of hip instability, and the treatment of static

TABLE 6-2.
Gait Analysis

Motion analysis	A system of hardware and software that documents the position of body parts in three-dimensional space. Allows assessment of deviations from normal. Augments observation in complex deformities and documents results.
Dynamic electromyogram	Determines the timing and length of muscle activity during the gait cycle. Out-of-phase or prolonged activity suggest pathogenic muscle activity. Does not give information about strength of contraction or force generated.
Force plate	A measuring platform that determines foot-floor reaction force in three dimensions. The loading characteristics of the foot can be determined.
Foot switches	Pressure sensitive devices attached to the foot or shoe. They allow timing for electromyograms, and multiple switches can be used to indicate the pattern of load bearing on the foot.
Energy expenditure	This is directly measured by oxygen consumption or indirectly measured with less accuracy from heart rate or body part motion analysis.

contracture or dynamic muscle imbalances that interfere with function.

Spinal deformity increases in incidence with greater severity of motor involvement. Ambulatory patients are affected only 3% or less of the time. Children with spastic quadriplegia have a reported incidence of scoliosis of up to 64%. Although significant scoliosis or kyphosis may occur in childhood, these deformities are usually supple and manageable by bracing. The severe fixed deformities that interfere with sitting posture usually do not develop and require treatment until preadolescence or adolescence.

Hip instability like spinal deformity is more likely with more severe motor involvement. Hip instability is rare in hemiplegics, common in diplegics, and likely (up to 75%) in quadriplegics. The treatment of hip instability is generally begun in childhood as the average age of dislocation of untreated hips is only 7 years of age. Treatment is safer and more certain when done early when normal acetabular development can be obtained. When treatment is delayed until severe acetabular dysplasia exists, treatment becomes more difficult and less certain of obtaining a stable, painless hip. Because of the persistence of muscular imbalance about the hip, treatment may be necessary at more than one time in some children.

Treatment of muscle imbalance, contractures, and rotational abnormalities is simpler in the nonambulatory than ambulatory patients. Maintaining good sitting posture may require Achilles tendon or hamstring lengthening any time from late childhood through adolescence. Much of the orthopaedist's efforts in cerebral palsy has been to improve the gait of ambulatory patients by treatment of muscle imbalances, contractures, and rotational deformities. Unless fixed contractures develop, which is rare, this treatment should be delayed until the child is 5 to 7 years old when the adult gait pattern is largely established. At that time, physician, parents, and therapist can usually agree that no significant change in gait pattern is occurring. This allows more accurate assessment of gait abnormalities and more predictable surgical results with fewer overcorrections and undercorrections. When surgical treatment is undertaken, all abnormalities should be corrected at one time. This has several advantages. The recovery of muscle strength after immobilization for children with cerebral palsy is prolonged (3 to 6 months). This probably results from impaired voluntary muscle control, which limits the rate at which strength can be regained. Performing all anticipated operations at one time allows one rather than several lengthy recovery periods. Furthermore, the costs to social, in-

tellectual, and emotional growth caused by time away from home and school are minimized. Also, the financial and emotional burden to families from surgery and hospitalization for their child is lessened. Finally, functional results are arguably improved by one-stage corrections, especially in the diplegic patients requiring ankle, knee, and hip procedures as the improved position of one joint after surgery is not compromised by continued deformity at an adjacent joint.

Spinal Deformity

Scoliosis in ambulatory patients is infrequent and in general is similar in curve pattern and treatment to idiopathic scoliosis. Progressive curves in skeletally immature patients should be braced. Curves that progress despite bracing or curves of 40 to 50 degrees in immature patients require stabilization by fusion with instrumentation. The natural history of scoliosis in ambulatory persons with cerebral palsy after skeletal maturity has not been elucidated. Follow-up of patients with scoliosis into adulthood seems prudent as small neuromuscular curves probably have more tendency to progress than idiopathic curves.

Scoliosis is much more common in the spastic

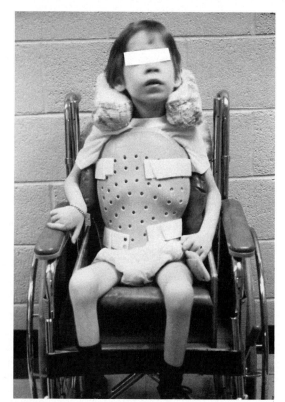

FIGURE 6-3. Child with spastic quadriplegia and scoliosis controlled in a thoracolumbosacral orthosis.

quadriplegic patients who are dependent on external support for sitting. Scoliosis often begins in childhood in these patients as a long C-shaped flexible curve with little vertebral rotation. With time, many curves become progressively severe and rigid. If curves become sufficiently severe, inability to sit ensues, with pain and pressure sores as less common problems. Bedfast children and adults are far more burdensome to care for, and the risks of aspiration and decubitus ulcers increase.

Scoliosis should be monitored clinically, and when detected serial radiographs should be done to monitor progression. Progressive curves in children are treated with body shells (total-contact thoracolumbosacral ortheses [TLSOs]) to control progression (Fig. 6-3). If the curve is controlled, this must be continued indefinitely. Except in the smallest curves, progression after skeletal maturity may occur in ce-

rebral palsy. In general, curves of less than 50 degrees progress more slowly after skeletal maturity than curves of greater magnitude, but there seems to be fairly great individual variation.

If curves progress despite bracing, surgery is considered. This is a difficult area as the decision to subject a severely involved child to the risks of a surgery of the magnitude of spinal fusion is not easily made by family members or physicians. If a curve progresses to 40 to 50 degrees, a careful discussion of the risks and benefits of spinal stabilization should be done. With curves of this magnitude, spinal stabilization can usually be accomplished by posterior surgery alone using segmental wiring (Luque technique) without the need for external immobilization. If curves are larger or more rigid, anterior diskectomy and fusion as well as posterior stabilization becomes necessary (Fig. 6-4). This increases the mortality and

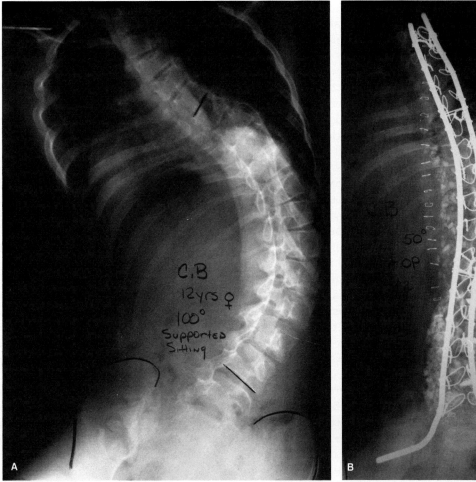

FIGURE 6-4. (A) Preoperative scoliosis radiograph of a 12-year-old girl with spastic quadriplegia cerebral palsy showing a 100-degree neuromuscular curve. (B) Immediate postoperative radiograph after anterior Dwyer and posterior Luque instrumentation and fusion.

morbidity of spinal stabilization. Curves can become sufficiently severe that adequate correction to restore sitting balance cannot be obtained or that, because of respiratory compromise from thoracic curve components, the risk of surgery is prohibitive. Custom seating is then used to maintain sitting as well and as long as possible.

Hip Stability

Hip subluxation and dislocation in cerebral palsy is a challenging problem. Disagreement exists as to when, how, and whether to intervene in the natural history of this problem. Untreated, hip dislocation occurs in up to 60% of children with spastic quadriplegia, 6% of diplegics, and is uncommon in hemiplegics. The reasons for treating hip instability in the ambulatory patient are to avoid pain and to maintain gait efficiency by avoiding leg length differences and weakness of abductors. The stated reasons for treating hip instability in dependent sitters include avoidance of pain, maintenance of sitting balance, minimization of decubitus ulcers, avoidance of fractures, and easing perineal care.

Retrospective studies of cerebral palsy patients with dislocated hips have not found any of these to be major problems. Sitting posture and decubitus ulcers are determined more by scoliosis and pelvic obliquity than hip status. Fractures are associated more with fixed contracture, although a small increased incidence in patients with hip dislocation has been reported. Perineal care is uncommonly a problem according to caretakers. Pain is reported in up to 52% of patients; however, severe, limiting pain is described in only 1% to 9%. Unfortunately these studies were all retrospective, and most were of institutionalized patients. Retrospective studies of dislocated hips automatically tend to select out the nonpainful hips. Furthermore, in the studies of institutionalized patients, 20% to 60% of these patients were bedfast. They may have been bedfast because of painful sitting.

Our experience is that both hip subluxations and dislocations may be painful. In a group of 25 preadolescent patients with sufficiently severe hip subluxation or dislocation to warrant acetabular osteotomy for coverage, fully 80% were painful preoperatively. Determination of the true incidence of pain would require a prospective study of a cohort of untreated patients with cerebral palsy. Most orthopaedists think that maintaining hip stability is worth the risks of treatment; because a significant percentage of dislocated hips do become painful, one

cannot distinguish hips that will be painful from those that will not, and no entirely satisfactory treatment for painful dislocated hips exists.

The treatment of subluxating hip varies with the age of the patient, the anatomy of the hip, and to some extent the ambulatory status of the child. The treatment options include bracing, adductor myotomy, or transfer with or without obturator neurectomy, varus derotation osteotomy of the proximal femur, and acetabular augmentation or redirection procedures.

Bracing alone is seldom a treatment of hip subluxation. Abduction bracing can be used in young children with spastic adductors to attempt to prevent contractures and to stimulate acetabular development. Bracing may be used postoperatively to avoid recurrent adduction contractures. After any procedure, soft tissue or bony, abduction bracing is appropriate if adduction contractures begin to develop.

Soft tissue procedures alone are generally indicated in children under age 5 with progressive subluxation or marked adductor tightness (less than 20 to 30 degrees of abduction of hips in extension). Children with poor ambulatory potential require adductor longus, gracilis, and sometimes adductor brevis myotomy as needed to obtain 40 to 50 degrees of abduction in extension (Fig. 6-5). Obturator neurectomy in addition to myotomy is widely recommended in nonambulatory patients but may increase the incidence of abduction contractures postoperatively. A tight iliopsoas may be a partial cause of hip dislocation by direct pressure over the medial hip capsule and can certainly inhibit full reduction of a subluxated hip. In children with poor ambulatory potential with hip subluxation, iliopsoas should be released if any significant hip flexion contracture exists.

Walking children or children with good ambulatory potential require a more cautious approach to adductor and iliopsoas surgery so as not to compromise strength necessary for ambulation. Subluxating hips in these patients should be treated with adductor longus, gracilis, and occasionally adductor brevis myotomy or transfer of the origin of adductor longus, brevis, and gracilis to the ischium. If release is chosen, the tenotomized muscles may be sutured to the fascia overlying adductor brevis. Anterior obturator neurectomy should rarely be done as excessive compromise of stance phase stability provided by the adductors may occur. If significant hip flexion contracture exists in patients with good ambulatory potential, iliopsoas should not be released as hip flexor power for advancing the limb in swing phase

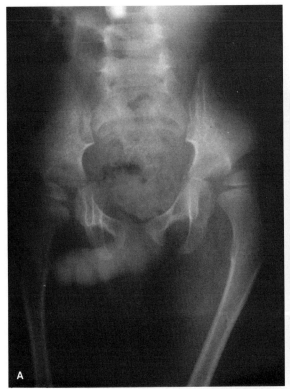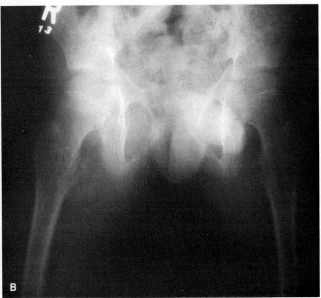

FIGURE 6-5. (A) Three-year-old boy with spastic quadriplegia, and right hip subluxation and left hip dislocation. (B) Seven years after adductor release, the hips are stable and well developed.

and climbing stairs may be compromised. Iliopsoas tightness may be treated by recessing the iliopsoas to the anterior hip capsule, Z-lengthening of the tendon, or fractional lengthening by cutting the fascial portion of the psoas muscle at the brim of the pelvis. It should be noted here that a good estimation of ambulatory potential can be made by 1 to 2 years of age by assessing the presence and absence of certain normal and abnormal postural reflexes.

Children with hip subluxation who are older than age 5 usually require bone surgery in addition to the soft tissue procedures previously described. If acetabular development is appropriate for age or if the patient is unusually young and has much potential acetabular growth remaining, a varus-derotational osteotomy is effective for obtaining hip stability (Fig. 6-6). Both femoral neck valgus and femoral anteversion have been implicated in the causation of hip instability. The suitability of varus derotational osteotomy (VDO) for repair of unstable hip can be assessed by taking a radiograph in abduction and internal rotation. If full reduction can be accomplished, VDO can be undertaken. Varus derotation is performed through an intertrochanteric osteotomy, which is then fixed with one of several internal fix-

ation devices or crossed pins supplemented with casting. In general, derotation of femoral anteversion is performed by externally rotating the distal fragment until only 20 to 30 degrees of internal rotation remains. In hips requiring varization, approximately 100 to 110 degrees of varus should be obtained in children younger than age 8 and 110 to 120 degrees should be obtained in children older than age 8.

Older children with subluxated/dislocated hips often have severe acetabular dysplasia in addition to the soft tissue contractures and femoral deformity. Reconstruction of these hips requires a procedure to augment or deepen the existing acetabulum. The Chiari pelvic osteotomy is effective in providing coverage and immediate stability for these hips (Fig. 6-7). Shelf procedures that place bone graft harvested from the pelvis onto the uncovered capsule can be used to augment the existing acetabulum. The occurrence of resorption 1 to 2 years after shelf incorporation has resulted in waxing and waning enthusiasm for these procedures. Recent technical modifications may improve the results of this type of procedure, which is flexible in the coverage obtainable, easy to perform, and has little operative morbidity. More complex redirectional osteotomies

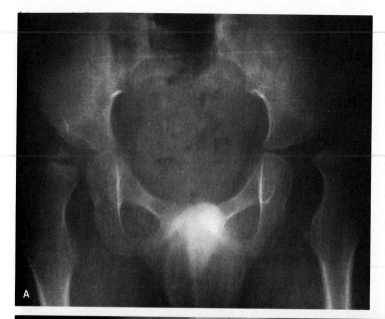

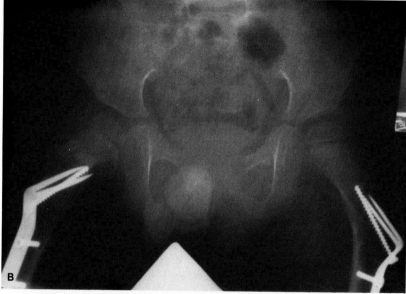

FIGURE 6-6. (A) Four-year-old boy with spastic quadriplegia and severe hip subluxation of the right hip and dislocation of the left. (B) One year after bilateral varus–derotational osteotomies of the proximal femur, the hips are satisfactorily reduced.

of the acetabulum may be indicated in the rare case of a congruent dysplastic hip. When severe subluxation or dislocation exist, combined procedure of soft tissue release, varus derotational osteotomy of the femur, and acetabular reconstruction are necessary to obtain and maintain hip stability.

If hip dislocation has been present for a long time, articular cartilage degeneration occurs and reconstruction may result in a painful degenerative hip. If long-standing dislocated hips are not painful, no treatment is indicated. The exception is if the adducted position of the leg prohibits adequate perineal care and sitting position. In this unusual circum-

stance, a subtrochateric abduction osteotomy of the femur gives improved position of the leg without complex hip reconstruction.

Three options exist for the painful hip with long-standing dislocation–resection arthroplasty, arthrodesis, and total joint replacement. Resection arthroplasty has become popular in recent years because of a modification of the girdlestone-type procedure described for painful, degenerative hips of nonspastic patients. A head and neck of femur resection alone in patients with spasticity often results in a proximal migration of the femur and recurrent pain when it abuts against the pelvis. Creation of

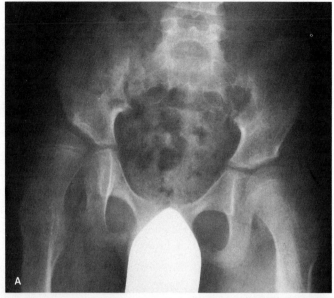

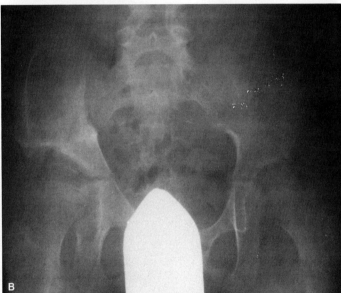

FIGURE 6-7. (A) Eleven-year, 8-month-old boy with spastic diplegia and right hip subluxation with acetabular insufficiency. (B) One year after Chiari osteotomy, the hip is stable and well covered.

muscle envelopes over the acetabulum and proximal femur can avoid this problem. The head and proximal femur to below the lesser trochanter are resected extra periosteally to minimize heterotopic ossification. The hip capsule, hip abductors, and iliopsoas are sutured across the acetabulum. The vastus lateralis then sutured over the end of the femur to prevent proximal migration and to create a muscle mass that articulates with the muscle mass created over the acetabulum. Traction for 3 to 6 weeks postoperatively is necessary until healing of the muscle envelopes is secure. This procedure results in a "floppy" hip that tends to lie in flexion and abduction, but is effective in reliev-

ing pain and allowing satisfactory sitting posture (Fig. 6-8).

Arthrodesis of the hip is an effective way of relieving pain but has two major drawbacks. First, achieving fusion is difficult in spastic patients. Second, a compromise hip position between sitting and lying posture is necessary. This makes seating more complicated.

Total hip replacement has been reported to be successful in relieving pain. Because of the likelihood of loosening requiring several revisions during a patient's lifetime, this procedure should be undertaken cautiously. Only ambulatory patients for whom a

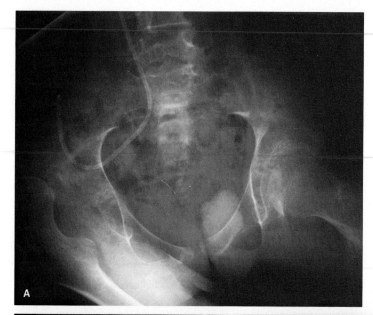

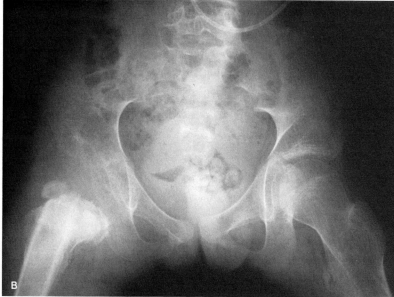

FIGURE 6-8. (A) Fourteen-year-old boy with spastic quadriplegia and a painful dislocated left hip. (B) One year after a proximal femoral resection and interpositional arthroplasty, the patient is pain-free. Note the distance maintained between the femur and pelvis by the interposed muscles.

stable, painless hip joint will improve function should be considered for this procedure.

Hip Adduction Deformity in Gait

Excessive hip adduction or scissoring during gait is identified by observing the thighs cross the midline during gait. Scissoring must not be confused with internal rotation of the entire limb coupled with excessive knee flexion. This combination of problems causes the knees to cross the midline during swing phase and may occur without significant hip adduction deformity. If true scissoring is present, adductor release or transfer as described in the section on hip instability should be performed.

Hip Internal Rotation Deformity

Internal rotation deformity of the entire limb is diagnosed by inward direction of the patellae during gait. If severe, clumsiness may ensue by one foot running into the other. Internal rotation can be unattractive cosmetically as well. Generally, excess femoral anteversion is present in addition to any muscle imbalance. Both soft tissue and bony surgeries have been described to correct this deformity. Adductor myotomy relieves mild intoeing in many patients and should be kept in mind if adductor surgery is necessary for other reasons. Anterior and distal transfer of the gluteus medius and minimus can give good results in the few patients meeting the criteria for this procedure. Lateral transfer of the medial hamstrings in the distal thigh can be effective in patients with overactive medial hamstrings as identified by dynamic EMGs.

Most surgeons think derotation osteotomy of the femur is the most predictable technique for relieving this deformity. Derotation may be performed at the intertrochanteric or supracondylar level in the femur with advantages described for both locations. Whichever level is chosen, care must be taken to ensure control of both fragments with internal fixation or pins-in-plaster as loss of position is all too frequent in spastic patients. Clinically, derotation should be accomplished with the preservation of 20 to 30 degrees of internal rotation.

Hip Flexion Deformity

If static hip flexion contracture is less than 15 to 20 degrees, sufficient compensation can occur through the lumbar spine so that treatment is unnecessary. Diplegic patients can be difficult to assess if the static contractures are borderline, and they have flexion at both the knees and hips during gait. Application of knee immobilizers in the clinic to minimize knee flexion contractures is helpful in determining whether the hip flexion deformity is primary or compensatory in these patients. Patients with dynamic knee flexion and little primary hip flexion deformity lose their excessive hip flexion when knee immobilizers are in place. Similarly, little hip flexion should be present during knee walking in these patients.

Treatment of a significant hip-flexion deformity is usually directed at the iliopsoas. As discussed previously, release of the iliopsoas in the ambulatory patient is unadvisable as limb advancement may be compromised. Lengthening or recession is appropriate for walking patients.

Knee Flexion Deformity

Normal hamstring tension allows extension of the knee with the hip flexed to 90 degrees to within 20 degrees of full extension (the popliteal angle). Even with significant hamstring contracture with the hip flexed, full knee extension is usually possible with the hip extended. Lack of full knee extension with the hip extended indicates knee capsule contracture in addition to muscle contracture.

Persistent knee flexion of more than 15 degrees in stance phase is usually an indication for hamstring surgery. The reason for performing surgery at relatively small amounts of contracture is the increase in quadriceps force necessary to maintain upright posture with increasing knee flexion in stance. Quadriceps fatigue with pain, limitation of walking tolerance, and progressive crouch may occur with knee flexion contracture.

The treatment of this deformity is lengthening of hamstring and rarely posterior knee capsulotomy in the cases with fixed-joint contracture. Hamstring lengthening is done by a Z-lengthening of the semitendinosus tendon and fractional lengthening of the semimembranosus and biceps femoris muscle. Fractional lengthening involves a V- or shallow S-shaped cut of the fascia overlying the muscle in one or two places, which then allows the underlying muscle to be spread. Management of the gracilis is somewhat controversial. Simple tenotomy has been routinely done as development of an extension contracture from tenotomy of this muscle is rare. Recent work, however, has suggested a significant role of the gracilis in initiating swing. Therefore, the extra few minutes required to Z-lengthen this tendon may be warranted. Routine lengthening of both medial and lateral hamstrings avoids the development of late external rotation deformity of the leg that may occur after medial hamstring lengthening alone.

Distal hamstring recession to the femur has been largely abandoned as an unacceptable incidence of extension contracture and recurvatum occur. Proximal hamstring release offers less control of length than distal lengthening in ambulatory patients. In nonambulatory patients with knee flexion, contractures that interfere with sitting proximal release can be considered; however, a patient occasionally develops severe lumbar lordosis, and this may be painful.

Knee Extension Deformity

Knee extension deformity is manifest in gait by limited swing phase flexion. This results in a stiff legged gait with reduced stride length and is usually accompanied by knee flexion contracture. On physical examination it is demonstrated by spastic resistance to passive knee flexion. Treatment should be considered if a significant inhibition of cadence and step length are present.

Treatment consists of release or transfer of the distal rectus femoris. Optimally, dynamic EMGs should be performed to document rectus femoris activity during swing phase without activity of the remaining quadriceps muscles before transfer surgery is performed. Although rectus surgery can be indicated by clinical examination alone, one would expect less consistent results than with EMG identification of nonphasic activity of only the rectus femoris.

Recent articles suggest that distal rectus femoris transfer is superior to release. Transfer may be done medially or laterally. Little effect on limb rotation occurs. This procedure can be performed simultaneously with hamstring lengthening with minimal risk of genu recurvatum developing.

Ankle Equinus Deformity

Equinus deformity of the ankle is the most common deformity requiring treatment in children with cerebral palsy. Many procedures have been devised of varying complexity to treat this deformity. The indications for surgery vary with the age of the patient and functional status.

In general, nonambulatory patients with equinus should be braced and have surgical lengthening if they cannot be held in a brace. Treatment is to maintain shoe ability and a plantigrade foot on the wheelchair foot rests to avoid pressure sores and discomfort.

Ambulatory patients must be considered more carefully for several reasons. Overlengthening of the Achilles tendon creates triceps surae weakness. This may result in a loss of restraint of ankle dorsiflexion as the center of gravity of the body moves anterior to the ankle. Unrestrained ankle dorsiflexion in stance causes compensatory knee and hip flexion to maintain upright posture. With gradual quadriceps fatigue, a progressive crouch posture may ensue. This significant complication, if recognized early, can be treated with an anterior floor reaction brace that restrains forward tibial motion. If diagnosed late, knee and hip flexion contractures develop and require surgical lengthening as well as bracing for the ankle.

A second concern with the ambulatory child with ankle equinus is the timing of surgery. Achilles tendon lengthening done before age 4 is more likely to recur and require reoperation than lengthening preferred later. For this reason, management of correctable equinus by bracing with an ankle foot arthrosis until after this age is generally appropriate. In the occasional young child with unbraceable equinus, Achilles tendon lengthening (TAL) is indicated if the lack of a stable base seems to interfere with overall motor skills progress.

Of the multiple techniques for TAL, two have become predominant. The sliding lengthening technique of White or Hoke consists of two or three incisions one half of the way through the Achilles tendon alternating on each side of the tendon. This technique can be done open or percutaneously with good results reported from both. Z-lengthening of the tendon is the other common technique. This can be used for any TAL and is probably superior to the sliding technique if a large amount of correction is required as sliding technique may result in rupture if too much lengthening is attempted. Care must be taken with the Z-lengthening more than with sliding technique to avoid overlengthening and triceps surae insufficiency. The proximal tendon should be stretched distally and sutured to the distal stump with the ankle in neutral. Immobilization recommendations vary from 3 to 6 weeks with a below- or above-knee cast. Authors report no problems with any of these techniques. Short immobilization with below-knee cast is probably more appropriate for sliding lengthening as rupture might occur with Z-lengthened tendons. The ankle should always be immobilized in neutral as immobilization in dorsiflexion may result in an overlengthened tendon.

The problems with leaving equinus untreated include metatarsalgia, ankle instability with sprains, and functional leg length discrepancy in the hemiplegic.

Equinovarus Deformity

Equinovarus can be a disabling problem because of ankle instability and the development of callosities and pain from weight bearing on the outside of the foot (Fig. 6-9). These feet are difficult to brace and often require surgical treatment.

Dynamic EMGs may be useful in obtaining consistently good surgical results. EMGs can help define the pathogenic muscle by identifying continuous, out-of-phase, or premature onset of muscle activity. Dynamic EMG cannot, however, measure the power of muscle contraction, and therefore the EMG results should be supported by clinical observation. Continuous posterior tibialis or anterior tibialis activity (with other muscles of the calf having normal phasic activity) are the most common patterns seen in the spastic equinovarus foot. Continuous posterior tibialis activity may be treated by a split transfer of one half of the tendon to the peroneus brevis. Anterior tibialis overactivity is treated by a split transfer of one half of the tendon to the cuboid or by transfer of the entire tendon to the third cuneiform. Out-of-phase activity of the posterior tibialis is not uncommon and may be treated by anterior transfer of the posterior tibialis tendon through the interosseous membrane to the third cuneiform. Several authors, however, have reported an unacceptable incidence of calcaneus

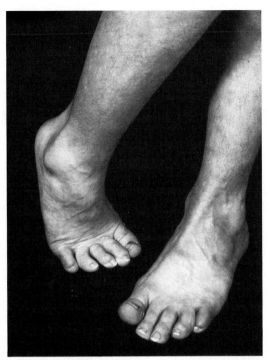

FIGURE 6-9. The right foot shows a marked equinovarus deformity seen commonly in spastic hemiplegia.

deformity developing after this procedure, and caution is warranted. Other patterns of abnormal muscle activity occur, and treatment plans may be adjusted based on the specific pattern found.

Similar judgments can be made on clinical grounds alone by careful observation. Visual inspection can often indicate the phase of anterior tibial activity. Also, the posterior tibial tendon causes more forefoot adduction as contrasted with foot supination

caused by anterior tibial overactivity. Good results have been reported by astute clinicians using clinical criteria alone.

Fixed deformity of the hindfoot and midfoot are treated in the preadolescent or adolescent child by bony procedures. Heel varus alone can be treated with calcaneal osteotomy. More commonly, a combination of hindfoot and midfoot deformities are present requiring a triple arthrodesis.

Valgus Deformity

Valgus deformity is common in patients with spastic diplegia and quadriplegia (Fig. 6-10). In young children valgus of the heel can be exacerbated by a tight tendon Achilles. Occasionally, in these rocker-bottom–type feet, a TAL turns an unbraceable valgus foot into a more flexible and braceable foot.

This deformity is difficult to brace but can be done in flexible feet if an excellent heel mold is obtained in the ankle-foot orthosis (AFO). Even with bracing this deformity tends to progress in many children. Most authors recommend surgical treatment for moderate to severe valgus feet in children older than ages 5 to 7. Soft tissue and tendon surgery (mainly peroneal tendon lengthening or transfer) has generally had an unacceptable incidence of failure or overcorrection. Most authors recommend some modification of the Grice extraarticular subtalar arthrodesis with or without peroneal tendon lengthening. This procedure has had a high rate of complications and failures in spastic patients in many surgeons' hands, although some authors report good results.

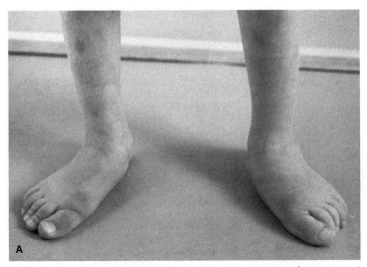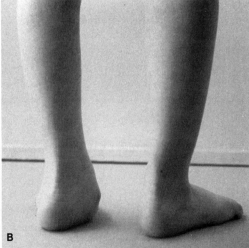

FIGURE 6-10. These are typical planovalgus feet commonly seen in spastic diplegia and quadriplegia.

We have not found the valgus foot to be a functionally limiting deformity in most children. Pain and pressure sores from the medial prominence of the talar head have rarely been observed by us. We therefore usually treat this as a benign deformity and brace with an AFO- or UCBL-type insert for partial correction in the moderate and severe deformity or if mild discomfort exists. For the few patients with severe deformity and pain, a triple arthrodesis in adolescence is satisfactory.

Upper Extremity

Surgical treatment of the upper extremity is relatively uncommon and is usually performed in patients with spastic hemiplegia. Three reasons for treatment exist—to improve function, to improve cosmesis, and to improve hygiene.

Functional improvement can be expected in relatively few patients. Requirements for improved functional results include normal intelligence; intact sensibility (especially stereognosis); voluntary control of pinch, grasp, and release; absence of tonic neck reflexes, and ability to cooperate with physical therapy. Generally, surgery is performed in later childhood when cooperation is possible and physical examination is accurate. Dynamic EMGs can be helpful in assessing appropriate transfer since no phase of activity change will occur after transplantation.

In the carefully selected patients, surgery at shoulder, elbow, forearm, wrist, and hand can be considered as necessary. Shoulder adduction and internal rotation is treated by subscapularis and pectoralis major release if mild and humeral osteotomy if severer. Limiting elbow flexion contracture can be released by lengthening of the biceps, lacertus fibrosis and brachialis. If severe, lengthening of the brachioradialis pronator teres and flexor slide may be necessary as well. Pronation of the forearm can be corrected by pronator teres release or transfer. Flexion deformities of the wrist and fingers are treated differently depending on severity. Mild deformities may respond to individual flexor muscle lengthening or flexor slide. Moderate deformities require wrist flexor transfer to wrist extensor often with flexor release as well. Severe deformities require multiple tendon lengthening or release. Arthrodesis of the wrist may be necessary. The thumb-in-palm deformity is disabling, and several techniques are available for correction depending on the specific nature of the deformity. Release of intrinsic contracture, tendon transfer about the thumb, and metacarpal phalangeal arthrodesis may be necessary singly or in combination. Postoperative rehabilitation and splinting is crucial to the success of the procedures.

In hemiplegics for whom improved function cannot be expected, tendon lengthening or release can significantly improve appearance, which is important to many patients. A flexor slide alone can often reduce flexion and pronation sufficiently for a improvement in self-image.

Quadriplegic patients may develop sufficient contractures of fingers, wrist, or elbow that maceration can occur at opposed skin surfaces. Releases to improve hygiene and permit splinting are occasionally indicated.

Nonorthopaedic Treatment

Physical Therapy

Physical therapy has been and will continue to be an integral part of the management of the cerebral palsy patient. The relation formed between the therapist and family is often strong and helps at multiple levels in family adjustment to life with a disabled child. The therapist is often the first health care worker to identify developing problems. Therapists are important in maximizing function through instructing families in positioning techniques and limb motion maintenance.

There are multiple schools of therapy for cerebral palsy, the most common being neurodevelopmental therapy. None of the approaches used has been shown to improve neurologic outcomes, although this is the goal of all schools. In general, an active, interested therapist using any approach can obtain equally good results. The program chosen should not, however, be so burdensome to the family that it increases family stress. It should be remembered that what is good for the family is generally good for the child.

Drug Therapy

Drug therapy attempts to decrease muscle tone pharmacologically have centered around three drugs—diazepam, baclofen, and dantrolene sodium. None has been generally useful as the extent of unwanted side effects overwhelms the limited benefits derived from their use. A few carefully selected patients can benefit from drug therapy with careful titration of dosage.

Neurosurgery

Several neurosurgical procedures have been devised to attempt to control the abnormal movements and spasticity of cerebral palsy. These include cerebellar stimulators and myelotomies. These procedures have not gained general acceptance as results are inconsistent and unpredictable.

Recently, a technically improved version of a procedure proposed in the early part of the century to control spasticity has become popular. Selective posterior rhizotomy as presently performed involves sectioning of 25% to 50% of the posterior rootlets from L2 through the upper sacral roots as needed. Which rootlets are sectioned is determined by a combination of preoperative clinical evaluation and abnormal EMG response to stimulation of individual rootlets. The goal of the procedure is to reduce spasticity by decreasing the spinal reflex arc that is under diminished central inhibition. The procedure will not improve fixed muscle contractures or bony deformities. The two major indications for this procedure are (1) the severely involved patient with spastic quadriplegia who cannot be handled or positioned satisfactorily because of severe spasticity, and (2) the relatively mildly affected ambulatory child with spasticity interfering with free joint motion in gait.

As envisioned, selective posterior rhizotomy and orthopaedic surgeries are complementary procedures. Rhizotomy is used to diminish spasticity and orthopaedic surgery for contractures and bony deformities. Patient selection seems key to the success of selective posterior rhizotomy. Ambulatory patients with only spasticity and without severe, underlying weakness are probably the ideal candidates. The indications and limitations of this procedure have yet to be established.

MYELOMENINGOCELE

Myelomeningocele is the most common serious congenital spine defect. It consists of a defect of the spinal cord, spinal nerves, meninges, and vertebral bodies. Typically, there is a large sac at the level of the defect containing the abnormal neural elements that have herniated from the vertebral canal (Fig. 6-11). This sac is covered by epidermis and attenuated meninges and is filled with cerebral spinal fluid as well as spinal cord. Less commonly, no sac exists with the spinal cord exposed; this is called myeloschesis or rachischisis. Another uncommon variant of these spinal dysraphisms is meningocele. A meningocele is a sac of cerebrospinal fluid (CSF) with meningeal covering without neural elements present in the sac. In the pure form, these patients are neurologically normal.

The typical myelomeningocele (MMC) produces flaccid paralysis, sensory loss, and autonomic dysfunction below the level of the lesion. Spastic muscles and isolated areas of cord function capable of reflex stimulation below the level of major cord disruption are commonly seen. Hydrocephalus develops in 70% to 90% of patients and is present by 1 month in 50% of affected children. An Arnold-Chiari malformation is commonly associated with MMC and is probably the cause of hydrocephalus in these cases. Arnold-Chiari malformation is a congenital anomaly of the hindbrain in which the cerebellar tonsils are displaced into the spinal canal, and the brain stem is elongated with resultant aqueductal abnormality. Other associated CNS anomalies are tethered cord, hydromyelia, syringomyelia, and diastematomyelia.

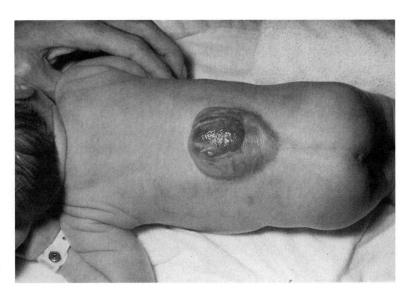

FIGURE 6-11. A 10-day-old girl with a myelomeningocele before repair.

Many other problems are caused by or associated with these malformations of the neural axis. They include mental retardation, congenital scoliosis and kyphosis, foot deformities, hip dislocation, bladder and bowel paralysis, hydronephrosis, hypospadias, kidney malformation, and imperforate rectum. Because of the multiple system involvement, a team approach to the care of these children is required. The team should include a neurosurgeon, orthopaedic surgeon, urologic surgeon, developmental pediatrician or pediatric neurologist, physical therapist, and social worker.

Epidemiology

The incidence of MMC varies with racial/ethnic background and geographic location. In the United State, the incidence is 1 per 1000 births with higher incidence in whites than blacks. The incidence is higher in Great Britain and varies from 2 to 4 per 1000 births. The incidence varies from 0.5 to 3 per 1000 in Australia and MMC is rare in Japan.

A clear trend toward decreasing incidence is apparent during the past 50 years worldwide. The reasons for this decline are unclear. Hypotheses to explain this decline include improved prenatal detection, improved maternal nutrition, and lessening of a predisposing environmental factor.

Etiology and Diagnosis

Genetics

Myelomeningocele is believed to have a multifactorial causation. That is, multiple genes plus an environmental influence are required to produce the phenotype. The evidence for a gene effect is the increased risk of a neural tube defect in a second child after one affected child has been born. This risk is about 5%. If two children with neural tube defects are born, the risk of a subsequent child's being affected is 10%. The second neural tube defect may be different from that of the first child. For example, after a child with MMC is born, another child may have anencephaly and vice versa.

The evidence for an environmental influence is the absence of identical twin concordance and the variation in incidence in the same genetic stock living in different parts of the world.

Pathologic Anatomy

Two hypotheses have been advanced to explain neural tube defects such as MMC: (1) failure of neural tube closures during embryogenesis, and (2) distention and rupture of the closed neural tube.

The neural tube begins as the flat neural plate. Differential growth rate of all cells in the plate result in curving that eventually forms a tube. This tube fuses dorsally beginning in the center and proceeding caudad and cephalad simultaneously. Complete fusion occurs with the first embryonic month. The most common cause of failure to close hypothesized is a vascular malformation resulting in inadequate nutrients for closure.

Rupture of a closed neural tube is hypothesized to occur because of excessive CSF pressure within the neural tube. Such excessive pressure would cause distention and rupture of the weakest areas of the tube that are the most recently closed. Cephalad rupture would result in anencephaly, and caudad rupture would cause MMC. The correct hypothesis and sequence of events is not yet certain, although the preponderance of the evidence supports the rupture of an already closed neural tube hypothesis.

Prenatal Diagnosis

Prenatal diagnosis of neural tube defects including MMC is often possible. Routine screening of maternal serum for α-fetoprotein is now done. High levels of α-fetoprotein are present in open neural tube defects because of leaking of this liver synthesized protein into the amniotic fluid. Correct analysis of levels is dependent on an accurate gestational age, which is obtained through ultrasound. If levels are abnormally high, amniocentesis may be elected to measure α-fetoprotein in the amniotic fluid. If this level is high, a neural tube defect is confirmed. Ultrasound can also directly identify neural tube defects in some cases. Combined use of ultrasound and amniocentesis for α-fetoprotein identifies 80% to 90% of neural tube defects prenatally.

Initial Management

Neurosurgical closure of the open spine is generally accomplished within 12 to 24 hours after birth. Delaying closure increases the risks of infection of the neural axis. If treatment of the open spine is withheld, most affected children die within 6 months, and nearly all die within a few years. Attempts to define children for whom active treatment should be withheld have been made on the basis of expected outcomes. A grossly enlarged head, complete paraplegia, high lesions, clinically evident spine deformity, and other gross congenital anomalies have been correlated with poor quality of life. At present, the issue of selection for treatment has been removed from the province of families and health care workers and placed in the political arena in the United States, rendering identification of newborns for whom active intervention might be withheld mute. In addition to closure of the spinal lesion, early shunting is frequently necessary for congenital or early developing hydrocephalus. Although active intervention is neurosurgical in the newborn period, other members of the health care team are called for initial evaluation of the patient and discussion with the family. Developmental pediatricians, physical therapists, urologists, and orthopaedists should all take this opportunity to begin the education of the family to what the future holds for their children.

Initial Orthopaedic Evaluation Management

The orthopaedist evaluates the infant in the nursery to assess neurologic level, spine deformity, contractures, foot deformities, and hip stability. Neurologic level is defined as the lowest nerve root that results in antigravity strength or better in muscles (Table 6-3).

Determining neurologic level is difficult in lumbar level patients in the newborn period. Repeated examinations are necessary, and a completely accurate level may not be obtained before the child is 2 to 3 years old when voluntary activity can be distinguished from reflex activity. Careful examinations are important as knee control through strong quadriceps is the key to long-term functional walking. Whether a child can be expected to be a functional walker has implications for treatment, mainly of the hip. Thoracic and sacral level patients can usually be identified early by a combination of physical examination and the level of the structural lesion. The neurologic level is important in formulating a treatment plan and in advising the family.

Spinal deformity is assessed clinically and radiographically. Congenital scoliosis or kyphosis must not

be overlooked because of the dominating presence of the spinal dysraphism.

Hip stability is assessed by clinical examination to find dislocatable hips. Limited hip abduction suggests a rare teratologic dislocation that can be confirmed by radiograph.

Contractures are confined to the lower extremity and usually consist of flexion and abduction contractures of the hip, flexion and occasionally extension contractures of the knee, and positional deformities of the foot such as calcaneovalgus. Structural foot deformities seen are clubfoot and congenital vertical talus.

Management in the first year of life involves observation, education, and intervention. The child is examined several times to refine assessment of neurologic level. Parents can be prepared for the range of bracing that will probably be required and the level of ambulatory function that can be expected. Spinal deformities are followed radiographically every 6 months.

An aggressive physical therapy is taught to the parents to reduce hip flexion and abduction contracture and knee flexion contractures. A hip-knee-ankle-foot orthosis may be prescribed for infants with severer contractures (usually lumbar levels) for nighttime use. Elimination of contractures through physical therapy at this time is important to avoid the need for surgical soft tissue release when it is time to start standing and for walking devices between 1 and 2 years of age.

Foot deformities are managed to allow a plantigrade foot at the time that standing and walking begin. Mild positional deformities are treated with serial casting or manipulation alone. A well-molded AFO is sometimes necessary to maintain foot position. Vertical talus is treated by early surgical correction. The common clubfoot deformity is treated with well-molded serial casts. Some feet can be corrected with casting. Those that require surgery have fewer problems with skin closure if casts have given partial correction. The clubfeet requiring surgery are treated with a radical posteromedial release or by talectomy. Posteromedial release should be radical with correction of all components of deformity. Talectomy is reserved for the severe, rigid deformity for which soft tissue release is thought to be inadequate. This can be the primary procedure or a salvage procedure for failed soft tissue procedures. Prolonged (4 to 6 months) plaster immobilization is required after talectomy, and continued bracing with an AFO is necessary to avoid loss of position after talectomy. Spastic muscle or muscles under reflex control only should be released rather then lengthened.

TABLE 6-3.
Muscles Present

Thoracic	Flail legs
L1-L2	Adductors and iliopsoas
L3	Quadriceps
L4	Quadriceps and medial hamstring
L5	Anterior tibialis
Sacral	All muscles except triceps surae toe flexors or foot intrinsics depending on sacral level

Management of the hips in MMC is controversial at all stages of development. If dislocatable hips are present at birth, the decision to treat is made on a neurologic level. For high-level patients without quadriceps function, the dislocations can be ignored since no functional impairment will occur. Dislocatable hips are rarely a problem in sacral level patients but if present should be treated as a routine congenital dislocation of the hip with a Pavlik harness. Lower lumbar level patients with active quadriceps present a dilemma. Typical treatment with flexion and abduction accentuates the tendency toward contracture. Three options are available: (1) treatment with Pavlik harness until hip stability is obtained followed by aggressive therapy to relieve contractures, (2) treatment with an abduction extension brace to maintain hip location and stimulate acetabular development without aggravating hip flexion contracture, and (3) ignoring the dislocatable hips and maintaining motion with the plan of leaving the hips out or surgically relocating them at a later time. The treatment program probably should be individualized and depends on the surgeon's experience and preference.

Orthopaedic Management at Walking Age and After

Ambulation

Management depends on neurologic level. Thoracic and high lumbar level patients (without quadriceps function) are begun in a standing program or wheelchair program depending on the philosophy of the treatment team. Little difference in outcome has been noted between patients who eventually use a wheelchair for mobility whether or not they spent their early years in a standing program. Both approaches have strong advocates. Most studies show few high-level patients who continue upright ambulation after adolescence.

Low lumbar level patients with strong quadriceps have a good potential for walking long term. Some of these patients can begin walking with just an AFO to control foot and ankle instability. Those patients with less hip and knee strength may require knee-ankle-foot orthoses or a period in a parapodium before they have sufficient strength to walk with less bracing. Sacral level patients generally begin walking at the normal time and require no bracing or an AFO.

Children who are candidates for a parapodium may require soft tissue releases if hip or knee contractures are excessive (greater than 20 to 30 degrees).

Walking ability can generally improve up to age 5, and less bracing may be possible with improvement in strength. Children who are nonfunctional walkers by ages 9 or 10 will use a wheelchair for mobility in later life.

High-level patients who start in a parapodium can be progressed as strength and control improves to more functional devices. A swivel base may be applied to the parapodium to allow ambulation using trunk rotation (Fig. 6-12). Between ages 2 and 4, a reciprocating gait orthosis may be considered to allow smoother and more rapid ambulation in some patients (Figs. 6-13 and 6-14).

Ambulation skills are primarily but not solely determined by neurologic level. Intelligence, hydrocephalus, contractures, and pelvic obliquity all have an effect on walking ability and bracing needs.

Spine Management

Congenital scoliosis should be managed in conventional fashion with a limited posterior fusion and occasionally AP hemiepiphysiodesis/hemiarthro-

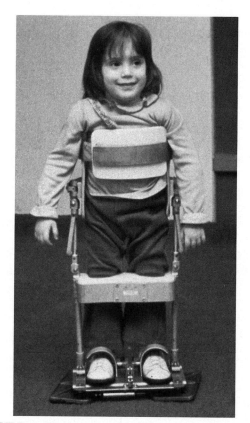

FIGURE 6-12. A young girl with myelomeningocele in a parapodium. Attached to the base is a swivel walker that allows mobility by trunk rotation.

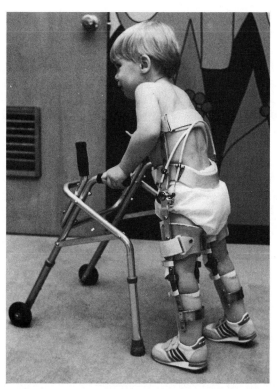

FIGURE 6-13. A young boy with high-level myelomeningocele in a reciprocating gait orthosis.

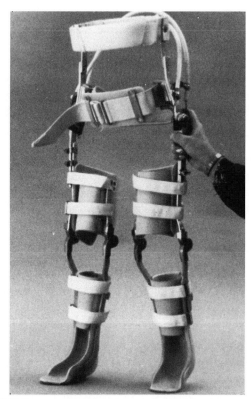

FIGURE 6-14. The reciprocating gait orthosis allows reciprocating gait through a cable system activated by trunk motion.

desis. Neuromuscular scoliosis develops in almost all thoracic level patients and occurs with decreasing frequency as the neurologic level decends. Bracing with total contact body shells (TLSOs) is used to control curves until sufficient trunk growth has occurred for definitive fusion. AP fusion is often necessary because of absence of posterior elements at the level of the lesion.

Kyphosis is often the severest and most difficult to treat spinal deformity. Kyphosis at the level of lesion can result in chronic ulceration. Treatment of this deformity when severe is kyphectomy. This is a major surgery with many complications and requires an experienced spinal surgeon. Care must be taken that a functioning ventriculoperitoneal shunt is present if cord transection is performed as acute increase in intracranial pressure may occur.

Hip Management

Radical soft tissue release is indicated if flexion or abduction contractures interfere with bracing limbs in a stable upright posture. Hip joint stability in thoracic and high lumbar lesions is unimportant. Patients with dislocated hips function equally well as patients with located hips. Sacral level patients rarely have problems with hip joint stability as the full complement of normal strength muscles are present about the hip.

Lower lumbar level hips generate the most controversy. Should dislocated hips be relocated? Should located hips be prophylactically stabilized by muscle transfer? Should a unilateral dislocation always be treated? At what age and which procedures should be done if hips are to be stabilized? Those questions are not as yet fully answered. Some physicians treating many patients with MMC aggressively seek to maintain hip joint stability in patients with good ambulatory potential, although little evidence exists that located hips improve walking ability or efficiency. A unilateral dislocation is almost always treated to avoid problems of limb length discrepancy and pelvic obliquity. Physicians at some centers think that established bilateral dislocations should go untreated while aggressively treating subluxating or prophylactically performing stabilizing muscle transfers. The major drawbacks to aggressive treatment are the difficulty in maintaining hip location despite multiple surgeries and the recognition that a stiff hip from multiple surgeries interferes with walking much more than a dislocated hip in these patients.

Treatment of subluxated/dislocated hips is directed at obtaining a stable concentric reduction with muscle strength balancing about the hip with as few procedures as possible, preferably only one. Weak abduction and extension is balanced by iliopsoas transfer to the greater trochanter or by external oblique transfer to the greater trochanter with tensor fasciae latae muscle recession posteriorly. Unopposed adductor power is treated with adductor release or transfer to ischium to augment extensor power. Varus derotation osteotomy and acetabular procedures (most commonly Pembertion or Chiari osteotomies or shelf procedures) are used as needed to obtain bony stability. Bone procedures without muscle balancing are in general doomed to failure as the deforming forces remain.

Leg Rotational Deformity Management

Rotational abnormalities are common in lumbar level patients. Rotational abnormalities in young children can be managed with a twister cable from a hip belt to shoes or foot orthoses. Correction cannot be expected, but control of rotation to optimize walking ability can be obtained. Femoral rotational abnormalities can be corrected with subtrochanteric derotational osteotomy, which is often performed at the time of hip stabilization. Tibial rotational deformities are treated in childhood with supramalleolar tibial osteotomy.

Knee Management

Surgical treatment of the knee is uncommonly necessary if aggressive therapy is performed early in life to eliminate contractures. Occasionally, posterior soft tissue releases are necessary to relieve residual flexion contractures. Rarely, anterior transfer of functioning hamstrings to augment quadriceps function is considered or quadriceps tendon lengthening to treat an hyperextension deformity is needed.

Foot and Ankle Management

The two major deformities that are treated in childhood are calcaneous deformity and valgus deformity of the hindfoot or ankle. Calcaneous can be a devastating deformity if untreated as the excessive weight bearing on the insensate heel results in intractable ulceration. This deformity occurs in low lumbar and occasionally high sacral lesions with strong ankle dorsiflexion and absent or weak plantar flexion. Posterior transfer of the anterior tibialis tendon through the interosseous membrane to the calcaneous with or without tendo Achilles tenodesis has been successful in avoiding and treating this deformity. Prophylactic transfer can be performed as soon as accurate muscle grading can be done, around 3 years of age. A higher percentage of functioning tendons can be expected if transfer is delayed until the patient is 4 or 5 years old; an argument can, therefore, be made for waiting if a severe deformity is not developing. Anterior tibialis not under voluntary control should be released rather than transferred since an equinus deformity often develops with time. Neglected calcaneocavus feet are treated with triple arthrodesis in preadolescence or adolescence.

Valgus deformity can result in unacceptable weight bearing causing pressure sores or difficulty with shoeing. One must distinguish between subtalar valgus and ankle valgus with a wedge-shaped epiphysis as either may exist or both may coexist. Standing radiographs of the ankle are necessary to assess ankle valgus. Ankle valgus is treated with osteotomy or medial physeal stapling with good results reported for both if proper indications are followed. Five to 10 degrees of overcorrection into varus are generally necessary to compensate for recurrences or for subtalar valgus. If valgus is confined to the hindfoot, extraarticular subtalar arthrodesis is commonly recommended, although the complication rate is high. Children near adolescence can be treated with a subtalar or triple arthrodesis depending on the conformation of the entire foot.

Final Comments

Although much orthopaedic surgery is geared to optimizing walking functioning, one must remain cognizant that independent, productive living is the goal for these patients. A strikingly high number of patients with good walking ability and normal intelligence fail to gain independence in living apart from their families and fail to gain regular employment. The entire team of treating physicians, therapists, and social workers should keep this goal foremost for patients for whom independence is a reasonable goal.

ARTHROGRYPOSIS MULTIPLEX CONGENITA

Arthrogryposis (curved joint) multiplex congenita (AMC) is a clinical syndrome characterized by multiple joint contractures present at birth. A dichotomy has developed in definition of this problem between orthopaedic surgeons, on the one hand, and child neurologists and geneticists, on the other. Child neurologists and geneticists view arthrogryposis as a physical sign that has multiple prenatal etiologies, including brain disease, spinal cord disorders, peripheral nerve disease, myopathy, connective tissue disease, and congenital skin disorders. Orthopaedists would exclude many of these disorders from the typical syndrome of arthrogryposis multiplex congenita.

The severly involved patient with this syndrome is born with equinovarus feet; knee flexion contracture; hip flexion contractures with or without hip dislocation; scoliosis; internal rotation contracture of the shoulders; elbow flexion contracture; wrist flexion, pronation, and ulnar deviation; and finger and thumb contractures. These typical deformities are not present in all patients. Upper and lower extremity involvement alone may present or may predominate. The deformities are usually symmetric and are accompanied by limitation of motion, muscle atrophy, and glossy skin with absent creases (Fig. 6-15). The reason for recognizing the different perspectives of orthopaedists, neurologists, and geneticists is to avoid communication problems that may arise in clinically assessing these children and also in understanding differences in etiology and pathogenesis presented in the literature of different specialities.

Etiology

The common thread of all disorders resulting in the physical sign of contracted joints with limited motion is limited movement of affected joints early in fetal life. More than 150 genetic and nongenetic conditions may produce this physical finding.

The most common cause of the syndrome designated AMC in the orthopaedic literature is absence of or decrease in numbers of anterior horn cells in the areas of spinal cord supplying affected body parts. This has been shown in numerous autopsy studies. Given the increase in incidence of new cases seen in the 1960s, and the recent decrease, an environmental factor (such as a virus) has been suggested as the cause of anterior horn cell death. A much smaller number of patients with the typical clinical syndrome have primary myopathic rather than neuropathic etiology. The classic neuropathic AMC seems to be a nongenetic disorder. Many other causes of arthrogryposis (the sign) have a genetic component including the myopathic type, which is often a variant of congenital muscular dystrophy, although nonprogressive myopathic AMC occurs.

Evaluation of all patients with arthrogryposis by a childrens neurologist and geneticist is appropriate. Work-up may include EMGs, nerve conduction velocity, muscle enzymes, MRI of the spinal cord and brain, and muscle or nerve biopsy. As specific a diagnosis as possible should be made in each patient with this sign for optimal treatment and for accurate prognostication and counseling of families.

The remainder of this section deals with the typical neuropathic clinical syndrome recognizing that firm boundaries are lacking, and multiple etiologies of even this typical pattern probably exist.

Initial Management

In addition to making a specific diagnosis, the initial evaluation involves the search for other congenital anomalies. Musculoskeletal anomalies such as

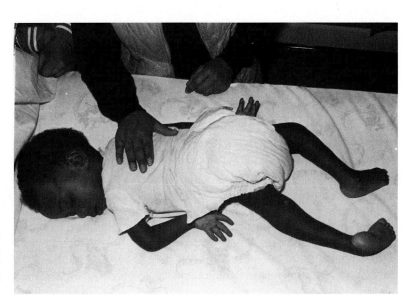

FIGURE 6-15. Nineteen-month-old boy with arthrogryposis multiplex congenital. Note equinovarus foot, knee and elbow flexion contractures, and wrist flexion and ulnar deviation.

Klippel-Feil syndrome, Sprengel deformities, and congenital scoliosis are seen. The most common nonskeletal deformities involve the genitourinary system, craniofacial deformities, and occasional cardiac defects.

Physical examination reveals the extent and severity of limb contractures. Radiographs are helpful in identifying teratologic congenital dislocation of the hip and in assessing scoliosis, which, though often present at birth, is rarely congenital in the sense that vertebral failure of formation or segmentation is present.

Active treatment in the first year of life consists mainly of correction of foot deformities and unilateral hip dislocation and vigorous physical therapy. The first year of life or so is the only time during which an increase in range of motion is likely to occur. Vigorous passive range of motion is begun before discharge from hospital and is taught to the family. Regular checkups to monitor progress and performance by a physical therapist are helpful in maintaining the program. Later in infancy, part-time splinting may be used to maintain new gains in motion. Occasionally, serial plaster casts are used to improve joint position such as severe knee flexion, but this technique should be used cautiously as loss of arc of motion may occur. Whatever range of motion is obtainable in the first year or so of life is likely to be the ultimate range of motion. Soft tissue releases and osteotomies later in life can change the arc through which the motion acts but rarely increase motion. Soft tissue releases are sometimes necessary in the first year of life if no progress is being made by physical therapy with a joint contracture (usually knee or hip) certain to limit function in the future.

Later Management

Foot Management

Clubfoot is the most common foot deformity and may present with varying amounts of equinus, varus, cavus, and adductus. The most predictable treatment of these extremely rigid feet is primary talectomy with concomitant posterior release as needed to obtain a plantigrade foot. Cast immobilization for about 4 months followed by indefinite bracing with an AFO is usually necessary to avoid recurrent deformity. Soft tissue releases are occasionally successful in milder feet but aggressive release with total correction is necessary to avoid recurrence.

Congenital vertical talus can be managed two ways. Because these feet are plantigrade and correc-

tion will not improve suppleness, some authors manage these expectantly and perform surgery (usually triple arthrodesis) in late childhood or adolescence if the prominent talar head causes skin problems or pain. Others recommend surgical correction in infancy followed by prolonged immobilization to maintain position.

Residual deformities in older children and adolescence are treated by bony surgery. Triple arthrodesis is used to correct residual hindfoot deformity, and midtarsal wedge osteotomies are useful in isolated cavus.

Knee Management

Because most children with AMC are upright walkers, knee flexion contracture is treated to obtain a stable lower extremity for weight bearing. Flexion contracture of more than 20 degrees in the young child is treated with hamstring lengthening or release and posterior knee capsulotomy with cruciate release as needed. Often the neurovascular bundle limits correction. If so, some increase in extension can be gained by serial casting after surgical release. Caution must be taken not to subluxate the knee joint during these maneuvers.

An extension osteotomy of the supracondylar area of the femur can effectively change the arc of motion and gain full extension. In young children, the deformity often recurs, requiring repeated osteotomy. For this reason, osteotomies should be delayed until near skeletal maturity if possible.

Extension contracture of the knee generally do not require treatment in ambulatory patients. Patients with significant hyperextension are treated with quadriceps lengthening and radical anterior knee release with prolonged postoperative bracing.

Hip Management

Both hip joint stability and contracture must be considered. Bilateral hip dislocations are usually high and stiff, and generally no treatment is recommended. Although stable relocation of both hips through open reduction is possible, the risks of creating a unilateral dislocation or of increasing hip stiffness through multiple operations have lead most authors away from aggressive management. Unilateral hip dislocation, however, should be reduced as unacceptable pelvic obliquity, and hence scoliosis may occur. Open reduction is usually necessary, and the medial approach has been reported to give less stiffness than the anterolateral approach in these hips.

Hip flexion contracture is the most difficult lower extremity contracture to correct. Radical soft tissue release often gives less correction than desired, and recurrence is common especially if there is residual knee flexion. Subtrochanteric femoral osteotomy corrects position, but recurrence is common if performed at an early age.

Spine Management

Scoliosis occurs in about 20% of patients. The curves are often present at birth, and most are noted by 5 years of age. The most common curve is thoracolumbar and is associated with hip contractures and pelvic obliquity. Treatment of pelvic obliquity can slow or halt progression in some mild curves. Some patients develop typical paralytic curves with a long C-shaped curve. Bracing is used to slow progression in the young child; however, many, if not most, require surgical spinal stabilization.

Lower Extremity Selection for Treatment

Not all patients with AMC will be ambulators. Identification of nonambulators is important as surgery to place lower extremity joints in a weight-bearing position may hinder sitting in this group of patients. Ambulators in general must have hip extensor strength of grade 4, quadriceps strength of grade 3, or crutchable upper extremities to substitute for weakness. Furthermore, those patients with weak quadriceps and hip extensors need to have less than 20-degree contracture at knee and less than 30-degree flexion contracture at hips so that bracing and crutches can be effective substitutes for the weak muscles.

Upper Extremity Management

Upper extremity surgery should be delayed until the child's functional abilities with the existing arm deformities are clear. Despite contractures, children often develop adaptive strategies that allow independence in activities of daily living. These strategies can be compromised by ill-conceived surgeries.

Shoulder and elbow deformities should be assessed together as both joints are responsible for the positioning of the hand in space. Getting the hand to the face and the perineurium are primary concerns with crutch usage and wheelchair usage being considered when appropriate.

Shoulder internal rotation deformity is most definitely treated with a proximal humeral derotation osteotomy in the older child. Soft tissue release of the pectoralis major, subscapularis, and shoulder capsule may be attempted in young children, but recurrence is frequent.

Flexion contracture of the elbow usually results in an acceptable position for function and does not require treatment. Extension contracture, however, prohibits getting the hand to the mouth, and correction on one side is often indicated. Posterior capsulotomy and triceps lengthening have been successful in gaining a flexed elbow. If adaptive changes in joint surface have occurred (usually not until adolescence) a supracondylar flexion osteotomy can be done. Flexion power to the elbow can be supplied by transfer of the triceps, pectoralis major, or Steindler flexor plasty depending on the pattern of weakness.

Wrist deformity is usually flexion, pronation, and ulnar deviation. If there is no or minimal hand function, this deformity can be accepted, and the backs of the hands are used in a pincer movement for grasp. If a functional hand exists, a proximal row carpectomy with or without fusion improves wrist position. Soft tissue release alone usually fails.

Hand function is difficult to improve by capsulotomies and tendon lengthening. Usually the fingers that seem to require these procedures are sufficiently stiff so that no significant functional benefit occurs. Correcting a thumb-in-palm deformity may often improve grasp capability. Adductor pollicis release and web space widening accomplish this goal.

MUSCULAR DYSTROPHIES

Definition

This group of disorders is defined by the documented or presumed etiology of primary muscle disease. Furthermore, they are hereditary disorders whose cardinal feature is progressive muscle degeneration and weakness. The explosion of knowledge occurring through the application of molecular biology techniques to hereditary conditions will probably alter and refine the classification schemes currently in use. Table 6-4 shows a conventional classification of the muscular dystrophies. This section discusses those disorders that most commonly present for orthopaedic evaluation.

Duchenne and Becker Muscular Dystrophy

These two forms of muscular dystrophy will be considered together because they have similar etiologies and evaluation, although the clinical courses of the

TABLE 6-4.
Muscular Dystrophies

Duchenne muscular dystrophy
Becker muscular dystrophy
Limb-girdle muscular dystrophy
Facioscapulohumeral muscular dystrophy
Myotonic dystrophy
Oculopharyngeal muscular dystrophy
Congenital muscular dystrophy
Distal muscular dystrophy

Becker type is much milder. Both types are generally X-linked recessive disorders; however, rare autosomal recessive Duchenne occurs. New mutations in mother or child account for 30% of Duchenne muscular dystrophy. Duchenne type occurs in 30 of 100,000 male births and Becker type is about one tenth as common.

Etiology

Discovery of the cause of these two disorders is a triumph of molecular genetics and molecular biology. Using genetic linkage techniques researchers identified the area of the X chromosome containing the defective gene. It was then possible to determine the product of this gene, which is a large protein called dystrophin. This protein seems to be a structural protein that is localized to the sarcolemma (surface membrane of muscle cells).

Dystrophin is absent in most patients with Duchenne muscular dystrophy and is structurally altered or reduced in patients with Becker muscular dystrophy. Both clinical and animal exceptions to a direct correlation of dystrophin levels and evident progressive muscular dystrophy exist, so that a complete understanding of causation is not yet in hand. Rapid progress in understanding the biochemical basis of these disorders can be expected, however.

The knowledge of gene location has greatly improved the ability to perform accurate and sensitive detection of carriers and affected individuals as well as prenatal diagnosis. The accuracy of prediction using these techniques is largely dependent on the type of gene abnormality presented (eg, deletion versus point mutation). These techniques have supplanted the present use of muscle biopsy for diagnosis and creatinine kinase assay for carrier determination in most cases.

Clinical Features

DUCHENNE MUSCULAR DYSTROPHY. A mild delay in walking often occurs, but a significant gait abnormality is not evident until age 3 or 4. Weakness of the hip girdle muscle precedes shoulder girdle weakness (Fig. 6-16). Distal muscles are clinically spared early in the disease. The initial gait disturbance consists of a waddling gait with increased lumbar lordosis. Difficulty climbing stairs and rising from the floor is noted. Weakness of the gluteus maximus results in Gower sign usually by age 5 or 6. This sign consists of the patient pushing off from the floor with his arms followed by pushing the trunk erect by stabilizing the arms against the anterior thigh.

Loss of muscle mass in the legs and shoulder girdle and diminished or absent reflexes are evident before age 10. Muscle enlargement (pseudohypertrophy) is seen in the calf and occasionally in the quadriceps and other individual muscles.

Fixed equinus or equinovarus of the feet and ankles develop, which help lock the knees in extension. There is increased lumbar lordosis with the arms carried posteriorly, which shifts the weight-bearing line posterior to the hip joint. This posture seems to be an attempt to decrease the stress on the weak quadriceps and gluteus maximus by shifting the weight

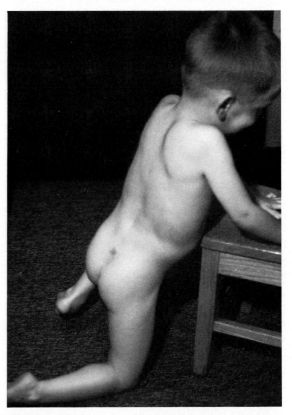

FIGURE 6-16. A 2½-year-old boy with Duchenne muscular dystrophy attempting to rise from the floor. He "climbs" up the chair using his arms because of weak lower extremities.

bearing line so that ligaments are used rather than muscle to maintain joint stability. This precarious balance is usually lost by age 9, and bracing is necessary to substitute for the weak quadriceps. Further ambulation often occurs until about 12 years of age by which time most patients require a wheelchair.

Teenage patients develop progressive weakness of arms and trunk muscles. Median age of death is 18 years, with only 25% reaching age 21. Death results from pulmonary compromise most often with cardiomyopathy being the primary cause of death in a small percentage. Pulmonary compromise can be hastened by scoliosis that often begins before ambulation ceases but may progress rapidly after wheelchair mobility is begun.

BECKER MUSCULAR DYSTROPHY. Becker muscular dystrophy resembles Duchenne but has a later onset of symptoms and much slower progression. Symptom onset is usually in the second decade. The age of onset and rate of progression is variable but runs true within a family. Most patients lose walking ability in the late teens or early 20s. Approximately 50% survive to 40 years of age.

Diagnosis

If the disease is suspected, assay of muscle enzymes is performed as these leak from the diseased muscle cells. Creatinine kinase is most useful and is elevated in Duchenne type and less elevated in Becker type and other muscular dystrophies. Muscle biopsy is used to confirm the diagnosis of myopathy but does not in general discriminate different types of muscular dystrophy. In many patients, the molecular assay for dystrophin gene abnormality is diagnostic. When biopsy is necessary, the muscle can be assayed for dystrophin, which is absent or reduced in these disorders. Improved diagnostic capabilities from peripheral blood using molecular genetic technique is to be expected in the near future. Muscle biopsy and EMGs are typical of myopathic disease but not diagnostic of a specific disorder.

Orthopaedic Treatment of Duchenne Muscular Dystrophy

Orthopaedic treatment consists of minimizing and treating contractures, bracing to compensate for weakness, and scoliosis management. Avoiding contractures consists of physical therapy, splinting, and positioning. The most common contractures are equinus of the ankles and abduction with flexion of the hips. Passive stretching programs have shown

limited benefits but are a standard part of most treatment programs. Night splinting with AFOs can significantly delay the onset of Achilles tendon contractures and minimize their severity. Similarly, a standing program and a platform to maintain neutral ankle position while sitting (especially at school) can minimize this contracture. AFOs alone should not be used in ambulatory patients while walking because falls will increase as a result of loss of compensatory knee extension.

Bracing with knee-ankle-foot orthoses can prolong walking when quadriceps weakness results in difficulty maintaining upright posture. If contractures are present, they must be surgically released. Choosing the timing for surgery can be difficult. When walking becomes labored and long leg braces are thought to be necessary, surgery should be done if significant contractures are present. Care must be taken with anesthesia as these patients are at increased risk for malignant hyperthermia.

Achilles tendon tightness is treated with percutaneous tenotomy, open TAL, or TAL and posterior tibial tendon transfer to the dorsum of the foot. Iliotibial band contracture is released by percutaneous tenotomy proximally and distally or by open Ober procedure proximally and Yount fasciotomy distally. Hip flexor release is also needed on occasion. Regardless of the specific procedure employed, mobilization must be rapid, and aggressive or loss of strength will preclude walking altogether. The patients are immobilized in a light cast and begun standing within 24 hours of surgery. Walking in parallel bars is to begin on day 2 or 3. By the fifth postoperative day, patients should be walking with a walker. Transition from casts to braces may necessitate a return to aggressive therapy to avoid loss of function.

Scoliosis develops in most (up to 95%) patients and usually progresses after upright walking ceases. Uncontrollable progression decreases respiratory reserve and can hasten pulmonary death. Furthermore, curves can become severe enough to prohibit sitting and can result in painful postures. For all these reasons, aggressive treatment of scoliosis is indicated. Brace treatment is not recommended as this method merely slows curve progression at best and may delay recognition of the need for surgery past the point where respiratory function is adequate to allow surgery. In general, progressive curves of more than 20 to 30 degrees should be surgically stabilized by segmental wiring techniques. Fusion to L5 is sufficient except in the severest curves with pelvic obliquity in which fusion to the sacrum may be necessary.

Limb-Girdle Muscular Dystrophy

Limb-girdle muscular dystrophies consist of several distinct disorders characterized by predominately proximal muscle weakness and autosomal recessive inheritance. Many cases appear to be sporadic. Autosomal dominant inheritance has rarely been reported. Symptom onset is usually in the second or third decades with difficulty climbing stairs and rising from the floor. Gower sign is present and weakness of all the gluteal muscles and iliopsoas are present. Progression is slow with backache a prominent complaint. Leg muscles become involved later, and the Achilles tendon often becomes contracted with resultant equinus or equinovarus. Many patients loose walking ability by age 30. Neck flexor and extensor weakness and weakness and atrophy of pectoral muscles, deltoid, biceps, and triceps develop. Serum creatinine kinase is elevated, and muscle biopsy and EMG show typical myopathic abnormalities. Surgical correction of lower extremity contractures, especially about the ankle and foot are sometimes necessary.

Facioscapulohumeral Dystrophy

This autosomal dominant muscular dystrophy varies widely in severity amongst affected individuals. Onset of symptoms varies between 5 and 25 years of age. Typically, onset of symptoms is toward the end of the first decade or the beginning of the second decade. Weakness is first apparent in facial muscles followed by the shoulder girdle with scapular winging and inability to elevate the arms. Weakness of biceps and triceps develops. Some patients develop more distal weakness of wrists and fingers. The most severely affected patients have leg involvement with foot drop. Scoliosis may develop and require surgical stabilization. Fusion of the scapula to the thorax improves shoulder motion in appropriately selected patients.

Myotonic Muscular Dystrophy

Myotonia is the inability to relax a contracted muscle in a normal time span. Limb muscle and fascial muscles are commonly involved and myotonia is exacerbated by cold and fatigue. Most conditions with myotonia are autosomal dominant and run a wide spectrum of age at onset and severity. These clinical disorders include myotonic muscular dystrophy, myotonic chondrodystrophy, paramyotonia congenita, and myotonia congenita.

Myotonic dystrophy occurs in 2 to 5 per 100,000 persons. Clinical findings may appear in neonates or develop in later childhood or adult life. Some patients have minimal findings throughout life. A wide spectrum of severity within a family is common. An affected neonate's mother may have mild signs of which she is unaware. This represents the genetic phenomenon of "anticipation."

An affected neonate may have arthrogryposis (the sign) or foot deformities alone. Facial weakness and difficulty with sucking and swallowing are common. Weakness of hip muscles causes gait disturbance in the second year of life and more distal weakness then ensues.

Presentation later in childhood is usually with the complaint of stiffness. Difficulty opening the clenched fist is typical. Percussion of tongue, thenar eminence, or deltoid often elicits myotonic contraction.

Adolescents often show ptosis and dysarthria as well as stiffness. Regardless of age of presentation, patients exhibit a large variation in rate of progression and amount of weakness. When clinically suspected, EMG and muscle biopsy are used to support the diagnosis. EMG show high frequency, periodic discharge with the classic "dive bomber" sound. Muscle biopsy is variable but often shows atrophy of type I muscle fibers and hypertrophy of type II fibers. Improved diagnosis and classification is likely in the near future using molecular genetic techniques. The gene for myotonic dystrophy is located in chromosome 19. Localization of the gene region on chromosome 19 with subsequent gene product identification seems likely.

Orthopaedic management usually consists of treating foot deformities and bracing to compensate for weakness. Neonates may have a rigid clubfoot deformity or a more supple deformity of equinus, cavus, or varus. Serial cast correction is attempted, but rigid deformities require posteromedial release before walking age. The supple deformities may be correctable with casts, but recurrence is common, and prolonged splinting or soft tissue release is often necessary. Older children and adolescents most commonly develop cavovarus deformities because of anterior compartment weakness. When supple, soft tissue procedures such as TAL with anterior tibial tendon transfer laterally, or anterior transfer of the posterior tibial tendon are indicated depending on pattern of weakness. Plantar releases may be needed for cavus. Bony procedures are reserved for rigid deformities in older patients.

Spinal Muscular Atrophy

Spinal muscular atrophy is a degenerative disorder of the anterior horn cells and cranial motor nerve nuclei. Autosomal recessive inheritance is the rule, although exceptions exist. A clinical spectrum of severity exists ranging from death before 2 years old to survival with walking ability into adulthood. In general, the earlier the onset of symptoms the severer and more rapid the progression. An infantile (Werdnig-Hoffman disease) and juvenile (Kugelberg-Welander disease) form are described, and subgroups of the infantile form have been defined to assist with prognostication and planning programs of management. A continuum of severity exists, however, with no clear boundaries between types and subtypes (Fig. 6-17).

Infantile Spinal Muscular Atrophy

GROUP I. This group demonstrates weakness within the first 2 months of life. Severe weakness of proximal muscle groups and intercostal muscles is present. Deep tendon reflexes are absent. Ability to sit, roll over, or stand is rare. Most of these children do not survive beyond 3 years of age.

GROUP II. These infants show stigmata of the disease between 2 and 12 months. Disease severity is less and progression is slower than in group one patients. Proximal muscle weakness is present and is greater in the lower extremities than upper extremities. Distal deep tendon reflexes may be present. Some children learn to sit but almost none walk. Death usually occurs by 7 years, but a few patients have a slowly progressive course and survive into the 20s.

GROUP III. Children in this group develop the disease between 1 and 2 years of age. Good head control and sitting ability are attained with some able to walk though with a waddling gait. Walking ability is usually lost by the second decade.

Juvenile Spinal Muscular Atrophy

Weakness develops between 2 and 17 years of age in this group. With later onset, loss of abilities is the presenting complaint, such as loss of ability to run, jump, and climb stairs foot over foot. Legs are affected before arms, with quadriceps weakness most evident early. Slow progression is the rule, with loss of walking ability occurring between 8 years of age and more than 20 years after symptom onset.

Diagnosis

Diagnosis of all types is made by EMG findings of denervation with fibrillation potentials and loss of motor units. Muscle biopsy shows neuropathic muscle atrophy.

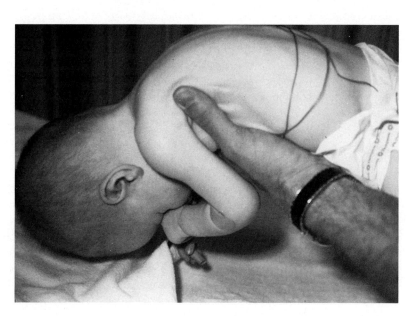

FIGURE 6-17. Five-month-old boy with Werdnig-Hoffmann–type spinal muscular atrophy. Weakness of neck and trunk muscles is shown.

Orthopaedic Management

Spinal deformity is the major orthopaedic problem and occurs in almost all children with infantile types and half the patients with juvenile-type spinal muscular atrophy. Curves are most commonly thoracolumbar, but thoracic spine involvement is often seen. Progressive curves can cause decreasing respiratory reserve, difficulty with seating, decubital ulcers, and pain. A spinal orthosis, usually of the total contact type, is used for early scoliosis to slow or halt progression until sufficient growth has occurred so that surgical spinal stabilization can be considered. A spinal orthosis is also indicated to maintain sitting posture in some patients without a structural scoliosis. A total contact orthosis can worsen respiratory status by adding external restrictive component in some children. These patients should be supported by trunk bolsters built into their wheelchairs.

As might be expected, the mortality and morbidity can be significant from spinal instrumentation and fusion in these patients. Mortality is most related to respiratory function; sufficient reserve to withstand surgery must be present. Morbidity is largely due to loss of functional abilities, which occurs in most patients, and problems with pseudoarthrosis and pain especially at the lumbosacral junction. A careful discussion of advantages and disadvantages must be made with each patient and family before surgery.

Contracture of hips, knees, and ankles can create problems of positioning and occasionally pain in wheelchair patients. Avoidance of severe contractures is best with a program of physical therapy and night splinting as needed. Radical soft tissue release is occasionally necessary if contractures interfere with positioning, cause pain, or result in ulcers about the foot.

Lightweight knee-ankle-foot orthoses may prolong walking in some patients with sufficient retained upper extremity strength to use crutches or a walker.

FRIEDREICH ATAXIA

This is the most common of the spinal cerebellar degenerative diseases. Autosomal recessive inheritance is most common but autosomal dominant and X-linked varieties occur. The variation in inheritance pattern suggests that more then one condition is subsumed under this clinical diagnosis.

Friedreich ataxia usually presents between 5 and 10 years of age, although adult onset may occur. Gait difficulty characterized by ataxia is the presenting complaint. The gait is wide based, lurching, and slow. The Romberg test is positive. Next to develop are upper extremity in-coordination and dysarthria. Cavus foot deformity is often present initially but if not almost always develops. Deep tendon reflexes are absent and variable amounts of weakness, atrophy, and upper motor neuron signs are present because of variable spinal cord degeneration. Gross and fine motor coordination and posterior column function (position sense and vibratory sense) are severely affected. Cerebellar dysfunction is probably the major cause of loss of walking ability, although weakness is contributory. Clawing of the hand is present in some patients because of intrinsic weakness. Scoliosis of varying severity occurs in almost all patients. Cardiomyopathy and diabetes mellitus are common associated disorders. Cardiac disease is the most common cause of death in affected persons. Loss of walking ability by age 30 and death before 40 years of age is typical.

Degeneration is widespread in the nervous system. The spinal cord is small with degeneration of the posterior columns, spinocerebellar tracts, and corticospinal tracts. Lumbar and sacral nerve dorsal roots and ganglia are decreased in number and show signs of degeneration. The cerebellum shows varying amounts and distributions of degeneration.

Diagnosis is made by the presence of typical clinical findings. Nerve conduction velocities show decrease in sensory nerve action potential with motor nerve sparing. Muscle biopsy shows neuropathic changes in muscle fibers.

Orthopaedic Management

The scoliosis in Freidreich ataxia seems to behave like idiopathic scoliosis in many respects. Curve patterns typical of idiopathic scoliosis are seen and progression depends on severity of curve and maturity of the patient. The effectiveness of brace treatment has been questioned, but bracing is probably appropriate for small, progressive curves in immature patients. Curves of less than 40 degrees at maturity do not require stabilization, whereas curves of more than 60 degrees should be stabilized. Forty- to 60-degree curves represent a gray area as in idiopathic scoliosis and surgical decisions are based on age, progression, and philosophy of the surgeon.

Foot deformity management is determined by pattern of weakness, severity of deformity, and age of the patient. AFOs are used in supple deformities in young patients to maintain position and to treat the occasional foot drop. Planter releases and calcaneal osteotomies are recommended for progressive cavovarus and cavus deformities before sufficient adaptive changes have occurred to make triple arthrodesis necessary. Despite soft tissue procedures, progression requiring fusion may be necessary.

It must be remembered that the immobilization period following spinal surgery or major foot surgery may result in loss of walking ability in a significant number of patients.

HEREDITARY MOTOR SENSORY NEUROPATHIES

These are a group of peripheral neuropathies in which signs and symptoms of motor nerve degeneration dominate the clinical picture. This is in contradistinction to the group of hereditary sensory neuropathies whose major manifestations are sensory with indifferences to pain resulting in foot ulceration and Charcot joints. The most common hereditary motor and sensory neuropathies (types I and II) show prominent peroneal weakness and atrophy and were previously called Charcot-Marie-Tooth disease.

TYPE I. This disorder presents in the first or second decade with foot deformity and clumsiness. Initially the foot deformity is supple with mild cavus and claw toes. With disease progression, there is increasing weakness of peronei and the ankle dorsiflexors. An increasingly severe cavovarus foot develops (Fig. 6-18). Equinus is present in varying degrees depending on the extent of anterior compartment weakness. Intrinsic wasting in the hands commonly develops. Peripheral nerves may be palp-

ably enlarged. Little sensory abnormality is present in childhood, but some loss of light touch and posterior column sensation develop in adulthood.

The disorder is inherited at an autosomal dominant trait. Nerve conduction velocity is slowed in all peripheral nerves.

TYPE II. The clinical characteristics are similar to type I disease except that much more wasting of the legs is present resulting in a "stork-leg" appearance (Fig. 6-19). Also, there is no hypertrophy of peripheral nerves. Severer weakness of the triceps surae muscles may result in a calcaneocavus deformity rather than the typical caneovarus deformity of type I and many type II patients.

This disorder is inherited by an autosomal dominant pattern. Motor nerve conduction velocities are normal or slightly slow with a reduction in amplitude of motor nerve action potentials in the affected legs.

TYPE III. This is a hypertrophic neuropathy occurring in infancy generally called Dejerine-Sottas disease. Delayed motor development is noted in infancy. Although walking skills develop, patients usually loose this ability in the 20s and 30s. Sensory deficit can be pronounced and enlarged peripheral nerves are often palpable. Cavus foot, drop foot, and scoliosis are common.

This disorder is uncommon and inherited as an autosomal recessive disorder. Nerve conduction velocity are extremely slow.

TYPE IV. This rare, autosomal recessive disease is commonly called Refsum disease. Elevated serum phytanic acid levels are diagnostic of this disease.

Onset of symptoms is in childhood or adoles-

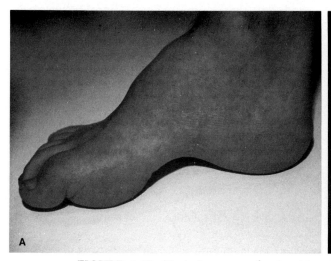
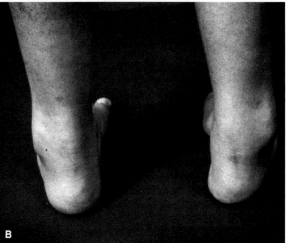

FIGURE 6-18. Typical cavovarus feet in a 14-year-old boy with Charcot-Marie-Tooth disease.

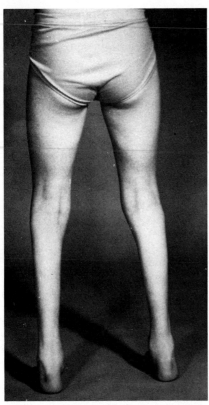

FIGURE 6-19. Typical "stork legs" in a patient with hereditary motor sensory neuropathy type II.

cence with both motor and sensory abnormalities. Associated problems include ataxia, deafness, cardiomyopathy, and lens opacity. Scoliosis, cavus, and equinus foot deformities may develop.

Other types of hereditary motor and sensory neuropathies have been classified but are similar to one of these four types with an associated finding of little concern to orthopaedic management. Molecular genetic investigation of these disorders will likely result in new classification in the coming years.

Orthopaedic Management

Type I and II disease have cavovarus foot as the common orthopaedic deformity. Because this problem affects most patients, we will consider only the treatment of cavovarus.

The pathogenesis of cavovarus deformity is uncertain. The two prominent theories are primary weakness of intrinsic muscles and primary weakness of extrinsic muscles. Regardless of the exact pathogenesis, the sequence of development of the deformity is clear. Fixed pronation of the forefoot develops first. This pronation is due to plantar flexion of the medial metatarsals, mainly the first. To set the pronated forefoot flat on the floor, the hindfoot must

slide into varus through the subtalar joint. The initially flexible hindfoot becomes fixed in varus with time. This deformity causes excessive weight bearing on the first metatarsal head and base of the fifth metatarsal. Furthermore, ankle instability with frequent inversion sprains may ensue.

Bracing is of little value in correcting or preventing progression in these disorders. An AFO is often necessary to treat foot drop in an otherwise corrected foot. Surgical treatment depends on the age of patient, pattern of muscle imbalance, severity of deformity, and, most important, on whether the hindfoot is flexible or fixed. Flexibility of hindfoot is assessed clinically by the Coleman block test. A block is placed under the heel and lateral foot so that the plantar flexed first metatarsal hangs free. If the hindfoot returns to neutral or valgus, it is supple. If varus remains, the hindfoot is fixed. Muscle balance is assessed by grading the ankle muscles and observing their apparent function in gait.

If the forefoot is fixed in pronation and the hindfoot is flexible, surgical treatment can usually correct the deformity without resorting to fusion. Occasionally, in a young child a radical plantar release followed by corrective serial casts may be sufficient. More commonly, the plantar-flexed first and sometimes second metatarsal must be elevated. This is done by dorsal lateral wedge osteotomies at the base of the metatarsal or by osteotomy of the first cuneiform. Transfer of the peroneus longus into the peroneus brevis can eliminate the tendency of the peroneus longus to flex and pronate the first metatarsal. The tight plantar structures are released by plantar fasciotomy alone or radical plantar release as needed. Clawing of great toe is reduced by recession of the extensor hallucis longus into the first metatarsal neck and suture of the stump of the extensor hallucis longus into the extensor hallucis brevis tendon or arthrodesis of the interphalangeal joint to prevent dropping of the distal phalanx. If lessor toe clawing is significant, the common toe extensors may be recessed.

If the hindfoot is rigid, a calcaneal osteotomy in addition to the preceding procedure may be satisfactory in cases of mild heel varus. More commonly, a triple arthrodesis is necessary, although the long-term results are less than perfect.

SYRINGOMYELIA

This is a degenerative disorder consisting of a slowly progressive cavity formation within the spinal cord. The cervical cord is most commonly affected followed

failed. No functional improvement was found because of hips being located. The worst function results by level were those having complications following hip surgery, mainly stiffness.

Bliss DG, Menelaus MD. The results of transfer of the tibialis anterior to the hell in patients who have a myelomeningocele. J Bone Joint Surg 1986;68A:1258.
A long-term follow-up of 46 transfers to avoid or treat the disabling calcaneus deformity resulting from triceps surae weakness. Several overcorrections requiring further surgery occurred, prompting the recommendation that spastic anterior tibial muscles not be transferred to the calcaneus.

Bunch WH, Hakala MW. Iliopsoas transfers in children with myelomeningocele. J Bone Joint Surg 1984;66A:224.
This article describes the results of iliopsoas transfer to the greater trochanter with adductor longus weakening. Good results with few complications are presented. The authors recommend this surgical procedure to balance muscle forces about the hip and maintain hip reduction.

Dias LS, Jasty MJ, Collins P. Rotational deformities of the lower limb in myelomeningocele. J Bone Joint Surg 1984;66A:215.
An excellent review of the treatment and complications of the common rotational deformities seen in ambulatory patients. Fifty children are described with 66 limbs treated. A significant number of complications occurred in tibial derotational osteotomies.

Feiwell E, Sahai D, Blatt T. The effect of hip reduction and function in patients with myelomeningocele. J Bone Joint Surg 1978;60A:169.
A study of 76 patients was done with 41 patients having had no surgery on the hip and 35 having had attempts to surgically stabilize the hip. No difference in functional abilities or pain was found regardless of whether the hip was located, subluxated, or dislocated. Complications from surgery occurred in 40% of patients. A level pelvis and free hip motion were important for function.

Hall P, Lindseth R, Campbell R, Kalsbeck J, DeSousa A. Scoliosis and hydrocephalus in myelocele patients: the effects of ventricular shunting. J Neurosurg 1979;50:174.
Progressive scoliosis may be due to shunt malfunction. The importance of neurologic examinations at each visit is stressed.

Hoffer MM, Feiwell E, Perry R, Perry J. Functional ambulation in patients with myelomeningocele. J Bone Joint Surg 1972;55A:137.
A review of 56 patients revealed no functional ambulators at the thoracic level and all functional ambulators at the sacral level. Lumbar level patient's walking abilities were affected by level (high versus low), age, mental retardation, lower extremity deformities, and social situation.

Hydemann JS, Gillespie R. Management of myelomeningocele kyphosis in the older child by kyphectomy and segmental spinal instrumentation. Spine 1986;12:37.
Short-term review of 12 patients treated by kyphectomy and segmental spinal instrumentation. The authors present a method of anterior fixation of the pelvis.

Lindseth RE. Treatment of the lower extremity in children paralyzed by myelomeningocele (birth to 18 months). AAOS Instruct Course Lect 1976;25:76.
A review of the early treatment of MMC with descriptive data on a large population of affected children. A simplified scheme for classifying the functional neurologic level is presented.

Lindseth RE, Stelzer L Jr. Vertebral excision for kyphosis in children with myelomeningocele. J Bone Joint Surg 1979;61A:699.
A method of kyphectomy is presented that allows continued growth of the remaining lumbar spine.

Malhotra D, Puri R, Owen R. Valgus deformity of the ankle in children with spina bifida aperta. J Bone Joint Surg 1984;66B:381.
A review of valgus deformity of the hindfoot that emphasizes that the valgus can exist in the ankle joint, subtalar joint, or both.

Mazur J, Menlaus MD, Dickens DRV, et al. Efficacy of surgical management for scoliosis in myelomeningocele: correction of deformity and alteration of functional status. J Pediatr Orthop 1986;6:568.
The authors evaluated the effect of spinal fusion in 49 patients with MMC. Combined anterior interbody fusion and posterior fusion and instrumentation to the sacrum gave the best results with respect to correction of the deformity; however, the ability to ambulate was adversely affected.

Mazur JM, Shurtleff D, Menelaus M, Colliner J. Orthopaedic management of high-level spina bifida. J Bone Joint Surg 1989;71A:56.
A superb interinstitutional study of two matched sets of patients: one group treated with early walking and the other with early wheelchair use. No major differences in activities of daily living were found. The early walkers were slightly more independent and had fewer fractures and pressure sores, but required more surgical procedures and hospitalization.

McMaster MJ. Anterior and posterior instrumentation and fusion of thoracolumbar scoliosis due to myelomeningocele. J Bone Joint Surg 1987;69B:20.
The author demonstrates improved posture and function in 21 of 23 patients with MMC scoliosis treated by anterior and posterior spinal instrumentation and fusion. Indications, operative techniques, and complications are discussed.

McMaster MJ. The long-term results of kyphectomy and spinal stabilization in children with myelomeningocele. Spine 1988;13:417.
A small series of 10 patients treated by kyphectomy and various forms of instrumentation for MMC kyphosis and followed for a mean of 7 years is presented. A long fusion from the midthoracic region to the sacrum was necessary to provide long-term stability and to prevent the development of thoracic lordosis. Operative techniques, risks, and complications are discussed.

Menelaus MB. The orthopaedic management of spina bifida cystica. New York, Churchill Livingstone, 1980.
An excellent single source for all aspects of the aggressive treatment of this disorder derived from a large clinical experience in Melbourne, Australia.

Menelaus MB. Talectomy for equinovarus deformity in arthrogryposis and spina bifida. J Bone Joint Surg 1971;53B:468.
This study followed 41 operations in 23 children an average of 2.5 years. Principles, indications, and techniques are discussed in this short follow-up that recommends talectomy for rigid neuromuscular clubfeet.

Osebold WR, Mayfield JK, Winter RB, Moe JH. Surgical treatment of paralytic scoliosis associated with myelomeningocele. J Bone Joint Surg 1982;64A:841.
Series discussing results and evolution of treatment of scoliosis in meningomyelocele.

Samuelsson L, Eklog O. Scoliosis in myelomeningocele. Acta Orthop Scand 1988;59:122.
Review of the prevalence, type, and magnitude of scoliosis in 163 patients with MMC. One hundred forty-three of the patients developed scoliosis, 21 (15%) of which were congenital in origin. Scoliosis severity increased with higher neurologic level (particularly above L3) and increasing age. Curve direction correlated with pelvic obliquity but not with hip discloation.

Sharrard WJW. The orthopaedic surgery of spina bifida. Clin Orthop 1973;92:195.
A general review of evaluation and treatment of MMC by an author with a large experience. Not all procedures described are popular now, but the approach is current.

Stillwell A, Menelaus MM. Walking ability in mature patients with spina bifida. J Pediatr Orthop 1983;3:184.
One third of high lumbar and thoracic level patients were community ambulators in this study. This is the only report with a large number of high level patients maintaining functional walking.

Trumble T, Banat JV, Roycroft JF, Curtis BH. Talectomy for equinovarus deformity in myelodysplasia. J Bone Joint Surg 1985;67A:21.

Nine patients had 17 feet corrected by talectomy. Follow-up averaged 7.4 years. Nearly all had good hindfoot correction, but one half had poor forefoot correction.

Yugue DA, Lindseth RE. Effectiveness of muscle transfers in mMyelomeningocele hips measured by radiographic images. J Pediatr Orthop 1982;2:121.
These authors recommend external oblique transfer to the greater trochanter and adductor transfer to the ischium to balance muscle forces about the hip. Good results are reported. The results of other procedures are described.

Arthrogryposis Multiplex Congenita

Daher YH, Lonstein JE, Winter RB, Moe JH. Spinal deformities in patients with arthrogryposis: a review of 16 patients. Spine 1985;10:609.
Literature review and results of management of a small group of patients with arthrogryposis.

Drummond DS, Cruess RL. The management of the foot and ankle in arthrogryposis in multiplex congenita. J Bone Joint Surg 1978;60B:96.
The range of treatment options is discussed. The use of primary talectomy in severe, rigid clubfoot deformities is emphasized. Follow-up to near skeletal maturity in most patients was available.

Drummond DS, MacKensie DA. Scoliosis in arthrogryposis: multiplex congenita. J Bone Joint Surg 1978;60B:96.
In 14 patients with scoliosis, both congenital scoliosis and long C-shaped curves were observed. Progression to severe and rigid curves was typical.

Gibson DA, Urs DNK. Arthrogryposis multiplex congenita. J Bone Joint Surg 1970;52B:494.
An excellent review of 114 patients treated during over a 15-year period. Multiple tables help organize the complex problems and treatment of these patients.

Herron LD, Westin GW, Dawson EG. Scoliosis in arthrogryposis: multiplex congenita. J Bone Joint Surg 1978;60A:293.
Scoliosis in 18 of 88 patients with AMC was found. The curves were commonly thoracolumbar and tended to progress early despite brace or cast treatment.

Hoffer MM, Swank S, Clark D, Teitge R. Ambulation in severe arthrogryposis. J Pediatr Orthop 1983;3:293.
This article outlines criteria for identifying nonambulators, which is important in developing a treatment plan for severely involved patients.

Lloyd-Roberts GC, Lettin AWF. Arthrogryposis multiplex congenita. J Bone Joint Surg 1970;52B:494.
A review of treatment and results in 52 patients. Treatment to gain functional range in the first year is emphasized. Soft tissue rather than bone procedures are recommended in the young child.

Menelaus MB. Talectomy for equinovarus deformity in arthrogryposis and spina bifida. J Bone Joint Surg 1971;53B:468.
An in-depth discussion of the indications, technique, and complications of talectomy. The results of 41 operations are reviewed, but follow-up is short (average of 2.5 years).

Williams P. The management of arthrogryposis. Orthop Clin North Am 1978;9:67.
An aggressive, early surgical approach is presented in detail.

Wynne-Davies R, Williams PF, O'Connor JCB. The 1960's epidemic of arthrogryposis multiplex congenita. J Bone Joint Surg 1981;63B:76.
This article describes the epidemiology of this disorder. Specifically, the high number of new cases presenting in the 1960s is documented. This suggests an environmental factor as part or all of the etiology.

Muscular Dystrophies

Bieber FR, Hoffman EP, Amos JA. Dystrophin analysis in Duchenne muscular dystrophy: use in fetal diagnostic and in genetic counseling. Am J Hum Genet 1989;45:362.
The use of dystrophin assay to identify an affected fetus and establish carrier status in the mother is presented. A discussion of the general use of dystrophin analysis is presented.

Brooke MH. A clinician's view of neuromuscular diseases. Baltimore, Williams & Wilkins, 1986.
A superb clincan's extensive experience with the muscular dystrophies and other neuromuscular disorders is detailed in this relatively short book.

Brooke MH, et al. Duchenne Muscular dystrophy: patterns of clinical progression and effects of supportive therapy. Neurology 1989;39:475.
A detailed analysis of 283 boys enrolled in a prospective study. Best available data on natural history and effects of intervention except surgery of lower extremities, which was not included in the analysis.

Gutmann DH, Fishbeck KH. Molecular biology of Duchenne and Becker's muscular dystrophy: clinical applications. Ann Neurol 1989;26:189.
A review of the research that lead to the identification of the defective gene product in Duchenne and Becker muscular dystrophy. Clinical implications are discussed.

Harper PS. Congenital myotonic dystrophy in Britain: I and II. Arch Dis Child 1975;50:505.
A description of congenital myotonic dystrophy. This disorder often requires treatment of foot deformities in infancy.

Hsu JD. The natural history of spine curvature progression in the nonambulatory Duchenne muscular dystrophy patient. Spine 1983;8:771.
When the curve progresses beyond 40 degrees, patients experience loss of sitting balance, decreased sitting tolerance, pain, decreased vital capacity, and need to use hands and arms to prop the body. Surgery is indicated to prevent these problems.

Kurz LT, Mubarak SJ, Schultz P, et al. Correlation of scoliosis and pulmonary function in Duchenne muscular dystrophy. J Pediatr Orthop 1953;3:347.
Forced vital capacity peaks at the age when standing ceases. It decreased by 4% each year and with each 10-degree increase in curvature. Early spinal instrumentation is indicated to slow rate of decline of forced vital capacity.

Miller F, Moseley CF, Koreska J, Levison H. Pulmonary function and scoliosis in Duchenne dystrophy. J Pediatr Orthop 1988;8:133.
Pulmonary function (forced vital capacity) declines most rapidly during adolescent growth spurt. Surgery does not influence the rate of pulmonary function deterioration.

Siegel IM. Diagnosis, management, and orthopaedic treatment of muscular dystrophy. AAOS Instruct Course Lect 1981;30:3.
A detailed review of the orthopaedic management of muscular dystrophy. Diagnostic information is largely outdated.

Smith AD, Koreska J, Moseley CF. Progression of scoliosis in Duchenne muscular dystrophy. J Bone Joint Surg 1989;71A:1066.
Longitudinal study of 51 boys with Duchenne muscular dystrophy followed until death without surgical treatment. All patients developed scoliosis, and severe curves led to difficulty sitting, skin breakdown, and pain. When the curve exceeded 35 degrees, the vital capacity usually was less than 40% of predicted. Spinal arthrodesis should be considered when walking becomes impossible.

Swaiman KF, Smith SA, Swaiman AF, eds. Progressive muscular dystrophies in pediatric neurology: principles and practice. St Louis, CV Mosby, 1989:1105.
A concise, readable review of clinical characteristics and diagnosis of these disorders.

Vignos PJ, Wagner MD, Kaplan JS, Spencer GE. Predicting the success of reambulation in patients with Duchenne muscular dystrophy. J Bone Joint Surg 1983;65A:719.
A detailed approach to the selection of patients for bracing and surgery is presented.

Weimann RL, Gibson DA, Moseley CF, Jones DC. Surgical stabilization of the spine in Duchenne muscular dystrophy. Spine 1982;8:776.
Results in 24 patients with Duchenne muscular dystrophy. Discussion of natural history, curve progression, and results of early surgery.

Spinal Muscular Atrophy

Apin H, Bowen JR, MacEwen GD, Hall JE. Spine fusion in patients with spinal muscular Atrophy. J Bone Joint Surg 1982;64A:1179.
A report of 22 surgical fusions. Bracing was ineffective in halting progression preoperatively. Several techniques were employed. A high rate of complications occurred.

Emery AEH. The nosology of the spinal muscular atrophies. J Med Genet 1971;8:481.
A dense review of the history and classification of these disorders with emphasis on the distinctions between these disorders and the progressive muscular dystrophies.

Evans GA, Drennan JC. Functional classification and orthopaedic management of spinal muscular atrophy. J Bone Joint Surg 1981;63B:516.
Fifty-four patients formed the basis of a functional grouping with differences in natural history and orthopaedic treatment among the groups. An explicit, detailed approach to the management of spine and lower extremity deformities is presented.

Schwentker EP, Gibson DA. The orthopaedic aspects of spinal muscular atrophy. J Bone Joint Surg 1976;58A:32.
Excellent review of orthopaedic problems in 50 patients with a mean age of 11.5 years. Scoliosis is the major problem with timing of surgery and complications discussed in detail. Loss of function is common after spinal stabilization. Release of lower extremity contractures is discussed.

Swaiman KF. Anterior horn cell and cranial motor neuron disease. In: Pediatric neurology: principles and practice. St Louis, CV Mosby, 1989:1086.
A brief, up-to-date review of the clinical characteristics, diagnosis, and pathology of these disorders.

Friedreich Ataxia

Cady RB, Bobeckko WP. Incidence, natural history, and treatment of scoliosis in Friedreich's ataxia. J Pediatr Orthop 1984;4:673.
This report on 42 patients found relentless progression even after skeletal maturity, suggesting a more typical neuromuscular scoliosis than suggested in the reference by Labelle and associates in patients with this disorder.

Chamberlain S, et al. Genetic homogeneity at the Freidreich ataxia locus on chromosone 9. Am J Hum Genet 1989;44:518.
Two populations with clinically different Freidreich ataxia (French Canadians and Acadians from Louisiana) were investigated by genetic linkage and found to have the same or nearly the same locus of gene abnormality on chromosome 9. This type of investigation will doubtless refine classification and improve prognostication in the future.

Labelle H, Tohme S, Duhaime M. Natural history of scoliosis in Friedrich's ataxia. J Bone Joint Surg 1986;68A:564.
A follow-up of 78 patients showing similar curve pattern and progression to that found in idiopathic scoliosis. No correlation of curve progression with weakness was found. Early age of disease onset and presence of scoliosis before puberty correlated with progressive curves. Virtually all patients had curves of 10 degrees or more.

Lovitt BL, Canale ST, Cooke AJ Jr, Gartland JJ. The role of foot surgery in progressive neuromuscular disorders in children. J Bone Joint Surg 1973;55A:1396.

This article reemphasizes the need for triple arthrodesis to obtain and maintain a stable foot in this disorder.

Makin M. The surgical management of Friedreich's ataxia. J Bone Joint Surg 1953;95A:425.
A review of 34 patients undergoing foot surgery with an average follow-up of 7.2 years. Good results are reported using subtalar or triple arthrodesis to stabilize the foot. Tendon transfers were used as needed for foot muscle balance and toe deformities.

Heredity Motor Sensory Neuropathies

Coleman SS. The cavo varus foot. In: Complex foot deformity in children. Philadelphia, Lea & Febiger, 1983.
A thoughtful and rational approach to treatment of cavo varus. It emphasizes the different treatment options available depending on whether the hindfoot is correctable or fixed in varus.

Jacobs JE, Carr CR. Progressive muscular atrophy of the peroneal type (Charcot-Marie-Tooth disease). J Bone Joint Surg 1950;32A:27.
Forty-five patients having had foot surgery are reviewed. Sixty-six good results and 23 unsatisfactory results were obtained using a combination of soft tissue and bony procedures.

Levitt RL, Canale ST, Cooke AJ, Gartland JJ. The role of foot surgery in progressive neuromuscular disorders in children. J Bone Joint Surg 1973;55A:1396.
Fifteen patients with Charcot-Marie-Tooth disease or Friedreich Ataxia with foot deformity were reviewed. Soft tissue and bone procedures other than triple arthrodesis failed to maintain correction.

Smith SA. Peripheral neuropathies in children. In: Swaiman KF, ed. Pediatric neurology: principles and practice. St Louis, CV Mosby, 1989:1110.
A brief review of the present classification of these disorders.

Wetmore RS, Drennan JC. Long-term results of triple arthrodesis in Charcot-Marie-Tooth disease. J Bone Joint Surg 1989;71A:417.
Thirty triple arthrodeses were followed an average of 21 years. Fourteen (47%) were considered poor results. Some bad results seem secondary to disease progression, but arthritis in adjacent joints and recurrent deformity were common. Attempts to maintain foot position without fusion seem warranted in light of these results.

Syringomyelia

Huebert HT, Mackinnon WB. Syringomyelia and scoliosis. J Bone Joint Surg 1969;51B:338.
A review of 43 patients with syringomyelia showed 27 (63%) with scoliosis. Site and severity of scoliosis is presented in tables. Risks of correction are noted.

Menezes AH, Smoker WRK, Dyste GN. Syringomyelia, Chiari malformations, and hydromyelia. In: Youmons J, ed. Neurological surgery, ed 3. Philadelphia, WB Saunders, 1990:1421.
A current review of the pathogenesis, diagnosis, and treatment of all types of syringomyelia and associated conditions—especially the Chiari malformation of the brain. Tables of symptoms and their frequency are helpful. Early treatment (less than 2 years of symptoms) gives much better outcomes.

Swaiman KF, ed. Anterior horn cells and cranial motor neuron disease. In: Pediatric neurology: principles and practice. St Louis, CV Mosby, 1989:1085.
A brief discussion of the pathogenesis and clinical characteristics of idiopathic syringomyelia.

Williams B. Orthopaedic features in the presentation of syringomyelia. J Bone Joint Surg 1979;61B:314.
A review of syringomyelia as it presents to the orthopaedist. Emphasis on pain, especially headache and neckache, as the initial symptom is made.

Turek's Orthopaedics: Principles and Their Application, Fifth Edition,
edited by Stuart L. Weinstein and Joseph A. Buckwalter.
J.B. Lippincott Company, Philadelphia, © 1994.

7

George S. Bassett

Idiopathic and Heritable Disorders

OSTEOGENESIS IMPERFECTA
ACHONDROPLASIA
PSEUDOACHONDROPLASTIC
    DYSPLASIA
SPONDYLOEPIPHYSEAL
    DYSPLASIA CONGENITA
DIASTROPHIC DYSPLASIA
METAPHYSEAL
    CHONDRODYSPLASIA
MULTIPLE EPIPHYSEAL
    DYSPLASIA

MORQUIO SYNDROME
NEUROFIBROMATOSIS
MARFAN SYNDROME
CONGENITAL LOWER LIMB
    DEFICIENCIES
PROXIMAL FEMORAL FOCAL
    DEFICIENCY
FIBULAR HEMIMELIA
TIBIAL HEMIMELIA

This chapter deals with a group of dissimilar disorders affecting the musculoskeletal system in either a generalized or regional fashion. Many of these conditions are associated with a variety of major medical problems in addition to the obvious orthopaedic abnormalities. Excluding the limb deficiencies, all of these conditions have a genetic basis. As is the case for all other areas of medicine and surgery, treatment is based on an accurate diagnosis and an understanding of the natural history of the disorder. Obtaining an accurate history and physical as well as analyzing appropriate radiographic studies is essential in the management of these disorders. Consultation with a clinical geneticist should be considered for most of these patients.

OSTEOGENESIS IMPERFECTA

Osteogenesis imperfecta is a group of genetic disorders affecting the connective tissues in a generalized fashion. The earliest clinical description of this disorder was given by Ekman in 1788 ("congenital osteomalacia"). Vrolik named this disorder "osteogenesis imperfecta." Looser distinguished two different types of osteogenesis imperfecta and described them as the "congenita" and "tarda" types. The classic triad of fragile bones, blue sclerae, and early deafness was described by Adair-Dighton in 1912. The predominant clinical manifestation of osteogenesis imperfecta is the increased susceptibility for fractures to occur. Apart from the osseous manifestations, individuals may also have blue sclerae, hearing deficiencies, peculiar dental abnormalities, growth disturbances, respiratory insufficiency, excessive sweating, and easy bruisability.

Attempts at classification have been fraught with the problem of extreme variability in both the phenotypic presentations and inheritance patterns of this group of disorders. The original division into congenita and tarda forms, based on age at presentation and severity of involvement, fails to consider the differing inheritance patterns. Furthermore, it is recognized that there is considerable overlap between these two forms with respect to age at presentation. There are some patients with the tarda form of osteogenesis imperfecta who have fractures at birth, whereas other patients with the severer congenita variety develop their first fractures after the neonatal period. Conversely, the classification system as proposed by Sillence divides osteogenesis imperfecta syndromes into four major groups (I through IV) with two of these groups transmitted as an autosomal dominant trait and the remaining two transmitted as an autosomal recessive trait. Within three of these groups, further subtypes have been delineated based on clinical and radiographic features. Despite these advances, geneticists still find it difficult to properly classify a given patient or pedigree. Nevertheless, the Sillence classification is the most widely used classification internationally and is extremely useful from both a counseling and treatment vantage point.

In the Sillence classification, type I is a milder form of osteogenesis imperfecta. It is transmitted as an autosomal dominant trait. Many of these patients have the classic Van der Hoeve syndrome with blue sclerae and significant early hearing loss in addition to the osseous changes. These patients typically develop fractures after reaching walking age, associated with falling episodes and other traumatic events. These fractures typically heal without deformity, and the incidence of fractures decreases in frequency after puberty. Radiographs reveal mild osteoporosis without severe deformity. Many of these patients have short stature, ligamentous laxity, mitral valve prolapse, and bruise easily. Type I patients are further divided into two subgroups based on the presence or absence of dentinogenesis imperfecta.

Sillence type II patients are the most severely involved with most infants dying in the perinatal period. These infants are extremely fragile and have multiple fractures in utero; growth retardation; micromelia; and an enlarged, soft cranium. Many infants are stillborn or delivered prematurely. Intracranial hemorrhage may result from attempts to deliver vaginally. Apart from multiple fractures at birth, these patients often have severe respiratory insufficiency resulting from involvement of the thoracic cage. Radiographically, the ribs have a beaded appearance from multiple in utero fractures. The long bones have a crumpled appearance with disruption of normal bony contours and severe osteoporosis. Type II is transmitted as either an autosomal dominant or recessive trait.

Sillence type III patients develop severe progressive deformities of the spine and extremities. By definition, according to the Sillence classification, this type is transmitted as an autosomal recessive trait. There are many patients, however, who are phenotypically identical to the type III patients originally described by Sillence with apparently normal pedigrees. Hence, their genetic defect is unknown and therefore cannot be classified as type III patients. Patients with type III osteogenesis imperfecta usually have in utero fractures secondary to severe osseous fragility. Many die in infancy and early childhood from respiratory insufficiency. Progressive deformities occur from multiple fractures with little or no antecedent trauma. Some patients have blue sclerae in infancy that changes to a normal white appearance with time. A severe growth disturbance is present in all patients, and most are nonambulatory.

Type IV patients may be distinguished from type I by their normal sclerae and severer osseous involvement. These patients have increased osteoporosis, bowing of the long bones, and increased susceptibility to fractures. Fractures may occur in utero, at birth, or with onset of walking. The rate of fractures usually decreases, however, with the onset of puberty. Many of these patients have short stature. This diminution in height is not as extensive as seen in the type III patients. Type IV patients are also subdivided into two groups based on the presence or absence of dentinogenesis imperfecta.

The osseous and connective tissue abnormalities in patients with osteogenesis imperfecta have been linked to a defect in type I collagen. Specific biochemical abnormalities of the type I collagen have been identified for all four groups of the Sillence classification. However, the defects identified thus far are variable, reflecting the heterogeneous genetic defect for osteogenesis imperfecta. The abnormalities include decreased secretion of normal procollagen, synthesis of abnormal $\alpha_1(I)$ and $\alpha_2(I)$ chains, and abnormal modifications of the procollagen in the extracellular spaces. These changes result in alterations

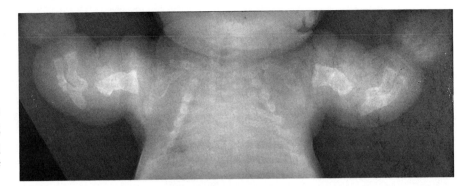

FIGURE 7-1. Osteogenesis imperfecta, type II (neonate). Osteoporosis with "crumpled" appearance of long bones and beading of the ribs from multiple in utero fractures.

in the cross-linking of the collagen fibrils. With current technology, specific deletions or insertions of alleles have been documented for certain genes. Specific abnormalities of type I collagen, however, have not been identified for every patient with osteogenesis imperfecta. This again emphasizes the heterogeneity of the osteogenesis imperfecta syndromes. In the future, we can anticipate that a classification scheme will eventually be developed incorporating not only clinical and radiographic data but biochemical abnormalities as well.

Despite the advances made at the molecular level, no systemic treatment of osteogenesis imperfecta is currently available. Pharmacologic and dietary alterations have been attempted without documented benefit. These include the use of vitamin C, calcium, phosphorous, vitamin D, calcitonin, and sodium fluoride.

Radiographic studies in patients with osteogenesis imperfecta demonstrate osteoporosis in all cases though it varies in its severity according to the type of osteogenesis imperfecta. Type I patients have minimal alteration in the overall structure of the bone. There is a decreased number and thickness of trabeculae in the cancellous bone with mild thinning of the cortices. In the severer forms, the cortices may be indistinct, and deformities of the overall shape of the bone are present. For instance, in type II patients, the tubular bones are short and wide. They have a crumpled appearance lacking normal modeling (Fig. 7-1). In type III, the diaphyses are characteristically narrowed with increased flaring and enlargement of the metaphyses and epiphyses. Typically, the long bones are deformed secondary to multiple fractures (Fig. 7-2). These patients often have irregular calcifications in the expanded regions of the tubular bones (popcorn-like appearance). Radiographs of the pelvis often demonstrate protrusio acetabuli. Changes in the spine are characteristic, including platyspondyly, biconcave vertebrae, and scoliosis of varying sever-

ity. Radiographs of the cranium demonstrate osteoporosis and the presence of multiple wormian bones. Some patients demonstrate flattening of the occiput (tam-o'-shanter skull), and, rarely, basilar impression may be present at the craniocervical junction (Fig. 7-3).

The most frequent problem faced by a patient with osteogenesis imperfecta is recurrent fractures of the long bones (Fig. 7-4). Though these patients are susceptible to fractures throughout their lifetime, the incidence of fractures tends to decrease after puberty. The age of onset of fractures is variable, dependent on the severity of the osteogenesis imperfecta. Fractures may be present at birth in the severer types or

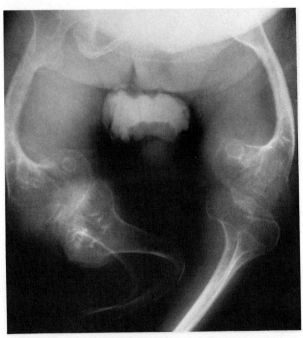

FIGURE 7-2. Osteogenesis imperfecta, type III (age 18 years). Severe angular deformities result from multiple fractures of the osteoporotic bone.

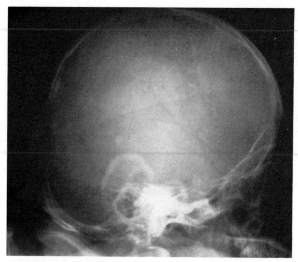

FIGURE 7-3. Osteogenesis imperfecta (age 29 years). Lateral skull radiograph demonstrates flattening of the occiput and multiple wormian bones.

develop at a later age particularly when walking commences. Fractures usually heal uneventfully with external immobilization, though angular deformities often result. Nonunions have been reported and are more common in the type III patients. These typically occur at sites of repeated fractures in patients with progressive deformities. The nonunions may be either hypertrophic or atrophic. Surgical treatment of nonunions is usually successful. This requires excision of the nonunion, autologous bone grafting, and intramedullary rodding.

Patients treated for fractures may develop a vicious cycle of recurrent fracture and deformity (Fig. 7-5). Increased osteoporosis frequently occurs after immobilization for a fracture predisposing the patient to subsequent refracture. This sequence may be interrupted or prevented to a certain extent by a combination of techniques including shorter periods of immobilization, the judicious use of custom-molded plastic orthoses, early weight bearing, physical therapy to improve muscle strength, and the use of standing frames or other mobility aids. Bowing or angular deformities often result in patients who have multiple fractures and may predispose the child to additional fractures. Surgical realignment using mul-

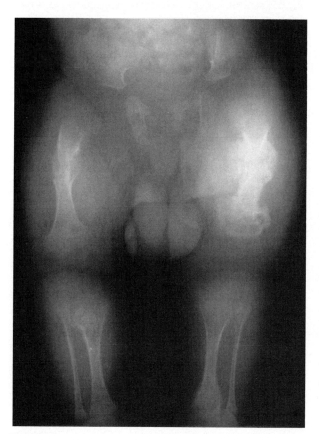

FIGURE 7-4. Osteogenesis imperfecta (age 3 months). Osteoporosis with multiple healing fractures.

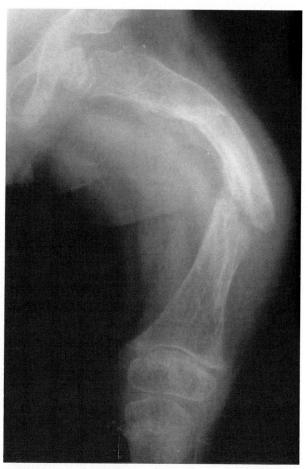

FIGURE 7-5. Osteogenesis imperfecta (age 1 year). Recurrent fractures typically develop through the diaphyses of long bones.

tiple osteotomies and intramedullary rodding often decreases the incidence of fractures secondary to the bowing. Intramedullary fixation may be achieved by either fixed rigid rods or, alternatively, by the use of the expandable Bailey-Dubow rod. The later device is a telescoping system that is inserted through the proximal and distal epiphysis of the long bone to be treated. With longitudinal growth of the bone, the Bailey-Dubow rod elongates internally decreasing the need for frequent reoperations for insertion of a longer rod. Nevertheless, complications occur frequently with either the fixed or the telescoping devices. Rod migration or disengagement of the Bailey-Dubow rod are the most frequent complications. Furthermore, intramedullary rodding with multiple osteotomies may not obviate the need for external support for those patients with severe disease.

The incidence of spinal deformities is high in patients with osteogenesis imperfecta. Fifty to 80% of patients, depending on their age and the severity of their disease develop scoliosis, kyphosis, kyphoscoliosis, or spondylolisthesis. Attempts at controlling curve progression by brace treatment have been generally unsuccessful. Progressive rib cage deformities have resulted from the use of spinal orthoses. These may further compound any pulmonary compromise produced by severe scoliosis. Hence, brace treatment should generally be avoided. Early surgical treatment should be considered for patients whose curves are 40 degrees or greater. Instrumentation complications are more frequent in this population of patients because of the softened lamina. Methylmethacrylate has been used with some success to improve the purchase and fixation of spinal hooks. Most patients require supplementary bank bone because of the diminished availability of iliac crest bone. Patients undergoing surgery need to be carefully monitored for the occurrence of hyperthermia, which is more frequent in these patients.

The orthopaedic surgeon involved in the care and treatment of patients with osteogenesis imperfecta needs to be aware of other potential medical problems. These patients are particularly prone to recurrent respiration infections, which is the major cause of death in osteogenesis imperfecta. Hearing losses are common, and patients should be screened routinely. Unfortunately, the hearing deficits are often irreversible. Dental problems are also frequent in patients with osteogenesis imperfecta. Dentinogenesis imperfecta leads to premature erosions and wear of both deciduous and permanent teeth. Good dental hygiene and follow-up is imperative. Children with osteogenesis imperfecta are more susceptible to diaphoresis and heat intolerance.

ACHONDROPLASIA

Achondroplasia is the most common form of short-limb, disproportionate dwarfism (Fig. 7-6). A single gene defect has been established for this disorder, and it is transmitted as an autosomal dominant trait. Most cases, however, are the result of a new random mutation. A paternal age effect has been noted for these sporadic cases. The fathers are frequently older than 36 years of age. The skeletal manifestations of achondroplasia are related to a defect in endochondral bone formation. Histologic and histochemical changes suggest an alteration in the normal processes of chondrocyte maturation, hypertrophy, and degeneration. The resulting growth disturbances are variable, affecting proximal limb segments to a greater extent than distal limb segments (rhizomelia). Appositional and periosteal bone formation are normal in achondroplasia.

Achondroplasia is recognizable at birth. There is

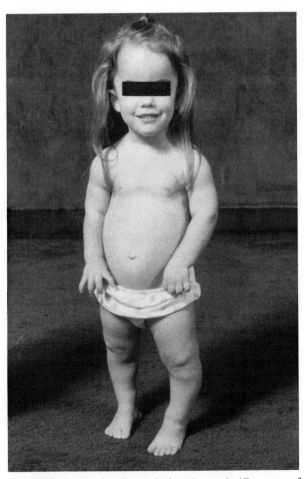

FIGURE 7-6. Achondroplasia (age 3 years). (Courtesy of the Department of Medical Education, Alfred I. duPont Institute, Wilmington, DE)

enlargement of the cranium associated with frontal bossing, midface hypoplasia, flattening of the nasal bridge, and prominence of the mandible. Both communicating and noncommunicating forms of hydrocephalus have been described in achondroplasia, which, for these patients, would explain their increased head circumference. Most patients, however, appear to have a true megalencephaly without evidence of a cerebrospinal fluid block. The foramen magnum is frequently narrowed in achondroplasia. The base of the skull develops by endochondral ossification, which is abnormal in this disorder. This narrowing has been associated with significant neurologic complications from compression of the brain stem. These include respiratory insufficiency, quadriparesis, and sudden death. Many patients have abnormalities in somatosensory-evoked potentials and yet are neurologically normal. Decompression of the foramen magnum is indicated for those patients with major neurologic findings, but prophylactic decompression in achondroplasia does not appear warranted. With growth and development, the foramen magnum enlarges, and the frequency of neurologic problems from compression in this region diminishes with time.

A variety of spinal deformities are common in the achondroplastic dwarf. Before walking age, a thoracolumbar kyphosis commonly occurs and is most noticeable when children begin to sit. This kyphosis may or may not completely reduce when the child is placed in the prone position (Fig. 7-7). Typically, there is a lordosis of the thoracic spine proximal to the kyphosis at the thoracolumbar junction. Though this kyphosis may measure greater than 80 degrees before walking age, spontaneous resolution typically occurs once independent ambulation is initiated (Fig. 7-8). Some degree of persistent kyphosis

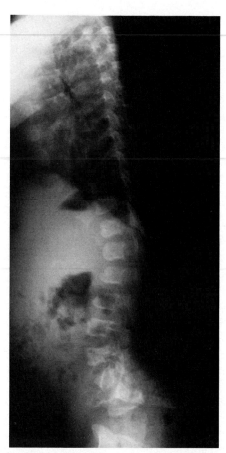

FIGURE 7-8. Achondroplasia (age 3 years). The kyphosis resolves once patient begins independent ambulation. There is posterior scalloping of the vertebral bodies with shortening of the pedicles. (Courtesy of the Department of Medical Education, Alfred I. duPont Institute, Wilmington, DE)

is present in approximately one fourth of adult achondroplastic dwarfs. The enlarged cranium, hypotonia, ligamentous laxity, and hip flexion contractures present in infants, and young children all have been implicated in the development of this kyphosis. Most children do not require treatment because spontaneous improvement is to be anticipated. Bracing may be indicated, however, for those young children with rigid curves or evidence of apical wedging. If a rigid 40-degree kyphosis persists beyond age 5, then combined anteroposterior (AP) fusion should be considered because further progression and neurologic compromise may result. Laminectomy alone is contraindicated and typically leads to rapid progression of the kyphosis.

The anatomy of the lumbar spine in achondroplasia gives rise to a high incidence of symptomatic lumbar spinal stenosis. Radiographically, there is narrowing of the interpedicular distances in the lum-

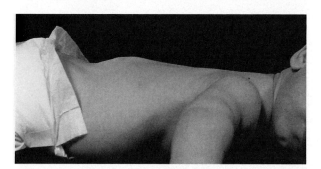

FIGURE 7-7. Achondroplasia (age 1 year). A thoracolumbar kyphosis persists in the prone position. (Courtesy of the Department of Medical Education, Alfred I. duPont Institute, Wilmington, DE)

bar spine increasing in severity from proximal to distal. In addition, the pedicles are shortened, further narrowing the canal in the sagittal plane. Lateral radiographs demonstrate posterior scalloping of the vertebral bodies (see Fig. 7-8). Computed tomographic (CT) imaging frequently reveals thickening of the lamina and inferior facets as well as intervertebral disk herniation. It is estimated that up to half of all achondroplastic adults develop neurologic symptoms from stenosis of the lumbar spine, including low back and leg pain, paresthesia, dysesthesia, weakness, or bowel and bladder incontinence. Patients with neurogenic claudication usually develop symptoms of aching pain or tiredness in the lower extremities with walking or standing. Symptoms frequently slowly progress and often include sensory disturbances as well as weakness. In the earliest phases of symptomatic spinal stenosis, the achondroplastic dwarf notices improvement in symptoms by squatting, which tends to flatten the increased lumbar lordosis. Patients with excessive thoracolumbar kyphosis are at increased risk for the development of neurologic signs, which may include posterior column dysfunction and upper motor neuron signs.

Conservative treatment of lumbar spinal stenosis for the achondroplastic patient includes weight reduction, reversal of hyperlordosis by pelvic tilt exercises, and stretching of hip flexion contractures. Unfortunately, the results of these measures are frequently unpredictable. Bracing has been used in some patients but imposes further restrictions on the patient's mobility, thus creating additional problems with respect to activities of daily living. Surgical treatment necessitates wide multilevel laminectomies extending from the low thoracic spine to the sacrum. The lateral recesses must be decompressed, and foraminotomies must be performed. It is important to maintain integrity of the facet joints by undercutting the inferior facets rather than performing a complete facetectomy to prevent postlaminectomy instability. Diskectomies should be performed as necessary. If instability develops, anterior interbody fusion is necessary. In addition, those patients with thoracolumbar kyphosis require anterior spinal fusion concurrently to prevent postlaminectomy kyphosis. An adequate posterolateral fusion following laminectomy is difficult to achieve because of the small size of the transverse processes. Spinal instrumentation in achondroplasia has been associated with a high incidence of spinal cord injury and should be avoided.

In the upper extremities, rhizomelic shortening is apparent. Typically, there is limitation of extension of the elbow averaging 20 to 30 degrees. Some patients have a posterior dislocation of the radial head, which further limits extension and supination. Generally, this dislocation is asymptomatic, and no treatment is necessary. Patients with achondroplasia typically have a "trident" hand characterized by a persistent space between the long and ring fingers. Hand function is generally normal in achondroplasia, and the functional limitations for these patients relate to the overall shortening of the extremity. Typically, their fingertips barely reach to the level of the greater trochanters, resulting in difficulties with personal hygiene and dressing.

Rhizomelic shortening is also present in the lower extremities. Radiographically, the pelvis is broad with a diminished vertical height. The iliac crest has a square appearance, and the superior acetabular roof is horizontal. Hip dysplasia is not a typical feature of achondroplasia. Hip flexion contractures develop in association with the hyperlordosis of the lumbar spine. True coxa vara is absent in achondroplasia, though overgrowth of the greater trochanters occurs because of normal appositional bone formation. There is metaphyseal flaring of the distal femora.

Genu varum is a typical finding in achondroplasia and, in severe cases, is associated with varus of the ankle. Radiographically, the fibulae are elongated with respect to the tibias (Fig. 7-9). This growth discrepancy between the tibia and the fibula has been implicated in the development of the genu varum deformity. Bracing has not been successful in correcting the deformities and has resulted in peroneal palsies. For those patients developing pain, gait disturbances, or progressive varus deformities, proximal tibiofibular osteotomies generally provide excellent symptomatic relief as well as a cosmetic improvement. In children and adolescents, these osteotomies may be performed through small incisions using opening-wedge techniques and long-leg cast immobilization.

Limb lengthening has been promoted with increasing frequency particularly in Europe for patients with achondroplasia. Increases in length up to 30 cm have been reported using newer methods of distraction and external fixation for the femora, tibias, and humeri. Apart from the possible cosmetic and functional benefits of these procedures, many other factors need to be weighed before recommending these procedures in achondroplasia for which symmetric shortening exists. These factors include the social, psychological, and economic issues involved in any procedure in which there is a multitude of potential major complications, a prolonged duration of treat-

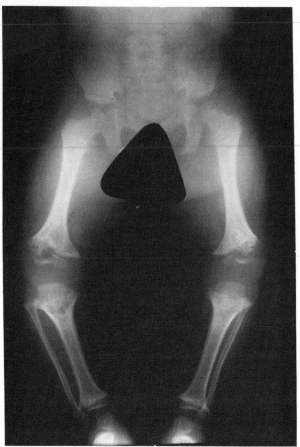

FIGURE 7-9. Achondroplasia (age 3 years). Genu varum deformity.

orders both in terms of the magnitude of skeletal involvement and the inheritance patterns. Most cases are inherited as an autosomal dominant trait, though autosomal recessive transmission has also been identified. Histologic alterations have been noted in biopsies of cartilage from patients with pseudoachondroplastic dysplasia. The cell columns of the physes are disorganized with a clumping of the chondrocytes. In the hypertrophic zone, peculiar cytoplasmic inclusions have been identified. Electron microscopic studies have established abnormalities in the rough endoplasmic reticulum. Furthermore, proteoglycan abnormalities have been identified by histochemical determinations.

Pseudoachondroplastic dysplasia is one of the short-limb disproportionate dwarfing conditions with rhizomelic involvement. In contrast to infants with achondroplasia, the diagnosis of pseudoachondroplastic dysplasia for new mutations is generally not made in the newborn period. The disturbance of growth found in this disorder is frequently not iden-

ment, and the lack of information regarding the long-term results of these procedures in short-statured individuals.

The epiphyseal cartilage is not significantly involved in achondroplasia; hence, osteoarthritis is not frequently observed in achondroplasia. Patients presenting with hip or knee pain should be carefully evaluated for other causes of pain, including lumbar spinal stenosis and radiculopathy.

PSEUDOACHONDROPLASTIC DYSPLASIA

Pseudoachondroplastic dysplasia is the preferred terminology given to a group of disorders with distinct clinical and radiographic features. It is characterized by moderate to severe changes involving the epiphyseal, physeal, and metaphyseal regions of tubular bones as well as changes in the spine. Considerable heterogeneity exists within this group of dis-

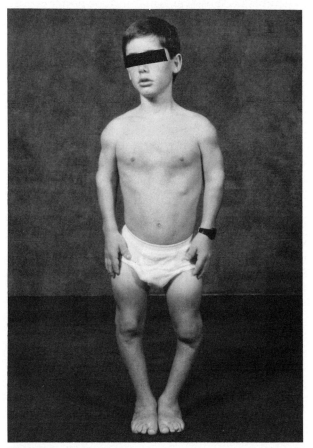

FIGURE 7-10. Pseudoachondroplastic dysplasia (age 14 years). (Courtesy of the Department of Medical Education, Alfred I. duPont Institute, Wilmington, DE)

tified until 2 or 3 years of age. Clinically and radiographically, the face and head have a normal appearance (Fig. 7-10).

Clinically, the spine has a normal appearance apart from an increased lumbar lordosis. Scoliosis may occur but is generally not severe (Fig. 7-11). A significant thoracolumbar kyphosis is less common in patients with pseudoachondroplasia. Radiographically, there is mild platyspondyly. The pedicles are not narrowed in the lumbar spine. In the sagittal plane, there is frequently anterior beaking of the vertebral bodies because of delayed ossification at the insertion of the annulus fibrosis. Odontoid hypoplasia may be present with concurrent atlantoaxial instability. If patients develop significant instability of the first and second cervical vertebrae, with or without signs of myelopathy, posterior atlantoaxial arthrodesis should be considered.

Extremity involvement is characterized by significant rhizomelic shortening and ligamentous laxity of all joints. The digits of the hands and feet have a short, broadened appearance lacking the normal distal tapering (Fig. 7-12). Pes planus is typically present though rarely symptomatic. This is accentuated in those patients who have a valgus angulation of their ankles. Ossification of the epiphyses is delayed in pseudoachondroplastic dysplasia. The articular surfaces of the major weight-bearing bones usually deform early, leading to incongruity and premature osteoarthritis. It appears that the delayed ossification of the cartilaginous epiphyses leads to a lack of osseous support for these articular surfaces. Hence, the cartilaginous epiphyses are more susceptible to deformation from normal mechanical forces crossing the articulations (Fig. 7-13).

The delayed ossification of the femoral heads may resemble bilateral Perthes disease. There is no evidence to suggest, however, that a true avascular

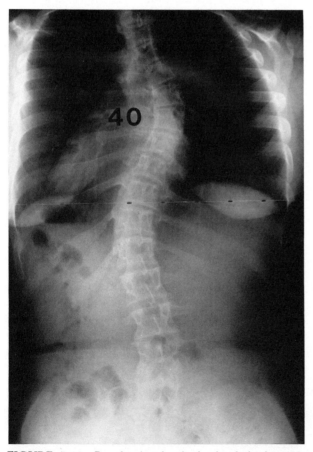

FIGURE 7-11. Pseudoachondroplastic dysplasia (age 20 years). Thoracic scoliosis is present. The interpedicular distance is not narrowed in the lumbar spine. (Courtesy of the Department of Medical Education, Alfred I. duPont Institute, Wilmington, DE)

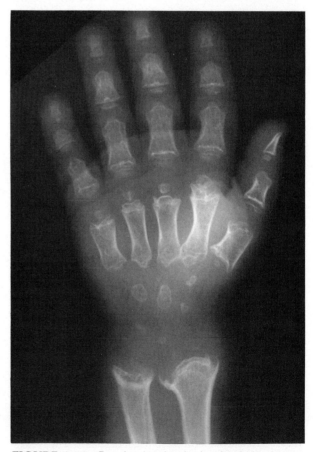

FIGURE 7-12. Pseudoachondroplastic dysplasia (age 4 years). There is a delay in ossification of the epiphyses and carpal bones. The metaphyses are flared, and distal tapering is absent. (Courtesy of the Department of Medical Education, Alfred I. duPont Institute, Wilmington, DE)

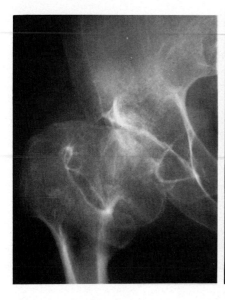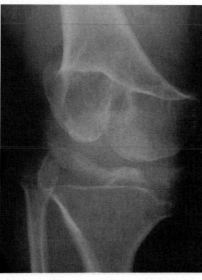

FIGURE 7-13. Pseudoachondroplastic dysplasia (age 35 years). Incongruity of the hip and knee. (Courtesy of the Department of Medical Education, Alfred I. duPont Institute, Wilmington, DE)

necrosis has occurred. In contrast to true bilateral Perthes, the deformities are typically symmetric, and there is evidence of generalized involvement of the entire skeletal system. Femoral head deformity is frequently evident in the adolescent age group with either flattening, extrusion, or subluxation of the femoral head. The phenomenon of hinge abduction may develop. With abduction of the hip, the deformed femoral head tends to lever out of joint, further leading to increased congruity as has been described for Perthes disease. Premature osteoarthritis in early adult years is a frequent sequelae in pseudoachondroplastic dysplasia. Patients with symptomatic subluxation or incongruity may benefit from a realignment osteotomy of the proximal femur. Preoperative evaluation should include arthrography. This usually demonstrates improved congruity with 15 to 20 degrees of flexion and adduction of the femur, whereas abduction of the femur usually does not improve the incongruity and leads to hinge abduction of the femoral head. In those circumstances in which congruity is improved arthrographically by valgus and adduction of the femur, a valgus-extension intertrochanteric osteotomy may be considered. Pelvic reconstruction is usually limited to so-called salvage procedures such as a shelf augmentation or the Chiari osteotomy. The more traditional reconstructive pelvic osteotomies, such as the Salter innominate osteotomy, are generally contraindicated in the skeletal dysplasias because a concentric reduction is not present preoperatively.

Patients with pseudoachondroplastic dysplasia typically have significant angular deformities of the lower extremities with severe involvement of the knees. The deformities may either be varus, valgus, or "windswept" with a varus deformity on one side and a valgus deformity on the contralateral side. When valgus deformities are present, hip pathology is typically severer secondary to subluxation. Angular deformities appear to result as a consequence of cartilaginous and osseous changes as well as the presence of ligamentous laxity. Pseudoachondroplastic dwarfs frequently develop severe deformities during short periods and have recurrent deformities after surgical realignment. Careful preoperative assessment is necessary to properly realign the mechanical axis through the hip, knee, and ankle. In particular, care must be taken to ensure that the plane of the knee and ankle joint following reconstruction is parallel to the ground. For instance, in a genu varus deformity, bowing is usually present in both the femur and the tibia, requiring osteotomies in both the distal femur and the proximal tibia (Fig. 7-14). Single-level osteotomies in the lower extremities can be satisfactorily performed through small incisions using no internal fixation and long-leg cast immobilization postoperatively. If dual-level osteotomies are required on the ipsilateral side, some internal fixation are necessary such as crossed pins or staples in addition to plaster immobilization.

SPONDYLOEPIPHYSEAL DYSPLASIA CONGENITA

Spondyloepiphyseal dysplasia congenita is a specific type of *spondyloepiphyseal dysplasia*. The latter term is a descriptive one used generically for any one of

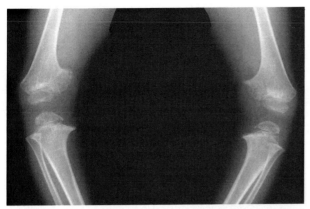

FIGURE 7-14. Pseudoachondroplastic dysplasia (age 5 years). Bowing of femurs and tibias with resultant genu varum. (Courtesy of the Department of Medical Education, Alfred I. duPont Institute, Wilmington, DE)

several intrinsic skeletal dysplasias that result in disproportionate dwarfism with primary involvement of both the epiphyseal centers of ossification and the vertebral column. Pseudoachondroplastic dysplasia is one type of spondyloepiphyseal dysplasia, as is chondrodysplasia punctata, spondyloepiphyseal dysplasia tarda, and the spondylometaphyseal dysplasias. It is important to establish an accurate diagnosis to provide proper genetic counseling, suitable information regarding the natural history of the disorder, and the potential for medical and orthopaedic abnormalities. In most circumstances, the orthopaedist would be prudent to seek consultation with a clinical geneticist experienced in the evaluation of patients with intrinsic skeletal dysplasias.

Spondyloepiphyseal dysplasia is transmitted as an autosomal dominant trait, though most cases are the result of a new mutation (Fig. 7-15). The diagnosis of spondyloepiphyseal dysplasia is usually made at birth. These newborn infants are short with obvious disproportionate involvement of the trunk. Their head circumference is normal, but the midface is flattened resulting in a prominent forehead. The eyes may be widely set, and typically a cleft palate is present. By adult life, more than 50% of these patients develop severe myopia or retinal detachment. Regular ophthalmologic examination during childhood is necessary to identify retinal pathology early.

Variability in the extent of skeletal abnormalities of both the spine and lower extremities is present in spondyloepiphyseal dysplasia congenita. Two clinical subgroups have been distinguished based on the severity of the coxa vara and the magnitude of spinal involvement. This differentiation may not be apparent until 3 to 4 years of age.

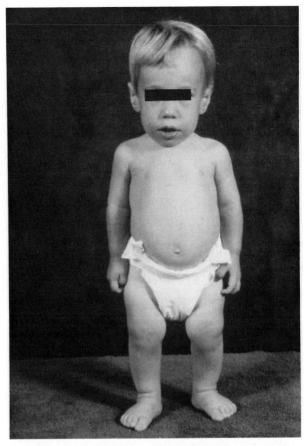

FIGURE 7-15. Spondyloepiphyseal dysplasia congenita (age 4 years). (Courtesy of the Department of Medical Education, Alfred I. duPont Institute, Wilmington, DE)

Clinically, examination of the thorax reveals a pectus carinatum in conjunction with an increased AP diameter of the chest. The neck is short. There is an increased lumbar lordosis associated with a protuberant abdomen and flexion contractures of the hips. Radiographic evaluation of the spine reveals varying degrees of platyspondyly. There is an increased AP diameter of the vertebral bodies with posterior wedging. Scoliosis or kyphoscoliosis often develops in late childhood and early adolescence (Fig. 7-16). Progressive curves measuring less than 40 degrees in the skeletally immature patient should be treated with bracing. Larger curves or curves progressing despite brace treatment should be considered for posterior spinal fusion with appropriate instrumentation. Spinal deformities in spondyloepiphyseal dysplasia congenita should not be allowed to progress while awaiting full skeletal maturation to achieve full spinal height.

These patients frequently have upper cervical abnormalities, including odontoid hypoplasia or an

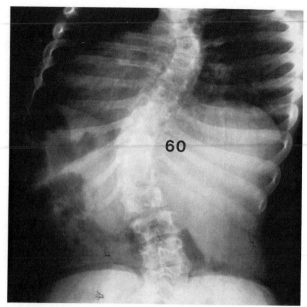

FIGURE 7-16. Spondyloepiphyseal dysplasia congenita (age 8 years). This scoliosis progressed rapidly during a 2-year period. (Courtesy of the Department of Medical Education, Alfred I. duPont Institute, Wilmington, DE)

os odontoideum. Lateral flexion–extension cervical radiographs may reveal atlantoaxial instability with either anterior, posterior, or combined instability (Fig. 7-17). This instability may lead to cervical myelopathy with symptoms of respiratory insufficiency, delayed motor development, and decreased walking endurance. MRI of the upper cervical spine in flexion and extension is useful to document cord compression. Patients with instability measuring more than 5 mm or evidence of a myelopathy usually require posteroatlantoaxial fusion. For most of these patients, the fusion needs to be extended to the occiput because the posterior ring of the atlas is small, and frequently a large synchondrosis exists. In the presence of an os odontoideum or posterior (extension) instability, the preferred surgical technique uses halo-cast or vest immobilization preoperatively without atlantoaxial wires. When these wires are used and tightened in the presence of posterior instability, the ring of C1 may be overreduced, thus compromising the cord anteriorly. Decortication should be performed carefully with a high-speed dental burr. Lower extremity abnormalities are common and usually severe in spondyloepiphyseal congenita. Typically, ossification of the capital femoral epiphysis is delayed, and a coxa vara is present. The coxa vara is often severe, leading to a progressive varus deformity and, in some instances, actual discontinuity of the femoral neck (Fig. 7-18). The predominately cartilaginous

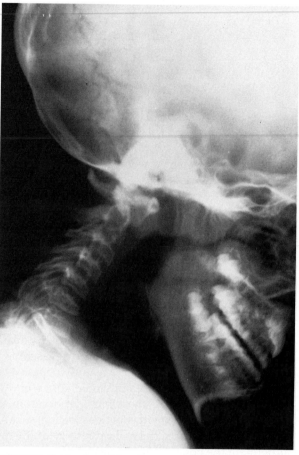

FIGURE 7-17. Spondyloepiphyseal dysplasia congenita (age 9 years). Odontoid hypoplasia with combined flexion and extension instability. (Courtesy of the Department of Medical Education, Alfred I. duPont Institute, Wilmington, DE)

femoral head usually deforms with lateral extrusion, incongruity, or subluxation. In those patients with ligamentous laxity and valgus alignment of the lower extremities, dislocation may develop. As in pseudoachondroplastic dysplasia, premature osteoarthritis is a frequent sequelae of this intrinsic skeletal dysplasia. Treatment of the coxa vara often requires a

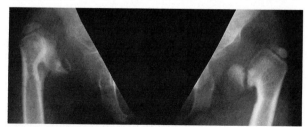

FIGURE 7-18. Spondyloepiphyseal dysplasia congenita (age 7 years). Severe coxa vara with subluxation. (Courtesy of the Department of Medical Education, Alfred I. duPont Institute, Wilmington, DE)

valgus extension osteotomy not only to correct the femoral neck-shaft angle but also to compensate for the presence of hip flexion contractures. Again, preoperative hip arthrography is extremely useful in planning the surgical approach to these patients.

Excessive valgus alignment of the knee is typically present, though an occasional patient has genu varum. Delayed ossification of the epiphysis of the distal femur and proximal tibia is also present, leading to deformity and incongruity. Realignment may be necessary for significant valgus deformities because of pain and progressive laxity of the medial collateral ligament of the knee. A varus supracondylar osteotomy should be considered for these patients, but preoperative evaluation must consider correction of deformities of the adjacent joints proximally and distally at the same time. Talipes equinovarus deformities may be present at birth and are be treated by traditional modalities of casting or surgery as the circumstances dictate.

DIASTROPHIC DYSPLASIA

Diastrophic dysplasia is characterized by extreme short-limb disproportionate dwarfism with characteristic abnormalities of the hands, feet, hips, and pinnae of the ears (Fig. 7-19). Frequently, significant abnormalities of the cervical spine or thoracolumbar spine are also present. This is a rare disorder transmitted as an autosomal recessive trait. Biopsies of physeal cartilage have identified abnormal collagen in the matrix between columns of chondrocytes. In addition, there appears to be decreased numbers of chondrocytes in all zones of the cell columns.

Diastrophic dysplasia is recognizable at birth. Although the head circumference is normal, there is a distinctive facial appearance, including a wide mouth, flaring of the nostrils, and broadening of the midportion of the nose. More than half the individuals with diastrophic dysplasia have a cleft palate. Eighty percent of the patients develop calcification and thickening of the cartilage constituting the pinnae of the ear. This so-called cauliflower deformity is not present at birth, but rather develops between the third to sixth week of life. Typically, an acute inflammatory reaction is observed with swelling and redness. The pinnae become thickened and hard. Lateral radiographs of the skull frequently show a superimposition of the calcified pinnae, which should not be confused with intracranial calcifications.

Some patients develop cervical kyphosis with the apex centered at the third, fourth, or fifth cervical

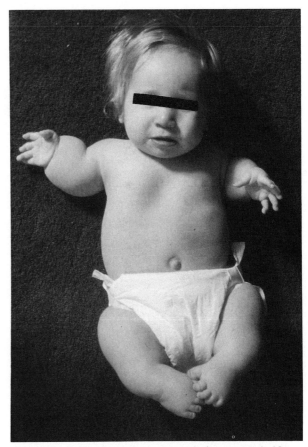

FIGURE 7-19. Diastrophic dysplasia (age 2 years). (Courtesy of the Department of Medical Education, Alfred I. duPont Institute, Wilmington, DE)

vertebrae (Fig. 7-20). The apical vertebrae are frequently wedge shaped anteriorly. Posteriorly, over these same segments, a spina bifida occulta is frequently present. Cervical kyphoses in excess of 90 degrees have resulted from this dangerous combination of posterior element dysraphism and anterior failure of formation. Unfortunately, the risk of quadriplegia is high in these patients with progressive cervical kyphosis. Therefore, all patients with diastrophic dysplasia should have lateral cervical spine radiographs obtained within the first year of life. For those patients with cervical kyphosis who are neurologically normal and not unstable, conservative treatment may be pursued. In the absence of instability on flexion–extension radiographs, resolution of the kyphosis may occur with extension bracing. If there is instability or evidence of neurologic involvement, however, surgical stabilization is warranted. This generally requires both anterior and posterior fusion with external immobilization such as a halo vest. MRI of the cervical spine in flexion and exten-

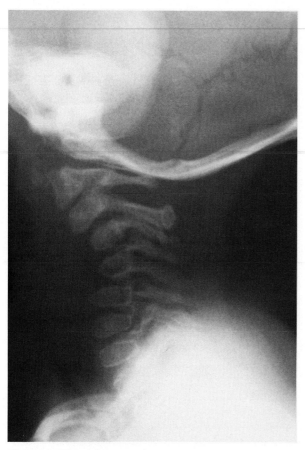

FIGURE 7-20. Diastrophic dysplasia (age 18 months). A lateral extension radiograph reveals persistent cervical kyphosis and hypoplasia of the third and fourth cervical bodies. (Courtesy of the Department of Medical Education, Alfred I. duPont Institute, Wilmington, DE)

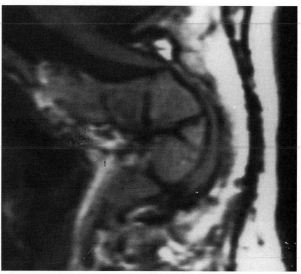

FIGURE 7-21. Diastrophic dysplasia (age 16 years). MRI reveals significant cord compromise secondary to severe cervical kyphosis in this paraparetic dwarf. (Courtesy of the Department of Medical Education, Alfred I. duPont Institute, Wilmington, DE)

sion has been extremely useful in assessing the possibility of spinal cord compromise (Fig. 7-21).

Kyphoscoliosis of the thoracolumbar spine is also common in diastrophic dysplasia as well (Fig. 7-22). At an early age, the curves are frequently small and flexible though curve progression is to be anticipated for those patients left untreated. Curves measuring greater than 100 degrees have developed in many patients, and these curves are typically extremely rigid. Attempts to obtain curve correction through distraction instrumentation at the time of fusion have been fraught with neurologic compromise. Bracing should be strongly considered for patients with small curves measuring 20 to 30 degrees while they are flexible. If curve progression occurs despite bracing, then surgical intervention should be considered for curves measuring 40 degrees or greater in the skeletally immature patient.

Diastrophic dwarfs have a characteristic "hitch-hiker thumb" deformity. The thumbs have a disproportionately shortened first metacarpal, which is also abducted and hypermobile. Another characteristic finding is symphalangism of the proximal interphalangeal joints of the fingers. The hands appear broad, short, and are often ulnarly deviated. Patients typically have bilateral rigid talipes equinovarus deformities that are extremely resistant to conservative casting techniques. The lower extremities in the newborn period are short, particularly in the thighs, and have bulky soft tissues. Casts frequently slide off and are difficult to mold. Most children with diastrophic dysplasia require surgical releases to correct the clubfoot deformities.

Shortening of the extremities occurs in a rhizomelic pattern. Other lower extremity abnormalities include limitation of motion of the hips and knees with severe flexion contractures measuring more than 45 degrees. Radiographically, the long bones are broadened with flaring of the epiphyseal and metaphyseal regions. The epiphyseal centers of ossification are also delayed in appearance, leading to eventual joint incongruity. A peculiar saucer-shaped defect of ossification is present in the femoral heads at an early age (see Fig. 7-22). Subluxation or even dislocation of the hips with growth and development is not unusual in diastrophic dysplasia. In general, reconstructive osteotomies about the hips are generally not feasible in light of the restriction of motion and presence of contractures. Attempts at soft tissue

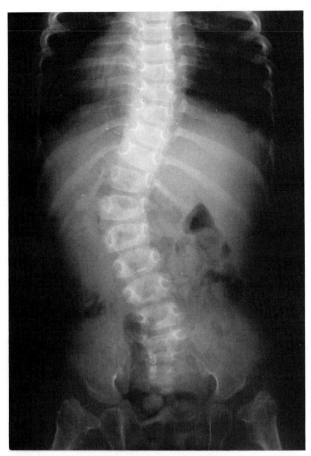

FIGURE 7-22. Diastrophic dysplasia (age 4 years). Progressive scoliosis has developed at an early age. Note the saucer-shaped defects in the femoral heads. (Courtesy of the Department of Medical Education, Alfred I. duPont Institute, Wilmington, DE)

release of flexion contractures of either the hips or knees are associated with a high recurrence rate. In addition to the knee contractures, increased genu valgus alignment may be present with patellar dislocations. Radiographically, the fibulae are usually disproportionately shortened with respect to the tibias in contrast to patients with achondroplasia. Premature osteoarthritis is a frequent sequelae of the severe epiphyseal abnormalities present in this condition.

METAPHYSEAL CHONDRODYSPLASIA

Metaphyseal chondrodysplasia is a generic term used to delineate a heterogeneous group of disorders with characteristic radiographic changes in the metaphyseal regions of tubular bones with normal-appearing epiphyses. Histologically, the most dramatic changes are observed in the proliferative and hypertrophic zones of the physes rather than in the metaphyses. Chondrocytes are clustered together rather than forming organized columns of cells. The zone of provisional calcification is narrow, and areas of unmineralized cartilage extend into the metaphyses. Electron microscopy has revealed granular participates within the rough surface endoplasmic reticulum. Therefore, the primary defect appears to reside primarily in the physes rather than in the metaphyses. Hence, metaphyseal chondrodysplasia is a misnomer histologically.

There are several different types of metaphyseal chondrodysplasias, the more common ones being the Schmid type and cartilage hair hypoplasia (McKusick type). These disorders are rarely recognized at birth unless there is a positive family history for a skeletal dysplasia. The diagnosis is generally made during childhood when these patients are referred for a variety of complaints including short stature, lower extremity pain, angular deformities, gait abnormalities, or increased lumbar lordosis. In general, the diminution in stature is mild in comparison with other dwarfing conditions. The Schmid type is transmitted as a autosomal dominant trait. The McKusick type is autosomal recessive and most frequently found in the Amish. The Schmid-type metaphyseal chondrodysplasia has been confused with disorders of vitamin D metabolism, such as vitamin D–resistant rickets.

Patients with the Schmid type have a clinically normal appearance. Head circumference and facial features are normal throughout life. Patients with cartilage hair hypoplasia have characteristically light-colored, sparse hair (Fig. 7-23). In addition, many patients with the McKusick type appear to have an alteration of cellular immunity with increased susceptibility to viral infections such as varicella. Megacolon and intestinal malabsorption frequently occur in these patients. Abnormalities of the chest wall are common in the metaphyseal chondrodysplasias, including enlargement of the costochondral junctions, Harrison grooves, and pectus excavatum (Fig. 7-24).

Abnormalities of the spinal column are generally mild in this group of disorders. Patients frequently have an increased lumbar lordosis and rarely a mild scoliosis. Odontoid hypoplasia has been reported and may be associated with atlantoaxial instability.

Patients with metaphyseal chondrodysplasia have short-limb disproportionate dwarfism with the lower extremities involved to a greater extent than the upper extremities. The growth disturbance is less

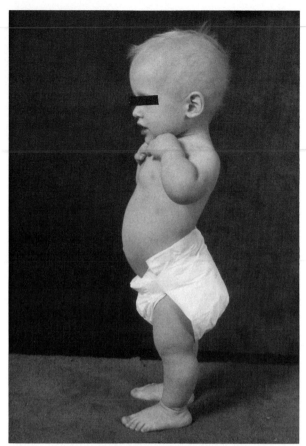

FIGURE 7-23. Metaphyseal chondrodysplasia, McKusick type (age 4 years). (Courtesy of the Department of Medical Education, Alfred I. duPont Institute, Wilmington, DE)

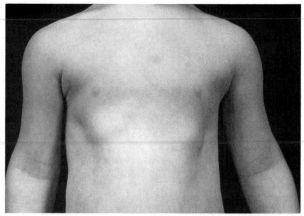

FIGURE 7-24. Metaphyseal chondrodysplasia, Schmid type (age 9 years). The costochondral junctions are expanded, associated with Harrison's grooves. (Courtesy of the Department of Medical Education, Alfred I. duPont Institute, Wilmington, DE)

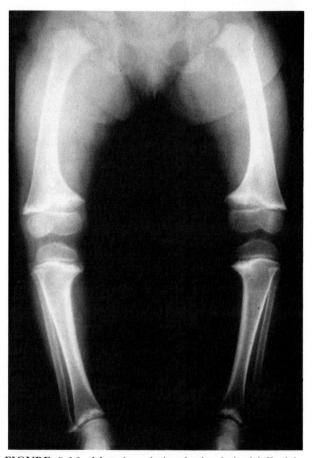

FIGURE 7-25. Metaphyseal chondrodysplasia, McKusick type (age 4 years). There is mild coxa vara and mild genu varum. Epiphyseal centers ossify normally. The physes are widened, and the metaphyses expanded. (Courtesy of the Department of Medical Education, Alfred I. duPont Institute, Wilmington, DE)

severe in patients with the Schmid type in comparison with those with cartilage hair hypoplasia. Involvement of the upper extremities is generally mild with excessive mobility noted in the fingers and wrists. Elbow flexion contractures are generally present but are usually mild. Expansion of the metaphyses of the tubular bones leads to a prominent appearance particularly for those joints where the muscle mass is diminished, such as the wrists and ankles.

The lower extremities are involved to a greater extent than the upper extremities. Bowing of the hips, knees, and ankles is typically present (Fig. 7-25). Radiographic evaluation reveals expanded metaphyses with areas of cyst formation representing islands of unmineralized cartilage. The fibulae are elongated with respect to the tibias. Bowing is generally present both in the femora and the tibias in contrast to achondroplasia. In addition, coxa vara is typically present in patients with metaphyseal chondrodysplasia. Rarely is the coxa vara progressive in patients with cartilage hair hypoplasia. Valgus osteotomy should be considered for patients who have evidence of progressive varus, a femoral neck-shaft angle of less than 100 degrees, or a triangular metaphyseal fragment of the inferior femoral neck.

The genu varum deformity may initially be severe—especially in those patients with the Schmid type. Spontaneous correction, however, frequently occurs during the first decade with observation alone. Therefore, realignment procedures should be delayed until it is determined that no further improvement is occurring. For those patients in whom corrective osteotomy is contemplated, careful preoperative assessment is necessary to determine the site of osteotomy because bowing is typically present in both the femora and the tibias. Aside from restoring a normal mechanical hip-knee-ankle axis, the plane of the knee and ankle joints must be parallel to the ground following surgery to ensure a satisfactory result. Varus deformities of the ankle do occur in both the Schmid and McKusick types and appears to be related to distal fibular overgrowth. In some patients, a corrective supramalleolar osteotomy is indicated.

MULTIPLE EPIPHYSEAL DYSPLASIA

Multiple epiphyseal dysplasia is one of the more common skeletal dysplasias resulting in mild diminution of stature associated with disproportionate limb shortening. Classically, two forms have been described based on the severity of skeletal involvement. The severe form (Fairbank) has been differentiated from the milder form (Ribbing). The described differences, however, are rather arbitrary, and the varying severity represents a spectrum of involvement. Multiple epiphyseal dysplasia is typically transmitted as an autosomal dominant trait though recessive forms have been described. A disturbance of endochondral ossification is observed histologically in both epiphyseal centers of ossification and regions of physeal growth. Abnormalities of both matrix and chondrocytes have been described.

Patients seek medical attention because of gait disturbances, lower extremity pain, stiffness, angular deformities, or short stature. Many patients, after initial evaluation, are referred to an orthopaedic surgeon for bilateral Perthes disease. Depending on the severity of the epiphyseal dysplasia, symptoms may develop as early as 4 or 5 years. It is not uncommon, however, for patients with milder forms to go unrecognized until young adult life. The disturbance of

longitudinal growth of the lower limbs leads to mild diminution of stature. Most patients are above the third percentile for standing height, however, so true dwarfism is not present. The appearance of the head and face is normal. Mild radiographic changes may be noted in the vertebral column consisting of mild end-plate irregularities in the thoracic region. Clinically, the spine is normal apart from a mild increased lumbar lordosis. Kyphosis or scoliosis is not typical.

The epiphyses of the upper extremities have variable involvement. There is a delay in the appearance of the ossification centers of both tubular bones as well as carpal bones. There may be distal ulnar overgrowth that leads to mild subluxation of the wrist. In patients with severe involvement, some irregularity and flattening does occur in the major joints of the upper extremity. Occasionally, there may be mild limitation of motion in the elbow or wrist. The short tubular bones of the hands are also involved, with maximal shortening present in the middle and distal phalanges. Patients rarely complain of any significant symptoms in the upper extremities.

Lower extremity complaints include angular deformities, restricted motion, and pain. The hips frequently are the site of the severest involvement in the lower extremities. Ossification of the capital femoral epiphyses is delayed (Fig. 7-26). This lack of osseous support for the growing cartilaginous femoral head results in early deformation. The femoral heads frequently have a mushroom-shaped appearance and develop flattening or extrusion as is seen in other skeletal dysplasias with epiphyseal involvement. Subluxation and hinge abduction may also occur. Premature osteoarthritis is an eventual sequelae for most patients (Fig. 7-27). Coxa vara may be present but is rarely severe as in spondyloepiphyseal dysplasia congenita. Radiographically, as ossification of the femoral head proceeds, the small irregular centers

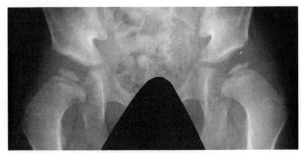

FIGURE 7-26. Multiple epiphyseal dysplasia (age 6 years). Ossification of the capital femoral epiphyses are symmetrically delayed in appearance. (Courtesy of the Department of Medical Education, Alfred I. duPont Institute, Wilmington, DE)

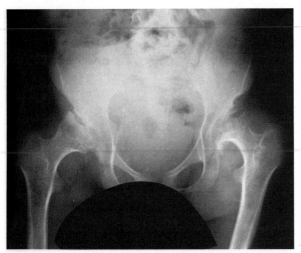

FIGURE 7-27. Multiple epiphyseal dysplasia (age 20 years). Severe premature osteoarthritis. (Courtesy of the Department of Medical Education, Alfred I. duPont Institute, Wilmington, DE)

of ossification gradually coalesce and become more confluent. These changes may mimic Perthes disease. In patients with multiple epiphyseal dysplasia, hip involvement is typically symmetric involving other epiphyses as well. In the patient with classic bilateral Legg-Calve-Perthes disease, the involvement is asymmetric and limited to the hips. Furthermore, in multiple epiphyseal dysplasia, the fragmented appearance of the femoral head is not related to resorption of previously formed bone but rather represents progressive coalescence of areas of irregular ossification. Conversely, in Perthes disease, there is radiographic loss of bone as resorption occurs before reossification.

Unfortunately, these classical differences, which have been used to distinguish patients with multiple epiphyseal dysplasia and bilateral Perthes disease, have been blurred by the recognition that avascular necrosis does occur in patients with multiple epiphyseal dysplasia. For those patients with multiple epiphyseal dysplasia in whom avascular necrosis develops, the appearance of the femoral heads becomes asymmetric (Fig. 7-28). Sequential radiographic imaging for these patients demonstrate changes of increased density followed by resorption and subsequent repair superimposed on irregular ossification centers. When avascular necrosis occurs in patients with multiple epiphyseal dysplasia, the femoral head will usually develop increased deformity compared with the nonnecrotic contralateral hip. The diagnosis of avascular necrosis has been facilitated by the use of MRI.

Unfortunately, patients with multiple epiphyseal dysplasia are predisposed to osteoarthritis in early adult life. Some patients benefit from realignment osteotomies of the hip to improve existing incongruity. Valgus-extension osteotomies may be considered for those patients who have improved congruity documented by arthrography when the hip is placed in adduction and flexion. Varus osteotomies usually are contraindicated because there is a relative coxa vara present in most of these patients. It must be understood, however, that there is little the orthopaedic surgeon can do that will change the natural history of an epiphyseal disturbance of growth. Patients with superimposed avascular necrosis usually have a worsened prognosis. Treatment should include range of motion, particularly abduction and internal rotation. Although no long-term results of

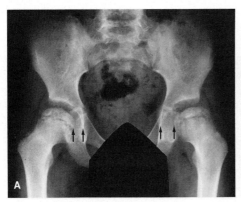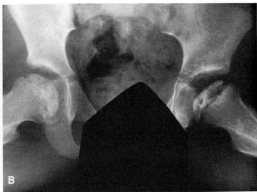

FIGURE 7-28. Multiple epiphyseal dysplasia (age 8 years). Avascular necrosis of the left hip is evidenced by apparent joint space widening, increased radiodensity, and resorption. Note the irregular ossification of the "normal" contralateral hip. (Courtesy of the Department of Medical Education, Alfred I. duPont Institute, Wilmington, DE)

treatment have been reported, it would appear prudent to consider containment modalities for those patients with superimposed avascular necrosis.

Angular deformities or incongruity of the knees and ankles is another frequent problem in patients with multiple epiphyseal dysplasia. Typically, the angular deformities are valgus rather than varus. Recurrence of deformity in the growing child is not uncommon following surgical correction. As in other realignment procedures, careful preoperative evaluation is necessary to determine the most appropriate site for osteotomy. The goal of surgery is to restore a normal mechanical axis through the hip, knee, and ankle. In addition, following realignment, the joint surfaces of the knee and ankle should be parallel to the floor.

MORQUIO SYNDROME

The Morquio syndrome is one type of lysosomal storage disease that is transmitted as an autosomal recessive trait. Otherwise known as mucopolysaccharidosis IV (MPS IV), specific enzymatic deficiencies have been identified that result in the accumulation of keratan sulfate in the connective tissues and urine. This abnormal accumulation of the mucopolysaccharide keratan sulfate results in several skeletal and extraskeletal abnormalities. MPS IV has been subdivided into two types based on clinical severity and the enzymatic defects. The severe form, type A, is due to a deficiency of N-acetylgalactosamine-6-sulfatase while in the milder form, type B, there is a deficiency of β-galactosidase activity in either cultured skin fibroblasts or white cells. In both types A and B MPS IV, there is an excess of keratan sulfate in the urine.

Patients with Morquio syndrome have severe short stature secondary to their short-trunk disproportionate dwarfism (Fig. 7-29). Because of the significant trunk involvement, these patients have been confused with spondyloepiphyseal dysplasia congenita. Morquio syndrome usually becomes evident by 1 to 2 years of age when patients develop clinical features of short stature, spinal deformities, excessive genu valgum, pes planus, or gait disturbances.

These patients have a characteristic facial appearance, including coarsened features, a broad mouth, and widely spaced teeth with discolored enamel. After 5 years of age, patients often develop corneal clouding evident by slit lamp examination. Patients may develop hearing loss, hepatomegaly, and significant aortic regurgitation. The life expec-

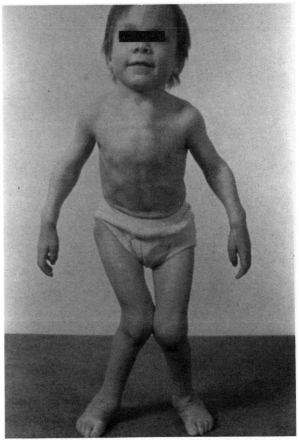

FIGURE 7-29. Morquio syndrome (age 7 years). (Courtesy of the Department of Medical Education, Alfred I. duPont Institute, Wilmington, DE)

tancies of these patients is generally shortened related to pulmonary complications from severe spinal or cardiac involvement.

Spinal deformities are common in patients with the Morquio syndrome. Virtually every patient with Morquio syndrome has dysplasia of the odontoid process, ranging from hypoplasia to complete absence of the base of the odontoid. Many of these patients have atlantoaxial instability (Fig. 7-30). This instability may be asymptomatic, or patients may present with neck pain, decreased endurance, progressive myelopathy, posttraumatic paresis, or sudden death. Symptoms often develop during late childhood or early adolescence. The diagnosis of atlantoaxial instability is made by lateral flexion–extension radiographs. Instability may be identified in flexion or extension. Cord compression may be further documented noninvasively by the use of flexion–extension MRI (Fig. 7-31). Atlantoaxial or occipitoaxial fusion is necessary for patients with instability. Preferably, patients usually undergo surgical

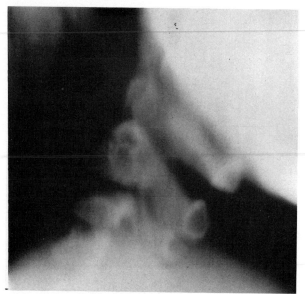

FIGURE 7-30. Morquio syndrome (age 9 years). A lateral extension tomogram of the cervical spine demonstrates odontoid hypoplasia and posterior instability. The ring of the atlas slides posteriorly over the body of the axis in extension. (Courtesy of the Department of Medical Education, Alfred I. duPont Institute, Wilmington, DE)

stabilization using postoperative halo-vest immobilization. Posterior wiring techniques may lead to overreduction of the atlas on the axis in the presence of an extension instability. Internal stabilization is not necessary to achieve a satisfactory arthrodesis in children. If the surgeon elects to use atlantoaxial wires

in the presence of extension instability, however, extreme care must be taken during surgery with intraoperative radiography to avoid overreduction and iatrogenic neurologic deficits. Unfortunately, neurologic signs and symptoms do not always resolve following successful surgical stabilization. Therefore, atlantoaxial fusion should strongly be considered for patients with radiographic evidence of significant instability even if the patient is completely asymptomatic.

Platyspondyly of the thoracolumbar spine is typically found in patients with the Morquio syndrome. In infancy, the vertebrae are flattened, gradually developing an ovoid appearance with progressive ossification and anterior beaking (Fig. 7-32). Kyphosis at the thoracolumbar junction frequently

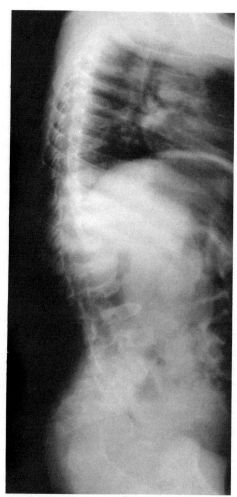

FIGURE 7-32. Morquio syndrome (age 10 years). Platyspondyly with anterior beaking and a mild kyphosis of the thoracolumbar junction. (Courtesy of the Department of Medical Education, Alfred I. duPont Institute, Wilmington, DE)

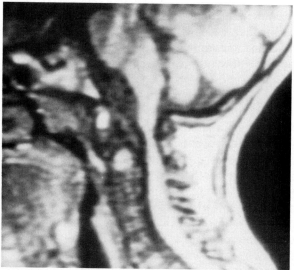

FIGURE 7-31. Morquio syndrome (age 9 years). MRI of this same patient reveals cord compression at the atlantoaxial level. (Courtesy of the Department of Medical Education, Alfred I. duPont Institute, Wilmington, DE)

develops. The apical vertebrae are often hypoplastic anteriorly, and patients may develop a progressive deformity. If thoracolumbar kyphosis is present, bracing is indicated for those patients with curves measuring 45 degrees or less. Combined AP spinal fusion is warranted for patients with curves progressing beyond this extent. Chest wall deformities are also common in patients with Morquio syndrome. These include pectus carinatum and significant flaring of the ribs.

A variety of extremity deformities may occur in patients with the Morquio syndrome. These patients have a significant ligamentous laxity that is most noticeable in the wrists, knees, and ankles. Volar subluxation of the carpus on the radius is typically found. When examined, considerable dorsal and volar instability may be present. Attempted stabilization by wrist arthrodesis historically has been unsuccessful. Symptomatic patients usually benefit from lightweight volar wrist splints. Ankle and subtalar joint laxity is also typical of Morquio patients. This is usually associated with severely pronated feet or pes planus. These foot and ankle deformities occur simultaneously with the development of genu valgum. The valgus alignment of the knees is often progressive and may result in grotesque deformities. In severe cases, the patellae may laterally dislocate with external rotation of the tibias on the femora. Radiographically, there appears to be underdevelopment of the lateral portion of the proximal tibial epiphysis. Realignment osteotomies are frequently necessary and may have to be repeated because of recurrent deformity if performed initially at an early age.

There is abnormal development of the hips in patients with the Morquio syndrome. The capital femoral epiphysis flattens early and becomes progressively deformed. In addition, the acetabular roof fails to ossify laterally and becomes progressively dysplastic. The natural history of these hips is incongruity, subluxation, with eventual dislocation (Fig. 7-33). This sequence of events may occur despite attempts at containment of the femoral head by pelvic osteotomies. It is important to recognize that gait disturbances in these patients may result from either upper cervical instability with myelopathy or lower extremity deformities.

NEUROFIBROMATOSIS

Neurofibromatosis is a multisystem disorder caused by an abnormal proliferation of cells from the neural crest. It is characterized by a wide variety of abnor-

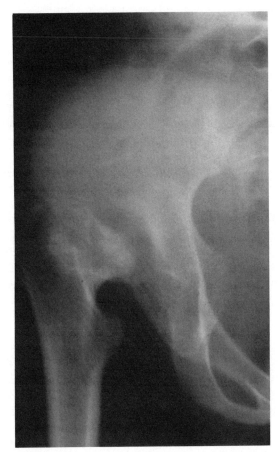

FIGURE 7-33. Morquio syndrome (age 12 years). This patient has severe incongruity of the hips with progressive subluxation. (Courtesy of the Department of Medical Education, Alfred I. duPont Institute, Wilmington, DE)

malities affecting the skin, soft tissues, skeleton, and central or peripheral nervous systems. Though previous descriptions of this disorder were reported before 1800, Von Recklinghausen, in 1882, was the first to demonstrate the neural origin of the cutaneous nodules and name them *neurofibromas*. For this reason, neurofibromatosis has been previously called Von Recklinghausen disease. Traditionally, two clinical forms of neurofibromatosis have been described, namely, peripheral and central types. The peripheral form consists of those patients who have the classic skin and skeletal abnormalities, whereas patients with the central type present with a variety of central nervous system neoplasms. It is now recognized, however, that there is considerable overlap because of the heterogenic manifestations of this disorder.

Current preferred terminology divides neurofibromatosis patients into two groups, NF-1 and NF-2, based on clinical presentation and genetic defect. Although both types are inherited as an autosomal dominant trait, a single gene defect for NF-1 has been located on chromosome 17, whereas the single gene defect for NF-2 has been localized to chromosome 22. NF-1 is the more common type of neurofibromatosis, with the classic cutaneous and osseous manifestations to be described further in this chapter. The diagnostic criteria includes two or more of the following: (1) at least six café-au-lait lesions measuring greater than 5 mm in diameter before puberty and greater than 15 mm in mature individuals; (2) at least two neurofibromas or one plexiform neurofibroma; (3) axillary or inguinal freckling; (4) at least two hamartomatous lesions of the iris (Lisch nodules); (5) optic gliomas; (6) characteristic skeletal lesions, including congenital tibial pseudarthrosis, hemihypertrophy, or spinal deformity; and (7) a positive history for NF-1. NF-2 is less common than NF-1 and is characterized by bilateral acoustic nerve tumors. These patients may also have a variety of other central nervous system neoplasms including meningiomas, ependymomas, gliomas, and so forth.

There is a variety of cutaneous manifestations in neurofibromatosis. The most common are café-au-lait spots. These lesions vary in size, shape, location, and number dependent on the age of the patient. Café-au-lait lesions are found in up to 90% of NF-1 patients. The presence of freckles in axillary (Crowe sign) or inguinal regions is distinctive for neurofibromatosis but occurs less frequently than café-au-lait spots. Large nevi may be present on the abdominal wall localized to one side and ending at the midline (nevus lateralis). These are frequently found in association with plexiform neurofibromata in the subcutaneous tissues. The latter may undergo malignant degeneration. Less commonly, verrucous hyperplasia is a classic but rare finding in patients with neurofibromatosis, characterized by a large area of skin overgrowth. These areas have a soft, velvety feel to palpation. Another rare but characteristic abnormality of the skin is elephantiasis neuromatosa. With this lesion, there is thickening and redundancy of the skin with a rough texture to palpation. Elephantiasis neuromatosa is frequently associated with overgrowth of the underlying bone.

The classic subcutaneous nodules (fibroma molluscum) are more typically found after puberty (Fig. 7-34). These soft, painless nodules are usually small and may be localized in a peripheral nerve distribution. Ultrastructural studies have identified the presence of Schwann cells and axons in these lesions, thus confirming their neural origin. Cutaneous fibroma molluscum generally are asymptomatic, and sarcomatous degeneration is rare. Neurofibromas

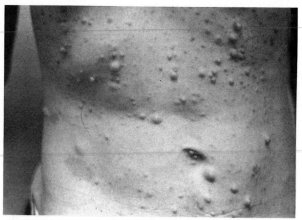

FIGURE 7-34. Neurofibromatosis (age 18 years). Multiple fibroma molluscum on the abdomen. (Courtesy of the Department of Medical Education, Alfred I. duPont Institute, Wilmington, DE)

may also develop in association with deep peripheral or autonomic nerves. These lesions may become large and cause mechanical compression of the vascular, tracheobronchial, esophageal, gastrointestinal, or genitourinary systems.

A variety of ocular abnormalities may occur, including ptosis, exophthalmos, and intraorbital or optic nerve tumors. Lisch nodules are small hamartomas of the iris, which may be identified by slit lamp examination.

There are myriad other extraskeletal abnormalities identified in neurofibromatosis, including hypertension secondary to either pheochromocytoma or renal artery stenosis, gastrointestinal bleeding, seizures, and a variety of benign and malignant neoplasms of the central nervous system. Up to half of the patients with neurofibromatosis have evidence of developmental delay, learning disability, or below-average intelligence. NF-1 patients have an increased predisposition for the development of other malignancies including thyroid carcinoma, leukemia, Wilms tumor, and soft tissue sarcomas.

Spinal deformities are the most common skeletal abnormality found in neurofibromatosis and are reported to occur in up to 60% of all patients. A typical neurofibromatosis curve is a short, sharply angulated curve involving the thoracic spine (Fig. 7-35). This dysplastic type of curve is generally progressive and responds poorly to brace management. These curves tend to be rigid with wedging of the apical vertebrae and are associated with rib changes, scalloping of the vertebral bodies, widening of intravertebral foramina, and significant rotation. High-volume myelography performed in patients with vertebral scalloping or

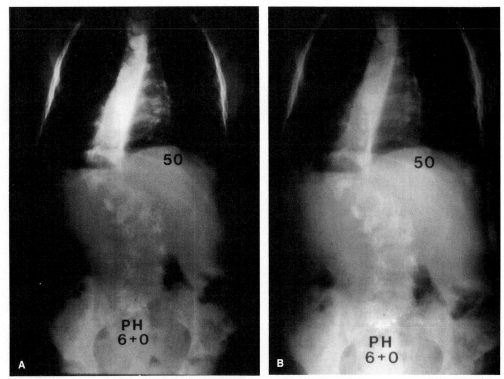

FIGURE 7-35. Neurofibromatosis (age 6 years). A progressive left thoracolumbar scoliosis (dysplastic type). (Courtesy of the Department of Medical Education, Alfred I. duPont Institute, Wilmington, DE)

widening of intravertebral foramina often demonstrates dural ectasia and intraspinal neurofibromas otherwise known as "dumbbell" tumors. Many dysplastic curves have also been found to have a significant kyphotic component to them. If left untreated, these kyphoscoliotic curves typically progress and cause severe deformities. These curves are associated with neurologic impairment secondary to cord compression (Fig. 7-36). Cervical spine abnormalities are not unusual in neurofibromatosis patients. These include dysplastic changes, loss of normal cervical lordosis, development of excessive cervical kyphosis, or instability. Other patients with neurofibromatosis have curvatures that resemble idiopathic curves with no evidence of dysplastic changes. Curves in these patients have a more favorable prognosis and may be treated according to traditional guidelines used for idiopathic scoliosis. Brace treatment of nondystrophic curves in neurofibromatosis should be used for curves ranging in magnitude from 20 to 40 degrees. For curves greater than 40 degrees or for those that progress despite brace treatment, posterior spinal fusion with instrumentation would be the treatment of choice. Though these curves generally behave in a fashion similar to

idiopathic curves, there is some evidence to suggest that these patients have a higher incidence of pseudarthroses. Hence, careful assessment of radiographs obtained at 6 months and 1 year following surgery including oblique projections is essential.

In general, brace treatment of the short, angu-

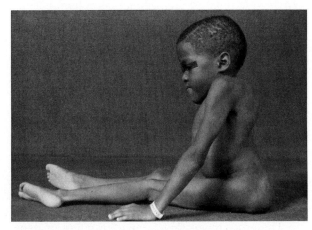

FIGURE 7-36. Neurofibromatosis (age 12 years). Severe kyphoscoliosis with paraplegia. (Courtesy of the Department of Medical Education, Alfred I. duPont Institute, Wilmington, DE)

lated dystrophic curves has not been successful. Many surgeons recommend posterior spinal fusion for curves measuring greater than 20 degrees. Patients with dystrophic scoliosis frequently develop pseudarthrosis despite meticulous surgical technique, including facet fusion, copious bone graft, and rigid internal fixation. Resorption of bone graft is not uncommon. Surgeons must be ready to augment the fusion mass at 6 months to 1 year if there is any evidence of a pseudarthrosis radiographically. Patients with kyphoscoliosis are at risk for the development of paraplegia with distraction instrumentation. The presence of intraspinal pathology, such as dural ectasia or intraspinal neurofibromas, should be evaluated by high-volume myelography before surgical intervention. Patients with kyphosis measuring greater than 50 degrees require combined anterior and posterior fusions to achieve satisfactory stabilization. Posterior spinal fusion alone with kyphosis measuring greater than 50 degrees has been associated with a high incidence of pseudarthrosis and curve progression. Prophylactic laminectomy should be avoided in the presence of kyphoscoliosis for this same reason.

Patients with severe kyphoscoliosis may present with paraplegia or respiratory insufficiency. The paraplegia is most commonly caused by a sharp, angulated, kyphotic deformity rather than to the presence of an intraspinal lesion. Preoperative myelography should be performed in both prone, supine, and lateral positions. Although MRI of the spine is less invasive, interpretation is much more difficult because of the magnitude of the three-plane deformity of the kyphoscoliosis. Anterior spinal decompression with fusion is indicated for those patients with anterior intraspinal neurofibromas or large, rigid curves associated with paraplegia. For those patients with more flexible kyphotic deformities and mild neurologic losses, preoperative halo-dependent traction may be considered. Currently, halo-wheelchair traction is preferable to halo-femoral or halo-pelvic traction. The judicious use of preliminary traction often leads to an improvement in neurologic signs as curve correction is obtained. However, progressive neurologic deterioration may complicate the use of traction. Exploration and augmentation of the posterior fusion mass should be considered at 6 months if there is any evidence of pseudarthrosis radiographically.

The other major skeletal manifestation of neurofibromatosis is congenital pseudarthrosis of the tibia, which occurs in up to 10% of these patients (Fig. 7-37). Neurofibromatosis has been documented

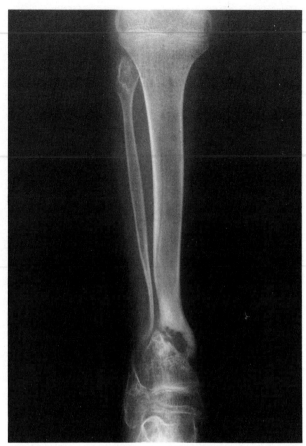

FIGURE 7-37. Neurofibromatosis (age 8 years). Congenital pseudarthrosis of the tibia.

in about half of patients who present with congenital pseudarthrosis of the tibia. This disorder is most commonly associated with anterolateral bowing of the tibia. A variety of radiographic changes are possible, occurring at the junction between the proximal two thirds and the distal one third of the tibia and fibula. Dysplastic changes in the tibia and frequently the fibula are most common. These include sclerosis of the medullary canal, narrowing of the diaphysis, and angular deformities with or without frank pseudarthrosis. Less commonly, patients have cystic lesions of the distal third of the tibia associated with fracture and eventual pseudarthrosis (Fig. 7-38). The anterolateral bowing of the tibia is generally evident by 1 year of age. Fractures generally occur by walking age though they may be present at birth. Less commonly, patients may have anterolateral bowing without other radiographic changes in the tibia or fibula. Pseudarthrosis may not occur in these patients until after a corrective osteotomy is performed.

When the diagnosis of anterolateral bowing and congenital pseudarthrosis of the tibia is made at an

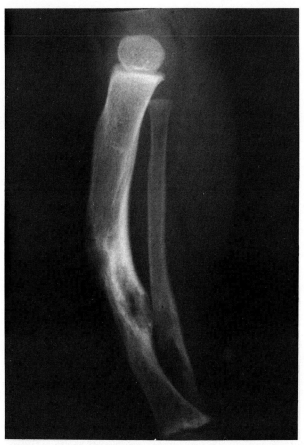

FIGURE 7-38. Neurofibromatosis (age 1 year). Cystic changes of the distal third of the tibia and fibula. This patient eventually fractured and developed a frank pseudarthrosis.

early age, the cutaneous stigmata and other skeletal abnormalities of neurofibromatosis may not be present. Biopsies of tissue removed from cystic lesions or pseudarthroses have rarely demonstrated neurofibromatosis tissue. Fibroblasts rather than neural elements are generally demonstrated histopathologically.

If the diagnosis of anterolateral bowing is made before fracture, the patient should be treated with a total contact, below-knee orthosis. Corrective osteotomy should not be preformed because of the high risk of postoperative pseudarthrosis. Once fracture and pseudarthrosis have occurred, patients often undergo multiple bone grafting procedures in an attempt to gain union. Rigid internal fixation has been difficult to achieve because of the softness of the bone and the typical distal location of the lesion. Treatment by electrical stimulation, whether by implantable electrodes or external coils, has been used with some success. There are no prospective randomized trials, however, comparing the use of electrical stimulation

to conventional bone grafting procedures in patients with neurofibromatosis and congenital pseudarthrosis of the tibia. The most promising surgical technique in recent years involves the free microvascular transfer of the contralateral fibula for refractory cases. Valgus deformity of the ankle may develop in the donor limb subsequent to the fibulectomy. Refracture following successful union of the pseudarthrosis site has also occurred following microvascular transfer. Further details regarding treatment of congenital pseudarthrosis of the tibia is covered in a subsequent chapter.

Other skeletal abnormalities may occur in neurofibromatosis. Pseudarthrosis of other long bones have been reported, including the radius, ulna, humerus, and femur. Skeletal overgrowth is not an infrequent finding in neurofibromatosis and generally occurs with hypertrophy associated with elephantiasis neuromatosa. Remodeling changes in the metaphysis or diaphyses of long bones may have a lytic or cystic appearance. However, these do not appear to be true cysts but rather represent erosive defects from contiguous soft tissue neurofibromas.

An exciting development in the field of medical imaging appears to be useful in localizing deep soft tissue tumors. Technetium-99m diethylenetriaminepentaacetic acid (^{99m}Tc DTPA), used frequently for the evaluation of renal function, has been found to accumulate in many neurofibromas measuring 1.5 cm or greater. The mechanism by which this accumulation occurs is not known at the present time. However, this scintigraphic imaging technique may be useful for the early diagnosis of neurofibromatosis as well as for localization of deep soft tissue masses.

MARFAN SYNDROME

The Marfan syndrome is a heritable disorder of connective tissue involving the ocular, cardiovascular, and skeletal systems. It is transmitted as an autosomal dominant trait (Fig. 7-39). Approximately one fourth of the cases are sporadic occurrences. These are spontaneous new mutations for which there appears to be a paternal age effect. The Marfan syndrome has traditionally been thought to be caused by a defect of either collagen or elastin, though no specific biochemical defect has been elucidated thus far. Within a given pedigree, considerable heterogeneity may be present. Affected family members may have widely differing clinical manifestations of the syndrome. In its classic form, the Marfan syndrome is unmistakable. A less involved family member, how-

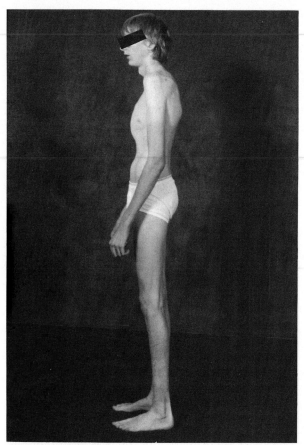

FIGURE 7-39. Marfan syndrome (age 18 years). (Courtesy of the Department of Medical Education, Alfred I. duPont Institute, Wilmington, DE)

ever, may go unrecognized until another relative is diagnosed. At the present time, there are no laboratory tests that confirm the diagnosis.

The most common ocular manifestation of the Marfan syndrome is ectopia lentis, which is a superior displacement of the lens. This subluxation may not be recognized unless a complete ophthalmologic evaluation is carried out with complete dilatation of the pupil and a slit lamp examination. Ectopia lentis occurs in more than half of involved patients. Other ocular manifestations include myopia, retinal detachments, and a flattened corneal shape as measured by keratometer.

Multiple cardiovascular abnormalities exist in patients with the Marfan syndrome and account for their generally shortened life expectancy. Mean age of survival is the fourth decade for Marfan patients. The most serious complication is dilatation of the aortic root and associated aortic regurgitation. Acute dissection of the ascending aortic aneurysm may occur. Mitral valve prolapse and mitral valve regurgi-

tation are the most common significant cardiac problems in children. Echocardiography has become a routine diagnostic tool in the evaluation and treatment of patients with the Marfan syndrome. Many patients are being treated with β-adrenergic–blocking agents in an attempt to delay the onset of serious cardiovascular abnormalities. In addition, these patients are at risk for bacterial endocarditis and therefore require antibiotic prophylaxis during their surgical procedures.

Other clinical extraskeletal manifestations of Marfan syndrome include dural ectasia and anterior meningoceles, which occur in over 60% of these patients' lumbosacral spines. These patients may be asymptomatic or present with radicular pain and evidence of neuropathy. Computed tomography (CT) has revealed widening of the neural canal, erosion of the pedicles, laminae, or vertebral bodies, and widening of neural foramina. Anterior meningoceles may become large and present as pelvic masses. Patients with the Marfan syndrome have an increased incidence of inguinal and femoral hernias. Recurrence following surgical repair is unfortunately common. Striae may be present on the trunk, thighs, or shoulders. Pulmonary dysfunction may occur and is usually related to severe scoliosis or pectus deformities. In addition, these patients also have an increased incidence of spontaneous pneumothoraces. Other distinctive but nondiagnostic features of patients with the Marfan syndrome include a high arched palate, protrusion of the lower jaw, and crowded dentition.

Patients with the Marfan syndrome must be distinguished from those with homocystinuria. Though these patients may have phenotypic features similar to the Marfan syndrome, patients with homocystinuria differ in that they are generally mentally retarded, have restricted joint motion, cavus foot deformities, and osteoporosis. In addition, the cyanide-nitroprusside test for homocystinuria is positive, whereas it is negative in the Marfan syndrome.

Diagnostic criteria for the Marfan syndrome differs according to whether the family history is positive for an affected relative. If there is a positive family history, the diagnosis of Marfan syndrome may be made based on positive features in at least two of the systems previously outlined. If there is a negative family history, the diagnosis requires skeletal abnormalities as well as positive features in two additional extraskeletal systems. The terms *Marfinoid* or *forme frust* should not be used for those patients who do not fulfill the necessary diagnostic criteria. The potential medical, emotional, physical, and economic consequences of this disorder are too great to allow for casual usage of these other terminologies. For those patients and families with Marfan syndrome, there is excellent medical and lay support through the National Marfan Foundation.

A variety of skeletal manifestations may be present in patients with the Marfan syndrome. Most characteristic is a tendency toward tall stature with limbs that are elongated out of proportion to the trunk height (dolichostenomelia). This is documented by either a smaller than normal upper-to-lower segment ratio or an arm span that is greater than the total body height by at least 7.5 cm. Patients frequently have arachnodactyly and ligamentous laxity. Steinberg has described a thumb sign that is positive in the Marfan syndrome. This is positive if the opposed thumb projects past the ulnar border of the hand when the patient is asked to make a fist. Alternatively, the wrist sign, described by Walker, may also be used to document the presence of arachnodactyly and ligamentous laxity. This test is positive if the distal phalanges of the thumb and little finger overlap when they encircle the opposite wrist.

The extremities are long and slender secondary to diminished muscle mass and a minimum of subcutaneous tissue. Hypermobility of joints is common, and many patients have recurrent instability of the patella, shoulder, sternoclavicular joint, or thumb. Generally there is increased genu valgum and at times genu recurvatum. The feet are long, narrow, and typically have a severe pes planus. The hindfoot is in valgus with collapse of the midfoot and prominence of the talar head medially.

Acetabular protrusio has been reported in up to half of patients with Marfan syndrome (Fig. 7-40). This occurs equally unilaterally or bilaterally. The incidence of scoliosis appears to be higher in patients

who have associated acetabular protrusio. Patients may be completely asymptomatic or have symptoms of pain and limitation of motion, particularly abduction.

Spinal deformities are a frequent finding in patients with the Marfan syndrome. Abnormalities include thoracic lordosis, scoliosis, thoracolumbar kyphosis, flat-back deformity, and spondylolisthesis (Fig. 7-41). These vertebral column abnormalities are frequently associated with pectus excavatum or pectus carinatum. Scoliosis is the most frequent musculoskeletal abnormality in patients with Marfan syndrome. There is a high predominance of double structural curve patterns, which begin in the infantile or juvenile age group (Fig. 7-42). Involvement in male patients is more common in the Marfan syndrome than in adolescent idiopathic scoliosis. In addition, back pain is a more frequent occurrence. Unfortunately, these curves tend to be rigid, steadily progressive, and poorly controlled by orthoses. Patients with curves that progress beyond 40 degrees despite bracing should be considered for posterior spinal fusion with autogenous bone graft and rigid internal fixation. Preoperative cardiac evaluation is critical and frequently determines whether a patient is a suitable candidate for extensive spine surgery.

A flat-back deformity secondary to decreased thoracic kyphosis and lumbar lordosis is often present in Marfan syndrome. These patients also frequently have associated pectus excavatum, which further narrows the AP diameter of the chest and reduces the vital capacity. Thoracic hypokyphosis may be present without coexisting scoliosis.

CONGENITAL LOWER LIMB DEFICIENCIES

Proximal femoral focal deficiency (PFFD), tibial hemimelia, and fibular hemimelia are the result of a disturbance of growth and development of the embryonic limb occurring by 3 to 7 weeks postconception. As early as 4 weeks, limb buds of mesenchymal tissue appear on the body wall. During the next 3 weeks, this mesenchymal tissue continues to grow and differentiate into a recognizable limb. This development occurs in a proximal to distal fashion, and, hence, the thigh, leg, and foot segments appear sequentially. The exact etiology for these limb deficiencies has not been specifically elucidated. Numerous factors have been implicated, including environmental influences, trauma, viral infections, ischemia, pharmacologic agents (eg, thalidomide),

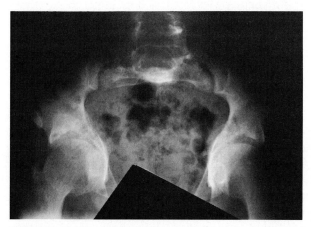

FIGURE 7-40. Marfan syndrome (age 14 years). Bilateral acetabular protrusio.

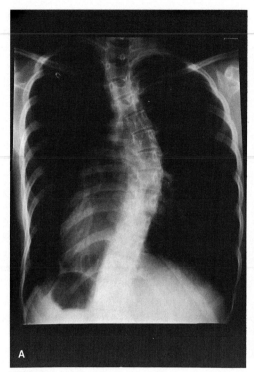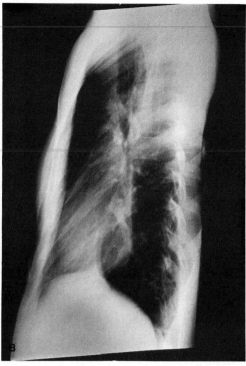

FIGURE 7-41. Marfan syndrome (age 15 years). Progressive thoracic scoliosis with significant lordosis.

and genetic influences. Except for thalidomide, none of these factors has been confirmed. From what is known regarding embryology of the human fetus, however, it appears that the insult or arrest in the development in the limb occurs during a narrow time frame.

Patients with PFFD, tibial hemimelia, or fibular hemimelia may have a variety of other associated anomalies. These may include congenital limb deficiencies of the upper extremities, syndactyly, scoliosis, genitourinary abnormalities, and congenital heart disease. In general, these limb deficiencies are not considered heritable. Patients with tibial hemimelia are a notable exception. Pedigrees have been reported, which demonstrates congenital deficiency of the tibia involving first-degree relatives.

PROXIMAL FEMORAL FOCAL DEFICIENCY

Congenital deficiencies of the femur have been variably classified by several authors. Proximal femoral focal deficiency, as defined by Aitken, represents a severe disturbance in the growth and development of the proximal end of the femur (Fig. 7-43). This disorder results in significant shortening of the limb, abnormalities of the hip joint, and may be associated with fibular hemimelia. Aitken has classified PFFD into four classes—A through D (Fig. 7-44). In class A, a femoral head is present with an adequate acetabulum. The femur is shortened, and there is evidence of significant coxa vara, though initially the femoral head and femoral shaft remnant appears separated. The cartilaginous neck eventually ossifies, though a pseudarthrosis is usually present at the subtrochanteric level. Class B is similar in that there is a femoral head and acetabulum radiographically. At the proximal end of the shortened shaft of the femur, a small bony tuft is present. In contrast to class A, at maturity, there is no osseous connection between the femoral head and the shaft of the femur in class B patients. In class C, there is no femoral head; hence, the acetabulum is poorly developed. The femoral shaft is shortened and, as in class B, a small tuft of bone is present at the proximal end of the shaft. For patients with class D deformities, there is no tuft of bone nor evidence of acetabular development. Femoral shortening is present, and many of these patients have bilateral involvement.

Other classifications have been proposed that include these proximal femoral focal deficiencies in

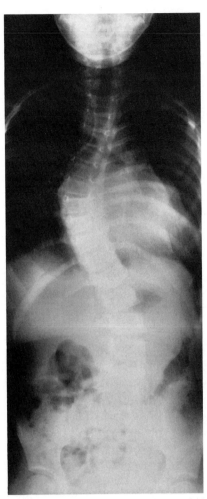

FIGURE 7-42. Marfan syndrome (age 2 years). A progressive left thoracic scoliosis in a juvenile patient.

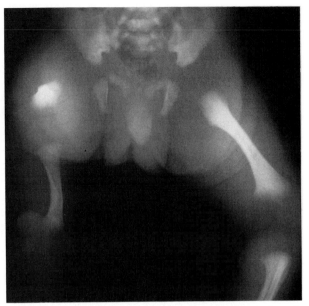

FIGURE 7-43. Proximal femoral focal deficiency (age 4 months). Associated with complete fibular hemimelia.

a spectrum of femoral growth disturbances. These classifications place the Aitken types at the severe end of a continuum, which includes hypoplastic femur, congenital coxa vara, and congenital short femur with coxa vara. These patients rarely have the distal anomalies of the ipsilateral limb that are present in patients with PFFD.

The Aitken classification of PFFD is determined by roentgenographic evaluation and not by clinical differentiation. The involved extremity in all four classes has a similar appearance. The affected thigh is shortened with the foot and ankle frequently at the level of the contralateral knee. The thigh is flexed, abducted, and externally rotated. The soft tissues have a bulky appearance. Frequently, there is an associated fibular hemimelia that may be either of the intercalary or terminal type, depending on the presence or absence of foot abnormalities. These patients may have a ball-and-socket ankle joint, extensive

tarsal coalitions, and absent rays at the lateral border of the foot. In addition, absence of the cruciate ligaments has been reported in patients with PFFD. Aitken has outlined four major biomechanical losses resulting from this type of deformity. These include limb length inequality, malrotation of the hip, inadequate proximal musculature, and potential instability of the hip. Treatment objectives must consider all of these abnormalities as well as the presence of any distal limb anomalies.

Patients with unilateral PFFD require prosthetic fitting to equalize limb lengths and promote inde-

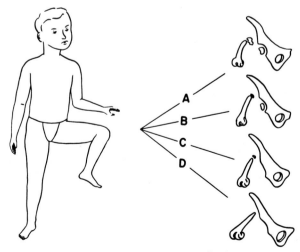

FIGURE 7-44. Aitken classification.

pendent ambulation. The initial prosthesis is usually fit at about 1 year of age when the patient shows an interest in standing. This prothesis may be fabricated to accommodate all the hip abnormalities previously mentioned, including abduction, flexion, external rotation, and any foot deformities that are present. This prosthesis is rigid and must control movements about the child's hip, knee, and ankle. Knee hinges are not used initially but are added to subsequent prostheses once the patient demonstrates good control in walking ability. If no surgery is performed, the knee hinge must be placed below the level of the foot on the involved side.

Surgical procedures have been used to improve both the cosmesis and function of the involved extremity. In patients with bilateral PFFD, no significant limb length discrepancy is usually present. Bilateral prosthetic fitting may be used to normalize these patients' short stature more. Usually, the patient does not use these prostheses in the home setting. Surgical procedures in bilateral cases are rarely indicated except in those incidences in which severe foot deformities interfere with independent ambulation or prosthetic fitting.

For those patients with unilateral PFFD, several factors need to be considered, once the decision has been made to improve prosthetic fit and function by a surgical reconstruction. One basic decision must address the issue of whether the patient is going to be treated as an above-knee or below-knee amputee. Most patients traditionally have been treated as an above-knee amputee because their lower extremity is so short and the anatomic knee joint is extremely proximal. In this circumstance, the patient's knee is stabilized by arthrodesis, and the foot is ablated. This may be accomplished by ankle disarticulation or preferably a Boyd amputation. In the Boyd procedure, the calcaneus is fused to the distal tibial. Therefore, the heel pad remains centered on the calcaneus, minimizing the tendency for posterior migration as occurs in a Syme amputation. Arthrodesis of the knee with accompanying foot ablation provides an excellent end-bearing stump as well as providing an adequate lever arm for fitting of the prosthesis. The knee should be fused in extension even though there is an associated hip flexion–abduction contracture. Generally, these contractures diminish with growth and ambulation.

Ultimate stump length for the above-knee amputee is another important consideration. Ideally, the final stump length should be 5 or 6 cm shorter than the contralateral normal femur. This allows for the use of an internal prosthetic knee joint. Careful pre-

operative planning should include determining of the percentage of growth inhibition as described by Amstutz as well as plotting data obtained from serial scanograms on either a Green-Anderson graph or a Mosely chart. Frequently, epiphysiodesis of the involved distal femur and proximal tibia is required for an appropriate-length stump.

Patients with unilateral PFFD whose foot and ankle are distal to the level of the contralateral normal knee may be considered for treatment as a below-knee amputee. The Van Nes rotation-plasty involves a 180-degree rotation of the distal tibia with accompanying foot and ankle. By rotating the distal tibia 180 degrees, the ankle joint becomes a knee joint with the foot acting as a proximal tibia. Motion of the foot and ankle then simulates flexion–extension of a knee joint. The knee is fused, and the limb is shortened to bring the ankle to the level of the contralateral knee. Important prerequisites include a normal foot and ankle, thus excluding most patients who have significant fibular hemimelia. Patients with hip joint instability are also excluded. Further considerations include a stable physiologic profile because this procedure results in increased cosmetic disfigurement. One further disadvantage has been a tendency for the limb to derotate in time when performed in the younger child.

The decision whether to treat hip instability or deformity is controversial in patients with unilateral proximal femoral deficiency. Some orthopaedic surgeons believe it is important to maintain or obtain stability of the hip joint in PFFD to facilitate ambulation and prosthetic fitting. These surgeons would, therefore, recommend establishing the Aitken class for each patient based on medical imaging techniques. Plain roentgenograms, arthrography, push-pull studies, and MRI have all been used to more accurately define the anatomy of the proximal femur and acetabulum. For those patients with Aitken class A involvement, valgus osteotomies of the proximal femur have been used to treat pseudarthroses and coxa vara. For class B patients, bone grafting with subtrochanteric osteotomy has been recommended in an attempt to achieve stability between the ossified femoral head fragment and shaft of the femur. For those patients with class C or class D involvement, iliofemoral arthrodesis has been used to achieve a stable proximal femoral-pelvic relation.

Many orthopaedic surgeons, however, do not believe that these procedures lead to any substantial improvement in the mechanics of walking or prosthetic fitting of patients with PFFD. Hence, in this approach, surgical procedures to achieve union or for correction of varus deformities is not advocated. In this instance, accurate differentiation of the deformity according to the Aitken classification is not necessary because the hip would be allowed to develop without active surgical intervention. The decision regarding treatment of hip deformities in PFFD remains controversial for patients with unilateral deformities. For patients with bilateral PFFD, however, most orthopaedic surgeons recommend a nonoperative approach unless foot ablation is necessary for ambulation or prosthetic fitting.

FIBULAR HEMIMELIA

Fibular hemimelia or *congenital deficiency of the fibula* are the terms used to describe a spectrum of abnormalities related to abnormal growth and development of the fibula. The fibula may be partially or completely absent (Figs. 7-45 and 7-46). The resultant limb deficiency is usually of the terminal type with associated foot abnormalities. Less commonly, an intercalary deficiency may occur with no significant

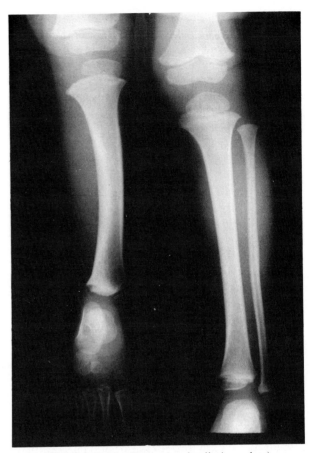

FIGURE 7-46. Fibular hemimelia (complete).

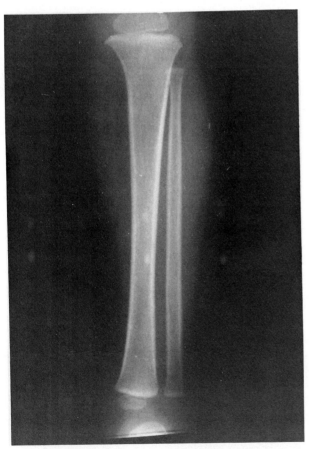

FIGURE 7-45. Fibular hemimelia (partial).

abnormalities proximally or distally. In general, however, fibular hemimelia is associated with a variety of anomalies of the entire limb. Femoral shortening is present in more than half the patients and is variable in severity. Many patients have milder degrees of femoral shortening related to congenital short femur and coxa vara, whereas other patients have severe shortening related to PFFD. Typically, there is increased valgus angulation of the knee with hypoplasia of the lateral femoral condyle. Patellofemoral joint abnormalities may be present, including hypoplasia of the patella, patella alta, or subluxation. Absence of the cruciate ligaments has been described with associated mild instability. Typically, there is a significant growth disturbance of the tibia ranging from a mild valgus angulation of the tibia in patients with partial absence of the fibula to severe anteromedial bowing in patients with complete absence of the fibula. The ankle mortise is in valgus because of deficiency of the lateral malleolus and angulation of the distal tibial physis and epiphysis. Lateral instability of the ankle is not uncommon. A ball-and-socket ankle has been classically described. A variety of foot abnormalities are found in association with fibular hemimelia. The severity of these abnormalities tends to correlate well with the severity of the deficiency of the fibula. In severe deficiencies, the foot is usually fixed in equinus and valgus. Typically, there is an absence of a portion of the lateral border of the foot, including tarsals, metatarsals, and phalanges. Tarsal coalitions involving the subtalar joint or pantalar joints is a frequent occurrence (Fig. 7-47).

Limb length inequality from shortening of the tibia and fibula is a universal finding in these patients. In general, the magnitude of tibial shortening is greatest for those patients with severer fibular deficiencies. The percentage of growth inhibition usually remains the same throughout growth and development, however. Therefore, a patient whose involved foot and ankle are at the midtibial level of the contralateral normal side at birth will maintain that relation at skeletal maturity unless there is surgical intervention.

Treatment considerations include management of the foot deformities as well as the limb length discrepancy. Is the foot plantigrade, or is it possible to obtain a plantigrade foot surgically? If the foot has significant lateral deficiency and is rigidly deformed, then surgical ablation of the foot is generally considered. This will be accomplished either by Boyd- or Syme-type amputation. For these patients, treatment of the tibial shortening is not required since they will be fit with a below-knee prosthesis unless they have an associated PFFD.

Treatment of limb length discrepancy should be considered for those patients who have an acceptable plantigrade foot and no associated PFFD. Epiphysiodesis of the contralateral extremity femoral or tibial lengthenings, or a combination of techniques, may be used for patients with a plantigrade foot. If the magnitude of the limb length discrepancy is too great, however, amputation of the foot with prosthetic fitting would remain the treatment of choice—especially for those patients with a rigid, deformed foot.

TIBIAL HEMIMELIA

Tibial hemimelia is a rare type of congenital limb deficiency. It is characterized by a partial or complete absence of tibia, an intact fibula, shortening of the leg, and bowing (Fig. 7-48). The congenital deficiency of the tibia may be intercalary with preservation of a relatively normal knee and foot. Alternatively, the deficiency may be terminal with associated absence of the medial portion of the foot. Characteristically,

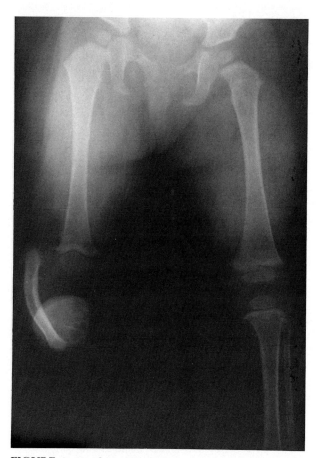

FIGURE 7-48. Complete tibial hemimelia (age 11 months).

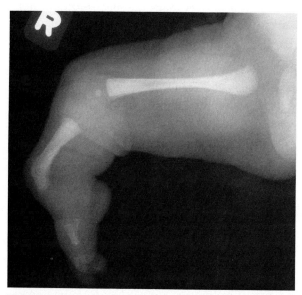

FIGURE 7-47. Fibula hemimelia (age 4 months). There are tibial bowing, shortening, fixed equinus, absence of the lateral border of the foot, and complete fibular hemimelia (terminal type).

patients with tibial hemimelia have a significant flexion contracture of the knee and a foot that is rigidly held in varus and supination. Other findings may include polydactyly and a skin dimple in the region of the knee. Congenital femoral shortening is frequently present on the ipsilateral side. Many patients have bilateral involvement as well as upper extremity abnormalities. Familial occurrences have been recorded.

Three general patterns of deformity have been reported for patients with congenital deficiencies of the tibia. The first pattern is complete absence of the tibia. In these patients, there is a flexion contracture of the knee in excess of 45 degrees in magnitude. The patella is usually absent, and there is no evidence of quadriceps function. The foot typically is in varus with supination. The medial rays of the foot are frequently missing. Radiographs reveal proximal migration of the head of the fibula. In infancy, the distal femoral epiphysis is frequently unossified. When there is complete absence of the tibia, the distal femoral ossific nucleus is delayed in appearance, and the overall width of the distal femoral condyles is reduced. Unless the proximal tibial portion is present, the distal femur does not develop normally and remains hypoplastic.

In the second group of patients, a portion of the tibia is present proximally but is absent distally. There is a knee articulation, including a patella, and usually some quadriceps function can be demonstrated. Proximal migration of the fibula still occurs along with a flexion contracture of the knee though usually not to the same extent as in patients with complete absence of the tibia. The foot deformities are similar to those seen in the first group of patients. Radiographs in infancy may or may not demonstrate ossification of the proximal tibia. The presence of a cartilaginous anlage of the tibia, however, may be inferred by normal development of the distal femur. In this group of patients, the width of the distal femoral epiphysis and metaphysis is normal as well as the extent of ossification.

The third pattern seen in patients with congenital deficiency of the tibia is a shortened tibia with diastasis of the distal tibiofibular syndesmosis. These patients usually have normal development of the proximal tibia, but proximal dislocation of the fibular head is still present. These patients have good quadriceps function. The foot is displaced proximally because of the diastasis and is held in an equinovarus position.

One last variation has been reported in patients with congenital deficiency of the tibia. In several incidences, the distal tibia was well formed but was deficient proximally. These patients had an unstable knee associated with proximal migration of the fibula and a varus foot deformity.

Several important factors need to be considered when making treatment decisions in patients with tibial hemimelia. What is the extent of the tibial deficiency, the adequacy of the quadriceps mechanism, the magnitude of shortening, and the severity of the foot deformities? In general, patients with a completely absent tibia are treated with a knee disarticulation. This provides an excellent end-bearing stump for prosthetic fitting. An occasional patient with complete deficiency may be considered for transfer of the fibular head into the femoral condylar notch as described by Brown. In successful cases, the fibula has been found to hypertrophy and substitute nicely for the absent tibia. Unless there is a well-developed quadriceps mechanism, however, the Brown transfer is doomed to failure because of progressive knee flexion contracture and instability. If the fibular transfer is successful, a Syme- or Boyd-type procedure is necessary to handle the associated foot deformity. For those patients with significant shortening of the femur in association with complete absence of the tibia, fusion of the fibula to the distal femur may be warranted to increase the length of the stump and provide a longer lever arm for prosthetic fitting.

Patients who have a portion of the proximal tibia present are treated with a proximal tibiofibular synostosis and ablation of the foot by either a Syme- or Boyd-type amputation. Below-knee amputations are to be avoided because of ensuing problems of stump overgrowth. Patients with partial absence of the tibia usually have a satisfactory quadriceps mechanism and hence can function nicely with a below-knee prosthesis following synostosis and Boyd amputation. Similarly, patients with distal diastasis of the tibiofibular syndesmosis usually have excellent range of motion and control of the knee. Foot and ankle abnormalities resulting from diastasis are usually treated by fusion of the calcaneus to the fibula. Alternatively, a Boyd amputation may be used for patients in whom excessive shortening is present. This, again, provides an excellent end-bearing stump to prosthetic fitting.

Annotated Bibliography

Osteogenesis Imperfecta

Albright JA. Management overview of osteogenesis imperfecta. Clin Orthop 1981;159:80.
This article reviews the major medical and orthopaedic problems of patients with osteogenesis imperfecta.

Benson DR, Donaldson DH, Millar EA. The spine in osteogenesis imperfecta. J Bone Joint Surg 1978;60A:925.
The incidence and severity of scoliosis is related to the age of the

patient. The incidence of spinal deformities in patients younger than 5 years was 26%, increasing to 80% of those older than 12 years.

Gamble JG, Rinsky LA, Strudwick J, Bleck EE. Non-union of fractures in children who have osteogenesis imperfecta. J Bone Joint Surg 1988;70A:439.
Twelve nonunions in 10 patients with osteogenesis imperfecta were analyzed. The authors discuss etiologic factors as well as treatment of the nonunions.

Gamble JG, Strudwick WJ, Rinsky LA, Bleck EE. Complications of intramedullary rods in osteogenesis imperfecta: Bailey-Dubow rods versus non-elongating rods. J Pediatr Orthop 1988;8:645.
Twenty-nine patients with osteogenesis imperfecta underwent 108 intramedullary roddings with rigid or expandable rods. With an average follow-up of 3 years, the complication rate was 69% for the Bailey-Dubow rods and 55% for the rigid rods.

Marini JC. Osteogenesis imperfecta: comprehensive management. Adv Pediatr 1988;35:391.
A geneticist provides a state-of-the-art monograph of the genetic, biochemical, radiographic, and clinical aspects of osteogenesis imperfecta.

Sillence DO. Osteogenesis imperfecta: an expanding panorama of variants. Clin Orthop 1981;159:11.
This article provides an extensive update of the original Sillence classification emphasizing the heterogeneity of this disorder.

Sillence DO, Senn AS, Danks DM. Genetic heterogeneity in osteogenesis imperfecta. J Med Genet 1979;16:101.
The authors outline the major clinical, genetic, and radiographic features that distinguish four major types of osteogenesis imperfecta (Sillence classification).

Wynne-Davies R, Gormley J. Clinical and genetic patterns in osteogenesis imperfecta. Clin Orthop 1981;159:26.
The authors discuss the problems inherent in classifying patients with osteogenesis imperfecta and suggest an alternative scheme based on clinical and genetic patterns.

Yong-Hing K, MacEwen GD. Scoliosis associated with osteogenesis imperfecta: results of treatment. J Bone Joint Surg 1982;64B:36.
The authors conducted a survey to determine the results of bracing and fusion for scoliosis in patients with osteogenesis imperfecta. One hundred twenty-one patients underwent treatment by 51 orthopaedic surgeons. The authors determined that bracing was ineffective for stopping progression. Complications following surgery for scoliosis were frequent, including excessive blood loss, pseudarthroses, and instrumentation problems.

Skeletal Dysplasias (General References)

Bassett GS, Scott CI. The osteochondrodysplasias. In: Morrissy RM, ed. Lovell and Winter's pediatric orthopaedics. Philadelphia, JB Lippincott, 1990:91.
This chapter covers in detail all of the major skeletal dysplasias with extensive bibliography.

Bethem D, Winter RB, Lutter L, et al. Spinal disorders of dwarfism: review of the literature and report of eighty cases. J Bone Joint Surg 1981;63A:1412.
An extensive retrospective review of 80 patients with disproportionate short stature and spinal deformities, including kyphosis, scoliosis, and atlantoaxial instability.

Kopits SE. Orthopaedic complications of dwarfism. Clin Orthop 1976;114:153.
Dr. Kopits is known for his vast experience in treating patients with various skeletal dysplasias. The insights presented in this article are based on his series of 248 patients with dwarfing conditions.

Stelling FH. The hip in heritable conditions of connective tissue. Clin Orthop 1973;90:33.
The author clearly elucidates and categorizes the wide range of hip abnormalities present in skeletal dysplasias.

Tolo VT. Spinal deformity in dwarfs. In: Bradford D, ed. The pediatric spine. New York, Thieme, 1985:338.
An excellently written chapter that describes the clinical and radiographic features of spinal deformities in dwarfing conditions and details the author's experience in both the conservative and operative management of these abnormalities.

Achondroplasia

Lutter LD, Langer LO. Neurological symptoms in achondroplastic dwarfs: surgical treatment. J Bone Joint Surg 1977;59A:87.
A detailed description of the spectrum of neurologic problems arising from spinal deformities in achondroplasia.

Lutter LD, Lonstein JE, Winter RB, Langer LO. Anatomy of the achondroplastic lumbar canal. Clin Orthop 1977;126:139.
A description of the anatomic variations of the lumbar spine in achondroplasia.

Maynard JA, Ippolito EG, Ponseti IV, Mickelson MR. Histochemistry and ultrastructure of the growth plate in achondroplasia. J Bone Joint Surg 1981;63A:969.
The authors have performed a detailed analysis of achondroplastic growth plates using histochemical studies and electron microscopy.

Morgan DF, Young RF. Spinal neurological complications of achondroplasia: results of surgical treatment. J Neurosurg 1980;52:463.
The results of spinal decompression performed in 17 achondroplastic patients for neurologic symptoms related to abnormalities of the spine are presented from a neurosurgical perspective.

Nehme AME, Riseborough EJ, Tredwell SJ. Skeletal growth and development of the achondroplastic dwarf. Clin Orthop 1976;116:8.
A comprehensive description of the anticipated "normal" growth and development in achondroplasia.

Ponseti IV. Skeletal growth in achondroplasia. J Bone Joint Surg 1970;52A:701.
A classic description of the growth disturbances present in achondroplasia based on histologic and radiographic observations.

Scott CI. Achondroplastic and hypochondroplastic dwarfism. Clin Orthop 1976;114:18.
An excellent review of the clinical features and medical concerns for patients with achondroplasia.

Pseudochondroplastic Dysplasia

Cooper RR, Ponseti IV, Maynard JA. Pseudoachondroplastic dwarfism: a rough-surfaced endoplasmic reticulum storage disorder. J Bone Joint Surg 1973;55A:475.
The authors describe important ultrastructural abnormalities in pseudoachondroplasia that clearly differentiate this disorder from other skeletal dysplasias.

Hall JG. Pseudoachondroplasia. Birth Defects 1975;11:187.
This is an excellent review of the genetic, clinical, and radiographic abnormalities present in pseudoachondroplastic dwarfism.

Kopits SE, Lindstrom JA, McKusick VA. Pseudoachondroplastic dysplasia: pathodynamics and management. Birth Defects 1974;10:341.
These authors discuss the management of cervical spine instability with myelopathy and lower extremity malalignment in pseudoachondroplasia.

Pedrini-Mille A, Maynard JA, Pedrini VA. Pseudoachondroplasia: biochemical and histochemical studies of cartilage. J Bone Joint Surg 1984;66A:1408.

The authors delineate the generalized histochemical changes present in the cartilage of pseudoachondroplastic dwarfs.

Spondyloepiphyseal Dysplasia Congenita

Harrod MJ, Friedman JM, Currarino G, Pauli RM, Longer LO Jr. Genetic heterogeneity in spondyloepiphyseal dysplasia congenita. Am J Med Gent 1984;18:311.
The authors summarize the variable inheritance patterns and clinical features emphasizing the heterogeneity of spondyloepiphyseal dysplasia congenita.

Spranger JW, Langer LO Jr. Spondyloepiphyseal dysplasia congenita. Radiology 1970;94:313.
This is a classic article detailing the clinical and radiographic features of spondyloepiphyseal dysplasia congenita.

Wynne-Davies R, Hall C. Two clinical variants of spondyloepiphyseal dysplasia congenita. J Bone Joint Surg 1982;64B:435.
Two groups of spondyloepiphyseal dysplasia congenita are recognized based on the severity of the coxa varu and the spinal deformities.

Diastrophic Dysplasia

Bethem D, Winter RB, Lutter L. Disorders of the spine in diastrophic dwarfism: a discussion of nine patients and review of the literature. J Bone Joint Surg 1980;62A:529.
Nine patients with diastrophic dwarfism were reviewed. Scoliosis was present in all patients with a strong tendency to progress and become rigid. Four of these patients had cervical kyphosis, which resolved in three.

Herring J. The spinal disorders in diastrophic dwarfism. J Bone Joint Surg 1978;60A:177.
In seven patients with diastrophic dysplasia, scoiosis was present and progressive in five. Cervical kyphosis developed in two patients.

Hollister DW, Lachman RS. Diastrophic dwarfism. Clin Orthop 1976;114:61.
This article reviews the main clinical and radiographic features of diastrophic dysplasia.

Walker BA, Scott CI, Hall JG, Murdoch JL, McKusick VA. Diastrophic dwarfism. Medicine 1972;51:41.
The authors have extensively analyzed 51 patients with diastrophic dysplasia and represents the largest series reported to date from one institution. Extensive demographic, clinical, and radiographic findings are presented.

Metaphyseal Chondrodysplasia

Kozlowski K. Metaphyseal and spondyloepimetaphyseal chondrodysplasia. Clin Orthop 1976;114:83.
This article summarizes the features that distinguish the major types of metaphyseal chondrodysplasias.

Maynard J, Ippolito EG, Ponseti IV, Mickelson MR. Histochemistry and ultrastructure of the growth plate in metaphyseal dysostosis: further observations on the structure of the cartilage matrix. J Pediatr Orthop 1981;1:161.
The authors detailed the extensive biochemical and ultrastructural abnormalities observed in metaphyseal chondrodysplasia differentiating this disorder from other skeletal dysplasias.

McKusik VA, Eldridge R, Hostetler JA, Ruangwit U, Egeland JA. Dwarfism in the Amish. II. Cartilage-hair hypoplasia. Bull Johns Hopkins Hosp 1965;116:285.
This classic article details the genetic, clinical, and radiographic features of 77 cases of cartilage-hair hypoplasia in the Old Order Amish.

Multiple Epiphyseal Dysplasia

Crossan JF, Wynne-Davies R, Fulford, GE. Bilateral failure of the capital femoral epiphysis: bilateral Perthes disease, multiple epiphyseal dysplasia, pseudoachondroplasia, and spondyloepiphyseal dysplasia congenita and tarda. J Pediatr Orthop 1983;3:297.
The authors have reviewed the clinical features and radiographs of 110 patients with various skeletal dysplasias and 25 patients with bilateral Perthes disease. The authors conclude that differentiation is feasible using plain roentgenograms.

Fairbank T. Dysplasia epiphysialis multiplex. Br J Surg 1947;34:325.
This is a classic article describing the clinical and radiographic features of multiple epiphyseal dysplasia.

Griffiths HE, Witherow PJ. Perthes disease and multiple epiphyseal dysplasia. Postgrad Med J 1977;53:464.
Five atypical cases of Perthes disease were analyzed. These patients were found to have an underlying intrinsic skeletal dysplasia.

Mackenzie WG, Bassett GS, Mandell GA, Scott CI. Avascular necrosis of the hip in multiple epiphyseal dysplasia. J Pediatr Orthop 1989;9:666.
Avascular necrosis of the capital femoral epiphysis mimicking Perthes disease was identified in 9 hips of 11 patients with multiple epiphyseal dysplasia.

Spranger JD. Epiphyseal dysplasia. Clin Orthop 1976;114:46.
This article reviews the clinical, genetic, and radiographic features of the epiphyseal dysplasias.

Morquio Syndrome

Blaw ME, Langer LO. Spinal cord compression in Morquio-Brailsford's disease. J Pediatr 1969;74:593.
Eight patients with Morquio syndrome were evaluated radiographically and found to have odontoid dysplasia. Spinal cord compression was identified in three of these patients.

Langer LO, Carey LS. The Roentgenographic features of the KS mucopolysaccharidosis of Morquio (Morquio-Brailsford disease). Am J Roentgenol 1966;97:1.
This classic article describes the roentgenographic abnormalities present in the Morquio syndrome.

Lipson SJ. Dysplasia of the odontoid process in Morquio's syndrome causing quadripresis. J Bone Joint Surg 1977;59A:340.
Based on their series of 11 patients with the Morquio syndrome, the authors conclude that all patients with MPS IV have odontoid dysplasia. Ten of these patients had atlantoaxial instability, and six had neurologic signs and symptoms. The authors suggest early prophylactic posterior cervical fusion in patients with the Morquio syndrome and odontoid dysplasia.

McKusick VA, Neufeld EF. Mucopolysaccharidosis IV (MPS IV, Morquio syndrome, keratansulfaturia), type A and B. In: Stanbury JB, ed. The metabolic bases of inherited disease. New York, McGraw-Hill.
This book chapter provides an excellent review of the clinical and radiographic features of the Morquio syndrome.

Neurofibromatosis

Anderson KS. Congenital pseudarthrosis of the leg: late results. J Bone Joint Surg 1976;58A:657.
The results of treatment of congenital pseudarthrosis of the tibia were reviewed in 46 patients. Neurofibromatosis was present in 37. A classification scheme is presented.

Crawford AH. Neurofibromatosis in children. Acta Orthop Scand 1986;57(Suppl 218):5.

This is an extensive review of the clinical and radiographic findings of 116 children with neurofibromatosis. Considerable emphasis is placed on the evaluation treatment of spinal deformities and congenital pseudarthrosis of the tibia.

Mandell GA, Herrick WC, Harcke HT, et al. Neurofibromas: location by scanning with Tc 99m DTPA: work in progress. Radiology 1985;157:803.
Sixteen patients with neurofibromatosis underwent bone scintigraphy. ^{99m}Tc DTPA was found to be useful in localizing the soft tissue tumors of neurofibromatosis.

Morrissy RT, Riseborough EJ, Hall JE. Congenital pseudarthrosis of the tibia. J Bone Joint Surg 1981;63B:367.
The authors present the results of treatment for 40 patients with congenital pseudarthrosis of the tibia. Twenty patients in their series had associated neurofibromatosis.

Winter RB, Lonstein JE, Anderson M. Neurofibromatosis hyperkyphosis: a review of 33 patients with kyphosis of 80 degrees or greater. J Spinal Disord 1988;1:39.
The natural history and results of treatment hyperkyphosis secondary to neurofibromatosis were reviewed in 30 patients. The kyphosis ranged in magnitude from 80 to 180 degrees. Six patients had paraparesis and six had respiratory distress.

Winter RB, Moe JH, Bradford DS, Lonstein JE, Pedras CV, Weber AH. Spine deformity in neurofibromatosis: a review of one-hundred-two patients. J Bone Joint Surg 1979;61A:677.
This landmark article reviews the Twin Cities experience in the evaluation and treatment of spinal deformity secondary to neurofibromatosis.

Yong-Hing K, Kalamchi A, MacEwen GD. Cervical spine abnormalities in neurofibromatosis. J Bone Joint Surg 1979;61A:695.
Fifteen of 56 patients with neurofibromatosis were found to have radiographic evidence of cervical spine abnormalities.

Marfan Syndrome

Pyeritz RE. The Marfan syndrome. Am Fam Physician 1986;34:83.
This article reviews the diagnostic criteria and clinical features of the Marfan syndrome.

Pyeritz RE, Fishman EK, Bernhardt BA, Siegelman SS. Dural ectasia is a common feature of the Marfan syndrome. Am J Hum Genet 1988;43:726.
Dural ectasia and widening of the lumbosacral spinal canal was found radiographically in 63 of 57 patients with Marfan syndrome.

Pyeritz RE, McKusick VA. The Marfan syndrome: diagnosis and treatment. N Engl J Med 1979;300:772.
This current concepts article succinctly summarizes the major abnormalities present in the Marfan syndrome based on the author's extensive experience in the evaluation and treatment of patients with this disorder.

Robins PR, Moe JH, Winter RB. Scoliosis in Marfan's syndrome: its characteristics and results of treatment in thirty-five patients. J Bone Joint Surg 1975;57A:358.
The authors have reviewed 64 patients with Marfan syndrome and found significant scoliosis in 35 patients. The Milwaukee brace treatment was generally unsuccessful because of the rigidity and severity of the curves. The authors recommend early operative intervention.

Wenger DR, Ditkoff TJ, Herring JA, Mauldin DM. Protrusio Acetabuli in Marfan's syndrome. Clin Orthop 1980;147:134.
Using radiographic measurements, the authors determined that protrusio acetabuli was present in more than 50% of the hips in 14 patients with the Marfan syndrome.

Proximal Femoral Focal Deficiency

Aitken GT. Proximal femoral focal deficiency: definition, classification, and management. In: Proximal femoral focal deficiency: a congenital abnormality. Washington, DC, National Academy of Sciences, 1969:1.
The classic article describing the clinical and radiographic features of proximal femoral focal deficiencies including classification and management.

Boden SD, Fallon MD, Davidson R, Mennuti MT, Kaplan FS. Proximal femoral focal deficiency: evidence for a defect in proliferation and maturation of chondrocytes. J Bone Joint Surg 1989;71A:1119.
A detailed radiographic and histologic analysis of a proximal femoral focal deficiency in a 21-week fetus.

Epps CH. Current concepts review: proximal femoral focal deficiency. J Bone Joint Surg 1983;65A:867.
An excellent review article describing the etiology, classification, and treatment of proximal femoral focal deficiency.

Hamanishi C. Congenital short femur. Clinical, genetic, and epidemiological comparison of the naturally occurring condition with that caused by thalidomide. J Bone Joint Surg 1980;62B:307.
The author describes 70 patients with 91 congenital short femoral deformities. A classification is presents suggested with PFFD comprising one end of the spectrum of congenital short femoral abnormalities.

Kalamchi A, Cowell HR, Kim KI. Congenital deficiency of the femur. J Pediatr Orthop 1985;5:129.
The authors present a classification scheme based on the clinical and radiographic analysis of 60 patients with 70 congenital deficiencies of the femur.

Kostuik JP, Gillespie R, Hall JE, Hubbard S. Van Ness rotational osteotomy for treatment of proximal femoral focal deficiency and congenital short femur. J Bone Joint Surg 1975;57A:1039.
This article describes the Van Ness rotationplasty, which uses the ankle joint of the shortened limb to control the knee joint of a prosthesis.

Steel HH, Lin PS, Betz RR, Kalamchi A, Clancy M. Iliofemoral fusion for proximal femoral focal deficiency. J Bone Joint Surg 1987;69A:837.
Iliofemoral fusion is described as a helpful procedure for patients with Aitken class C and D hips to promote stability and prosthetic fitting.

Fibular Hemimelia

Achterman C, Kalamchi A. Congenital deficiency of the fibula. J Bone Joint Surg 1979;61B:133.
The authors have reviewed 97 limbs in 81 patients with congenital deficiencies of the fibula. A classification scheme has been proposed with recommendations for treatment.

Bohne WHO, Root L. Hypoplasia of the fibula. Clin Orthop 1977;125:107.
The authors discuss the clinical findings in 14 patients with fibular hemimelia and the results of surgical treatment.

Hootnick D, Boyd NA, Fixsen JA, Lloyd-Roberts JC. The natural history and management of congenital short tibia with dysplasia or absence of the fibula. J Bone Joint Surg 1977;59B:267.
Forty-three patients with fibular hemimelia were reviewed. The authors note that the relative difference in growth between the affected leg and the contralateral normal leg stays relatively constant throughout growth. This observation allows for early predication of ultimate limb length discrepancy in these patients.

Westin GW, Sakai DN, Wood WL. Congenital longitudinal deficiency of the fibula. J Bone Joint Surg 1976;58A:492.
Follow-up of the Syme amputation as the definitive treatment for the equinovalgus foot deformities and severe shortening present in patients with fibular hemimelia.

Tibial Hemimelia

Brown FW. Construction of a knee joint in congenital total absence of tibia (paraxial hemimelia, tibia). J Bone Joint Surg 1965;47A: 695.
This is the classic description of the fibular transfer for complete absence of the tibia.

Jones D, Barnes J, Lloyd-Roberts GC. Congenital aplasia and dysplasia of the tibia with intact fibula: Classification and management. J Bone Joint Surg 1978;60B:31.
Based on their review of 20 patients with 29 affected limbs, the authors propose a classification scheme with recommendations for treatment.

Kalamchi A, Dawe RV. Congenital deficiency of the tibia. J Bone Joint Surg 1985;67B:581.
A revised classification scheme is presented dividing patients with tibial hemimelia into three groups based on radiographic appearances. Results of treatment of 21 patients with 24 affected limbs is presented.

Jayakumar SS, Eilert RE. Fibular transfer for congenital absence of the tibia. Clin Orthop 1979;139:97.
The results of the Brown procedure are presented in six patients. Satisfactory results may be achieved if there is a strong quadriceps muscle is present. Otherwise, a significant flexion contracture will recur following surgery.

Turek's Orthopaedics: Principles and Their Application, Fifth Edition,
edited by Stuart L. Weinstein and Joseph A. Buckwalter.
J.B. Lippincott Company, Philadelphia, © 1994.

8

Joseph A. Buckwalter

Musculoskeletal Neoplasms and Disorders That Resemble Neoplasms

CLINICAL PRESENTATION
  Pain
  Swelling or a Mass
  Loss of Function
  Incidental Discovery
INITIAL EVALUATION
DISORDERS THAT CAN
   RESEMBLE NEOPLASMS
  Bone Disorders
  Soft Tissue Disorders

BENIGN NEOPLASMS
  Benign Bone Neoplasms
  Benign Soft Tissue Neoplasms
MALIGNANT NEOPLASMS
  Malignant Bone Neoplasms
  Malignant Soft Tissue Neoplasms
METASTATIC NEOPLASMS
SUMMARY

Compared with other disorders of the musculoskeletal system, neoplasms and some lesions that resemble neoplasms present particularly difficult diagnostic and treatment problems. The locations, tissue origins and compositions, clinical presentations, and behaviors of these lesions vary greatly. They may appear in any region of the musculoskeletal system; consist of or involve almost any tissue, including bone, cartilage, fibrous tissue, bone marrow, lymphoid tissue, nerve, blood vessel, and lymphatic vessel; and arise in patients of any age. They may destroy normal tissue and cause dramatic signs and symptoms, including intolerable pain, massive swelling, severe disability, and pathologic fracture; or they may have little affect on normal tissues and remain asymptomatic. They vary in natural history from lesions that spontaneously regress to those that rapidly spread and lead to death despite early diagnosis and aggressive treatment. Despite their diversity, benign and malignant neoplasms and lesions that resemble neoplasms can have similar clinical presentations and appearances on imaging studies.

Many of the lesions that can resemble neoplasms occur frequently, cause minimal discomfort or disability, and can be treated without surgery or left untreated. Musculoskeletal neoplasms present more complex problems. Because they are rare, few physicians have extensive experience with these problems; because these neoplasms vary in presentation and clinical course, physicians cannot apply a standardized approach to each patient with symptoms, signs, or imaging studies

TABLE 8-1.
Common Musculoskeletal Disorders That Resemble Neoplasms and Benign Neoplasms

Disorders That Resemble Neoplasms		Disorders That Resemble Benign Neoplasms	
Bone	*Soft Tissue*	*Bone*	*Soft Tissue*
Diffuse osteopenia caused by metabolic bone disease	Muscle contusions, tears, and hematomas	Osteomas	Lipomas
Stress fractures	Myositis ossificans	Osteoid osteomas	Hemangiomas
Brown tumors of hyperparathyroidism	Nodular fasciitis	Osteoblastomas	Glomus tumors
Osteomyelitis	Traumatic fat necrosis	Osteochondromas	Lymphangiomas
Simple bone cysts	Traumatic neuromas	Endochondromas	Neurilemomas
Aneurysmal bone cysts	Soft tissue abscesses	Periosteal chondromas	Solitary neurofibromas
Bone necrosis	Ganglia	Chondroblastomas	Neurofibromatosis
Bone islands	Intramuscular myxomas	Chondromyxoid fibromas	Desmoid tumors
Paget's disease		Giant cell tumors of bone	Elastofibromas
Fibrous cortical defects and nonossifying fibromas		Desmoid tumors	Giant cell tumors of tendon sheath
Fibrous dysplasia		Hemangiomas	Pigmented villonodular synovitis
Infantile cortical hyperostosis		Histiocytosis	Synovial chondromatosis

that suggest the presence of a musculoskeletal neoplasm. In many instances, optimal care requires a multidisciplinary group of physicians, including orthopaedists, radiologists, pathologists, oncologists, and radiation therapists. For these reasons, orthopaedists and other specialists with experience in the treatment of malignant and aggressive benign neoplasms of the musculoskeletal system should provide the definitive care for most patients with these rare complex problems.

Patients with musculoskeletal neoplasms are not always easily distinguished from patients with disorders that resemble neoplasms when they first seek medical attention. Musculoskeletal neoplasms and disorders that resemble neoplasms often come to the patient's or physician's attention because of nondiagnostic symptoms, signs, and abnormalities on imaging studies; as a result, most patients with musculoskeletal neoplasms first present to physicians other than orthopaedists with special experience in the treatment of these problems. These physicians must determine whether a lesion is present and then decide if they should recommend observation and symptomatic treatment, further laboratory and imaging studies, referral for further evaluation, and possible treatment or immediate treatment.

To provide an overview of the information necessary to identify musculoskeletal neoplasms and disorders resembling neoplasms and make initial de-

cisions concerning diagnosis and treatment, this chapter first reviews the clinical presentation of these disorders. Subsequent sections summarize the more common disorders that resemble neoplasms, benign neoplasms of the musculoskeletal tissues, primary malignant neoplasms of the musculoskeletal system, and metastatic neoplasms of the musculoskeletal system. Tables 8-1 and 8-2 list the most common musculoskeletal disorders that resemble neoplasms, benign and malignant primary musculoskeletal neoplasms, and malignant neoplasms that metastasize to the musculoskeletal system.*

CLINICAL PRESENTATION

Bone and soft tissue neoplasms or musculoskeletal lesions that resemble neoplasms usually come to the attention of the patient or physician because of pain or vague discomfort, swelling, or loss of musculoskeletal function. Less frequently, physical examination or an imaging study performed for other reasons incidentally shows the presence of a musculoskeletal lesion.

---

* *The sources included in the bibliography provide more detailed information concerning the diagnosis and treatment of these lesions.*

TABLE 8-2.
Common Malignant Musculoskeletal Neoplasms and Metastatic Neoplasms

Malignant Neoplasms		Metastatic Neoplasms
Bone	*Soft Tissue*	
Myelomas	Liposarcomas	Breast
Lymphomas	Malignant fibrous histiocytomas	Prostate
Ewing sarcomas	Fibrosarcomas	Lung
Osteosarcomas	Synovial cell sarcomas	Kidney
Chondrosarcomas	Neurosarcomas	Thyroid
Fibrosarcomas	Rhabdomyosarcomas	Gastrointestinal tract
Malignant fibrous histiocytomas	Malignant vascular tumors	Ovary
Malignant vascular tumors	Epithelioid sarcomas	Cervix
Adamantinomas	Clear cell sarcomas	Pancreas
Chordomas		

Pain

Pain is usually the first indication of the presence of a neoplasm, but the type and pattern of pain varies. Musculoskeletal lesions can cause symptoms that range from excruciating, sharply localized pain to vague discomfort or a sense of fullness, weakness, abnormal sensation, or stiffness; but not all musculoskeletal lesions cause symptoms. Some aggressive benign neoplasms invade or destroy substantial regions of normal tissue before the patient has pain; some malignant neoplasms may reach large size or metastasize widely before the patient experiences significant discomfort. When aggressive benign or malignant musculoskeletal neoplasms cause pain, patients commonly describe the pain as a progressive deep aching that may interfere with normal activities, awaken them at night, or interfere with sleep. Often, rest does not relieve the pain, and occasionally the pain may be referred to a location distant to the tumor. For example, a tumor about or involving the hip may cause pain extending down the thigh to the knee or pain limited to the knee. A tumor of the cervical spine may cause pain radiating down the arm, and neoplasms of the lumbar spine or pelvis may cause discomfort in the buttock, thigh, or leg. Because of referred pain, the physician may perform an extensive examination and evaluation of a site distant from the tumor before examinations of another region shows the lesion. For example, it is not unusual for a patient with a lesion of the middle or proximal femur to complain of knee pain and therefore have extensive studies of their knee before radiographs of the proximal femur reveal the presence of the lesion responsible for their symptoms.

Swelling or a Mass

Many soft tissue neoplasms and some bone neoplasms cause easily detected diffuse swelling or firm, discrete, easily palpated, well-defined masses. Others produce only a slight increase in limb circumference. Infrequently, the reaction of normal tissues to a neoplasm near or involving a synovial joint causes a joint effusion, or bleeding into or around a small tumor produces a hematoma; but some neoplasms do not produce a mass, swelling, or effusion detectable by physical examination. Tumors confined within bone cannot be palpated, and deep soft tissue tumors may produce little or no increase in limb circumference. This is a particular problem with deep soft tissue tumors of the thigh, hip, and shoulder. These lesions can reach substantial size without producing an easily palpated mass, particularly in obese or muscular patients. Intrapelvic, intraabdominal, and intrathoracic neoplasms extending from musculoskeletal tissues may also grow to large size before they cause signs and symptoms. For these reasons, lack of a palpable mass or measurable swelling does not eliminate the possibility of a musculoskeletal neoplasm.

Loss of Function

Most patients with musculoskeletal tumors detect the presence of the tumor because of pain or swelling, or both. Occasionally, patients with musculoskeletal tumors present with a primary complaint of loss of musculoskeletal function. The loss of function associated with tumors may result from pain, neurologic deficit, a pathologic fracture, or a joint contracture or restriction of joint motion. Neurologic deficits due to tumors may progress slowly, as in a patient with a slowly growing soft tissue sarcoma of the posterior thigh that gradually compresses the sciatic nerve. Alternatively, the neurologic deficits may occur acutely, as in the sudden compression of the spinal cord or nerve roots that results from rapid enlargement of a primary or metastatic spinal tumor.

Physicians should suspect the presence of a neoplasm or a lesion resembling a neoplasm in any patient that fractures a bone after minor trauma. Some of these patients report that they had pain at the site of the fracture before the injury. Plain radiographs often show some radiographic irregularity of the bone near the fracture site or in other parts of the bone, but these irregularities occasionally are difficult to identify or the neoplasm may have caused a diffuse decrease in bone mass and density instead of a localized abnormality. For this reason, even when the radiographs do not show any bone irregularity, patients who suffer a fracture after minimal trauma should be carefully evaluated for the possible presence of a neoplasm.

Incidental Discovery

Evaluations performed for other reasons occasionally show abnormalities caused by a previously unsuspected neoplasm. Physical examination may detect the presence of soft tissue or bone mass, subtle neurologic deficit, or slight increase in limb circumference. Plain radiographs or other imaging studies, such as computed tomographic (CT) scans, magnetic resonance imaging (MRI) studies, or bone scans ordered to evaluate an acute injury or some other process, may show abnormalities like bone defects or destruction, new bone formation, soft tissue distortion or swelling, or increased uptake of radioactive tracer that suggest the presence of a bone or soft tissue neoplasm.

INITIAL EVALUATION

When a physician suspects that a patient may have a musculoskeletal neoplasm, he or she should perform a systematic initial evaluation. If the patient has symptoms, the physician should determine the duration and type of symptoms and the conditions or activities that alleviate or exacerbate the symptoms. The physical examination should include careful inspection and palpation for tenderness, masses, or

swelling; measurement of limb circumference, joint motion, and muscle strength; and assessment of neurologic and vascular function. In most instances, the initial evaluation of bone lesions and some soft tissue lesions should include plain radiographs.

Based on the results of the initial evaluation, the physician may be able to decide if the patient has a lesion that resembles a neoplasm, a benign neoplasm, a malignant primary musculoskeletal neoplasm, or a metastatic neoplasm. The physician must decide if the patient needs further diagnostic evaluation, including laboratory and imaging studies, referral to a physician with special experience in the care of patients with musculoskeletal neoplasms, or immediate treatment. Conditions associated with musculoskeletal neoplasms that require immediate treatment include severe pain, pathologic fracture or impending pathologic fracture, and a progressive neurologic deficit or impending neurologic deficit.

DISORDERS THAT CAN RESEMBLE NEOPLASMS

Musculoskeletal disorders that can resemble neoplasms occur more frequently than neoplasms. The symptoms, signs, and imaging studies of some metabolic bone diseases, musculoskeletal injuries, infections, developmental disorders, and diseases of unknown etiology may closely resemble neoplasms. For example, stress fractures can mimic bone-forming neoplasms; osteomyelitis and Ewing sarcoma often are difficult to distinguish based on the history, physical findings, and plain radiographs; and myositis ossificans can resemble a sarcoma.

Bone Disorders

Diffuse Osteopenia Caused by Metabolic Bone Disease

Metabolic bone diseases, most commonly osteoporosis, osteomalacia, and various forms of hyperparathyroidism, decrease bone density and strength in almost all parts of the skeleton and thereby increase the probability of fracture. In some patients, multiple myeloma produces similar diffuse bone changes, and some pathologic fractures associated with nonneoplastic causes of osteopenia may be difficult to distinguish from pathologic fractures due to metastatic carcinoma.

Vertebral compression fractures, collapse or

wedging of vertebral bodies, in patients with osteopenia occur frequently and can present especially difficult diagnostic problems. Common nonneoplastic conditions that cause osteopenia and predispose older patients to vertebral compression fractures include osteoporosis and osteomalacia; but neoplasms, especially multiple myeloma and metastatic carcinoma, may produce similar clinical, physical, and radiographic findings. Many vertebral compression fractures associated with nonneoplastic causes of osteopenia require only symptomatic treatment, but untreated vertebral fractures due to neoplastic disease can cause progressive pain and neurologic deficits.

The presence of osteopenia due to metabolic bone disease may come to the attention of the physician because of a pathologic fracture or because radiographs taken for evaluation of another problem show decreased bone density. Clinical evaluation and standard laboratory tests can help identify the probable cause of diffuse osteopenia in many patients. Well-nourished elderly people with diffuse osteopenia but normal blood counts, erythrocyte sedimentation rates, serum calcium, and serum phosphorus usually have osteoporosis, but they may also have osteomalacia, and a bone biopsy may be necessary to make a definitive diagnosis. An elevated serum calcium and depressed serum phosphorus suggests the possibility of hyperparathyroidism, and elevation of the erythrocyte sedimentation rate and anemia suggest the possibility of neoplastic disease, particularly myeloma.

Stress Fractures

Stress or fatigue fractures, a disruption of bone or localized osteoblastic reaction of bone without apparent disruption of the cortex, usually cause pain and may cause radiographic changes that closely imitate bone-forming neoplasms. They occur in children, adults, and the elderly. In children, stress fractures may closely resemble osteosarcomas; in older people, stress fractures may closely resemble metastatic tumors. Biopsies of stress fractures usually show cellular tissue with extensive new bone formation that may be difficult to distinguish from tissue that forms part of benign and malignant bone-forming neoplasms.

Stress fractures presumably result from fatigue failure of bone or localized reaction of bone to repetitive loading. Common sites include the metatarsals, the tibia and fibula, the femur, the pelvis, and the lamina of the lumbar vertebrae. Stress fractures often occur in young active people with normal bone but also may present in patients with osteopenia due osteoporosis, osteomalacia, or other causes and in patients with neoplasms. The pain associated with a stress fracture usually increases with activity and decreases with rest. In the early phases of a stress fracture or stress reaction of bone, plain radiographic studies may not show any abnormalities, but a bone scan shows increased uptake at the site of new bone formation. At later stages, plain radiographs may or may not reveal a fracture line but usually show periosteal new bone formation that often extends as a line into the medullary cavity of the bone. Stress fractures usually heal with restriction of activity or immobilization.

Brown Tumors of Hyperparathyroidism

Patients with hyperparathyroidism can develop localized expansile destructive bone lesions, brown tumors, that mimic neoplasms or diffuse bone resorption similar to neoplastic and nonneoplastic osteopenia. The focal destructive lesions usually occur within the diaphyses or metaphyses of long bones, where they resorb the medullary cancellous bone and expand and thin the bone cortex. They may reach large size, leading to pathologic fractures. Because of their radiographic appearance and because they consist of multiple giant cells as well as hemorrhage and fibrous tissue, brown tumors can be mistaken for giant cell tumors of bone. Unlike patients with giant cell tumors, patients with hyperparathyroidism often have a history consistent with hyperparathyroidism and radiologic changes indicative of diffuse bone resorption, and they usually have elevated serum calcium, depressed serum phosphorus, and elevated parathormone. The bone disease associated with hyperparathyroidism usually resolves after successful treatment of the cause of the excessive parathyroid hormone.

Osteomyelitis

Osteomyelitis, infection of bone usually due to bacteria, can cause pain, systemic symptoms, physical findings, and radiographic changes (bone destruction combined with new bone formation and prominent periosteal reaction) that closely resemble benign lesions, including osteoid osteomas and eosinophilic granulomas, and malignant neoplasms, particularly Ewing sarcoma, lymphomas, and osteosarcomas (Figs. 8-1 through 8-3). Histologic examination of infected bone shows inflammatory cells, necrotic bone, and often new bone formation (Fig. 8-4). Although

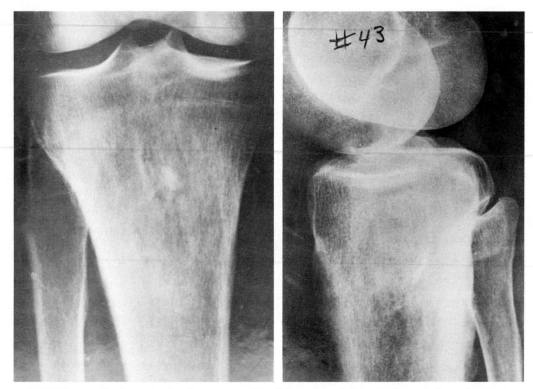

FIGURE 8-1. Radiographs showing osteomyelitis of the proximal tibia with irregular bone destruction and formation.

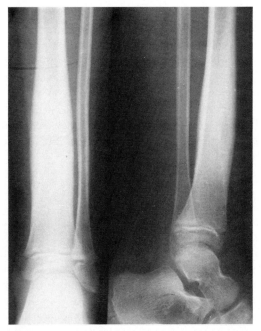

FIGURE 8-2. Radiographs showing osteomyelitis of the distal tibia. Periosteal new bone increases the diameter and density of the bone.

some patients with osteomyelitis have significant systemic symptoms, including fever, weight loss, and fatigue, others have minimal symptoms.

Typically, hematogenous osteomyelitis involves the metaphyses of long bones, but it may appear in any location. Definitive diagnosis of osteomyelitis depends on culture of the infecting organism because biopsies of infected bone often show nonspecific inflammation along with regions of new bone formation that could result from infection by a variety of organisms, and these same processes may be found near some bone neoplasms. In addition to antibiotic therapy, treatment of bone infections usually requires surgical debridement.

Treatment may not eradicate the infection in some patients, and they may develop chronic draining sinuses. Some of these patients, after years of drainage from the infection, develop carcinomas in the sinus tract. These malignancies can cause a change in the amount or odor of the drainage, bloody drainage, a friable vascular enlarging mass, and bone destruction. Treatment of these carcinomas often requires amputation.

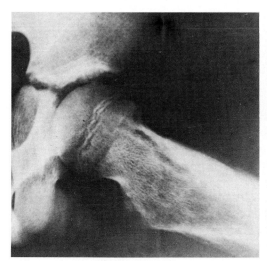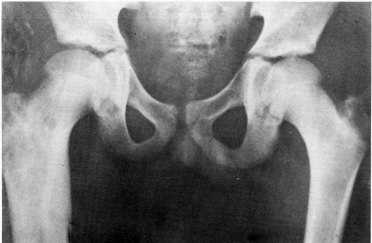

FIGURE 8-3. Radiographs showing osteomyelitis of the proximal femur with bone destruction.

Simple Bone Cysts

Simple, or unicameral, bone cysts consist of fluid-filled cavities within bone lined by a thin layer of fibrous tissue. They may cause considerable expansion of bone and thinning of the bone cortex; they often cause pathologic fractures; and occasionally they cause extensive bone destruction and resemble a neoplasm.

They occur most commonly in patients younger than 15 years of age. About half of them develop in the proximal end of the humerus. Other common sites include the proximal femur and the proximal and distal tibia. Most bone cysts come to the attention of the physician because of pathologic fracture. Others may be discovered incidentally when radiographs are taken for other reasons.

Radiographically simple cysts commonly appear as symmetric lucent lesions of bone metaphyses (Fig. 8-5), although as the bone grows away from the cyst, the lesion may come to lie in the diaphysis. Unicameral cysts that present as symmetric lytic expansile lesions of the proximal humerus or proximal femur in young children do not closely resemble muscu-

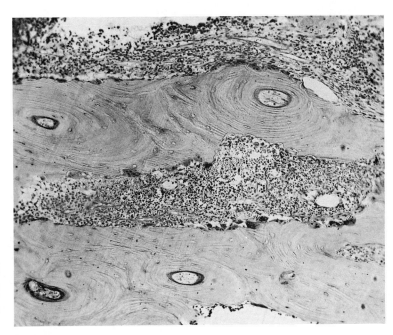

FIGURE 8-4. Light micrograph of infected bone. Inflammatory cells fill the marrow space, and osteoclasts resorb necrotic bone. The absence of osteoclasts indicates that the bone is necrotic.

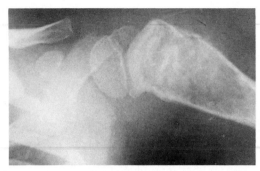

FIGURE 8-5. Radiograph showing a simple bone cyst of the proximal humerus with a pathologic fracture. Notice the symmetric metaphyseal location of the cyst.

loskeletal neoplasms; however, cysts in other locations and cysts that lack these characteristic radiographic features may mimic other musculoskeletal lesions, including aneurysmal bone cysts, fibrous dysplasia, enchondromas, and even osteosarcomas, especially cysts that have fractured, leading to formations of fracture callus. With skeletal growth and maturation, simple cysts heal; but during growth, large cysts can cause multiple pathologic fractures. These fractures may cause skeletal deformity, especially when they occur in the proximal femur. Most fractures through simple cysts heal rapidly with closed treatment. Treatments of simple cysts include observation or restriction of activity until the cyst heals, steroid injections, and curettage and bone grafting.

Aneurysmal Bone Cysts

Aneurysmal bone cysts consist of blood-filled cavities contained by nonendothelialized fibrous septa that may include giant cells and areas of osteoid and woven bone formation (Figs. 8-6 and 8-7). Radiographs often show marked expansion of the involved bone, cystic bone destruction, and periosteal new bone formation (Fig. 8-8), abnormalities similar to those caused by aggressive neoplasms, including giant cell tumors, primary malignant neoplasms, and some types of metastatic neoplasms. In many instances, the lesion rapidly destroys the original bone cortex and is contained only by a thin rim of periosteal new bone.

Aneurysmal bone cysts usually involve the metaphyses of long bones or the posterior elements of the vertebrae, but they can occur almost anywhere in the skeleton, including the pelvis and the scapula. About 85% of the patients with aneurysmal bone cysts present before 20 years of age. The most common symptoms are pain and swelling, and many lesions are tender on palpation of the involved bone. Aneurysmal bone cysts can grow rapidly and frequently cause pathologic fractures. They often occur in association with other bone lesions, including fibrous dysplasia, giant cell tumors, simple bone cysts, eosinophilic granulomas, nonossifying fibromas, chondroblastomas, osteoblastomas, and some malignant lesions, including osteosarcomas. They can grow rapidly, and when located in the spine, they may cause neurologic compromise. These lesions may

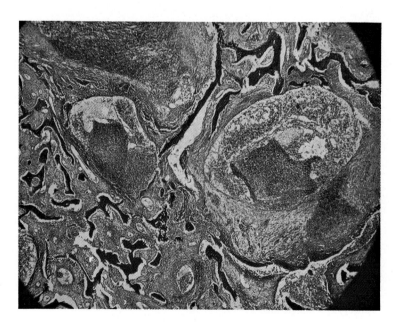

FIGURE 8-6. Light micrograph of an aneurysmal bone cyst. Reactive bone and fibrous tissue surround blood-filled cavities.

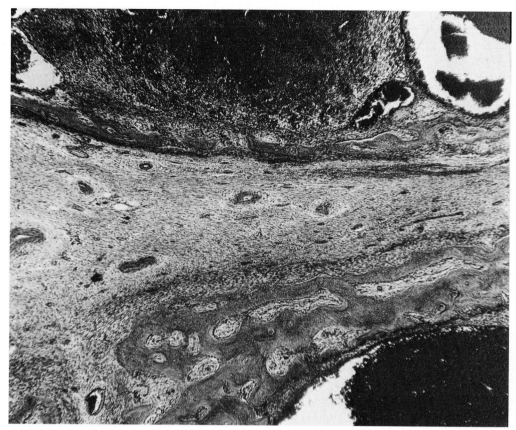

FIGURE 8-7. Light micrograph of an aneurysmal bone cyst. Notice the fibrous tissue and bone that form the wall of a blood-filled cavity.

stop expanding after reaching a certain size and begin to ossify, or they may regress spontaneously; but definitive diagnosis frequently requires a biopsy, and they commonly cause so much bone destruction that they require treatment. Treatments of aneurysmal bone cysts include curettage and bone grafting and resection.

Bone Necrosis

Bone infarcts occur frequently, and many may remain undetected. In some patients, they cause pain and radiographic abnormalities, including areas of irregular increased density within the medullary canal, that may resemble bone neoplasms, particularly enchondromas and chondrosarcomas. Bone necrosis may occur after traumatic or surgical interruption of the blood supply to a portion of the bone or in association with multiple other conditions, including corticosteroid therapy, radiation therapy, and sickle cell anemia. Necrosis also occurs in the absence of any underlying medical condition or known cause.

Common sites of necrosis include the femoral head, femoral condyle, talus, carpal navicular, and metaphyses of the long bones, especially the humerus, femur, and tibia; but the process occurs in almost any region of the skeleton. Necrosis of small regions of bone marrow does not significantly weaken the bone, although it may cause pain; but necrosis of load-bearing subchondral regions and subsequent vascular invasion and resorption of necrotic bone can lead to structural collapse, particularly in the femoral head, humeral head, and talus. Degenerative joint disease develops after collapse of the articular surface. Rarely, malignant tumors, especially malignant fibrous histiocytomas, appear in or near bone infarcts, especially the idiopathic metaphyseal infarcts of the long bones.

Metaphyseal bone infarcts usually require only symptomatic treatment, but subchondral infarcts that cause articular surface collapse often require surgical reconstruction. The indications and long-term results of surgical procedures intended to revascularize or decompress large areas of subchondral bone necrosis are controversial.

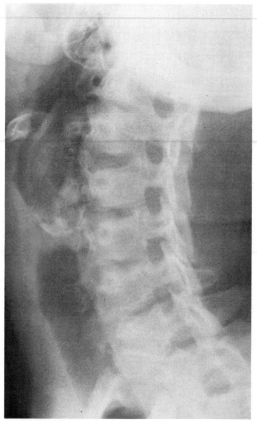

FIGURE 8-8. Radiograph showing an aneurysmal bone cyst of the cervical spine. The aneurysmal bone cyst in the body of the C4 vertebra produced an unusually large soft tissue mass that extends along the anterior aspects of the bodies of C3, C4, and C5.

Bone Islands

Bone islands consist of mature lamellar bone and look like islands of cortical bone within the medullary cavity. On radiographic studies, they appear as rounded lesions, usually of less than 2 cm, located within cancellous bone. Occasionally, they resemble osteoblastic metastasis. Because they are asymptomatic, bone islands usually are identified as incidental findings on plain radiographs or other imaging studies. They do not require treatment.

Paget Disease (Osteitis Deformans)

Paget disease, an idiopathic disorder characterized by increased bone resorption and bone formation, produces bone lesions that can cause pain, deformity, and occasionally fracture along with striking radiographic abnormalities. Histologic examination of pagetoid bone shows an irregular or mosaic pattern of bone formation and fibrovascular tissue filling the marrow spaces (Color Fig. 8-1). It may occur in only one bone (monostotic Paget disease) or in multiple bones (polyostotic Paget disease). It varies in severity from isolated asymptomatic bone lesions to crippling deformities of multiple bones. The clinical presentation of Paget disease and the radiographic abnormalities may resemble some neoplasms, especially metastatic carcinoma.

Paget disease rarely occurs before 20 years of age, and most patients are older than 50 years of age. It can affect any part of the skeleton, although it appears in the pelvis, femur, skull, tibia, and spine more frequently than in other locations, and it is one of the few disorders that causes bone enlargement. Patients may present with bone pain, deformity, or pathologic fracture, or a lesion of Paget disease may be detected as an incidental finding on an imaging study.

Radiographically, Paget disease proceeds through three phases: a purely lytic phase, a mixed lytic and blastic phase, and a blastic phase (Fig. 8-9). The early bone lysis results from extensive osteoclastic bone resorption. The blastic changes correspond to a decrease in bone resorption and increase in formation of new dense bone with an irregular mosaic pattern (see Color Fig. 8-1). The earliest lytic phase of Paget disease often appears radiographically as a wedge-, flame-, or V-shaped region of bone lysis at one end of a long bone. Later, the cortical bone and medullary trabeculae become more dense, enlarged, and irregular. Eventually, in some regions, the bone becomes extremely dense, obliterating the areas of lysis.

Pagetoid bone lacks the strength of normal bone. As a result, it deforms and fractures more easily. Patients with Paget disease may develop primary bone malignancies in the pagetoid bone, including osteogenic sarcomas that spread rapidly and have an extremely poor prognosis. Increasing localized pain, a mass, radiographic evidence of bone destruction, and extension of a lesion outside the bone cortex (Figs. 8-10 and 8-11) or a pathologic fracture suggest the possibility of a malignant neoplasm.

Fibrous Cortical Defects and Nonossifying Fibromas

Fibrous cortical defects (metaphyseal fibrous defects) and nonossifying fibromas consist of fibroblasts arranged in whirled bundles with scattered giant cells and regions of histiocytes. They appear radiographically as sharply circumscribed, radiolucent, markedly eccentric, or entirely intracortical lesions of long bones. Except for rare pathologic fractures, they do not cause pain; and unless they have grown to un-

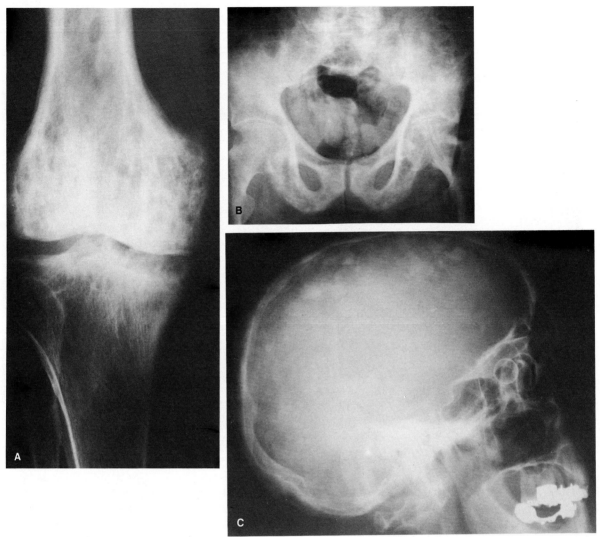

FIGURE 8-9. Radiographs showing the lytic and blastic changes of Paget disease. **(A)** Paget disease of the distal femur. **(B)** Paget disease of the pelvis. **(C)** Paget disease of the skull.

usual size or have led to a pathologic fracture, the diagnosis can usually be made based on their distinctive radiographic appearance.

These lesions are commonly discovered incidentally on plain radiographs. They rarely appear in children younger than 2 years of age or in people older than 20 years of age. They develop in the metaphysis near the physis, and as the bone grows, they gradually become located in the diaphysis. Within a few years of diagnosis, they begin to fill in with normal bone or completely disappear. Most authors refer to large fibrous defects that extend into the intramedullary region of the bone as *nonossifying fibromas*; they refer to similar lesions confined to the cortical bone as *fibrous cortical defects* or *metaphyseal fibrous defects*. Because these lesions heal spontaneously,

they do not require treatment unless they have weakened the bone to the extent that a pathologic fracture has occurred or is likely to occur.

Fibrous Dysplasia

Fibrous dysplasia, dysplastic bone formation consisting of irregularly arranged bone trabeculae in bland fibrous tissue (Color Fig. 8-2), is among the most common lesions of bone. It can weaken bone and lead to pathologic fractures, and it may produce a radiographic appearance that resembles a neoplasm. In some patients, it involves a single bone (monostotic fibrous dysplasia), but in others, it involves many bones (polyostotic fibrous dysplasia). The severity of the disorder ranges from isolated small lesions that remain asymptomatic to lesions

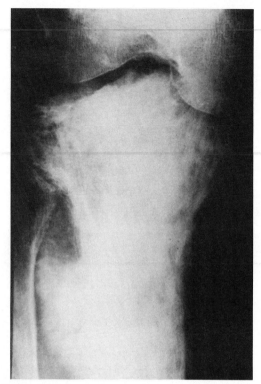

FIGURE 8-10. Radiograph showing a tibial osteogenic sarcoma in an area of pagetoid bone. The neoplasm has disrupted the cortex and formed a mass outside the bone.

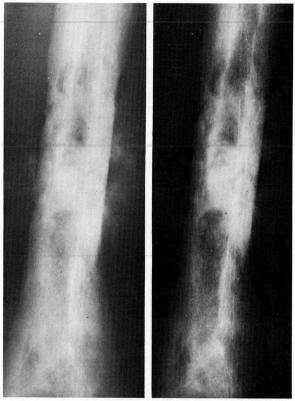

FIGURE 8-11. Radiograph showing a femoral osteogenic sarcoma in an area of pagetoid bone. The neoplasm has formed new bone and extended outside the bone cortex.

that cause repeated pathologic fractures and deformity of multiple bones. Although most authors consider fibrous dysplasia a developmental disorder rather than a neoplasm, regions of fibrous dysplasia can enlarge, destroying or expanding normal bone, and the lesions frequently recur after curettage and bone grafting.

Fibrous dysplasia usually comes to the attention of a physician because of pathologic fracture (Fig. 8-12), skeletal deformity, or an incidental abnormality on plain radiographs. Radiographs show regions of fibrous dysplasia as circumscribed areas of decreased bone density that often look like ground glass. Because fibrous dysplasia can thin and expand the cortex concentrically or eccentrically, the lesions may resemble unicameral or multilocular cysts (Fig. 8-13).

Fibrous dysplasia commonly affects the ribs. Other bones that frequently have regions of fibrous dysplasia include the tibia, femur, and maxilla. When fibrous dysplasia involves the proximal femur, the resulting weakening of the bone may lead to progressive deformity of the proximal femur, referred to as a *shepherd's crook deformity* (Fig. 8-14).

The lesions of fibrous dysplasia appear during childhood and may progressively enlarge. They become less active or inactive at skeletal maturity, but they can grow even in adults. Occasional lesions heal spontaneously. In some patients, polyostotic fibrous dysplasia occurs in association with precocious puberty and darkly pigmented skin lesions, a disorder called *Albright syndrome*. Several reports have described the appearance of malignant tumors in regions of fibrous dysplasia, although given the large number of people with fibrous dysplasia, malignant transformation occurs rarely. Most patients with small regions of fibrous dysplasia do not develop symptoms, but people with large regions of fibrous dysplasia may require treatment for pathologic fractures and progressive or potentially progressive skeletal deformity.

Infantile Cortical Hyperostosis (Caffey Disease)

Infantile cortical hyperostosis, a rare idiopathic disorder that causes rapid periosteal new bone formation, occurs most frequently in children younger than 6 months of age. Common sites include the diaphyses of long bones, the ribs, the mandible, and

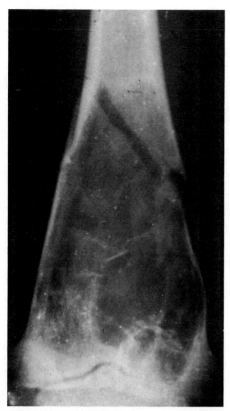

FIGURE 8-12. Radiograph showing a pathologic fracture of the distal femur through a region of fibrous dysplasia.

the scapula. Fever, leukocytosis, and an increased erythrocyte sedimentation rate often accompany the periosteal new bone formation. Irritability, fever, tenderness of the involved bones, and palpable swelling of the periosteum precedes radiographic changes. Once new bone formation begins, radiographs show multiple layers of periosteal new bone (Fig. 8-15). The clinical presentation and radiographic changes may resemble osteomyelitis, syphilis, vitamin A toxicity, vitamin C deficiency, trauma, and malignant tumors, especially Ewing sarcoma. The patient may have alternating remissions and exacerbations, but eventually the disorder resolves and the bones remodel to a normal shape.

Soft Tissue Disorders

Muscle Contusions, Tears, and Intramuscular Hematomas

Muscle contusions and tears may result in soft tissue masses that resemble neoplasms. The hemorrhage that results from these injuries can cause swelling and may form a mass, and muscle that retracts from the site of a tear may also form a mass. Initially, the muscle damage, inflammation, and hemorrhage cause pain and may cause weakness. As

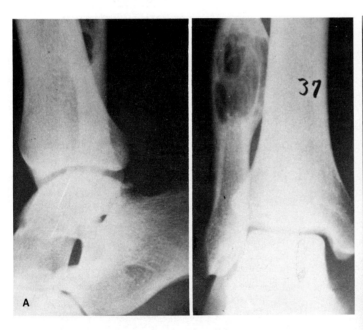

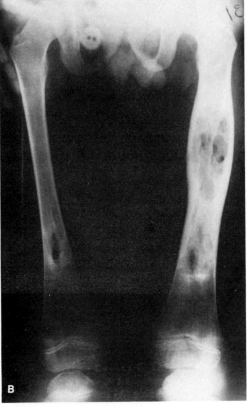

FIGURE 8-13. Radiographs showing fibrous dysplasia. (A) Fibrous dysplasia of the distal fibula. (B) Fibrous dysplasia of the femurs.

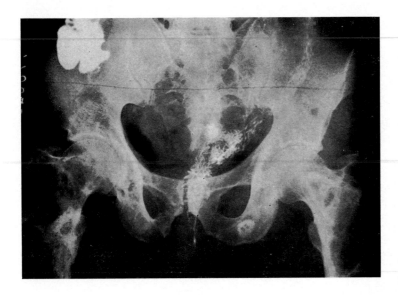

FIGURE 8-14. Radiograph showing fibrous dysplasia of the proximal femur producing a shepherd's crook deformity.

the tissue heals, the pain resolves, but a mass may remain.

Muscle contusions result from direct trauma that ruptures blood vessels and damages muscle cells. Common sites of muscle contusions include the deltoid, brachialis, biceps, and quadriceps. Muscle tears usually result from contraction of the muscle against resistance. Common sites of muscle tears include the hamstrings, quadriceps, and biceps. Muscle tears of-

ten occur in the region of the muscle tendon junction, but this junction extends over a large portion of the length of some muscles so that the tears do not necessarily occur at the ends of the muscle tendon units. Common sites of muscle tears include the biceps, hamstrings, and quadriceps.

Most intramuscular hematomas gradually resolve, but some become organized and remain as firm intramuscular masses. These organized hematomas

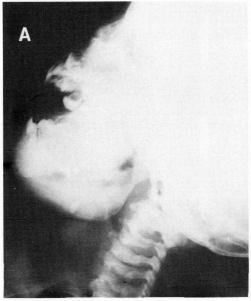

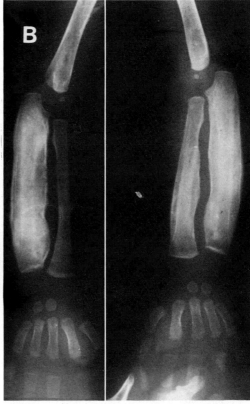

FIGURE 8-15. Radiograph showing characteristic laminations of subperiosteal new bone about the mandible (**A**) and the forearm bones (**B**).

may mimic intramuscular neoplasms on physical examination and on imaging studies, including MRI and ultrasound studies. Most patients can identify a specific traumatic episode followed by pain, swelling, weakness, and ecchymosis, but not all patients have a definite history of trauma. In patients with muscle tears, physical examination often shows a muscle defect or retraction of the muscle. In the absence of a history of trauma, deep intramuscular hematomas may be difficult to distinguish from neoplasms without performing a biopsy. Muscle tears and intramuscular hematomas generally can be treated by restriction of activity.

Myositis Ossificans

Occasionally, single or repetitive blunt muscle trauma causes myositis ossificans, formation of benign bone, cartilage, and fibrous tissue within contused muscle. This poorly understood condition begins after muscle damage with hemorrhage and inflammation. During the initial stages, it causes pain or tenderness along with diffuse swelling and may be confused with malignant soft tissue tumors, parosteal osteosarcomas, or benign lesions, including nodular fasciitis. As the inflammation subsides, pain and tenderness decrease, but a firm mass containing bone usually remains.

Myositis ossificans most frequently occurs in adolescents and young adults. Common sites include the quadriceps, adductors of the thigh, deltoid, and brachialis. Mineralization begins within the lesion about 4 to 6 weeks after injury and proceeds from the periphery toward the center. Microscopic examination generally reveals a distinct zonal pattern reflecting gradations of cellular maturation (Fig. 8-16). The inner regions of the lesion contain immature, rapidly proliferating fibroblasts along with inflammatory cells and occasionally some giant cells. A zone of poorly defined osteoid trabeculae with fibroblasts and osteoblasts surrounds this region, and in the peripheral areas, the osteoid mineralizes, and mature lamellar bone may appear. Radiographically, the lesions initially consist of an area of soft tissue swelling that becomes progressively mineralized and eventually contains bone. Initial treatment of myositis ossificans includes restriction of activity and efforts to prevent loss of joint motion.

Nodular Fasciitis

Nodular fasciitis or pseudosarcomatous fasciitis consists of a proliferation of fibroblasts, capillaries, and inflammatory cells that produce a tender soft tissue mass, most often in the subcutaneous tissues,

but occasionally within muscle. It develops most commonly in adolescents and young adults and may enlarge rapidly. The cause of this rare disorder remains unknown, but it appears to be an inflammatory process instead of a neoplasm. Excision of the mass usually is sufficient to prevent local recurrence and provides a definitive diagnosis.

Traumatic Fat Necrosis

Blunt trauma to subcutaneous fat can cause cell death, hemorrhage, and inflammation. In some instances, as the inflammation subsides, it leaves a firm plaque-like mass consisting of scar tissue and fat that may persist long after the injury. A history of injury and the subcutaneous location of the mass usually suggest the diagnosis of traumatic fat necrosis.

Traumatic Neuromas

Partial or complete transection of a peripheral nerve causes a proliferation of nerve tissue that can form firm, usually mobile, nodules. These traumatic neuromas may grow to moderate size and can cause significant discomfort. A history of trauma or previous surgery and paresthesia in the region of the mass, or the production of paresthesia by palpation or percussion of the mass, help establish the clinical diagnosis of posttraumatic neuroma. But neuromas that develop in the site of previous surgical resection of a soft tissue neoplasm may be difficult to distinguish from recurrent tumor without biopsy.

Soft Tissue Abscesses

Soft tissue abscesses produce masses that may resemble neoplasms. These uncommon lesions develop by direct extension of infection from other structures, including bones and joints, or from open wounds. They rarely result from hematogenous spread of organisms. Most bacterial soft tissue abscesses cause exquisite tenderness, erythema, and fever, but some abscesses caused by common bacteria and most tuberculous abscesses (cold abscesses) cause minimal tenderness and may not produce significant systemic symptoms. These more indolent abscesses may be difficult to distinguish from neoplasms without a biopsy. Treatment of musculoskeletal soft tissue abscesses includes tissue cultures, surgical drainage, and antibiotics.

Ganglia

Soft tissue ganglia, masses consisting of fibrous tissue surrounding unilocular or multilocular cysts filled with translucent fluid or gelatinous myxoid tis-

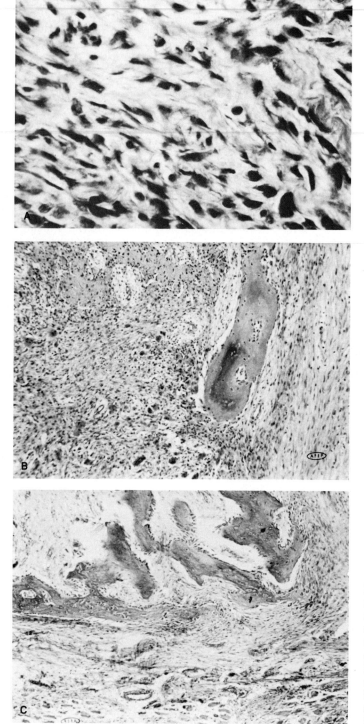

FIGURE 8-16. Light micrographs of myositis ossificans. (A) The cellular inner zone illustrates numerous cells with occasional atypical mitotic figures and variations in size and shape of the cells. The histologic appearance is sarcomatous. (B) The middle zone shows osteoid formation with a fibrovascular background. The cellular pattern is uniform. (C) The outer zone illustrates mature, well-oriented peripheral bone. The fibrous stroma appears more mature than at the center of the lesion. (Courtesy of Dr. William Bacon)

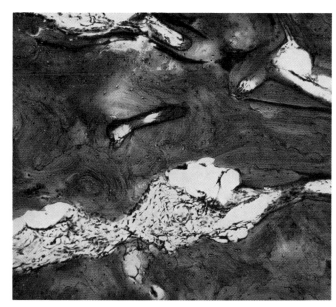

COLOR FIGURE 8-1. Light micrograph showing pagetoid bone. The thick trabeculae have an irregular or mosaic structure instead of the normal lamellar structure. Fibrovascular tissue replaces the marrow.

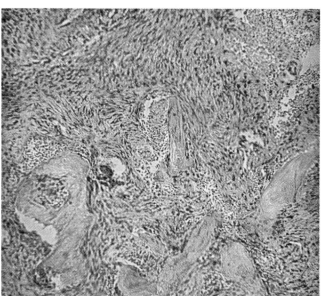

COLOR FIGURE 8-2. Light micrograph of fibrous dysplasia. The lesion consists of woven bone trabeculae surrounded by a fibrous tissue stroma. Unlike other bone-forming lesions, fibrous dysplasia contains few if any recognizable osteoblasts.

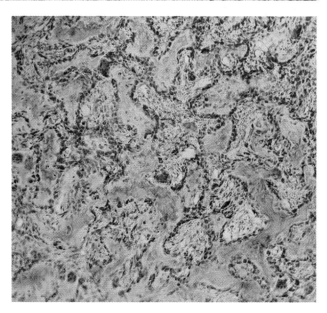

COLOR FIGURE 8-3. Light micrograph of an osteoid osteoma. The lesion consists of abundant osteoid, osteoblasts, fibroblasts, and blood vessels.

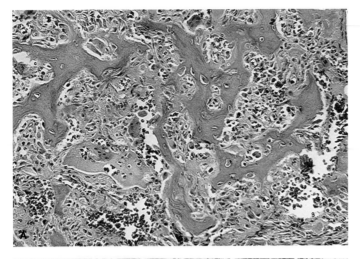

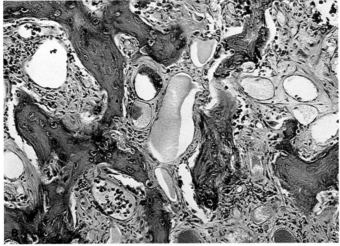

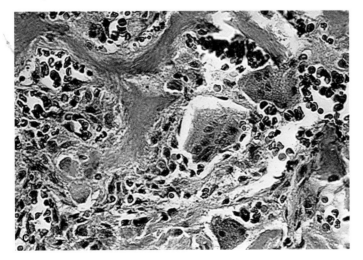

COLOR FIGURE 8-4. Light micrographs of osteoblastomas. (A) A low-magnification micrograph shows osteoblasts, fibrous tissue, and blood vessels surrounding trabeculae formed by neoplastic osteoblasts. (B) Thin-walled blood vessels form a significant part of the lesion. (C) A high-magnification micrograph shows the osteoblasts that form the trabeculae and multinucleated osteoclasts.

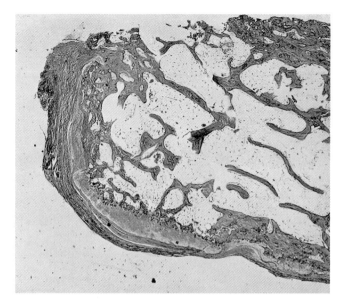

COLOR FIGURE 8-5. Low-magnification light micrograph of an osteochondroma consisting of a bony stalk covered by a layer of hyaline cartilage. A fibrous tissue capsule covers the cartilage.

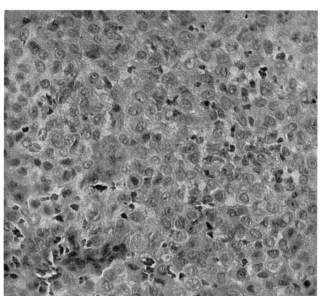

COLOR FIGURE 8-6. Light micrograph of a chondroblastoma. The lesion consists of densely packed round and polyhedral cells with large vesicular nuclei and giant cells.

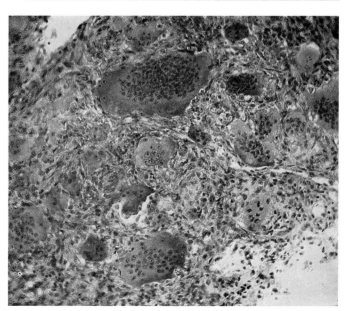

COLOR FIGURE 8-7. Light micrograph of a giant cell tumor. The lesion consists of multiple giant cells, fibroblast-like stromal cells, and blood vessels.

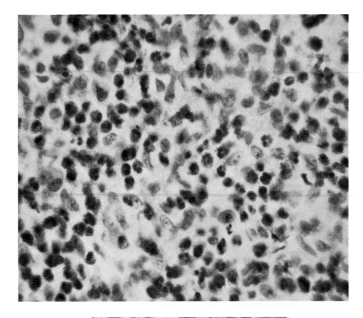

COLOR FIGURE 8-8. Light micrograph of an eosinophilic granuloma. The lesion consists primarily of histiocytes and eosinophils.

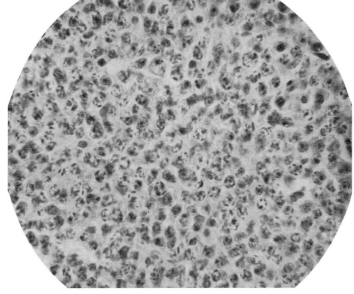

COLOR FIGURE 8-9. Light micrograph of a myeloma. The neoplasm consists of plasma cells with round, eccentrically placed nuclei. Within the nuclei, the chromatin forms dark clumps, usually arranged around the periphery of the nuclear membrane like the hour markers on a clock face.

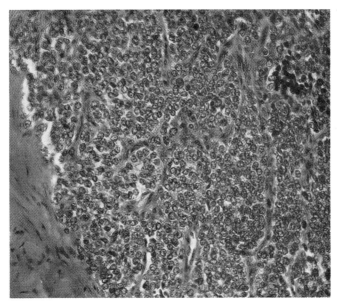

COLOR FIGURE 8-10. Light micrograph of histiocytic lymphoma of bone (reticulum cell sarcoma). These lesions consist of densely packed round cells and often closely resemble Ewing sarcomas when examined by routine light microscopy.

COLOR FIGURE 8-11. Light micrographs showing Ewing sarcoma. (**A**) Low-magnification light micrograph of a Ewing tumor. Sheets of densely packed, dark-staining cells invade between bone trabeculae. (**B**) High-magnification light micrograph of a Ewing sarcoma. The lesion consists of densely packed round cells with prominent nuclei and meager cytoplasm.

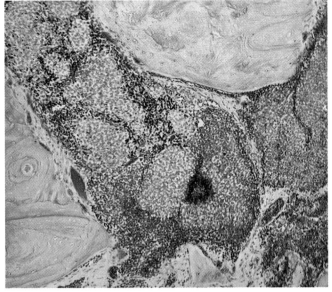

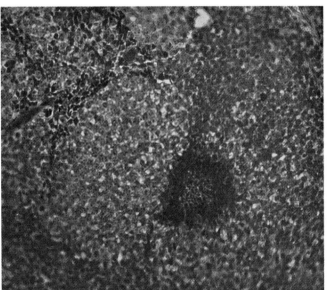

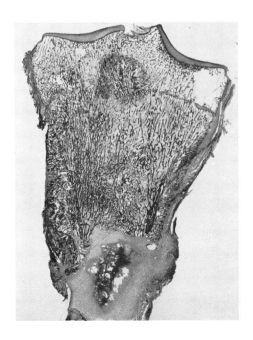

COLOR FIGURE 8-12. Ewing sarcoma of the proximal tibia. The neoplasm has caused intraosseous bone destruction and has broken through the cortex, elevating the periosteum.

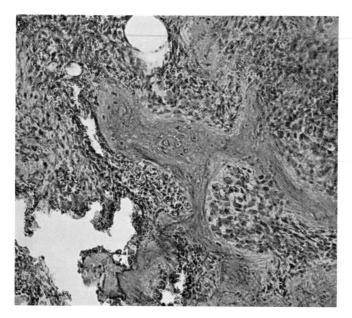

COLOR FIGURE 8-13. Light micrograph of an osteosarcoma. The lesion consists of pleomorphic cells forming poorly organized immature bone.

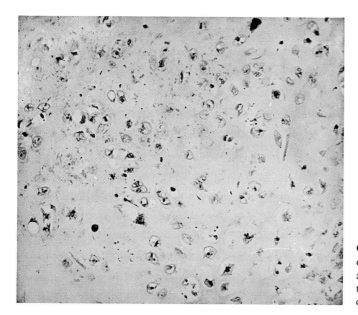

COLOR FIGURE 8-14. Light micrograph of a chondrosarcoma, showing the malignant chondrocytes and the matrix they have synthesized. The cellular features of malignancy include pleomorphism, increased cell density, and binucleated cells.

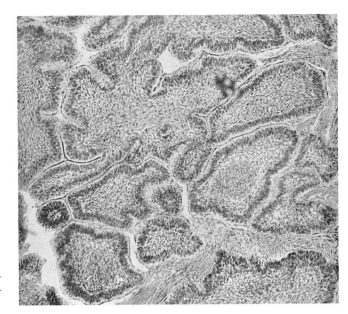

COLOR FIGURE 8-15. Light micrograph of an adamantinoma. The neoplasm consists of islands of epithelium-like cells surrounded by fibrous tissue.

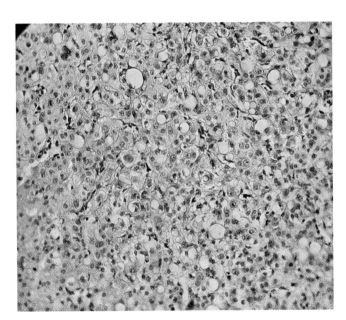

COLOR FIGURE 8-16. Light micrograph of a chordoma. The neoplasm consists of large polyhedral cells formed into epithelium-like cords, clusters, and sheets. The cells have abundant cytoplasm and well-defined nuclei.

sue, occur in patients of almost any age. They usually lie in a superficial location adjacent to or attached to synovial joints or tendon sheaths, most commonly near the wrist, hand, and knee. Ganglia, especially those that develop near the knee, occasionally grow to large size and dissect through the deep soft tissues of the limbs. Enlargement of the limb or swelling caused by these unusual ganglia may suggest the presence of a neoplasm. Although aspiration can remove the fluid from a ganglion, surgical resection is the most predictable method of eradicating these lesions.

Intramuscular Myxomas

Intramuscular myxomas consist of solid tissue formed from an abundant gelatinous myxoid matrix containing few cells and occasional cystic areas that resemble ganglia. Myxomas produce firm, usually mobile intramuscular masses that occur most frequently in patients between 40 and 70 years of age. They may enlarge slowly, or they may remain unchanged for many years; but because of their deep intramuscular location, they cannot be easily distinguished from soft tissue sarcomas by clinical evaluation. Physicians usually recommend removal of intramuscular myxomas to prevent enlargement and make a definitive diagnosis.

BENIGN NEOPLASMS

Benign neoplasms of bone and soft tissue occur more commonly than malignant neoplasms. All these benign lesions result at least in part from cell proliferation and matrix synthesis that produce new tissue, but their behavior varies considerably. Some do not grow relentlessly. Instead, they enlarge to a certain size, usually during skeletal growth, and then remain unchanged indefinitely; thus, they might be considered developmental disorders rather than neoplasms. Lesions that follow this pattern include osteochondromas, enchondromas, and some lymphangiomas and hemangiomas. Other benign lesions, including giant cell tumors of tendon sheath, elastofibromas, and pigmented villonodular synovitis, may represent inflammatory or reactive disorders; but some lesions, like giant cell tumors of bone and osteoblastomas, behave like neoplasms.

Because of the differences in their behavior, these benign proliferative lesions require different treatments. Most osteochondromas and enchondromas should be left untreated; but others, like giant cell

tumors and osteoblastomas, usually require surgical removal. These benign neoplasms and some others aggressively invade and destroy normal tissue and may be difficult to distinguish from malignant neoplasms. Some of these lesions may be capable of metastasizing despite their benign histologic appearance; in particular, rare patients with giant cell tumors and chondroblastomas have developed lung lesions with the benign histologic appearance of the primary bone neoplasm.

Benign Bone Neoplasms

Osteomas

Osteomas, like bone islands, consist of mature bone. They form on endosteal and periosteal bone surfaces, most commonly in the mandible, the flat bones of the skull, and the tibia, in adolescents and young adults. On plain radiographs, they appear as dense nodules of bone. Patients may notice a firm bony mass, or the lesion may be detected as an incidental finding on plain radiographic studies. They generally do not require treatment.

Osteoid Osteomas

Osteoid osteomas consist of a central region, or nidus, less than 2 cm in diameter, containing osteoblasts forming large volumes of disorganized osteoid, capillaries, and occasional osteoclasts (Color Fig. 8-3). A larger region of reactive new bone formation that matures to become dense lamellar bone surrounds the central region. A thin rim of granulation tissue may separate the central osteoid-forming region from the dense reactive bone.

Radiographs show some osteoid osteomas as small, spheric, dense regions rimmed by a thin lucent ring within a larger region of dense mature bone. Other osteoid osteomas appear only as small lucent areas surrounded by dense bone. Occasionally, the increased density of the reactive bone hides the central lesion on plain radiographs. In these instances, CT usually shows the central lucency.

Most osteoid osteomas occur in children, adolescents, or adults younger than 30 years. They can cause considerable pain, usually worse at night. Typically, aspirin provides excellent pain relief. Osteoid osteomas occur most frequently in the diaphyses and metaphyses of the long bones, but they can develop in almost any part of the skeleton. When they involve bone near synovial joints, they can cause joint effusions, muscle spasm, and joint contractures.

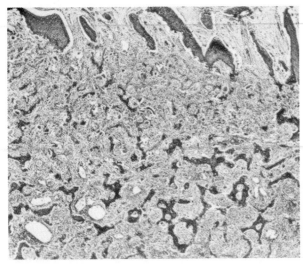

FIGURE 8-17. Low-magnification light micrograph of an osteoblastoma shows bone trabeculae formed by the neoplastic cells.

The pain due to an osteoid osteoma may eventually resolve spontaneously, and therefore patients may be treated symptomatically, but most lesions are treated by surgical excision.

Osteoblastomas

Like the central region of an osteoid osteoma, osteoblastomas consist primarily of osteoblasts, osteoid, and blood vessels. (Fig. 8-17 and Color Fig. 8-

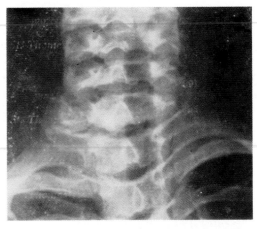

FIGURE 8-18. Radiograph of an osteoblastoma. The neoplasm has expanded the right transverse process of C7. It appears as a lucent area with surrounding rim of bone. (Dahlin DC. Bone tumors. Springfield, IL, Charles C Thomas, 1957)

4). They are larger than osteoid osteomas, that is, larger than 2 cm in diameter, and they can expand and destroy bone as well as form new bone. Radiographically, they usually appear as lucent lesions surrounded by a thin rim of reactive bone (Figs. 8-18 through 8-20). In many of these neoplasms, the central lucent area contains small areas of mineralization.

Most osteoblastomas occur in patients younger than 30 years of age and cause pain, but the pain is usually less severe than that associated with an os-

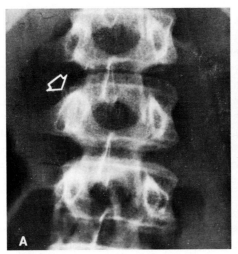
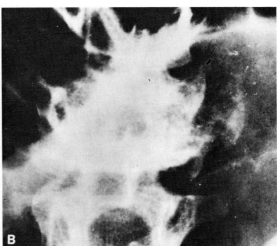

FIGURE 8-19. Radiographs of a spinal osteoblastoma. (A) The right pedicle of L2 appears to be slightly enlarged, and the margin of the L2 vertebral body is indistinct. (B) At a later stage, expanding combined osteolytic and ossifying mass involves the right portion of the posterior arch, including lamina, pedicle, and transverse process, and also the right half of the body of L2. A soft tissue mass extends outward toward the right, is sharply circumscribed by a calcific shell, and contains mottled opacities of new bone. (Pochaczevsky R, et al. The roentgen appearance of benign osteoblastoma. Radiology 1960;75:429)

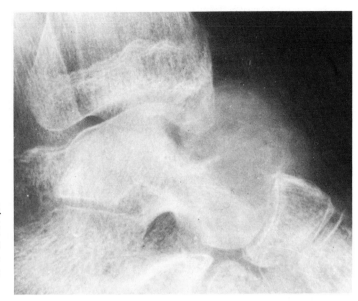

FIGURE 8-20. Radiograph of an osteoblastoma. An osteolytic, expanding tumor has eroded the cortex of the talus and has extended outward. It is circumscribed by a thin shell of bone. Scattered, minute opacities throughout the tumor represent new bone. (Pochaczevsky R, et al. The roentgen appearance of benign osteoblastoma. Radiology 1960;75:429)

teoid osteoma. They usually involve the metaphyses or diaphyses of long bones or the vertebrae (see Figs. 8-18 and 8-19). The differential diagnosis of an osteoblastoma usually includes osteosarcoma and may include giant cell tumor and osteoid osteoma.

The behavior of osteoblastomas varies from slow enlargement to rapid aggressive growth that resembles the behavior of an osteosarcoma. Occasionally, they cause pathologic fractures. Surgical resection or meticulous curettage eradicates most osteoblastomas.

Osteochondromas

Osteochondromas or osteocartilaginous exostoses, the most common benign bone tumors, consist of benign cartilage and bone. They form a bony base or stalk and a cartilage cap that projects from normal bone, usually in the region of a physis (Color Fig. 8-5). A fibrous tissue capsule or a bursa typically covers the cartilage. Osteochondromas may develop from proliferation of cartilage-forming periosteal cells, or alternatively they may result from a defect in the fibrous tissue surrounding a physis, and therefore represent a developmental disorder instead of a neoplasm. Common locations of osteochondromas include the metaphyses of the proximal tibia, the distal femur, the distal tibia and fibula, the proximal femur, and the proximal humerus. They also can develop from flat bones of the pelvis and from the scapula.

Study of plain radiographs usually can establish the diagnosis of an osteochondroma: the bony base of the lesion extends directly from normal bone, and the normal bone cortex and cancellous bone pass di-

rectly into the bone of the osteochondroma (Fig. 8-21). Most patients have solitary osteochondromas, but some have a hereditary disorder that causes multiple osteochondromas. This disorder, hereditary multiple osteocartilaginous exostoses, is transmitted as an autosomal dominant trait with a high degree of penetrance and can cause significant skeletal deformity and disability.

Osteochondromas commonly present as solitary or multiple firm, fixed, asymptomatic bony masses. Most patients recognize their presence before 20 years of age. Severely affected people with multiple lesions often develop considerable skeletal deformity. During skeletal growth, the lesions enlarge, sometimes rapidly. When skeletal growth ceases, most osteochondromas stop enlarging. Because the cartilage component of osteochondromas enlarges the lesion and the bone component forms by enchondral ossification, growing osteochondromas typically have a large cartilaginous component. As the lesions mature, the cartilage component decreases, and eventually most osteochondromas in adults consist primarily of bone.

Occasionally, osteochondromas fracture through their bony stalk or develop a soft tissue bursa. In these instances, they may cause pain. Enlargement of the osteochondromas may cause nerve compression or skeletal deformity. Rarely, chondrosarcomas develop in osteochondromas that undergo malignant degeneration during adult life, especially in patients with multiple osteochondromas. Malignant transformation occurs more frequently in osteochondromas of flat bones, particularly the pelvis and scapula,

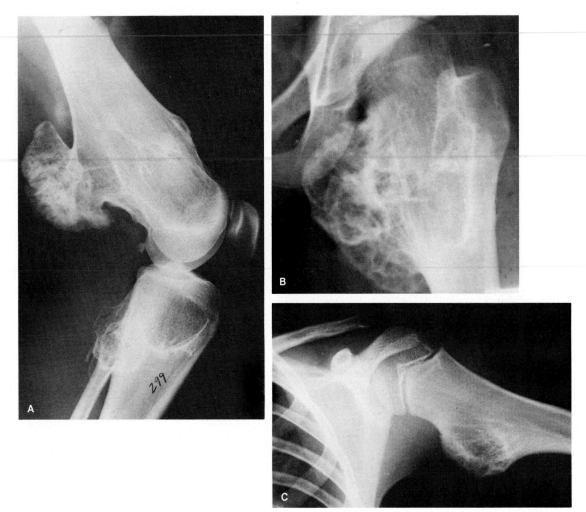

FIGURE 8-21. Plain radiographs showing typical osteochondromas of long bone metaphyses. The bony bases of the lesions extend directly from normal bone, and the medullary cavity of the normal bone extends into the lesion. Plain radiographs do not show the cartilage portion of an osteochondroma, so the lesions may be much larger than the plain radiographic images. (**A**) Osteochondromas of the distal femoral and proximal tibial metaphyses. (**B**) An osteochondroma of the proximal femoral metaphysis. (**C**) An osteochondroma of the proximal humeral metaphysis.

and should be suspected when an osteochondroma causes pain or enlarges in an adult. Treatment of osteochondromas consists of surgical resection if they cause pain due to fracture or bursa formation or if they cause nerve compression, limitation of joint motion, or significant skeletal deformity.

Enchondromas

Enchondromas consist of benign hyaline cartilage masses formed in the medullary cavities of otherwise normal bones. They frequently occur in the bones of the hands and feet but may appear in almost any part of the skeleton, including the large long

bones of the limbs, especially the femur, tibia, and humerus. Radiographs show the lesions as centrally placed or occasionally slightly eccentric, circumscribed, lucent regions. They often resemble bone infarcts or occasionally fibrous dysplasia. During skeletal growth, the lesions may slowly enlarge. After completion of normal growth, they cease to enlarge and frequently develop multiple areas of mineralization that give the lesion a stippled appearance on plain radiographs. Occasionally, enchondromas weaken the bone sufficiently to cause a pathologic fracture, and rarely chondrosarcomas develop in enchondromas. Because enchondromas usually remain asymptomatic and do not enlarge after skeletal maturity, a lesion that causes pain or enlarges in an adult strongly suggests the possibility of malignant transformation.

Some patients have multiple enchondromas that can cause severe deformity and stunting of growth and increase the probability of a lesion becoming a chondrosarcoma, a condition named *Ollier disease.* Rarely, multiple enchondromas occur in association with multiple hemangiomas, a condition named *Maffucci syndrome,* that also increases the probability of the patient developing a chondrosarcoma. Unless they cause pathologic fractures or show signs of malignant transformation, enchondromas generally do not require treatment.

Periosteal Chondromas

Periosteal chondromas, subperiosteal lesions consisting primarily of hyaline cartilage, occur less frequently than osteochondromas and enchondromas. They form between the cortical bone and overlying periosteum, often creating a shallow depression in the bone surface and a smooth bulge of periosteum-covered cartilage that projects into the soft tissues (Fig. 8-22). Radiographs show a scalloped depression in the bone cortex and may show a faint image of a soft tissue mass that contains small, speckled regions of calcification.

Presumably, periosteal chondromas develop from proliferation of cartilage-forming periosteal cells. They occur most frequently in the proximal humeral metaphysis, phalanges, metacarpals, and metatarsals. They usually present as a solitary painless mass detected by the patient or as an incidental finding on a plain radiograph. Most patients are young or middle-aged adults. Periosteal chondromas can slowly enlarge, but they have not been shown to cause significant damage to normal tissues. Most surgeons treat periosteal chondromas by resection.

Chondroblastomas

Chondroblastomas consist of regions or "islands" of densely packed polyhedral cells called *chondroblasts,* regions of chondrocytes forming a cartilage matrix, and regions of more fibrous tissue (Fig. 8-23 and Color Fig. 8-6). In some regions, the cartilage matrix mineralizes, creating a distinctive "chicken wire" pattern of mineralization; other regions may contain large numbers of giant cells. Chondroblastomas usually involve the epiphyses of long bones in patients with open physis. Radiographs typically show an eccentric epiphyseal lucent area that may contain punctuate calcifications. A sclerotic bony

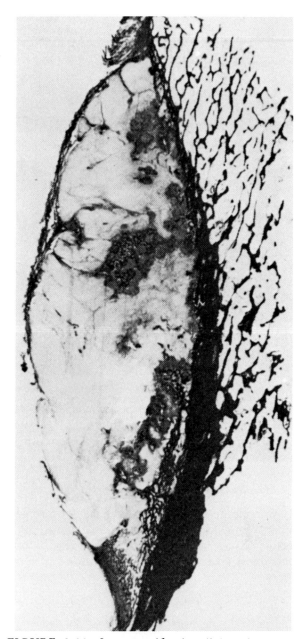

FIGURE 8-22. Low-magnification light micrograph showing a periosteal chondroma of the proximal humerus. The hyaline cartilage lesion has caused a shallow depression in the bone cortex and bulges into the soft tissues.

boarder often surrounds the lucent area. The lesions rarely involve more than half the epiphysis and only occasionally extend into the metaphysis.

They occur most commonly in the proximal humeral epiphysis, but they have been found in multiple other sites. Most patients present with pain and local tenderness. Occasionally, they may have swelling, limitation of joint motion, joint effusions, and joint contractures. Curettage and bone grafting cures

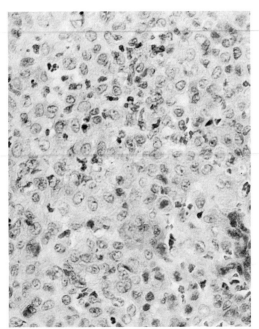

FIGURE 8-23. Light micrograph of a chondroblastoma. The lesion consists of densely packed round and polyhedral cells.

most chondroblastomas, but occasionally these lesions recur in the bone and even in the soft tissues after this treatment. Rarely, chondroblastomas metastasize to the lungs.

Chondromyxoid Fibromas

Chondromyxoid fibromas, rare benign cartilage tumors consisting of fibrous, cartilaginous, and myxoid tissues in variable proportions (Fig. 8-24), occur most commonly in the metaphyses of long

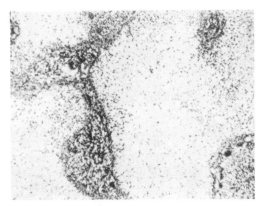

FIGURE 8-24. Light micrograph showing a chondromyxoid fibroma. The lesion consists of lobules of myxoid, cartilage-like matrix surrounded by vascular fibrous tissue. The cell density of the lobules increases toward their peripheries.

bones, especially the tibia, although the lesions may also occur in the pelvis and scapula. Radiographs show eccentric regions of decreased bone density, often with smooth sclerotic margins (Fig. 8-25). Most chondroblastomas present in older adolescents and young adults. They may be discovered as an incidental finding on a plain radiograph or because of mild to moderate pain. In some locations, they form a palpable mass, but they rarely cause pathologic fractures. Treatment by curettage or resection usually eradicates the lesion.

Giant Cell Tumors of Bone

Giant cell tumor of bone, a neoplasm consisting primarily of osteoclast-like giant cells, fibroblast-like stromal cells, and blood vessels (Color Fig. 8-7), occurs in the epiphyseal–metaphyseal regions of long bones. Common sites include the tibial plateau, the femoral condyle, the distal radius, and the humeral head. Radiographs demonstrate radiolucent, usually

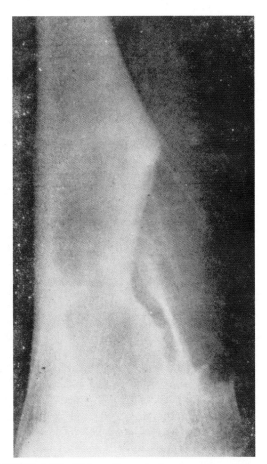

FIGURE 8-25. Plain radiograph showing a chondromyxoid fibroma. The lesion creates an eccentric lucency with smooth margins in the metaphysis.

eccentric, expansile lesions that cause thinning or fracture of the cortex (Fig. 8-26). The differential diagnosis of giant cell tumor includes aneurysmal bone cysts, chondroblastomas, brown tumors of hyperparathyroidism, and nonossifying fibromas. The radiographic appearance of extremely aggressive giant cell tumors can resemble a sarcoma.

Most patients with giant cell tumors are between 20 and 40 years of age. Unlike chondroblastomas, most giant cell tumors occur after physeal closure in the involved bone. Giant cell tumors can cause pain, swelling, and pathologic fracture, and aggressive lesions can cause extensive destruction of normal tissue. Rarely, giant cell tumors appear in multiple sites or produce lung metastases that consist of tissue consistent with a benign giant cell tumor. Most orthopaedic surgeons treat giant cell tumors by curettage or excision.

Desmoid Tumors of Bone

Desmoid tumors of bone consist of dense benign fibrous tissue. These rare lesions can behave like low-grade malignant neoplasms and may be mistaken for fibrosarcomas. They can aggressively destroy bone and invade surrounding soft tissues. Although they do not metastasize and their behavior varies among patients, they frequently recur unless excised with a margin of normal tissue.

Desmoid tumors can affect people of almost any age, but most appear in patients younger than 30 years. They may cause aching pain, swelling, and rarely, pathologic fractures. Radiographically, they appear as lytic regions of bone, and occasionally they may produce bone expansion. Treatments include wide excision when possible and, in some patients, radiation therapy and chemotherapy.

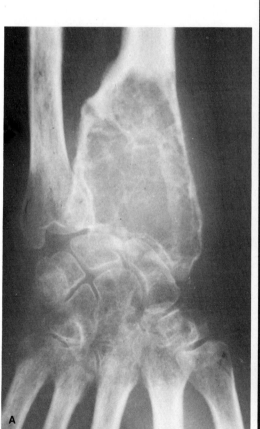
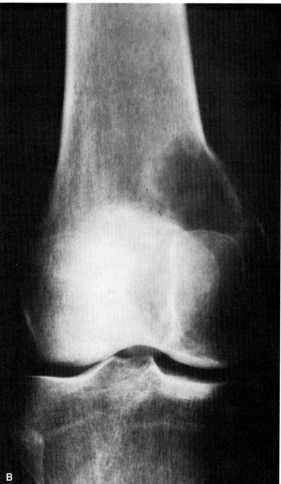

FIGURE 8-26. Radiographs of giant cell tumors. (**A**) A giant cell tumor of the distal radius that has destroyed bone and expanded the cortex. (**B**) A giant cell tumor of the distal femur. Bone destruction and expansion of cortex by the eccentric lesion can be seen.

Hemangiomas

Hemangiomas consist of collections of blood vessels within bone (Fig. 8-27), often within vertebral bodies. They may represent a developmental disorder or a neoplasm. Generally, they remain within the medullary cavity. Radiographs show regions of a generalized decrease in bone density containing abnormally prominent bone trabeculae. Most of these lesions remain asymptomatic and are detected as an incidental finding on plain radiographs; but in at least a few patients, vertebral hemangiomas have been associated with pain and possibly neurologic deficits.

Histiocytosis

The bony lesions of histiocytosis consist of histiocytes along with variable numbers of eosinophils, lymphocytes, and neutrophils (Fig. 8-28 and Color Fig. 8-8). They cause bone destruction and frequently bone reaction that mimics benign and malignant neoplasms as well as osteomyelitis. They can lead to pathologic fractures, and in children these lesions may cause collapse of a vertebral body, called vertebra plana (Fig. 8-29). Radiographs of the lesions vary from sharply circumscribed, round or oval lucent regions to extensive permeative bone destruction (Fig. 8-30).

The age at diagnosis and severity of the disease separate histiocytosis into three overlapping disorders: two disorders, Letterer-Siwe disease and Hand-Schüller-Christian disease, involve multiple tissues and affect young children; and one disorder, eosinophilic granuloma, involves only bone and affects older children and young adults. Because Letterer-

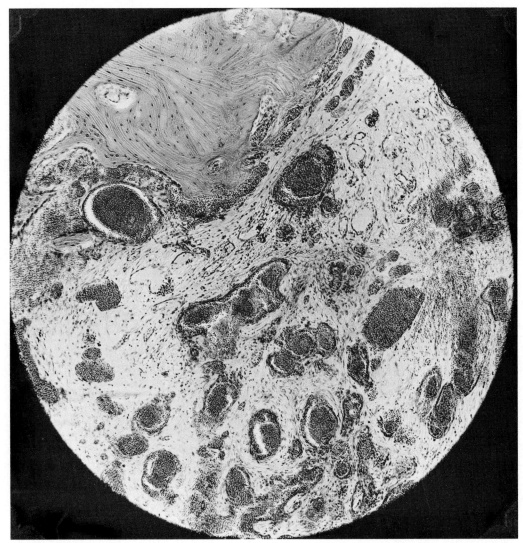

FIGURE 8-27. Light micrograph of a hemangioma in bone. The lesion consists of blood vessels and fibrous tissue.

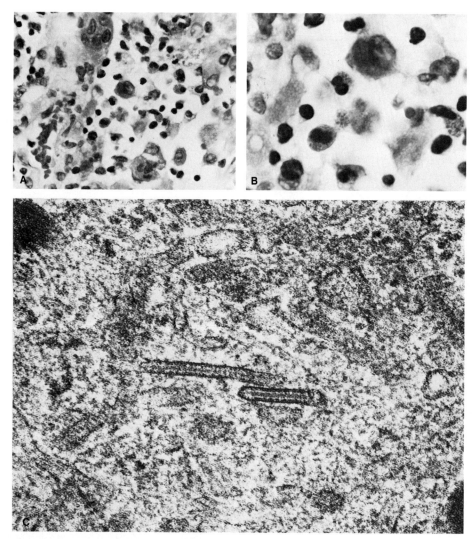

FIGURE 8-28. Cytologic features of histiocytosis X. **(A)** Smear of aspiration specimen shows an admixture of abundant histiocytes, containing either single or multiple nuclei. These nuclei often contain lipid-filled vacuoles and hemosiderin-like pigment. Also shown are eosinophils, lymphocytes, and neutrophils (×460). **(B)** Higher magnification. The histiocytes are irregularly shaped with ill-defined outlines, and they contain an eccentric, large, indented, finely creased nucleus with delicate chromatin, surrounded by abundant, delicate, pink-staining cytoplasm that contains granular material. The histiocytes sometimes have a loose syncytial appearance, often possess long cytoplasmic processes, and appear to fuse to form giant cells (×1150). **(C)** Ultramicroscopic features of histiocytosis X shows characteristic Langerhans granules. The electron micrograph shows the tubular inclusions within the cytoplasm of a typical histiocyte of eosinophilic granuloma. These are invariable features of this disease. They may be found in any condition in which the pathologic process is associated with a reactive histiocytosis (×140,000). (Katz R, Silva EG, de Santos LA, et al. Diagnosis of eosinophilic granuloma of bone by cytology, histology, and electron microscopy of transcutaneous bone-aspiration biopsy. J Bone Joint Surg 1980;62A:1284)

Siwe disease and Hand-Schüller-Christian disease cause severe systemic illness in young children, patients rarely present to physicians because of skeletal involvement alone. In contrast, patients with eosinophilic granulomas usually seek medical attention because of bone pain or pathologic fracture or because of bone lesions discovered as incidental abnormalities on plain radiographs.

Most patients with Letterer-Siwe disease, the most severe form of histiocytosis, present at younger than 2 years of age with an acute onset of the disease that may include hepatosplenomegaly, lymphadenopathy, rash, bleeding diathesis, anemia, and occasionally exophthalmos and diabetes insipidus. Patients with Hand-Schüller-Christian disease, the more chronic form of disseminated histiocytosis,

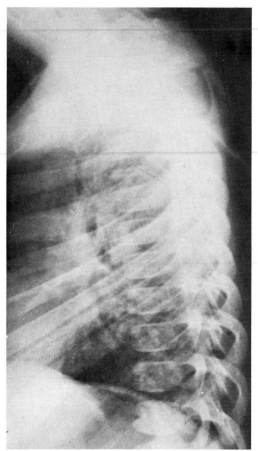

FIGURE 8-29. Radiograph showing an eosinophilic granuloma that has caused collapse of the T5 vertebral body. These lesions usually resolve spontaneously, and if a sufficient period of growth remains, the vertebral body regains normal size.

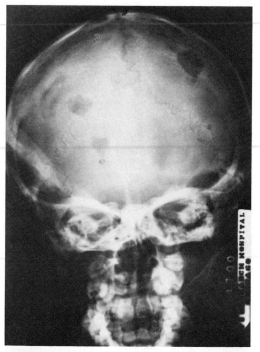

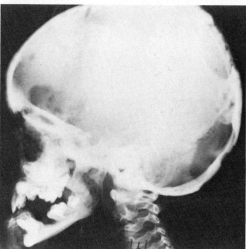

FIGURE 8-30. Radiographs showing disseminated histiocytosis (Hand-Schüller-Christian disease) involving the skull. The lesions have created circumscribed lytic bone defects.

usually present before 5 years of age and may develop otitis media, diabetes insipidus, exophthalmos, fever, hepatosplenomegaly, lymphadenopathy, anemia, and disturbances of liver function. These disseminated forms of the disease have a high mortality rate despite treatment.

Eosinophilic granuloma, the mildest form of histiocytosis, appears in children, adolescents, and young adults, although most patients present before 10 years of age. The symptoms may include localized aching pain. Eosinophilic granulomas of long bones generally occur in the diaphyses and can stimulate a periosteal reaction that makes them resemble osteomyelitis or Ewing sarcoma. Patients may have a solitary lesion, multiple lesions simultaneously, or a succession of lesions over years. Occasional patients who present with an isolated bone lesion develop Hand-Schüller-Christian disease. Eventually, eosinophilic granulomas involving bone heal spontaneously, but establishing the diagnosis, relieving pain, or preventing pathologic fracture may require

intervention before this occurs. Curettage of eosinophilic granulomas usually leads to their resolution, and steroid injections also may cause these lesions to heal.

Benign Soft Tissue Neoplasms

Lipomas

Lipomas, benign neoplasms consisting of mature fat, are the most common neoplasm. They rarely develop in people younger than 20 years of age and become more frequent with age, reaching their peak incidence in the fifth and sixth decades. They occur in the superficial subcutaneous tissues and in the deep soft tissues. Superficial lipomas occur most frequently in the back, shoulder, neck, and proximal regions of the arms and legs. Lipomas that develop deep to the muscle fascia (usually within muscle) can occur in almost any muscle but appear most frequently in the large muscles of the limbs, back, and pelvis.

Most patients recognize lipomas because of the presence of an asymptomatic, slowly growing, mobile soft tissue mass. Occasionally, large lipomas compress peripheral nerves, causing pain and rarely neurologic deficits. Plain radiographs show lipomas as distinct radiolucent masses. Left untreated, some lipomas become so large that they make it difficult for patients to find clothing that fits. Surgical excision successfully removes most lipomas.

Hemangiomas

Hemangiomas consist of abnormal collections of blood vessels. It is not clear if they result from a disturbance in tissue development or neoplasia. They occur most frequently in the skin and subcutaneous tissue, where they form soft masses with a blue tinge. These superficial lesions may be present at birth or develop during childhood and adolescence. The appearance of these lesions usually is diagnostic.

The more rare, deep soft tissue or intramuscular hemangiomas are more difficult to diagnose and may resemble malignant neoplasms. They consist of blood vessels, fibrous tissue, and often at least some fat. They may appear in any muscle, but they most commonly involve the muscles of the lower extremity, particularly the thigh muscles. They do not cause skin discoloration unless they extend into the subcutaneous tissues. Over 80% of these lesions first appear in people younger than 30 years. Often, they present as slowly enlarging soft tissue masses; many patients have pain or vague discomfort in the region of the hemangioma for years before diagnosis. Small deep lesions may be difficult to identify without performing an MRI study of the involved muscle. Although many hemangiomas remain confined to muscle, these lesions can extend into bone or surround nerves and blood vessels.

Complete surgical excision offers the best treatment of small lesions, if the surgery does not compromise limb function. Reformation of a mass at least the size of the original lesion often follows partial excision. In most instances, radical surgery is not appropriate because these lesions do not metastasize; they have not been shown to become malignant even

in patients with large lesions, and they generally do not enlarge after skeletal maturity.

Rarely, a patient is born with a hemangioma that extends throughout the soft tissues of an extremity. This disorder, congenital hemangiomatosis, increases the circumference and length of the involved extremity and may cause significant deformity. During childhood, the discrepancy in size between the normal and involved extremities may increase, and in some patients, amputation may be appropriate.

Glomus Tumors

Glomus tumors consist of capillary-sized blood vessels surrounded by layers of polygonal cells called pericytes. Fine, unmyelinated nerve fibers run between the blood vessels. These tumors occur in young adults and usually form soft vascular masses no more than a few millimeters in diameter. Patients with glomus tumors characteristically report episodes of intense pain in the region of the tumor. Many of these episodes follow minor trauma. The tumors have been found in multiple locations, but they typically develop in the nail beds of the fingers and toes, where they may be seen through the nail as small blue nodules. Surgical resection eradicates most glomus tumors.

Lymphangiomas

Lymphangiomas, masses formed primarily from lymphatic vessels and lymphoid aggregates, rarely affect the musculoskeletal system. Most lymphangiomas that involve the trunk and limbs occur in the superficial tissues of the axilla or upper extremity. It is not certain if these lesions form by neoplastic proliferation of lymph vessels or represent hamartomas or lymphangiectasis. They are benign but may enlarge, possibly by accumulation of fluid.

These lesions usually become apparent in newborns or infants: over 50% present at birth and over 90% present by 2 years of age. Parents or physicians recognize the presence of lymphangiomas because of the appearance of a fluctuant soft tissue mass that may enlarge and then decrease in size. The lesions rarely cause pain at rest but may be associated with discomfort after trauma to the lesion or exercise. Large lymphangiomas may cause disfigurement or interfere with musculoskeletal function. Surgical excision can cure small lesions, but attempts to surgically excise large lesions frequently leads to complications, including infection and wound healing problems.

Neurilemomas (Benign Schwannomas)

Neurilemomas, consisting of benign encapsulated proliferations of nerve sheath cells, occur at all ages but reach a peak incidence in patients between the ages of 20 and 50 years. They most commonly develop in the larger nerves of the head, neck, and flexor surfaces of the upper and lower extremities. They grow slowly and rarely cause pain or neurologic deficit unless they become large. Palpation or compression of a neurilemoma usually causes paresthesia. Malignant transformation of a neurilemoma occurs rarely if at all. Because neurilemomas tend to expand within a nerve sheath without infiltrating between nerve fibers, they often can be removed without sacrificing nerve fibers, and surgical excision usually eliminates the lesion.

Solitary Neurofibromas

Solitary neurofibromas and neurilemomas share many clinical and histologic features, and some solitary neoplasms of nerve sheath cells cannot be clearly classified. Presumably, they both originate from the same cell type, the Schwann cell, but theoretically, neurilemomas consist of a more homogeneous population of cells and have distinct capsules. They both can develop from major nerves and therefore can have similar clinical presentations, but unlike neurilemomas, neurofibromas also develop from

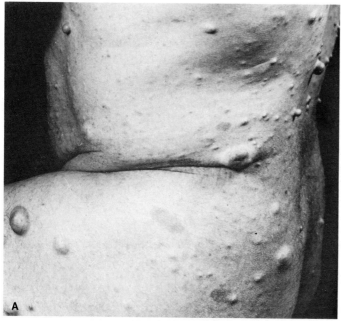

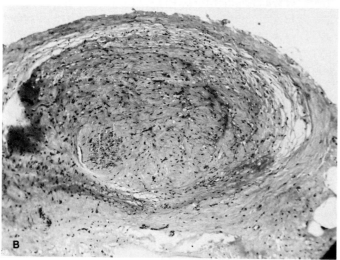

FIGURE 8-31. Neurofibromatosis. **(A)** Typical multiple subcutaneous tumor nodules. These nodules are composed of nerve tissue covered by areolar tissue and skin. **(B)** Low-power magnification of enlarged nerve fiber removed from a plexiform neurofibromatous mass. (McCarroll HR. Clinical manifestations of congenital neurofibromatosis. J Bone Joint Surg 1950;32A:601)

small, unmyelinated nerves, and in some instances, it is difficult to identify a clear relation between a neurofibroma and a nerve. Neurofibromas also tend to grow between and around individual nerve fibers rather than compressing or displacing them like neurilemomas. This often makes it difficult to resect a neurofibroma without causing neurologic damage.

Isolated neurofibromas occur most frequently in people between the ages of 20 and 30 years and appear as superficial lesions in the dermis or as deeper soft tissue masses. They usually remain asymptomatic and may grow slowly, but they may cause a neurologic deficit; few solitary neurofibromas become malignant. Surgical excision usually cures these solitary neurofibromas.

Neurofibromatosis (Von Recklinghausen Disease)

Neurofibromatosis, a genetically determined disorder, causes neurofibromas (Figs. 8-31 and 8-32), acoustic neuromas, café-au-lait spots on the skin, and skeletal deformities, including scoliosis, kyphosis, pseudarthroses, and asymmetric enlargement of limbs (Fig. 8-33). Neurofibromatous tissue may form discrete masses, like those seen in patients with solitary neurofibromas, or it may form plexiform neurofibromas, diffuse lesions that extend throughout normal structures without definite margins.

Neurofibromatosis follows an autosomal dominant inheritance pattern with a high degree of penetrance, but about half the patients present as new mutations. The severity of neurofibromatosis varies among patients: some have only café-au-lait spots and may or may not have neurofibromas; others have extensive disfiguring neurofibromas and severe skeletal deformity (Figs. 8-34 and 8-35). In severely affected people or people with a family history of neu-

rofibromatosis and the cutaneous or skeletal manifestations of the disorder, the diagnosis is apparent at birth. In other people, multiple neurofibromas appear during childhood or adolescence and progressively enlarge.

In addition to the problems caused by skeletal deformities, patients with neurofibromatosis have a high risk of developing a malignant neoplasm. People who have had the disease for a prolonged period, usually more than 10 years, have the greatest risk. Rapid enlargement of a neurofibroma or increasing pain in a neurofibroma suggest the possibility of malignant change. Despite radical surgical excision and aggressive adjunctive treatment, the prognosis for patients with malignant schwannomas and neurofibromatosis remains poor.

Desmoid Tumors

Like desmoid tumors of bone, desmoid tumors of soft tissues consist of dense proliferating fibrous tissue. These lesions do not metastasize, but they can aggressively invade normal tissues, including bone; and occasionally they develop in multiple sites. They rarely affect infants or the elderly and occur most commonly in people between the ages of 25 and 35 years. They usually present as firm, painless masses. With time, they may cause discomfort and even nerve compression and muscle weakness. Large lesions can restrict joint and muscle tendon unit motion. The tumors usually have a deep location, most frequently in the musculature of the shoulder, followed by the chest wall, back, and thigh. They usually lie within or involve muscle, but they can extend along fascial planes and appear in multiple sites in a limb.

Although untreated desmoid tumors usually continue to grow and invade normal tissue, they do not follow a predictable pattern of behavior. Their

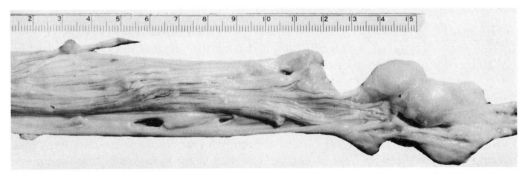

FIGURE 8-32. Neurofibromatosis. Multiple involvement of nerve roots at cauda equina. The patient died at 42 years of age of sarcomatous degeneration of a neurofibroma of the brain. (Courtesy of Pathology Department, Mount Sinai Hospital, Chicago)

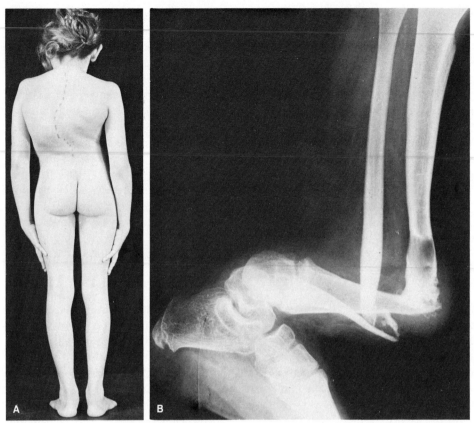

FIGURE 8-33. Neurofibromatosis. (**A**) Congenital thoracic scoliosis in a child. The angulation is acute and usually rapidly progressive and disabling. Fusion should be done promptly. (**B**) Pseudarthrosis of tibia at site of a cystic lesion. (McCarroll HR. Clinical manifestations of congenital neurofibromatosis. J Bone Joint Surg 1950;32A:601)

aggressiveness has led some authors to call them well-differentiated fibrosarcomas; but an occasional desmoid tumor ceases growing or even spontaneously regresses. If possible, these tumors should be treated by wide surgical excision, but in many locations, this is difficult, and with less than a wide excision, the lesions frequently recur. For this reason, radiation therapy and chemotherapy have been used to treat desmoid tumors along with surgical excision.

Elastofibromas

Elastofibromas consist of ill-defined, firm masses of fibrous tissue containing elastic fibers appearing in the soft tissue between the scapula and chest wall of elderly people. Elastofibromas may result from repetitive mechanical trauma rather than a neoplastic process, but this hypothesis has not been proved. These lesions cause few symptoms with the exception of mild tenderness, pain, and occasional restriction of scapulothoracic motion. They do not generally adhere to the skin and usually can be palpated in the lower subscapular area deep to the rhomboid and latissimus dorsi muscles, where they lie firmly fixed to the chest wall. These lesions grow slowly and can be treated by surgical excision.

Giant Cell Tumors of Tendon Sheath

Giant cell tumors of tendon sheath (also called xanthoma of tendon sheath and benign fibrous histiocytoma) consist of proliferations of multinucleated giant cells, inflammatory cells, histiocytes, and fibroblasts. They develop in or near synovial-lined joints, bursae, and tendon sheaths and may represent a reactive inflammatory process or a benign neoplasm. They occur at any age but most frequently develop in people between the ages of 30 and 50 years; they most commonly appear in the hand and less commonly in the foot, ankle, and knee. Physical examination shows firm, small, lobulated masses fixed to deep soft tissues, especially tendon sheaths. Occasionally, they erode bone. They may grow slowly and recur after surgical excision.

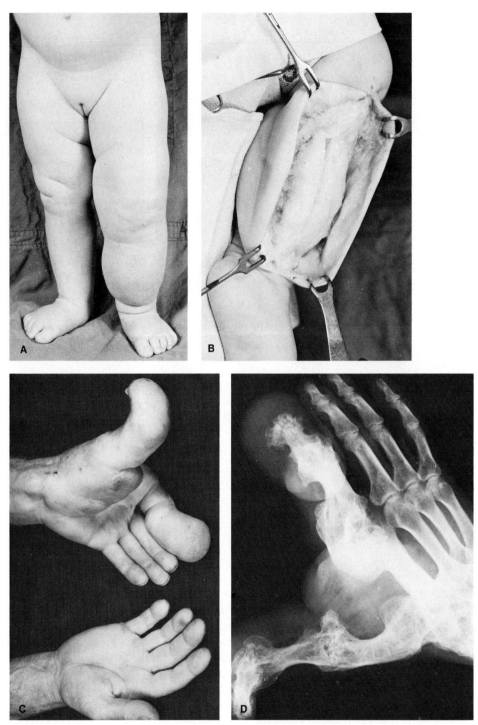

FIGURE 8-34. Neurofibromatosis. (**A**) Diffuse soft tissue hypertrophy and increased length of the lower extremity. (**B**) A typical tumor mass of hypertrophied soft tissue is exposed at operation. It is not encapsulated and is superficial to the deep fascia. (**C** and **D**) Hypertrophy of the left thumb and index finger and corresponding portion of the hand. (McCarroll HR. Clinical manifestations of congenital neurofibromatosis. J Bone Joint Surg 1950;32A:601)

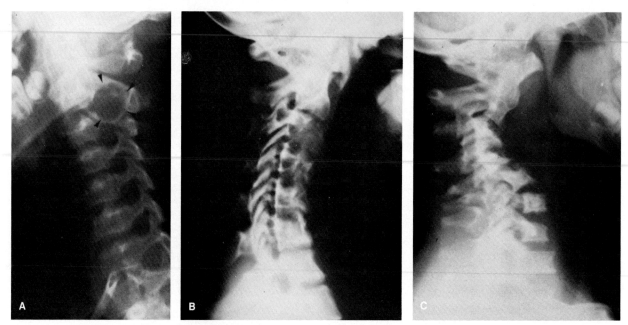

FIGURE 8-35. Cervical spine abnormalities in neurofibromatosis. Various deformities can develop in early life and are often asymptomatic at first. They occur more frequently in the patient with scoliosis, especially when the curve is short, sharp, and dysplastic and has a kyphotic element. Even in a patient with a severely deformed cervical spine, the changes are generally long-standing, fixed, and relatively stable, as demonstrated by flexion–extension roentgenograms. This spine may be injured by ill-advised cervical traction or manipulation and handling of the patient during induction of anesthesia or attempted correction of the scoliosis. (A) Enlarged foramina and dysplasia of posterior elements. (B) Fixed reversal of cervical lordosis. (C) Gross cervical kyphosis with subluxation in asymptomatic patient. (Yong-Hing K, Kalamchi A, MacEwen GD. Cervical spine abnormalities in neurofibromatosis. J Bone Joint Surg 1979;61A:695)

Pigmented Villonodular Synovitis

Pigmented villonodular synovitis consists of proliferating synovial tissue containing histiocytes, fibroblasts, multinucleated giant cells, and capillaries that can destroy dense fibrous tissue, form soft tissue masses, and invade bone. Like giant cell tumor of tendon sheath, pigmented villonodular synovitis may represent a reactive inflammatory process or a benign neoplasm. It occurs most commonly in adolescents and young adults and usually occurs in large synovial joints, including the knee, hip, and ankle, although it also occurs in smaller synovial joints and in tendon sheaths and bursae. Most patients present with a swollen joint and give a history of recurrent joint effusions. Radiographs may show degenerative joint disease and periarticular bone destruction. Occasionally, it forms solitary or multiple soft tissue nodules near a joint that closely resemble giant cell tumors of tendon sheath. Pigmented villonodular synovitis is usually treated by resection of the involved tissue.

Synovial Chondromatosis

Synovial chondromatosis consists of hyaline cartilage nodules within synovium and synovial joint cavities. It occurs most frequently in young adults and usually involves large joints. Patients present with pain, joint locking and catching, and an enlarging mass. Most patients develop multiple loose fragments of cartilage within the joint, but in some people the proliferating chondrocytes form an enlarging mass in the periarticular tissues. Radiographs show speckled calcification within the joint and, in some instances, in the soft tissues around the joint. Treatment of synovial chondromatosis includes synovectomy, removal of cartilaginous loose bodies, and resection of any cartilaginous masses.

MALIGNANT NEOPLASMS

Primary malignant musculoskeletal neoplasms occur much less frequently than benign lesions, and unlike benign lesions, malignant neoplasms have the capacity to cause disseminated disease and death. Some malignant neoplasms develop in or near previously existing benign lesions, including osteochondromas (especially in patients with hereditary multiple exostoses), enchondromas (especially in patients with Ollier disease and Maffucci syndrome), fibrous dysplasia (especially in patients with polyostotic fibrous dysplasia), chronic draining osteomyelitis, bone infarcts, Paget disease, and neurofibromas (especially in patients with neurofibromatosis). In some instances, the development of a malignant neoplasm presumably results from expression of preexisting malignant potential. This may explain the appearance of malignant neoplasms in patients with Ollier disease and neurofibromatosis. In other lesions, development of a malignant neoplasm presumably results from an alteration in the originally normal cells near the lesion. This may explain the development of malignant lesions in patients with chronic draining osteomyelitis or bone infarcts.

Malignant neoplasms of bone vary in their clinical presentation. For example, myelomas frequently present as bone pain without a mass or swelling and generalized weakness in elderly debilitated people, whereas osteosarcomas commonly present as sharply localized bone pain and a mass in children and adolescents without systemic symptoms. Treatment of these neoplasms also varies from systemic chemotherapy and radiation therapy used for myelomas to the combinations of systemic chemotherapy and surgery used for many osteosarcomas.

In contrast to malignant bone neoplasms, most malignant neoplasms of the soft tissues vary less in clinical presentation and treatment. Most present as a mass that sometimes causes pain. When possible, most physicians recommend wide excision of these neoplasms as the primary treatment. In some patients, chemotherapy and radiation therapy may also be helpful.

Malignant Bone Neoplasms

Myelomas

Myeloma, the most common malignant neoplasm of bone, consists of malignant plasma cells showing variable degrees of differentiation (Color Fig. 8-9). The disease rarely occurs before the fifth decade of life. In many patients, the malignant cells extend throughout the marrow, so marrow aspiration provides diagnostic tissue. Most patients have moderate to severe anemia, an elevated erythrocyte sedimentation rate, and abnormal serum protein electrophoresis and immunoelectrophoresis. Occasionally, patients present with a solitary focus of myeloma cells referred to as a *plasmacytoma*. These patients usually develop diffuse disease after a latent period of as long as 5 to 10 years.

Most patients with myeloma complain of bone pain that may be diffuse or localized to regions of bone destruction. Because the disease often involves the vertebra, patients with myeloma often have back pain and vertebral compression fractures. In addition, many affected people have systemic symptoms, in-

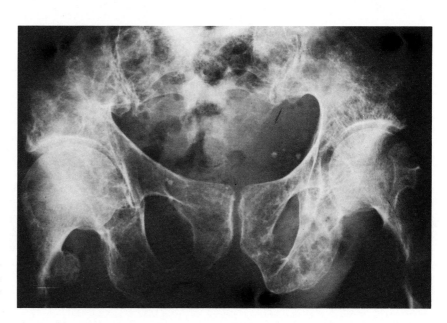

FIGURE 8-36. Radiograph showing the multiple round bone defects in the pelvis of a patient with multiple myeloma.

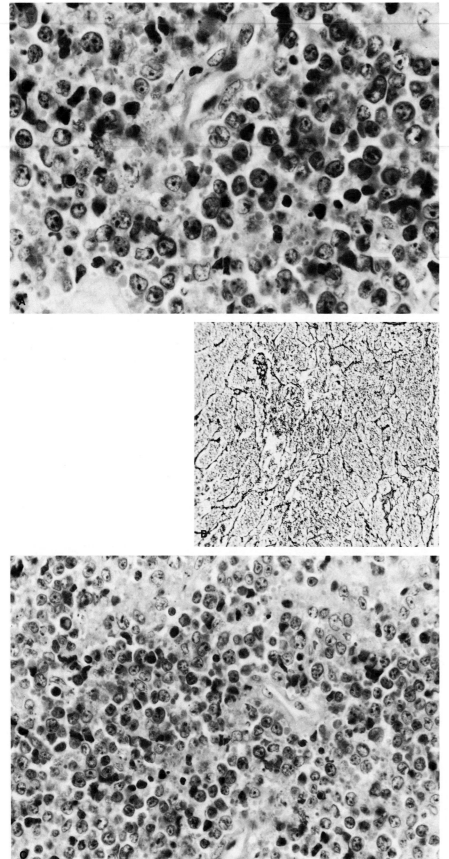

FIGURE 8-37. Light micrographs of a histiocytic lymphoma of bone. (**A** and **B**) Routine light micrographs show the population of round cells that form the neoplasm. (**C**) Treatment of a histologic section of the neoplasm with a silver stain shows the network of fine matrix fibers (reticulum fibers) that confirm the diagnosis of lymphoma of bone (reticulum cell sarcoma). (Courtesy of Dr. A. G. Huvos)

cluding weakness, easy fatigability, and weight loss. The radiographic features of myeloma vary from single or multiple discrete, sharply defined, punched-out areas of bone destruction, often in the skull and pelvis (Fig. 8-36), to diffuse osteopenia that can be difficult to distinguish from osteopenia due to metabolic bone diseases. In the early stages of myeloma, radiographs may not show any changes. Bone reaction to myeloma occurs rarely, and bone scans may not show increased tracer activity. Pathologic fractures due to myeloma commonly occur in the vertebral bodies but may occur in any part of the skeleton. Radiation can effectively treat localized myeloma, and chemotherapy may result in improvement in some patients.

Lymphomas

Lymphomas of bone, consisting primarily of malignant histiocytes (Color Fig. 8-10), present most commonly in middle age. The histologic appearance of these histiocytic lymphomas, also called reticulum cell sarcomas, frequently resembles that of Ewing sarcomas, but the lymphomas contain a network or reticulum of fine matrix fibers that appear as thin dark threads when stained with a silver or reticulum stain (Fig. 8-37).

Bone lymphomas cause pain as they enlarge or cause pathologic fractures. Radiographs often show extensive permeative, destructive lesions that in some patients extend through most of the bone. The regions of bone destruction have an irregular appearance that blends with normal bone. Occasionally, plain radiographs appear normal; in these patients, a bone scan or MRI usually shows the lesion in the bone. Most isolated lymphomas of bone are treated with radiation and, in some instances, surgical resection. Chemotherapy is used for patients with systemic disease.

Ewing Sarcomas

Ewing sarcoma, a highly malignant tumor of bone, consists of densely packed, distinctive small round cells of uncertain origin (Color Fig. 8-11). It occurs more frequently in males and primarily in patients younger than 25 years. The tumor may appear in any bone, or even in the soft tissues, but most Ewing sarcomas present in the bones of the pelvis or lower extremities. The tumor usually causes pain and may enlarge rapidly to produce significant soft tissue swelling and occasionally pathologic fractures.

Commonly, radiographs show a diffuse permeative destructive lesion that stimulates a striking periosteal reaction (Fig. 8-38). In long bones, Ewing sarcoma usually initially involves the diaphysis, but it

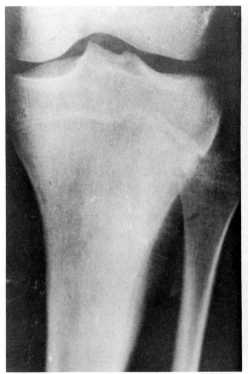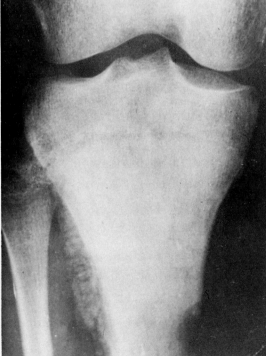

FIGURE 8-38. Radiographs of Ewing sarcoma of the tibia in two patients. Diffuse bone involvement and a prominent periosteal reaction can be seen.

may extend from one metaphysis to the other; in flat bones, it can involve the entire bone. The radiographic appearance of Ewing sarcoma may resemble osteomyelitis, lymphoma, osteosarcoma, eosinophilic granuloma, and metastatic tumor. In many patients, the tumor has broken through the bone cortex and periosteum and invaded the soft tissues at the time of diagnosis (Color Fig. 8-12). Some patients with Ewing sarcoma have systemic symptoms, including fever and generalized weakness, and laboratory abnormalities, including an elevated sedimentation rate and anemia. Treatment of Ewing sarcoma includes chemotherapy and, in some patients, radiation and surgical resection.

Osteosarcomas

The presence of malignant cells producing osteoid or bone identifies a neoplasm as an osteosarcoma (Color Fig. 8-13). The matrix of a typical osteosarcoma consists primarily of osteoid that may or may not mineralize, but some osteosarcoma cells synthesize a cartilaginous or fibrous matrix instead of osteoid, and some of these tumors form large vascular channels. Most osteosarcomas develop in the metaphyses of long bones, especially the femur (Fig. 8-39), tibia, and humerus, although osteosarcomas have been found in almost every part of the skeleton. Less commonly, osteosarcomas develop on the surface of the bone (periosteal osteosarcomas) and in the soft tissues next to bone (parosteal osteosarcomas). An extremely rare type of osteosarcoma develops in muscle or other soft tissues at a distance from bone (extraosseous osteosarcomas).

Osteosarcomas that arise within bone cause progressively increasing pain. At the time of diagnosis, many of these neoplasms have extended through the bone cortex and have produced a firm soft tissue mass (see Fig. 8-39). Despite extensive involvement of bone and bone destruction, they rarely cause pathologic fractures. These neoplasms occur most frequently in the second decade of life, although they may occur at any age, and they may develop in association with Paget disease or after radiation therapy. Osteosarcomas associated with Paget disease or radiation therapy characteristically have a worse prognosis than osteosarcomas that develop in the absence of preexisting lesions.

Radiographically, osteosarcomas typically appear as regions of permeative bone destruction and irregular new bone formation (Fig. 8-40); although, because the tumor osteoid does not always mineralize, occasional osteosarcomas do not produce radiographic evidence of new bone formation. The bone

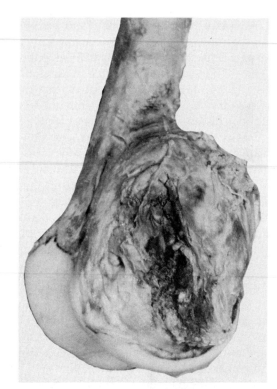

FIGURE 8-39. Photograph of an osteosarcoma of the distal femur. The neoplasm has broken through the bone and formed a large soft tissue mass.

destruction caused by osteosarcomas containing large vascular channels, telangiectatic osteosarcomas, may resemble the bone changes seen in aneurysmal bone cysts. Other osteosarcomas mineralize so densely that they appear as sclerotic masses (Fig. 8-41).

Osteosarcomas that originate within bone almost always behave aggressively. They rapidly destroy normal bone, invade and destroy soft tissue, and frequently metastasize to the lungs within 2 years of diagnosis. Treatment of osteosarcomas that originate within bone consists of surgical resection if possible and chemotherapy.

Periosteal osteosarcomas develop on the outer cortical surface of long bones, most often in young adults. They erode the cortex, producing a shallow cavity and reactive periosteal new bone formation around their margins. Some periosteal osteosarcomas produce radiographic changes that resemble a periosteal chondroma, but the osteosarcomas tend to create a more irregular bony margin that suggests the presence of a malignant neoplasm. As a periosteal osteosarcoma grows, it extends into the soft tissues, and ossification may appear within the enlarging mass. Eventually, the lesions grow into the medullary cavity. Patients with periosteal osteosarcomas often present after they notice a firm, fixed, slowly enlarg-

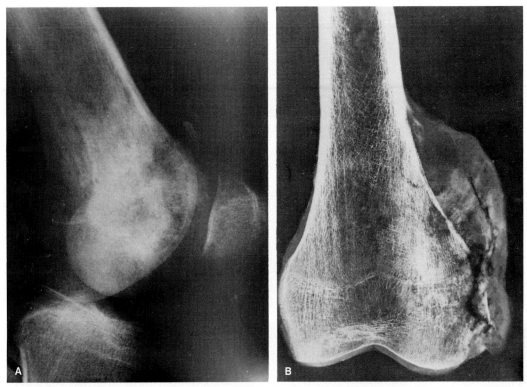

FIGURE 8-40. Radiographs of a distal femoral osteosarcoma. (**A**) Lateral view of the distal femur showing the irregular bone destruction and bone formation that gives the bone a mottled appearance. (**B**) Anteroposterior view of the distal femur after removal of the soft tissues. This view shows how the neoplasm has broken through the bone to form a soft tissue mass. New bone formation is seen in the soft tissue mass.

ing mass. Most of these neoplasms are treated like osteosarcomas that develop within bone.

Parosteal osteosarcomas, osteosarcomas that arise in the soft tissues adjacent to bone (Fig. 8-42), generally have a better prognosis than periosteal osteosarcomas and the more common osteosarcomas that develop within bone. Almost all reported parosteal osteosarcomas have involved the femur, humerus, or tibia, with the most frequent site being the posterior distal portion of the femur (Fig. 8-43). These tumors often grow slowly over a period of years, and the patient may notice swelling but relatively little discomfort. Radiographs show that the tumor contains dense mineral deposits, lies adjacent to the bone, and often has grown at least partially around the circumference of the bone (see Fig. 8-43). Plain radiographs or CT may show a border of soft tissue between the tumor and underlying bone. The differential diagnosis usually includes myositis ossificans, periosteal osteosarcoma, osteosarcoma originating in bone, and osteochondroma. Wide excision usually eradicates the tumor.

Extraosseous osteosarcomas produce soft tissue masses that usually contain regions of ossification.

They tend to occur in young adults near the shoulder and pelvis. These rare tumors are usually treated by surgical resection and, in some patients, with adjuvant chemotherapy.

Chondrosarcomas

Chondrosarcomas, malignant tumors consisting primarily of chondrocytes and a cartilaginous matrix (Color Fig. 8-14), may develop in the region of an enchondroma or osteochondroma or more commonly in areas of the skeleton with no known preceding cartilage lesion. Chondrosarcomas occur most frequently in adults and the elderly and appear most commonly in the pelvis, scapula, humerus, femur, and tibia. Patients with hereditary multiple exostoses, Ollier disease, and Maffucci syndrome have a particularly high risk for malignant transformation of a cartilaginous lesion.

Chondrosarcomas vary considerably in their behavior: some enlarge rapidly, aggressively invade normal tissue, metastasize, and cause death, but many others enlarge slowly, cause little damage to adjacent tissues, and metastasize after many years

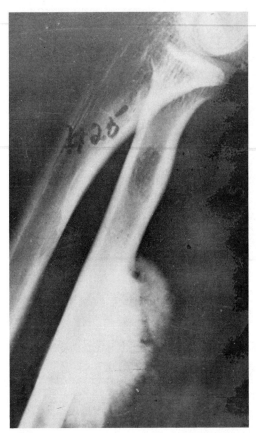

FIGURE 8-41. Radiograph showing an osteosarcoma of the radius. This neoplasm has extended into the soft tissues, and its high concentration of mineral gives it a radiodense appearance.

or fail to metastasize. They also vary in their histologic appearance from lesions that resemble normal hyaline cartilage to lesions consisting of poorly differentiated cells that fail to produce a typical hyaline cartilage matrix. These differences in the histologic appearance of chondrosarcoma have led to the classification of these neoplasms into three grades based on their degree of resemblance to normal hyaline cartilage (Fig. 8-44). Although some relation exists between the histologic appearance of the tumors and their behavior, the grade of the tumor alone does not allow reliable prediction of its behavior. Rare malignant lesions that form cartilage and appear to be forms of chondrosarcomas include mesenchymal chondrosarcomas, dedifferentiated chondrosarcomas, and clear cell chondrosarcomas.

Chondrosarcomas may arise within the bone, a central chondrosarcoma, or from the surface of the bone, a peripheral chondrosarcoma. Plain radiographs usually show evidence of bone destruction in the area of the lesion as well as mineralization within the tumor (Fig. 8-45). Peripheral chondrosarcomas may resemble osteochondromas on plain radiographs, although they commonly show at least some bone destruction and irregular calcification. MRI studies and, in some instances, CT scans of these lesions may show increased thickness of cartilage, suggesting the presence of malignancy. Because plain radiographs usually do not show the cartilage component of these neoplasms, the tumors may be con-

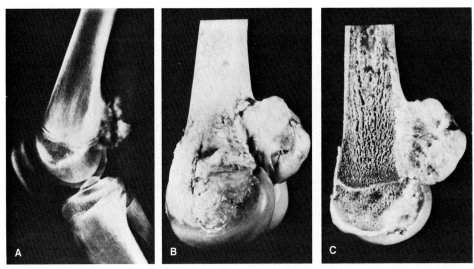

FIGURE 8-42. Grade I lesion of parosteal osteogenic sarcoma. (A) Roentgenogram shows an irregular ossified mass with prominent lucency indicating a large amount of fibrous and cartilaginous tissue. The subjacent cortex is sclerotic. (B) Typical external appearance. This is the most common location of the tumor on the posterior aspect of the distal end of the femur at the popliteal area. (C) Sagittal section shows that this tumor merges imperceptibly with the cortex along its entire base. The underlying cortical bone is thickened. (Ahuja SC, et al. Juxtacortical (parosteal) osteogenic sarcoma. J Bone Joint Surg 1977;59A:632)

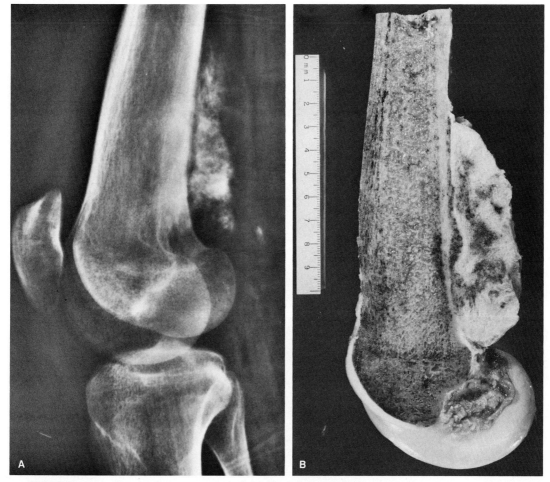

FIGURE 8-43. Parosteal osteosarcoma of the distal femur. (**A**) Roentgenogram shows a nonhomogeneous tumor with the highly diagnostic, broad linear lucency between the osseous neoplasm and the underlying cortex. Note the spiculated margin. (**B**) Sagittal section of the gross specimen shows that the tumor is merged only focally to the underlying cortex distally. Elsewhere, the tumor is separated from the cortex by a thickened band of periosteal fibrous tissue. (Ahuja SC, et al. Juxtacortical (parosteal) osteogenic sarcoma. J Bone Joint Surg 1977;59A:632)

siderably larger than they appear on the radiographs. Central chondrosarcomas appear as regions of bone destruction and often contain regions of calcification (Fig. 8-46). Frequently, they extend further in the medullary cavity than the plain radiographs suggest. When they break through the bone cortex, they can form large soft tissue masses. They usually do not cause significant reactive bone formation.

Most chondrosarcomas eventually cause pain, but some cause little or no discomfort despite reaching large size. Peripheral chondrosarcomas and central chondrosarcomas that extend into the soft tissues form firm, fixed masses. In some patients, a mass may have been present for years before they seek medical attention. Intrapelvic chondrosarcomas in particular can grow to large size until they cause symptoms, or they are detected as an incidental find-

ing on an imaging study. Wide surgical excision offers the best possibility of cure; radiation and chemotherapy have not proved to be effective primary methods of treatment for chondrosarcomas.

Fibrosarcomas

Fibrosarcomas are one of the most uncommon malignant bone tumors. Like fibrosarcomas of soft tissue, they consist primarily of fibroblasts and a collagenous matrix. They occur over a wide age range and may appear in any part of the skeleton. Most of them cause pain, and some cause swelling. They may occur in association with Paget disease, fibrous dysplasia, and bone infarcts or after radiation therapy. Radiographs show irregular, mottled bone destruc-

(text continues on page 330)

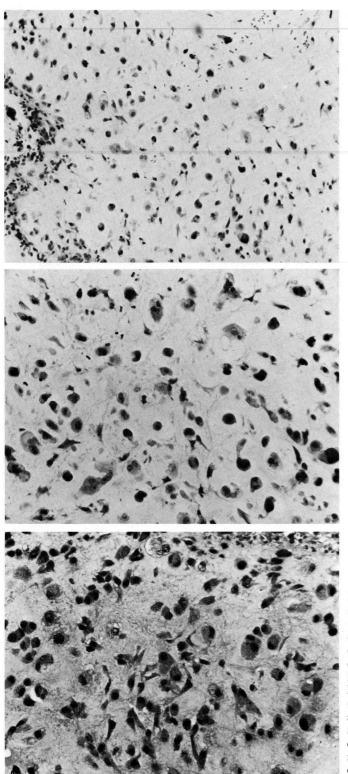

FIGURE 8-44. Light micrographs showing the variability in the histologic appearance of chondrosarcomas. (**A**) The histologic appearance of grade I and grade II chondrosarcomas. (*Top* and *center*) Grade I changes include increased cell density and increased variability in cell size, shape, and staining. (*Bottom*) Grade II changes include more advanced cellular pleomorphism. (**B**) The histologic appearance of grade III chondrosarcomas. (*Top* and *center*) Dedifferentiation toward fibrosarcoma at the periphery of chondrosarcomatous lobules. (*Bottom*) Lobules of malignant cartilage penetrate bone, demonstrating the ability of these lesions to destroy normal bone. (Dahlin DC, Salvador AH. Chondrosarcomas of bones of the hands and feet: a study of 30 cases. Cancer 1974;34:755)

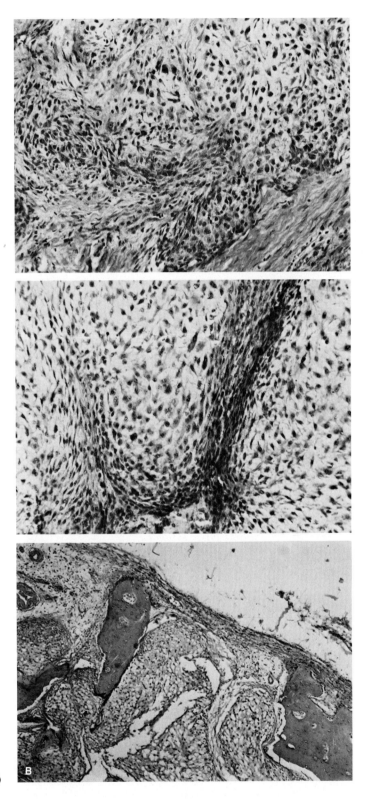

FIGURE 8-44. (*Continued*)

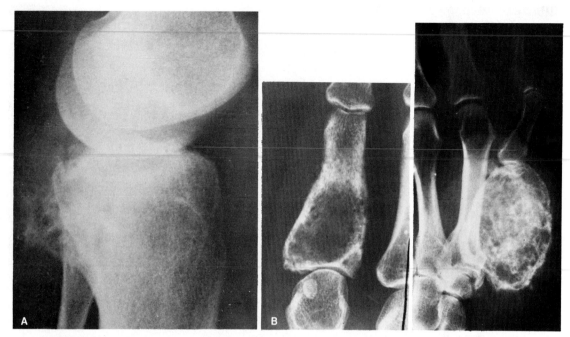

FIGURE 8-45. Plain radiographs of chondrosarcomas. (A) Plain radiograph of a chondrosarcoma of the proximal tibia. Notice the mineralization with the neoplasm and the irregularity of the bone. (B) Plain radiographs of chondrosarcomas in the hand. (*Left*) Chondrosarcoma of the proximal phalanx. The lesion has destroyed the medullary bone and invaded the cortical bone. (*Right*) A chondrosarcoma of a metacarpal has invaded the soft tissues.

tion with occasional regions of reactive new bone formation around the periphery. Wide surgical excision is the accepted treatment, although adjuvant chemotherapy has been used for some patients.

Malignant Fibrous Histiocytomas

Malignant fibrous histiocytomas, highly malignant tumors consisting of the same cell types found in malignant fibrous histiocytomas of soft tissues (giant cells, fibroblasts, and histiocytes), rarely affect bone. They may appear in patients of any age and have been reported in association with Paget disease and bone infarcts as well as after radiation therapy. Patients usually complain of pain, and radiographs show irregular bone destruction. When possible, wide surgical excision offers the best probability of cure. Chemotherapy has been used for some patients as well.

Malignant Vascular Tumors

All malignant vascular tumors contain capillaries formed by malignant cells, but they vary in their predominant cell type. In hemangioendotheliomas, capillary endothelial cells appear to be the predominant cell type; in hemangiopericytomas, pericytes

appear to be the predominant cell type. Hemangioendotheliomas occur more frequently in bone than soft tissue, whereas hemangiopericytomas occur more frequently in soft tissue than in bone. The term *angiosarcoma* is sometimes used to refer to all types of malignant blood vessel–forming neoplasms, but it may also refer to the most malignant forms of hemangioendothelioma and hemangiopericytoma.

Malignant vascular tumors have appeared in most regions of the skeleton, and in some instances, highly malignant vascular tumors have occurred in multiple sites within the skeleton simultaneously. They usually produce pain, and radiographs show evidence of bone destruction. Surgical resection appears to be the most appropriate treatment. Radiation therapy or chemotherapy may be beneficial in some instances.

Adamantinomas

Adamantinomas, rare neoplasms consisting of islands or strands of epithelial-like cells surrounded by fibrous tissue (Color Fig. 8-15), usually occur in long bones, primarily the tibia. They tend to follow a prolonged course and occur most frequently between late adolescence and middle age. Lesions of

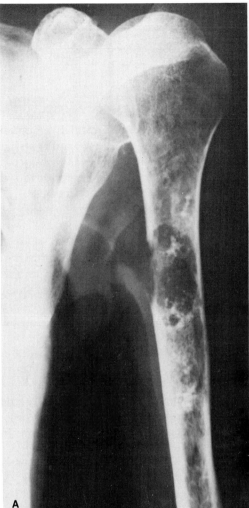

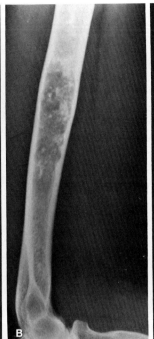

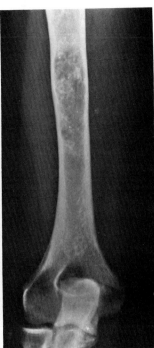

FIGURE 8-46. Plain radiographs showing central chondrosarcomas. These lesions cause bone destruction and often produce regions of mineralization. (A) A central chondrosarcoma of the humerus showing an irregular area of central bone destruction with mineralization and erosion of the inner bone cortex. (B) Radiographic features include osteolysis, scalloping erosion of inner cortex, central areas of calcification, and no reactive bone formation about the periphery.

the tibia often produce a palpable mass, and most adamantinomas cause mild to moderate discomfort. Radiographically, they appear as a region of irregular bone destruction involving primarily the cortex; and in some patients, the lesion may be confined to the cortex of the bone. Wide resection of the tumor appears to offer the best treatment.

Chordomas

Chordomas consist of malignant notochordal cells (Color Fig. 8-16) and may appear anywhere in the spine, but they appear most frequently in the sacrococcygeal region or at the base of the skull. They rarely occur in people younger than 30 years. Most of these neoplasms grow slowly and come to the attention of the patient because of pain and, less frequently, bowel dysfunction or neurologic symptoms. Radiographs of chordomas typically show irregular

midline bone destruction and, in some instances, bone expansion without appreciable bone reaction. Small lesions are often difficult to see on plain radiographs because of overlying shadows. The location of these lesions makes treatment difficult, but, if possible, wide excision offers the best opportunity for controlling the tumor.

Malignant Soft Tissue Neoplasms

Malignant soft tissue neoplasms, like fibrosarcomas and neurosarcomas, are named for their presumed cell of origin; however, for many of these lesions, such as synovial cell sarcomas and epithelioid sarcomas, the cell of origin is uncertain. Other soft tissue sarcomas may consist of undifferentiated cells that cannot be identified with a specific tissue. Although soft tissue sarcomas differ in cell type, they have similar clinical presentations, appearances on imaging studies, and treatment. They usually present as firm masses that may or may not cause pain or other symptoms. Imaging studies, especially MRI, can show the size and anatomic location of a soft tissue neoplasm, but these studies cannot be relied on to distinguish different histologic types of neoplasms or, in most instances, distinguish benign neoplasms from malignant neoplasms. Treatment of soft tissue sarcomas consists of wide surgical resection when possible and use of chemotherapy and radiation therapy in some patients.

Liposarcomas

Liposarcomas, malignant tumors of fat cells that have a variable histologic appearance, are the most common soft tissue sarcoma. They frequently reach large size and have a peak incidence in people between 40 and 60 years of age. Most liposarcomas of the extremities lie deep within the soft tissues, especially in the quadriceps muscle and popliteal fossa. Other common locations include the shoulder and the leg. Patients usually first detect liposarcomas because they notice a mass or an increase in size of part of the limb.

Malignant Fibrous Histiocytomas

Malignant fibrous histiocytoma, the most common malignant soft tissue tumor of late adult life, like the more rare malignant fibrous histiocytoma of bone, consists of malignant fibroblasts and histiocytes as well as giant cells and occasionally inflammatory cells. Most soft tissue malignant fibrous histiocytomas present as painless enlarging masses in people between the ages of 50 and 70 years. They occur most frequently in the deep soft tissues of the lower extremity.

Fibrosarcomas

Soft tissue fibrosarcomas, like fibrosarcomas in bone, consist of malignant fibroblasts. They may occur in patients of any age but appear most frequently in people between 30 and 55 years of age. They may occur anywhere in the body but occur most often in the lower extremity, especially the thigh. Usually, they lie deep within the soft tissues and present as an enlarging mass. Only rarely do they cause significant discomfort before reaching large size. Occasionally, fibrosarcomas arise in tissues that have previously been treated with radiation or in burn scars.

Synovial Cell Sarcomas

Despite their name, the cells forming synovial cell sarcomas have not been shown to originate from synovium. Many synovial cell sarcomas consist of two morphologically distinct cell types—epithelial-like cells that assume a cuboidal or columnar form and fibroblast-like spindle cells. The combination of these two cell types creates a distinctive biphasic pattern: the spindle cells surround islands and strands of epithelial cells. Some synovial cell sarcomas do not contain both cell types and therefore are referred to as monophasic synovial cell sarcomas.

Synovial cell sarcomas occur most frequently in people between 15 and 35 years of age and rarely appear in people older than 50 years of age. They usually present as discrete masses or diffuse swelling, and they often cause some discomfort and may be tender. Plain radiographs show scattered small areas of calcification in many synovial cell sarcomas. Because these neoplasms generally grow slowly, many patients have symptoms for years before biopsy or excision demonstrates the presence of the tumor. Synovial sarcomas appear most frequently in the extremities, usually in periarticular regions or near tendon sheaths, bursae, and joint capsules. Despite their frequent proximity to these structures, synovial cell sarcomas rarely occur within joints, tendon sheaths, or bursae.

Neurosarcomas

Neurosarcomas (also referred to as malignant schwannomas and neurofibrosarcomas) usually arise from peripheral nerve sheaths or from neurofibromas. Most of these tumors occur in patients between 20 and 50 years of age. They usually present as enlarging masses that may or may not cause pain. Patients with neurofibromatosis (von Recklinghausen disease) have a significantly increased risk of malignant schwannomas; and some series indicate that patients who develop malignant schwannomas in association with neurofibromatosis have a worse prognosis than patients who develop these tumors but do not have neurofibromatosis. Like other soft tissue sarcomas, surgical excision offers the best treatment for this disorder. Unfortunately, some of the tumors assume a diffuse form that makes wide resection almost impossible.

Rhabdomyosarcomas

Rhabdomyosarcomas usually arise in or near skeletal muscle and consist of cells closely related to the cells that form myofibers. They are the most common soft tissue sarcoma of children and adolescents, but they occur in people of almost any age. Most of these tumors present as enlarging deep masses closely associated with muscle. They rarely cause pain or tenderness. Combinations of surgical excision, radiation therapy, and chemotherapy are frequently used for many patients with rhabdomyosarcoma.

Malignant Vascular Tumors

Malignant vascular neoplasms account for only a small portion of soft tissue sarcomas. Like malignant vascular neoplasms of bone, malignant vascular tumors of soft tissue form capillaries and vary in their predominant cell type (as discussed previously, hemangiopericytomas occur more frequently in the soft tissues than in bone, and hemangioendotheliomas occur more frequently in bone than in soft tissue).

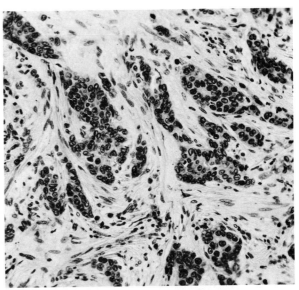

FIGURE 8-48. Light micrograph showing a metastatic carcinoma of the breast. The lesions consist of islands of neoplastic epithelial cells surrounded by reactive fibrous tissue.

Some types of malignant vascular neoplasms arise in the superficial soft tissues and skin and therefore may present as a superficial mass, but others develop in the deep soft tissues and closely resemble the other soft tissue sarcomas.

Epithelioid Sarcomas

Epithelioid sarcomas consist of malignant round cells presumably of mesenchymal origin, inflammatory cells, and capillaries. These neoplasms occur most commonly in young adults and often develop in the hand or foot, although they have been found in most regions of the musculoskeletal soft tissues. They usually present as small tender masses that may be fixed to tendon sheaths, periarticular tissues, and fascia. Because their clinical presentation differs from most soft tissue neoplasms and because of the inflammatory cells in the lesion and the often unremarkable appearance of the round cells, these neoplasms frequently are mistaken for nonspecific inflammatory processes, even after biopsy and recurrence. Treatment of these lesions is wide excision when possible.

Clear Cell Sarcomas

Clear cell sarcomas consist of large malignant cells with clear cytoplasm resembling swollen chondrocytes. These neoplasms most frequently occur in older adolescents and young adults and usually

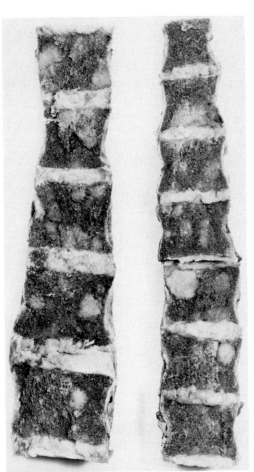

FIGURE 8-47. Thoracic and lumbar vertebrae with multiple metastases from a carcinoma of the breast. The roughly spherical metastatic lesions have replaced bone marrow in part of every vertebral body.

present as a slowly growing, fixed mass. Like epithelioid sarcomas, clear cell sarcomas may involve periarticular tissues and fascia, and treatment is wide excision when possible.

METASTATIC NEOPLASMS

Skeletal metastases of carcinomas occur far more frequently than primary bone malignancies. The malignant cells grow within the bone, replace normal bone marrow, and frequently cause bone destruction (Fig. 8-47), although some metastases stimulate bone formation. Nearly all malignant tumors have shown the ability to metastasize to bone; but carcinomas of the breast, lung, and prostate produce over 80% of bone metastases, and about half of patients with breast, lung, or prostate cancer eventually develop bone metastases. Renal cell cancers, gastrointestinal cancers, gynecologic cancers, and thyroid cancers also commonly involve bone. Examination of skeletal metastases usually shows cells like those in the pri-

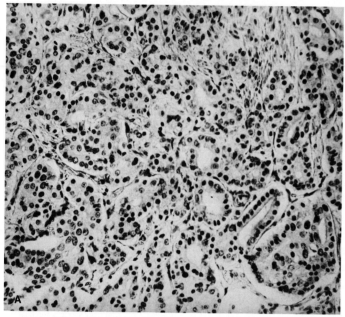

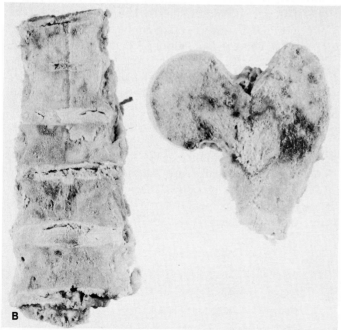

FIGURE 8-49. Metastatic carcinoma of the prostate gland. (A) Light micrograph showing metastatic carcinoma of the prostate gland. The lesion consists of gland-forming epithelial cells. (B) Metastases of prostatic carcinoma to the vertebral body and femur.

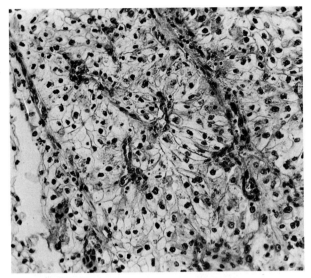

FIGURE 8-50. Light micrograph of metastatic carcinoma of the kidney.

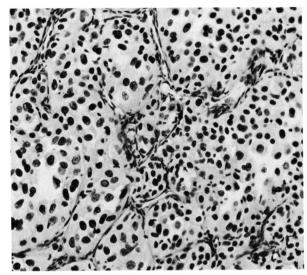

FIGURE 8-52. Light micrograph of metastatic carcinoma of the lung.

mary neoplasm (Figs. 8-48 through 8-53). Soft tissue sarcomas and primary malignancies of bone seldom metastasize to bone.

Metastatic bone lesions cause pain and frequently cause pathologic fractures (Figs. 8-54 and 8-55). They occur most frequently in the vertebrae, pelvis, ribs, and proximal appendicular skeleton (Figs. 8-56 and 8-57) and seldom occur in the hands or feet or in the musculoskeletal soft tissues. Although bone metastases occur primarily in adults of middle age or older, they occasionally affect younger adults, and neuroblastomas can involve bone in children. Most patients

with bone pain or pathologic fractures due to skeletal metastases have a known primary malignant neoplasm, but some patients present with skeletal metastases as the first indication of the primary malignancy. For this reason, the possibility of metastatic carcinoma should be investigated in middle-aged and older patients with bone lesions. In some of these patients, biopsy of the bone lesion shows a poorly differentiated metastatic carcinoma, and physical examination, imaging studies, and laboratory studies do not find the primary lesion.

Although plain radiographs often demonstrate

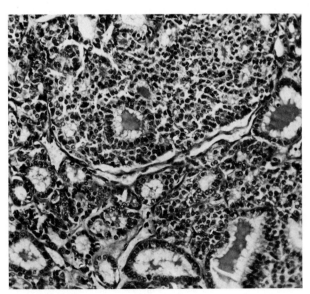

FIGURE 8-51. Light micrograph of metastatic carcinoma of the thyroid gland.

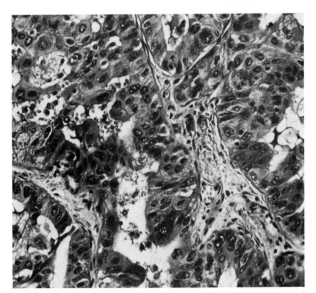

FIGURE 8-53. Light micrograph of metastatic carcinoma of the pancreas.

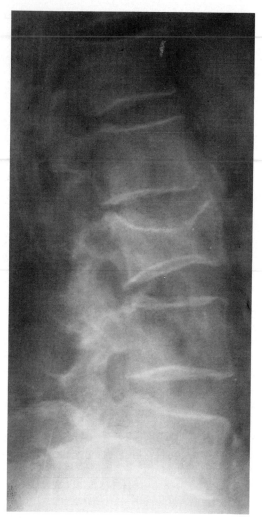

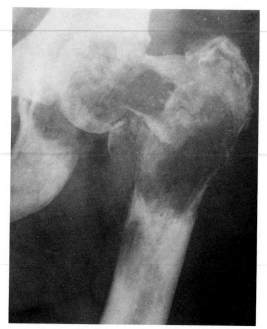

FIGURE 8-55. Radiograph showing a pathologic fracture of the proximal femur caused by metastatic lung carcinoma.

FIGURE 8-54. Radiograph showing a pathologic compression fracture of a vertebral body caused by metastatic breast carcinoma.

bone destruction with areas of reactive new bone formation in patients with metastatic disease, the tumor must destroy a substantial portion of the bone, estimated to be 30% to 50%, before a plain radiograph shows an abnormality. For this reason, radioisotope scanning offers a more sensitive method of detecting metastatic disease, although it may not show rapidly destructive lesions or bone destruction due to multiple myeloma and, in some instances, renal cell carcinomas. If plain radiographs and radionuclide imaging fail to adequately demonstrate the bone abnormalities in a patient with metastatic disease, CT and MRI may provide more detailed information. Although most metastases destroy bone, some metastatic neoplasms, especially metastases from carcinomas of the prostate and breast, can

stimulate bone formation and therefore appear as regions of increased bone density.

Treatment of metastatic disease of the skeleton can help preserve musculoskeletal function and relieve or prevent pain. It includes prophylactic internal fixation of involved bones to prevent fracture and relieve pain, internal fixation of pathologic fractures, amputation when other treatments would be inadequate, radiation therapy, and for some neoplasms, chemotherapy and hormonal therapy.

SUMMARY

Lesions that resemble benign neoplasms, primary malignant neoplasms, and metastatic neoplasms (see Tables 8-1 and 8-2) can involve all parts of the musculoskeletal system. They vary in clinical behavior from developmental disturbances of the musculoskeletal tissues that resolve spontaneously, to benign neoplasms that, left untreated, destroy bone and soft tissue, to highly malignant neoplasms that cause death despite aggressive treatment.

Partially because neoplasms of bone and soft tissue occur infrequently, many physicians, including orthopaedists, may not suspect neoplastic disease in a patient with vague discomfort, swelling, loss of musculoskeletal function, or incidentally discovered

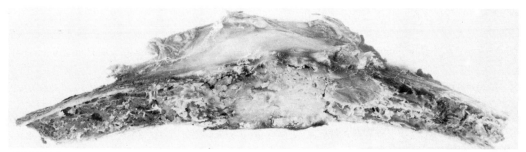

FIGURE 8-56. Metastatic carcinoma of the rib. The neoplasm has extended through the bone cortex into the soft tissues.

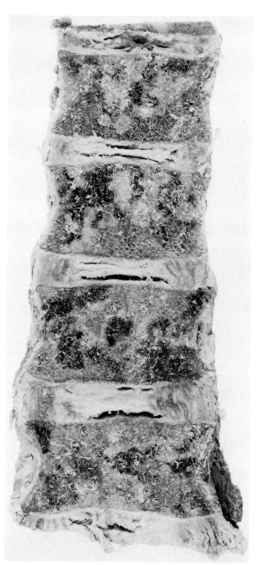

FIGURE 8-57. Metastases from a prostatic carcinoma to the spine. The dark areas consist of remaining bone marrow. The neoplasm has spread through most of the bone in all of the vertebrae shown.

and unexplained physical findings or abnormalities on imaging studies. Because common benign lesions of the musculoskeletal system may initially resemble malignant lesions, even when a physician identifies the presence of a musculoskeletal abnormality, he or she may not consider the possibility of malignant disease; and even if the physician considers the possibility of malignant disease, distinguishing neoplasms from nonneoplastic lesions can be difficult when the patient is first seen by a physician. For example, synovial sarcomas have been initially diagnosed and treated as ganglia, and osteosarcomas have been initially diagnosed and treated as stress fractures.

For these reasons, patients with symptoms, signs, or abnormalities on imaging studies that suggest the presence of a musculoskeletal neoplasm should have a careful initial evaluation. Based on this evaluation, the physician must decide if the patient can be treated symptomatically or observed or if the patient should have further laboratory and imaging studies, referral, or immediate treatment. Conditions requiring immediate treatment include pathologic fractures or impending pathologic fractures, neurologic deficits or impending neurologic deficits, and uncontrolled pain. In most instances, the definitive evaluation and biopsy of a lesion that may be malignant should be performed by an orthopaedist with experience in the management of these problems.

Annotated Bibliography

Enneking WF. Musculoskeletal tumor surgery. New York, Churchill Livingstone, 1983.
The author reviews the clinical presentation and surgical treatment of bone and soft tissue neoplasms. The first section of the book discusses the presentation, natural history, and staging of musculoskeletal neoplasms. The second section explains how different

anatomic locations affect the presentation, progression, and treatment of these neoplasms, and the last section covers specific types of neoplasms.

Enzinger FM, Weiss SW. Soft tissue tumors. St Louis, CV Mosby, 1988.
The authors provide in-depth discussions of benign and malignant neoplasms of the musculoskeletal soft tissues and lesions of the soft tissues that resemble neoplasms.

Milgram JW. Radiologic and histologic pathology of nontumorous diseases of bones and joints. Northbrook, IL, Northbrook Publishing, 1990.
This book presents clear illustrations of the plain radiographic, gross, and microscopic appearances of nonneoplastic diseases of the skeleton, traumatic injuries, and the response of the tissues to implants.

Mirra JM. Bone tumors: clinical, radiologic, and pathologic correlations. Philadelphia, Lea & Febiger, 1989.
This detailed text presents the clinical, radiologic, and pathologic characteristics of bone tumors. The author also summarizes the course and treatment of each neoplasm.

Sim FH, ed. Diagnosis and management of metastatic bone disease: a multidisciplinary approach. New York, Raven Press, 1988.
The authors of this book provide an excellent review of the diagnosis and treatment of metastatic bone disease. They include discussions of clinical findings, laboratory tests, imaging studies, and biopsy in the sections on diagnosis. The chapters devoted to treatment include the general principles of surgical and nonsurgical management and the specific approaches to metastases in different parts of the skeleton and to particular types of metastatic neoplasms.

Wold LE, McLeod RA, Sim FH, Unni KK. Atlas of orthopaedic pathology. Philadelphia, WB Saunders, 1990.
This well-illustrated atlas summarizes the symptoms, signs, radiographic features, pathologic features, differential diagnosis, and treatment of orthopaedic tumors and lesions that resemble tumors.

III

Regional Disorders of the Musculoskeletal System

9

Eric T. Jones
Philip Mayer

Turek's Orthopaedics: Principles and Their Application, Fifth Edition,
edited by Stuart L. Weinstein and Joseph A. Buckwalter.
J.B. Lippincott Company, Philadelphia, © 1994.

The Neck

TORTICOLLIS
  Differential Diagnosis
  Clinical and
    Radiographic
    Features
  Treatment
  Rotatory Subluxation of
    Childhood
  Clinical Features
  Treatment
  Spasmodic Torticollis
STIFF NECK
  Clinical Features
  Radiographic Studies
  Natural History

DEGENERATIVE AND
  HERNIATED
  INTERVERTEBRAL
  DISK DISEASE
  Incidence
  Clinical Features
  Cervical Radiculopathy
  Myelopathy
  Roentgenographic
    Features
  Computed Tomographic
    Scans
  Myelography
  Diskography
  Other Diagnostic Studies
  Local Injection
  Pathoanatomy
  Treatment

KLIPPEL-FEIL
  SYNDROME
  Clinical Findings
  Radiographic Findings
  Associated Conditions
  Treatment
JUVENILE RHEUMATOID
  ARTHRITIS
  Clinical Features
  Etiology
  Natural History
  Treatment
RHEUMATOID
  ARTHRITIS
  Clinical Features
  Natural History
  Treatment
  Complications of
    Treatment

TORTICOLLIS

Torticollis, or wry neck, a common clinical symptom and sign found in a variety of situations, is a rotational deformity of the upper cervical spine that causes a turning and tilting of the head (Fig. 9-1). The head is tilted to the involved side and the chin rotated to the opposite side. This is most often seen in the newborn period. It is often associated with deformity of the head (plagiocephaly). If torticollis is present in the newborn period, the usual cause is congenital muscular torticollis. Roentgenograms of the cervical spine, however, should be obtained to exclude other less common congenital conditions, such as fixed or bony torticollis resulting from Klippel-Feil syndrome, or other anomalies of the atlantoaxial portion of the cervical spine.

Torticollis may also be seen following a childhood upper respiratory tract

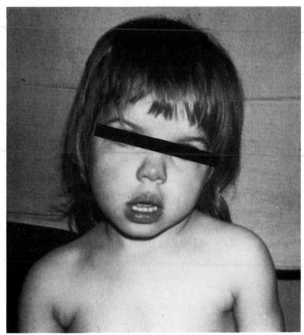

FIGURE 9-1. Torticollis is head tilt with rotation. Congenital muscular torticollis and rotatory subluxation of the atlas on the axis are the two most common causes in children. Facial asymmetry is present.

illnesses. When torticollis is present after the newborn period one should be highly suspicious of a problem in the upper cervical spine as 50% of the rotation of the cervical spine occurs at C1-C2. Therefore, conditions that would cause a rotational deformity are likely present at the atlantoaxial level.

Congenital Muscular Torticollis (Congenital Wry Neck)

Congenital muscular torticollis is usually discovered in the first month of life. It presents as unilateral tightness of the sternocleidomastoid muscle. There

may be a palpable mass (tumor) that is generally nontender, firm to soft and mobile beneath the skin, and attached to or located within the body of the sternocleidomastoid muscle. This mass often enlarges during the 4 to 6 weeks of life and then gradually decreases in size. By 4 to 6 months of age, the mass is usually absent, and the only clinical findings that may remain are the contracture of the sternocleidomastoid muscle and the torticollic posture with the head tilted toward the involved side and the chin rotated toward the opposite shoulder.

Differential Diagnosis

The etiology of torticollis is diverse, and identifying the cause can pose a difficult diagnostic problem. Radiographs are often difficult to obtain because the mastoid overlies the upper cervical spine. A radiograph of the cervical spine taken as a lateral to the skull can image the atlantoaxial region where the problem usually exists.

If congenital muscular torticollis is not present, there may be an odontoid anomaly, C1-C2 instability, Klippel-Feil syndrome, and so forth (Table 9-1). All children with torticollis should be evaluated with roentgenograms to exclude bony abnormality or fracture. Roentgenographic evaluation may be difficult in any child with a rotational deformity, but this is particularly true in the neonate.

Clinical and Radiographic Features

If torticollis is noted in the weeks following delivery, the usual cause is congenital muscular torticollis. If the child is less than 2 months of age, the palpable lump usually is diagnostic. Congenital muscular torticollis is painless, is associated with a contracted sternocleidomastoid muscle, and is unaccompanied

TABLE 9-1.
Differential Diagnosis of Torticollis

Congenital	Neurologic	Inflammatory	Traumatic
Congenital muscular torticollis	Ocular dysfunction	Lymphadenitis of the neck	Fractures, subluxations, dislocations of the cervical spine, particularly C1-C2
Klippel-Feil syndrome	Syringomyelia	Spontaneous hyperemic atlantoaxial rotatory subluxation	
Basilar impressions	Spinal cord or cerebellar tumors (posterior fossa)		
Atlantooccipital fusion			
Pterygium colli (skin webs)	Bulbar palsies		
Odontoid anomalies			

by any bony abnormalities or neurologic deficit. Any findings of pain or neurologic deficit should lead one to seek out other causes. Soft tissue problems are less common and include abnormal skin webs or folds (pterygium colli). Tumors in the region of the sternocleidomastoid include brachial cleft cyst and teratomas, which are rare but should be considered.

In later childhood, bacterial or viral pharyngitis and involvement of the cervical nodes is the primary cause of torticollis. Spontaneous atlantoaxial rotatory subluxation may follow an acute pharyngitis. Radiographic confirmation is difficult, and computed tomographic (CT) scans and magnetic resonance images (MRIs) may be necessary for diagnosis. If torticollis goes untreated for more than several weeks, there may be secondary soft tissue deformities that result in fixed rotatory subluxation.

Traumatic causes should be considered and excluded as part of the evaluation. Torticollis most commonly follows injury to the C1-C2 level. Fractures of the odontoid may not be apparent in the initial radiographic views; if a high index of suspicion is present, special radiographic studies should be undertaken. Children with bone dysplasias, such as Morquio disease, spondyloepiphyseal dysplasia, and Down syndrome, have a high incidence of C1-C2 problems and should be evaluated if torticollis is present.

Neurologic problems, particularly space-occupying lesions of the central nervous system, such as tumors of the posterior fossa or spinal column and syringomyelia, may be accompanied by torticollis. Generally, there are additional neurologic findings such as long tract signs, weakness in the upper extremities, and hearing or visual problems that may also cause head tilt.

Pathoanatomy

Congenital muscular torticollis is believed to be caused by local trauma to the soft tissues of the neck just before or during delivery. These children often have had breech or difficult forceps deliveries. Torticollis can occur after otherwise normal delivery, however, and has been reported following cesarean section. The fibrosis in the muscle may be due to venous occlusion and pressure on the neck in the birth canal because of cervical and skull position. The persistent clinical deformity is probably related to the ratio of fibrosis in the muscle to the remaining functional muscle. If sufficient normal muscle is present, it usually stretches with growth, and the child does not develop torticollis. In three of four children, the lesion is on the right side. Up to 20% of these children have congenital dysplasia of the hip associated with torticollis.

Natural History

If the condition is not treated, considerable cosmetic deformities of the face and skull can result, including asymmetry of the eyes and ears. Flattening of the face on the side of the contracted sternocleidomastoid may be impressive and is due to the position of the head when the child sleeps. If the child sleeps prone, it is more comfortable to have the affected side down. The face on the affected side remodels to conform to the surface. In children who sleep supine, the modeling of the contralateral aspect of the skull is evident.

Treatment

Excellent results can be obtained in most patients with stretching exercises. The exercises include positioning the ear opposite the contracted muscle to the shoulder and also stretching the chin to the shoulder on the opposite side. When adequate stretching has been obtained in the neutral position, these maneuvers should be repeated with the neck extended. Other measures include positioning of crib toys so the sternocleidomastoid are stretched when trying to reach and grasp. If exercises are unsuccessful, surgical resection may be required to release a portion of the tendon at the clavicular attachment. Surgery is usually performed before school age. Asymmetry of the skull and face corrects as long as adequate growth potential remains after the deforming force of the sternocleidomastoid is removed. The results of surgery are usually good with a low incidence of complications and recurrence, although some children require a repeat procedure during adolescence. Severer deformities may require both proximal and distal sternocleidomastoid release.

Rotatory Subluxation of Childhood

A common condition present in children is C1-C2 rotatory subluxation or C1-C2 rotatory displacement (rotatory subluxation of childhood; Fig. 9-2). This condition may occur following trivial trauma or a viral upper respiratory tract inflammatory condition but can also occur following tonsilectomy or other oral pharyngeal surgery. Grisel syndrome is not a

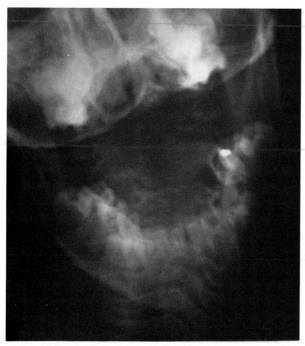

FIGURE 9-2. Rotatory subluxation, C1 on C2. This open mouth view is consistent with atlantoaxial rotatory subluxation. There is tilt of the skull as well as a shift of the lateral masses of C1 on C2, with overlap of the lateral mass of C1 on C2 on the left side. Cineradiography or dynamic CT scan is the best method to confirm fixed rotatory subluxation of C1 on C2.

cervical infection but a rotatory displacement of C1-C2 secondary to local inflammation, which can allow capsular or synovial interposition of tissue at the atlantoaxial level.

Clinical Features

Symptoms and signs of rotatory subluxation include local muscle spasm, torticollis, and pain on cervical motion. Usually the range of motion is not significantly altered, but motion is uncomfortable if moved from the torticollic position. This condition occurs most commonly in children 3 to 12 years of age. There is no spasm or contracture of the sternocleidomastoid muscle. The sudden onset of torticollis in this age group or in adults should lead to radiographs of the upper cervical spine. If these are not rewarding, further radiographic studies should be done in this area to look for the cause of torticollis.

If the torticollis develops rather slowly, one should consider either some type of central nervous system tumor or a visual abnormality. As children compensate for various abnormal vision-related

problems, they may tilt their head to be more comfortable with the image.

Treatment

In most cases, the torticollis resolves in a few days with or without treatment. Occasionally, it becomes fixed and requires treatment. Most patients are in between these extremes and may require antiinflammatory medication, soft collar, or head halter traction to resolve the torticollis. Treatment should be persistent and early to avoid the fixed rotatory problem. If the torticollis becomes fixed, in situ fusion is indicated.

Spasmodic Torticollis

This is an uncommon condition that may be present in adults with painful spasms producing a wry neck deformity. Radiographic studies are normal. The cause is idiopathic; however, electromyelographic studies show involvement of many muscles in the area, including the sternocleidomastoid, trapezious, and splenious. This condition is resistant to the usual forms of treatment, including surgery. Often these patients have concomitant or develop severe psychiatric disturbances.

Treatment consists of intradural section of the spinal accessory nerves and the first three anterior cervical nerve roots. Minimal involvement on one side and severe involvement on the other may require nerve root section on one side only. When the pain is intense and bilateral and many muscles are at fault, section of the fourth anterior cervical nerve root may be added without fear of compromising diaphragmatic function. Postoperatively, neck function is weak but the patient's painful spasms have improved.

Neuritis of the spinal accessory nerve can present much like spasmodic torticollis (Fig. 9-3). This condition is, however, temporary and usually resolves in a few weeks with application of heat, rest, and, occasionally, local injection of the spinal accessory nerve.

STIFF NECK

A stiff neck may be caused by trauma or can follow exposure to direct cool air on the neck. There are multiple causes for neck stiffness, and many of these

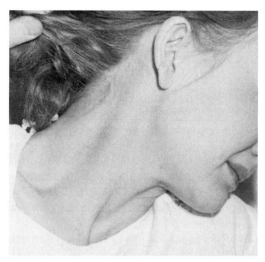

FIGURE 9-3. Acute torticollis due to neuritis of the spinal accessory nerve. The severely painful spasms were unilateral, temporary, and relieved by infiltration of the nerve with a local anesthetic. In contrast, spasmodic torticollis is bilateral, persistent or intermittent, and unaffected by injection of the nerve.

problems may come from the degenerative processes discussed later. Patients may present with torticollis that lasts for several days or more. A significant amount of discomfort is commonly associated with any motion of the cervical musculature leading one to rotate the thorax with the head. This condition is more commonly seen in adolescents and young adults than in older patients. The exact etiology is variable and often not identified. Causes can include muscle spasm, early disk herniation, multiple sclerosis, rheumatoid arthritis, primary or metastatic neoplasm, and vertebral osteomyelitis.

Clinical Features

Symptoms may last for only a few days to a few weeks. The area of discomfort may be the entire neck but is usually located in the paraspinous muscles posteriorly and in the occipital area. Often patients are tender to palpation and with any passive or active motion is painful. Lying down, using traction or cervical collars, or employing other measures to relax the cervical muscles are the only methods that tend to give any relief from the complaint. There may be associated symptoms such as nausea, dizziness, or headache that accompany the neck discomfort. Patients with this problem are usually obvious because when they turn their head, they turn their entire body, or they may use their hands for support of

their head with any active movement. Pain may be referred to the scapula, occipital area, or the shoulders, and there may be diffuse tenderness in the area of the trapezius.

Radiographic Studies

Following a history and physical examination, radiographic evaluation should include anteroposterior (AP) and lateral flexion–extension radiography to evaluate the bony portions of the cervical spine. Early with muscle spasm, there is loss of cervical lordosis as seen in the lateral cervical spine radiograph. There is little movement of the cervical spine on motion studies, which are often not helpful in evaluating for stability or injury because patients guard the spine against attempts at motion. Depending on history and physical examination, other studies (eg, myelogram or MRI) may be important to arrive at the exact diagnosis for a stiff neck.

Natural History

Depending on the cause of the problem the condition usually is self-limiting and responds to rest and antiinflammatory agents. The problem may clear without treatment. If one of the more significant degenerative, infectious, or neoplastic processes are found, treatment should be appropriate to that condition.

In general, if all early studies and physical examination are within normal limits, treatment usually consists of application of heat, nonsteroidal antiinflammatory medication, and a soft collar or supine cervical traction to relax cervical musculature.

DEGENERATIVE AND HERNIATED INTERVERTEBRAL DISK DISEASE

Degenerative problems of the cervical spine generally occur in the middle or later years of life. Cervical disk degeneration may lead to radiculopathy or myelopathy. Although an acute cervical disk herniation causes symptoms resembling those of an acute lumbar disk herniation (ie, radiculopathy, pain, motor, and sensory deficits), the clinical picture resulting from chronic cervical disk degeneration may be confusing. Several terms are commonly used to describe the degenerative cervical spine. The most appropriate term is *cervical spondylosis;* other synonyms are *osteoarthritis, osteoarthrosis, chronic herniated disk, chondroma,* and *spur formation.*

Incidence

Kelgren found that 82% of people age 55 and older have radiographic evidence of cervical degeneration. Degeneration of cervical disks is associated with aging. Disk disease is a deteriorative process that may produce pain. DePalma reported that in people older than 70 years, 72% had severe radiographic abnormalities. Rothman found myelographic abnormalities were common in asymptomatic patients. Abnormalities were seen in 21% of cervical myelograms, 24% of lumbar myelograms, and 8% of lumbar and cervical myelograms. Thus, no clear correlation exists between radiographic changes and symptoms. The most frequently involved level is C5-C6 followed by C6-C7, and C4-C5. Upper-level (occiput-C3) involvement is uncommon.

Clinical Features

Patients usually present with either pain or neurologic dysfunction (ie, radiculopathy or myelopathy). Radiculopathy is pain in the distribution of a nerve root and may be associated with or without neck pain, sensory deficit, and motor deficiency. Spinal cord compression may cause a myelopathy with involvement of the upper and lower extremities with mixed upper and lower motor neuron lesions.

Pain production is multifactorial. Nerve roots may be directly compressed. Osteophytes, which develop as a reaction to the process of degenerative disk disease extending across the posterior and posterolateral aspect of the vertebral bodies, may cause direct compression. An inflammatory component of the neuroelements may be a more significant cause of pain than actual mechanical changes. Studies have shown that compression of a normal nerve root results in paresthesia while compression of an inflamed root results in pain.

The spondylitic spine may be hypermobile, resulting in instability. This can usually be identified on lateral flexion and extension radiographs. AP movement of one vertebral body on another of 3.5 mm or greater in the adult is considered abnormal. Traction (horizontal) osteophytes are the result of hypermobility.

Spinal cord compression occurs when the dimensions of the spinal canal become compromised by bone or soft tissue hypertrophy. Hyperextension in the spondylitic cervical spine may cause inward bulging of the posterior ligamentum flavum. The cord may be further compromised by disk protrusion. Ischemic changes of the spinal cord may result from compression of its blood supply as the vessels pass through the pia mata. Additionally, the vertebral artery, which ascends through an osseous canal formed by the foramen transversarium in the transverse processes of the sixth to the second cervical vertebra, may be compressed.

Arthrosis of the facet joints in the spondylitic cervical spine may be a source of a dull, aching pain or lancinating pain secondary to direct nerve root compression. Additional mechanical sources of pain are microfractures in the vertebral bodies and pseudarthrosis of the cervical spine.

The differential diagnosis of neck pain must include tumors such as osteoid osteomas of the glenoid or a Pancoast (superior sulcus) tumor in the apex of the lungs. Additional causes of neck pain are direct compression of nerve roots, compressive lesions of the brachial plexus, compression of the vertebral artery and cervical sympathetics, degenerative osteoarthrosis involving the posterior facet joints, or degeneration of the disks anteriorly with subsequent instability or protrusion.

Vertebral artery compression must be considered in the differential diagnosis and may result in vertebral artery syndrome. The symptoms are intermittent in nature and include headaches, vertigo, tinnitus, and momentary loss of consciousness particularly when associated with extension or rotation maneuvers of the head and neck. The patient may experience dizziness, ataxia, headaches, nystagmus, and visual aberrations. Vertebral artery compression syndrome resulting by ingrowth of osteophytes from the lateral aspect of the vertebral bodies are more common than realized.

Thoracic outlet syndrome may cause neck pain. The patient may experience supraclavicular pain with radiation to the arm increased by use of the arm. There may be a history of paresthesia, particularly in the ulnar distribution, and blanching or coldness of the fingers. Physical examination may reveal tenderness about the brachial plexus and a positive Adson test in which patients place their hands on the thighs in a sitting position, turn the head to the side, and inhale deeply, resulting in a reproduction of the symptoms.

Posterior head and neck pain may result from greater occipital nerve neuralgia in which the posterior primary ramus of the C2 nerve becomes irritated or inflamed. Physical examination may reveal subjective paresthesia to percussion. The patient may

TABLE 9-2.
Cervical Radiculopathy: Differential Diagnosis

Carpal tunnel syndrome
Ulnar nerve compression palsy
Tardy ulnar palsy
Thoracic outlet
Cervical pain syndrome
Brachial plexopathy
Shoulder soft tissue and articular pain syndromes
Shoulder hand syndrome
Infection and inflammation
Developmental abnormalities
Vascular malformations
Neoplasms

experience limited neck motion, and symptoms may be reproduced by vertical loading or by maintaining the neck in extension.

Cervical Radiculopathy

Cervical radiculopathy is most common between ages 40 and 70. The onset of pain is insidious, and there may or may not be a history of trauma. The location of pain varies with the nerve root involved. Referred pain and soreness in the intrascapular region via the dorsal ramus of C6, or suboccipital headache sec-

ondary to greater occipital nerve involvement may occur (Tables 9-2 and 9-3). The pain of cervical radiculopathy may be described as dull, aching, boring, and related to neck motion. It may or may not be related to sneezing or coughing.

Myelopathy

Cervical myelopathy secondary to chronic disk degeneration with posterior osteophyte formation is the most common cause of spinal cord dysfunction in patients older than 55 years. The patient may present with a stooped wide-based or somewhat jerky gait and complain of weakness in the hands (see Table 9-3).

The clinical examination often reveals signs of upper motor neuron involvement in the lower extremities and lower motor neuron involvement in the upper extremities. In other words, the lower extremities are spastic with increased deep tendon reflexes and a positive or upgoing Babinski test. The upper extremities show weakness and atrophy without spasticity. There are several proposed mechanisms to describe the pathophysiology of cervical myelopathy. Anterior compression of the spinal cord results from posterior osteophytes. Posterior compression may result by infolding of the ligamentum flavum particularly in extension. Nutritional and vascular involvement with decreased blood supply through

TABLE 9-3.
Cervical Radiculopathy

Nerve Root	Disk Level	Sensory and Pain Symptoms	Motor and Reflex
C3	C2-C3	Pain and numbness in back of neck, especially around ear	No changes; electromyelographic findings only
C4	C3-C4	Pain and numbness in back of neck; radiation to intrascapular area and down anterior chest	No changes; electromyelographic findings only
C5	C4-C5	Pain radiating from side of neck to supraspinous shoulder; numbness chevron or middeltoid (axillary nerve) area	Deltoid weakness; shoulder abduction; biceps reflex
C6	C5-C6	Pain lateral arm and forearm, into thumb and index; numbness tip of thumb and first dorsal interosseous muscle	Weak biceps, elbow flexion and supination; wrist extension; brachioradialis reflexes
C7	C6-C7	Pain middle of forearm to long finger; index and ring may be involved	Triceps elbow extension; finger extension, wrist flexion; triceps reflex
C8	C7-T1	Pain medial forearm to ring and little fingers; numbness ulnar side of ring finger and little finger	Triceps elbow extension, finger flexion at metacarpophalangeal joints and distal joints; reflex—none
T1	T1-T2	Medial arm	Finger intrinsics, dorsal interrossei, abduction, and palmar interrossei adduction; reflex—none

the spinal arteries resulting in ischemic changes to the spinal cord has been identified.

Roentgenographic Features

Plain radiographs of the spine provide a clue to the level or levels of spine disease that may be responsible for the radicular syndrome in cervical spondylosis. Studies should include AP, bilateral obliques, lateral, odontoid open mouth, and lateral flexion and extension views (Fig. 9-4). One should look for evidence of foraminal encroachment, vertebral malalignment, sclerosis, facet joint subluxation, osteophyte protrusions, and ossification of the posterior longitudinal ligament. Further evaluation may include MRI, myelography using water-soluble contrast followed by contrast-enhanced CT scanning. An extension lateral view taken during the myelogram may illustrate infolding of the ligamentum flavum and dynamic encroachment in the spinal canal.

Computed Tomographic Scans

High-quality CT scans are extremely useful in assessing the size of the neuroforamina, which are normally 5 to 8 mm in vertical diameter. Scans must be performed using thin overlapping slices, appropriate bone windows, and reconstructions in the parasagittal plain to show the neuroforamina in profile.

Myelography

For many investigators, water-soluble contrast myelography in combination with CT scanning remains the securest way of defining root sleeve pathology (Figs. 9-5 and 9-6). It must be remembered that myelography does not define the most lateral component of the neuroforaminal encroachment because the subarachnoid space does not extend out to the full extent of the neuroforamen along with the nerve

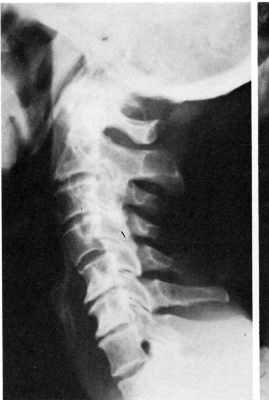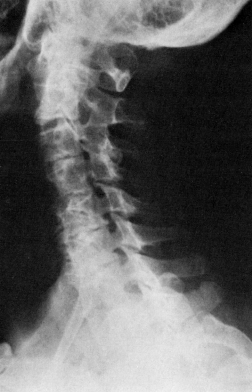

FIGURE 9-4. Degenerative arthritic changes in the cervical spine following loss of disk material particularly between C5 and C6. However, the oblique view shows spur formation encroaching on the intervertebral foramina from C3 to C7, which can cause nerve root symptoms.

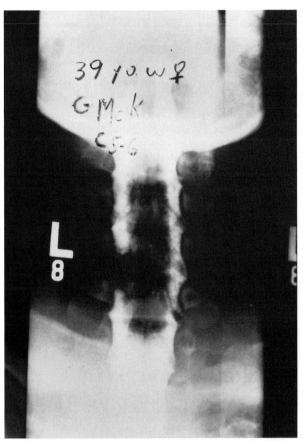

FIGURE 9-5. Cervical myelogram demonstrating herniated disk with left C5-C6 nerve root compression.

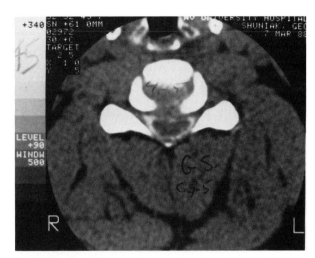

FIGURE 9-6. Postmyelogram-enhanced CT scan demonstrating herniated C4-C5 disk.

roots. Myelography with flexion and extension views can demonstrate dynamic cord compression related to bulging of the posterior longitudinal ligament and ligamentum flavum, or to spinal instability.

Diskography

The internal structure of the disk can be outlined by injecting it with a radioopaque substance, thus obtaining a cervical diskogram (Fig. 9-7). Distinctive diskogram determinations are dynamic tension on injection, the actual diskogram appearance on radiograph, and the reproduction of pain response. In the cervical spine, reproduction of clinical symptoms with injection is more important than the actual interpretation of the diskogram. Diskography is not a routine diagnostic procedure. It is important, however, to recognize that abnormal diskograms and pain produced locally and at a distance by injecting can be demonstrated in some asymptomatic people. The percentage of false-positive examinations increases

with advanced age. The procedure itself, therefore, is not infallible proof of an abnormal symptom. Accuracy of the various modalities is variable: clinical examination, 43%; plain radiographs, 46.5%; myelography, 45.6%; and diskography, 91%. Combined clinical examination and plain radiographs together have an accuracy rate of 61%.

Other Diagnostic Studies

Electrodiagnostic studies are most useful in establishing the diagnosis particularly by documenting the distribution of involvement. Nerve conduction studies can indicate that the nerve lesions are axonal rather than demyelinated. Conduction velocities within the involved nerve are normal or reduced in proportion to the degree of axonal loss.

Electromyography is a motor study not a sensory study. It takes 4 to 28 days for electromyelographic (EMG) changes to develop in acute radiculopathy. One third of patients have abnormalities in only the arm muscles, one third are abnormal in only the paraspinal muscles, and one third have electrical abnormalities in both paraspinal and arm muscles. The EMG is an electronic extension of the physical examination.

Local Injection

In older patients with multiple levels of abnormality shown on radiologic and other imaging studies in whom cervical radiculopathy cannot be localized,

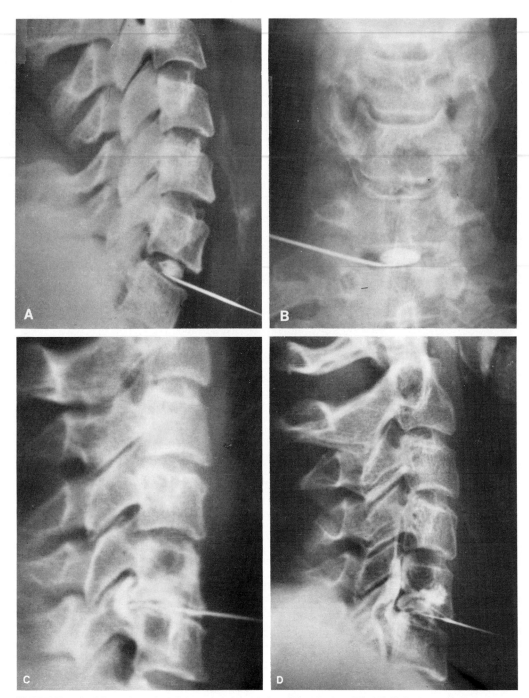

FIGURE 9-7. Normal cervical diskograms: lateral view (**A**); AP view (**B**). (**C**) "Mushroom" diskogram.
(Dye around the posterior osteophyte beneath the posterior longitudinal ligament.) (**D**) Massive posterior
disk rupture. (**E** and **F**) Examples of unilateral disk rupture.

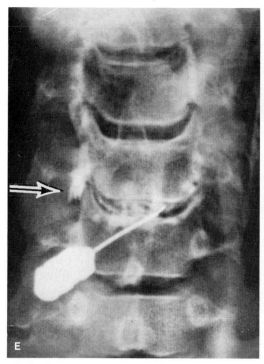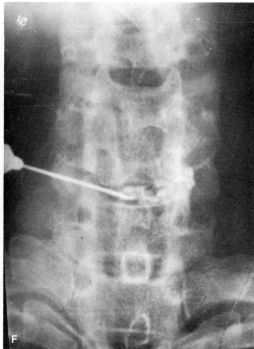

FIGURE 9-7. (*Continued*)

injection of local anesthetic into the interspace under fluoroscopic control and injections of local anesthetic into the facet joints may be useful in localizing the pain syndrome.

Pathoanatomy

Several factors should be considered in cervical disk degeneration, including physical stress, biochemical abnormalities, genetic defects, psychophysiologic effects, and autoimmune processes.

Biochemical changes precede structural changes. With aging, there is decreased water content of the disk and diminished water binding capacity. Collagen, the main structural component of the disk, increases, and its orientation and pattern change with age. These and other biochemical changes lead to a loss of the gel behavior of the nucleus and a loss of the desired biomechanical properties of the annulus, which becomes weakened and inelastic. Radiographically, this is manifested by gradual narrowing of the cervical disk space, sclerosis of the vertebral bodies, and the presence of osteophytes.

Deterioration of a cervical disk may result in acute nuclear herniation, annular protrusion or bulging, and diffuse degenerative changes. Degenerative changes commonly seen include osteophytes, both anterior and posterior, fissures in the disks, nuclear extrusion, abnormality and sclerosis at the joints of Luschka, foraminal narrowing, rounding of the anterosuperior vertebral bodies, and disk space narrowing.

The neuroforamen may be compromised as the disk space narrows. Encroachment into the neuroforamina may be caused by the joints of Luschka (oncovertebral joints), products of disk (78%), or hypertrophic or subluxed facet joints. Osteophytes may develop posteriorly and extend across the entire width of the vertebral body as a protuberant ridge. Additionally, the posterior longitudinal ligament may become hardened or calcified. Hypertrophy of the ligamentum flavum may also occur, which, on hyperextension, results in a rigid encroachment or bulging into the spinal canal with resultant compression on the posterior aspect of the thecal sac. The average spinal canal diameter between C3 and C6 is 17 mm. Degenerative changes in the cervical spine may result in a decreased canal diameter, thus reducing the space available for the cord (SAC). A SAC of 11 mm or less implies spinal cord compression.

Treatment

Conservative management of patients with neck pain involves the use of rest and splinting. Often a soft cervical collar is adequate to provide gentle support.

Philadelphia collars and other rigid cervical collars are frequently not well tolerated. Gentle traction using 5 to 10 lb with a head halter and a neutral position of flexion–extension to open up the neuroforamina may be of value. Traction applied in either flexion or extension may aggravate the patient's pain problem. Salicylates and the application of hot moist packs may be effective.

Surgical treatment for radiculopathy is usually indicated if there has been a documented failure of appropriate nonoperative treatment or if there is progressive neurologic deficit with a radiculopathy. Options are anterior or posterior decompression with or without fusion (Fig. 9-8).

The surgical treatment for cervical myelopathy resulting from degenerative spondylosis is controversial. Options are anterior decompression via corpectomy, diskectomy, and fusion versus posterior complete laminectomy and decompression. More recently, open door hinged laminoplasty, in which the lamina is cut on one side and hinged on the other side to create a flap-type opening and thus expand

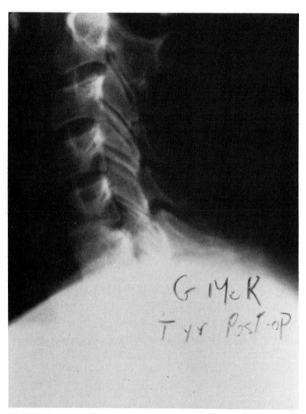

FIGURE 9-8. One-year postoperative lateral cervical radiograph demonstrating C5-C6 interbody fusion for a C5-C6 herniated nucleus pulposus and C6 radiculopathy.

the spinal canal, has been gaining favor. Open-door laminoplasty for multiple-level decompression seems to prevent postoperative swan-neck–type deformities, which sometimes occur after extensive multilevel posterior laminectomies.

KLIPPEL-FEIL SYNDROME

Klippel-Feil syndrome includes all individuals with congenital fusion of the cervical vertebra whether it be two segments or the entire cervical spine. The incidence is less than 1% of the population.

The etiology is unknown; however, embryologically congenital cervical fusion represents a failure of the normal segmentation of the cervical somites during the the 3rd to 8th week of life. There can be congenital blocked vertebrae with complete fusion of two or more adjacent vertebral bodies or a congenital bar with partial fusion of two or more vertebra. This syndrome is usually most apparent in children in the posterior elements and radiographically may appear as a bar between the bones (Fig. 9-9). The embryologic abnormality is not limited to the cervical spine.

Children with Klippel-Feil syndrome, even those with minor cervical fusions, may be at risk for other less apparent but serious defects in the genitourinary, nervous, and cardiopulmonary systems. Many have hearing impairment. These hidden abnormalities may be far more detrimental to the child's general well-being than the deformity of the neck.

Clinical Findings

Most patients appear normal without any abnormal clinical appearance. There is, however, a classic syndrome triad that includes a low posterior hairline, a short neck, and limitation of head and neck motion. The limitation of motion is predominantly in lateral side bending. Despite severe congenital fusion, many with this syndrome are able to maintain a deceptively good range of motion. Associated conditions, which are commonly seen when congenital cervical fusion is present, include Sprengel deformity, scoliosis, deafness, synkinesis, and hand, renal, and cardiac deformities. Individuals with this syndrome may present because of an incidental radiologic finding or in association with the work-up of other conditions or because of cosmetic concerns about their neck web or low hairline.

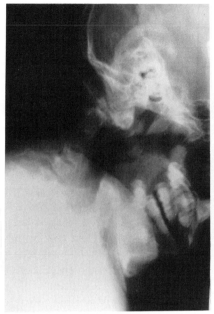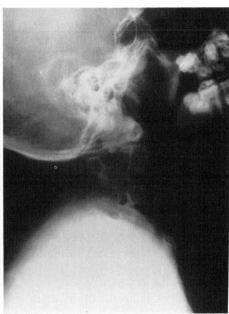

FIGURE 9-9. Lateral flexion–extension radiographs of a 10-year-old child with occipital and shoulder pain. There is fusion of C2–C4 (Klippel-Feil syndrome), the odontoid is absent, and motion of C1 on C2 is abnormal.

Radiographic Findings

The fixed bony deformities often times prevent classic positioning for AP, lateral, and oblique views of the cervical spine. Often there are overlapping shadows from the mandible, occiput, and mastoid areas. Lateral flexion–extension views, CT scans, and other studies may be necessary to fully evaluate the cervical spine deformity. If pain is present (as may be evident in older patients with this problem), serial lateral flexion–extension views may be necessary to evaluate for segmental instability with blocked motion at other levels. Other special studies, such as cineradiography, CT scans, and MRIs, may be necessary in certain situations.

If fusion is suspected in a child, it may be evident on flexion–extension views; however, there may be persistent cartilaginous end-plates, which look as if they are normal disk spaces. As the vertebral body completes its ossification, the fusion often becomes obvious.

Usually, no neurologic problems are associated with Klippel-Feil syndrome; however, there can be radiculopathy, myelopathy, quadriplegia, and sudden death from abnormal motion in the neck.

Associated Conditions

Scoliosis or kyphosis is commonly associated with this syndrome. Spinal deformity may be present in up to 60% of patients with Klippel-Feil syndrome.

There is a 20% incidence of renal abnormalities reported in patients with congenital scoliosis. Usual evaluation of Klippel-Feil syndrome includes an ultrasound of the kidneys and, if there is any doubt about a diagnosis, an intravenous pyelogram.

Treatment

Treatment, in general, is directed at the symptoms that may be associated with Klippel-Feil syndrome. Few children are symptomatic, and most patients who develop symptoms are in at least the second or third decade of life. Usually patients with Klippel-Feil syndrome can be expected to lead a normal, active life with only minor restrictions. Many of the severely involved patients may require fusion of abnormally mobile levels.

JUVENILE RHEUMATOID ARTHRITIS

Cervical spine involvement in juvenile rheumatoid arthritis (JRA) is usually limited to polyarticular and systemic JRA. The major problem associated with the cervical spine in JRA is slow, progressive, clinical stiffness and anatomic fusion of segments of the cervical spine. The usual reason to evaluate this problem early is to provide cervical protection during the active stage of the disease to direct the iatrogenic fusion of segments to a position of function.

Involvement of the cervical spine in JRA is common, with an occurrence of 60% to 70% in patients with the disease. Radiographic evidence of cervical spine abnormalities have been found in 27% to 80% of children with JRA.

Clinical Features

Neck pain is a frequent complaint in children with JRA. The pain is characteristically in the posterior area of the neck, radiating up into the occipital area and down into the shoulders and is worse with any motion of the head and neck. Usually the pain and loss of motion occur before the radiographic abnormalities, although severe neck pain is not common in the juvenile form of this disease.

Signs of neurologic change, either radicular, compressive, or myelopathic, are rare. They may occur in those few children with C1-C2 instability or with one motion segment following spontaneous fusion above and below.

Etiology

As in joint destruction in other anatomic areas, there is inflammation of synovial tissues with spread to involvement of the supporting ligamentous structures around the cervical spine. Synovial joints in the cervical spine include the posterior apophyseal joints, which rapidly become ankylosed with developing arthrosis, and the area around the odontoid both in the anterior articulation with the ring of C1 as well as with the transverse ligament. This results in the radiographic apple core odontoid.

The upper cervical spine may be involved in JRA just as in adult rheumatoid arthritis. Early changes consist of erosion of the odontoid or the so-called apple core odontoid. There may be apparent C1-C2 instability because of narrowing of the odontoid from this process. There is erosion of the odontoid at the level of the synovial membrane with the transverse ligament.

With long-standing rheumatoid disease, C1-C2 instability may be evident because of attrition or fracture of the odontoid. There may also be collapse of the C1-C2 facet area laterally, resulting in torticollis or abnormal positioning.

The most common problem in juvenile arthritis is apophyseal joint ankylosis resulting from inflammatory disease of the facet joints (Fig. 9-10). There may be decreased height secondary to this fusion if

it occurs when the growth plates are still open. Spontaneous fusion usually has no associated neurologic problems. There may be decreased size of the vertebral body, but the spinal canal is not compromised. Subluxation and instability may be a problem because of segmental fusion and abnormal motion occurring at fewer mobile levels.

Natural History

The ankylosis of the apophyseal joints in the cervical spine, particularly the joints between the second and third cervical vertebrae, is considered characteristic of JRA. As these areas fuse, the mechanical cervical pain improves but results in an inability to move the neck. This may result in instability if there are levels between fused segments that become hypermobile. The usual course of the cervical spine disease parallels the systemic course of the disease and also usually correlates with the severity of involvement of the individual patient. The stiffness of the cervical spine usually results in stiffness in extension and is a common early finding in polyarticular or systemic onset juvenile arthritis. Severe neck pain or torticollis is not common. When a severe amount of pain or torticollis is present, one must seek either a fracture or infection as the cause of that complaint.

Treatment

The treatment for cervical spine involvement in JRA consists of splinting the neck in a functional position. The patient should be encouraged to sleep without a pillow or in a position with a small amount of flexion. A cervical collar, either hard or more commonly soft, is the usual treatment method. Occasionally, surgical treatment for instability is required to further fuse areas of the cervical spine. Rarely, atlantoaxial subluxation requiring surgery may be present.

RHEUMATOID ARTHRITIS

Involvement of the cervical spine in adults with rheumatoid arthritis varies significantly from the juvenile counterpart. Stiffness is the rule in JRA, whereas looseness and instability is frequently a problem in adults who have cervical spine involvement. The most significant problems occur at occiput-C1 and C1-C2. Only rarely is there fusion of the subaxial spine as in JRA. Atlantoaxial subluxation is probably the most common and significant manifestation of involvement of the cervical spine. Its inci-

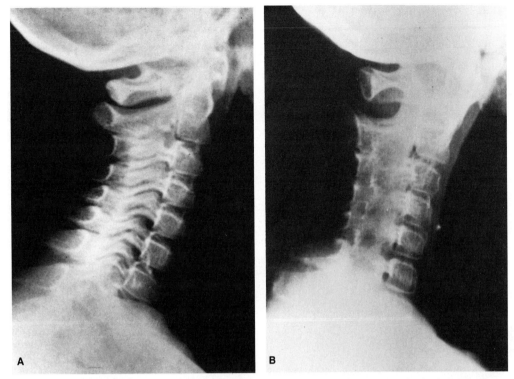

FIGURE 9-10. (A) Radiograph of a 9-year-old child with neck pain and polyarticular juvenile rheumatoid arthritis, illustrating early sclerotic change in posterior cervical joints. (B) Radiograph of the same patient 13 months later shows complete ankylosis of the apophyseal joints of the cervical spine typical of juvenile arthritis.

dence has been estimated to be somewhere between 25% to 60% of patients with rheumatoid arthritis. About 33% of patients with rheumatoid arthritic involvement demonstrate C1-C2 subluxation on flexion–extension radiographs. The severer the disease, the severer the involvement of the cervical spine.

Clinical Features

Neck pain is a frequent complaint in rheumatoid arthritic patients regardless of the radiographic findings. The presentation may be from the instability with pain on movement as well as peripheral nerve, cord, or brain-stem involvement. Another less common manifestation of instability is vertebral artery insufficiency resulting from intermittent mechanical blockage. It is sometimes difficult in more debilitated patients to identify true weakness; however, evidence of spasticity may become evident. Complaints of electric shock-like sensations are considered good evidence that the instability is clinically significant.

Atlantoaxial subluxation is usually best seen on the lateral flexion view (Fig. 9-11). The atlantodental interval (ADI) is measured from the anterior surface of the odontoid to the posterior surface of the anterior ring of C1 (see Fig. 9-11A). Flexion–extension views can identify how much motion is present at that level. The ADI is thought to be abnormal when greater than 3 mm in an adult and greater than 4 mm in a child. MRI flexion extension views may also be helpful in identifying instability and cord compression.

Similar measurements can be made for translocation of the odontoid into the foramen magnum. This is usually done by measuring the McGregor line as well as the Chamberlain line to determine the degree of odontoid projection (Fig. 9-12). The line drawn across the foramen magnum described by McRae should be well above the tip of the odontoid process. This disease is a systemic disease, so nearly all elements of the cervical spine are involved, including the bone ligaments, capsules, and so forth. Further changes can occur if the patient has been using steroids. The severity of cervical spine involvement usually parallels the severity of the disease.

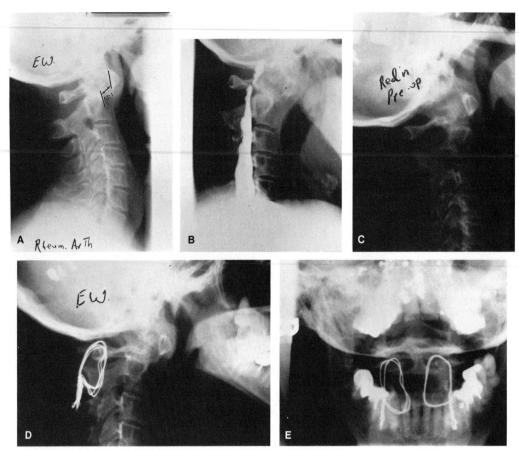

FIGURE 9-11. (**A**) C1-C2 instability, adult rheumatoid arthritis with forward subluxation of C1 on C2. (**B**) Myelogram in flexion, adult rheumatoid arthritis, demonstrating C1-C2 instability. (**C**) Pre-operative reduction in extension, adult rheumatoid arthritis, exhibiting C1-C2 instability. (**D**) Post-operative Brooks-type fusion, C1-C2 with reduction. (**E**) AP view, C1-C2, Brooks fusion.

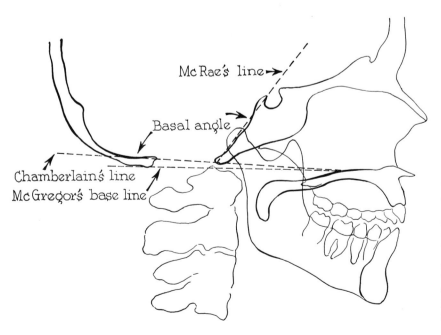

FIGURE 9-12. Measurement of platybasia and basilar invagination. Normally, the tip of the odontoid may lie slightly above the Chamberlain line. Displacement of the rim of the foramen magnum to a considerable degree above the McGregor line indicates basilar impression. The McRae line lies along the plane of the clivus. It normally subtends an angle with the Chamberlain or McGregor baseline not exceeding 145 degrees. A more obtuse angle indicates platybasia. (McGregor M. The significance of certain measurements of the skull in the diagnosis of basilar impression. Br J Radiol 1948;21:171)

Natural History

The natural history of involvement of the upper cervical spine is somewhat controversial. Several studies have shown that surgical management of this problem is associated with a high incidence of complications. More recent studies, however, suggest that when surgical intervention is necessary for pain, instability, or neurologic deficit, that the surgery is relatively safe (see Fig. 9-11*C* through *E*). These patients usually have systemic involvement, and a mortality rate for C1-C2 fusion has been reported as high as 25% to 40%. Five-year studies of untreated patients with atlantoaxial instability found that long track signs developed in one third of those with anterior subluxation and in half of those with protrusion of the odontoid into the foramen magnum.

Treatment

A protective soft collar or firm collar may help provide some degree of stability. A firm Philadelphia collar may give excellent support and be well tolerated by the patient. Often, however, there may be skin sensitivity and difficulty in using the collar, but it is the initial form of treatment in most patients.

The indications for surgical intervention are usually neurologic deficit; however, pain and instability play a role, particularly early in a patient who does not have severe systemic disease. The infection and complication rates in these debilitated patients are high. Postoperative management should consist of halo vest; however, the reconstruction of the spine should provide as much stability as possible to minimize the length of time necessary in a halo.

Successful surgery usually does relieve the patient's complaint and provides stability and halts progressive neurologic injury. There may be significant anesthetic problems associated with surgery in these patients.

Complications of Treatment

The mortality rates from surgery on the cervical spine, particularly the upper cervical spine in patients with rheumatoid arthritis, range as high as 50%. These patients have a high incidence of failure of fusion and a tendency to resorb bone graft. Infection rate and difficulty with postoperative immobilization are other significant problems in the treatment of this condition.

Annotated Bibliography

Torticollis

Coventry MB, Harris LE. Congenital muscular torticollis in infancy: some observations regarding treatment. J Bone Joint Surg 1959;41A:815.
This is an excellent classic review of thirty-five patients with congenital muscular torticollis. The physical and pathologic findings and treatment with follow-up are well recorded.

Ling CM, Low YS. Sternomastoid tumor and muscular torticollis. Clin Orthop Relat Res 1972;86:144.
This article discusses the clinical features and results of treatment of congenital muscular torticollis. There is follow-up on 66 of 150 patients with this condition.

MacDonald D. Sternomastoid tumor and muscular torticollis. J Bone Joint Surg 1969;51B:432.
This article evaluates the relation between the sternomastoid tumor and congenital muscular torticollis. It reviews the etiology and pathogenesis of the condition and presents the cases of 152 children with torticollis.

Wycis HT, Moore JR. The surgical treatment of spasmodic torticollis. J Bone Joint Surg 1954;36A:119.
This article describes the surgical treatment for spasmodic torticollis and discusses the differential diagnosis and how to arrive at the diagnosis of true spasmodic torticollis.

Rotatory Subluxation

Phillips WA, Hensinger RN. The management of atlanto-axial subluxation in children. J Bone Joint Surg 1989;71A:664.
This is a retrospective review of 23 children treated for atlantoaxial rotatory subluxation. In children seen less than 1 month after, the onset of symptoms the subluxation was able to be reduced either spontaneously or with traction. Of the other 7 children seen more than a month after the onset of symptoms, 3 eventually needed C1-C2 fusion. Dynamic CT scans made in maximum rotation to each side proved to be an excellent method of documenting the presence of rotatory subluxation.

Degenerated and Herniated Intervertebral Disc Disease

Cervical Spine Research Society Editorial Committee. Cervical spine. 2nd ed. Philadelphia, JB Lippincott, 1989;599.
Chapter 11 is divided into sections, each written by different experts in the field of cervical spine. It presents an informative discussion of the pathophysiology, an algorithm for diagnosis of neck pain, and a full discussion of therapeutic modalities, operative and nonoperative.

Wienir MA. Spinal segmental pain and sensory disturbance. Spine 1988;2.
This journal issue presents practical approaches to the diagnosis of patients presenting with local and limb symptoms of pain, numbness, parasthesia, and dysesthesia. The problems of diagnosis of local, musculoskeletal, orthopaedic, rheumatologic, and vascular conditions are not addressed but rather those entities affecting the neurostructures are emphasized. There is an excellent discussion of physical examination, electrodiagnostic techniques, and other diagnostic modalities.

Robinson RA, Southwick WO. Surgical approaches to the cervical spine. AAOS Instruct Course Lect 1960;17:299.
An excellent review of the classic approaches to the cervical spine.

Holt S, Yates PO. Cervical spondylosis and nerve lesions. J Bone Joint Surg 1966;48B:704.

This article presents a clear discussion of cervical spondylosis and associated nerve root injuries.

Simeone FA, Rothman RH. Cervical disc disease, ed 2. In: The spine. Philadelphia, WB Saunders, 1982:444.

This excellent, multiply-authored chapter gives a complete and reliable description of cervical degenerative disease, including pathophysiology, clinical presentation, diagnostic evaluation, and therapeutic modalities.

Klippel-Feil Syndrome

Hensinger RN, Lang JE, MacEwen GD. Klippel-Feil syndrome: a constellation of associated anomalies. J Bone Joint Surg 1974;56A:1246.

This is an evaluation of 50 patients with Klippel-Feil syndrome to evaluate associated anomalies. Less than half had the classic triad, more than half had scoliosis, and a third had renal anomalies. All patients with Klippel-Feil syndrome were found to be at risk for having other serious but less apparent anomalies including the Sprengel deformity, impairment of hearing, and congenital heart disease.

Pizzutillo PD. Klippel-Feil syndrome. In: Baily RW, ed. The cervical spine. Philadelphia, JB Lippincott, Philadelphia, 1983:174.

This chapter is the best single reference for reviewing Klippel-Feil syndrome. The triad of short neck, low posterior hairline, and limited range of motion, as well as other clinical findings in Klippel-Feil syndrome are discussed thoroughly. The history, embryology, associated problems, natural history, and treatment are also discussed.

Juvenile Rheumatoid Arthritis

Hensinger RN, DeVito PD, Ragsdale CG. Changes in the cervical spine in juvenile rheumatoid arthritis. J Bone Joint Surg 1968;68A:189.

This article sought evidence of disease in the cervical spine in 121 patients with juvenile rheumatoid arthritis. The authors reported that clinical stiffness and radiographic changes occurred most commonly in patients with polyarticular-onset disease and system-onset disease. Despite extensive roentgenographic involvement of the cervical spine, neck pain was not a common complaint.

Espada G, Babini JC, Maldonado-Cocco JA, Garcia-Morteo O. Radiologic review: the cervical spine in juvenile rheumatoid arthritis. Semin Arthritis Rheum 1988;17:185.

This is a good radiographic review of involvement of the cervical spine in juvenile rheumatoid arthritis. The most common radiographic abnormality found was apophyseal joint fusion, with paraspinal calcifications and growth disturbance being next in frequency. About 20% of patients in this study of 120 had atlantoaxial subluxation or odontoid erosion.

Rheumatoid Arthritis

Halla JT, Hardin JG, Vitek J, Alarcon GS. Involvement of the cervical spine in rheumatoid arthritis. Arthritis Rheum 1989;32:652.

This article summarizes the radiographic involvement of the cervical spine in rheumatoid arthritis and focuses on the use of special studies such as CT and MRI in evaluating these patients both for patterns of involvement as well as in treatment.

Turek's Orthopaedics: Principles and Their Application, Fifth Edition,
edited by Stuart L. Weinstein and Joseph A. Buckwalter.
J.B. Lippincott Company, Philadelphia, © 1994.

10

Edward V. Craig

The Shoulder and Arm

BIRTH PALSY

Birth palsy is a paralysis of part or all of the upper extremity from trauma to the brachial plexus, usually occurring during a difficult or prolonged labor and delivery. The mechanism is presumably forced separation of the interval between the head and shoulder, either by bending the head while the shoulder is held behind the pubic symphysis or by bending the infant's body to one side away from the head during a breech delivery while the head is fixed behind the pubis. Usually, large fetal size and undiagnosed cephalopelvic disproportion contribute to the necessity for manipulation during delivery, which may lead to the plexus trauma. Other factors besides breech position that may contribute include excessive maternal sedation, which may require instrumentation for delivery, or infant hypotonia.

With improvements in obstetric techniques during the past 25 years, including enlarging the indications for cesarean section, the incidence of trauma to the brachial plexus has decreased significantly. Recently, the incidence has leveled off and is about 2 in 1000 live births. Likewise, the severity of the injuries appears to be decreasing.

The nerve lesions range from slight stretching (neuropraxia), which is accompanied by edema and temporary loss of nerve conduction and is associated with early recovery, to complete rupture of the nerve (neurotmesis), with no hope for recovery. The upper plexus is more commonly involved and is usually at the fifth and sixth cervical roots (Erb palsy), with resultant weakness in the deltoid, biceps, brachialis, supinator, supraspinatus, and infraspinatus. This weakness of the abductors and external rotators leads to overpull by the adductors and internal rotators (subscapularis, pectoralis major), resulting in shortening and contracture of these anterior structures.

Total plexus involvement is the second most common injury. The extremity is usually limp, with loss of deep tendon reflexes, loss of Moro reflex, Horner syndrome due to involvement of the cervical sympathetic nerves, and diaphragmatic paralysis from phrenic nerve injury. Because this is generally a root avulsion injury, the prognosis for recovery is poor.

In the rare injury to the seventh and eighth cervical roots (Klumpke paralysis), there is weakness of the hand and wrist flexors as well as of the hand intrinsic parts, resulting in a clawhand deformity.

Clinical Features

Initially, the infant lies with the extremity limp at the side. Typically, there is no spontaneous movement of the extremity from the shoulder to fingertip. Swelling in the area of the shoulder girdle may be present and may reflect concomitant traumatic injuries to the clavicle or humeral physis. The infant usually cries when any attempt to move the extremity passively is undertaken. Within a few hours or days, recovery begins, as swelling diminishes and sensitivity of the limb improves. With gradual resolution of the edema surrounding the nerve roots, the plexus recovers, nerve conductivity returns, and muscle activity ensues. Although most children recover spontaneously and fully, there may be residual paralysis. In Erb palsy, the typical paralysis involves the abductors and external rotators of the shoulder, the flexors of the elbow, and the supinators of the forearm, resulting in the so-called waiter's tip position, with the shoulder held in adduction and internal rotation, the elbow extended, and the forearm pronated. Usually, atrophy and thinning of the deltoid muscle occur, and the humeral head may rest in an inferiorly or posteriorly subluxated position.

Radiography of the neck and both upper extremities should be performed because associated injuries are common, including fractures of the clavicle and proximal humerus. Fractures of the clavicle can usually be identified by crepitation over the clavicle and sometimes palpation of the free ends of the broken bone. Fractures through the humeral epiphysis may be more difficult to diagnose since the humeral epiphysis is not ossified at birth. Normally, however, the humeral ossification center lies in the superior and medial position relative to the upper end of the humeral shaft. Any deviation may be a clue to the presence of an epiphyseal separation. It is not unusual, however, for the first clue to concomitant bony fracture to be the appearance of a mass or lump 2 weeks after injury, which is, in fact, callus formation of a healing fracture.

The radiographic features associated with birth palsy may change in time as asymmetric muscle pull and fixed contracture lead to secondary bone changes in the shoulder girdle. The humeral head fixed in an internally rotated and posteriorly subluxated position may erode the posterior glenoid. Eventually, secondary degenerative changes and frank glenohumeral arthritis can occur (Figs. 10-1 and 10-2). The acromion and coracoid process often are elongated and hooked, and the scapula may be hypoplastic.

A number of other radiographic studies were found to be useful in evaluating birth injuries. Ultrasonography is used to identify the presence of the humeral head in the glenoid when there is a question of associated dislocation of the shoulder. It has also been useful in identifying some fractures around the shoulder. If there is a question of whether the unos-

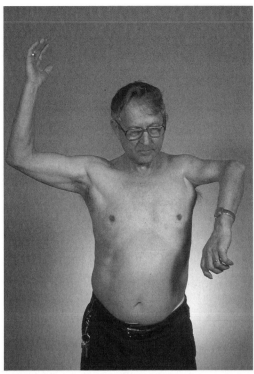

FIGURE 10-1. A 62-year-old patient with history of Erb palsy. The internal rotation contracture of the arm is so severe that, with any elbow flexion, the patient's hand hits against his rib cage.

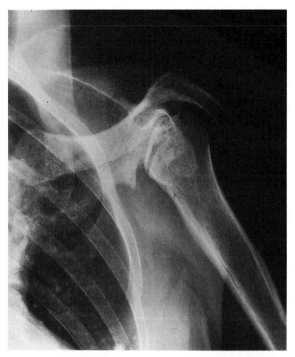

FIGURE 10-2. Radiograph of the patient shown in Figure 10-1 with deformity of coracoid, flattening of the humeral head, and secondary arthritic changes of the glenohumeral joint.

sified humeral head is located in the glenoid, arthrography may be considered. Another radiographic study that is used to evaluate the severity of the nerve injury is myelography, although its usefulness is limited because it has not been specific in identifying the extent of nerve root pathology. Magnetic resonance imaging (MRI) may be useful in evaluating root avulsion. An electromyogram (EMG) of the associated muscles of the shoulder girdle may be useful to document nerve recovery, or as the child gets older and consideration is made for reconstruction, it may identify muscles that are available for tendon transfer.

Treatment

Although there is no uniform appreciation of the "true" natural history of brachial plexus birth injury, it appears from recent studies that 80% to 95% of children with upper extremity neurologic dysfunction from a brachial plexus injury at birth obtain normal or near normal function. It also appears that 92% of these patients recover within 3 months after the injury, and thus no operation is ordinarily performed earlier than that. The outlook for the Klumpke type

of paralysis is much less optimistic than that for the Erb type.

Even though outlook for most infants is favorable regarding return of function, some natural history studies suggest the following: (1) patients who have biceps function before 3 months of age have an excellent prognosis for normal recovery; (2) patients who have their first evidence of biceps function between 3 and 6 months of age often achieve near-normal function; and (3) absent biceps function or absent EMG evidence of the biceps function after 6 months of age worsens the outlook because it often indicates that the nerves were transected.

Early after discovery of the nerve injury, treatment is aimed at preventing deformity, relaxing the weakened muscles, and avoiding further tension on the brachial plexus. With the Erb type of paralysis, the patient should be positioned in external rotation and abduction of the shoulder. Daily physical therapy is useful and consists of moving all the joints of the extremity through a full range of motion three times daily and massaging the muscle to help preserve muscle tone. Splinting and therapy should be continued for an indefinite period, until the child reaches the age to be able to cooperate with a surgical reconstruction aimed at restoring function.

Recent advances in nerve surgery technology and microsurgery have made possible early brachial plexus exploration and possible repair of disrupted nerves. Since the prognosis for return of function is so poor if the biceps has not returned within 6 months of the injury, and since this often is indicative of nerve transection, surgical exploration of the brachial plexus may be considered at this time. If the nerve is transected, nerve grafts or direct nerve repair is possible and, if successful, increases the likelihood for return of muscle function that would otherwise never be innervated.

After nerve repair, recovery usually takes from 18 to 24 months. If recovery is incomplete, late reconstructive surgery may still be considered.

When muscle recovery after the injury is incomplete, the functional limitation of an adduction, internal rotation contracture at the shoulder, extension contraction of the elbow, and pronation deformity of the arm can be considerable. The main functional disability caused by this contracture is inability to reach the mouth. If no bony deformity exists to limit the movement, and if hand function is unimpaired and elbow flexion is either present or reconstructable, release of the internal rotation contracture alone is considered. This often restores the ability for the shoulder to be externally rotated. If the external rotators remain weak, however, the internal rotation deformity usually recurs. In this situation, muscle restoration is attempted, providing active external rotation. One of the procedures used to improve function is a combination of the Sever and L'Episcopo procedures, which consists of an open release of the contracted anterior shoulder capsule and division of the subscapularis and pectoralis major muscles, thus permitting external rotation. After this, the teres major and latissimus dorsi muscles with their tendinous attachments can be transferred from their positions as internal rotators of the shoulder to the outside of the humerus, permitting active external rotation. If fixed bony deformity does not permit external rotation, even with tendon transfers, an osteotomy of the humerus may be considered. In this procedure, the humerus is osteotomized, or cut, below the level of the deltoid insertion, and the whole humerus is externally rotated, putting the extremity in a better functional position.

For cases in which paralysis of the elbow does not permit active elbow flexion because of loss of the brachialis and biceps, a number of tendon transfers were described to restore elbow flexion (flexorplasties). These muscles must be strong enough to supply active flexion of the elbow. Among the muscles that have been transferred are the pectoralis major, the triceps, the latissimus dorsi, and the flexor pronator mass of the forearm.

In some patients, despite weakness of elbow flexion, a flexion deformity of the elbow may develop. Ordinarily, a significant flexion contracture of the elbow is compatible with useful function. If a flexion contracture has developed and is greater than 50 to 60 degrees, however, consideration is given to release of the tight structure, including the anterior capsule of the elbow and the biceps brachialis.

When growth has ceased in the older child, if paralysis of the deltoid and the rotator cuff tendons leaves an unstable, weak, and flail shoulder girdle, arthrodesis, or fusion, of the shoulder may be considered to restore stability, power, and improved function.

Successful arthrodesis of the shoulder eliminates external and internal rotation of the shoulder since these motions occur through the glenohumeral joint. Movement of the shoulder girdle is possible through scapulothoracic motion, however, and a patient with arthrodesis of the shoulder often has the ability to reach the forehead, opposite axilla, belt, and side pocket. As a prerequisite for a successful arthrodesis, scapula muscles, especially the trapezius, must be present and strong since they provide the motor power for shoulder girdle motion.

In the unusual situation of late glenohumeral arthrosis that follows a brachial plexus palsy, if the glenohumeral joint is painful and the pain is disabling for the patient, total shoulder arthroplasty (total shoulder replacement) may be considered to resurface the glenohumeral joint. Although the joint can be resurfaced to eliminate pain from glenohumeral arthrosis, however, movement and stability of the arthroplasty depend on adequately balanced and functioning muscles of the shoulder girdle.

DEGENERATIVE DISEASE OF THE ACROMIOCLAVICULAR JOINT

The joint between the lateral margin of the clavicle and medial aspect of acromion is classified as a *diarthrodial joint*. Between these two joint facets is a fibrocartilaginous intraarticular disk, which can vary in size and shape. As with any joint, the acromioclavicular joint may be subject to normal effects of aging, degeneration, or trauma, or it may be part of generalized inflammatory arthropathy, such as rheumatoid arthritis. Marked variability in the plane of the joint can occur, and it is estimated that the angle between the two facets may, in part, determine the tendency of the joint to deteriorate with age because shear forces of obliquely oriented joints appear to be more disruptive to cartilage than pure compressive forces between two joints that directly face one another.

As the arm is elevated above shoulder level, the clavicle rotates. The acromioclavicular joint is stabilized by a series of ligaments, including the acromioclavicular ligaments and coracoclavicular ligaments (conoid and trapezoid ligaments). The acromioclavicular ligaments reinforce the acromioclavicular joint capsule and blend with fibers of deltoid and trapezius fascia. They appear to be important primarily for stability of the joint against anterior and posterior displacement. Thus, patients who have traumatic disruption of the acromioclavicular ligaments alone may have an excessive amount of motion in the anteroposterior (AP) plane, while little change is seen in the superoinferior plane. By far the most important ligamentous structures stabilizing the acromioclavicular joint are the conoid and trapezoid ligaments. These ligaments run from the inferior surface of the clavicle to the base of the coracoid process of the scapula. It appears that traumatic rupture of the coracoclavicular ligaments is predominantly responsible for the wide separation seen in some patients with traumatic acromioclavicular separation. Acromioclavicular joint separations are thus classified by the extent of severity of the ligamentous injury. Lower grades of acromioclavicular separation imply that the acromioclavicular ligaments are disrupted, while the coracoclavicular ligaments are intact. Higher degrees of acromioclavicular separation suggest disruption of all stabilizing structures between the clavicle and scapula. Because of the wider displacement between acromion and clavicle, the higher degrees of acromioclavicular separation are usually the most obvious clinically.

Epidemiology

With normal aging, the intraarticular disk undergoes degeneration, and this degeneration precedes degenerative changes in the cartilaginous surfaces. Degeneration of the acromioclavicular joint appears related to normal aging since cartilage loss and subsequent radiographic changes are common as patients get older. Not all acromioclavicular joint degeneration may be symptomatic, however, and since this is the age group in which other disorders of the shoulder occur, distinguishing between these conditions and acromioclavicular joint degeneration may be difficult. A recent study that compared radiographic findings with actual pathologic findings in 108 cadaver acromioclavicular joints showed that early osteoarthritic or degenerative changes were

frequently missed by radiographs. Many joints that show loss of cartilage and radiographic evidence of degenerative changes may not be clinically painful. Although the extent of joint degeneration is usually equal bilaterally, a recent study suggested that arthritic changes were more common on the right side than the left. In a study of 620 joints, clinical symptoms became more frequent with increasing age and with radiographic progression of arthrosis.

Painful arthritis of the acromioclavicular joint may also accompany rheumatoid arthritis. In one recent series of patients with rheumatoid arthritis and painful shoulders, acromioclavicular joint pain and tenderness were present in about one third of the patients. It is important to distinguish the many causes of pain in the rheumatoid shoulder, especially since newer methods of joint replacement arthroplasty have become such an effective treatment for the arthritis of the glenohumeral joint. Some patients, however, may have pain that originates predominately in the acromioclavicular joint, and these patients may benefit from either therapeutic injection or surgical resection of the acromioclavicular joint without addressing the changes in the glenohumeral joint.

Pathology in the acromioclavicular joint probably is most important as it relates to disease and degeneration of the rotator cuff. The supraspinatus tendon travels directly inferior to the acromioclavicular joint as the arm is elevated overhead. Any arthritic changes in the joint that may produce distally projecting osteophytes may contribute to mechanical wear on the underlying subacromial bursa and rotator cuff, eventually contributing to subacromial impingement of this tendon with degeneration and cuff rupture. Thus, in most patients with a rotator cuff tear, the acromioclavicular joint should be evaluated. It may be necessary to resect this joint in part or in total as a step in the surgical repair of a rotator cuff tear. In some patients with cuff tears, glenohumeral joint fluid may actually dissect out into the subacromial bursa, and concomitant erosion of the inferior joint capsule by the high-riding humeral head may permit glenohumeral joint fluid to dissect directly into the acromioclavicular joint. This may present as a mass over the top of the acromioclavicular joint, which transilluminates and clearly is fluid-filled. This mass is called an *acromioclavicular joint ganglion* (Fig. 10-3). In fact, however, when this transparent fluid mass is found over the top of the acromioclavicular joint, it usually represents significant underlying rotator cuff pathology or tearing (Fig. 10-4).

Posttraumatic acromioclavicular arthroses may also occur, particularly after acromioclavicular joint

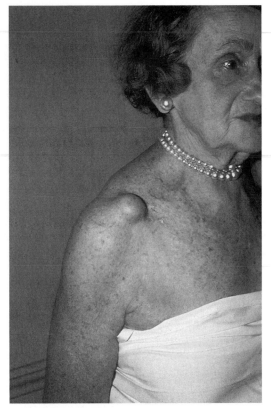

FIGURE 10-3. Acromioclavicular joint ganglion. Although this ganglion may appear as an innocuous collection of fluid over the acromioclavicular joint, it usually reflects an underlying rotator cuff tear, with glenohumeral joint fluid dissecting through the subacromial space and into the acromioclavicular joint.

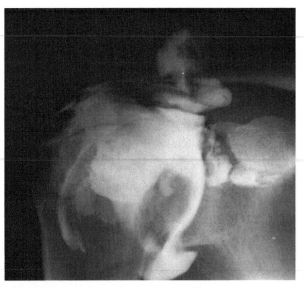

FIGURE 10-4. A corresponding arthrogram showing radiographic dye in the glenohumeral joint, in the subacromial space, and up through the acromioclavicular joint, forming the so-called geyser sign.

Clinical Features

With loss of the articular cartilage and degeneration of the clavicular and acromial facets of acromioclavicular joint, there is ordinarily accompanying synovitis of the joint. This may produce a painful shoulder. The patients who have painful degeneration of the acromioclavicular joint usually specifically localize their pain to this joint. The pain is most pronounced when using the arm above shoulder level, reaching across the chest (adduction) or reaching up behind the back, the positions which maximize the contact between acromial and clavicular facets. The patient may have pain when lying on the involved side and thus may be awakened from sleep at night. Throwing and racket sports are usually difficult, and workers who use their arms above shoulder level may be particularly disabled. A dull aching may be felt in addition to the sharp pain centered over the acromioclavicular joint. This aching may occur even with the arm at the side.

On examination of the patient, asymmetric swelling of the acromioclavicular joint may occur as a result of synovitis or osteophytes. Usually, direct tenderness is centered over the acromioclavicular joint. Because hard pressure over a normal acromioclavicular joint may even be uncomfortable, it is often useful to compare the symmetry of the discomfort while palpating both acromioclavicular joints simultaneously. Asymmetric tenderness localized to the

separations or intraarticular fractures. Posttraumatic changes in the distal clavicle also may be reflected by osteolysis, or bone resorption, of the distal clavicle. The entity of osteolysis was described more than 50 years ago. It is seen most commonly in patients whose activities involve repeated athletic activities or work above the shoulder level. This is seen frequently in weightlifters and is called *weightlifter's clavicle*. When the shoulder is subject to this repeated microtrauma, minute fractures may occur in the distal clavicle. In response, the hyperemia of injury and synovial hyperplasia may produce resorption of bone. Bone resorption of the distal clavicle in response to trauma may be greater than the other parts of the body because of the tremendous vascularity of the distal clavicle. Osteolysis of the clavicle is most commonly unilateral; however, bilateral resorption of the distal clavicle can occur in other disease entities, such as hyperparathyroidism, rheumatoid arthritis, and scleroderma.

acromioclavicular joint is the hallmark of symptomatic degeneration of the acromioclavicular joint. This pain is usually exaggerated by adducting the arm across the chest.

With acromioclavicular joint degeneration, weakness of the shoulder is unusual, and the glenohumeral joint range of motion is not usually affected. A useful clinical test to isolate the acromioclavicular joint as a source of pathology in the painful shoulder is the injection of lidocaine or an equivalent local anesthetic directly into the acromioclavicular joint. Relief of pain after injection as the arm is put through a range of motion is diagnostic. This may also help to predict the possible response to surgical excision of the joint and may even be therapeutic if steroid is added to the area.

Radiographic Features

An AP view of the acromioclavicular joint alone usually demonstrates pathologic degenerative change in the acromioclavicular joint. Unless there is a slight superior tilt to the x-ray beam, however, the acromioclavicular joint may be superimposed on the spine of the scapula, and the pathology in the joint can be missed (Fig. 10-5). Thus, a 15-degree cephalic tilt view is usually the best radiographic view for pathologic changes to be demonstrated in the acromioclavicular joint.

With degenerative joint disease of the acromioclavicular joint, it is typical to see joint space narrowing, osteophyte formation on either the superior or inferior aspect of the distal clavicle, and cystic changes in the distal clavicle (Fig. 10-6). These radiographic features usually occur late in the disease,

however, and may not be present in earlier cases of symptomatic inflammation of the joint. In patients with weightlifter's clavicle, there is usually osteopenia, osteolysis, and tapering of the distal clavicle.

Bone scan and computed tomography (CT) scan may help in the diagnosis of acromioclavicular arthritis if the plain radiographs are unclear or if differentiation between degeneration localized to this joint and other diseases is important. Infection and neoplastic lesions may also affect the distal clavicle, and these other radiographic studies may help to rule out these processes.

Although weighted views to distract the clavicle and the acromion may be helpful for traumatic separation of the acromioclavicular joint, they are not helpful in radiographic evaluation of acromioclavicular joint degeneration.

Natural History

The natural history of untreated acromioclavicular degeneration is unknown. It appears that the joint is prone to cartilage loss and disk degeneration as a natural part of the aging process, and many patients with degenerative acromioclavicular joint radiographically may not have symptoms. Only symptomatic acromioclavicular joint degeneration needs treatment.

Treatment Recommendations

Because pain from a clinically symptomatic degenerated acromioclavicular joint is usually caused by associated symptomatic inflammation within the

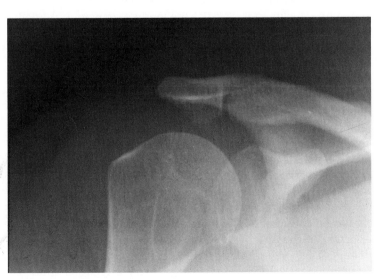

FIGURE 10-5. AP view of the right shoulder gives little bony detail of the right acromioclavicular joint.

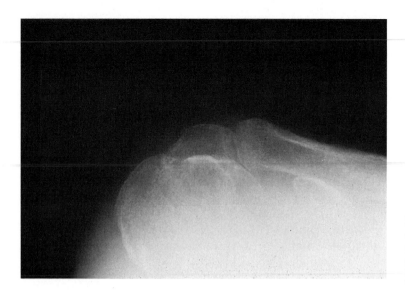

FIGURE 10-6. Angling the beam 15 to 20 degrees shows the acromioclavicular joint free of surrounding bone and, in this patient, severe narrowing consistent with acromioclavicular joint arthritis.

joint, nonoperative treatment ordinarily includes some nonsteroidal antiinflammatory medication. A course of nonsteroidal medication for 3 to 6 weeks often brings the symptoms under control, thus solving the problem. Although there is little role for specific muscle rehabilitation in the treatment of acromioclavicular joint degeneration, it is possible for secondary stiffness of the glenohumeral joint to develop. Thus, taking the arm through a complete range of motion daily appears to be a useful treatment adjunct to avoid stiffness. If secondary stiffness of the glenohumeral joint has occurred as a result of the acromioclavicular joint degeneration, there may be a role for specific range of motion exercise of the shoulder to eliminate this stiffness.

If antiinflammatory medications do not provide enough relief of symptoms, consideration should be given for an intraarticular cortisone injection into the acromioclavicular joint. Because the joint capacity is only 1 to 2 mL, there is often little ability to inject a large amount of fluid within this joint. It is essential to make certain that the fluid is being injected directly into the symptomatic joint, and palpating the point of maximal tenderness to ensure the location of the injection appears to be important. Acromioclavicular joint space may be narrowed with the joint degeneration, making penetration with the needle challenging. With osteolysis and associated bone resorption, however, it is usually not difficult to palpate the acromioclavicular joint space.

If nonoperative treatment fails, surgical treatment should be considered. The most effective surgery is resection of the distal end of the clavicle, which is done distal to the important coracoclavicular ligaments to avoid producing clavicular instability. As with all surgical treatment, careful patient selection

is essential. This procedure is usually done as an open procedure directly centered over the acromioclavicular joint, with careful repair of the deltoid muscle to the trapezius fascia. Distal clavicle excision usually produces a space about 2 cm between clavicle and acromion, which does not appear to be a functional disability to the shoulder.

Although it is commonly done as an open procedure, arthroscopic resection of the distal clavicle has been described. Adequate bone resection is possible arthroscopically, although the precise extent of bone resection may be more difficult to judge than when this procedure is done as an open procedure. Whether it is done arthroscopically or as an open procedure, success of surgery depends on patient selection and adequate bone removal.

Complications of Treatment

The complications of surgical resection of the distal clavicle are generally related to poor patient selection, inadequate clavicle excision to relieve symptoms, or bone fragments left behind in the acromioclavicular joint space. In addition, overly generous excision of the clavicle medial to the coracoclavicular ligaments may produce acromioclavicular joint instability with concomitant symptoms similar to a chronic acromioclavicular separation.

DEGENERATIVE ARTHRITIS OF THE GLENOHUMERAL JOINT

Degenerative disease of the glenohumeral joint, although less common than degenerative arthritis of either the hip or the knee, is not infrequently seen.

Osteoarthritis is the most common form of articular cartilage degeneration. Osteoarthritis is usually described as *primary*, in which no specific cause is identified, or *secondary*, due to specific factors that can be identified, such as trauma, endocrinopathies, or long-standing rotator cuff arthropathy. Although these rigid classifications are probably somewhat arbitrary, it is useful to consider this breakdown in arthritis of the shoulder because various types of degenerative arthritis in the shoulder have different radiographic presentations, behave differently clinically, and have different responses to operative and nonoperative treatment.

Epidemiology and Etiology

The etiology of primary osteoarthritis of the shoulder is unknown. As with osteoarthritis of other joints, however, various hypotheses have been proposed to explain the occurrence. These generally can be grouped into two basic categories: excessive stress on normal tissue and inadequate chondrocyte response to normal forces.

It is believed that the enzymes synthesized by chondrocytes may be early mediators in the pathogenesis of osteoarthritis and cartilage breakdown. It is known that fatigue strength of articular cartilage changes and decreases with age. It may be that genetic and constitutional factors that change the stress distribution and force across the joint may change the strength of the articular cartilage and may change the biochemical response to articular cartilage insult. These things may, to various degrees, combine to underlie the cause of primary osteoarthritis. In the shoulder, with an intact rotator cuff, the maximal joint reactive force occurs at the point of greatest contact between the humeral head and glenoid. An estimate of the joint reactive force is that in 90 degrees of abduction, the joint reactive force approaches body weight across the glenohumeral joint. Thus, although it is not thought of as a weight-bearing joint, considerable forces are transmitted across the shoulder.

Clinical Features

Onset of the symptoms of degenerative arthritis of the shoulder is often gradual, becoming more intense as months go by. Ultimately, the patient may complain of almost constant pain, aggravated by any movement of the shoulder. Simple tasks, such as brushing teeth, may be impossible because of the incapacitating pain. Although some patients with ra-

diographically advanced osteoarthritis may not have many symptoms, most patients with severe radiographic osteoarthritis are incapacitated by pain. Although activity aggravates the pain, it is common to have pain at rest and pain at night, interfering with sleep. The pain is commonly felt down the outside of the arm and into the scapular region. Because of cartilage loss and osteophyte formation around the shoulder joint, the patient may have a sense of grating as the arm is moved, and the grating may be audible as well as palpable. Usually, the patient has limited use of the arm because of stiffness and pain. Movements that require rotation of the glenohumeral joint (reaching overhead, perineal care, reaching up behind the back) are often most affected.

On examination, there is often deep or hard crepitus. This is usually palpable and is distinguished from the softer crepitus often present in the subdeltoid bursal area. Joint line tenderness is typical, and this is usually more easily palpated along the posterior joint line than the anterior. Passive range of motion is typically limited because of capsular tightness, joint incongruity, intraarticular loose bodies, or pain inhibition. Although active motion usually is painful, there is usually not a great discrepancy between active and passive motion in most patients with primary osteoarthritis, and many of these patients have near-normal muscle strength. Some mild muscle atrophy of the deltoid may occur if the patient has avoided using the arm for a long period of time because of pain.

Radiographic Features

Radiographic features of primary osteoarthritis of the shoulder are classic. These features include joint space narrowing, indicating cartilage loss, sclerosis at the point of maximal contact between the humeral head and glenoid, and cysts in the subchondral area of both humeral head and glenoid. The radiographic feature most commonly seen with primary osteoarthritis is a circumferential osteophyte of the humeral head. This is most prominent anteriorly and inferiorly (Fig. 10-7). Because the osteophytes are at the margin of the articular surface of the humeral head, they can cause apparent enlargement in the humeral head and are the reverse of the typical marginal erosions seen with rheumatoid arthritis. The radiographic findings are usually easily seen in the AP view. Loose osteocartilaginous bodies may be present. An axillary view may identify asymmetric wear on the glenoid, with posterior wear of the glenoid more common than anterior wear (Fig. 10-8).

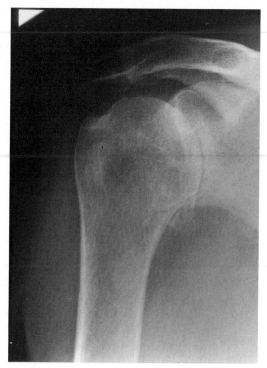

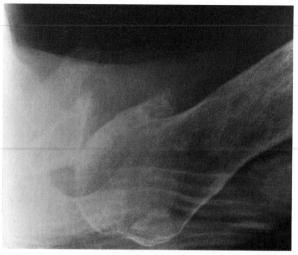

FIGURE 10-8. Axillary radiographic view. There is asymmetric posterior wear of the glenoid fossa with resultant posterior subluxation of the humeral head. This finding is common in primary osteoarthritis of the shoulder.

FIGURE 10-7. Primary osteoarthritis of the shoulder. There is joint space narrowing, sclerosis of the humeral head, and a large inferior osteophyte, which is a classic radiographic finding. The osteophyte is, in fact, circumferential.

A CT scan may be helpful in determining the precise extent of the glenoid and humeral head wear, which is important if surgery is considered (Fig. 10-9).

Treatment Recommendations

In osteoarthritis that is symptomatic, a trial of anti-inflammatory medication is warranted.

In painful osteoarthritis, there is little role for specific physical therapy exercises. Although maintaining muscle tone may be useful, the pain produced by forced movement of an incongruous humeral head on the glenoid usually precludes effective use of range-of-motion exercises.

Although intraarticular injections may play a role in the nonoperative treatment of some glenohumeral arthritides, repeat injections in the glenohumeral joint should be discouraged because they are rarely effective over the long term, may introduce infection, and may weaken the otherwise healthy tendinous structures.

If a patient fails nonoperative management of glenohumeral arthritis and is otherwise a good sur-

gical candidate, surgical treatment should be considered. The surgical alternatives that were described for this condition include joint debridement, osteotomy, humeral head resection, arthrodesis, and total shoulder replacement arthroplasty.

The results of joint debridement in the glenohumeral joint are disappointing. Although joint debridement can remove cartilage debris and loose bodies and partial synovectomy can remove some of

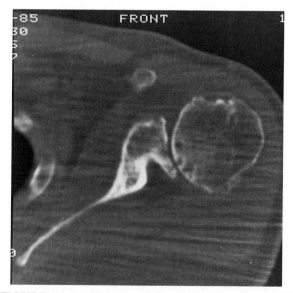

FIGURE 10-9. CT scan and glenohumeral arthritis. A CT scan can help to define the area of wear. In this patient, there is an osteophyte on the glenoid as well as cystic changes in the humeral head. Joint space narrowing is also evident.

the inflamed tissue, if nothing is done to alter the arthritic process, scarring may diminish motion further, and the symptoms usually recur quickly.

The role of osteotomy, or redirecting the humeral head articular surface to a different area of the glenoid, has been described. This procedure has been successful in early degenerative joint disease in some other joints, but there is little information on osteotomies around the shoulder. The few reports that have surfaced suggested that pain relief is highly variable and motion is not changed.

Humeral head or glenoid resection has been described for the treatment of arthritis. Removal of the humeral head, however, includes removal of an important lever arm for action of the rotator cuff muscles, and weakness of the arm is typical after this procedure, as are lost motion and variable pain relief.

Arthrodesis has had a long history of success in treating some shoulder problems. A successful arthrodesis certainly eliminates the pain caused by an

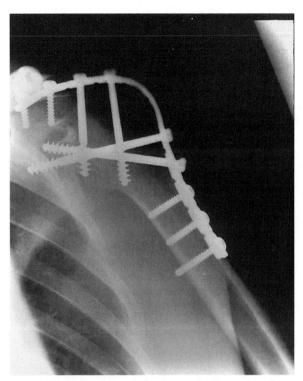

FIGURE 10-11. Internal fixation typically used to fuse a glenohumeral joint. A plate extends from the spine of the scapula along the proximal humerus, aiding in the compression of the humerus and the glenoid while fusion occurs.

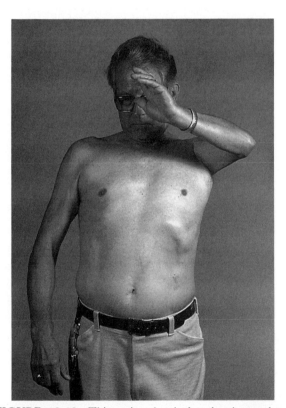

FIGURE 10-10. This patient has had a glenohumeral arthrodesis. Although glenohumeral joint motion is eliminated with a successful arthrodesis, there is some arm movement through the scapula thoracic area. A patient with a successful glenohumeral arthrodesis is usually able to touch the level of nose or mouth through the scapula thoracic motion. Glenoid rotation, however, is eliminated with a glenohumeral joint arthrodesis.

incongruous glenohumeral articulation. Some motion remains in the shoulder girdle because of movement of the scapula on the thorax. Patients with a shoulder arthrodesis can generally feed themselves because they can reach their mouth, they can often fix their hair by bending the neck, and they may be able to do heavy activity if the scapular muscles are strong (Figs. 10-10 and 10-11). A successful arthrodesis of the shoulder, however, permanently eliminates rotation externally and internally, all of which occurs through the glenohumeral joint. Thus, the patient is unable to use the arm above shoulder level, is unable to reach behind, and may have difficulty with some aspects of perineal care. Many patients find this to be a disability. This is particularly problematic with arthritis of the shoulder because many arthropathies are bilateral, and many of the patients are older patients. Since immobilization is usually required for successful arthrodesis, this can be additionally problematic in the elderly population. Nevertheless, there are clearcut indications for glenohumeral arthrodesis, most noticeably pain and loss of cartilage from active infection, arthritis accompanied by significant muscular or nerve deficits, and failed arthroplasty of the shoulder.

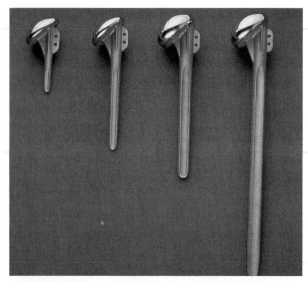

FIGURE 10-12. A typical proximal humeral replacement consists of a ball that articulates with a plastic glenoid. An intermedullary stem aids in fixation.

In 1951, the first humeral head replacement procedure was performed by Neer for treatment of a proximal humeral articular surface fracture. Since then, humeral head replacement alone has been used in a variety of reconstructive procedures, and it certainly can be considered for use without a glenoid component in some forms of arthritis. In 1971, a matching polyethylene glenoid component was used for the first time in the United States as the first total shoulder replacement arthroplasty. Today, total shoulder replacement arthroplasty is a highly successful treatment for arthritis of the glenohumeral joint. Patients predictably have excellent pain relief, with well over 90% of patients having either no or only minor pain after successful shoulder arthroplasty. The most common shoulder arthroplasty consists of a humeral component that goes down the intramedullary canal of the humerus and substitutes

for the arthritic humeral head (Fig. 10-12). A matching polyethylene glenoid component (Fig. 10-13) has the same radius of curvature of the humerus, and thus the prosthesis shows minimal constraint, requires minimal removal of bone, resurfaces the arthritic joint, and allows the patient's own muscles to move the prosthesis (Fig. 10-14). As with other joint replacements, total shoulder replacement has made a tremendous difference in the quality of life in most patients on whom it is performed (Fig. 10-15).

The primary indication for shoulder replacement is incapacitating pain from glenohumeral joint arthritis. Although passive range of motion of the shoulder may be restored by meticulous intraoperative techniques of surgery and by specific attention to the postoperative rehabilitation, active range of motion of the shoulder depends on the strength of the patient's muscles to move the implant. Thus, in most patients who have strong rotator cuff and deltoid muscles, such as patients with osteoarthritis, the potential to reestablish normal range of motion of the shoulder exists (Fig. 10-16). In most patients who may have permanently weakened muscles, such as in some patients with large rotator cuff tears, some rheumatoid patients, or patients who have had multiple surgical procedures, although pain relief after total shoulder replacement is still predictable, the amount of active range of motion may be highly variable. Thus, the function of the shoulder after total shoulder replacement is almost solely dependent not only on the technical aspects of the surgical procedure but also on the success of the rehabilitation and, most importantly, on the quality of the muscles moving the shoulder. Thus, the role of rehabilitation in total shoulder replacement is critical.

The complications after shoulder arthroplasty are relatively few. Since most components are usually anchored to bone with an acrylic cement, long-term evaluation is necessary to assess the risk of mechanical failure of the implant parts. Experience with the

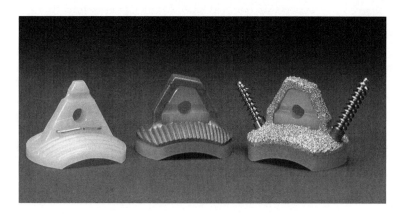

FIGURE 10-13. A matching glenoid component for total shoulder system. Various types of glenoids are available, depending on the particular need of the patient.

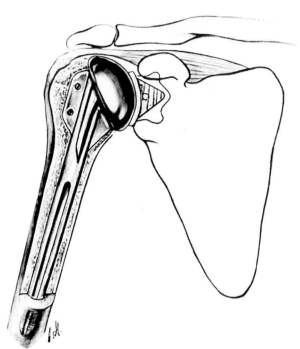

FIGURE 10-14. A total shoulder arthroplasty (humerus and glenoid in place). With elimination of the pain through resurfacing of the arthritic joint, the muscles providing motion for the glenohumeral joint can be rehabilitated successfully.

unconstrained shoulder arthroplasty has included only minimal evidence of mechanical failure, mechanical breakage, clinical loosening, and need for revision surgery.

OSTEONECROSIS

Osteonecrosis, or avascular necrosis, may occur in the glenohumeral joint as well as in other joints. This occurs as the blood supply to the humeral head is interrupted, leading to loss of the subchondral bone support, collapse of the humeral head, joint incongruity, and secondary degenerative changes on the glenoid. Osteonecrosis of the shoulder may occur throughout all age groups.

A number of diseases have been implicated in the etiology of osteonecrosis, or at least associated with it. In many cases, however, steroid use as part of the medical treatment of these conditions make it difficult to separate out the osteonecrosis caused by systemic use of steroids from the disease process itself. Implicated conditions have included alcoholism, sickle cell disease, decompression sickness, Gaucher disease, renal or other organ transplantation, systemic lupus erythematosus, and gout. If no other specific cause can be identified, osteonecrosis usually is thought of as idiopathic. In addition, osteonecrosis may occur as the result of trauma to the shoulder, particularly with certain types of proximal humeral fractures.

Clinical Features

The clinical features of osteonecrosis of the shoulder depend to a great extent on the stage at which the osteonecrosis is seen. Early on in osteonecrosis, there may be pain from the shoulder or associated synovitis without collapse of the humeral head and joint incongruity. Pain with motion of the shoulder or limitation of range of motion secondary to synovitis and soft tissue stiffness may thus occur in the earlier stages. Once the radiographs show collapse of the humeral head with late osteonecrosis, the clinical findings are similar to osteoarthritis of the shoulder. Because extensive joint incongruity and osteophyte formation are not typically present in osteonecrosis

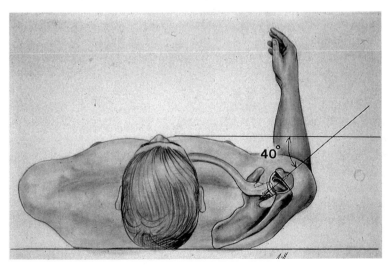

FIGURE 10-15. A total shoulder replacement in place, showing the position of the glenoid and the humeral head viewed from above.

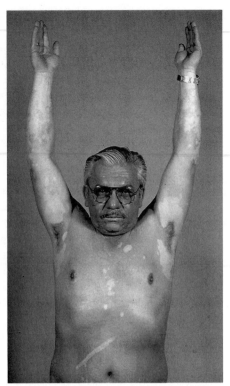

FIGURE 10-16. A patient who has primary osteoarthritis of the shoulder after bilateral total shoulder replacements. Because the rotator cuff and deltoid muscles are typically normal in primary osteoarthritis, the potential exists for near full range of motion of the shoulder.

of the shoulder, however, limitation of passive motion may not occur until late in the disease process. Typically, the patient with late osteonecrosis and collapse of the humeral head with secondary glenoid arthritis may have deep grating. Restriction of joint motion may occur. Muscle strength is ordinarily preserved with osteonecrosis of the shoulder, unless the disease that has played some role in the etiology has an associated myopathy, such as in patients with some collagen vascular diseases or in patients who were on systemic steroids.

Radiographic Features

The radiographic features of osteonecrosis of the shoulder depend almost entirely on the stage at which the disease is seen. The earliest stage of osteonecrosis is a preradiologic stage, in which the plain radiographs are normal. Bone scanning or MRI, however, shows changes within the humeral head. As the disease progresses, there are radiologic

changes of osteoporosis, perhaps osteosclerosis, or some combination of the two. A crescent sign develops, indicative of a fracture through the abnormal subchondral bone. In the humeral head, this is usually located superior and central. As the disease continues to progress, there may be collapse of the subchondral bone with deformity of the humeral head (Fig. 10-17). A separate osteocartilaginous flap may develop. The later stages of osteonecrosis may show all the previous changes in the humeral head, with the glenoid showing significant erosion and wear.

Other imaging studies that are used for radiographic diagnosis of osteonecrosis include bone scanning and MRI. These are most helpful early in the disease process, before there are clearcut radiographic changes. Once the radiographic changes have occurred, they are usually classic for osteonecrosis of the shoulder.

Other diagnostic studies may be necessary if the cause of the osteonecrosis is unclear.

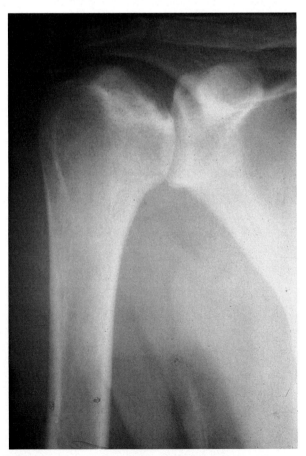

FIGURE 10-17. Osteonecrosis of the shoulder with collapse of the humeral head and sclerosis underneath the area of collapse.

Pathoanatomy

Although the etiology of osteonecrosis is multifactorial, the pathologic findings at surgery are typical. Often, a loose cartilage flap is seen with underlying collapse of the subchondral bone. This is thought to be caused by loss of the blood supply for a time sufficient to result in cellular death in the area of the humeral head. Although compromise of blood supply to bone tissue may be important to pathologies, other factors may be involved. Elevated vascular pressure and delayed emptying of the intraosseous spaces were found in hips of patients who have osteonecrosis and are thought to be a possible mechanism of osteonecrosis production and the rationale for core decompression that has been described for the hip.

Typically, intraoperatively, the soft tissue of the rotator cuff and biceps tendon around the humeral heads are normal. An associated synovitis may be seen within the joint and may be dramatic.

Natural History

The natural history of osteonecrosis of the shoulder is variable. Although interruption of the blood supply to the humeral head may produce radiographic changes typical of osteonecrosis, there is variable collapse of the subchondral bone. When there is minimal collapse of the subchondral bone, the patient may have relatively few symptoms. If the disease progresses to collapse of the subchondral bone, there is subsequent joint incongruity of the humeral head. Eventually, the wear of this incongruous humeral head on the glenoid surface destroys the cartilage of the glenoid. The symptoms of the patients usually depend on the amount of joint incongruity and associated synovitis.

Treatment and Recommendations

As with any form of arthritis, patients with tolerable symptoms of osteonecrosis of the humeral head should probably be treated nonoperatively. Symptom progression may not occur. Symptom progression is much more likely once the later stages of osteonecrosis with collapse of the humeral head have occurred. Patients with substantial symptoms in association with the late stages of osteonecrosis and collapse of the humeral head or the glenoid should be considered for surgical treatment.

For cases in which surgical treatment for osteo-

necrosis of the hip is considered, core decompression and drilling has been described as one of the surgical alternatives to take away the high intravenous pressure within the femoral head. Almost no information is available on the efficacy of core decompression for early osteonecrosis of the shoulder. If nonoperative treatment consisting of nonsteroidal antiinflammatory medications and isometric exercises to maintain muscle tone fails, then surgical treatment should be considered.

With collapse of the humeral head and an incongruous humeral head, it is reasonable to consider arthroplasty of the shoulder. If the disease in the humeral head has progressed, but not to the point at which there is associated glenoid cartilage loss, humeral head arthroplasty alone without resurfacing the patient's glenoid may be satisfactory, and excellent results were reported with hemiarthroplasty alone in this disease (Fig. 10-18). With osteonecrosis of longer standing and associated glenoid cartilage loss, however, total shoulder replacement is probably the most effective procedure.

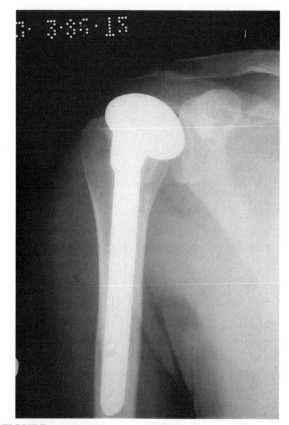

FIGURE 10-18. Because the pathology was confined to the humeral head and glenoid wear had not yet occurred, a successful proximal humeral replacement was performed for osteonecrosis. The glenoid was not replaced.

The results of total shoulder replacement for osteonecrosis of the shoulder are excellent and have approached the results of this procedure for osteoarthritis. The pain relief is usually predictable, as with other forms of glenohumeral arthritis. Since the muscles of the rotator cuff and deltoid are usually normal in osteonecrosis, the functional results and active motion in patients with osteonecrosis typically are similar to those in patients with osteoarthritis. The myopathy associated with the disease process that caused the osteonecrosis, however, may limit the active motion of the shoulder.

RHEUMATOID ARTHRITIS

As with other joints, rheumatoid arthritis of the shoulder usually occurs as part of a generalized rheumatoid disease. Work on the epidemiology and etiology of rheumatoid arthritis of the shoulder mirrors the research on disease etiology in other joints. The pathologic changes in the shoulder with rheumatoid arthritis, however, can be variable. Although all tissues are affected by the disease, certain tissues are involved to a greater degree in some patients, while other tissues may be damaged in other patients.

Pathoanatomy

Neer classified shoulder involvement in rheumatoid arthritis as *dry, wet,* or *resorptive,* with the possibility of *low-grade, intermediate,* or *severe* changes within each group. In the dry form, there is marked tendency for loss of the joint space, periarticular sclerosis, bone cysts, and stiffness. In the wet form, there is exuberant synovial disease, with marginal erosions and intrusion of the humeral head into the glenoid. The outstanding feature of the resorptive type is bone resorption.

The subacromial space may develop an isolated primary bursitis. In most instances, however, when the bursa is extensively affected, other shoulder structures are usually also affected.

Clinical Features

As is typical of a systemic disease that may affect both bone and soft tissues, rheumatoid arthritis may affect many of the structures around the shoulder girdle. Thus, the causes of shoulder pain in rheumatoid arthritis are multiple. Each area must be examined carefully. Cervical spine involvement in rheumatoid arthritis can manifest as referred shoulder pain. In addition, although glenohumeral joint involvement in rheumatoid arthritis is typical, the spectrum of involvement of the shoulder may be large. It is typical to have disease in the acromioclavicular joint, which may be a significant factor in the shoulder pain. If primary bursitis of the rheumatoid shoulder occurs, rotator cuff disease usually is present. The scapulothoracic and sternoclavicular joints may also be involved in the disease of the rheumatoid patient.

The clinical features of rheumatoid arthritis are highly variable. Some patients may have a surprising amount of radiographic destruction in the shoulder without many clinical symptoms. When the patients are symptomatic from the rheumatoid disease, pain is almost always the chief complaint. In rheumatoid arthritis, this is usually combined with a degree of functional loss, the extent of which usually depends on the status of the soft tissues. Often, the difficult problem with the rheumatoid shoulder is associated hand and elbow involvement, making use of the entire extremity difficult. Generalized muscle wasting may be seen around the shoulder (Fig. 10-19). Muscular or skin effects of systemic steroids may be present, and the skin is typically thin, with easy bruisa-

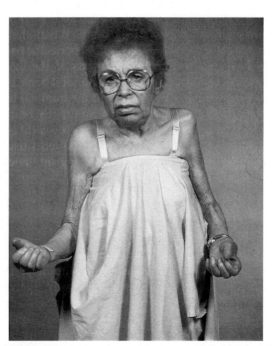

FIGURE 10-19. A patient with rheumatoid arthritis, bilateral shoulder disease, and bilateral elbow and hand disease. The condition of the muscles (rotator cuff and deltoid) is highly variable in rheumatoid arthritis. With marked weakness of the rotator cuff and deltoid, even though shoulder replacement can eliminate pain, active motion may be limited by the muscle disease.

bility and ecchymosis. Typically, tenderness along the posterior joint line and deep crepitation are present. Because of the extent of superficial tendon and bursal involvement, there is often a softer crepitus, which can be felt just beneath the deltoid. Exuberant bursal inflammation may even produce a mass effect, which may mimic a neoplasm of the shoulder.

Range of motion is typically limited in the shoulder in the rheumatoid patient but may be difficult to assess because of the extent of muscle weakness and other involvement in the same extremity. Active motion may be affected more than passive motion, particularly if the patient has a steroid myopathy or if there is an associated rotator cuff tear, which occurs in about one third of rheumatoid patients. Acromioclavicular joint tenderness may be present.

It may be difficult to evaluate muscle strength in the rheumatoid patient because pain can impede muscle strength testing. In addition, peripheral neuropathy can accompany rheumatoid arthritis, and cervical spine disease can also lead to secondary muscle weakness if there is associated cervical radiculopathy. An EMG may be necessary to define the extent of nerve involvement. The cervical spine must be assessed carefully because both pain and instability of the spine are not infrequent.

Radiographic Features

The radiographic features of rheumatoid arthritis are highly variable. In some patients, the glenohumeral joint may appear to be normal or show only mild osteopenia (Fig. 10-20). With continued proliferative synovitis, marginal erosions typically occur, and these may be extensive. As cartilage is lost, bony destruction usually occurs. Later, as the disease progresses, there may be significant central glenoid bone loss with actual loss of the bone stock of the glenoid. The humeral neck may impinge on the glenoid border and show a secondary indentation (Fig. 10-21). Loss of the rotator cuff may allow the humeral head to ride superiorly, and secondary thinning of the acromion and even acromial fracture may occur. Wear into the coracoid process with coracoid fracture may occur.

It is unusual to require extensive imaging studies in the rheumatoid patient. With extensive bone loss, however, a CT scan may better define the extent of bone involvement and residual bone, particularly if arthroplasty of the shoulder is being considered (Fig. 10-22).

Treatment Recommendations

As with other joints affected by rheumatoid arthritis, there may be extensive radiographic joint destruction in the rheumatoid shoulder that is way out of proportion to the extent of symptoms and the functional deficit. The usual nonoperative means of treating rheumatoid arthritis of other joints is useful for treating rheumatoid arthritis of the shoulder. If there is an inflammatory flare-up of the rheumatoid arthritis with little bony joint destruction, exercises of the shoulder may be used to maintain range of motion

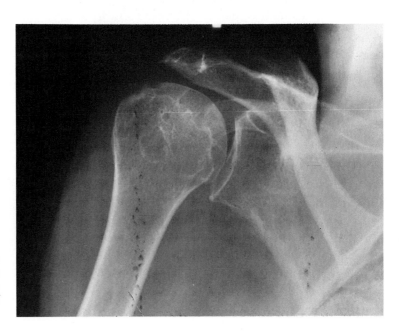

FIGURE 10-20. Rheumatoid arthritis of the shoulder with marginal erosion, cystic changes in the humeral head, pathology in the acromioclavicular joint, and reasonable preservation of the glenohumeral joint space.

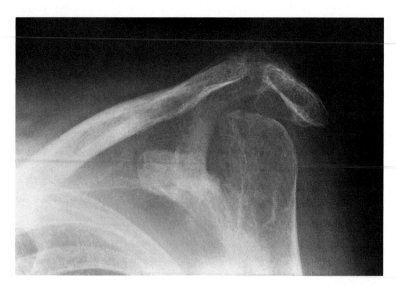

FIGURE 10-21. More severe destruction of the glenohumeral joint in rheumatoid arthritis. There is marked collapse of the humeral head, medial and central glenoid wear, and a fracture of the acromion.

and avoid secondary stiffness. Likewise, if there is isolated arthritis of the acromioclavicular joint or predominant bursitis without much glenohumeral joint destruction, an injection of cortisone in the subacromial space or into the acromioclavicular joint may be considered. Although it may be considered, an injection of cortisone directly into the glenohumeral joint certainly carries with it some of the same problems as injecting the glenohumeral joint in an osteoarthritic shoulder.

If nonoperative treatment fails in rheumatoid arthritis, then surgical treatment should be considered. In many patients with rheumatoid disease, surgical treatment of the shoulder is delayed because other joints take priority or because misinformation has suggested that joint replacement in the shoulder is less successful than in other joints. A long delay in treating the rheumatoid patient with arthroplasty of the shoulder, however, carries certain risks. Although pain relief may be excellent in the rheumatoid shoulder, there may be such soft tissue destruction, particularly in the rotator cuff, that function and strength may be severely limited. In addition, the disease process may destroy so much bone that it may make the shoulder replacement a technically much more difficult operation than implant surgery performed earlier in the disease process.

For the symptomatic joint that is destroyed by rheumatoid arthritis, the most predictable surgical treatment is that of a total shoulder arthroplasty. As with other joints treated by total replacement, pain relief in the shoulder is usual. Attention must be paid to the cervical spine, to associated acromioclavicular joint disease, to associated rotator cuff pathology, and to distal extremity involvement of the arthritis. If the rotator cuff muscles and tendons are healthy, strong, and without extensive degeneration and tearing, the functional results of shoulder replacement with active and passive range of motion can be excellent. More extensive soft tissue disease, such as larger rotator cuff tears, or long-standing muscle atrophy or myopathy may impair the return of active motion after total shoulder replacement.

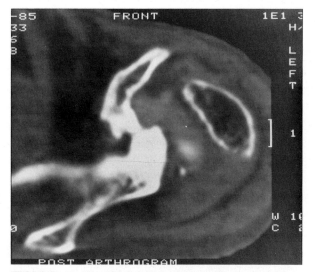

FIGURE 10-22. CT scan in a patient with rheumatoid arthritis shows a marked loss of the humeral head with severe wear in the glenoid. In this patient, there was not enough glenoid bone to support a prosthesis, and the humeral replacement was used alone.

POSTTRAUMATIC ARTHRITIS

By definition, posttraumatic arthritis of the shoulder occurs after a major traumatic insult to the shoulder. This is most often a fracture of the proximal humerus involving the articular surface of the humeral head with joint incongruity and secondary cartilage erosion of both the humeral head and the glenoid. In addition, some patients who had recurrent dislocations of the shoulder with or without surgical repair can develop secondary degenerative changes in the glenohumeral joint.

Clinical Features

The clinical features of the patient with posttraumatic arthritis are similar to those patients with other forms of degenerative arthritis of the shoulder. Pain is the predominant feature. Usually, the patient loses passive range of motion, owing to either joint incongruity, scarring from the previous trauma, or malunion of previous fracture fragments. Active motion depends on the degree of pain and soft tissue integrity but often is similar to passive range of motion. Previous trauma, if it involved a dislocation of the shoulder, may have involved associated nerve injury, so that it is particularly important to assess the nerve status around the shoulder girdle, especially the axillary and musculocutaneous nerves. An EMG may be necessary for this.

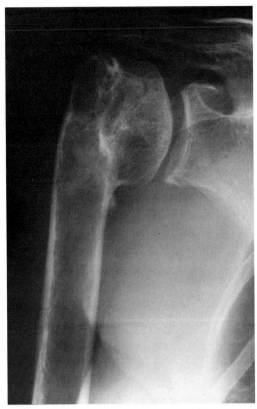

FIGURE 10-23. Posttraumatic arthritis. There was a fracture of the greater tuberosity and surgical neck of the humerus, with malunion of the humeral head in a varus position.

Radiographic Features

Radiographic features reflect the cause of the traumatic injury. If the arthritis is due to joint incongruity from a proximal humeral fracture, there may be associated malunion of tuberosities or the humeral head, nonunion of the proximal humerus, secondary joint collapse with avascular necrosis, or loose intraarticular bodies (Fig. 10-23). If the arthritis is secondary to multiple dislocations of the shoulder, there may be radiographic evidence of old dislocations of the shoulder, such as a Hill-Sachs lesion (impression defect in the humeral head), or glenoid bone loss in the direction of the instability. If there was previous surgery for either fracture or dislocation, hardware may be present in the glenohumeral joint that is evident radiographically.

Because the anatomy is usually distorted in posttraumatic arthritis, it is often advantageous to use additional studies to assess the relation of the humeral head to the shaft, the humeral head to the glenoid, and the tuberosities with attached rotator cuff to the humeral head. This may necessitate tomography, CT scan, or MRI evaluation of the shoulder.

Treatment Recommendations

As with other forms of glenohumeral arthritis, a trial of nonoperative treatment for symptomatic improvement of pain is warranted. This may include a combination of gentle exercises, antiinflammatory medications, or both. Usually, intraarticular injections have little use in posttraumatic arthritis.

If nonoperative treatment fails, operative treatment is indicated. If malunion or nonunion of the fracture exists without associated arthritis, then restoring the anatomy of the shoulder toward normal may adequately relieve pain without the need for arthroplasty. Bone grafting of a nonunion, osteotomy and repositioning of the bone with internal fixation, and lysis of scar tissue with tendon lengthening are all procedures that may be done instead of arthroplasty if there is good glenoid or humeral cartilage. Often, however, with posttraumatic changes, frank arthritis is present. If so, arthroplasty of the shoulder is usually the best solution. Because most posttraumatic arthritis involves extensive glenoid and humeral head destruction, total shoulder replacement is usually the most predictable form of treatment.

As with other forms of total shoulder replacement arthroplasty, the intraoperative technical challenges are great because of the extensive scar tissue, distorted anatomy, and associated soft tissue injury. With attention to the details of surgery, however, the results of total shoulder arthroplasty for posttraumatic arthritis are good for pain relief. The range of motion may be limited somewhat by extensive scarring and fixed contracture of soft tissues, but pain relief is usually associated with significant functional improvements and gratified patients.

CUFF TEAR ARTHROPATHY

In the early 1980s, the orthopaedic literature described an extensive collapse of the humeral head with glenohumeral joint destruction associated with a massive, untreated, full-thickness tear of the rotator cuff of long duration. This entity was given the name *cuff tear arthropathy*. In the rheumatology literature, this same entity was called *Milwaukee shoulder*.

Etiology

The etiologic mechanism of cuff tear arthropathy is unclear. Some investigators think that a combination of nutritional factors, mechanical factors, and perhaps crystalline deposits with collagenase release into the joint is responsible for both destruction of the glenohumeral joint and the soft tissue of the rotator cuff.

The functions of the rotator cuff are to stabilize the humeral head against the glenoid, to rotate the humeral head in the glenoid, and to help to provide a watertight compartment, which may be important for the nutrition of healthy articular cartilage. A massive rotator cuff tear of long duration may compromise the watertight compartment and impact on the cartilage nutrition and may lead to instability of the glenohumeral joint with secondary trauma of the cartilage.

Cuff tear arthropathy does not occur in every patient with an untreated rotator cuff tear. In fact, it is estimated that about 3% to 4% of untreated large rotator cuff tears eventually develop arthritis of the glenohumeral joint.

Clinical Features

The clinical features of patients with cuff tear arthropathy are usually typical since there is usually an associated rotator cuff tear of long duration. The patient often has a long history of shoulder pain. The patient may have been told of bursitis in the past, may have been told of irritation of the rotator cuff, and may have been given multiple injections of steroids. By definition, cuff tear arthropathy involves a massive tear of the rotator cuff, so there are usually features that are typical of both glenohumeral arthritis and long-standing rotator cuff disease (Fig. 10-24). The pain is often incapacitating and may require narcotics for relief. Limitation of passive range of motion may occur because of the secondary joint incongruity. Active motion is usually severely restricted because of the combination of pain, joint incongruity, and extensive large tendon tearing, and this is reflected in marked weakness of the arm (Fig. 10-25).

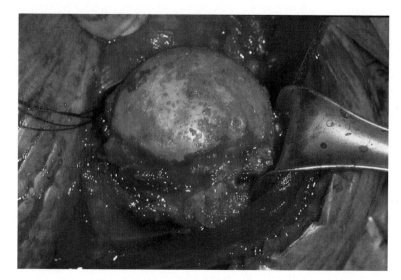

FIGURE 10-24. Intraoperative photograph of cuff tear arthropathy showing complete loss of articular cartilage of the humeral head (and the glenoid). In addition, no rotator cuff is visible because of a massive tear of the rotator cuff.

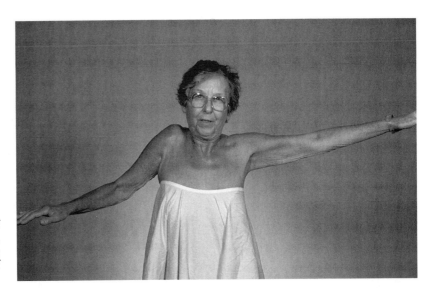

FIGURE 10-25. A patient with cuff tear arthropathy of the right shoulder. The patient has little ability to elevate the arm above shoulder level because of a severe massive rotator cuff tear.

Associated acromioclavicular tenderness and disease usually are present, and a tremendous amount of subdeltoid bursal swelling may be caused by the long-standing rotator cuff deficiency. An associated long head of biceps rupture may be present, along with marked atrophy around the shoulder girdle because of the long-standing associated rotator cuff tear.

Radiographic Features

Early in the disease process, the radiographic features usually reflect a long-term rotator cuff tear before humeral head collapse. Often, a diminished acromiohumeral interval, sclerosis in the area of greater tuberosity, and acromioclavicular joint arthritis are seen (Fig. 10-26). Subacromial spur formation may occur. These changes are all typical of the associated rotator cuff tear. Eventually, there may be collapse of the humeral head, with gross joint destruction in combination with the radiographic features of cuff insufficiency (Figs. 10-27 and 10-28).

Because the presence of a torn cuff is usually not in doubt with this entity, arthrography or MRI scan are typically not necessary to assess the integrity of the rotator cuff, which probably can be suggested by the significant changes in the radiograph. A CT scan, however, may be useful to assess the extent of bone destruction.

If there is any question about the integrity of the rotator cuff with associated arthritis, then some means of assessing the cuff integrity, whether arthrography, ultrasonography, or MRI evaluation, may be warranted.

Treatment Recommendations

Many investigators believe that cuff arthropathy has a direct relation to a large, full-thickness rotator cuff tear of long duration. This is one argument for surgical repair of documented symptomatic full-thickness rotator cuff tears. Before the humeral head collapse and significant joint incongruity, there is

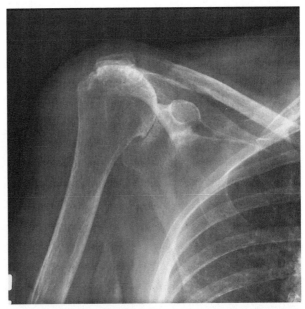

FIGURE 10-26. Radiographic appearance of cuff tear arthropathy. Because of the loss of the depressor activity of the rotator cuff (due to a massive rotator cuff tear), there is high riding of the humeral head, which directly articulates with the undersurface of the acromion. There is narrowing of the glenohumeral joint as well.

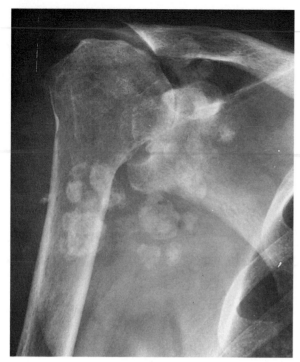

FIGURE 10-27. Cuff tear arthropathy with covering of the undersurface of the acromion and undersurface of the clavicle, diminution of the acromiohumeral interval, medial superior wear of the glenoid, and several osteocartilaginous loose bodies in the glenohumeral joint.

usually a stage of precollapse of the humeral head, which is typically accompanied by a mild to moderate loss of articular cartilage of the humeral head, a massive rotator cuff tear, and associated signs of subacromial impingement. At this stage, decompression

of the rotator cuff and surgical repair of the tendon are usually adequate for pain relief. If there is joint destruction with incongruity and collapse and deformity of the humeral head, however, surgical repair of the rotator cuff may not provide enough pain relief because the glenohumeral arthritis often contributes significantly to the pain. When the patient is severely symptomatic from cuff tear arthropathy, it is reasonable to consider a shoulder replacement arthroplasty. Pain relief remains the predominant indications for total shoulder replacement, and this is the main indication for performing the operation in cuff tear arthropathy. At the time of the total shoulder replacement, the rotator cuff may be repaired or reconstructed, and associated pathology either in the acromioclavicular joint or acromion may be treated. Few large series are related to shoulder arthroplasty for cuff tear arthropathy. In those series that were published, the pain relief was good and paralleled that resulting from arthroplasty performed for other degenerative conditions around the glenohumeral joint. By definition, however, there are massive soft tissue deficits in cuff tear arthropathy with a large tear of the rotator cuff, so the repair often has permanent weakness. This impacts on the active motion that the patient may achieve after surgery. Although shoulder replacement arthroplasty and cuff repair usually provide effective maintenance of rotation below shoulder level, the ability of the patient to raise the arm above shoulder level depends on the strength of the reconstructed tendons and may be variable. Some have suggested that humeral head arthroplasty be used without addition of a glenoid,

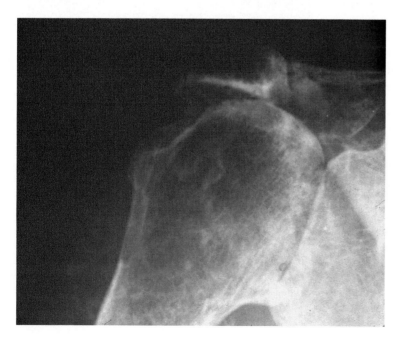

FIGURE 10-28. Cuff tear arthropathy with collapse and disorganization of the glenohumeral joint. There is an osteophyte on the undersurface of acromion, disease in the acromioclavicular joint, and collapse of the humeral head.

and the relief of pain appears to be equally good as a result of this procedure.

IMPINGEMENT SYNDROME AND ROTATOR CUFF TEAR

Unlike the hip joint, in which there is a deep socket to contain the femoral head and thus provide significant stability of the joint, the humeral head articular surface is about four times that of the glenoid socket in surface area. The glenoid socket depth may be changed slightly by the fibrocartilaginous labrum at the periphery, but in general, the humeral head rests against the glenoid. This lack of joint constraint permits range of motion but sacrifices bony stability. The relatively nonconstrained bony surfaces, a frail scapula that moves synchronously with the glenohumeral joint, capsular ligament structures that also allow motion, and an active musculotendinous cuff providing the mobility all are significant contributors to glenohumeral motion. Although elevation of the arm above shoulder level is contributed to both by glenohumeral joint motion and scapulothoracic motion (about 120 degrees of glenohumeral joint motion and 60 degrees of scapulothoracic motion for every 180 degrees of total arm elevation), all rotation comes through the glenohumeral joint. The glenohumeral ligaments and capsule of the shoulder act in some fashion to help stabilize the shoulder in certain positions of the arm, but the predominant stability in the glenohumeral joint occurs from the centering effect provided by the musculotendinous or rotator cuff. The rotator cuff muscles consist of the subscapularis, which originates on the inner surface of the scapula and inserts on the lesser tuberosity of the humerus; the supraspinatus, which originates in the supraspinatus fossa and inserts on a facet of the greater tuberosity; the infraspinatus, which originates in the infraspinatus fossa and inserts on the facet on the greater tuberosity; and the teres minor, which originates just beneath the infraspinatus and also inserts on the greater tuberosity.

The rotator cuff probably has three functions:

1. It *rotates the humeral head* as the deltoid muscle elevates the arm. As the arm is elevated overhead, without external rotation, the prominence of the greater tuberosity is blocked by the lateral acromion. External rotation of the humerus allows the greater tuberosity to clear underneath the acromion and thus allows full forward elevation of the arm. Most of the power for external rotation of the humerus comes from the infraspinatus mus-

cle, with a smaller component contributed by the teres minor. Thus, for external rotation and strong use of the arm above shoulder level, a functioning infraspinatus is usually necessary, and tears that involve this muscle are particularly devastating. The subscapularis is an internal rotator of the humerus. Other muscles can also internally rotate the humerus, so the subscapularis probably functions most effectively as one of the stabilizers of the humeral head in the glenoid. The supraspinatus not only contributes to the abduction of the arm but also probably provides a static restraint to superior migration of the humeral head.

2. It *stabilizes the humeral head* against the glenoid. As tension on the rotator cuff is developed, the humeral head is centered in the glenoid. This provides a dynamic fulcrum for the powerful deltoid muscle to elevate the arm. As the deltoid pulls the humeral head upward, the rotator cuff functions to center and depress the humeral head to permit the arm to be used above shoulder level. With nerve injury involving the muscles to the rotator cuff or a large rotator cuff tear, the deltoid acts unopposed, and effective depression and centralization of the humeral head in the glenoid does not occur.

3. It *provides a relatively watertight compartment*, which may be important for the nutrition of the articular surfaces of both the humeral head and the glenoid.

The biceps tendon should also be considered when considering rotator cuff anatomy. The tendon of the long head of the biceps runs in the bicipital groove and crosses the top of the humeral head to insert on the superior aspect of the glenoid. It lies between the subscapularis and the supraspinatus and is essentially immediately adjacent to the supraspinatus. Because of the unique anatomic position of the biceps tendon adjacent to the rotator cuff, any mechanical factors that affect wear on the rotator cuff ordinarily affect the biceps tendon as well, so it is common for disease of the biceps tendon to occur in conjunction with disease of the rotator cuff tendons. In addition to its importance as an elbow flexor and supinator of the forearm, an important role of the biceps tendon is to act as an adjunctive stabilizer of the humeral head. A recent cadaver study noted significant migration superiorly of the humeral head on sectioning the biceps tendon, suggesting that this tendon acted along with the rotator cuff to effectively depress and stabilize the humeral head.

Thus, normal synchronous movement of the arm above shoulder level is contributed to by a series of muscle groups. The scapula must be stabilized and then rotated along the chest wall as the arm is elevated forward. The glenohumeral joint must be stabilized and moved. The deltoid, particularly the anterior and middle deltoid, is the prime mover of the arm, but the rotator cuff effectively externally rotates the humerus and the glenoid, stabilizes and depresses the humeral head against the glenoid, and, aided by the biceps tendon, effectively acts to center the humeral head on the glenoid so the deltoid can move the humerus.

Because the rotator cuff is so critical to the stability and motion of the glenohumeral joint, it is commonly affected by trauma, wear and tear of aging, and external mechanical factors.

The rotator cuff ordinarily is covered by a thin film of bursal tissue, the subdeltoid or subacromial bursa. Factors that impact on the rotator cuff thus may also impact on the bursa, and inflammation of both structures often occurs in conjunction. As the arm is elevated forward, the rotator cuff tendons pass underneath the coracoacromial arch, which is composed of the coracoacromial ligament and the most anterior one third of the acromion. In addition, the supraspinatus also passes directly under the acromioclavicular joint as the arm is elevated overhead. Any anatomic changes, either in the coracoacromial ligament, the anterior acromion, or the acromioclavicular joint, that change the local anatomy may impact on the rotator cuff. The space through which the rotator cuff passes, the subacromial space, is ordinarily narrow, and any factors that diminish the space available for the rotator cuff to pass, whether external mechanical factors (spur) or internal tendinous factors (swelling), may create an environment in which there is less room for the rotator cuff to move and may contribute to tendon disease.

Tears of the rotator cuff are extremely common in cadaver studies, with most cadaver studies suggesting that 20% to 35% of cadavers may have an associated rotator cuff tear, with about one third of these tears being full-thickness tears and two thirds of the tears being partial-thickness tears. Tears of the rotator cuff are common in cadaver studies, but it is impossible to know what the incidence of clinical symptoms for rotator cuff tearing is in the general population. Rotator cuff tears appear to be the most common cause of shoulder pain in patients older than 40 years of age. They appear to affect men and women equally and appear equally to involve dominant and nondominant arms. Thus, it is unclear whether trauma plays a significant role in producing rotator cuff tears.

Etiology

The etiology of rotator cuff tearing is probably multifactorial. Most rotator cuff tears begin at the insertion of the supraspinatus tendon on the greater tuberosity. As the tears enlarge, they extend posteriorly to involve the infraspinatus and teres minor or anteriorly to involve the subscapularis. Several investigators referred to this area of the supraspinatus insertion on the greater tuberosity as the *critical area* because most rotator cuff tears begin here. A number of investigators studied the vascular anatomy of the rotator cuff and demonstrated a dearth of vasculature in this critical area of the supraspinatus, suggesting that perhaps hypovascularity of the tendon may contribute to an intrinsic degeneration of the tendon and eventual tearing. It may also contribute to poor repair potential once the rotator cuff tear begins. Trauma is thought in some instances to play a role in rotator cuff tearing, but it is unclear precisely what role this is since about half of the patients with rotator cuff tears have no history of trauma, and many patients who present with rotator cuff tears after a traumatic episode have some history of shoulder pain before the traumatic injury. A relation exists, however, between a traumatic anterior dislocation that occurs for the first time in a patient older than 40 years of age and a torn rotator cuff.

Normal aging is also thought to be a contributing factor to tearing of the rotator cuff. Newer radiographic studies show some signs of degeneration in the tendon in otherwise asymptomatic patients.

The role of subacromial impingement is thought to be critical in the development and progression of full-thickness tears of the rotator cuff. It is logical to assume that any pathologic process that decreases the space between the rather rigid coracoacromial arch and the greater tuberosity of supraspinatus insertion may result in impingement or mechanical squeezing of the rotator cuff and bursa between these two hard structures. The subacromial space is normally between 1 and 1.5 cm wide. For many years, it has been known that pathologically there appears to be matching lesions on the undersurface of the anterior acromion and the greater tuberosity in patients who have full-thickness tears of the rotator cuff. In the normal anatomic position, the supraspinatus insertion into the greater tuberosity is located just anterior to the anterior acromion. As the arm is brought up in forward elevation, the usual arc in which the arm is used for most activities, the supraspinatus insertion passes directly under the anterior acromion and the coracoacromial arch. It is thought that mechanical alterations in the anterior acromion (such as spurring) or changes in the rigidity of the coracoacromial ligament may result in decreased pliability of these structures, which may begin to compress the rotator cuff as the arm is brought up into forward elevation. This has been termed *subacromial impingement*. Cadaveric studies demonstrated that the morphology of the acromion may contribute to the development of impingement syndrome. Some acromions may be flat, curved, or hooked. A hook on the anterior edge of the acromion is highly correlative with full-thickness tears of the rotator cuff. Thus, most rotator cuff tears are thought to be mechanical in nature and due to subacromial impingement. It is not clear, however, whether subacromial impingement is a primary factor or whether it may result from intrinsic changes in the rotator cuff tendon, allowing superior migration of the humeral head from the rotator cuff weakness. It is thus controversial whether impingement is the initiating cause or merely a contributing factor in rotator cuff degeneration and tearing.

Thus, the etiology of rotator cuff tears is probably multifactorial. Local anatomic features, such as acromial morphology, may narrow the coracoacromial arch, causing mechanical impingement of an aging tendon with poor repair potential. Once the fibers of the rotator cuff fail, there is an increase in the amount of tension on the remaining intact cuff fibers. Thus, it is not unusual for a small tear to gradually enlarge as more and more tendinous fibers of cuff insertion fail sequentially. Although this may not cause an increase in symptoms, the failure of increasing numbers of cuff fibers usually causes an increase in weakness.

Clinical Features

The patient with subacromial impingement syndrome is typically older than 40 years of age. The patient usually has a history of pain, particularly with use of the arm above chest or shoulder level. This may be reflected by pain in sporting activities, such as racket sports, work activities that require use of the arm above shoulder level, or household tasks such as reaching to the top of a shelf. It may affect the dominant or nondominant side. The history is initially typical in that in the earlier stages, tendon inflammation is usually reversible with rest. As this disease progresses, pain often occurs whenever the arm is used above shoulder level there is pain, but with the arm used near the side, there is often much less pain. Reaching up behind the back may aggra-

vate the symptoms. In earlier stages of impingement, prolonged attempts to rest the arm may produce secondary stiffness in the shoulder, and the patient may present with predominantly a frozen shoulder syndrome. As the disease progresses with fixed tendon swelling, thickening and inflammation of the subacromial bursa, and irritation of the rotator cuff, the symptoms may not be reversible, and the patient may complain of pain with the arm at rest. Typically, the pain is felt down to the area of the deltoid insertion, but there may be some radiation of the pain into the scapula or even to the base of the neck from the shoulder. If the impingement syndrome continues over a period long enough for the rotator cuff to tear, the patient may also notice weakness, particularly when using the arm above shoulder level. With a large tear, the patient may be unable to raise the arm at all (Fig. 10-29). Activities such as combing the hair, brushing the teeth, and reaching to open a car door may cause severe pain if the tendon tear is large. Pain may be significant at night and may awaken the patient from a sound sleep. The patient may no-

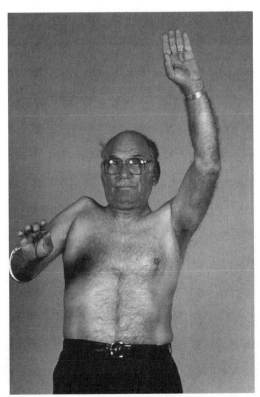

FIGURE 10-29. A patient with a full-thickness tear of the rotator cuff. Because of the loss of head depression caused by a lack of a rotator cuff, the deltoid acts unopposed, and a shrugging type of movement of the arm exists if the patient tries to elevate the arm overhead.

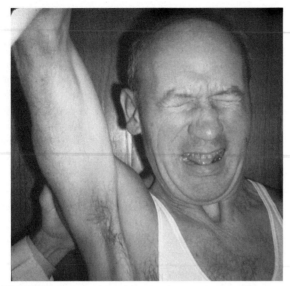

FIGURE 10-30. A positive impingement sign. The examiner's hand is on the superior scapula, and the affected arm is elevated in the overhead position. As the rotator cuff area contacts the coracoacromial arch, a reproduction of the pain is evident. Elimination of this pain with a subacromial injection of lidocaine solidifies the diagnosis.

tice a clicking or popping as the torn tendon edge and thickened subacromial bursa pass under the coracoacromial ligament.

On examination of the patient, the specific signs relate to the stage of impingement. In the earlier stages of tendon inflammation or mechanical impingement, the physical signs have more to do with mechanical irritation of the rotator cuff than with tendon failure. In the earlier stages of impingement,

there is typically pain as the arm is brought into full forward elevation, causing the greater tuberosity to contact the coracoacromial arch; this has been called the *impingement sign* (Fig. 10-30). A painful arc may be felt the arm is lowered from the fully overhead position and the rotator cuff merges from under the coracoacromial arch. This typically occurs between 80 and 120 degrees of forward elevation. Diffuse tenderness to palpation of the shoulder may be present. Often, the thickened subacromial bursa may produce soft crepitus that is felt immediately under the deltoid. Associated acromioclavicular joint tenderness may be present because there is often an overlap between acromioclavicular joint disease and rotator cuff impingement. With tendon inflammation and impingement, there is typically pain as the arm is abducted to the side (Fig. 10-31), particularly if the abducted arm is slightly internally rotated (Fig. 10-32). This may reproduce the patient's symptoms. Internal rotation up behind the back may aggravate the pain. Although the strength of the arm is usually unaffected when the arm is tested, if the tendon is in continuity, pain may inhibit the muscle contraction and may make strength testing difficult. The patient may "let go" during strength testing because of pain, mimicking actual muscle weakness or tendon fiber failure.

A helpful diagnostic test for the presence of subacromial impingement is the impingement injection test. In this test, 10 mL of 1% lidocaine (Xylocaine) is injected directly beneath the acromion into the subacromial space. The arm is then brought through a range of motion and the impingement sign, painful

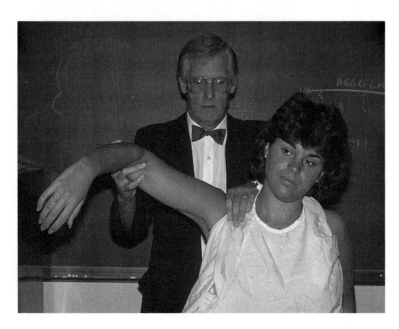

FIGURE 10-31. A patient with impingement syndrome has pain as the arm is abducted.

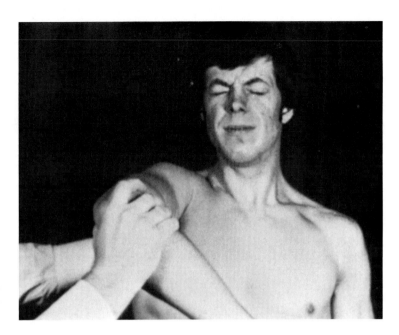

FIGURE 10-32. Impingement syndrome. Abduction and internal rotation of the arm results in closer contact of the rotator cuff with the coracoacromial arch and reproduction of the pain.

arc, and other signs are retested. If the patient reports that with the subacromial space anesthetized the pain is gone, this is virtually diagnostic for subacromial impingement.

With actual rotator cuff tearing, several other signs may be noted. Atrophy of the infraspinatus and supraspinatus fossa may be viewed from behind due to the tearing of the rotator cuff and associated lack of use of the cuff muscles. With rotator cuff tearing, there is often a discrepancy between active and passive motion. It is important, however, not to wait for weakness of the arm overhead or a discrepancy between active and passive motion before considering a diagnosis of a full-thickness tear of the rotator

cuff because many small tears present predominantly as a painful shoulder without much associated weakness. Perhaps the best clinical sign of a full-thickness tear of the rotator cuff is weakness of external rotation (Figs. 10-33 and 10-34). With the arm at the side and the elbow flexed to 90 degrees, the patient is asked to resist internal rotation by the examiner by contracting the external rotators. When there is a full-thickness tear of the rotator cuff, there often is a giving way on the affected side, indicating weakness of external rotation. Even in isolated tears of the supraspinatus, there is often measurable weakness of external rotation, perhaps because the rest of the external rotators function inefficiently

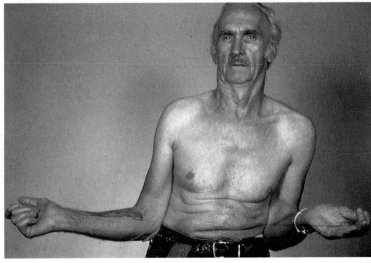

FIGURE 10-33. Full-thickness tear of the rotator cuff in the left shoulder of a patient. Although active external rotation on the right appears normal, there is inability to initiate external rotation on the left, owing to the involvement of the infraspinatus and teres minor with the tear.

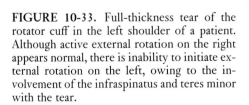

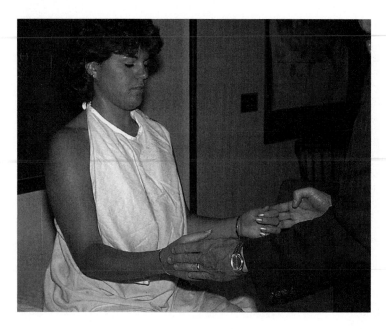

FIGURE 10-34. With smaller tears, the clinical finding of weakness of external rotation may be more difficult to elicit, and the external rotation strength should be compared with the nonsymptomatic side.

without a functioning supraspinatus. An associated rupture of the long head of the biceps tendon may also occur with a full-thickness tear of the rotator cuff. With a large tear of the rotator cuff, the patient may be unable to initiate flexion of the arm or abduction of the arm at all. The powerful deltoid muscle acts unopposed since the torn rotator cuff is not effectively able to depress or stabilize the humeral head against the glenoid. The shoulder appears to shrug as elevation is attempted. This is a classic finding with a large rotator cuff deficiency but is usually not present with smaller tears or in earlier stages of rotator cuff fiber failure.

Radiographic Features

Because of the mechanical nature of rotator cuff disease and subacromial impingement, plain radiographs may be helpful to look for signs of mechanical impingement. Sclerosis or actual spur formation may be seen on the undersurface of the anterior acromion. Cystic changes or bone reaction may be seen in the area of supraspinatus insertion of the greater tuberosity. Both these are usually demonstrable on an AP view of the shoulder (Fig. 10-35). Since acromioclavicular joint disease is common with subacromial impingement syndrome, there may be narrowing, spur formation, or cystic changes in the acromioclavicular joint. A lateral view may be helpful to show the encroachment of the subacromial spur into the space normally occupied by the supraspinatus, the supraspinatus outlet (Fig. 10-36). Large or massive

rotator cuff tears may demonstrate a decrease in acromiohumeral interval. The sensitivity of this finding is increased by stress views, in which the active deltoid contraction causes superior humeral migration, normally prevented by the head-depressing function

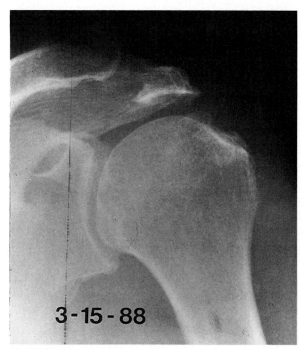

3-15-88

FIGURE 10-35. Radiographic changes in a patient with subacromial impingement. There is sclerosis on the undersurface of the acromion, an anterior acromial spur tracking toward the coracoid process, and reactive bony changes in the area of the greater tuberosity (rotator cuff insertion site).

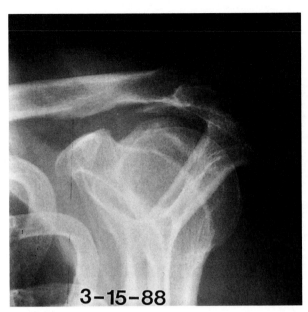

FIGURE 10-36. An outlet lateral. The anterior acromial spurs seen tracking toward the coracoacromial ligament take up the space ordinarily occupied by the supraspinatus as it passes toward its insertion.

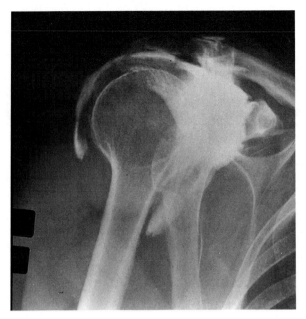

FIGURE 10-37. A positive arthrograph with dye in the glenohumeral joint and also in the subacromial space. This is diagnostic of a full-thickness tear of the rotator cuff.

of an intact cuff. The supraspinatus outlet radiographic view may be a helpful study to evaluate not only the presence of a spur but also the acromial shape. This view is a lateral view in the scapula plane, with the beam directed caudally about 5 to 10 degrees. The subacromial space as measured by the acromiohumeral interval is usually 9 to 10 mL thick. A space of less than 6 mL was usually considered pathologic. With the most severe long-standing rotator cuff tears, there may be complete abolition of the acromiohumeral interval, with rounding of the undersurface of the acromion matching in arc the rounding of the humeral head and greater tuberosity. In the latest stages, arthritis may develop (see Cuff Tear Arthrography).

Because plain radiography gives only indirect evidence of the presence of rotator cuff disease or tearing, other imaging studies have been the mainstay for a diagnosis of rotator cuff tear.

Single- and double-contrast arthrography are the gold standard and are highly accurate tests for the diagnosis of full-thickness tearing of the rotator cuff. In a single-contrast arthrogram, dye is injected into the glenohumeral joint, and the arm is exercised. If there is a full-thickness tear of the rotator cuff, once the arm is exercised, the dye may be seen to leak out into the subacromial space, outlining not only the glenohumeral joint but also the subacromial space (Fig. 10-37). The addition of air with dye (double-

contrast arthrography) may help to define better the size of the rotator cuff tear. The arthrogram is accurate in defining the presence or absence of a full-thickness tear of the rotator cuff in patients who did not have previous surgery. Up to three quarters of patients who undergo a shoulder arthrography may experience at least moderate discomfort 1 to 2 days after a shoulder arthrogram.

In patients who are sensitive to dye, pneumoarthrography may be considered. The injection of air alone is a difficult study to interpret unless the exposure is precise.

Subacromial bursography, or injection of dye into the subacromial bursa, is thought to be helpful for the diagnosis of some rotator cuff tears or with bursal side partial-thickness tears. Subacromial bursograms are difficult to interpret and have limited clinical usefulness.

Because of some of the difficulties of shoulder arthrography, such as pain, poor patient acceptance, and invasiveness, several noninvasive studies have been done to assess the rotator cuff. In the early 1980s, ultrasonography was described as a means of assessing rotator cuff integrity. The advantages of this procedure are that both shoulders can be imaged in about 15 minutes, the procedure is noninvasive and thus carries no risk to the patient, and there is a high degree of patient acceptance because the study is short and painless. Several studies reported encouraging results with ultrasonography in terms of the accuracy of rotator cuff tear diagnosis. The ability to image abnormalities of the anatomy dynamically and the relative inexpensiveness of this study add to its attractiveness. The accuracy of this study was improved with modern equipment and the addition of dynamic scanning. Ultrasonography was reliable in detecting larger full-thickness tears in most reports but less valuable in detecting defects of less than 1 cm or partial-thickness tearing. Operator dependency was noted to be a drawback to this diagnostic modality. In ultrasonographic studies, bones are seen as bright echogenic contours. Muscles are homogeneously hypoechogenic. Ultrasonographic changes indicative of tendon tearing include an actual discontinuity in the normal homogeneous echogenicity of the cuff, lack of visualization of a segment of the cuff, or significant focal thinning of the rotator cuff (Figs. 10-38 and 10-39).

In recent years, the use of MRI has increased to evaluate the rotator cuff. The advantages of MRI include the precise anatomic detail provided by the study, the fact that it is also noninvasive, with no known risk to the patient, and the ability to identify associated muscle atrophy, quality of remaining tendon tissue, and precise localization of the torn tendons. MRI appears to require less operator dependence than ultrasound. It produces readily understandable images of the bone and soft tissue. Partial- and full-thickness tears may be differentiated, and the extent of the tear can be visualized. As the rotator cuff is imaged with T1 and T2 relaxation

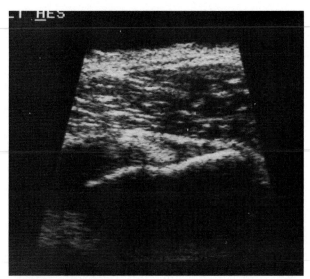

FIGURE 10-39. With a torn rotator cuff, the layer of supraspinatus tapering toward the greater tuberosity is absent. There is an echogenic focus, which is the torn edge of tendon. In addition, the deltoid sags to fill in the area left vacant by the torn rotator cuff.

times, fluid that has a high signal intensity can precisely define the location and presence of the rotator cuff tear and the precise position of the retracted tendon edge (Fig. 10-40). Most studies indicated that MRI is highly sensitive in detecting a full-thickness

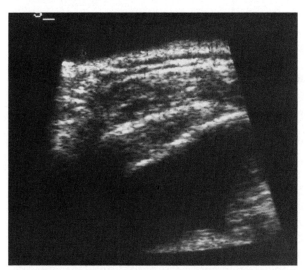

FIGURE 10-38. A normal shoulder ultrasound. The rotator cuff layer is seen adjacent to the dark bone of the humeral head. The supraspinatus is seen to taper toward its insertion on the greater tuberosity.

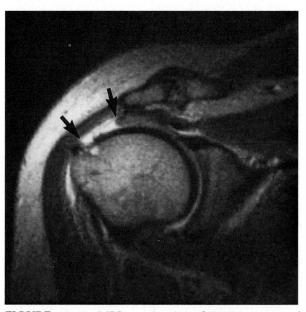

FIGURE 10-40. MRI scan showing a full-thickness tear of the rotator cuff. The arrows outline the extent of tear, and high-signal intensity indicates fluid, which tracks from the glenohumeral joint into the subacromial space. This is a tear in the supraspinatus and is easily identifiable between two arrows.

tear of the rotator cuff. The drawbacks to MRI imaging are that it is expensive, is time-consuming (the study takes 45 minutes), and may be difficult for claustrophobic patients. Although its expense may limit its widespread use in the evaluation of rotator cuff tears, it is clearly the most highly sensitive study available for viewing the precise anatomy of soft tissue around the shoulder.

Pathoanatomy

In patients who are operated on for subacromial impingement, there is often a tremendous amount of thickened edematous subacromial bursa seen directly above the rotator cuff tendon. This bursa may be seen to "catch" as the arm is elevated under the coracoacromial arch. Direct visualization of the rotator cuff may actually suggest that the cuff has little room as it passes under the coracoacromial arch. The anterior acromion may be seen to be overhanging, and a spur may actually impact on the supraspinatus insertion as the arm is raised overhead. Matching eburnation or sclerosis may be seen at the area of supraspinatus insertion. In patients who have rotator cuff tears, an actual tendon defect may be seen, which is typically located at the insertion at the supraspinatus tendon but may extend to involve all the tendons of the rotator cuff. In chronic cases, the tendon edges are smooth and rounded-off. The tendon edge may be retracted far by the associated pull of the muscle. On entering the subdeltoid space, joint fluid is usually readily encountered, attesting to the lack of integrity of the rotator cuff to keep the joint fluid enclosed. Associated changes in the acromioclavicular joint and biceps tendon may also be seen.

Natural History

Rotator cuff pathology appears to occur as a progressive process. Initially, the impingement of the rotator cuff tendons produces tendon inflammation, bursal inflammation, and swelling. As repeated episodes of tendon inflammation and swelling continue, there is fixed tendon and bursal thickening from subacromial impingement. As this process continues untreated, bony spurs may form on the undersurface of the acromion and may appear to form in the substance of the coracoacromial ligament. Gradually, as the coracoacromial arch is narrowed, there may be fraying and fiber failure of the supraspinatus tendon. This may start as an partial-thickness tear, but even-

tually all the tendon fibers of the supraspinatus fail, and a full-thickness tear, or hole, in the rotator cuff develops (Fig. 10-41). As the arm continues to be used, the rest of the tendons of the rotator cuff appear to have a more difficult time taking the loads applied to the shoulder, and it is not uncommon for smaller tears to gradually enlarge, leading to further weakness of the arm (Fig. 10-42). This may be analogous to a hole in the carpet, which when walked over, gradually enlarges. Eventually, all the tendons of the rotator cuff may be involved in a massive rotator cuff tear. If this rotator cuff tearing is associated with joint instability and trauma, arthritis of the joint may develop, as indicated with cuff tear arthropathy.

Treatment Recommendations

In the absence of rotator cuff tearing, nonoperative treatment is undertaken for all patients with subacromial impingement syndrome. In the early stages of tendon inflammation, the mainstays are rest or activity modification, antiinflammatory medications, gentle stretching exercises if there is associated stiffness, and strengthening exercises of the rotator cuff. The most effective strengthening exercises are usually isometric exercises with the arm near the side, away from the position of impingement. The idea behind strengthening exercises is to help increase the muscle

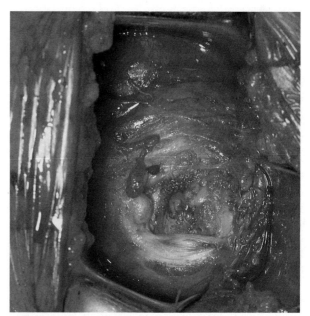

FIGURE 10-41. An operative photograph of a torn rotator cuff. This is a small defect, measuring about 2 cm at its greatest diameter.

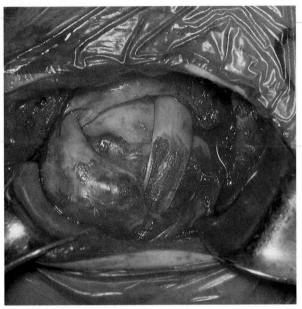

FIGURE 10-42. A large rotator cuff tear with a defect that is at least 4 cm. The biceps tendon, although inflamed, is seen entering the bicipital groove. The retracted supraspinatus and infraspinatus leave a bare humeral head.

tone of the head depressors and thus help actively increase the subacromial space.

If the antiinflammatory medication and exercises do not give satisfactory relief, there may be a role for a subacromial injection of corticosteroids. This is usually performed by combining the cortisone compound with procaine (Novocain) for injection directly into the subacromial space. Since the steroid compounds may impede tendon metabolism and temporarily weaken the tendons, it is usually important to avoid strenuous exercises of the shoulder for a period of 10 days to 2 weeks after injection of corticosteroid.

Some patients with documented subacromial impingement syndrome who do not have an associated rotator cuff tear remain symptomatic despite the treatment with exercise, antiinflammatory medication, and steroid injection. These patients may be candidates for surgical treatment of the impingement lesions. Surgical treatment for the impingement syndrome without rotator cuff tearing is intended to enlarge the space for the rotator cuff tendons to pass. In some patients, resection of the coracoacromial ligament alone without associated bony surgery may be adequate surgical treatment. If an anterior acromial spur or an overhanging anterior acromion is present, however, an anterior acromioplasty is usually required for complete decompression of the rotator cuff tendons (Fig. 10-43).

Proper patient selection is important. It is important to evaluate the patient to be certain that the signs and symptoms are consistent on repeated evaluations. After a prolonged period of nonoperative treatment, operative alternatives should be considered. In addition to coracoacromial ligament and anterior acromioplasty, abnormal bursal tissue is usually removed. In patients who have associated acromioclavicular joint disease, distal clavicle excision may be warranted. Since its introduction in 1972, open anterior acromioplasty for impingement with an intact rotator cuff has been consistently associated with good results if the indications for surgery are sound. Pain relief has been reported to be satisfactory in more than 90% of patients. Limitation of motion or strength seldom is a problem before or after surgery if attention is paid to the postoperative rehabilitation. For surgical success, adequate bone removal from the entire undersurface of the anterior acromion is essential. In 1984, arthroscopic (closed) acromioplasty was first described as an alternative to open anterior acromioplasty. This procedure has the advantages of any arthroscopic approach, including avoiding an

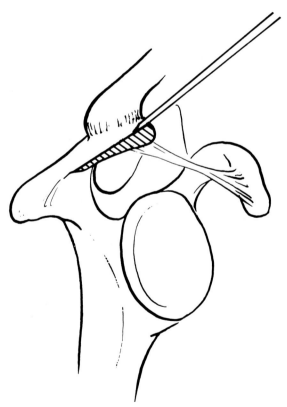

FIGURE 10-43. An anterior acromioplasty removes the undersurface of anterior acromion (and the overhanging anterior acromial spur). In addition, the coracoacromial ligament is removed. This removes the impingement wear.

incision, minimizing deltoid injury, facilitating rehabilitation, shortening postoperative recovery, and being performed as an outpatient procedure. It has been shown in the laboratory that adequate bone removal can be achieved. Arthroscopic acromioplasty has the same indications as an open procedure. As in open acromioplasty, adequate bone removal is important for the success of surgery. A few series have reported results approaching those of open acromioplasty. This technique is demanding, is more difficult technically than open anterior acromioplasty, and depends on adequate hemostasis. Results of arthroscopic acromioplasty appear to be good in impingement syndrome or in patients with partial-thickness rotator cuff tears, but results are unsatisfactory in patients with full-thickness tears. Complications of this technique include inadequate or inappropriate bone removal, excessive bleeding, acromial fracture, and instrument breakage. If there is a full-thickness tear of the rotator cuff, open surgery is the treatment of choice.

With a documented full-thickness tear of the rotator cuff, while a trial of antiinflammatory medications may be warranted with gentle exercises, if symptoms continue, surgical treatment is usually preferable, and thus most investigators favor surgical repair of symptomatic full-thickness rotator cuff tears. The goals of repair are to provide dynamic stability, to restore the strength of external rotation, to improve head depression (reestablishing the force couple with the deltoid), and to seal the synovial cavity for articular nutrition. Tendon repair is accompanied by an anterior acromioplasty to decompress the rotator cuff and increase the space for the repaired tendon to pass. Although pain relief may be provided by the acromioplasty, cuff repair is thought to be important for restoring strength and functional activities. Usually, small and medium-sized tears are repaired by tendon-to-tendon and tendon-to-bone techniques (Figs. 10-44 and 10-45). Larger tendon tears are more difficult to repair. A number of muscle transfers, grafts, and synthetic implants have been advocated for adjunctive treatment in larger tears, but the results of these have not been uniformly encouraging.

The surgical results of rotator cuff repair are better when the repair is accompanied by adequate decompression of the subacromial space. Pain relief is reasonably good (85% to 95%) independent of the size of the tendon tear. Return of strength relates to the extent of tendon tearing, tissue scarring, and associated muscle atrophy. The larger and more extensive the tear, the weaker the patients generally are postoperatively and the less active motion they ordinarily obtain. The good results of surgery do not appear to deteriorate with time.

Patient compliance in a postoperative rehabilitation program is critical for the success of surgery. The trend in postoperative rehabilitation is for early

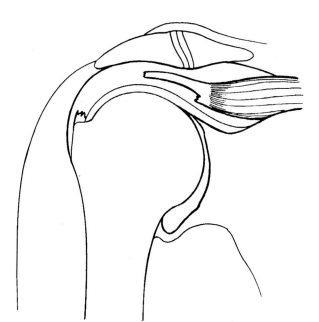

FIGURE 10-44. Diagramatic representation of a supraspinatus tear. The torn edge of the supraspinatus is retracted, almost to the level of the glenoid.

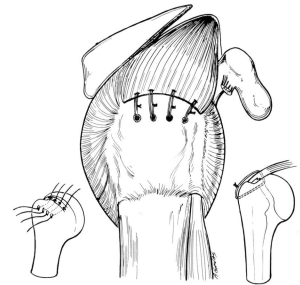

FIGURE 10-45. Method of rotator cuff repair. The torn edges of the rotator cuff tendon are advanced into the bone and anchored with sutures, which go through the bone.

passive movement to restore joint flexibility while protecting the tendon repair. When the tendon is adequately healed to bone, active motion may be initiated. Some surgeons advocate postoperative support in a brace. Once the tendon is adequately healed and active, to minimize the risk of rerupture, resistive exercises to increase the endurance and strength may be added.

Complications of Treatment

Few complications have been reported with the nonoperative treatment of impingement syndrome and rotator cuff tearing. Although there is potential for complications of steroid injections, including introduction of infection, reported incidents of this are few. Since steroids do impair the metabolism of the tendon, however, repeated steroid injections should be avoided, particularly if there is a documented full-thickness tear of the rotator cuff. The complications of surgical treatment may include deltoid muscle avulsion if the deltoid was detached, postoperative stiffness if rehabilitation was problematic, or continued weakness if a large tendon tear was present or if the quality of the repaired tissue is poor.

BICEPS TENDINITIS

The anatomic position of the biceps tendon is in the bicipital groove adjacent to the rotator cuff tendons. A portion of the biceps tendon is intraarticular, and thus inflammatory changes in the long head of the biceps may accompany other conditions that inflame the synovial lining of the shoulder. This is due to an extension of the glenohumeral synovial lining around the tendon in the bicipital groove for varying distances. In the superior part of the groove, the tendon is located in the same impingement area as the supraspinatus and may be involved along with the rotator cuff tendons in the subacromial impingement syndrome. In fact, most cases of biceps tendinitis are secondary to other shoulder abnormalities, and isolated biceps tendinitis in the absence of other abnormalities is extremely unusual. For this reason, a surgical tenodesis, or sewing the biceps into the groove, has limited value.

The same mechanical impingement process that may lead to fraying and tearing of the supraspinatus tendon may also cause inflammation, fraying, and eventual tearing of the long head of the biceps tendon. Thus, if a patient presents with a spontaneous rupture of the long head of the biceps muscle, the

clinical picture is classic. The muscle belly is bunched in a typical "Popeye" configuration. Although the biceps is an elbow flexor and supinator, when a patient presents with a long head of the biceps rupture, the focus should not be on associated weakness or limitations of elbow flexion but rather on associated symptomatology of the shoulder (Fig. 10-46). The patient should be questioned about associated shoulder problems, and, if necessary, investigative studies should be obtained to assess the adequacy and integrity of the rotator cuff. A high percentage of patients who present with a spontaneous rupture of the long head of the biceps have an associated rotator cuff tear.

For inflammatory problems in the biceps tendon, the treatment is similar to that of inflammation of the rotator cuff. If there is spontaneous rupture of the long head of the biceps tendon, little is to be gained by attempted repair in the bicipital groove. If

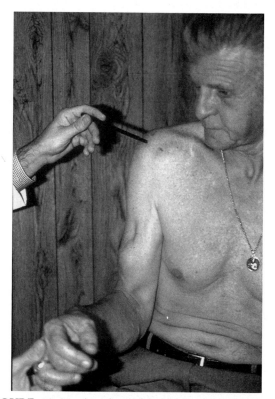

FIGURE 10-46. A patient with a spontaneous rupture of the long head of biceps. This most often results from subacromial impingement and is frequently accompanied by a full-thickness tear of the rotator cuff. In this patient, the clinician points to the area of pain, suggesting that the rotator cuff is involved. A spontaneous rupture of the long head of biceps should make the clinician focus on the area of the rotator cuff as the source of pathology.

this is accompanied by a tear of the rotator cuff, however, surgery should be directed toward treatment of the associated rotator cuff tear.

If during surgery for impingement syndrome, the biceps tendon is found to be flattened or inflamed, it may be left intact and decompressed by anterior acromioplasty. If it is torn or displaced from the groove at the time of surgery, tenodesis of the biceps tendon may be performed as part of the overall procedure on the rotator cuff.

THE ACROMIOCLAVICULAR JOINT IN IMPINGEMENT SYNDROME

The acromioclavicular joint plays an important role in the impingement syndrome. The supraspinatus muscle and tendon pass directly under the acromioclavicular joint as the arm is brought into the arc of forward elevation when used overhead. Any arthritic changes in the acromioclavicular joint may lead to spurring at the margins of the joint. Inferior spurs may take up space in the subacromial area and may contribute to the impingement of the rotator cuff tendons and associated rotator cuff tearing. Therefore, all patients who present with rotator cuff disease and impingement should be evaluated for associated acromioclavicular joint degeneration or arthritis. Many of these patients have clinical tenderness and radiographic signs consistent with degeneration of the acromioclavicular joint.

If the patient has isolated acromioclavicular joint disease, antiinflammatory medications or injections may be appropriate. In patients who undergo surgical treatment for rotator cuff impingement or tearing, the distal clavicle may be excised in part or in total, as part of the overall surgical treatment of the rotator cuff pathology.

FROZEN SHOULDER

A *frozen shoulder* is a glenohumeral joint with pain and stiffness that cannot be explained on the basis of joint incongruity. Many conditions can produce restricted active range of motion, but it is the restriction to passive range of motion that is the hallmark of this disease. Although some have attempted to make a distinction between the entities of frozen shoulder and adhesive capsulitis, it is generally thought that frozen shoulder and adhesive capsulitis are interchangeable terms.

Epidemiology

Frozen shoulder syndrome has a tendency to occur during the fifth to seventh decades and appears to affect women more frequently than men. Bilateral involvement occurs in 10% to 40% of cases. Once the syndrome resolves, frozen shoulder generally does not recur in the same shoulder, unless there are other predisposing factors, such as ongoing tendinitis or diabetes mellitus.

Etiology

The specific etiology of frozen shoulder syndrome is unknown. Although some think that an inflammatory component leads to stiffness in the shoulder, the exact nature and role of inflammation is uncertain. In general, any process that leads to the patient gradually restricting range of motion can lead to secondary contracture of the soft tissue and painful stiffness. Frozen should syndrome has many causes. Among the most common are cervical spine degenerative disease or radiculopathy, subacromial impingement syndrome, acromioclavicular arthritis, posttraumatic bursitis, and inflammatory synovitis of the shoulder. Frozen shoulder has also been recognized in association with other medical problems, such as cardiothoracic surgery. In addition, certain medical conditions appear to be associated with a particularly resistant form of frozen shoulder syndrome. The most common of these is diabetes mellitus.

In the classic description of adhesive capsulitis there are three clinical phases: (1) a painful phase, (2) a phase of progressive stiffness, and (3) a thawing phase with gradual return of motion.

Clinical Features

In general, the clinical picture in frozen shoulder is one of insidious onset of generalized aching discomfort about the shoulder. This is usually poorly localized and may radiate down the arm to the elbow. Usually, no precipitating cause is specifically remembered. Since many patients experienced traumatic episodes with variable degrees of severity, it is not unusual to get a history of some trauma to the shoulder before the progressive stiffness. Increasing shoulder discomfort is associated with a rather slowly progressive shoulder stiffness. Thus, a vicious cycle tends to occur. As the shoulder progressively gets

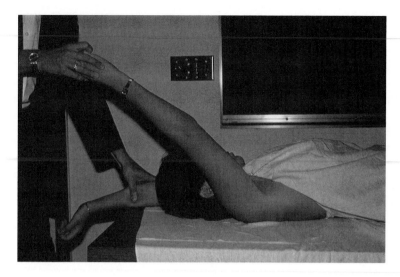

FIGURE 10-47. Frozen shoulder syndrome with limitation of passive forward flexion.

stiff, the patient voluntarily restricts the range of motion, leading to more stiffness. The more stiffness, the more pain. The pain is often worse at night and frequently interferes with the patient's sleep. External rotation of the humerus appears to be the motion that is lost first, and the limitation may be subtle. As the pain and restricted motion increase, the patient becomes more functionally disabled. Reaching behind the back to reach the back pocket, to reach into the back seat of a car, to fasten a bra strap, or to reach into an overcoat become particularly troublesome. Eventually, the patient may lose the ability to reach in front, and personal hygiene may be affected by the restriction of internal rotation.

The hallmark of the clinical examination on the patient with frozen shoulder is a restriction of passive range of motion, particularly in forward flexion, external rotation, abduction, and internal rotation (Figs. 10-47 through 10-49). Often, a solid endpoint is painful as the limit to the motion is reached. It is essential to compare passive motion to the contralateral nonpainful side because some patients may have mild symmetric limitations of range in certain positions, which may not be painful. The key to the diagnosis is asymmetric limitation of passive range of motion, which is painful. Typically, active motion is affected only to the extent that passive motion is, and there is not usually a discrepancy between active and passive ranges of motion. This distinguishes the frozen shoulder syndrome from other syndromes that

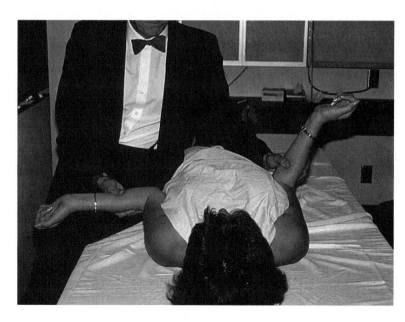

FIGURE 10-48. A patient with frozen shoulder with limited passive range of motion in external rotation, measured with the arm near the side.

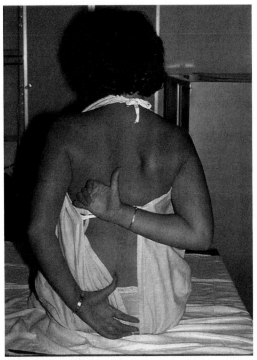

FIGURE 10-49. The same patient as shown in Figure 10-49 with a frozen shoulder and with limitation of internal rotation. Painful stiffness in these three directions, in the absence of joint incongruity, is typical of frozen shoulder syndrome.

are painful and in which active motion may be limited, such as rotator cuff impingement and tearing. On clinical examination, other associated findings may give a clue to the etiology of the syndrome. For instance, tenderness on motion of the neck or reflex changes suggests cervical spine problems as a cause. Tenderness over the acromioclavicular joint suggests degeneration or synovitis in this joint as an etiologic mechanism. Pain with resistance to rotation when the arm is to the side suggests tendinitis as an underlying mechanism. The differential diagnosis of frozen shoulder syndrome is somewhat limited and includes other entities that cause restriction of motion and pain in the shoulder. The most serious of these is a locked posterior or anterior dislocation, which causes restriction of passive motion, is also painful, and may be missed unless adequate radiographs are obtained.

Subacromial impingement and rotator cuff disease may mimic the frozen shoulder syndrome. The pain of subacromial impingement is usually worse with the arm at shoulder level and above, and there is typically not the solid painful endpoint with the arm at the side as the arm is rotated externally and internally. In addition, the pain of subacromial im-

pingement syndrome is often relieved with an injection of lidocaine (Xylocaine) into the subacromial space. Degenerative arthroses of the glenohumeral joint may cause painful stiffness, but in most situations the diagnosis is clear if adequate radiographs are obtained. Primary acromioclavicular joint disease is usually characterized by localized tenderness to the acromioclavicular joint and radiographic abnormalities.

Although many disease processes may cause some limitation of motion of the shoulder by pain in one plane, it is characteristic of a frozen shoulder syndrome to have limitations in many planes.

Radiographic Features

Plain radiographs of the shoulder are usually unremarkable. Depending on how long the syndrome has existed, the limitation of motion by the patient over a prolonged period may produce mild osteopenia radiographically. Frozen shoulder syndrome can be produced by either primary or secondary malignancy in the glenohumeral joint, and thus every patient who presents with a stiff and painful shoulder should have proper radiography of the shoulder.

A number of additional studies may be helpful in evaluating frozen shoulder syndrome. Blood work is usually normal. Some investigators indicated a relation between a hot bone scan and frozen shoulder syndrome, but there does not appear to be a consistent abnormality on bone scan. Some investigators used shoulder arthrography as a means of making a diagnosis. As capsular contracture progresses, the amount of contrast medium that a shoulder can imbibe is also limited. In addition, there is usually obliteration of the axillary fold by arthrography.

Injections may be helpful to elucidate the etiology, but they are ordinarily not helpful in making the diagnosis of frozen shoulder syndrome.

Some investigators suggested there is a role for arthroscopy in the evaluation or treatment of frozen shoulder syndrome. The role of arthroscopy in the evaluation or treatment of the syndrome needs to be better defined, but at this time, it does not appear to be particularly helpful in establishing the clinical diagnosis of frozen shoulder syndrome.

Natural History

The natural history of adhesive capsulitis has been described as typically lasting 18 to 24 months. Reeves described some restriction in shoulder motion in more than half of patients in a 5- to 10-year follow-up, despite functional improvement. Binder, in a prospective study, noted that 90% of patients did not regain the minimal range of motion when matched for age and sex with a control group 6 months after diagnosis.

It is thought that all patients get better without attention to treatment of their frozen shoulder syndrome if they are left alone, but the amount of disability and pain caused by this syndrome is highly variable, and many patients are not willing to wait the many months or years to see whether this syndrome will resolve by itself.

Treatment Recommendations

Most patients with frozen shoulder syndrome are treated nonoperatively. Because it may result from a variety of acutely painful conditions of the shoulder, such as tendinitis, impingement, calcific tendinitis, or traumatic irritation of the bursa, prevention may play a role in avoiding secondary stiffness of the shoulder. Simple measures, such as taking an arm through a complete range of motion once daily in the shower, may prevent secondary stiffness and contracture of the soft tissue before the syndrome becomes full-blown.

Although antiinflammatory medications may play a role, it is more typical to add a mild analgesic along with the exercises prescribed for the restricted range of motion.

The hallmark of treatment of frozen shoulder is a rehabilitation program aimed at eliminating the stiffness in the shoulder. Exercises are usually prescribed in planes that are the most stiff, such as forward flexion, external rotation, internal rotation, and abduction. Many of these exercises can be done by the patient several times a day without the assistance of a physical therapist. A formal program of physical therapy, however, in which the physical therapist passively does some stretching in addition to the patient's own use of exercise, can be helpful. Ordinarily, the patient notices that as the shoulder stiffness is eliminated by the stretching exercises, the improvement in pain parallels the improvement in motion. It is not unusual for frozen shoulder to take many months to resolve, despite aggressive and adequate physical therapy or a home exercise program. The addition of heat also may help in the home exercise program.

In some patients, there is a plateau on the exercise program, with continued stiffness and continued pain in the shoulder. This group of patients may benefit from a closed manipulation under general anesthesia. At the time of manipulation, many times the adhesions can be felt to break by the surgeon. Manipulation during anesthesia is accompanied by some risk, however, including the rare complication of humeral fracture or rotator cuff tear. For this reason, it is reserved for those who fail nonoperative treatment.

If there is high risk of fracture of the humerus, such as might occur in an osteopenic patient or an elderly patient with a frozen shoulder, then consideration rarely is given for an open release of adhesions to restore flexibility for an open operative approach.

SPRENGEL DEFORMITY

Sprengel deformity is a congenital high scapula caused by a failure of the scapula to descend from its origin as a cervical appendage. Sprengel deformity is the most common congenital anomaly of the shoulder. Thus, it is a permanent elevation of the shoulder girdle.

Etiology

The etiology of Sprengel deformity is unknown. Whatever factors cause this deformity clearly are operative during early embryonic life, especially during the development of the cervical spine and upper limb buds and during the subsequent descent of the limb buds. Before the third gestational month, the embryonic tissues form both the cervical spine and then the upper limb buds at about the level of C5. The limb buds then descend to the level of the thorax, usually the T5 level. Failure to descend results in the permanently high shoulder girdle. The undescended scapula is the most obvious manifestation of the problem, but because the development of the cervical spine is occurring at the same time, many other abnormalities are associated with Sprengel deformity. These include scoliosis, rib and vertebral abnormalities, clavicular abnormalities, muscular hypoplasia, (especially trapezius), renal abnormalities, torticollis, and cervical spine anomalies. Thus, Sprengel deformity is really a deformity of the cervicothoracic spine and shoulder girdle. In half of cases, an omovertebral body, consisting of bone, cartilage, or fibrocartilage, connects the superior angle of the scapula to the cervical spine. Because of the abnormal inferiorly directed glenoid and variant attachments of the scapula, shoulder abduction is limited, adding functional impairment to the cosmetic deformity.

Clinical Features

Sprengel deformity has varying clinical presentations due to the variety of associated deformities. In most instances, the primary deformity is cosmetic. The shoulder is higher than the opposite side when this is a unilateral deformity. A lump is often noted in the web space of what appears to be a short neck. The scapula is shaped like an equilateral triangle and is hypoplastic. It is also rotated so that the inferior pole of the scapula abuts against the thoracic spine, while the superior medial angle of the scapula is rotated anteriorly over the chest. The clavicle is usually straight since the impetus for the clavicle to curve to accommodate the great vessels is not there without scapular descent. The omovertebral connection may be palpable as a chondroosseous bar. Scapulothoracic motion may be severely limited by multiple soft tissue and bony connections binding the scapula to the thoracic structures. Although scapulothoracic motion may be limited, glenohumeral motion is usually normal. Total elevation of the arm may be incomplete because of the rotation and tilt of the scapula. With the glenoid facing inferiorly, there may be a block to the usual full abduction and forward elevation of the arm, which is normally a combined glenohumeral and scapulothoracic motion. Pain is generally absent. The deformities in the scapular area usually are noted during infancy or early childhood.

The associated clinical conditions are significant for several reasons:

1. Parents and patients must be made aware that many of these deformities persist even after surgical correction of the undescended scapula.
2. Any tethering of the cord should be ruled out before considering spinal scoliosis straightening.
3. Rib cage abnormalities may predispose these patients to thoracic outlet syndrome after scapular operations.
4. Before any surgical procedure, kidney and renal status must be assessed.

Radiographic Features

Radiographically, the changes are typical and include elevation and significant rotation of the scapula with decreased length of the medial border. Inferior direction of the glenoid is typical, and the acromion may be prolonged.

The rest of the radiographic features may be related to associated anomalies, including scoliosis, Klippel-Feil syndrome, spina bifida, and diastematomyelia. Scoliosis is found in nearly half of patients. Rib abnormalities, including synostosis, absence, duplication, and cervical ribs occur in about 38% of patients. Klippel-Feil syndrome is found in about 29%, spina bifida in 19%, and diastematomyelia in 3% of patients.

CT scan may be useful for identification of the location and nature of the omovertebral communication.

Pathologic Findings

In about half of patients, an omovertebral connection exists between the spinus process, lamina, or transfer process of the lower cervical spine, usually C6, and the superior medial angle of the scapula. The connection is a chondroosseous bar, the morphology of which is variable. It was shown to have diarthrodial joints, cartilaginous connections, fibrous bands, and solid bony unions. The connections to the cervical spine occasionally can even reach the base of the occiput of the skull. Associated errors in segmentation are represented by wedged and fused cervical and thoracic vertebrae, hemivertebrae, and fused ribs, all of which are responsible for the frequently associated scoliosis.

Treatment Recommendations

Treatment is undertaken for cosmetic reasons only. If severe function of the shoulder is restricted, restoration of position of the scapula may improve the function.

Although advocated in the past, early passive stretching and active exercises have not been found to alter the natural course of the deformity. Conservative measures have been recommended, such as padding the contralateral shoulder to improve the symmetry when the patient is dressed.

In general, surgery is indicated in those children with significant functional and cosmetic abnormalities. The usual age for such procedures is between 3 and 7 years.

Operative treatment in general includes operations to release, resect, or relocate the scapula. The ideal surgical candidate is someone between 3 and 8 years of age with moderate to severe deformity, although surgical correction in patients as young as 18 months or as old as 15 years has been reported. In general, early operative intervention in the most severe deformities gives the best results.

Before considering surgical treatment, it is imperative that preoperative evaluation include a thorough history, physical examination with radiographic evaluation of the cervical and thoracolumbar spine, and renal ultrasound or intravenous pyelogram to rule out associated abnormalities. The glenohumeral and scapulothoracic motion should be measured, and standing AP and lateral radiographs should be included.

The number of surgical procedures has been identified. Historically, there are two types of surgical treatment: procedures that attempt to improve cosmesis by resecting abnormal bony prominences and those that attempt to lower the scapula by mobilizing it from its abnormal attachments and then reattaching the muscles with the scapula in a more normal position.

The Schrock, Green, Jennopoulos, and Klisic procedures divide and reattach scapular muscles at their scapular insertion.

The most popular operation for this is the Woodward procedure. This involves resection of the supraspinus portion of the scapula, with detachment of the vertebral origins of the muscles. Relocation and derotation of the scapula are performed, with suturing of the detached muscles further caudally on the vertebral spinus process. Further temporary fixation of the relocated scapula may be achieved by suturing the inferior pole of the scapula to a rib and the medial border to a vertebral spinus process using large, absorbable suture material, so that the superior border of the scapula is at an equal level to the normal opposite side. Good to excellent results are reported in 80% of patients.

Complications of this procedure include winging of the scapula and brachial plexus palsy; the latter may be due to compression of the plexus between the deformed first rib or a cervical rib and the abnormally straight clavicle. Osteotomy or morcellation of the clavicle or osteotomy of the coracoid may be necessary to prevent this complication.

In some patients in whom the deformity is not severe, or in patients older than 8 years of age, some investigators advocate simple excision of the superior angle of the scapula and any omovertebral communication to give improved function and cosmesis.

Annotated Bibliography

Bigliani LU. Shoulder: trauma. In: Fitzgerald RH, ed. Orthopaedic knowledge update II. Park Ridge, IL, AAOS, 1987.
This chapter deals with many aspects of shoulder trauma, including fractures and fracture dislocations of the proximal humerus, fractures of the humeral shaft, fractures of the scapula, fractures of the clavicle, glenohumeral instability, acromioclavicular instability, and neurovascular injuries in adult and pediatric patients. This is a good update and overview of aspects of shoulder and glenohumeral joint trauma.

Bigliani LU, Flatow EL, Craig EV. Shoulder: reconstruction. In: Poss R, ed. Orthopaedic knowledge update III. Park Ridge, IL, AAOS, 1990.
This is an extensive review of current knowledge of basic sciences related to the articular surfaces, the static restraints of the glenohumeral joint, and the muscles stabilizing the glenohumeral joint. There is a description of the state of the art of glenohumeral arthroplasty, rotator cuff disease and its treatment, glenohumeral joint arthrodesis, and diseases of the acromioclavicular joint and biceps tendon. In addition, calcific tendinitis, suprascapular nerve entrapment, frozen shoulder, and controversies related to diagnosis and treatment of disorders of the glenohumeral joint are updated.

Cofield RH. Shoulder: reconstruction. In: Fitzgerald RH, ed. Orthopaedic knowledge update II. Park Ridge, IL, AAOS, 1987.
This chapter reviews shoulder reconstruction. Among the topics summarized are current research relative to the glenohumeral joint; advances in diagnosis, such as ultrasonography, computed tomography, arthrography, and arthroscopy; and the treatment of impingement syndrome, rotator cuff tears, and cuff tear arthropathy. Arthritis of the acromioclavicular and glenohumeral joints is also reviewed, as are current methods of diagnosis and treatment of these conditions.

Galinat BJ, Warren RF. Shoulder: trauma-related instability. In: Poss R, ed. Orthopaedic knowledge update III. Park Ridge, IL, AAOS, 1990.
In this review, the authors give a broad overview of the current status of diagnosis and treatment of glenohumeral instability, acromioclavicular joint separations and dislocations, fractures of the proximal humerus, humeral shaft, and clavicle, and nerve injuries around the shoulder. Current controversies regarding shoulder arthroscopy and treatment of acromioclavicular joint injuries are also described.

Goldberg BM. Arthritis. In: Fitzgerald RH, ed. Orthopaedic knowledge update II. Park Ridge, IL, AAOS, 1987.
Included in this overview are sections on normal joint physiology, experimental models of osteoarthritis and how they relate to development of osteoarthritis in humans, and the etiology and treatment of rheumatoid arthritis, gout, juvenile rheumatoid arthritis, ankylosing spondylitis, chondrocalcinosis, and infectious arthritis.

Gristiani AG, Webb LX. Shoulder and humerus reconstruction. In: Asher MA, Garland JJ, Lovell WW, Sarmiento A, Stauffer RN, eds. Orthopaedic knowledge update I. Chicago, AAOS, 1984.
The authors describe the current state of the art regarding diagnostic techniques and arthroscopy of the shoulder, glenohumeral disease and reconstruction, acromioclavicular joint reconstruction, total shoulder replacement arthroplasty, and other reconstructive procedures of the shoulder, such as osteotomies, arthrodesis, and scapulothoracic fusion. In addition, muscle flap reconstruction is reviewed.

Koman LA. Upper extremity: pediatric reconstruction. In: Poss, R, ed. Orthopaedic knowledge update III. Park Ridge, IL, AAOS, 1990.
The author presents an overview of upper extremity pediatric reconstruction, including embryology, localized disorders of the

shoulder, radial deficiencies, hypoplastic thumbs, ulnar deficiencies, and central deficiencies. The authors review congenital radioulnar synostosis, Madelung deformity, congenital pseudarthrosis of the forearm, syndactyly, polydactyly, macrodactyly, and congenital amputations. In addition, the treatment of generalized disorders, such as cerebral palsy and arthrogryposis, is considered.

Neviaser RJ. Shoulder and humerus: trauma. In: Asher MA, Garland JJ, Lovell WW, Sarmiento A, Stauffer RN, eds. Orthopaedic knowledge update I. Chicago, AAOS, 1984.
This is a consideration of trauma to the shoulder and humerus, including such issues as brachial plexus injuries, disorders of the rotator cuff and biceps tendon, glenohumeral instability, chronic unreduced dislocations, and fractures of the humeral shaft and the nerve injuries associated with them.

Nissenbaum M. Shoulder and humerus: pediatric. In: Asher MA, Garland JJ, Lovell WW, Sarmiento A, Stauffer RN, eds. Orthopaedic knowledge update I. Chicago, AAOS, 1984.
Pediatric upper extremity problems such as congenital anomalies, Spreagel deformity, congenital pseudarthrosis of the clavicle, infection, traumatic conditions, deltoid contracture, neuromuscular diseases, and rheumatoid arthritic problems are considered.

Ruby LK. Pediatric reconstruction. In: Fitzgerald RH, ed. Orthopaedic knowledge update II. Park Ridge, IL, AAOS, 1987:192.
Among the topics sumarized in this review are the treatment and diagnosis of radial clubhand, the congenital undescended scapula, acquired congenital amputations, radial and ulnar ray deficiencies of children, birth palsies (diagnosis and treatment), and some tumors and infections that appear in children.

Schurman DJ. Arthritis. In: Poss R, ed. Orthopaedic knowledge update III. Chicago, AAOS, 1990.
In this review, the author reviews concepts of normal joint physiology, etiology of osteoarthritis and inflammatory arthropathies, and current knowledge of the pathogenesis of crystalline arthritis and infectious arthritis.

Turek's Orthopaedics: Principles and Their Application, Fifth Edition,
edited by Stuart L. Weinstein and Joseph A. Buckwalter.
J.B. Lippincott Company, Philadelphia, © 1994.

11

Roy A. Meals

The Elbow and Forearm

**CONGENITAL RADIAL HEAD
   DISLOCATION**
**CONGENITAL RADIOULNAR
   SYNOSTOSIS**
PANNER DISEASE
**OSTEOCHONDRITIS DISSECANS
   OF THE ELBOW**
TENNIS ELBOW
OLECRANON BURSITIS

**NERVE ENTRAPMENTS
   AROUND THE ELBOW**
Ulnar Nerve
Median Nerve
Radial Nerve
RHEUMATOID ARTHRITIS

CONGENITAL RADIAL HEAD DISLOCATION

Dislocation of the proximal radius from its capitellar articulation on the humerus is the most commonly occurring congenital anomaly around the elbow (Fig. 11-1). Most often, the radial head is dislocated posterior to the humerus, but anterior and lateral dislocations also occur. The incidence is similar in males and females, as is the involvement of the left and right limbs in unilateral cases. The deformity may be noted at birth but sometimes goes undiscovered for many years.

Controversy exists over whether the observed dislocations are truly developmental anomalies or actually result from unrecognized trauma early in life. For instance, the pulled elbow of infancy, often referred to as nursemaid's elbow, results from longitudinal traction on the upper limb, leading to minor capsular and ligament tears and radial head subluxation or dislocation. If this injury is unrecognized and untreated, the resultant clinical and radiographic pictures may eventually resemble those of dislocations that are developmental in origin. Congenital radial head dislocation is often associated with conditions that result in a shortened ulna, such as ulnar ray deficiency, multiple exostoses, and enchondromatosis. Other radiographic findings that suggest a congenital or ancient traumatic cause include a convex contour to the proximal end of the radius and a long narrow neck, an absent or hypoplastic capitellum, an abnormal ulnohumeral articulation, and a prominent medial epicondyle. Further evidence for a congenital cause includes bilateral elbow involvement, the presence of other congenital anomalies, a familial occurrence, irreducibility by closed means, and a dislocation

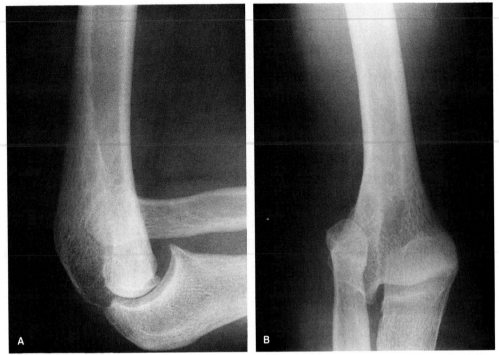

FIGURE 11-1. In congenital radial head dislocation, the proximal end of the radius is rounded, the radial neck is not tapered, the capitellum is malformed, and the humeroulnar portion of the elbow articulation shows minor abnormalities.

seen at birth or without known trauma. Conversely, normally shaped articular surfaces, the presence of soft tissue calcifications, and evidence of a previous ulnar fracture all suggest a traumatic cause.

Acquired radial head dislocation can also occur in cerebral palsy, Erb palsy, and arthrogryposis multiplex congenita. Forearm tumors, such as osteochondroma, can also push the radial head out of location. The cause in these patients can be determined easily. Other patients require careful evaluation to determine whether the cause is congenital or traumatic.

Because congenital radial head dislocations are frequently associated with other congenital anomalies, a thorough evaluation is indicated when a radial head dislocation is diagnosed. Associated anomalies include radial and ulnar deficiencies, lower limb anomalies, scoliosis, generalized types of skeletal dysplasia, and Fanconi anemia.

Despite a rather dramatic radiographic and clinical appearance of congenital radial head dislocation, elbow flexion and extension are only minimally limited, and forearm pronation and supination are restricted by about half. What limitations are present do not change significantly with growth. Loss of full supination is most likely to be the only disabling re-

striction. This precludes palm-up activities, such as accepting coins in the open hand. Pain is rarely associated and, when present, is usually an exertion-related ache.

Thus, treatment is generally not necessary. Pain and appearance can be improved with radial head excision, but this should not be considered until skeletal growth is complete because earlier removal of the proximal radius growth plate may alter additional forearm growth, disturbing the balance of the distal radioulnar joint. Motion is generally not improved by radial head excision because the contracted periarticular soft tissues cannot be effectively released.

CONGENITAL RADIOULNAR SYNOSTOSIS

Bony union between two adjacent bones occurs as a congenital anomaly at various sites in the upper extremity. The most common of these coalitions around the elbow occurs between the proximal radius and ulna, preventing forearm rotation.

During fetal development, longitudinal segmentation of the anlage destined to become the radius and ulna begins distally and proceeds proximally. A genetic influence or teratogenic insult at this time interrupts the normal separation of the proximal ends of the radius and ulna. Radioulnar synostosis occurs as an isolated anomaly in two thirds of cases, but it may also be associated with hip dysplasia, clubfoot, hand anomalies, and various central nervous system, cardiac, and chest wall anomalies (Fig. 11-2). Radioulnar synostosis is frequently seen in fetal alcohol syndrome. Thus, other congenital anomalies should be sought when radioulnar synostosis is noted. Familial occurrences are rare. Bilateral involvement is common.

A child born with radioulnar synostosis is frequently at least 1 year of age before the absence of forearm rotation is noted by the family. Functional difficulties include holding a pencil, eating with a spoon, drinking from a glass, and accepting small objects, such as dry cereal, in the palm. Difficulties are accentuated in patients with bilateral involvement and when the forearms are fixed in extreme pronation.

On examination, slightly diminished elbow extension and markedly increased wrist rotation are common. The wrist hypermobility partially compensates for the loss of forearm rotation. The forearm is usually fixed in a moderately pronated position. Radiographs show a bony coalition between the radius and ulna proximally, extending distally for a variable distance. The radial head may be dislocated.

Indications for treatment are related to the fixed position of the forearm. When the forearm is fixed in mild pronation, the patient can adapt well except for taking coins in the palm or doing pull-ups, and surgery usually is not helpful. When the forearm is fixed in full pronation, the functional disability is greatly increased, and these patients benefit from having their forearms repositioned in a more useful and aesthetic position.

Various techniques have been tried in an effort to restore forearm rotation; however, they have not been successful because of the extensive bony and soft tissue involvement as well as postoperative scarring. The limited goal of a rotational osteotomy places the forearm in a more functional fixed position, and this procedure is useful for the severely pronated cases. For unilateral involvement, the best functional and aesthetic position to achieve at surgery is 0 to 20 degrees of pronation; for bilateral cases, the dominant limb should be placed in 20 degrees of pronation and the nondominant limb in neutral rotation.

Vascular compromise with risk of compartment syndrome is a well-recognized complication of forearm rotational osteotomy. Thus, the osteotomy should be fixed with percutaneous Kirschner wires so that, if necessary, they can be removed quickly in the recovery room to reduce the stretch on the vessels. Likewise, any derotation of greater than 85 degrees should be performed in two stages.

PANNER DISEASE

Osteochondrosis of the capitellum, also known as Panner disease, is a localized lesion of the subchondral bone in the distal humerus that affects the congruity of the overlying cartilage (Fig. 11-3). It occurs most often in the right elbow in 5- to 11-year-old boys and during the period when the capitellar epiphysis is actively ossifying. The cause is unclear but is probably related to vascular alterations in the epiphysis. Injury is not implicated in the etiology.

Presenting complaints are usually pain and limited elbow extension. Tenderness and swelling over the lateral aspect of the elbow are noted on examination. Mild synovial thickening and joint effusion may be present.

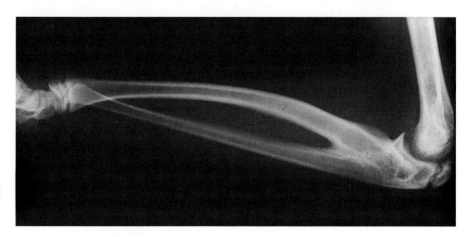

FIGURE 11-2. Bony coalition between the proximal radius and ulna is present in congenital radioulnar synostosis.

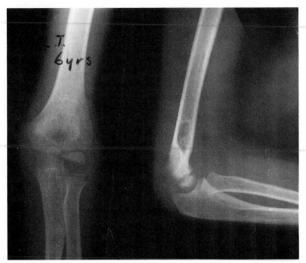

FIGURE 11-3. Panner disease: osteochondritis of the capitellum.

Radiographs show patchy areas of sclerosis and lucency, giving the appearance of fragmentation. The radial head may show advanced skeletal maturity, presumably because of the local reactive hyperemia.

Treatment is directed at preventing collapse and secondary arthritic changes at the radiocapitellar joint. A long arm cast immobilizes the elbow for 3 to 4 weeks until the acute inflammation subsides, and then protected motion is started. Complete healing and reconstitution of the capitellum takes 1 to 3 years, and a residual elbow flexion contracture may be permanent.

Panner disease has been compared with Legg-Calvé-Perthes disease of the hip because they occur in identically aged boys and the radiographic findings are similar. Collapse and deformity in Panner disease, however, are seen far less commonly in the capitellum than in the femoral head.

OSTEOCHONDRITIS DISSECANS OF THE ELBOW

Osteochondritis dissecans of the capitellum is a disease mainly of teen-aged boys (Fig. 11-4). A large segment of cartilage and underlying bone develops avascular necrosis and then becomes partially or completely detached. The condition is 10 times more common in males than in females. It has been seen in patients as young as 5 and as old as 44 years of age, but two thirds of patients are between 9 and 15 years of age. Both elbows are involved in 15% of cases. When unilateral, the elbow in the dominant limb is affected six times as often as the one in the nondominant limb. Occasionally, a patient has identical osteochondral involvement in the knees and possibly other joints.

The etiology of osteochondritis dissecans is unclear. Genetics, trauma, and ischemia have all been implicated. Multiple family members, both in the

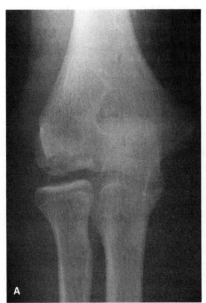
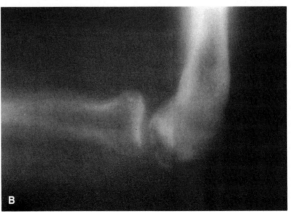

FIGURE 11-4. Fragmentation of the capitellum in teen-aged boys, characteristic of osteochondritis dissecans, can be noted on routine radiographs (**A**), but the extent is more fully seen on tomograms (**B**).

same generation and in sequential generations, are sometimes affected. Even so, the overall evidence for a genetic cause is weak. Repetitive trauma may be a causative factor because the osteochondritis dissecans is seen most often in athletically vigorous throwers and usually in the dominant limb. Forceful extension and pronation of the elbow causes marked compression and shearing forces to be transmitted from the radial head to the capitellum. This may cause separation of a segment of the incompletely ossified capitellum. Further forceful activity precludes healing. The possibility of an ischemic etiology is raised mainly because of the histologic appearance of the bone–cartilage fragment. Changes typical of bone infarction due to interruption of the intraosseous arterial blood supply are present.

Elbow pain is the most common presenting complaint. Poorly localized, it is exacerbated by throwing and relieved by rest. Loss of elbow extension is common, and loss of elbow flexion and forearm rotation can also occur. Lateral elbow tenderness and crepitation with elbow motion may also be noted.

Early radiographic changes include a crater in the articular surface of the capitellum with a sclerotic margin of subchondral bone. In unilateral cases, the radial head adjacent to the affected capitellum is larger than the one in the uninvolved limb, and the proximal radial epiphysis closes earlier. These findings are presumably related to a reactive hyperemia caused by the joint inflammation. If the central fragment becomes dislodged, one or more calcific loose bodies are noted in the joint, and the capitellum has an irregular, flattened appearance. If left untreated, deterioration of the radiocapitellar articulation is progressive.

Computed tomography with radioopaque dye in the joint can help determine whether the central fragment is loose in the crater. Arthroscopy may also be useful for this purpose as well as for removing loose bodies. A general survey of the articular surfaces is also an advantage of arthroscopy.

Multiple epiphyseal dysplasia may give a radiographic appearance similar to osteochondritis dissecans, but it is an inherited disorder affecting many articulations, so the resemblance is only superficial.

The type of treatment is dictated by the state of the central fragment in the crater. If the radiographic and arthroscopic studies show that the fragment is securely seated and the articular contour is undisturbed, preventative measures are appropriate. Casting for a few weeks should allow resolution of the inflammation and thereby reduce pain. Thereafter, the patient can gently move the elbow to restore mo-

tion, but forceful and rapid movements are to be avoided. The patient should have radiographs periodically over several years to ensure that the fragment remains in place and that healing is progressing. Half of undisplaced lesions may eventually displace.

If the fragment is loose but still in the crater, efforts at securing it surgically may immobilize it sufficiently for healing to occur.

If the fragment has been displaced out of the crater, removal, rather than replacement, is indicated because the displaced fragment becomes distorted and the crater becomes partially filled with scar. Removal of the loose body usually does not restore full motion. Radial head excision may be required if the arthritic changes are advanced.

The prognosis for osteochondritis dissecans of the capitellum is generally good. A gradual loss of extension may occur, and some residual pain, especially if a displaced fragment is present, can be expected. Catching and locking also occur more often in patients with displaced fragments, especially if the displaced fragments are not removed.

TENNIS ELBOW

The term *lawn-tennis elbow* was coined over 100 years ago and has been used to label a variety of symptoms in and around the elbow. To be specific, the term *tennis elbow* should be reserved for tendonitis of the forearm muscles arising from either the lateral or medial epicondyles of the humerus.

Lateral epicondylitis is far more common than medial epicondylitis. Rarely, both sides are affected simultaneously. Both lateral and medial epicondylitis occur in people of either gender generally between 30 and 50 years of age; and despite its nickname, epicondylitis is most commonly related to activities other than tennis. Repeated forceful wrist and finger movements produce an overuse syndrome at the origins of the stressed muscles. Onset of symptoms is gradual. Other athletic activities that produce symptoms include throwing sports, swimming, and golf. Forceful, repetitive wrist motions are also required in occupations such as carpentry, plumbing, and meat cutting, and these people are at risk. Not particularly forceful, but prolonged, rapid activities, such as sign language interpretation, can also cause symptoms.

The pathologic lesion is a chronic tear in the origin of the extensor carpi radialis brevis on the lateral epicondyle or in the flexor–pronator tendon origin on the medial epicondyle. Chronic granulation tissue, fibrinoid degeneration, and edematous tendon fibers are noted. The tears vary in size from microscopic to gross rupture.

Pain and tenderness centered at the epicondyle usually have a gradual onset and often follow a period of unusually vigorous activity. At first, the symptoms are present only during forceful activity, but as the inflammation progresses, symptoms may be noted with light self-care activities or even at rest.

Examination of the elbow elicits tenderness immediately distal to the epicondyle, and pain is increased both with resisted wrist movements and passive stretching of the involved motor units. Thus, resisted wrist flexion reproduces symptoms at the medial epicondyle. Particularly with the elbow extended, resisted wrist extension or passive wrist and finger flexion stress the fibers originating from the lateral epicondyle. Elbow motion is not restricted. Tenderness over the radial neck several centimeters distal to the lateral epicondyle suggests radial nerve entrapment, which can coexist with or mimic lateral epicondylitis. The tests to diagnosis radial tunnel syndrome are described later in this chapter. Radiographs rule out intraarticular pathology and reveal any calcification in the inflamed tendons.

Treatment decisions are affected by the duration, intensity, and resultant disability associated with the symptoms. For early symptoms associated only with stressful activity, temporary avoidance of the repetitive trauma, combined with oral nonsteroidal antiinflammatory medication, may be curative. If symptoms recur, the patient's technique for performing the causative activity may be faulty. A change of technique or equipment may be helpful in prevention. Racket weight, size, and handle diameter, for example, are factors to be considered in affected tennis players.

For more advanced symptoms that also occur with light functional activities, addition of a forearm support band and a cortisone injection into the inflamed area can be considered (Fig. 11-5). The band helps relieve symptoms probably by cushioning the forearm muscles and blunting the tension exerted on their proximal attachments. One or two cortisone injections may hasten resolution of the inflammation; further injections are unlikely to be curative and weaken the tendons.

Surgery is required for less than 10% of patients with tennis elbow. These individuals have disabling, long-standing symptoms resistant to nonoperative management. In the past, tendon repair or lengthening, annular ligament sectioning, and radial nerve decompression were among the recommended treatments. Although they all provided some success, they were directed at different sources of pathology than

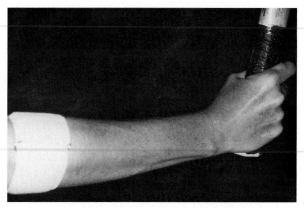

FIGURE 11-5. Trial of a forearm support band is a useful conservative treatment for lateral epicondylitis.

what is currently thought to be the cause. Surgical removal of the chronic granulation tissue and repair of any longitudinal tears in the tendon origins usually provide relief. Postoperative rehabilitation should extend for 3 to 6 months, with gradual, graded return to the previously traumatic activity.

The most common complication of surgical treatment is persistent symptoms, and this appears to be less frequent now that a specific site of pathology has been identified and a specific procedure devised to correct it.

OLECRANON BURSITIS

A bursa is a synovial lined pouch that facilitates gliding of adjacent tissues over one another. The olecranon bursa allows the skin to move easily over the olecranon and triceps insertion.

The bursa may become inflamed for a variety of reasons, including chronic repetitive trauma, acute trauma, rheumatoid arthritis, gout, and pseudogout. In addition to one of these causes, or as a primary cause itself, infection can also give rise to symptoms.

The most common cause of olecranon bursitis is probably repetitive trauma with direct pressure on the olecranon. It has been called miner's elbow and student's elbow for this reason. Acute blunt trauma, such as falling on the tip of the flexed elbow, can cause hemorrhage and subsequent inflammation. Nontender, pitting edema is often present in cases of recent onset.

Synovial proliferation in rheumatoid arthritis may affect bursae as well as joint and tendon sheaths. Probably as a secondary phenomenon, the olecranon bursa may communicate with the arthritic elbow joint.

Infection can occur in bursae previously inflamed from other causes as well as in previously normal bursae. Bacteremia and local cellulitic or pustular lesions may allow microorganisms access to the bursa. In rheumatoid arthritis, bacteria may spread from the bursa to the joint or from the joint to the bursa if a communication is present.

The distended bursa may be painless, particularly if trauma is responsible. Elbow flexion stretches the dorsal tissues and may elicit pain, thereby restricting further flexion. Bursae acutely inflamed from infection or gout are painful. About one third of patients with infected olecranon bursae have an inflamed bursa from another cause that secondarily becomes infected.

Although bursitis is a soft tissue lesion, radiographs should be obtained (Fig. 11-6). Bone spurs are present in about one third of affected elbows, and because they are larger than those seen in unaffected elbows, they may be a causative factor. The radiographs also may reveal osteomyelitis. A sinogram looking for communication with the joint or an arthrogram looking for communication with the bursa may help in planning treatment for a patient with rheumatoid arthritis and olecranon bursitis. Infection isolated to the bursa likely causes pain only at the extremes of motion, but a septic joint usually is painful with any attempted motion.

The first diagnostic steps are to determine the cause and to determine whether the bursa is septic. The clinical examination alone does not always differentiate infected bursae from those inflamed from other causes. Aspirated bursa fluid should be examined for white cells, crystals, and bacteria and cultured for microorganisms.

A low cell count and negative Gram stain suggest a nonseptic cause. Any underlying inflammatory process, such as gout, should be treated, and the bursa should be completely drained and compressed with a soft bandage. A steroid injection may assist with resolution of the inflammation once infection has been ruled out with certainty. Acute traumatic bursitis usually resolves spontaneously and requires no treatment. Repeated episodes of chronic traumatic bursitis can sometimes be prevented by padding the elbow to diffuse transmission of the mechanical forces. An infected bursa can initially be treated with aspiration and antibiotics. Intravenous antibiotics and repeated aspiration may be required if regional or systemic findings of infection are evident. Surgical drainage may be required if the infection is resistant to less invasive therapy.

Surgical excision of the bursa is required for repeated bouts of bursitis that interfere with functional activities and for chronically draining and infected bursae, particularly when olecranon osteomyelitis is present. Excision is fraught with difficulties, however, and should be performed only when thorough nonoperative treatment has failed. Persistence or recurrence of the bursa, chronically draining sinuses, and other wound healing problems are the commonly encountered postoperative problems.

NERVE ENTRAPMENTS AROUND THE ELBOW

Considering that three major nerves within a compact skin envelope cross a joint that not only flexes 150 degrees but also rotates 160 degrees, irritation and entrapment occur remarkably infrequently. The ulnar nerve is the most commonly affected, perhaps because of its location on the convex surface of the flexed elbow and its associated vulnerability to blunt trauma. The radial and median nerves are less commonly affected, but their involvement can be equally disabling. Physiologically, pressure on the nerve diminishes capillary perfusion, and the ischemic portion of the nerve does not repolarize normally, resulting in development of a conduction delay or block. This causes a vague aching in the general region of the compression. If the pressure is related to tight fascia of an adjacent muscle, exertional activity of that muscle may cause worsening of the symptoms. The irritated portion of the nerve may be sensitive to light tapping with paresthesia experienced in its normal sensory distribution. Edema fluid accumulates, heightening the magnitude of the entrapment.

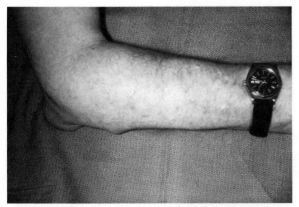

FIGURE 11-6. Olecranon bursitis causes a tender enlargement over the subcutaneous portion of the proximal ulna. It must be distinguished from rheumatoid nodule formation, which generally occurs along the subcutaneous border of the ulna more distally.

Nerve entrapments around the elbow must be differentiated from entrapments more proximally, such as cervical radiculopathy and thoracic outlet syndrome, and ones more distally, such as carpal tunnel syndrome. Brachial plexus neuritis and various tendonitis syndromes also have to be considered in the diagnosis.

Ulnar Nerve

Compression on the ulnar nerve at the elbow is known as cubital tunnel syndrome because the nerve passes through a fibroosseous canal behind the medial epicondyle en route from the arm to the forearm (Fig. 11-7). The patient notes a deep, aching sensation; if compression is severe or prolonged, he or she may also note paresthesia and hypesthesia in the ring and little fingers and loss of fine motor control in the fingers. It is important to determine whether the ulnar portion of the hand's dorsum is numb or tingling because the involvement of this area, along with the ring and little fingers, locates the problem proximal to the branching of the dorsal sensory branch of the ulnar nerve in the forearm. If the compression is at the wrist, conduction problems in the ulnar nerve cause symptoms in the ring and little fingers, but the dorsum of the hand is unaffected because the dorsal sensory nerve has already branched off. The patient may note increased symptoms when the elbow is acutely flexed. The condition has been called stock broker's elbow because of the need to hold the elbow in a flexed position when using the telephone. The patient should be asked about any trauma to the elbow, even in the distant past. Occasionally, an elbow injury in childhood with gradual progression of a cubitus valgus deformity results in cubital tunnel syndrome many years later. This condition is called tardy ulnar palsy.

On examination, the range of motion and the varus–valgus alignment of the elbow should be compared with the opposite side. The ulnar nerve should be checked for tenderness and sensitivity to light tapping in the cubital tunnel. Even healthy ulnar nerves are subject to paresthesia when forcefully struck—the source of the "funny bone"—so examination requires a light tap with the fingertip and comparison of the patient's response to similar stimulation of the opposite side. The ulnar nerve should be palpated while the elbow is flexed and extended. The patient's symptoms may result from a loosely tethered nerve riding back and forth over the medial epicondyle during elbow motion. Asking the patient to fully flex the elbows and hold the limbs still for a minute may reproduce or intensify the paresthesia in the digits. This elbow flexion test is analogous to the Phalen wrist flexion test for carpal tunnel syndrome.

Sensation in the fingertips should be tested, and comparisons between index and little finger on the affected side and between both little fingers should be made. In the palm, the ulnar nerve supplies the interosseous muscles, the hypothenar muscles, two lumbrical muscles, and the adductor pollicis. Weak-

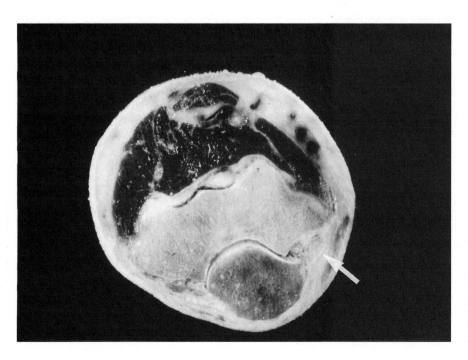

FIGURE 11-7. In a cross section taken through the distal humerus and the olecranon process of the ulna, the arrow indicates the location of the ulnar nerve behind the medial epicondyle. Ulnar nerve compression at this level is best relieved by surgical excision of the medial epicondyle. This allows the nerve to take a more gently directed course from the arm into the forearm.

ness of pinch and grip may therefore be noted; in severe, long-standing neuropathies, wasting of the intrinsic muscles occurs. This is usually most evident when examining the dorsal aspect of the first web. The normal convex bulk of the first dorsal interosseous muscle is absent, and the contours of the first and second metacarpals are much more evident. The fingers may assume abnormal and characteristic postures because of the inactivity of the small, ulnar innervated muscles. The ring and little fingers "claw" through hyperextension at the metacarpophalangeal joint and partial flexion at the interphalangeal joints. This posture is not seen in the index and middle fingers because these lumbricals are innervated by the median nerve, and although the interosseous muscles are palsied, the lumbricals alone are capable of preventing the claw posture. Pinch power of the thumb is diminished. When pinch is attempted, the thumb collapses into an abnormal posture of hyperflexion at the interphalangeal joint and hyperextension at the metacarpophalangeal joint.

The differential diagnosis of cubital tunnel syndrome includes nerve dysfunction from any cause. Conditions such as syringomyelia, thoracic outlet syndrome, brachial plexus palsy, and diabetic peripheral neuropathy must be considered. A careful history and physical examination can generally eliminate these less likely diagnoses.

The diagnosis of cubital tunnel syndrome can be confirmed by nerve conduction velocity and electromyogram studies. The conduction velocity is slowed across the elbow, and the electromyogram may show partial denervation of the intrinsic muscles, depending on the severity and duration of the compression. If the patient relates a history of elbow trauma or if a cubitus valgus deformity is evident, radiographs should be obtained.

If symptoms are mild and of recent onset, avoidance of the aggravating flexed elbow position may allow healing. People who use the telephone for long periods should get a shoulder cradle for the hand piece. A splint that holds the elbow in a moderately extended position and that does not apply any pressure directly on the nerve may be useful at night to eliminate habitual posturing of the elbow in flexion during sleep. Cortisone injections into the canal are without a rational basis because there is no tenosynovium there for the antiinflammatory medication to shrink.

Several operations have been used when the conservative treatments have failed. Release of the fascia over the nerve is simple and may fully relieve symptoms in some patients. It does not, however, address the acute bend the nerve takes around the flexed elbow, so many patients have persistent symptoms. A more extensive procedure is anterior transposition of the nerve, either into a subcutaneous position or into a submuscular position beneath the origin of the flexors and pronator arising from the medial epicondyle. This procedure has the advantage of relieving any compression on the nerve from the medial epicondyle, but the dissection and mobilization deprive the nerve of its segmental blood supply, and faulty wound closure may recompress the nerve. The basic pathophysiology of cubital tunnel syndrome is nerve ischemia. Therefore, it is illogical to perform a procedure that even temporarily reduces nerve nutrition even further or risks compressing the nerve with a different structure. For these reasons, the preferred treatment is removal of the medial epicondyle. The pronator and flexor muscle origins are unaffected by the bone removal, the mesoneurium is not disturbed, and the acute turn of the ulnar nerve in the flexed elbow is relieved. If a patient has tardy ulnar palsy with a marked cubitus valgus deformity, anterior transposition is preferable to medial epicondylectomy because only the transposition can relieve nerve tension over the deformed skeleton.

After operation, the patient can expect fairly prompt relief of the aching, gradual improvement in sensation, and diminution of paresthesia but probably not any recovery of intrinsic muscle function. Thus, the procedure should be performed before severe muscle wasting has developed. Patients with compression of ulnar nerve fibers at other sites, such as cervical spine, thoracic outlet, or wrist, and patients with diabetic neuropathy do not recover as promptly or as completely as those with otherwise healthy ulnar nerves.

The main risks of surgery are persistent or even worsening of symptoms related to continued nerve irritation. These risks are minimized with the medial epicondylectomy compared with the other available procedures.

Median Nerve

Compression syndromes involving the median nerve around the elbow are far less common than cubital tunnel syndrome. The median nerve runs a deeper course and passes immediately anterior to the axis of elbow flexion and extension. Fascial bands cross the nerve at several levels and can cause compression symptoms. Compression of the median nerve occurs more commonly in women and occurs over a wide span of ages.

The compression may elicit numbness and paresthesia in the lateral three and one half digits, similar to carpal tunnel syndrome. In addition, the thenar area of the palm may be numb. Because the median nerve branch that supplies this area on the thenar eminence does not pass through the carpal tunnel, numbness here suggests that the source of neuropathy is proximal to the wrist. The patient usually does not have a discrete pattern of sensory change, however, or does not have any sensory change at all. Instead, the patient may complain only of a vague ache on the anterior aspect of the proximal forearm or distal arm, perhaps related to exertional activity. Inciting activities often involve repetitive gripping or pronation, or both. Hammering, ladling food, and practicing the serve in tennis are examples. Night waking with paresthesia, so common with median nerve compression at the wrist, is not seen with compression more proximally.

Tenderness along the course of the nerve should be sought, and tapping over the tender area may cause a tingling sensation in the median innervated digits. Strength of the median innervated muscles in both the forearm and thenar area should be tested and compared with the opposite side. The median nerve may be compressed beneath the fascia of the biceps above the elbow. This fascia is called the lacertus fibrosus. If symptoms increase during the maneuver of resisted elbow flexion and supination, which tightens the lacertus fibrosus, this source of compression is suggested. Further distally, the nerve may be compressed as it runs through or beneath the pronator teres. Increased symptoms during resisted forearm pronation while gradually extending the elbow suggest this site for the entrapment. Another site of possible involvement is beneath the fascial origin of the flexor digitorum superficialis. This band is tightened during resisted middle finger flexion, and an increase of symptoms during this test should be noted.

The anterior interosseus nerve is a branch of the median nerve in the proximal forearm that supplies the flexor pollicis longus, the flexor digitorum profundus to the index finger, and the pronator quadratus (Fig. 11-8). It does not suppy sensory fibers to any skin areas. Compression of this median nerve branch therefore shows a characteristic alteration of pinch posture with absent flexion at the distal joints of the thumb and index finger, but sensation is normal.

Median nerve conduction velocity may be slowed, but this test is far less accurate for compressions around the elbow than it is at the wrist. An

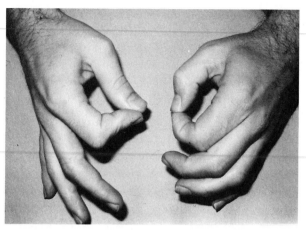

FIGURE 11-8. Anterior interosseous syndrome is characterized by palsy of the pronator quadratis, flexor digitorum profundus to the index finger, and flexor pollicis longus. When forceful pinch is attempted, weakness in the latter two muscles causes a collapse of the distal joints of the index finger and thumb into an extended position.

electromyogram may show denervation, and this test is accurate confirmation for anterior interosseous nerve compression. Even though the electromyogram and nerve conduction studies may identify a median nerve lesion in only 15% to 20% of patients with compression around the elbow, they should be obtained to distinguish other peripheral nerve problems that may have similar symptoms.

The vague symptoms and subtle physical findings, along with the likelihood of nonconfirmatory electrical studies, make the diagnosis difficult. Some patients may be misdiagnosed as having carpal tunnel syndrome and have persistent symptoms after carpal tunnel release. Others may be suspected of malingering disease or of being neurotic.

Initial treatment for median nerve compression around the elbow should consist of rest and oral nonsteroidal antiinflammatory medication. If symptoms are not relieved, surgical decompression should be considered. Despite any tentative localization of the site of compression on the preoperative physical examination, the nerve should be explored in the distal third of the arm, through the elbow area, and into the proximal third of the forearm, relieving any fascial constraints. Surgical incisions in the antecubital area often leave unsightly scars, and the patient should be advised of this possibility.

Postoperative recovery may be slow and incomplete. Tendon transfers should be considered for persistent disabling weakness of the palsied muscles.

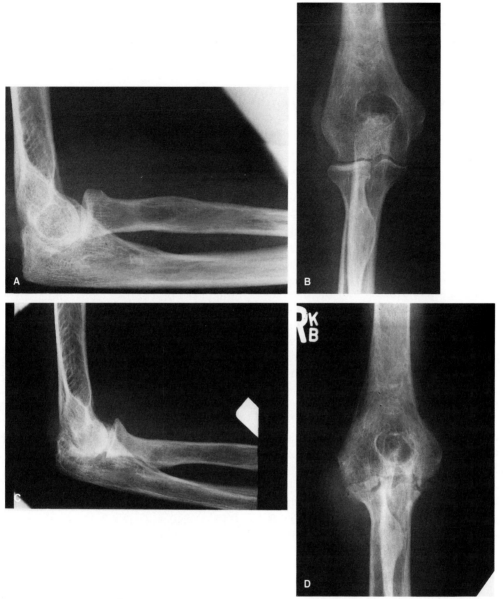

FIGURE 11-9. Significant rheumatoid destruction in this elbow occurred over a 3-year period. In the initial films (**A** and **B**), the joint appears normal except for slight anterior subluxation of the radius on the capitellum. In the later films (**C** and **D**), cartilage loss is noted both in the radial capitellar joint and in the ulnar trochlear portions of the joint, along with further deformity of the radial head.

Radial Nerve

Compression of the radial nerve in the elbow area is far less common than compression of the ulnar nerve. In addition, the symptoms, physical findings, and diagnostic studies can be nonspecific, making the diagnosis difficult.

Immediately after crossing the radiocapitellar portion of the elbow joint, the radial nerve divides into superficial and deep branches. The superficial

branch continues directly distally under cover of the brachioradialis to provide sensation on the dorsum of the thumb and index finger. The deep branch curves around the radius, passes through the supinator muscle, emerges on the dorsal forearm, and becomes the posterior interosseous nerve. The common site of compression is a fibrous leading edge of the supinator muscle, and the nerve is indented here as it passes to the dorsal side of the forearm. A fibrous band in the proximal portion of the extensor carpi radialis brevis may also irritate the nerve, and at times a crossing vessel may indent and compress the nerve.

Sensory changes are not a normal part of radial nerve compression because compression on the radial nerve proximal to its bifurcation is rare and the deep branch of the radial nerve does not contain any cutaneous sensory fibers. In severe cases of radial nerve compression, patients may complain of loss of dexterity with such finger extension activities as typing and piano playing, and wrist and finger extension is weak on examination. In these patients, the diagnosis is relatively easy, and compression of the radial nerve in the proximal forearm needs to be differentiated only from more proximal causes of neuropathy. For less severe compressions, contraction of overlying muscles may increase the pain. Thus, resisted forearm supination with the elbow flexed, resisted wrist extension, and resisted middle finger extension should all be tested. Full passive pronation of the forearm and flexion of the wrist may also tighten the responsible fascia. Most commonly, however, the neuropathy is not sufficiently severe to cause discernible weakness or even an increase in pain with muscle contraction, but just a vague, diffuse ache in the proximal forearm. The only consistently positive physical finding is tenderness of the nerve as it passes around the radial neck. This site, unfortunately, is only several centimeters distal to the lateral epicondyle, so radial tunnel syndrome may be misdiagnosed as tennis elbow. To make matters worse, tennis elbow and radial tunnel syndrome can coexist.

Conservative treatment consists of rest, nonsteroidal antiinflammatory medication and use of a wrist cock-up splint. The splint holds the wrist extended and diminishes activity in the extensor carpi radialis brevis. Theoretically, immobilization of the forearm in supination would relax the fibrous portion of the supinator over the deep branch of the radial nerve, but this treatment for any length of time proves to be a greater disability itself than the symptoms from the nerve compression. If lateral epicondylitis is thought to coexist, then cortisone injection into the extensor origin should be considered. If symptoms persist, the nerve should be explored and decompressed. The nerve can be approached through a short brachioradialis-splitting incision or a long extensile exposure across the antecubital crease. The former leaves less skin disfigurement. The latter offers more extensive exposure of the nerve.

Many patients get complete and prompt relief, but some wait many months before maximal benefit is noted, and even then, some aching may persist.

RHEUMATOID ARTHRITIS

In patients with rheumatoid arthritis, at least one third eventually show involvement of their elbows. Even so, elbow involvement to a degree of major functional limitation that requires surgical consideration is much less common than involvement of other joints. When pain and loss of motion do occur, however, the resultant disability is profound (Fig. 11-9).

Intraarticular synovial proliferation gradually destroys the cartilage surfaces and underlying bony supports. Crepitation is followed by progressively limited motion and progressively severe deformity as the joint architecture is destroyed. The rheumatoid synovitis also weakens the supporting ligaments. Laxity of the annular ligament allows the radial head to subluxate anteriorly because of the unopposed pull of the biceps, and laxity of the medial collateral ligament, particularly in concert with

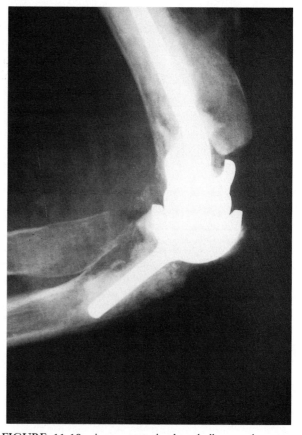

FIGURE 11-10. A nonconstrained total elbow replacement has been performed for rheumatoid arthritis. The patient's natural ligaments provide support for this resurfacing type of arthroplasty.

bony destruction, allows instability in the medio-lateral plane.

Even if the patient's hand function is well preserved, limited painful elbow motion greatly restricts placement of the hand and thereby greatly diminishes the patient's independence. Furthermore, the upper limbs in patients with rheumatoid arthritis are often called on for weight-bearing responsibilities because a cane, crutch, or walker may be needed for ambulation. In these cases, the importance of a stable, pain-free elbow is magnified.

On examination, elbow flexion extension range and forearm rotation range are measured. Crepitation noted during elbow flexion and extension may be coming from either the radiocapitellar or ulnotrochlear component of the joint, but crepitation noted during forearm rotation is coming from arthritic changes in the radiocapitellar joint. Any tenderness, synovial thickening, and joint instability are noted. When the examination is carefully performed, the radiographs basically confirm the physical findings regarding the degree of rheumatoid involvement.

The diagnosis of rheumatoid elbow involvement is straightforward, but the findings must be put in context of the patient's general disease, weight-bearing requirements, and activity level.

Like other rheumatoid joint involvement, synovitis at the elbow should first be managed my medical means. If concerted trials of oral medications do not control the synovium, an occasional intraarticular steroid injection may focus sufficient antiinflammatory power to quiet the inflammation.

Surgical synovectomy is the next step in treatment if the synovium remains inflamed. The synovectomy is usually performed through a lateral approach in combination with a radial head excision. Removal of the proximal radius not only improves forearm rotation by relieving radiocapitellar impingement but also allows improved surgical access to other portions of the joint and enhances the thoroughness of the synovectomy. Elbow synovectomy is useful for healing rheumatoid destruction and is most effective when performed before bone deformity and ligament laxity are pronounced. Even if performed later, when moderately severe changes are noted in the medial half of the joint, the results can be surprisingly good and long-lasting.

For severely disabling elbow involvement, total joint replacement is the accepted treatment (Fig. 11-

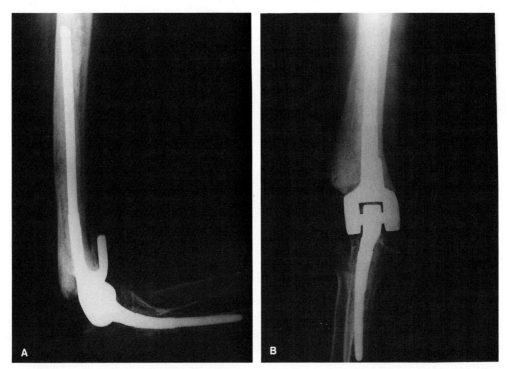

FIGURE 11-11. Because of markedly deficient distal humeral bone, a semiconstrained type of arthroplasty has been performed in this elbow. The metallic stems of the humeral and ulnar components are fixed to bone with methyl methacrylate cement. Together, the components function as a loose hinge.

10). Fascial arthroplasty was performed before the development of total elbow replacement, but the predictability of a good result is now better with total joint arthroplasty. The only current indication for a fascial arthroplasty is in a previously infected joint. Elbow arthrodesis is not used because, even though it would relieve pain, the functional impairment due to extremely limited hand placement would be profound.

Two types of total elbow replacement are available, and the choice depends on the degree of bone and ligament destruction. When the overall bone architecture and ligament supports are fairly well preserved, a resurfacing type of arthroplasty is preferred. This consists of a metal humeral component simulating the natural bony contour of the trochlea and a polyethylene component simulating the natural contour of the proximal ulna (Fig. 11-11). The radial head is excised and not replaced. Thus, smooth, gliding surfaces are restored, and elbow stability depends on the natural integrity of the ligaments. For more severe bone and ligament destruction, a hinge type of arthroplasty is preferred. This depends only on secure stem fixation into the medullary canals of the humerus and ulna. Pain relief is consistently achieved using either type of prosthesis. More motion is consistently recovered when using a hinged prosthesis than a resurfacing prosthesis. With the hinged implant, the soft tissue release can be more complete.

Complications related to total elbow arthroplasty are multiple and significant. Ulnar nerve palsy and delayed wound healing may be noted shortly after surgery. Joint dislocation for the resurfacing type of arthroplasty, implant loosening for the hinge type of arthroplasty, and infection for both types all lead to surgical failure. Careful surgical management minimizes all these problems. The patient also needs to avoid forceful and impact-related activities to preclude mechanical failure. The patient also must request antibacterial prophylaxis when undergoing dental or surgical procedures to minimize the risk of an infecting bacteremia.

Annotated Bibliography

Congenital Radial Head Dislocation

Kelly DW. Congenital dislocation of the radial head: spectrum and natural history. J Pediatr Orthop 1981;1:295.
Twenty-four patients with congenital radial head dislocations all were noted to have some limitation of wrist motion as well as limitation of forearm and elbow motions. Two thirds of the patients had other anomalies, but four patients had unilateral elbow involvement as an isolated anomaly.

Mardam-Bey T, Ger E. Congenital radial head dislocation. J Hand Surg 1979;4:316.
Fifty patients with 77 affected elbows were reviewed for symptoms, functional limitations, diagnostic features, and treatment results. Nearly 50% of patients also had other anomalies in the affected extremity, and 70% had anomalies elsewhere. Pain and loss of motion were minimal.

Congenital Radioulnar Synostosis

Green WT, Mital MA. Congenital radioulnar synostosis: surgical treatment. J Bone Joint Surg 1979;61:738.
Thirteen patients underwent rotational osteotomy, and results were assessed. Recommended position for the nondominant forearm is 20 to 35 degrees of supination. The other limb can then be left in considerable pronation.

Simmons BP, Southmayd WW, Riseborough EJ. Congenital radioulnar synostosis. J Hand Surg 1983;8:829.
Thirty-three patients underwent rotational osteotomy for radioulnar synostosis. Function and appearance were generally improved. Recommended positions for the forearms are 10 to 20 degrees of pronation for the dominant limb and neutral rotation for the other.

Panner Disease

Omer GE Jr. Primary articular osteochondroses. Clin Orthop 1981;158:33.
All the osteochondroses, including Panner disease, are reviewed with respect to incidence, pathophysiology, symptoms, and treatment. Osteochondrosis of the capitellum causes much less deformity and disability than osteochondrosis of the second metatarsal head, presumably because of the body weight–bearing forces exerted on the latter.

Panner HJ. An affection of the capitellum humeri resembling Calvé-Perthes' disease of the hip. Acta Radiol 1927;8:617.
These two cases are Panner's original observations of osteochondrosis of the capitellum. Boys aged 9 and 11 noted mild loss of motion and minimal pain. Radiographs showed a "curious flossiness and diminution of the osseous center of the capitellum humerii."

Osteochondritis Dissecans of the Elbow

Mitsunaga MM, Adishian DO, Bianco AJ Jr. Osteochondritis dissecans of the capitellum. J Trauma 1982;22:53.
Fifty-seven patients with 66 elbows affected by osteochondritis dissecans were followed an average of 14 years after treatment. Twenty-five loose-body excisions were performed, with 60% excellent results. All the patients with displaced fragments who did not undergo surgery had pain at follow-up. About half of the remaining patients had residual pain. Continued catching and locking symptoms also occurred more often in patients with displaced fragments and most often in those who did not have displaced fragments removed.

Tennis Elbow

Heyse-Moore G. Resistant tennis elbow. J Hand Surg 1984;9B:64.
In an anatomic and clinical study, the author showed that the origin of the extensor carpi radialis brevis from the lateral epicondyle and the superficial portion of the supinator are blended and inseparable. Thus, a surgical opening of the supinator fascia has the same effect on relieving undue tension on the lateral epicondyle as sectioning the origin of the extensor carpi radialis brevis. This anatomic observation may help explain the confusion in differentiating the diagnosis, treatment, and outcome of lateral epicondylitis from radial tunnel syndrome.

Nirschl PR, Pettrone FA. Tennis elbow: the surgical treatment of lateral epicondylitis. J Bone Joint Surg 1979;61A:832.
Eighty-eight patients operated on for tennis elbow uniformly demonstrated immature fibrous and vascular tissue in the origin of the extensor carpi radialis brevis. Excision of the granulation tissue and repair of the tendon origin gave consistently good results.

Olecranon Bursitis

Canoso JJ. Idiopathic or traumatic olecranon bursitis: clinical features and bursal fluid analysis. Arthritis Rheum 1977;20:1213.
Thirty patients with idiopathic olecranon bursitis were studied. Most had previous local trauma. The bursal fluid was serosanguineous, and the mucin clot test was fair to poor. White blood cell count averaged 878/μL. Glucose, total protein, and C3 complement concentrations averaged 80%, 60%, and 60% of the serum values, respectively.

Viggiano DA. Septic arthritis presenting as olecranon bursitis in patients with rheumatoid arthritis. J Bone Joint Surg 1980;62A:1011.
Three patients with rheumatoid arthritis whose elbow septic arthritis initially presented as olecranon bursitis are discussed. An abnormal communication between the olecranon bursa and the joint may result from rheumatoid destruction of the normal articular capsular supports. In such cases, an acute flare of the patient's rheumatoid arthritis may be difficult to distinguish from an infection.

Nerve Entrapments Around the Elbow

Goldberg BJ, Light TR, Blair SJ. Ulnar neuropathy at the elbow: results of medial epicondylectomy. J Hand Surg 1989;14A:182.
Medial epicondylectomy provides a predictable result for cubital tunnel syndrome. Symptomatic improvement is nearly universal, and strength is improved in over half of patients. The completeness of recovery is directly related to the degree of the compression before operation.

Hartz CR, Linscheid RL, Grause RR, Daube JR. The pronator teres syndrome: compressive neuropathy of the median nerve. J Bone Joint Surg 1981;63A:885.
Clinical findings, electrodiagnostic testing, and treatment results for 39 patients with median nerve compression around the elbow are reviewed. Forearm aching, hand weakness, and index and thumb numbness were the common symptoms. Electrical testing rarely identified the exact compression site. The patients generally responded to surgical decompression.

Johnson RK, Spinner M, Shrewsbury MM. Median nerve entrapment syndrome in the proximal forearm. J Hand Surg 1979;4:48.
The syndrome occurs more commonly in women than in men. Age and handedness are not predisposing factors. Three stress tests are described to localize the site of compression at the biceps fascia, at the pronator teres, or at the flexor digitorum superficialis arch. The pronator teres is the most common site of compression.

Moss SH, Switzer HE. Radial tunnel syndrome: a spectrum of clinical presentations. J Hand Surg 1983;8:414.
The anatomy and sites of compression along with the clinical presentations and treatment results in 15 patients are reviewed. Surgical decompression relieved the symptoms of popping, paresthesia, and paresis in all but one of the patients.

Ogata K, Manske PR, Lesker PA. The effect of surgical dissection on regional blood flow to the ulnar nerve in the cubital tunnel. Clin Orthop 1985;193:195.
In an experimental study using nonhuman primates and the hydrogen washout technique, anterior transposition of the ulnar nerve at the elbow was associated with a significant decrease in local nerve blood flow for at least 3 days. Blood flow changes were not noted with medial epicondylectomy or simple unroofing of the nerve.

Werner C. Lateral elbow pain and posterior interosseous nerve entrapment. Acta Orthop Scand 1979;174(Suppl):1.
The diagnosis and treatment of radial nerve compression in the proximal forearm are thoroughly reviewed. The findings are contrasted with those of tennis elbow.

Rheumatoid Arthritis

Copeland SA, Taylor JG. Synovectomy of the elbow in rheumatoid arthritis: the place of excision of the head of the radius. J Bone Joint Surg 1979;61B:69.
Nearly all patients experienced pain relief, and two thirds regained elbow motion after elbow synovectomy. The results were no different whether the radial head was excised or retained.

Goldberg VM, Figgie HE III, Inglis AE, Figgie MP. Current concepts review: total elbow arthroplasty. J Bone Joint Surg 1988;70A:778.
Anatomic and biomechanical considerations, indications and contraindications, implant types, results, and complications are all discussed. With appropriate patient selection and surgical technique, pain relief is consistently achieved, and motion may be improved. Results continue to improve as more is learned about implant design, positioning, and fixation.

Low WG, Evans JP. Synovectomy of the elbow and excision of the radial head in rheumatoid arthritis. South Med J 1980;73:707.
Even in advanced stages of rheumatoid involvement, elbow synovectomy provided good pain relief and an increased motion arc.

Turek's Orthopaedics: Principles and Their Application, Fifth Edition,
edited by Stuart L. Weinstein and Joseph A. Buckwalter.
J.B. Lippincott Company, Philadelphia, © 1994.

12

Roy A. Meals

The Wrist and Hand

RADIAL DEFICIENCY
THUMB HYPOPLASIA AND
  APLASIA
ULNAR DEFICIENCY
MADELUNG DEFORMITY
CONGENITAL TRIGGER THUMB
POLYDACTYLY
SYNDACTYLY
CAMPTODACTYLY
CLINODACTYLY
ACQUIRED TRIGGER FINGER
DE QUERVAIN TENOSYNOVITIS
CARPAL TUNNEL SYNDROME

ULNAR NERVE ENTRAPMENT
  AT THE WRIST
GANGLION
DUPUYTREN CONTRACTURE
KIENBÖCK DISEASE
OSTEOARTHRITIS
RHEUMATOID ARTHRITIS
  Wrist
  Metacarpophalangeal Joints
  Interphalangeal Joints
  Thumb
  Tendon
  Rheumatoid Nodules

RADIAL DEFICIENCY

Defective formation and development of the limb bud early in fetal life results in an anomalous limb. Such a defect can be either longitudinally or transversely oriented on the limb bud. Transverse defects lead to limb shortening with absence of the hand or a more proximal portion of the limb. Longitudinal defects lead to abnormalities and absences either on the preaxial (radial) or postaxial (ulnar) border of the limb. Although familial cases do occur, most are sporadic and are related to some chemical or other environmental insult, usually unknown, early in development.

When the preaxial portion of the limb is affected, the radius and thumb are hypoplastic or absent along with corresponding anomalies of the radial forearm muscles and neurovascular elements. This defective development causes a characteristic bowing of the forearm and radial deviation of the hand on the end of a well-formed ulna. This condition has been likened to clubfoot and therefore called *radial club hand*. It occurs about once per 100,000 births, and involvement can be either unilateral or bilateral. Multiple other anomalies, including cardiac septal defects, tracheo-esophageal fistulas, anal atresia, renal and vertebral defects, and aplastic anemia, are frequently associated and must therefore be specifically sought (Fig. 12-1).

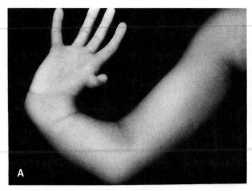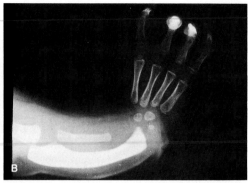

FIGURE 12-1. (A) In radial aplasia, the muscles of the forearm displace the unsupported hand into radial deviation. Thumb hypoplasia or absence is common. (B) Another patient with radial club hand shows characteristic radial deviation, a hypoplastic radius, bowing of the ulna, and an absent first ray.

The degree of limb abnormality is variable, and the conditions of the thumb and the radius are not linked. The radius can be well-formed and the thumb completely absent, for example, or the radius can be absent and the thumb only slightly hypoplastic. Overall, the limb is short, and the hand is unstable and radially deviated on the ulna because of insufficient radial support. Finger joint contractures are common. Elbow flexion may also be restricted. The functional disability resulting from radial club hand is proportional to the degrees of elbow stiffness, deviation of the wrist, and hypoplasia of the thumb that are present. When the wrist and hand are completely unstable on the distal radial border of the ulna, contraction of the finger flexor muscles augments the deformity because it draws the hand into further radial deviation rather than providing strong grasp.

Treatment should also be proportionate to the degree of involvement. Those patients with only a mild shortening and bowing of the radius and with a functional thumb need no treatment at all. For partial absence of the radius with moderate radial deviation of the hand, serial casting followed by night splinting until maturity may suffice. For subtotal and total absences of the radius, surgical centralization of the carpus on the distal ulna positions the hand so that the finger flexor and extensor tendons can function at maximal efficiency. If the ulna is bowed more than 30 degrees, a corrective osteotomy further improves the limb alignment. The surgery is best performed at about 6 months of age after as much passive correction as possible has been achieved by serial casting. Waiting longer invites fixed soft tissue contractures, which are difficult to overcome. By the

time a patient with an uncorrected radial club hand has reached adulthood, functional patterns have been firmly established. At that point, it generally is more disabling to have the hand repositioned and to modify firmly ingrained patterns of use. Another important contraindication to surgery is the presence of inadequate elbow flexion. Even when the elbow is stiff in extension, the shortened, bowed forearm and the radially deviated carpus allow placement of the hand near the face and mouth. Realigning the hand on the forearm precludes this important function when the elbow cannot adequately flex.

The centralization surgery releases the contracted soft tissues radially, tightens the flexor and extensor carpi ulnaris tendons on the ulnar side, and holds the corrected position of the carpus on the end of the ulna with a Kirschner wire for about 8 weeks. Thereafter, the wrist is splinted continuously until 6 years of age, and at night until growth is complete. The same longitudinal wire holding the corrected carpal alignment on the ulna can secure a wedge osteotomy in the ulna when that is required for further straightening.

The most common complication of centralization is failure to achieve a lasting improvement in position. The causes are inadequate release of soft tissue contractures, incomplete reduction and fixation of the carpus on the ulna, insufficient distal advancement of the transferred tendons to counter the deforming forces, and patient noncompliance with postoperative splint use. Pin tract infections are occasionally encountered. They can usually be managed with antibiotics, avoiding premature pin removal and loss of reduction.

THUMB HYPOPLASIA AND APLASIA

Incomplete development of the thumb can occur in conjunction with more proximal defects of preaxial limb development. It can also occur as an isolated anomaly. The spectrum of observed abnormalities varies from slight hypoplasia with excellent function to complete absence of the thumb and associated carpal bones.

The mildly hypoplastic thumb needs no treatment. If thenar muscles are absent or incompletely formed so that opposition is limited, a tendon or muscle transfer can restore this important function. When the hypothenar musculature is well formed, transferring the abductor digiti minimi across the palm on its proximal neurovascular pedicle provides excellent thumb opposition and thenar contour. Moderately hypoplastic thumbs are distally based, lack multiple muscles, and have spindle-like skeletal support. Severely hypoplastic thumbs lack any muscle control, have only vestigial skeletal support, and may be attached only by a narrow skin pedicle. They are appropriately called *floating thumbs.* Patients without thumbs develop unique prehensile patterns with their other digits. For the patient with an untreated radial deficiency and an absent thumb, grasp and manipulation of small objects is commonly performed between the two most ulnar digits because these are the closest to horizontal work surfaces. For a patient with a normally formed forearm but absent thumb, the radial digits can be brought close to horizontal surfaces by pronating the forearm, and small object manipulation is more often performed between the two most radial digits. Over time, the index ray shows some spontaneous tendency for pronation and opposition to the middle digit.

Depending on the degree of thumb hypoplasia, a decision must be made whether to attempt to correct the deficiencies or to ablate the ray and pollicize the index finger. Tendon and muscle transfers are usually successful when the skeleton is adequate, but when the bone is severely deficient, conversion to a four digit hand provides the best functioning and appearing hand. For complete aplasia, the decision to pollicize the index finger is easier because no vestigial thumb is present to give false hope of providing five functional digits.

Toe-to-hand microsurgical transfers for thumb construction in congenital absences has been considered, but the procedure is long and tedious and risks vascular failure. More important, the function of a transferred toe is inadequate because the necessary tendons and nerves in the forearm to control the transfer are generally deficient. Thus, pollicization of the index ray is the preferred treatment.

Pollicization entails shortening, rotating, and abducting the index ray while leaving its neurovascular supply intact and reattaching available intrinsic muscles. This allows the index ray to look and function like a thumb. Most of the index metacarpal is discarded. The index metacarpophalangeal joint becomes the carpometacarpal joint of the new thumb. The index proximal and distal interphalangeal joints become the metacarpophalangeal and interphalangeal joints, respectively, of the new thumb.

Vascular compromise with loss of the pollicized index ray would be a disastrous complication in an already severely compromised hand. Careful intraoperative management of the vascular pedicles and close postoperative monitoring are necessary. Removal of stitches and derotation of the pollicized digit may be required if vascular compromise is suspected.

ULNAR DEFICIENCY

Just as an insult to the radial aspect of the limb bud early during fetal development can lead to radial deficiencies, an insult to the postaxial or ulnar aspect can lead to ulnar deficiencies. These occur less commonly than radial deficiencies, at the rate of 1 to 4 per 1 million births. In contrast to radial deficiencies, which are frequently associated with visceral anomalies, ulnar deficiencies are not associated with visceral anomalies but instead with other musculoskeletal abnormalities. These include spina bifida, proximal femoral focal deficiency, fibular aplasia, clubfoot, and defects in the opposite upper extremity.

The clinical picture reflects the shortened or absent ulna and the generalized insult to the postaxial portion of the limb bud. The ulnar digits are hypoplastic or absent, and the remaining digits are frequently webbed. The thumb is routinely hypoplastic or absent. Why this and other abnormalities on the preaxial side of the limb occur is not known. The hand is deviated medially on the forearm, but usually only to a slight degree. The elbow is variably affected, with the defects ranging from instability to ankylosis. An internal rotation deformity of the humerus may be present that positions the shortened, bowed forearm and hand at rest near the posterior axillary line (Fig. 12-2).

The treatment is directed at preventing or correcting joint instability and limb malposition. Although the cause is controversial, growth of the distal

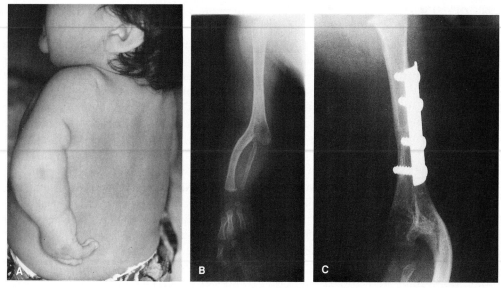

FIGURE 12-2. (A) A marked internal rotation deformity of the limb is characteristic of ulnar aplasia. The hand typically rests near the posterior axillary line, and it is poorly positioned for functional activities. (B) Ulnar aplasia may include fusion of the radius with the lateral humerus, a residual hypoplastic ulna, and missing rays. (C) A derotational osteotomy of the humerus has been performed to provide a more functional upper extremity by repositioning the hand in front of the trunk.

radius may cause additional bowing. Some believe that the ulnar margin of the distal radius epiphysis is affected and grows more slowly than the radial margin. Others think that the fibrocartilaginous anlage of the ulna tethers longitudinal growth on the ulnar side. Resection of the anlage may be required for severe or progressive ulnar deviation of the carpus on the radius, increased radial bowing, or dislocation of the radial head. Corrective osteotomy of the radius and creation of a one-bone forearm when the radial head is fully dislocated may improve limb stability and hand placement. A derotational osteotomy of the humerus repositions the hand in front of the trunk. Syndactyly releases improve the function and appearance of the webbed fingers.

MADELUNG DEFORMITY

Madelung deformity is a growth retardation on the ulnar and anterior portions of the distal radius epiphysis (Fig. 12-3). Madelung described this painful deformity of the wrist over 100 years ago without the aid of radiographs. This differential growth compared to the radial and posterior portions of the radius epiphysis causes an anterior and ulnar bowing of the distal forearm with subsequent loss of extension and radial deviation of the wrist. The distal ulna epiphysis is unaffected, so the ulna grows straight and becomes

prominent dorsally as it outgrows the defective radial epiphysis. When the limb is viewed laterally, the hand and wrist lie in a plane anterior to the forearm.

The deformity is a genetic disorder, and a hereditary form is transmitted in an autosomal dominant manner. Overall, the deformity is much more common in females, and it is usually bilateral. It is frequently diagnosed during adolescence. Generalized skeletal dysplasia is often present to some degree, with short stature and other defects of normal cartilage and bone development being common. Distortions of the normal distal forearm anatomy that can simulate Madelung deformity occur with epiphyseal injuries and syndromes such as Turner, Miller, dyschondrosteosis, and diaphyseal aclasis.

Persistent pain and extreme deformity are indications for treatment. The pain is usually associated with impingement of the carpus against the ulna as the carpus gets wedged in the gap between the radius and ulna. The degree of deformity is variable, so the choice of surgery must be individualized. Epiphysiodesis of the distal ulna and the radial portion of the distal radius has been used in younger patients when significant growth potential remains. Distal ulna resection in older patients may be all that is required for mild deformity. For severe deformity, a biplane wedge osteotomy of the distal radius with ulnar shortening or distal ulna excision is used when growth is complete or nearing completion. After sur-

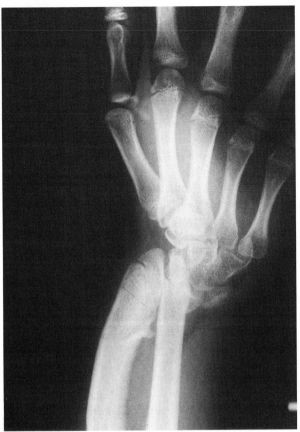

FIGURE 12-3. Madelung deformity results from differential growth of the lateral and posterior portions of the distal radius epiphysis. The ulna continues to grow straight and forces the hand and wrist anterior to the forearm.

gery, most patients note increased strength and decreased pain but little change in overall wrist and forearm motion.

CONGENITAL TRIGGER THUMB

A size discrepancy between a flexor tendon and its surrounding fibroosseous canal can impede normal gliding of the tendon and produce locking of the primary joint controlled by that tendon. In infants and young children, this mechanical impedance is seen frequently in the thumb and rarely in other digits. The thumb interphalangeal joint is usually fixed in flexion and cannot be passively extended even with considerable force. Snapping from a fully extended to a fully flexed position, a common finding in the adult form of stenosing tenosynovitis, is uncommonly seen in the infantile form.

The occurrence is generally sporadic, although siblings and sequential generations of family mem-

bers can be affected (Fig. 12-4). Some patients have bilateral involvement, but not necessarily to the same degree. The etiology is unknown, and although trigger thumbs can be noted at birth, the condition is not clearly genetic in origin. Thickening of the sheath and the underlying flexor pollicis longus tendon account for the mechanical blockage.

The average age when the condition is noted is 2 years. Perhaps it is present at birth but overlooked until the child develops functional pinch patterns that demonstrate the loss of motion. A nodule is palpable at the proximal flexion crease of the thumb, and with full metacarpophalangeal joint extension, a bulge from the thickened sheath and tendon can be seen under the skin. The affected area is not tender.

Thirty percent of trigger thumbs noted at birth resolve spontaneously by 1 year of age, so there is no rush to operate. A lower spontaneous resolution rate in older infants warrants waiting perhaps 6 months before recommending surgery. Children older than 3 years of age with trigger thumbs should have the constricting annular pulley released when diagnosed to avoid permanent stiffness or abnormal bone development at the interphalangeal joint.

The patient requires a brief general anesthetic to allow release of the constricting band. Both digital nerves are in close proximity to the pathology and must be protected. Use of absorbable sutures in the skin precludes the need for eventual suture removal.

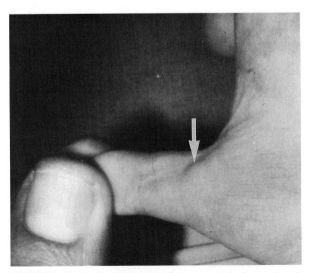

FIGURE 12-4. Examination of a congenital trigger thumb usually reveals a palpable nodular thickening at the proximal flexion crease of the thumb. The nodule is formed from the thickened flexor tendon sheath and underlying tendon enlargement.

POLYDACTYLY

Polydactyly means extra digits, and this condition is classified as either preaxial, central, or postaxial (Fig. 12-5). Preaxial polydactyly involves duplication of the thumb. Postaxial polydactyly involves duplication on the ulnar border of the hand. Syndactyly often occurs with duplication of the central rays, leading to the term *central polysyndactyly*.

Syndactyly and polydactyly are the two most common congenital anomalies seen in the hand. Depending on the population studied, one may be more common than the other. Hand surgeons generally do not see the full scope of polydactyly because the vestigial postaxial duplication attached only by a small skin pedicle is often tied off in the newborn nursery by the obstetrician or pediatrician.

Preaxial polydactyly occurs once per 12,000 live births and does not have a strong racial variation. The spectrum of thumb duplication ranges from a slightly broadened nail and distal phalanx to a fully duplicated phalangeal and metacarpal skeleton and all associated digital nerves and tendons.

Thumb triplication can occur. Nearly all thumb duplications are sporadic occurrences, although familial incidence is known. Associated anomalies do not occur nearly as frequently as with postaxial polydactyly, but a general evaluation is still warranted because musculoskeletal and visceral anomalies are associated along with hematopoietic and nervous system disorders.

The thumbs may not be identically sized, and in unilateral cases, both parts are generally slightly hypoplastic compared with the opposite thumb. More for appearance than function, the less well-formed digit is usually removed, using its tissue elements as necessary to construct ligaments, to centralize tendons, and to improve pulp contour and bulk. The most common complication of thumb duplication surgery is joint instability from inadequate construction of ligaments.

Although duplication of the central digits can occur without associated syndactyly, it is rare. More likely, the duplicated rays are fused to adjacent digits. Bilateral involvement is frequent, and girls are affected more than boys. Autosomal dominant inheritance is common, and associated anomalies are usually restricted to polydactyly and syndactyly of the toes.

Central polysyndactyly is one of the most vexing problems in congenital hand surgery. The bones are frequently malformed, and transversely oriented phalanges, triangular-shaped phalanges, and side-to-side coalitions are common. Tendon, nerve, and arterial anomalies abound, and sophisticated intraoperative decision making is required to plan the best solution to the specific anomalies encountered. Thus, the formation of a normally contoured and supple five-digit hand is far more complex than simply removing the extra digital tissue and recessing the webs.

The bones of all affected central digits may be spindle-like and unsuitable for supporting the soft tissues on a separated digit. In these cases, preservation of a fused central digital mass or reduction to a four-digit hand provides a more functional hand than when the elusive goal of five normal digits is rigidly pursued.

Postaxial polydactyly is the most common type of polydactyly, occurring eight times more commonly than preaxial and central polydactyly. In blacks, the

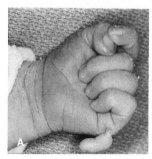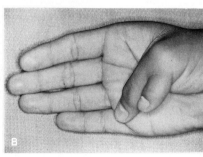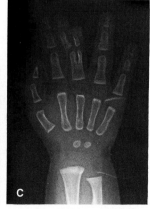

FIGURE 12-5. (A) Postaxial polydactyly is most commonly manifested by a small hypoplastic digit, which requires only ligation in the newborn nursery. (B) Preaxial polydactyly affects the thumb. The hypoplastic radial portion can be removed for improved appearance. (C) Central duplication is the least common form of polydactyly and is frequently associated with syndactyly.

incidence of postaxial supranumerary digits is 1 per 300 live births compared with 1 per 3000 in whites. In blacks, postaxial polydactyly is an autosomal dominant inherited trait and occurs as an isolated anomaly. In other races, a wide spectrum of associated congenital anomalies occurs in conjunction with postaxial polydactyly, so a thorough patient evaluation is in order. Associated anomalies have been noted in the musculoskeletal, genitourinary, digestive, circulatory, and nervous systems as well as in chromosome configuration.

The treatment depends on the degree of duplication. For the very small, poorly formed extra digit, ligation in the newborn nursery is appropriate. For the larger digit that may share a joint, nerve, tendon, or artery with its mate, more complex surgery when the child is 6 to 12 months old is required.

SYNDACTYLY

Syndactyly means joined digits or webbed fingers, and in some populations, it is the most common congenital anomaly that occurs in the upper limbs.

Syndactyly is usually related to a failure of differentiation. During the sixth and seventh weeks of gestation, the hand develops five ridges and terminal digit buds, which grow distally and separate from one another (Fig. 12-6). If this normal separation fails to occur, the digits remain webbed. This failure of differentiation occurs sporadically perhaps 80% of the time and is familial in the remainder of cases. It occurs once in about 2000 births, it is present bilaterally as often as not, and it occurs more frequently in boys. For no known reason, the first postaxial cleft in both the hands and feet is the one most commonly affected. In the hands, this is the interval between the middle and ring fingers, and in the feet, the interval between the second and third toes. In the hand, the fourth, second, and first intervals are progressively less commonly affected.

Syndactyly is classified as complete or incomplete and as simple or complex. Complete syndactyly is present when the webbing comes to the tips of the joined digits. In incomplete syndactyly, the web extends distally farther than normal but stops short of the fingertips. Complex syndactyly involves coalition of bone in the joined digits, and so-called simple syndactyly, although it does not involve bone, may involve ligaments, tendons, nerves, and arteries.

At the point of fetal development when the digital webs normally recede, many other organ systems are also at critical stages of development, so it is not surprising that many congenital anomalies in a variety of organ systems are associated with syndactyly. Thus, when syndactyly is noted at birth, a thorough evaluation searching for other anomalies is indicated. Two common syndromes involving syndactyly are Apert and Poland syndromes.

Apert syndrome, technically known as *acrocephalosyndactyly*, is a premature fusion of the cranial sutures associated with complex syndactyly of all five digits. The cranial synostosis causes a characteristic cranial deformity with frontal bossing and bulging, wide-set eyes. The complex syndactyly produces a common nail and a spoon-shaped hand. The proximal interphalangeal joints are incompletely formed or absent, resulting in marked digital stiffness.

Poland syndrome is the occurrence of limb hypoplasia with simple, usually incomplete syndactyly and absence of the ipsilateral pectoral muscle. As in Apert syndrome, the proximal interphalangeal joints are incompletely formed, and the small hand with webbed digits has been described as a "mitten hand." The absent pectoral muscle can be associated with more pronounced chest wall defects, such as pectus deformities and hypoplastic breast. The affected limb can have more pronounced hand deformities than syndactyly, such as absence of the central digits or even absence of the entire hand. Poland syndrome is more common in boys and more common on the right than the left. It is thought to be due to a vascular insult early during gestation when the limb bud and chest wall development are dependent on end-artery circulation, and transient ischemia causes the observed deformities.

Syndactyly is also commonly associated with cardiac problems and other skeletal abnormalities, such as facial defects. Less common associations with a diverse range of congenital anomalies abound.

A developmental type of syndactyly is seen in congenital constriction band syndrome. Here, digital formation and web recession occur normally, but later in fetal development, a portion of the amniotic sac becomes twisted around one or more limb parts, causing vascular compromise. If the ischemia is complete, an amputation ensues. If the ischemia is less severe, a deep scar band forms around the limb or digit. Digits with varying degrees of ischemia may heal to one another, creating an intrauterine, post-traumatic syndactyly. Small sinuses at the bases of the digits can almost always be observed. These are the normal web spaces that have been secondarily closed distally. *Acro* means distal, and so the syndactyly seen with congenital constriction band syndrome is appropriately termed *acrosyndactyly*. The digits are frequently misshapen with distorted, mis-

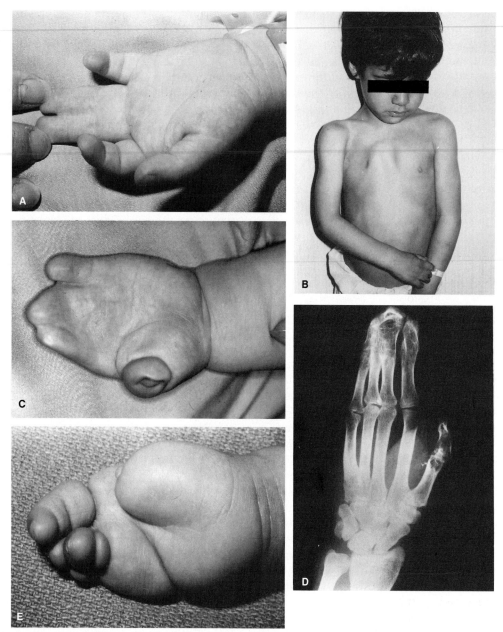

FIGURE 12-6. (A) The middle and ring fingers are most commonly affected in syndactyly. The coalition here does not involve bone and does not extend to the fingertips. It is therefore termed *simple, incomplete syndactyly*. (B) Poland syndrome includes absence of the pectoral musculature and general hypoplasia of the ipsilateral limb with simple syndactyly. (C) A spoon-shaped hand is characteristic of Apert acrocephalosyndactyly. (D) In Apert syndrome, the distal phalanges are joined, the interphalangeal joints are absent or poorly formed, and the fourth and fifth metacarpals are joined. (E) Several of the digits are joined distally, hence the descriptive term *acrosyndactyly*. In congenital constriction band syndrome, the digits form normally but are later damaged by encircling amniotic bands.

placed nubbins and have been described as having the appearance of dripped candle wax.

From whatever cause and regardless of what other congenital anomalies are present, hand function and appearance can generally be improved by separation of the joined digits. This, however, requires a complex preoperative and intraoperative decision-making process because the anomalies of skin, arteries, tendons, ligaments, joints, and bone rarely allow construction of a normally functioning and appearing hand.

Zig-zag incisions are made in the web, and local flaps are developed and closed over the exposed deep tissues. These oblique incisions break up the line of contracture of the postoperative scars and minimize development of secondary flexion contractures or other angular deformities of the digits. Careful planning is required to form a new web with a natural contour and at the appropriate, more proximal location. The natural web is concave on its distal margin, the dorsal surface slopes toward the palm as it extends distally, and the margin is even with the midportion of the proximal phalanges. Various local flaps have been designed to achieve these goals. Even when deep structures are not involved, there is not enough skin in the web to cover the exposed surfaces of the adjacent digits once the space is created. The need for skin grafting must therefore be anticipated. An elliptical piece of full-thickness skin is taken laterally from a groin crease to cover areas on the digits not covered by local flaps. The donor area can be closed as a straight-line incision, and the resultant scar is relatively inconspicuous.

Even in so-called simple syndactyly, the digital arteries and nerves may branch abnormally, complicating creation of a new web space. If the common digital nerve branches in an abnormally distal location, it can be teased apart into its component proper digital nerves. The division is brought sufficiently proximally so that it does not interfere with the skin rearrangement. A distally bifurcating digital artery must be divided, depriving one digit or the other from that blood supply. Thus, creation of web spaces on both sides of a digit should be staged at least 6 months apart with a great effort taken to preserve at least one digital artery to every digit to minimize risk of vascular compromise.

For complex syndactyly and in webbed fingers containing anomalous, triangular-shaped or transversely oriented phalangeal elements, skeletal alignment and stability must be addressed at the time of syndactyly release. Bone excision and corrective osteotomies may be required. In some cases, ablation of the bone from an entire central ray and use of that skin to reconstruct the remaining digits results in improved function and better appearance.

Surgical correction should be performed after sufficient growth has occurred to allow visualization and surgical manipulation of the affected tissues but before the child has acquired fully developed functional patterns. Results are best when surgery is deferred until at least 18 months of age. Earlier surgery may be indicated if a short border digit is tethering and thereby deforming the normal longitudinal growth of an adjacent digit. If multiple webs are involved, staged surgery should be planned to release the thumb and the third web at the first procedure and the second and fourth webs at the second. This completes the reconstruction in two procedures spaced 6 months apart, and the patient can use the thumb after the first operation.

Taking these surgical precautions into consideration results in only the rare occurrence of digital necrosis after syndactyly release. Scar contracture with secondary deformity is probably the most common postoperative complication. Parents should be advised that joints that appear stable before operation may be stabilized only by an adjacent, joined digit and that secondary correction of angular deformities may be required. Because the scarred skin incisions in the newly created web space do not grow as rapidly as uninjured tissue, some distal creep of the web can be anticipated during growth spurts. Therefore, the patient should be followed until growth is complete. An irksome complication of skin grafting is growth of pubic hair in the skin grafts. This can be avoided by taking the skin graft sufficiently laterally to be out of the area that will eventually be hair-bearing.

CAMPTODACTYLY

Camptodactyly means bent finger, and the term refers specifically to a nontraumatic flexion deformity of the proximal interphalangeal joint of the little finger (Fig. 12-7). To a mild degree, it occurs in about 1% of the population, it is commonly bilateral but not necessarily to an equal degree. Two forms are evident. One appears in infancy and affects males and females equally. The other appears during early adolescence and usually affects females. The former is more common. Its occurrence is usually sporadic, although an autosomal dominant inheritance is occasionally seen. Camptodactyly is seen in a variety of rare congenital syndromes and may be mistaken for posttraumatic joint stiffness, Dupuytren contracture, or muscle imbalance from injured tendons or nerves.

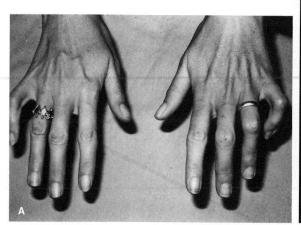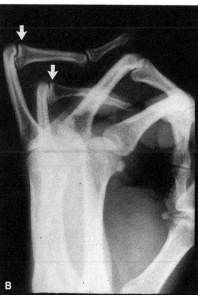

FIGURE 12-7. (A) *Camptodactyly* means "bent finger." This congenital nontraumatic flexion deformity must be distinguished from boutonniere deformity, ulnar nerve palsy, and other causes of joint contracture. (B) Articular changes at the proximal interphalangeal joints are characteristic of camptodactyly and are presumably related to growth alterations secondary to the contracture.

A variety of anatomic anomalies have been implicated as causes of camptodactyly. A short flexor superficialis or profundus tendon, anomalous or absent intrinsic muscles, skin contracture, and abnormal ligamentous support have all been described. The bony changes are most likely secondary to anomalies in the soft tissues.

The flexion contracture of the proximal interphalangeal joint is often progressive during growth, and when pronounced, may interfere with keyboard and gripping activities. It is not tender and therefore usually not noted until it hinders activity.

Because camptodactyly is usually not disabling and because the operative treatments are not particularly successful in consistently correcting the contracture, surgery should be recommended cautiously. If the deformity is both passively and actively correctable, a release of the flexor digitorum superficialis may relieve the imbalance. If passive joint extension is preserved but active extension is weak, then the superficialis insertion is transferred dorsally into the extensor mechanism. If a fixed flexion contracture is present, arthrodesis or extension osteotomy may be considered.

CLINODACTYLY

Clinodactyly is an angular deformity of a digit in the plane of the palm (Fig. 12-8). Although it may involve any digit, the usual deformity is a radial deviation of the little finger through the middle phalanx. Clinodactyly is associated with many congenital syndromes, and thus its presence warrants a thorough patient evaluation. Chromosomal disorders (especially mongolism), craniofacial syndromes, Holt-Oram syndrome, and myositis ossificans progressiva are among the related conditions.

Kirner deformity is a radial and anterior bowing of the distal phalanx of the little finger that gives a hooked appearance to the fingertip both clinically and radiographically. It is far less commonly associated with other congenital abnormalities and so must be distinguished from clinodactyly.

Once associated congenital anomalies have been evaluated, the crooked digit of clinodactyly is usually only of cosmetic concern; for minor angulation deformities, the risks of correction outweigh the benefits. A wedge osteotomy can be performed for pronounced deformities, and the surgical risks are joint stiffness and bone nonunion.

ACQUIRED TRIGGER FINGER

Stenosing tenosynovitis of the digital flexor tendons is known as trigger finger because of the snapping observed when the patient actively flexes or extends the interphalangeal joints (Fig. 12-9). A slightly enlarged area of the tendon fails to glide smoothly in and out the proximal end of the fibroosseous tendon

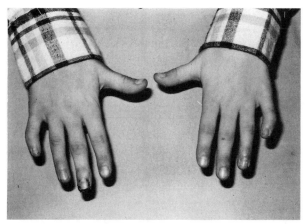

FIGURE 12-8. Clinodactyly is a congenital, angular deformity of the little finger in the medial–lateral direction.

sheath, but rather catches and then gives way, resulting in the observed snapping or triggering. This mechanical impedance is similar to pulling a knotted rope through a section of pipe.

Trigger finger is the most common tendon entrapment syndrome in the hand and wrist and is the most common diagnosis in many hand surgery practices.

It most often occurs in the thumb, middle, and ring digits, but can affect any of the fingers. In most cases, the etiology is unknown, but many patients with a trigger finger sooner or later develop identical symptoms in another digit, suggesting a congenital predisposition. It may be the related to general connective tissue tone because people who get trigger fingers are also likely to get other entrapments like de Quervain tenosynovitis and carpal tunnel syndrome. Trauma may also be implicated because a contusion to the palm or a sprain of the thumb meta-

carpophalangeal joint may initiate symptoms of triggering. Patients with diabetes appear to be predisposed to developing trigger digits, and here the link may be the mild, generalized palmar connective tissue thickening that results in narrowing of the tendon sheath. Likewise, tendon triggering is occasionally seen beneath palmar fascia contracted from Dupuytren disease. Whether the relation is causal or only coincidental is only speculative. Tenosynovial thickening is common in rheumatoid arthritis, but actual triggering from this etiology is unusual. Rather, the tendons move through the fibroosseous canals with a palpable and sometimes even audible crepitation as multiple small synovial enlargements move past the opening of the flexor tendon sheath.

Affected patients usually complain of painful, dysrhythmic finger motion as the proximal interphalangeal joint catches in midposition with attempted flexion or extension. A superficial assessment may conclude that the pathology involves the joint, but smooth, painless passive joint motion and absence of tenderness rules out joint pathology. Sometimes, the triggering is painless. A subtle variation that is more difficult to diagnosis occurs when there is enough inflammation to cause painful motion but not enough to cause the catching and giving way. In this instance, the flexor tendon and sheath are tender to palpation over the metacarpal head, and a pea-like nodule can be felt gliding back and forth through the tender area when the patient moves the affected finger. Because patients with trigger digits are predisposed to other entrapment syndromes, the diagnosis is confirmed if asymptomatic nodules can be palpated in other fingers.

The symptoms of trigger finger occasionally resolve spontaneously, perhaps to recur in one digit or

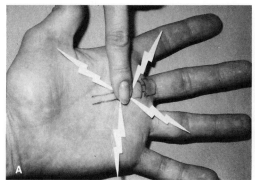 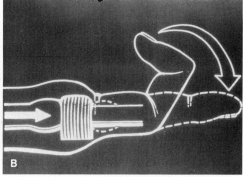

FIGURE 12-9. (A) Physical examination of a digit with stenosing tenosynovitis (trigger finger) reveals tenderness over the flexor tendon sheath at the level of the metacarpal head. Often, a small nodule can be palpated. (B) In trigger finger, the enlarged area of the tendon does not glide smoothly within the flexor tendon sheath. A snapping is noted as the digit pops from a fully extended to a fully flexed position.

another some months later. If the nodule becomes sufficiently large that tendon gliding is fully blocked, then the proximal interphalangeal joint is fixed in either an extended or flexed position, risking permanent joint stiffness.

Once a tendon begins triggering, an inflammatory cycle is established in which the continued mechanical irregularity generates inflammation with every excursion of the tendon, and the inflammation generates more swelling to accentuate the mechanical incongruity. Thus, the first step in treatment is to break the inflammatory cycle. An injection of a long-acting cortisone-type drug into the involved sheath counters the inflammation and cures about half of trigger digits. If necessary, a second injection a month or more later brings the cure rate into the 95% range, leaving few that require surgery. If two injections have not solved the triggering, it is unlikely that further injections will, and additional injections risk weakening the tendon with subsequent tendon rupture.

At surgery, the proximal 10 to 15 mL of the fibroosseous canal is incised longitudinally to allow the thickened tendon to glide without restraint. When done under local anesthesia, the surgeon can observe the pathology by asking the patient to flex and extend the digits. The opening of the sheath is deemed sufficient when triggering is no longer noted. Intact portions of the fibroosseous canal distally effectively prevent bow-stringing of the released tendon. After operation, the patient should begin moving the finger right away to prevent tendon adhesions at the surgical site.

Digital nerve laceration is a known complication of trigger digit release. In the thumb, the nerves are especially vulnerable because they lie closer to the anterior midline of the digit and are in closer proximity to the constricting tendon sheath.

DE QUERVAIN TENOSYNOVITIS

De Quervain disease is entrapment of the abductor pollicis longus and extensor pollicis brevis tendons as they pass beneath the extensor retinaculum at the radial styloid. This is the most common tendon entrapment in the hand and wrist after trigger finger. The extensor retinaculum holds the tendons close to the skeleton as they pass from the forearm to the hand, and normally the tendons glide smoothly through the fibroosseous canal. The first dorsal compartment contains the tendons of the abductor pollicis longus and extensor pollicis brevis, and tendon thickening or sheath narrowing from a variety of causes can impede smooth tendon gliding. This impedance stimulates inflammation with attendant pain and swelling. This swelling may further accentuate the impedance. Repetitive, forceful radial deviation of the wrist with abduction and extension of the thumb is the most common cause of de Quervain tendonitis. Mothers of infant children, for example, stress the tendons in the first dorsal compartment when they lift their babies. Compared with carpal tunnel syndrome, which may occur late in pregnancy and is probably related to fluid retention, de Quervain tendonitis of early motherhood appears to be purely mechanical in origin. Although rare during pregnancy, mothers of adopted infants and grandmothers may also develop the condition when caring for the baby. Vocational and avocational activities unrelated to infant care may also incite symptoms. Furthermore, blunt trauma to the radial styloid may be the initiating event, whereby the resultant swelling mechanically restrains tendon gliding, and subsequent thumb and wrist motions perpetuate inflammation (Fig. 12-10).

Pain with wrist and thumb movements is the most common complaint. Catching and giving way, a hallmark of trigger finger, is not seen in de Quervain tendonitis, probably because there is not a sharp, free edge to the wrist extensor retinaculum as there is with the finger flexor tendon sheath.

The inflamed sheath overlying the tendons thickens and forms a visible and bone-hard mass at the radial styloid. Resisted extension and abduction of the thumb may produce pain at the entrapment site; but this finding is inconsistent because other muscles, not passing through the first dorsal compartment, also provide these same thumb movements. The best test for diagnosing de Quervain tendonitis is the Finkelstein test. The patient is asked to place the thumb in the palm and close his or her fingers over it: this puts the thumb in maximal adduction and flexion. The physician then gently moves the patient's wrist into ulnar deviation. This maneuver causes maximal distal excursion of the abductor pollicis longus and extensor pollicis brevis tendons and incites sharp pain at the radial styloid when the first dorsal compartment is inflamed. Trapeziometacarpal arthritis, radioscaphoid arthritis, scaphoid nonunion, and bony abnormalities of the distal radius are the main considerations in the differential diagnosis and must be evaluated radiographically.

Avoidance of aggravating activities may be all that is necessary to relieve symptoms because working mothers often relate that their symptoms flare on the weekends when they are providing more of their

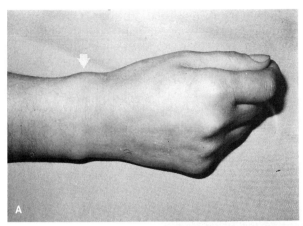
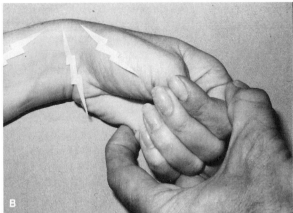
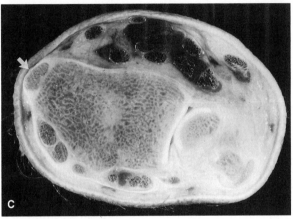

FIGURE 12-10. (A) De Quervain tendinitis causes a tender and bone-hard thickening of the extensor retinaculum over the first dorsal compartment. (B) The Finkelstein test is performed by asking the patient to grasp his or her thumb and then move the wrist into ulnar deviation. Pain over the radial styloid process is characteristic of de Quervain tenosynovitis. (C) In this cross section through the distal radial ulnar joint, the arrow highlights the first dorsal compartment. Pain occurs in de Quervain tenosynovitis when the tendons of the abductor pollicis longus and the extensor pollicis brevis become entrapped here.

infant's care. Immobilization in a cast or splint may be used to enforce rest, but the resultant encumbrance to overall hand function may make such treatment more disabling than the underlying tendonitis.

An injection of a long-acting cortisone-like preparation into the sheath often reduces the inflammation and breaks the cycle of inflammation and friction. Great care must be taken to ensure that the steroid is injected within the sheath and not subcutaneously because, in the more superficial location, it may cause skin hypopigmentation. If symptoms persist or recur a month or more after the first injection, a second injection may fully resolve the symptoms. Once pain is relieved, several more months will pass before the visible swelling from the thickened sheath subsides.

One or two injections relieve symptoms in 90% to 95% of patients. For those few with persistent pain,

further injections are unlikely to relieve the entrapment and also risk tendon rupture. If symptoms persist after two injections, surgical unroofing of the first dorsal compartment should provide relief. A transverse incision over the apex of the thickening gives adequate exposure and leaves the least disfiguring scar. The superficial radial nerve lies between the skin incision and the sheath and is the source of most complications related to release of the first dorsal compartment. A neuroma here can be severely disabling, and therefore any sharp or blunt injury to the superficial radial nerve is to be assiduously avoided.

At surgery, the sheath is opened longitudinally, exposing the tendons. More commonly than not, the abductor pollicis longus has multiple tendon slips, so the exposed tendons must be inspected to ensure they include the small extensor pollicis brevis, which may run in a separate sheath that is located slightly more dorsally within the first dorsal compartment. If the extensor pollicis brevis is not specifically sought and released, it may be a source of persistent symptoms. After operation, the thin, intact fasciae on the distal forearm and dorsum of the hand prevent undue mobility.

CARPAL TUNNEL SYNDROME

The median nerve can become compressed as it passes through its investing fibroosseous canal at the wrist. The compression can cause paresthesia and hypoesthesia on the radial side of the hand and weakness of the thenar muscles. This condition is known as carpal tunnel syndrome. Females are more commonly affected than males, and although it can occur at any age, at least half of patients are between 40 and 60 years of age.

The carpal tunnel is bound on three sides by wrist bones and on the anterior side by the dense transverse carpal ligament. Passing through the canal and deep to the median nerve are one flexor tendon to the thumb and two to each of the other digits, for a total of nine. The ligament covering the roof of the canal retains the nerve and tendon contents and redirects their courses into the hand as the wrist changes position. This canal is rigidly constructed, so an increased volume of tissue or fluid within its confines cannot expand the walls but rather increases pressure. This additional pressure on the median nerve diminishes capillary circulation, and the nerve becomes ischemic (Fig. 12-11).

An increase in the volume of the contents of carpal canal can occur for a variety of reasons. For example, carpal tunnel syndrome is frequently diagnosed during the third trimester of pregnancy and is related to fluid retention. Swelling from a Colles fracture can also compress the nerve. Rheumatoid tenosynovitis, myxedema, anomalous muscle bellies, tumors, and amyloid deposits are also occasionally implicated as causes. The nerve can also become ischemic without a particular increase in volume. This most commonly occurs while performing forceful finger flexion activities with a flexed wrist. Here, the tensed flexor tendons compress the nerve against the transverse retinacular ligament, restricting its capillary blood flow. Fortunately, most forceful activities, hammering for instance, are usually performed with the wrist extended. In this situation, the tendons exert pressure on the dorsal, bony wall of the carpal canal rather than on the median nerve. Simultaneous wrist

and finger flexion activities known to cause carpal tunnel syndrome include holding a car's steering wheel and holding a stack of books under one's arm. Many occupational activities that prompt faulty wrist posturing in flexion are also implicated in development of median nerve compression symptoms.

Once the above etiologic factors have been explored, however, the etiology of the nerve ischemia in most patients remains unexplained. These patients have idiopathic carpal tunnel syndrome. This condition occurs most frequently in middle-aged to older women, suggesting a hormonal influence.

Whatever the etiology of nerve ischemia in the carpal canal, only moderate compression is required to produce symptoms when the nerve is already diseased from another etiology. For example, the patient may have nerve fiber compression more proximally, at the cervical spine, thoracic outlet, or elbow. In these instances, less pressure is needed at the wrist to produce carpal tunnel symptoms. This is called *double crush syndrome*. A peripheral neuropathy from diabetes, alcohol, or other causes, even when subclinical, also predisposes the patient with a mildly ischemic median nerve at the wrist to carpal tunnel syndrome. Chronic renal dialysis patients frequently develop carpal tunnel symptoms. Peripheral neuropathy, amyloid deposition, and vascular steal from an arteriovenous shunt in that limb can all be implicated as causative factors in these patients.

Symptoms noted in early carpal tunnel syndrome are tingling in the fingers and a vague ache in the wrist. The entire median nerve distribution in the digits does not have to be involved, and the ache may radiate proximally as far as the neck. The tingling frequently causes night wakening and may be relieved by shaking the hand and moving the fingers. The night symptoms are almost pathognomonic for carpal tunnel syndrome and may be caused by a redistribution of extracellular water during recumbency. If the ischemia increases in severity, intermittent numbness in the median nerve distribution may occur and may gradually become constant. The median innervated thenar muscles also are affected, first with weakness and eventually with muscle atrophy and loss of thumb opposition. With progressive loss of sensation and fine motor control, the patient notices clumsiness and a tendency to drop objects.

On physical examination, sensibility in the median nerve distribution should be tested and compared to that in the little finger and to that in the opposite hand. Because there may be some crossover of sensory innervation between the median and ulnar nerves in the middle and ring fingers and because

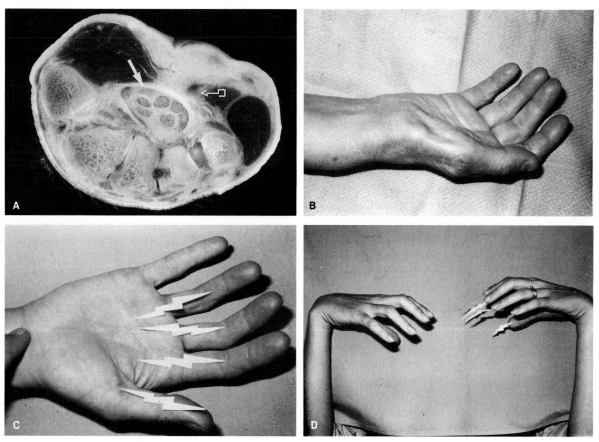

FIGURE 12-11. (A) At the level of the metacarpal bases, the median nerve (*closed arrow*) lies beneath the dense transverse carpal ligament. Tenosynovitis in the adjacent tendons can cause carpal tunnel syndrome. The ulnar nerve (*open arrow*) lies more superficially in a less well-defined tunnel. (B) Severe carpal tunnel syndrome causes wasting of the median innervated thenar musculature. Note the flattening of the normally convex thenar contour. (C) Tinel sign is elicited by gently tapping over the median nerve just proximal to the carpal canal. A positive test elicits paresthesia in the thumb, index, middle finger, and radial half of the ring finger. (D) The Phalen wrist flexion test is positive for carpal tunnel syndrome when paresthesia appears or increases in the median nerve distribution within 1 minute.

the radial nerve may innervate the sides of the thumb pulp, the most valuable information comes from testing the index and little fingers. Monofilament testing and vibratory sensation are the most sensitive tests, with two-point discrimination and light touch being diminished only with long-standing and at least moderately severe compression.

The contour, bulk, and function of the thenar muscles should be examined. Any wasting is noted as a flattening of the normally convex thenar contour. With long-standing median nerve compression, thenar muscle atrophy leaves a concave contour to the first metacarpal area. The patient should be asked to touch the thumb to the tip of the little finger while the examiner palpates the thenar muscle contraction and watches for efficient opposition. During opposition, the thumb pulp should be held well away from

the palm with the plane of the thumb nail parallel to the plane of the palm. In carpal tunnel syndrome, the muscles innervated by the median nerve in the forearm should be functioning properly. Thus, the possibility of a more proximal nerve compression should be considered by testing the strength of the flexor pollicis longus, flexor digitorum profundus to the index, flexor digitorum superficialis, and flexor carpi radialis.

In patients presenting with symptoms suggestive of carpal tunnel syndrome, gentle tapping over the course of the median nerve through the carpal canal usually elicits paresthesia in the thumb, index, middle, and ring digits. This is called the Tinel test. Another important test is the Phalen wrist flexion test. Patients are asked to hold their forearms vertical and let their wrists fall naturally into full flexion. This position increases pressure on the median nerve, and an increase in paresthesia within 1 minute is considered a positive test.

To rule out other causes of nerve irritability, the physician should inquire about numbness or tingling in the feet; palpate for nerve tenderness in the neck, axilla, and antecubital areas; and test for cervical nerve root compression, thoracic outlet syndrome, and median nerve compression around the elbow.

Electrodiagnostic testing quantitates the severity of the nerve dysfunction and may aid with the diagnosis of carpal tunnel syndrome. Median nerve conduction times through the carpal canal are measured in milliseconds and are normally less than 4.5 for motor conduction and 3.5 for sensory conduction. About 75% of the nerve fibers must be conducting abnormally before a change is noted in the conduction velocity, so an early or mild nerve compression may show normal conduction testing. A mild carpal tunnel syndrome usually shows an abnormal sensory conduction but a normal motor conduction time. A moderate compression may show a several millisecond delay in both times, and a severe compression may show an absence of sensory conduction and a near doubling of motor conduction time. Median nerve conduction velocity in the forearm assesses the general health of the nerve more proximally. If a peripheral neuropathy is suspected, perineal nerve conduction velocity should be obtained. On electromyogram testing, the median-innervated thenar muscles are often abnormal, but the median-innervated muscles in the forearm test normal.

Treatment of carpal tunnel syndrome is directed at relieving pressure on the nerve and thereby eliminating the ischemia. Because the nerve is additionally compressed in the extremes of both flexion and extension, night splinting is an important first treatment step in mild and moderate cases. A splint that holds the wrist in a neutral position is worn to bed and allows the nerve maximal circulation for the period of sleep. If the patient has daytime activities that exacerbate symptoms, the splint may be useful then as well. Work and hobbies that require forceful, repetitive, and prolonged wrist flexion should be modified whenever possible. Although vitamin B_6 treatment has been advocated, its usefulness for treatment of carpal tunnel syndrome is unproved.

An injection of corticosteroid into the carpal canal may be curative for early and mild symptoms. This medication accelerates resolution of any inflammatory tenosynovial thickening and thereby provides more space and less pressure on the nerve. Splinting and injection are more likely to be effective in patients with mild symptoms for less than 6 months. Even if the injection has only a temporary effect, a positive response helps confirm the diagnosis and indicates that the patient will respond favorably to carpal tunnel release.

Patients with advanced compression have measurable loss of sensation, visible thenar wasting, and marked slowing on nerve conduction testing. They are unlikely to respond completely to splinting and injection treatment. Carpal tunnel release should be considered sooner for these patients than for those with less pronounced findings.

Surgical release of the transverse retinacular ligament allows the contents of the carpal canal to expand into a larger space and thereby diminishes nerve pressure and ischemia. The procedure is routinely performed under local or regional anesthesia. The incision is designed to visualize the nerve throughout its course in the carpal tunnel while minimizing skin scarring and risk of injury to small cutaneous nerves in the palm. Once the canal is open, the tendons and deep surface of the canal should be palpated to avoid overlooking a mass or bony protuberance. If the external epineurium appears scarred and constrictive, it should be opened to facilitate expansion of the compressed nerve. An internal neurolysis is generally considered to be mettlesome and ineffective in additionally decompressing the nerve. After operation, the wrist is splinted in slight extension for several weeks to allow for skin healing and to prevent the contents of the carpal canal from bow-stringing anteriorly. Subsequently, the transverse carpal ligament has scarred sufficiently to resume its retinacular function.

Patients frequently indicate that the tingling and night symptoms subside almost immediately after carpal tunnel release. The hyperesthesia generally continues to abate over many months. Patients who had severe, long-standing sensory changes before operation may experience a painful, hyperesthetic phase of healing for several months during their recuperation. This is caused by the small, unmyelinated fibers that conduct pain regenerating faster than the larger, myelinated fibers that conduct the more sophisticated sensory modalities. Such patients should be advised of this eventuality before surgery and reassured that it is temporary when it occurs. Thenar muscle strength and bulk recover slowly if at all, and if useful opposition is absent, a tendon transfer for restoration of this important function should be considered.

The most common complication of carpal tunnel release is persistent symptoms. This may be related to a double crush syndrome, a peripheral neuropathy, or an incompletely decompressed carpal canal. The symptoms generally subside spontaneously as healing is completed. Neuromas in the surgical site continue to be bothersome and are best avoided by strategic location of the incision. Reflex sympathetic dystrophy is rare, but this potentially devastating complication should be treated promptly with stellate ganglion blocks.

ULNAR NERVE ENTRAPMENT AT THE WRIST

Compression neuropathy of the ulnar nerve can occur at the wrist, but it occurs there far less commonly than ulnar nerve compression at the elbow or median nerve compression at the wrist.

The ulnar nerve passes down the forearm between the muscle bellies of the flexor carpi ulnaris and flexor digitorum profundus. The dorsal sensory branch arises about 10 cm proximal to the wrist and passes around the ulna to supply sensation to the skin on the dorsum of the hand. The main ulnar nerve continues distally with the ulnar artery, and they cross into the palm between the pisiform and the hook of the hamate. A thin fascial layer lies over the nerve and artery at this level, and the dense, transverse carpal ligament lies beneath it. Nerve entrapment at this level results in numbness and tingling in the little and ulnar half of the ring fingers and, if severe, wasting of the ulnar innervated intrinsic muscles. These symptoms may coexist with symptoms of carpal tunnel syndrome.

The onset of symptoms may be related either to a single blow or to repetitive trauma to the hypothenar area. Using the heel of the hand as a hammer for such activities as replacing hubcaps, for instance, can contuse the nerve and generate a local inflammatory process. Local irritation and swelling with nerve compression may also result from fracture of an adjacent carpal bone, especially the hook of the hamate. A mass, such as a ganglion, in the base of the canal or a disturbance in the ulnar artery running through the canal, such as an aneurysm or thrombosis, may also compress the nerve.

On examination, the nerve may be tender in the proximal palm, and paresthesia in the ulnar distribution may be elicited by lightly tapping along its course. Sensation should be tested in the little finger and compared to the index finger and to the opposite little finger. If the skin on the dorsal ulnar surface of the hand is numb, the problem is proximal to the origin of the dorsal sensory branch, and evidence of ulnar nerve compression at the elbow should be carefully sought. A positive Allen test for slow or absent filling of the hand through the ulnar artery suggests an arterial thrombosis or aneurysm that may be the cause of the neuritis. The intrinsic muscles should be examined for weakness and wasting, but positive findings do not differentiate between compression at the wrist and compression at the elbow. To complicate matters, the nerve may be compressed at both the elbow and wrist, an example of a double crush syndrome. Nerve conduction velocity studies help localize the site of compression. The differential diagnosis includes all other sources of neuropathy, ranging from more proximal sites of compression and metabolic causes, such as diabetes or alcohol, to central nervous system problems, such as syringomyelia.

Primary treatment should include discontinuation of any repetitive trauma to the hypothenar area and administration of nonsteroidal antiinflammatory medication. Surgical unroofing of the ulnar tunnel at the wrist is indicated for resistant cases. If compression is concurrently present at the elbow, both sites can be released surgically during the same operative session. Prompt relief of the ache, gradual improvement in sensation, and doubtful improvement in motor control are normally noted postoperative changes.

GANGLION

A ganglion in the musculoskeletal system is a spherical accumulation of fluid produced from an adjacent joint capsule or tendon sheath. A ganglion in the nervous system refers to a collection of nerve cell bodies, and the two meanings are totally unrelated. In the sense that tumor means swelling, the ganglion is the most common tumor in the hand. It is not a neoplasm because it is acellular, and it is not a cyst because the collection of clear, viscous fluid is not contained within an endothelial cavity. Rather, the enlarging volume of fluid tends to gradually push normal adventitial tissue away, and as this tissue is stretched, a pseudocyst enclosing the fluid is formed. The content of the pseudocyst is hyaluronic acid, a mucopolysaccharide normally present in synovial fluid. Although the etiology of ganglion formation is unclear, an injury to the wrist capsule or flexor tendon sheath, usually unrecognized, may cause the production of abundant quantities of hyaluronic acid. The most common locations for these lesions are the radial aspects of the wrist, both dorsally and anteriorly; and in both these locations, they arise from the wrist joint capsule (Fig. 12-12). Another common presentation is in the midline of the finger at its proximal flexion crease, and here it arises from the flexor tendon sheath. Mucous cysts occur at the base of the nail and result from joint capsule irritation on an underlying osteophyte. Histologically and chemically, distal interphalangeal joint mucous cysts and ganglions at other locations are identical.

Ganglions can occur at any age, but most are seen in people between 20 and 50 years old. Women are affected twice as often as men. Some patients notice the rapid development of a painless lump and are justifiably concerned about the possibility of malignancy. Sometimes, the mass develops almost overnight. In such cases, the likelihood of the mass being a ganglion is good because solid tumors rarely grow this quickly. Other patients notice pain with limitation of wrist motion as the presenting symptom, and only weeks or months later does an associated mass appear. Onset in some cases is related to a specific wrist sprain or similar acute injury. Dorsal wrist ganglions may produce pain by stretching the posterior interosseous nerve as it gives sensory innervation to the dorsal wrist capsule. The pain at times is noted to radiate up the forearm. Grip strength may be diminished because of pain.

With flexor tendon sheath ganglions, patients usually note local tenderness with gripping a steering wheel, briefcase handle, or similar object, and local palpation reveals a hard, spherical mass at the site of tenderness. The patient may notice that the mass waxes and wanes in size, perhaps related to activity. This behavior makes the diagnosis of ganglion more certain because a solid neoplasm is not likely to act in this way.

On examination, ganglions may feel remarkably firm depending on the pressure of the contained hyaluronic acid. Ganglions are generally fixed to the deep tissue, but the overlying skin is freely mobile. These pseudocysts are usually spherical, but may be

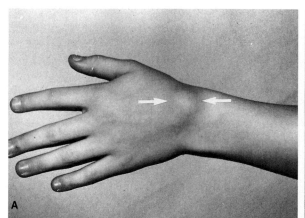
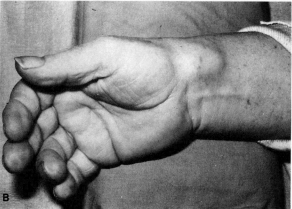
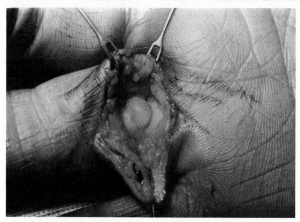

FIGURE 12-12. (A) The most common location of a ganglion is on the dorsal wrist over the scapholunate joint. (B) Another common location for a ganglion is on the radial aspect of the wrist anteriorly. Careful examination is necessary to distinguish a ganglion in this location from a radial artery aneurysm. (C) A ganglion at the base of the finger arises from the flexor tendon sheath. These are palpable but not visible on physical examination.

multilobed if a strand of intervening connective tissue restricts spherical development. Limitation of wrist motion should be noted. Transillumination with a penlight in a darkened room lends evidence to the fluid-filled nature of these tumors. Lesions presenting on the anterior aspect of the wrist may appear to be pulsatile because they distort the course of the radial artery and may transmit its pulse. Thus, an Allen test for competency of the radial artery should be performed.

If the described points of history and physical examination give reasonable certainty that the mass is a ganglion, a needle aspiration can confirm the diagnosis and at times prove to be curative. Aspiration of anterior wrist ganglions should not be attempted because a large-gauge needle perforation of the radial artery could produce significant complications. For presumed ganglions in other locations, the area should be first anesthetized with a small quantity of local anesthetic, and a large gauge needle is inserted into the mass. The hyalauronic acid contents can be viscous, and direct positive digital pressure over the mass in addition to negative pressure on the syringe may be necessary to withdraw the fluid. Recovery of clear, thick, jelly-like fluid confirms the diagnosis. Aspiration is curative about half the time and is equivalent to the more dramatic household treatment of bashing the mass with a book. Presumably, the reason that half of ganglions do not recur after decompression is that the underlying area of joint capsule or tendon sheath producing the fluid has become quiescent. Although cortisone injections have been advocated to achieve this end medically, their efficacy is unproved.

Once the diagnosis is confirmed by aspiration, surgical excision is not mandatory even if the mass recurs. Reasons for excision include pain, unsightly appearance, or failure to aspirate any characteristic fluid. The critical part of the surgery is not removing the mass itself but rather removing the area of joint capsule or tendon sheath that produces the fluid. Because the involved sheath or capsule area appears grossly normal, an incomplete excision is possible, leading to recurrence in about 5% of ganglion operations. Recurrence is the most common complication and is appropriately dealt with by excision of a wider area of capsule or sheath.

DUPUYTREN CONTRACTURE

Dupuytren disease is an inflammation and subsequent contracture of the palmar aponeurosis and corresponding connective tissue supports in the fin-

gers. It is seen six times more commonly in men than in women, and age of onset is usually around 50 years. It becomes progressively more common with increasing age. The collagen composition, myofibroblast activity, and various enzyme levels are altered in the affected fascia, but the exact molecular cause and mechanism remain unclear (Fig. 12-13).

A familial predisposition is frequently evident, particularly in patients whose ancestors came from northern Europe. Dupuytren fasciitis is common in Ireland, Wales, Scotland, England, and the Scandinavian countries, and it is postulated that the genetic trait responsible for the condition emanated from an ancient Celt. Thus, Dupuytren contracture is seen in other areas of the world with strong Anglo-Saxon racial origins, Australia for example. It is less common in southern Europe and essentially nonexistent in Africa and Asia. Because of the diverse ancestral origins of many Americans, Dupuytren contracture is seen at a moderate frequency compared with northern Europe.

In addition to inheriting the trait for palmar and digital fasciitis, other predisposing factors appear to accentuate the likelihood of significant clinical manifestations. Dupuytren contracture is seen more commonly in patients with alcoholic cirrhosis and other forms of chronic liver disease and in patients with seizure disorders taking antiseizure medication. These people are known to have decreased prostaglandin E levels. Further research may prove that prostaglandin E inhibits ATPase, which appears to be an important factor in myofibroblast contraction.

Controversy exists regarding the role of trauma in the development of Dupuytren disease. Although microtrauma to the fascia may initiate an overactive myofibroblast repair response in a predisposed pa-

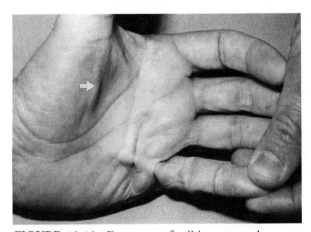

FIGURE 12-13. Dupuytren fasciitis commonly causes contracture in the ring and little fingers. Bands in the first web area are common but rarely limit motion.

tients, symptomatic Dupuytren contracture is as common in sedentary workers as in people with heavy manual occupations. There is also no predilection for the dominant hand. A correlation between Dupuytren contracture and diabetes has been sought, but the relation remains uncertain because diabetes and Dupuytren disease both tend to occur with increasing frequency in older people and hence their association may only be coincidental.

Dupuytren contracture in the palm and digits may occasionally be associated with similar types of fasciitis at other body sites. Thickening over the extensor surfaces of the proximal interphalangeal joints are known as *knuckle pads*. Fasciitis in the shaft of the penis is known as *Peyronie disease*. Fasciitis in the plantar aponeurosis on the sole of the foot is known as *lederhosen disease*. An individual with the onset of diffuse Dupuytren involvement in the hands and other sites at an early age is said to have *Dupuytren diathesis*, a strong predisposition to manifest significant changes.

The first thing a patient with Dupuytren fasciitis may notice is a tender thickening in the distal palm, most likely on the ulnar side. Usually within a few months, the acute inflammation resolves, and the tenderness subsides. A longitudinal band may then gradually develop and shorten to create a contracture of the metacarpophalangeal and interphalangeal joints. At this point, the developing contracture is painless. As finger extension is lost, the patient has difficulty with flat hand activities, such as face washing, putting the hand in a pocket, shaking hands, and clapping. The progression of the contracture is unpredictable, with perhaps no apparent contractile activity for months or years, and then without explanation, several joints rapidly lose extension.

Occasionally, digital contracture of the proximal interphalangeal joint precedes palmar involvement and contracture of the metacarpophalangeal joint. Without the characteristic pretendonous cords present in the palm, the diagnosis of Dupuytren contracture in these patients is more difficult, particularly if their family history is negative. Distal interphalangeal joint contractures are seen only rarely and then in conjunction with severe contractures at the more proximal joints. Thumb involvement causing functional loss of motion is also unusual.

The natural history is difficult to generalize because patients with Dupuytren diathesis may have already had several operations before reaching the age of 40 years, and faintly palpable, asymptomatic bands are common in octogenarians. Several years usually pass between the first appearance of a tender nodule and the development of a symptomatic metacarpophalangeal or proximal interphalangeal joint contracture. In general, about half of patients followed for more than 5 years show progression and extension of the fasciitis. Severe, long-standing contractures may fix the metacarpophalangeal and proximal interphalangeal joints in 90 degrees of flexion and hold the pulp of the digit in constant contact with the palm.

Dupuytren disease may masquerade as a posttraumatic contracture of the proximal interphalangeal joint when there is no involvement in the palm. Usually, a tight band, well anterior to the tendon sheath, can be palpated and can verify the etiology as Dupuytren disease rather than residual stiffness from trauma. A diffuse mild palmar fasciitis is seen in patients with a recent hand injury or Colles fracture. This appears to be a reactive fasciitis from the inflammation of injury, and it generally softens without contracting joints once the original injury is well healed.

Treatment in all forms, including massage, splinting, and injections, has been tried since Baron von Dupuytren first described operating on the contracture in 1832. Steroid injections into the inflamed nodule may have some effect on quieting the early process, but this is unproved. Over the 150 years that this condition has been recognized and treated, the only treatment that has met with any wide success is surgery. Operating on the mere presence of a nodule or cord in the palm when contracture is absent has proved futile because the inflammation generated by the surgical injury promotes stiffness and accelerates the contraction of adjacent, unoperated fascia.

Metacarpophalangeal joint contractures, even when severe and long-standing, are relatively easy to relieve with release or excision of the contracted palmar fascia. The superficial, longitudinal fibers of the palmar fascia are involved in the process, but the deeper, transverse fibers are not, and the neurovascular bundles in the palm lie completely beneath the palmar aponeurosis. Thus, surgery for metacarpophalangeal joint problems is appropriate when the patient has significant functional disability related to the contracture, and this surgery can be performed with relatively little risk to the underlying digital nerves and arteries. Usually, excision of the contracted fascia is performed, but a limited transection of the affected tissue can improve hand function in a patient unsuitable for a more extensive procedure.

The anatomic considerations in the digit make Dupuytren contracture of the proximal interphalangeal joint a much more difficult surgical problem than contracture of the metacarpophalangeal joint. The contracted fascia may lie superficial to the flexor tendon sheath, but portions of the diseased tissue may lie behind the neurovascular bundles or even spiral densely around them. In this case, the digital nerve may be drawn out of its normal location into the midline of the digit. Inflammation created by surgical excision of the contracted tissue is tolerated poorly in the digit compared with the palm, and recurrent proximal interphalangeal joint contracture is a significant risk. This occurs not necessarily from residual or recurrent Dupuytren fascia, but merely from surgical scarring. Thus, proximal interphalangeal joint involvement is best approached when the contracture is only 25 or 30 degrees and progressing, as opposed to waiting until the contracture becomes functionally disabling. When the proximal interphalangeal joint contracture is approached surgically, not only the contracted fascia but also any potentially contractible fascia should be removed. This minimizes risk of recurrence. Operation for contracture in a scarred, previously operated digit is difficult and potentially unrewarding.

Special care must be taken in planning skin incisions and skin closure to ensure that adequate skin coverage is present and that the surgical skin scars will not contract in such a way as to create a recurrent joint contracture. For mild degrees of joint contracture where the overlying skin appears ample and supple, zig-zag incisions from the palm extending into the digit provide satisfactory exposure. Subsequent skin wound healing contracts the skin in the same oblique, zig-zag pattern, precluding a shortened longitudinal scar and skin tightness. For more severe contractures, the skin is usually opened longitudinally in the midline of the digit, and at closure, is it converted to Z-plasties. This diverts the longitudinal orientation of the incision and brings additional skin into the anterior midline. When the skin in the distal palm is densely adherent and dimpled by the underlying contracted fascia, a transverse skin incision may be left open after surgery to heal by wound contraction over several weeks. Alternatively, the area can be skin grafted.

A carefully orchestrated postoperative program for recovery of motion is paramount to a good result. This is one example in hand surgery in which the treatment may be only half completed on exit from the operating room. The other half occurs over the following weeks as the patient maintains the motion recovered at surgery. The second half of the treatment may be the most difficult because it requires a high degree of patient compliance and because neither doctor, patient, nor hand therapist can actually see the inflamed deep tissues. The progressively more vigorous active and passive motions required must be carefully administered and monitored to ensure that the exercises do not generate disabling inflammation.

The most significant intraoperative complication of Dupuytren surgery is digital nerve laceration. This more commonly occurs in the finger than in the palm because of the proximity of the contracted tissue and the derangements of the normal anatomy here. The digital nerve should be clearly identified from one end of the surgical exposure to the other. Thus, if a nerve laceration has occurred, it is recognized and repaired. Even when the nerve remains in continuity, patients frequently note hyperesthesia and paresthesia in the digit for weeks or even months after surgery. The disturbed sensation is attributed to the traction and partial devascularization of the nerve during surgery. The patient should be made aware of this likelihood before surgery along with the risk of nerve division.

A more devastating early complication of Dupuytren surgery is vascular compromise. Even though the digital arteries may remain in continuity, the manipulation and stretching may cause vasospasm. This most commonly occurs after release of severe, long-standing proximal interphalangeal joint contractures. Thus, the patient, particularly if he or she smokes or has other risk factors, must me made aware before surgery of the possibility of tissue loss.

The most common early postoperative complication of Dupuytren fasciectomy is hematoma formation. The resultant pressure on skin flaps may jeopardize their viability. Hemostasis, loose skin closure, and limb elevation all diminish the risk of this complication. Prompt recognition and evacuation are appropriate treatment once a hematoma appears.

The most common late postoperative complication is residual or recurrent joint contracture. Sometimes, full digital extension is restored, but flexion, which was full before surgery, is lost. This is caused by inadequate postoperative mobilization of the surgically injured digit. Conversely, proximal interphalangeal joint extension, which was full for a matter of months after operation, is gradually lost. This is usually related to incomplete excision of all the potentially contractible tissue. Sometimes, previously uninvolved areas of the hand rapidly become contracted. This is perhaps coincidental to the surgical timing but perhaps stimulated by the surgically created inflammation. In an effort to circumvent this complication, total palmar fasciectomy has been tried, excising not only the presently contracted fascia but also the potentially contractible tissue. Unfortunately, the hand slowly and incompletely recovers from this massive surgical dissection.

Reflex sympathetic dystrophy can occur after Dupuytren excision, causing severe pain, erythema, and swelling with resultant unwillingness to mobilize the injured digits. Prompt recognition and treatment of this potentially devastating complication, usually with stellate ganglion blocks, is critical to a successful outcome.

KIENBÖCK DISEASE

In 1910, Robert Kienböck was the first to describe avascular necrosis and collapse of the lunate, and the condition bears his name. It generally occurs in 20- to 40-year-old people.

The lunate has a variable blood supply, with one or two nutrient vessels entering through both the dorsal and palmar poles. The proximal pole is relatively avascular. Patients may recall a specific forced hyperextension injury of the wrist after which symptoms were first noted. In these cases, a fracture of the lunate in the plane of the palm, not readily apparent on radiography, disrupts the blood supply. Other patients may not recall a specific traumatic event but may relate a forceful, chronic activity, such as dirt-biking or tennis, which may create microfractures in the lunate and likewise disrupt the blood supply. The third predisposing factor is the relative length of the ulna compared with the radius. Usually, the distal articular surfaces of the radius and ulna are level, and they share the support of the lunate, which straddles the distal radioulnar joint. This level alignment of the distal radius and ulna articular surfaces is known as *neutral ulnar variance*. In some people, the ulna is slightly shorter than the radius, so the lunate is only partially supported. This is known as *negative ulnar variance*. Studies have shown that a disproportionate number of patients with Kienböck disease have negative ulnar variance. It is thought that in this anatomic configuration, the lunate is subject to additional bending forces over the prominent edge of the radius. The risk of lunate fracture is therefore increased, and a fracture adversely affects the intraosseous blood supply. Although the etiology of Kienböck disease is somewhat speculative, the three predisposing factors in some combination are probably responsible for avascular necrosis of the lunate (Fig. 12-14).

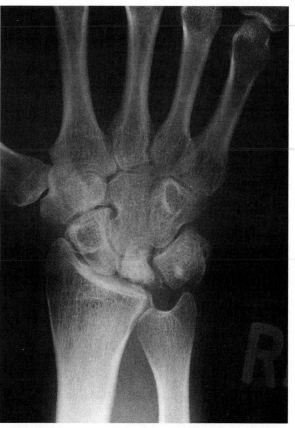

FIGURE 12-14. The short ulna exposes the lunate to additional stress, and microfractures can disrupt the lunate's blood supply. The resultant avascular necrosis with eventual sclerosis and collapse of the lunate is known as Kienböck disease.

The patient almost always presents with wrist pain of several months duration. The pain may be associated with some loss of wrist motion and the presence of slight dorsal thickening related to a reactive synovitis. Physical examination confirms the loss of motion and identifies tenderness over the lunate. The lunate can be palpated in the dorsal midline of the wrist along an imaginary line between the tips of the radial and ulnar styloid processes.

Radiographs show a spectrum of findings depending on the duration of the avascular necrosis and the degree of secondary changes. The earliest radiographic change of Kienböck disease is increased density of the lunate compared with the surrounding carpal bones. Bone turnover does not occur in the necrotic portion of the lunate, so it is denser than normal, and the surrounding bones may also be somewhat osteopenic from disuse related to pain. As the necrotic lunate loses its normal strength, it collapses from the compressive forces between the capitate distally and the radius proximally. This collapse leads to a sclerotic and flattened appearance of the lunate on radiograph. In long-standing untreated cases, proximal migration of the capitate and other derangements in intercarpal architecture are noted. When the lunate collapses and remains untreated, diffuse intercarpal and radiocarpal osteoarthritis slowly develops over a number of years. A bone scan shows increased activity in the lunate even before the additional density of the lunate or any collapse is noted on radiograph, and a scan should be obtained on patients with undiagnosed chronic wrist pain to investigate the possibility of Kienböck disease as early as possible.

If avascular necrosis of the lunate is diagnosed before collapse has occurred, immobilization could theoretically allow the avascular portions of the bone to revascularize and heal. A trial of casting for several months may therefore be tried for these early cases. External fixation with distraction has been considered to relieve the lunate of compressive forces during immobilization, but its effectiveness is unproved.

A number of surgical procedures have been devised to address the collapsed lunate before secondary osteoarthritic changes in the surrounding joints have occurred. The most straightforward is lunate excision. This relieves pain, possibly because of an unavoidable partial wrist denervectomy that occurs during excision. Follow-up studies show that over 5 or more years the capitate migrates proximally into the void created by the lunate excision, resulting in carpal collapse and osteoarthritis. Interposition of fascia or a lunate-shaped silicone spacer has been tried in an effort to prevent the carpal collapse, but the forces within the wrist are too great, and the interposition material is compressed or extruded. Synovitis may also complicate silicone interposition surgery as minute wear particles from the artificial implant stimulate a foreign-body inflammatory response. Other surgical procedures have been devised to bring a new blood supply to the lunate, either as a direct vascular pedicle implanted into the bone or as a vascularized bone graft transported on a pedicle of pronator quadratus muscle. Although the idea is appealing, the procedure remains experimental.

The best methods of preventing lunate collapse are ones that redirect compressive forces away from the vulnerable lunate. Various intercarpal fusions have been used to transmit compressive forces from the metacarpals and distal carpal row through the scaphoid and into the radius, for instance, rather than the normal path through the capitate and lunate and into the radius. Although these intercarpal fusions

may unload the lunate and prevent eventual carpal collapse, they invariably limit wrist motion.

The same goal of redirecting compressive forces away from the lunate can be achieved by altering the relative lengths of the radius and ulna. Either a slight lengthening of the ulna or a slight shortening of the radius effectively shifts the compressive pattern away from the lunate and radius toward the triquetrum and ulna. For patients without negative ulnar variance, a wedge osteotomy of the distal radius, which tilts its articular surface and redirects the forces, may prove useful. Mechanically, radial shortening and ulnar lengthening have the same effect on transmission of forces across the carpus. The lengthening procedure has the disadvantage of requiring a bone graft to fill the gap in the ulnar osteotomy. Thus, the radial shortening osteotomy is the generally preferred procedure. The osteotomy is secured with a plate and screws, and impact activities must be avoided for several months until the radius is healed.

Because the distal radioulnar joint is affected by either radial shortening or ulnar lengthening, secondary arthritic changes may eventually develop. Likewise, the additional force transmitted after operation through the triquetrum into the ulna may damage cartilage and ligament structures on the ulnar side of the wrist.

The patient with Kienböck disease should know that the carpal mechanics can never be completely restored to normal and that some ongoing degenerative changes are inevitable. Only a wrist arthrodesis can permanently halt further changes. Most patients, however, prefer to avoid this solution, at least as a first procedure, because of the associated total loss of wrist motion.

OSTEOARTHRITIS

The manifestations of osteoarthritis in the hand are seen frequently in older populations, but the problem is infrequently disabling. The most commonly involved joints are the distal interphalangeal joints and the trapeziometacarpal joint (Fig. 12-15). A thorough discussion of the etiology and pathophysiology of osteoarthritis is presented in Chapter 6.

At the distal interphalangeal joints, the debris of cartilage destruction is extruded to the low-pressure areas at the joint margins where it coalesces to form osteophytes (Fig. 12-16). These characteristic bone spurs dorsoradially and dorsoulnarly are Heberden nodes. Bone spurs of identical cause form less fre-

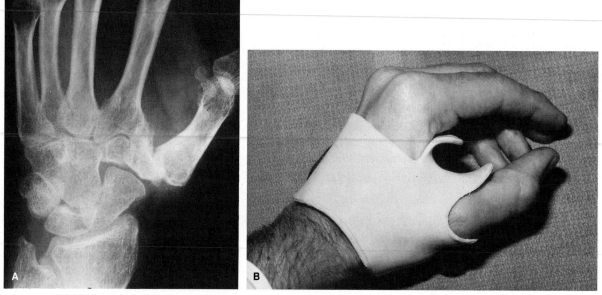

FIGURE 12-15. (A) Osteoarthritis at the carpometacarpal thumb joint results from joint subluxation and incongruity with resultant cartilage. (B) This splint partially immobilizes the damaged trapezio-metacarpal joint and may reduce symptoms in patients with mild to moderately severe osteoarthritis at the thumb base.

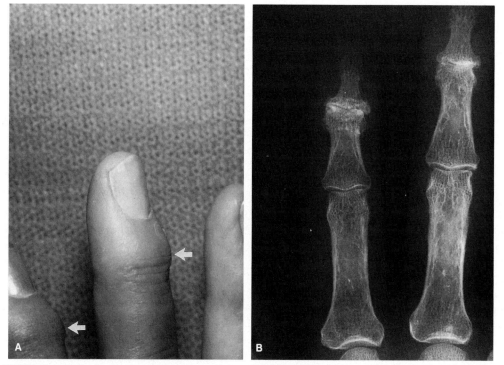

FIGURE 12-16. In osteoarthritis, the cartilage of the distal interphalangeal joints is destroyed, but that of the proximal interphalangeal joints and metacarpophalangeal joints usually is spared. Osteophytes in the distal interphalangeal joints are called Heberden nodes.

quently at the proximal interphalangeal joints and are known as Bouchard nodes.

As the osteoarthritis progresses, pain with forceful pinch activities intensifies, the osteophytes gradually enlarge, and the joint becomes increasingly tender and swollen. Motion is restricted as capsular fibrosis develops and as the osteophytes get large enough to mechanically block full-joint excursion. Fibrous or bony ankylosis may follow, at which time the joint becomes painless.

The osteophyte may irritate the joint capsule in such a way that a mucous cyst is formed. These subcutaneous collections of fluid at the base of the nail are identical chemically and histologically to ganglions. They may exert enough pressure on the nail matrix to cause a shallow groove in the nail. The thinned skin over the cyst may also break open, exposing the distal interphalangeal joint and risking infection.

Nonsteroidal antiinflammatory medications and temporary splinting of an acutely inflamed joint may relieve symptoms. Excision of large Heberden nodes is not particularly successful because it does nothing to alter the underlying pathology, and the surgical scar itself may remain tender. If the pain is disabling, arthrodesis of the distal interphalangeal joint in a slightly flexed position restores forceful, pain-free pinch. Successful treatment of a mucous cyst requires removal of the underlying osteophyte to prevent recurrence.

The symptoms produced by osteoarthritis at the base of the thumb may be more difficult for both patient and doctor to localize. The patient may have a vague, activity-related ache in the wrist or palm. The doctor may mistake the findings for carpal tunnel syndrome or de Quervain tendonitis. Certain activities forcefully load the trapeziometacarpal joint, and if the patient acknowledges pain with twisting jar lids, wringing out washcloths, or pushing car door handles, then tenderness at the trapeziometacarpal joint should be specifically sought. Motion is generally not restricted, but pulling, pushing, or translating the metacarpal on the trapezium causes pain if the joint capsule is inflamed. Radiographic findings vary according to the severity of the osteoarthritis. Early changes are slight joint incongruity and metacarpal subluxation radially on the trapezium. This results in reduced joint contact area and increased forces across the curved joint surfaces. Joint space narrowing, subchondral bone sclerosis, and osteophyte formation are noted radiographically.

If joint subluxation is diagnosed before cartilage destruction has occurred, reconstruction of the supporting ligaments precludes the natural evolution to degenerative arthritis. After joint destruction has commenced, ligament reconstruction alone does not provide suitable pain relief. Nonsteroidal antiinflamatory medication and fabrication of a custom-molded short opponens splint may relieve inflammation and provide sufficient immobilization to quiet the symptoms. If not, arthroplasty or arthrodesis should be considered. Trapeziometacarpal arthrodesis provides a strong, stable thumb with remarkably good motion because the subtrapezial joints can still move. This procedure is preferred in young people who make forceful demands on their thumbs and whose arthritis is clearly limited to the trapeziometacarpal joint. Isolated deterioration of that joint after an untreated fracture dislocation of the first metacarpal base is such an indication. For the much more commonly encountered idiopathic arthritis at the thumb base in middle-aged women, the subtrapezial joints are more likely to have clinical or subclinical changes, and a trapeziometacarpal arthrodesis in these patients places additional stresses on these joints and hastens their destruction. Thus, arthroplasty is preferred.

A variety of arthroplasty techniques have been described for trapeziometacarpal arthritis using silicone rubber spacers or local tissue. Over time, shear stresses abrade small wear particles from the silicone implants, and the immune system reacts with a foreign-body inflammatory response known as silicone synovitis. Because the techniques using only local tissue have an identical outcome to those incorporating a silicone implant with respect to pain relief, motion preservation, and strength enhancement, and because they do not carry the risk of silicone synovitis, they are preferred. Partial or complete resection of the trapezium is followed by filling the void with a rolled-up segment of tendon or fascia or by allowing the hematoma naturally to convert to a cushion of scar tissue during the 6-week postoperative immobilization period. The results appear to be the same, although conceptually the patient may find removing a bone and actively replacing it with something easier to comprehend than leaving a void that the body deals with on its own.

Complications of excisional and fascial arthroplasties include damage to the superficial radial nerve at the base of the thumb and residual stiffness in the thumb or other digits. These are best avoided by careful adherence to details of intraoperative and postoperative management.

RHEUMATOID ARTHRITIS

The manifestations of rheumatoid arthritis in the wrist and hand are protean; in its advanced state, the disease can devastate the patient's ability to perform even self-care activities, adversely affecting quality of life. Not only are all the joint surfaces and supporting ligaments at risk for destruction by intra-articular synovium, tendons also can be destroyed by rheumatoid tenosynovium. Various patterns of stiffness, instability, loss of motion, and pain are thereby produced.

Like rheumatoid arthritis elsewhere, findings in the hands and wrists are remarkably symmetric, but an identical deformity may be more irksome in the dominant limb because of its increased functional activity. Although the sites of synovial inflammation and tissue destruction may be symmetric, the increased functional demands placed in the dominant limb may also hasten the occurrence of deformity compared with the nondominant side (Fig. 12-17).

Prevention of functional loss requires a dual approach. The first is a direct assault on the diseased synovium itself, and the second is to protect the af-

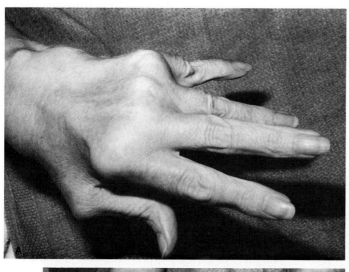

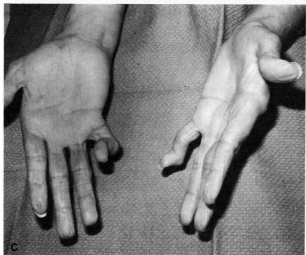

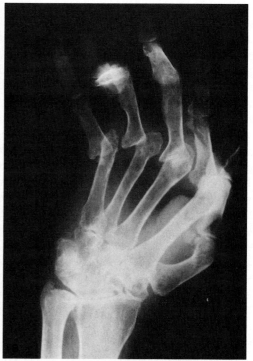

FIGURE 12-17. (A) Characteristic rheumatoid soft tissue deformities include prolific synovitis at the wrist and metacarpophalangeal joints, Z-collapse of the thumb, and extensor tendon ruptures to the ring and small fingers. (B) Collapse deformities in rheumatoid arthritis often form a Z-collapse pattern. Note the ulnar shift of the carpal bones, radial deviation of the wrist, intercarpal fusions, and metacarpophalangeal joint subluxations with ulnar drift of the digits. (C) Although rheumatoid changes in the hand are often symmetric, a boutonniere deformity is noted in the right little finger, and a swan-neck deformity in the left little finger.

fected cartilage, ligaments, and tendons from further destruction.

In most instances, the synovium can be controlled by medications. Useful drugs include nonsteroidal antiinflammatory medications, hydroxychloroquine, gold, prednisone, and methotrexate. The effective use of such medications is in the rheumatologist's domain. If the synovium has been persistently resistant to vigorous medical management, then a surgical synovectomy before adjacent tissue destruction has occurred is often effective at halting the disease locally.

Even if the synovium is not completely controlled by medical or surgical means, deformity and dysfunction can be prevented or at least delayed by minimizing stress on the tissues at risk. All patients with rheumatoid arthritis should learn and routinely practice means of joint protection. For example, jar lids should be twisted off with the left hand and replaced with the right hand to avoid stressing the vulnerable radial collateral ligaments at the metacarpophalangeal joints.

Corrective splinting may also aid joint protection as well as enhance function, but when carried to extremes, splints can restrict activity and be difficult for the arthritic patient to self-apply and remove. Other assistive devices may facilitate specific activities of daily living. Special key handles, jar openers, car door openers, door latch handles, and similar environmental modifications may greatly improve the patient's independence.

When the above nonoperative means have failed to maintain necessary hand function, surgery should be considered. The best surgical results are obtained when performed shortly after the nonoperative means have failed. Late surgery, when fixed joint contractures, marked bone resorption, muscle atrophy, and tendon ruptures have occurred, can at best be palliative. Thus, a close working relation between the medical and surgical arthritis specialists is paramount to maintaining and restoring maximal limb function.

Wrist

Synovium in the radiocarpal and intercarpal joints weakens the supporting wrist capsular ligaments and leads to eventual anterior subluxation and ulnar shift of the carpus on the forearm bones. Weakening of the ligaments supporting the distal radius and ulna allow the distal ulna to subluxate dorsally. This deformity limits forearm rotation and risks extensor tendon rupture on the sharp dorsal edge that may develop on the distal ulna. Reconstructive options include arthrodesis and arthroplasty. Arthrodesis corrects any wrist–forearm deformity but permanently stiffens the wrist. Silicone implant wrist arthroplasty restores alignment and preserves a limited range of motion, but the implant may eventually break. If this occurs, revision to an arthrodesis is generally indicated. With either arthrodesis or arthroplasty, the subluxated distal ulna needs to be addressed, usually by distal resection.

Metacarpophalangeal Joints

Classically, the metacarpophalangeal joints in rheumatoid arthritis subluxate anteriorly and deviate toward the ulna. This prohibits effective opening of the fingers away from the palm and effective pinching against the thumb. Joint synovectomy and soft tissue realignment can restore metacarpophalangeal joint function when performed before the development of fixed flexion contracture and marked cartilage destruction. For the more advanced deformities, silicone implant arthroplasty realigns the digits and restores a 40- to 50-degree arc of active motion.

Interphalangeal Joints

The proximal interphalangeal joint of the index finger is subject to marked medial bending forces from the thumb and is best arthrodesed when it is painful and deformed. The proximal interphalangeal joints of the middle, ring, and little fingers are subject to fewer mediolateral forces, and silicone implant arthroplasties can restore a useful arc of motion. Synovial proliferation with joint destruction is unusual at the distal interphalangeal joints, but joint deformities do occur at this level from tendon imbalances. A boutonniere deformity is one such imbalance. It causes a flexion contracture at the proximal interphalangeal joint and a secondary hyperextension deformity at the distal interphalangeal joint. A swan-neck imbalance results in the opposite configuration: hyperextension of the proximal interphalangeal joint and flexion of the distal joint. Tendon rebalancing procedures can at times restore a more normal alignment and functioning of the joints, and if not, arthrodesis in a partially flexed position is helpful.

Thumb

The metacarpophalangeal and interphalangeal joints of the thumb are frequently involved in rheumatoid arthritis, and the mediolateral stresses to which the thumb is habitually exposed hasten deformity and loss of function. Thumb deformities are particularly disabling when they occur in conjunction with ulnar drift of the other digits. Functional grasp and pinch in such instances may be virtually impossible. If the joint surfaces are reasonably well preserved, collateral ligament tightening and extensor tendon rebalancing can position the thumb joints more favorably. For more advanced destruction, arthrodesis of the interphalangeal joint and arthroplasty of the metacarpophalangeal joint are appropriate.

Tendons

Proliferation of the synovium covering the tendons in the carpal canal, in the digital flexor sheaths, or beneath the extensor retinaculum first produces local swelling, tenderness, and mechanical restraint to smooth tendon gliding. In the digital flexor sheaths, the prolific tenosynovium can cause triggering, but more commonly, crepitation is palpated as the affected tendons glide in and out of the sheaths. In the carpal canal, synovial thickening can cause increased pressure on the median nerve, leading to symptoms of carpal tunnel syndrome. At the dorsal wrist, the extensor tendon synovium is squeezed out from beneath the dorsal retinaculum proximally and distally, leading to a dumbbell-shaped mass.

If the proliferation is not controlled, the synovium begins to invade the tendons and weaken them. This phenomenon is evident on physical examination, particularly on the dorsum of the wrist, when the synovium, which previously was a sessile mass, begins to glide proximally and distally with active finger extension and flexion. A surgical tenosynovectomy is indicated at this point because if unattended, the tendons rupture. A tendon rupture is a dire warning that disaster is imminent. Tenosynovectomy and reconstruction of a single ruptured tendon can have a reasonably favorable outcome. If delayed until multiple tendon ruptures have occurred, the reconstructive options are limited and can salvage only a limited portion of the previous motion. On the dorsum of the wrist, the extensor tendons to the little finger are frequently the first to rupture. On the flexor surface, the flexor pollicis longus and the flexor digitorum profundus to the index are at greatest risk.

Rheumatoid Nodules

Subcutaneous nodules may interfere with hand function and comfort when they occur on the pulp pads of the digits or on the ulnar border of the forearm. They can be excised, but because of their infiltrative nature, excision is usually incomplete and recurrence is common.

Annotated Bibliography

Radial Aplasia, Thumb Hypoplasia, and Aplasia

Bayne LG, Klug MS. Long-term review of the surgical treatment of radial deficiencies. J Hand Surg 1987;12A:169.
A radiologic classification and preferred method of carpal centralization are provided along with long-term results on 101 radial deficiencies in 64 patients. The treatment goal is to centralize the carpus on the distal ulna for improved appearance and function yet retain wrist motion. Ninety-five percent of patients treated with the specified technique achieved satisfactory or good results.

Buck-Gramcko D. Pollicization of the index finger: methods and results in aplasia and hypoplasia of the thumb. J Bone Joint Surg 1971;53A:1605.
The author details his vast operative experience in reconstruction of thumb aplasia and hypoplasia. His preferred surgical timing is at 1 year of age to give the new thumb the longest possible period to develop and therefore provide the most natural result.

Lamb D. Radial club hand: a continuing study of sixty-eight patients with one hundred seventeen club hands. J Bone Joint Surg 1977;59A:1.
A thorough literature review covering embryology, genetics, associated anomalies, anatomy, function, and treatment is followed by the author's own extensive experience with the condition. He describes his techniques for overall patient management, including elbow mobilization, carpal centralization, and index pollicization.

Ulnar Aplasia

Broudy AS, Smith RJ. Deformities of the hand and wrist with ulnar deficiency. J Hand Surg 1979;4:304.
Twenty patients with ulnar deficiency were reviewed. In eight, the ulna was entirely absent. Hypoplastic, webbed, and absent digits were universal. The ulnar anlage was not routinely removed in 16 patients, and progressive deformity did not occur.

Madelung Deformity

Nielson JB. Madelung's deformity: a follow-up study of 26 cases and a review of the literature. Acta Orthop Scand 1977;48:379.
Symptoms developed between ages 8 and 14, and half of these patients underwent ulna shortening or distal resection with or without radius wedge osteotomy at an average of 10 years after the onset of symptoms. Symptoms often spontaneously resolve, so a period of observation is warranted. The history of Madelung deformity along with its etiology and pathogenesis is discussed.

Ranawat CS, DeFiore J, Straub LR. Madelung's deformity: an end-result study of surgical treatment. J Bone Joint Surg 1975;57A:772.
Six female and two male patients had 15 involved wrists. Their ages ranged from 12 to 26. Forearm rotation was painful and limited

in all but two of the affected wrists. Mild deformities when painful were treated with distal ulna resection. Severe deformities were treated with biplane osteotomy of the radius and distal ulna resection.

Congenital Trigger Thumb

Dinham JM, Meggit BF. Trigger thumbs in children: a review of the natural history and indications for treatment in 105 patients. J Bone Joint Surg 1974;56B:153.
The 131 trigger thumbs in this series were first noted at an average age of 2 years, ranging from birth to 11 years. Thirty percent of those noted at birth resolved spontaneously within 12 months, thus there should be no rush to operate. A lower spontaneous resolution rate in older infants warrants waiting 6 months. Children older than age 3 should have surgical release when first diagnosed to avoid permanent fixed contracture of the thumb interphalangeal joint.

Polydactyly and Syndactyly

Cheng JCY, Chan KM, Ma GFY, Leung PC. Polydactyly of the thumb: a surgical plan based on ninety five cases. J Hand Surg 1984;9A:155.
Preaxial polydactyly is the most common congenital hand anomaly occurring in the Chinese population of Hong Kong. The authors present a comprehensive analysis of the types of thumb duplication seen and the respective treatment recommendations. Carefully performed removal of the extra tissues with construction of stable ligaments for the remaining joints gave good results.

Ruby L, Goldberg MJ. Syndactyly and polydactyly. Orthop Clin North Am 1976;7:361.
Polydactyly and syndactyly along with their classifications and associated syndromes are reviewed. The authors review treatment recommendations for the various functional and cosmetic problems associated with the different manifestations.

Toledo LC, Ger E. Evaluation of the operative treatment of syndactyly. J Hand Surg 1979;4:556.
Children less than age 2 and those with major associated anomalies had less satisfactory results from syndactyly surgery than those having surgery after age 2 and those with isolated simple syndactyly. Full-thickness skin grafting yielded better results than split-thickness grafts.

Poland Syndrome

Gausewitz SH, Meals RA, Setoguchi Y. Severe limb deficiencies in Poland's syndrome. Clin Orthop 1984;185:9.
Ten patients are presented with absent pectoral muscle and ipsilateral upper limb deficiencies that are severer than the hypoplasia and syndactyly seen with classical Poland syndrome. A classification for Poland syndrome based on the wide range of limb deficiency that may occur is presented.

Ireland DCR, Takayama N, Flatt AE. Poland's syndrome: a review of forty-three cases. J Bone Joint Surg 1976;58A:52.
Poland syndrome includes absence of the proximal interphalangeal joints and simple, usually incomplete, syndactyly. The limb is generally hypoplastic. Associated chest wall defects include absent pectoral muscles, hypoplastic breast, and pectus deformities. Syndactyly release improves the appearance and function of the hand.

Apert Syndrome

Hoover G, Flatt AE, Weiss MW. The hand and Apert's syndrome. J Bone Joint Surg 1970;52A:878.
Clinical and radiographic findings along with treatment recommendations are based on experience with 20 patients. When referred

early, syndactyly release should be performed in the first and fourth webs bilaterally by age 1. Six months later, removal of the middle finger phalanges and use of the skin to reconstruct the index and ring fingers provides better sensation and skin coverage than trying to preserve a five-digit hand.

Camptodactyly and Clinodactyly

Engber WD, Flatt AE. Camptodactyly: an analysis of sixty-six patients and twenty-four operations. J Hand Surg 1977;2:216.
Nonoperative treatments such as splints and stretching exercises reduced the flexion contractures in only 20% of patients. Operative treatment is individualized according to patient age, presence of bony changes at the proximal interphalangeal joint, and the presence of associated anatomic anomalies.

Poznanski AK, Pratt GB, Manson G, Weiss L. Clinodactyly, camptodactyly, Kirner's deformity and other crooked fingers. Radiology 1969;93:573.
This review article thoroughly covers the clinical appearance, radiographic presentation, and associated syndromes and diseases found with various types of congenitally crooked fingers.

Trigger Finger

Fahey J, Bollinger J. Trigger finger in adults and children. J Bone Joint Surg 1954;36A:1200.
The etiology, clinical presentation, histopathology, and treatment recommendations for trigger digits in children and adults are compared. In children, only operative treatment has proved effective. In adults with recent onset of symptoms, a trial of conservative treatment is advised.

De Quervain Tendinitis

Arons MS. de Quervain's release in working women: a report of failures, complications and associated diagnoses. J Hand Surg 1987;12A:540.
In 16 patients referred for persistent problems following a de Quervain release, 23 associated diagnoses and 14 complications were noted. Trigger digit, tennis elbow, tendinitis, and carpal tunnel syndrome were among the other diagnoses. Neuritis of the superficial radial nerve, tendon subluxation, scar problems, and reflex sympathetic dystrophy constituted the complications. An appropriate diagnostic and treatment regimen minimizes persistent symptoms and complications after surgery.

Leao L. De Quervain's disease: a clinical and anatomical study. J Bone Joint Surg 1958;40A:1063.
The results of 27 cadaver dissections and the clinical courses of 29 patients are presented. The abductor pollicis longus usually has more than one tendon slip in the first dorsal compartment. De Quervain disease is occupationally related in many patients.

Carpal Tunnel Syndrome

Green D. Diagnostic and therapeutic value of carpal tunnel injection. J Hand Surg 1984;9A:850.
Eight milligrams of dexamethasone acetate was injected into 281 wrists considered to have carpal tunnel syndrome on clinical evaluation. Over 80% achieved temporary relief for an average of more than 3 months. The patients receiving benefit from injection universally did well with carpal tunnel release surgery. Even two thirds of the patients not receiving benefit from the injection did well with eventual carpal tunnel release.

Phalen G. The carpal tunnel syndrome: seventeen years' experience in diagnosis and treatment of 654 hands. J Bone Joint Surg 1966;48A:211.

All aspects of carpal tunnel syndrome in the author's vast personal experience are discussed. The wrist flexion test (Phalen test) is performed by asking the patient to hold the forearms vertically and allow the wrists to drop into complete flexion. Reproduction or worsening of symptoms within 1 minute is considered to be a positive test. The test may be negative in wrists with advanced degrees of median nerve compression.

Ulnar Tunnel Syndrome

Shea JD, McClain EJ. Ulnar nerve compression syndromes at and below the wrist. J Bone Joint Surg 1969;51A:1095.
The anatomy, pathophysiology, etiology, diagnosis, and treatment of ulnar nerve compression syndromes in the hand and wrist are discussed. Proximal lesions before the branching of the ulnar nerve will cause both motor and sensory changes. More distally located compressions will cause either motor or sensory changes depending on which branch is affected.

Ganglion

Angelides AC, Wallace PF. The dorsal ganglion of the wrist: its pathogenesis, gross and microscopic anatomy and surgical treatment. J Hand Surg 1976;1:228.
Surgical excision of 500 dorsal wrist ganglions included removal of the portion of dorsal wrist capsule attached to the ganglion stalk. This resulted in a 99% cure rate during a 4-month to 25-year follow-up.

Nelson CL, Sawmiller S, Phalen GS. Ganglions of the wrist and hand. J Bone Joint Surg 1972;54A:1459.
Five hundred forty-three patients with ganglions on their wrists and hands were studied. Their ages ranged from 4 to 89, with 80% occurring between 20 and 50 years old. Results of various treatments are compared. Dissipation of the fluid with or without injection of steroid or hyaluronidase gave recurrence rates of 33% to 88% compared with about 10% for surgical excision.

Dupuytren Contracture

McFarlane R. The current status of Dupuytren's disease. J Hand Surg 1983;8:703.
The author reviews the current research and mechanisms of contraction in Dupuytren disease. The preliminary statistical data from more than 800 patients collected internationally indicates a positive family history in one fourth of patients, a surgical complication rate of 19%, and a postoperative recurrence or extension of the disease in 21%.

Skoog T. Dupuytren's contracture with special reference to aetiology and improved surgical treatment: its occurence in epileptics: notes on knuckle pads. Acta Chir Scand 1948; 139(Suppl):1.
This classic treatise thoroughly reviews the entire condition, including incidence, sites of involvement, natural history, and treatment.

Kienböck Disease

Almquist E, Burns J Jr. Radial shortening for the treatment of Kienböck's disease: a five to ten year follow-up. J Hand Surg 1982; 7:348.
Eleven of 12 patients had long-term pain reduction following radial shortening for Kienböck disease that had not preoperatively progressed to radiocarpal and intercarpal arthritis. Relief of rest pain was dramatic, although some pain with forceful activities persisted. Wrist and forearm motions were preserved. Ten patients showed radiographic evidence of lunate revascularization. No carpus showed progressive collapse.

Gelberman R, Salamon P, Jurist J, Posch J. Ulnar variance in Kienböck's disease. J Bone Joint Surg 1975;57A:674.
A racial variation exists for the relative length of the ulna compared with the radius, and a relation of that measurement to the occurrence of Kienböck disease is apparent. A short ulna, however, must not be considered the primary etiologic factor.

Osteoarthritis

Amadio PC, Millender LH, Smith RJ. Silicone spacer or tendon spacer for trapezium resection arthroplasty: comparison of results. J Hand Surg 1982;7:237.
Twenty-five patients undergoing trapezium excisional arthroplasty for carpometacarpal arthritis were compared with 25 patients undergoing silicone replacement arthroplasty for the same condition. When pain relief, thumb motion, and strength were assessed 1 to 9 years postoperatively, the results for the two groups were nearly identical.

Swanson AB, Swanson G. Osteoarthritis in the hand. J Hand Surg 1983;8:669.
This review article covers pathophysiology, incidence, classification, clinical and radiographic findings, and treatment recommendations.

Rheumatoid Arthritis

Millender L, Sledge C, eds. Symposium on rheumatoid arthritis. Orthop Clin North Am 1975;6:601.
The diagnosis and medical management of rheumatoid arthritis as well as radiologic findings and surgical planning are discussed. Various experts then cover specific anatomic regions and individual deformities and detail relevant reconstructive techniques.

Nalebuff E. Rheumatoid hand surgery: update. J Hand Surg 1983;8: 678.
One fourth of all arthritis surgery is performed in the hand. The available and useful procedures can be classified as synovectomy, tenosynovectomy, tendon reconstruction, arthroplasty, and arthrodesis. Appropriately timed surgery aids greatly in maintaining and restoring useful hand function.

Turek's Orthopaedics: Principles and Their Application, Fifth Edition,
edited by Stuart L. Weinstein and Joseph A. Buckwalter.
J.B. Lippincott Company, Philadelphia, © 1994.

13

Stuart L. Weinstein

The Thoracolumbar Spine

SPINAL DEFORMITY

Deformities of the spine may occur either in the coronal or sagittal plane. All deformities of the spine are classified according to the magnitude and the direction of the curvature, the location of its apex, and the etiology. Curvature of the spine may be associated with many conditions (Table 13-1). The language used to describe the various aspects of spinal deformity is often confusing (Table 13-2).

General Considerations

In any patient presenting with a spinal deformity, it is incumbent on the examining physician to try to ascertain the etiology because this has bearing on the natural history of the condition and has implications for treatment. The etiology may be determined on the basis of a careful history, complete physical examination, and appropriate radiographic studies. The patient and family should be asked how the curve was detected (eg, school screening, observation by a friend or health care worker, apparent body asymmetry) and their impression about whether the curve is static or progressive. Idiopathic scoliosis in children is not a painful condition. If the patient gives a history of back pain associated with the deformity, other sources should be considered; Scheuermann kyphosis, spondylolysis, spondylolisthesis, and spinal or spinal cord tumor must be ruled out. Symptoms of shortness of breath, physical limitations, and psychosocial effects possibly caused

TABLE 13-1.
SRS Classification of Spine Deformity

SCOLIOSIS

Idiopathic
  Infantile (0–3 years)
    Resolving
    Progressive
  Juvenile (4 years to puberty onset)
  Adolescent (puberty onset to epiphyseal closure)
  Adult (epiphyses closed)
Neuromuscular
Neuropathic
  Upper motor neuron lesion
    Cerebral palsy
    Spinocerebellar degeneration
      Friedreich
      Charcot-Marie-Tooth
      Roussy-Lévy
    Syringomyelia
    Spinal cord tumor
    Spinal cord trauma
    Other
  Lower motor neuron lesion
    Poliomyelitis
    Traumatic
      Spinal muscular atrophy
      Myelomeningocele (paralytic)
    Dysautonomia (Riley-Day)
    Other
  Myopathic
    Arthrogryposis
    Muscular dystrophy
      Duchenne (pseudohypertrophic)
      Limb-girdle
      Facioscapulohumeral

    Congenital hypotonia
    Myotonia dystrophica
    Other
Congenital
  Failure of formation
    Partial unilateral (wedge vertebra)
    Complete unilateral (hemivertebra)
      Fully segmented
      Semisegmented
      Nonsegmented
  Failure of segmentation
    Unilateral (unilateral unsegmented
      bar)
    Bilateral (bloc vertebrae)
  Mixed
  Associated with neural tissue defect
    Myelomeningocele
    Meningocele
    Spinal dysraphism
      Diastematomyelia
    Other
Neurofibromatosis
Mesenchymal
  Marfan
  Homocystinuria
  Ehlers-Danlos
  Other
Traumatic
  Fracture or dislocation (nonparalytic)
  Postradiation
  Other

Soft tissue contractures
  Postempyema
  Burns
  Other
Osteochondrodystrophies
  Achondroplasia
  Spondyloepiphyseal
    dysplasia
  Diastrophic dwarfism
  Mucopolysaccharidoses
  Other
Tumor
  Benign
  Malignant
Rheumatoid disease
Metabolic
  Rickets
  Juvenile osteoporosis
  Osteogenesis imperfecta
Related to lumbosacral
    area
  Spondylolysis
  Spondylolisthesis
  Other
Thoracogenic
  Postthoracoplasty
  Postthoracotomy
  Other
Hysterical
Functional
  Postural
  Secondary to short leg
  Due to muscle spasm
  Other

KYPHOSIS

Postural
Scheuermann disease
Congenital
  Defect of segmentation
  Defect of formation
  Mixed
Paralytic
  Poliomyelitis
  Anterior horn cell
  Upper motor neuron
Myelomeningocele
Posttraumatic
  Acute

Chronic
Inflammatory
  Tuberculosis
  Other infections
  Ankylosing spondylitis
Postsurgical
  Postlaminectomy
  Postexcision (eg, tumor)
Postradiation
Metabolic
  Osteoporosis
  Senile

  Juvenile
  Osteogenesis imperfecta
  Other
Developmental
  Achondroplasia
  Mucopolysaccharidoses
  Other
Tumor
  Benign
  Malignant
    Primary
    Metastatic

(continued)

TABLE 13-1.
(Continued)

LORDOSIS
Postural
Congenital
Paralytic
  Neuropathic
  Myopathic
Contracture of hip flexors
Secondary to shunts

(Winter RB. Spinal problems in pediatric orthopaedics. In: Morrissy RT, ed. Lovell and Winter's pediatric orthopaedics. Philadelphia, JB Lippincott, 1990:697–698)

TABLE 13-2.
Glossary of Scoliosis-Related Terms

Adolescent scoliosis: spinal curvature developing after onset of puberty and before maturity

Adult scoliosis: spinal curvature existing after skeletal maturity (closure or epiphyses)

Apical vertebra: vertebra most deviated from the vertical axis of the patient

Cervical curve: spinal curvature that has its apex between C2 and C6

Cervicothoracic curve: spinal curvature that has its apex at C7 and T1

Compensation: accurate alignment of the midline of the skull over the midline of the sacrum

Compensatory curve: curve (which can be structural) above or below a major curve that tends to maintain normal body alignment

Congenital scoliosis: scoliosis due to congenital anomalous vertebral development

Double structural curve (scoliosis): two structural curves in the same spine, one balancing the other

Double thoracic curve (scoliosis): two structural curves, both having their apex within the thoracic spine

End vertebra: the most cephalad vertebra of a curve whose superior surface or the most caudad vertebra whose inferior surface tilts maximally toward the concavity of the curve

Fractional curve: curve that is incomplete because it returns to the erect position; its only horizontal vertebra is its caudad or cephalad one

Full curve: curve in which the only horizontal vertebra is at the apex

Gibbus: sharply angular kyphos

Infantile scoliosis: spinal curvature developing during the first 3 years of life

Juvenile scoliosis: spinal curvature developing between the skeletal ages of 4 years and the onset of puberty

Kyphos: abnormal kyphosis

Kyphoscoliosis: lateral curvature of the spine associated with either increased posterior or decreased anterior angulation in the sagittal plane in excess of the accepted normal for that area

Lordoscoliosis: lateral curvature of the spine associated with an increase in anterior curvature or a decrease in posterior angulation in the sagittal plane in excess of normal for that area

Lumbar curve: spinal curvature that has its apex from L2 to L4

Lumbosacral curve: spinal curvature that has its apex at L5 or below

Major curve: most apparent curve and usually the most structural curve

Nonstructural scoliosis: spinal curvature without structural characteristics (see *Structural curve*)

Pelvic obliquity: deviation of the pelvis from the horizontal in the frontal plane

Primary curve: the first or earliest of several curves to appear; usually, but not necessarily, the most structural curve

Structural curve: segment of spine with a fixed lateral curvature; not necessarily the major or primary curve; identified radiographically in supine lateral side-bending or traction films by the failure to demonstrate normal flexibility

Thoracic curve (scoliosis): curve with the apex between T2 and T11

Thoracolumbar curve: spinal curvature that has its apex at T12 and L1 or at the interspace between these vertebrae

(Winter RB. Spinal problems in pediatric orthopaedics. In: Morrissy RT, ed. Lovell and Winter's pediatric orthopaedics. Philadelphia, JB Lippincott, 1990:697)

by the curvature should be noted. The timing of reaching developmental milestones should be recorded. A careful family history must be obtained seeking out any history of neurologic or congenital conditions that may be associated with the curvature.

Treatment decisions and probabilities of curve progression depend on the patient's growth potential, so it is important to assess maturity historically. The age at onset of pubic hair, axillary hair, breast budding, and menarche should be noted. (Fig. 13-1). Finally, details of any previous treatment for the condition should be noted.

Each patient should have a general physical examination, paying particular attention to the patient's body habitus and any evidence of congenital abnormalities in the face, palate, ears, upper extremities, and heart. The skin should be inspected for neurofibromas or café-au-lait spots indicative of neurofibromatosis. The skin over the sacral area should be examined for evidence of hair patches, dimpling, pigmentation changes, nevi, and lipomas, which may be associated with spinal dysraphism. Secondary sex characteristics, including breast development and the presence of pubic and axillary hair (graded according to the Tanner scale), must be noted. Limb lengths should be measured to rule out limb length inequality. Sitting and standing height should also be measured. A complete neurologic examination must also be performed. Any abnormality indicative of an associated neurologic condition should be further investigated by a neurologist, and possible further diagnostic studies—such as a spinal cord magnetic

resonance imaging (MRI), electromyography (EMG), and nerve conduction velocities—should be considered. Abnormalities detected that suggest a syndrome may require genetic consultation.

Spinal deformity is suspected by the presence of body asymmetry (Fig. 13-2). The patient should be examined from both the front and the back, looking for asymmetry in shoulder height, waistline, chest, scapular height, and prominence. The relation of the thorax to the pelvis should be noted. Spinal compensation can be measured by dropping a plumb line from the spinous process of C7 and measuring the distance it falls from the midgluteal cleft.

Rotational asymmetry is best detected on the Adams forward bend test. The test is performed by having the patient stand with the feet together and the knees straight. The patient bends forward at the waist with the arms dependent and the hands held with palms opposed (Fig. 13-3). The rotational asymmetry is best assessed by viewing the patient from in front. Any leg length inequality should be compensated for by placing an appropriate-sized block underneath the short leg. The patient should be assessed in three positions to observe the thoracic, thoracolumbar, and lumbar spine (Fig. 13-4). The patient should also be viewed from the side to assess any abnormal increases in thoracic or thoracolumbar kyphosis and any evidence of failure to reverse the normal lumbar lordosis.

If on physical examination the patient has evidence of a structural scoliosis, a standing posteroanterior (PA) unshielded upright radiograph of the

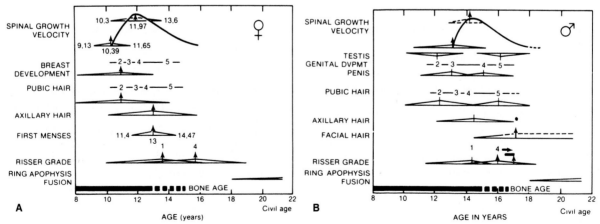

FIGURE 13-1. (A) The relation of spinal growth velocity to maturity landmarks and the events of puberty in girls. (B) The relation of spinal growth velocity to maturity landmarks and the events of puberty in boys. (Modified from Trever S, Kleinman R, Bleck EE. Growth landmarks and the evolution of scoliosis: a review of pertinent studies on their usefulness. Dev Med Child Neurol 1980;22: 675–684)

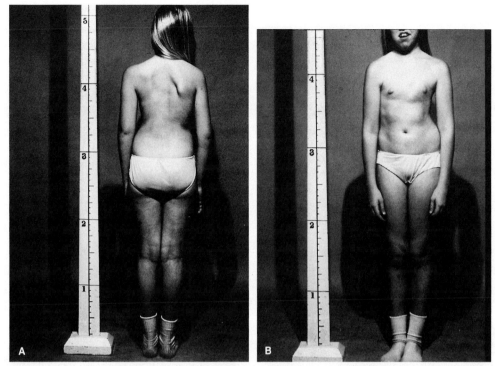

FIGURE 13-2. (A) A patient with a typical right thoracic curve as viewed from the back. The left shoulder is lower, and the right scapula is more prominent. The thorax is shifted to the right with a decreased distance between the right arm and the thorax. Because of the shift in the thorax to the right, the waistline is altered with the left iliac crest appearing higher. This crest asymmetry is apparent, not real. (B) A patient with a typical right thoracic curve as viewed from the front. The left shoulder appears lower. The thorax is shifted to the right with a decreased distance between the right arm and the thorax. The left hip appears more prominent secondary to the rightward shift of the thorax.

spine is ordered. The entire spine, as well as iliac crests, must be included on the radiograph so that no curves are missed and skeletal maturity can be assessed. If the patient has complaints of pain or signs of a sagittal spinal deformity, a standing, full-length lateral radiograph of the spine is also ordered.

The radiographs are assessed for any congenital abnormalities in the vertebral bodies, ribs, and pelvis. All curves are assessed for magnitude (Cobb measurements), direction (direction of the curve convexity), location (eg, thoracic lumbar, thoracolumbar, double major, double thoracic), and pedicle rotation (Fig. 13-5). Maturity is assessed by the Risser sign (Fig. 13-6). Additional diagnostic and radiographic studies may be indicated if other than idiopathic scoliosis is suspected.

Assessment of patients with spinal curvature depends on the probabilities of curve progression. These probabilities are based on the natural history of the specific curve, which depends on its etiology, pattern, magnitude, and associated sagittal plane deformity.

This natural history must be considered in relation to the patient's growth potential as determined by history, physical assessment of skeletal maturity, and radiographic assessment of maturity (ie, Risser sign, ossification of vertebral apophyses, wrist film for bone age assessment, or a combination of these tests).

Scoliosis

Scoliosis is a descriptive term that refers to a lateral curvature of the spine. The scoliosis may be structural or nonstructural. A nonstructural scoliosis corrects or overcorrects on supine side-bending radiographs or traction films. A structural scoliosis is a fixed lateral curvature with rotation. On radiograph, the spinous processes in a structural curve rotate to the curve concavity. On a supine side-bending radiograph or a traction radiograph, a structural curve lacks normal flexibility. Many conditions are associated with structural scoliosis (see Table 13-1). The most com-

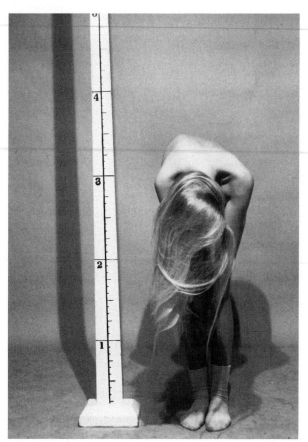

FIGURE 13-3. A patient with a typical right thoracic curve as viewed from the front on the forward bend test. Note the right thoracic prominence.

mon structural curvature has no known cause and is referred to as *idiopathic scoliosis.* Examples of non-structural curvatures include scoliosis secondary to limb length inequality or scoliosis secondary to a herniated nucleus pulposus with nerve root irritation causing a list. If the primary problem is corrected (eg, the limb length inequality), the scoliosis resolves.

The various etiologies of scoliosis are related to different natural histories. These varying natural histories profoundly influence the effect of the curvature on the patient's life and the indications for treatment.

Idiopathic scoliosis is the most common type of structural scoliosis. This type of scoliosis has a genetic predisposition, and although many etiologic theories have been proposed, the cause remains unknown.

Idiopathic scoliosis is subclassified into three groups by age at onset of the conditions: infantile (0 to 3 years of age), juvenile (3 to 10 years of age), and adolescent (older than 10 years of age but before

maturity). Although these subtypes may represent a continuum of the same condition, their natural histories differ. Therefore, these three subtypes of idiopathic scoliosis are considered separately.

Infantile Idiopathic Scoliosis

Infantile idiopathic scoliosis is a structural spinal deformity detected during the first 3 years of life. It accounts for less than 1% of all cases of idiopathic scoliosis in the United States. It is more commonly seen in Europe, especially Great Britain. Most of these curves develop within the first 6 months of life, with the left lumbar curve pattern being the most common. Epidemiologic and associated problems include older maternal age, increased incidence of inguinal hernias among relatives, and association with congenital heart disease (2.5%), congenital hip dysplasia (3.5%),

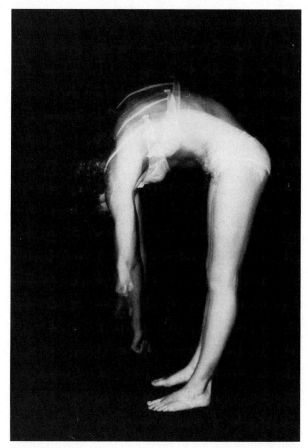

FIGURE 13-4. Forward bend test: three positions are required to observe the thoracic, thoracolumbar, and lumbar levels of the spine.

and developmental problems, particularly mental retardation (13%). Intrauterine molding is thought to be an etiologic factor because 83% of patients have plagiocephaly, and more than half have evidence of

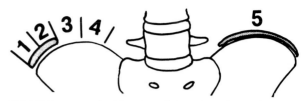

FIGURE 13-6. Ossification of the epiphysis usually starts at the anterosuperior iliac spine and progresses posteriorly. The iliac crest is divided into four quarters, and the excursion or stage of maturity is designated as the amount of progression.

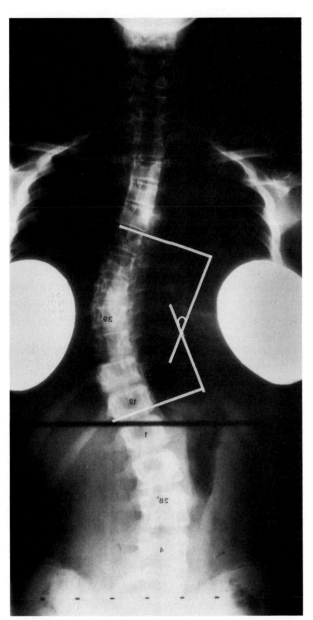

FIGURE 13-5. Curve measurements (Cobb method). (1) Apparent perpendicular is erected from the end plate of the most caudal vertebrae, whose inferior end plate tilts maximally to the concavity of the curve (inferior end vertebrae). (2) A perpendicular is erected from the end plate of the most cephalad vertebrae, whose superior end plate tilts maximally to the concavity of the curve (superior end vertebrae). The curve value is the number of degrees formed by the angle of intersection of these perpendiculars, in this case 39 degrees.

rib-molding deformities. Natural history studies indicate that 85% of the curves regress spontaneously, particularly if the curve onset was before 12 months of age. Fifteen percent of the curves may progress, often leading to severe deformities. Compensatory curves are generally not seen in patients with infantile idiopathic scoliosis.

The differential diagnosis in this age group (0 to 3 years) includes congenital scoliosis and scoliosis of a neuromuscular etiology or intraspinal pathology (eg, syringomyelia). Careful neurologic examination is imperative. Radiographs rule out congenital spinal abnormalities.

If the patient can sit or stand, upright PA and lateral radiographs should be obtained. The Cobb angle and the rib–vertebral angle difference should be measured (Fig. 13-7). If the rib–vertebral angle difference is greater than 20 degrees, the curvature is likely progressive. With measurements of less than 20 degrees, the curve is likely to resolve. All patients must be followed by serial radiographic examination, calculating the Cobb angle and the rib–vertebral angle difference at each visit. In progressive curves, the convex side rib head is overlapped by the shadow of the vertebral body. This radiographic sign indicates a progressive curve. Curves that maintain a Cobb angle of less than 35 degrees have a high likelihood of resolution. Compensatory curves are not common in patients with infantile idiopathic scoliosis. The development of a compensatory curve is a bad prognostic sign that indicates a probable curve progression (Fig. 13-8).

Observation is indicated for curves with less than a 25-degree Cobb angle and less than a 20-degree rib–vertebral angle difference. The patient should be reevaluated in 4 to 6 months with a repeat standing radiograph of the spine. With resolution of the curvature, the patient can be followed at 1- to 2-year intervals. In curves with a 25- to 35-degree Cobb

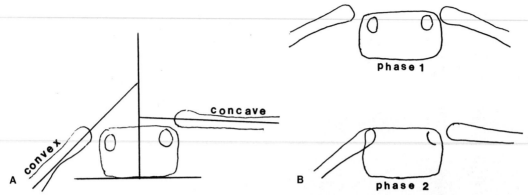

FIGURE 13-7. (A) The rib–vertebral angle difference is calculated by subtracting the convex value from the concave value at the thoracic curve apical vertebra. (B) Phase changes at apical vertebra. Phase 2 appearance denotes probable progression.

angle and with a rib–vertebral angle difference of 25 degrees, repeat clinical and radiographic evaluation at 4- to 6-month intervals is warranted. If the Cobb angle increases by 5 to 10 degrees with or without changes in the rib–vertebral angle difference, treatment is indicated.

Initial treatment for a progressive curve is serial casting to correct the deformity followed by the use of a Milwaukee brace (cervical-thoracic-lumbar-sacral orthosis) to maintain correction. In the infantile patient, the corrective cast usually needs to be applied with sedation or under general anesthesia. The casts are worn for 6 to 12 weeks and are serially changed until maximal correction is obtained. A Milwaukee brace is then fabricated and worn full-time (22 to 23 hours per day) for 2 to 3 years to maintain the correction obtained by casting. If correction is maintained, the patient may be gradually weaned from the brace. If progression occurs, full-time orthotic use must be reinstituted. With rapid curve progression or progression despite bracing, complete neurologic evaluation should be repeated. An MRI looking for intraspinal pathology should also be considered.

If curve progression continues despite the use of an orthotic, subcutaneous distraction spinal instrumentation without fusion followed by bracing is indicated. The rod can then be lengthened periodically to allow for growth with a formal posterior spinal fusion and instrumentation at maturity.

Juvenile Idiopathic Scoliosis

Juvenile idiopathic scoliosis is a lateral curvature of the spine that presents after 3 years of age but before the adolescent growth spurt. Patients classified as having juvenile idiopathic scoliosis may actually have late-onset infantile idiopathic scoliosis or early-onset adolescent idiopathic scoliosis. This group of patients accounts for about 20% of all idiopathic scoliosis patients.

Juvenile idiopathic scoliosis occurs more commonly in girls, with right thoracic curves accounting for about two thirds of all curve patterns. Double major curves (right thoracic and left lumbar) and thoracolumbar curves follow in frequency.

Juvenile adolescent idiopathic curvatures may progress and cause severe deformity. Some may progress relentlessly from onset, but others may be stable or progress slowly until the adolescent growth spurt when rapid progression ensues. Unlike infantile curves, juvenile idiopathic scoliosis curvatures do not resolve spontaneously.

The indication for treatment is a progressive curve of 25 degrees or more. The rib–vertebral angle difference has not been shown to be prognostic in these patients. Curves rarely progress more than 1 degree per month. Therefore, if the patient has a curve of less than 20 degrees, follow-up evaluation in 6 to 8 months is appropriate. Treatment is indicated for progression of at least 10 degrees.

If the curve is between 20 and 25 degrees at detection, follow-up evaluation clinically and radiographically should be obtained in 5 to 6 months, with treatment indicated for a greater than 5-degree increase in curve. For curves greater than 25 degrees, because of the high probably of progression, treatment should begin immediately.

If the curve is flexible, as determined by clinical evaluation and in some cases by supine side-bending radiographs, orthotic treatment is indicated in an at-

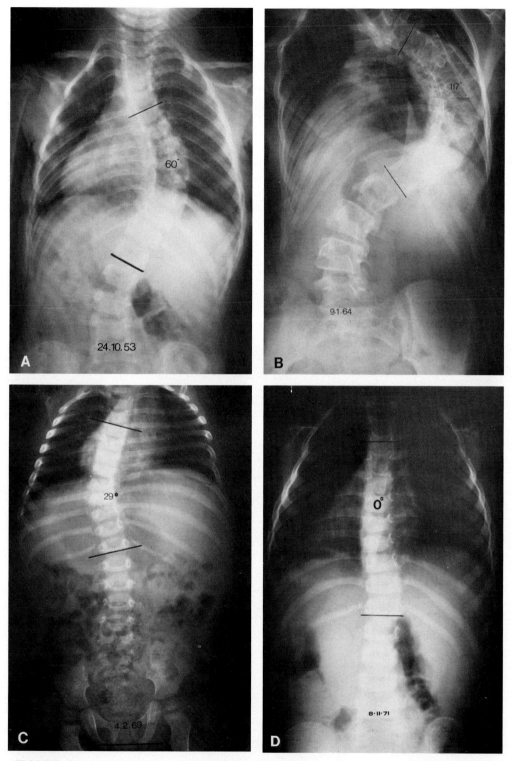

FIGURE 13-8. (A) Progressive type of infantile idiopathic scoliosis, early radiograph. Curve measures 60 degrees. (B) Late radiograph showing marked increase of primary curve and developing secondary curves. (C) Resolving type, early radiograph. Curve measures 29 degrees. No secondary curve. (D) Resolving type, later radiograph. Curve reduced to zero. (Courtesy of Dr. J.I.P. James)

tempt to prevent further progression. If the curve is rigid, serial cast correction, much like that recommended for infantile idiopathic scoliosis, is warranted before fitting the patient with a Milwaukee brace. The orthosis is worn on a full-time basis for several years until curve correction is achieved. Then, weaning may begin and continue as long as curve correction is maintained. The brace is then worn at night only until the patient reaches skeletal maturity (ie, Risser grade 4 or 5, or no spinal growth for the previous 18 months).

If the curve progresses rapidly or cannot be controlled by casting or an orthosis, careful neurologic examination and possible evaluation by MRI (looking for brain and intraspinal pathology) should be considered. If curve progression continues despite casting or bracing, distraction instrumentation without fusion should be considered (Fig. 13-9). After surgery, the

patient continues in an orthosis. The distraction device is lengthened with skeletal growth until the patient reaches puberty, when posterior spinal fusion and instrumentation are performed.

Adolescent Idiopathic Scoliosis

Adolescent idiopathic scoliosis is structural curvature of the spine presenting at or about the onset of puberty and before maturity. Adolescent idiopathic scoliosis accounts for about 80% of cases of idiopathic scoliosis. The etiology is unknown. The prevalence (ie, occurrence in the at-risk population, children 10 to 16 years of age) of adolescent idiopathic scoliosis is about 2% to 3%. Although there is an overall female predominance for the condition (3.6:1); the prevalence in males and females is equal in small-magnitude curves (10 degrees). With increasing curve

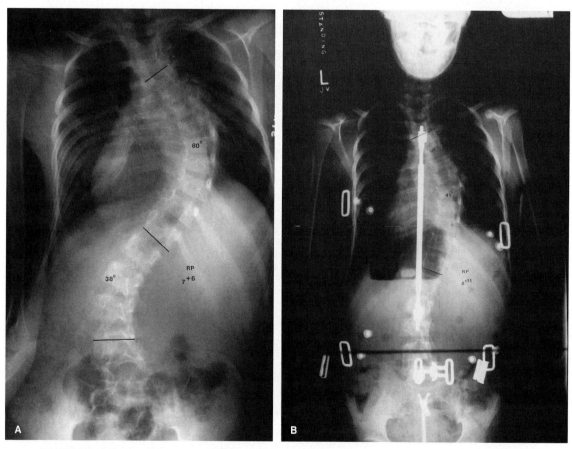

FIGURE 13-9. (A) Juvenile idiopathic scoliosis in a 7½-year-old boy with an 80-degree thoracic curve that progressed despite bracing. (B) Same patient at age 8 years and 11 months. Curve is maintained at 41 degrees with distraction instrumentation and fusion at hook sites. Patient is wearing TLSO external support. Definite surgery is planned at puberty.

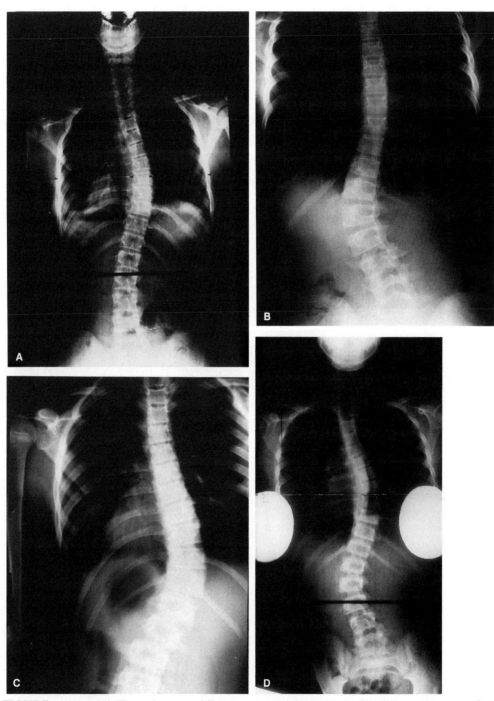

FIGURE 13-10. (A) Thoracic curve. Ninety-percent right convexity involving an average of six vertebrae: apex—T8, T9; upper end vertebrae—T5, T6; lower end vertebrae—T11, T12. (B) Lumbar curve. Seventy-percent left convexity involving an average of five vertebrae: apex—L1, L2; upper end vertebrae—T11, T12; lower end vertebrae—L3, L4. (C) Thoracolumbar curve. Eighty-percent right convexity involving an average of six to eight vertebrae: apex—T11, T12; upper end vertebrae—T6, T7; lower end vertebrae—L1, L2. (D) Double curve. Ninety-percent right thoracic convexity and left lumbar convexity. Thoracic component, average five vertebrae: apex—T7; upper end vertebrae—T5, T6; lower end vertebrae—T10. Lumbar component, average five vertebrae: apex—T2; upper end vertebra—T11; lower end vertebra—L4.

magnitude, there is an overwhelming female predominance (curves greater than 30 degrees; female predominance 10:1).

Four major curve patterns are seen in adolescent idiopathic scoliosis (Fig. 13-10). Because most thoracic curve patterns are convex to the right, a child presenting with a left convex thoracic curve should be examined carefully for a neurologic deficit. In this situation, neurologic consultation and MRI scanning should be considered because of the high association of intraspinal pathology with this curve pattern. Also, a history of rapid progression of an adolescent curvature should alert the physician to consider similar diagnostic evaluations.

Initial radiographic evaluation includes PA and lateral radiographs of the entire spine taken in the standing position. At follow-up visits, only PA radiographs are usually necessary. It is important to minimize the radiation that the patient receives over time. Radiographs should be taken only when necessary for treatment decisions. Appropriate technique should be used to avoid the need for repeat films. Other radiation protection measures include beam collimation, antiscatter grids, beam filtration, high-speed film, intensifying screens, gonadal and breast shields, and PA as opposed to anteroposterior (AP) projections. The use of the PA projection avoids radiation to the developing breast tissue, which is radiosensitive. Special radiographic views, such as side-bending radiographs, are rarely indicated unless the patient is being considered for surgical management. Each radiograph is measured for the Cobb angle, rotation, and ossification of the iliac apophysis (Risser sign).

Treatment of any condition is an attempt to alter the natural history of that condition. It is important to understand the natural history of untreated adolescent idiopathic scoliosis with regard to curve progression, effect on pulmonary function, back pain, mortality, psychosocial problems, and effect of and on pregnancy.

Most treatment decisions are based on curve progression or the probability of curve progression. Most information available on curve progression is from studies of girls, particularly those with thoracic curves. The factors that influence the probability of curve progression in the immature patient include growth potential factors, such as age, gender, and maturity, and curve factors, such as type and magnitude. Double-curve patterns have a greater tendency for progression than single-curve patterns. Curves detected before menarche have a much

TABLE 13-3.
Probabilities of Progression Based on Curve Magnitude and Age

Curve Magnitude at Detection (Degrees)	Age		
	10–12 y	*13–15 y*	*16 y*
<19	25%	10%	0%
20–29	60%	40%	10%
30–59	90%	70%	30%
>60	100%	90%	70%

(Nachemson A, Lonstein JE, Weinstein SL. Prevalence and natural history: committee report. Scoliosis Reasearch Society, 1982)

greater chance of progression than those detected after menarche. With increasing age at detection, there is a decreasing risk of curve progression. The larger the curve magnitude at detection, the greater the chance of progression; the lower the Risser grade at curve detection, the greater the risk of progression. The risk of progression for boys is about one tenth that of girls with comparable curves.

The risk of curve progression decreases with increasing skeletal maturity. Large-magnitude curves, however, may continue to progress after maturity (Table 13-3). Many curves continue to progress throughout the patient's life. In general, curves less than 30 degrees at maturity tend not to progress regardless of the curve pattern. Many curves greater than 30 degrees, and particularly thoracic curves greater than 50 degrees, continue to progress.

The generally accepted incidence of backache in the general population is about 60% to 80%, although the incidence varies considerably. The incidence of back pain in patients with scoliosis is comparable to that in the general population. Scoliosis patients, however, often have an increased incidence of frequent or daily backache compared with the general population. Patients with lumbar and thoracolumbar curves, particularly those with lateral listhesis or translatory shifts (Fig. 13-11) at the lower end of their curves, tend to have a slightly greater incidence of backache than patients with other curve patterns. Back pain in adult patients with scoliosis is not always related to the curvature; it may emanate from the counter-curve below, or it may be discogenic, neurogenic, or facet joint related.

With regard to pulmonary function, only in thoracic curves is there a direct correlation between decreasing vital capacity and FEV_1 with increasing curve

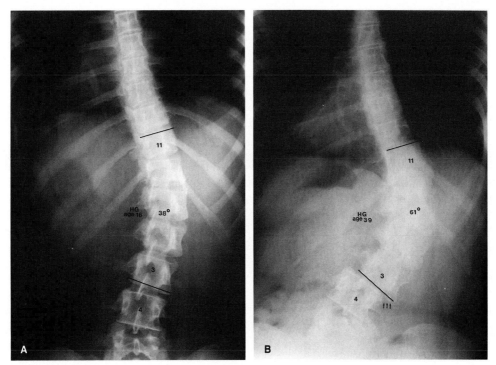

FIGURE 13-11. (**A**) Sixteen-year-old girl with a 38-degree right lumbar curve from T11 to L3. Her skeletal maturity is assessed as grade 5 on the Risser scale. (**B**) At 39 years of age, her right lumbar curve has increased to 61 degrees. Note the translatory shift of L3 on L4 (*arrows*). (Weinstein SL. The natural history of scoliosis in the skeletally mature patient. In: Dickson JH, ed. Spinal deformities, vol 1. Philadelphia, Hanley & Belfus, 1987:199)

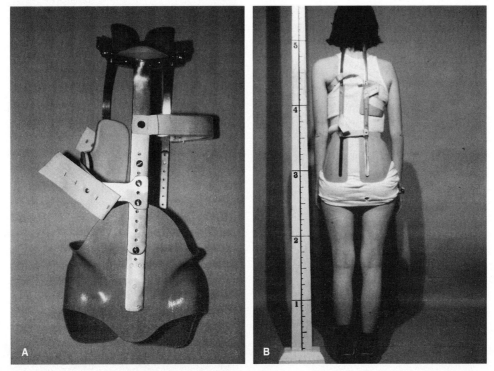

FIGURE 13-12. Milwaukee brace (CTLSO). The brace was developed in the late 1940s (**A**, frontal view of bone). Despite its widespread use, few long-term studies are available that evaluate the results of treatment (**B**, view from behind with patient wearing brace). In addition, most studies fail to document curve progression; thus, it is uncertain whether those patients braced would have had continued progression had they not been braced. There are no published prospective controlled studies on bracing.

severity. In all other curve patterns in idiopathic scoliosis, there is no direct correlation between curve magnitude and limitation in pulmonary function. Most patients with adolescent idiopathic scoliosis have loss of the normal thoracic kyphosis. This loss of thoracic kyphosis (hypokyphosis) further diminishes pulmonary function associated with increasing curve severity.

Patients do not die from adolescent idiopathic scoliosis. The only patients at risk are those with high-angled (greater than 100 degrees) thoracic curvatures. In these patients, mortality rates are significantly increased because of secondary cor pulmonale and right ventricular failure.

The cosmetic deformity of scoliosis may be associated with psychosocial concerns. There is, however, no correlation between the location or degree of the curvature and the extent of the psychosocial effects. Some adults with moderate to severe deformity may have severe psychosocial problems.

Scoliosis has no adverse effects on pregnancy. The reproductive experiences of scoliotic women are the same as those of nonscoliotic women. Whether pregnancy causes curve progression is unknown, with evidence being present on both sides of the issue.

Few patients with adolescent idiopathic scoliosis ever require active treatment (less than 10%). It is important to individualize all treatment decisions, taking into consideration the probabilities of progression based on the curve magnitude, skeletal and sexual maturity of the patient, and age of the patient. The general indications for treatment are a progressive curve of 25 degrees or more in a skeletally immature patient. In a skeletally immature patient with a curve of less than 19 degrees, curve progression of least 10 degrees should be documented before instituting treatment. If the curve is between 20 and 29 degrees, progression of least 5 degrees should be documented before instituting treatment. If a curve on initial evaluation is over 30 degrees, because of the high probability (over 90%) of progression, no documentation of progression is necessary, and treatment should be initiated immediately. Because curves rarely progress at more than 1 degree per month, follow-up appointments can be scheduled accordingly (ie, for a 15-degree curve in a skeletally immature girl, follow-up reevaluation is in 10 months).

The standard of nonoperative treatment for adolescent idiopathic scoliosis has been the Milwaukee brace. Despite widespread use, few long-term studies have evaluated the results of treatment with the Milwaukee brace (Fig. 13-12). In most of the studies performed, curve progression was not documented; thus, it is uncertain whether those patients braced would have had continued progression had they not been braced.

No published prospective studies have been done on bracing. Reviews of the few studies that are available show that bracing appears to alter the natural history of curve progression. It is generally accepted that the curve progression can be arrested in 85% to 90% of at-risk patients. The most common response to bracing is a moderate amount of correction while the brace is worn, with slow, steady progression of the curve back to the original magnitude after weaning from the brace. Occasionally, maintenance of correction obtained in the brace occurs in some patients who achieve at least a 50% reduction in their curvature during the course of treatment. The brace is worn 22 to 23 hours a day and is removed only

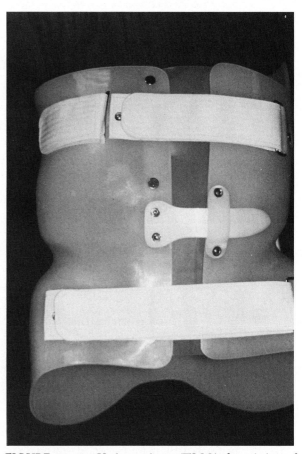

FIGURE 13-13. Underarm brace (TLSO): frontal view of one model.

for bathing or sporting activities. When the patient reaches skeletal maturity (ie, Risser grade 4, or no spinal growth over an 18-month period), the patient is gradually weaned out of the brace. The brace is used on a part-time basis followed by nighttime use only so long as no increases in curvature are noted. Bracing is ineffective in curves greater than 40 degrees.

Although full-time bracing has been the standard, many physicians are choosing part-time bracing programs and using under-arm orthoses (Fig. 13-13) because of compliance problems. An under-arm brace (thoracic-lumbar-sacral orthoses, TLSO) is generally acceptable for use in curves with an apex of T8 or below. Electrical stimulation was used in the past but has been shown to be ineffective.

Surgical treatment is indicated if the patient has evidence of curve progression despite bracing or has a curve magnitude that would be unsuccessfully treated by a brace (ie, greater than 45 to 50 degrees and skeletally immature). In the adult patient with adolescent idiopathic scoliosis, indications for surgical treatment include pain unresponsive to nonsurgical treatment and documented curve progression.

Surgical treatment of adolescent idiopathic scoliosis involves a posterior spinal fusion in combination with one of the various forms of spinal instrumentation (Fig. 13-14). The purpose of the procedure is to obtain a spinal fusion. Instrumentation is used to correct the deformity and prevent bending of the fusion mass. The standard surgical procedure for the treatment of adolescent idiopathic scoliosis is spinal fusion in conjunction with a Harrington spinal distraction rod (Fig. 13-15). The Harrington rod is used in combination with various other implants and fixation devices. Over the past few years, other implantation devices have been introduced for the correction of spinal curvatures. These devices allow for correction of the sagittal in addition to the coronal plane deformity (see Fig. 13-14).

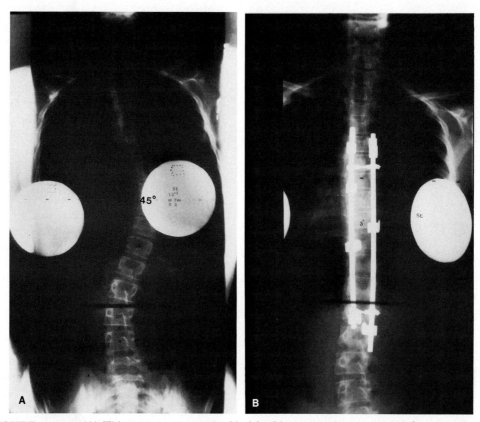

FIGURE 13-14. (A) Thirteen-year, 1-month-old girl with a curve that progressed from 23 to 45 degrees despite bracing. (B) After spinal fusion and Cotrel-Dubousset instrumentation, the same patient's curve measures 3 degrees.

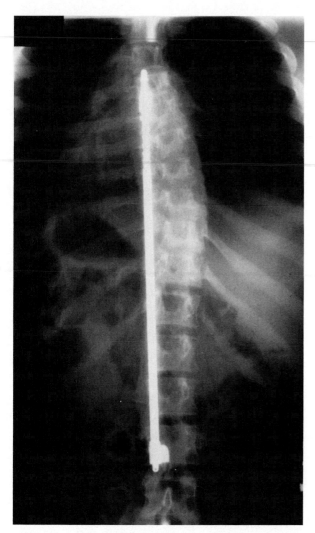

FIGURE 13-15. Spinal fusion for progressive idiopathic scoliosis using Harrington distraction instrumentation.

CONGENITAL SPINAL DEFORMITY

Congenital spinal deformities are due to abnormalities of vertebral development. These may result in scoliosis, kyphosis, lordosis, or combinations of these. Deformities may be of three structural types: failure of formation (eg, hemivertebrae); failure of segmentation (eg, unilateral unsegmented bar); or combinations of defects of segmentation and formation (Figs. 13-16 and 13-17). The resultant deformity is related to the location and type of the congenital anomaly and to the growth potential of the unaffected segments; for example, a lateral segmentation defect causes a pure scoliosis, a posterolateral segmentation defect causes a lordoscoliosis, and an an-

terior failure of segmentation causes a kyphosis. With defects of formation, any portion of the vertebrae may be hypoplastic or absent. Absence of a vertebral body causes a pure kyphosis, and presence of the posterolateral portion of the vertebrae causes a kyphoscoliosis. Failure of formation of various portions of the posterior elements results in spina bifida.

Isolated congenital vertebral abnormalities are not thought to have genetic implications. Patients with congenital scoliosis may, however, have other associated congenital abnormalities. The most frequently affected systems are the genitourinary, cardiac, and spinal cord. Some syndromes (eg, VATER syndrome) are also associated with congenital vertebral abnormalities. Many congenital spine deformities are discovered only incidentally on radiographs taken for other reasons, and some are associated with severe deformities noted at birth.

Progressive, untreated congenital spinal anomalies may produce severe functional and cosmetic deformities. If the deformity is associated with kyphosis, spinal cord compression and paralysis may occur. Early detection and careful follow-up of these patients is imperative.

All patients with congenital spinal deformity must have a careful and detailed neurologic examination. Up to 20% of patients have associated spinal dysraphism (eg, tethered cord, diastematomyelia, dural lipoma). Subtle physical findings, such as limb atrophy or mild foot abnormalities, may be the only evidence of spinal dysraphism. The skin should be inspected over the spine, looking for hair patches, dimpling, cyst formation, and hemangiomas, which are often associated with a spinal dysrhaphic condition. The chest wall should be examined for any evidence of defects or asymmetry.

About 15% of patients with congenital scoliosis have associated cardiac abnormalities. Any cardiac abnormality detected should be evaluated by a cardiologist.

All patients with congenital spinal deformity should have a urologic evaluation. Twenty to 40% of patients with congenital spinal abnormalities have an associated abnormality in the genitourinary tract. Six percent of these genitourinary tract abnormalities are potentially life-threatening. Renal ultrasound is generally sufficient to provide a screening test for genitourinary tract abnormalities. Evaluation of the lower tracts, however, may require excretory or retrograde urograms. The kidneys are also seen well on the MRI.

Spinal abnormalities are best demonstrated in

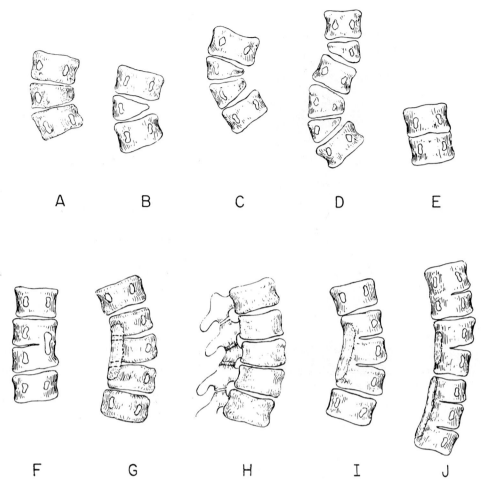

A   B   C   D   E

F   G   H   I   J

FIGURE 13-16. Scoliosis anomalies. (A) Unilateral failure of vertebral formation, partial (wedged vertebra). (B) Unilateral failure of vertebral formation, complete (hemivertebra). (C) Double hemivertebra, unbalanced. (D) Double hemivertebra, balanced. (E) Symmetric failure of segmentation (congenital fusion). (F) Asymmetric failure of segmentation (unsegmented bar). (G) Asymmetric failure of segmentation (unsegmented bar involving posterior elements only, anteroposterior view). (H) Asymmetric failure of segmentation, oblique view showing intact disk space and lack of segmentation confined to the posterior elements (surgically easy to divide). (I) Unsegmented bar involving both the disk area and posterior elements (a very difficult surgical problem to divide this). (J) Multiple unsegmented bars, unbalanced. (Winter RB, Moe JH, Eilers VE. Congenital scoliosis: a study of 234 patients treated and untreated. J Bone Joint Surg 1968;50A:1)

infancy on supine AP and lateral radiographs. These films provide the best detail of the congenital abnormalities (Fig. 13-18). It is important to pay attention to the sagittal plane deformity because many patients with congenital scoliosis may have accompanying kyphosis or lordosis. A baseline lateral radiograph should be obtained to assess any associated lordosis or kyphosis. Sagittal plane deformity may progress without progression of the scoliosis. Follow-up radiographs can be taken in the standing position

(when possible) and measured by the Cobb angle to follow curve progression.

Each radiograph should be evaluated for gross abnormalities, such as hemivertebrae or nonsegmented vertebrae. The ribs should be examined for congenital abnormalities, and all pedicles should be counted, disk spaces examined, and growth potential assessed. The prognosis for congenital deformities depends on the presence of asymmetric growth. Pedicular widening may be a sign of diastemato-

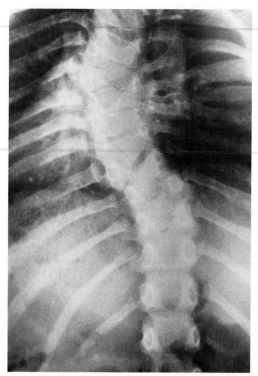

FIGURE 13-17. Congenital scoliosis. The ribs on the concave side are misshapen and fused. The seventh thoracic vertebra is wedged.

myelia, especially in patients with cutaneous or clinical manifestations of spinal dysraphism. Polytomography may be helpful in defining some congenital lesions, particularly in older patients. MRI is indicated if the patient has any evidence of spinal dysraphism. Patients with severe scoliosis may require myelographic enhanced computed tomographic (CT) scanning to better define any intraspinal pathology.

The natural history of congenital spinal deformities relates specifically to the location of the abnormality (eg, thoracic, thoracolumbar, lumbar spine), the type of abnormality (eg, unilateral unsegmented bar, hemivertebrae) and the patient's spinal growth potential. In general, about half of all congenital spine anomalies have significant enough progression to require treatment. By counting the number of growth centers, as represented by the pedicles on the concave and convex sides of the curve, as well as examining the quality of the disk spaces between vertebrae, the physician can estimate the probability of curve progression. If there is greater growth potential in the convexity of the curve than the concavity, progression is certain. The worst prognosis for progression of congenital anomalies is the unilateral unsegmented bar opposite to a convex hem-

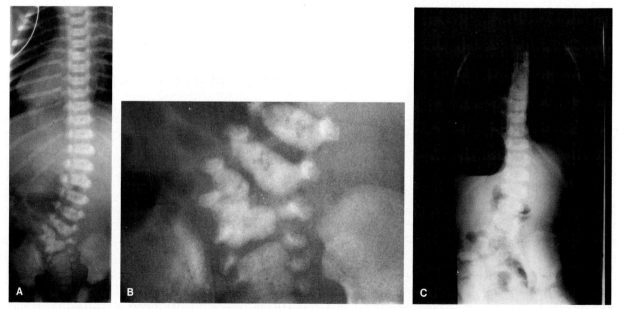

FIGURE 13-18. Eight-day-old boy with lumbosacral hemivertebrae. Radiographs of newborns generally provide the best detail of congenital spine abnormalities. (A) Spine film. (B) Coned-down view of lumbosacral junction. (C) Standing film at 2 years of age; because of progression of curve and pelvic obliquity, patient underwent excision of hemivertebra.

ivertebrae; this is followed by the unilateral unsegmented bar and the double-convex hemivertebrae (see Fig. 13-16).

The prognosis for progression in patients with hemivertebrae is difficult to predict in that there are three types of hemivertebrae: fully segmented (worst prognosis), semisegmented, and nonsegmented (most benign). The younger the patient at the age of detection, the more likely the patient is to have a progressive deformity. If a congenital anomaly is detected at an older age or only incidentally, it rarely causes significant problems.

Stable, nonprogressive curves require only observation until skeletal maturity. Patients with congenital spinal deformity should be followed with radiographs every 6 months during the first 3 years of life. If the curve remains stable, follow-up can be on a yearly basis until the adolescent growth spurt, when repeat evaluations every 6 months may be warranted.

Congenital spinal deformities tend to be rigid; therefore, bracing is generally not a treatment option. The Milwaukee brace, however, can be used in certain situations, particularly in long, flexible curves or compensatory curves above or below congenital abnormalities.

Progression of the curve regardless of the patient's age is an indication for surgical stabilization. In certain instances in which the natural history is well known (eg, unilateral unsegmented bar opposite a convex hemivertebrae), surgical stabilization is indicated without documentation of progression. The standard method of surgical stabilization is posterior spinal fusion without instrumentation. The deformity is then corrected by a plaster cast. This type of treatment is at times (particularly in the young patient) associated with bending of the fusion mass. Promising results have been reported with combination anterior hemiepiphysiodesis and posterior hemiarthrodesis, even demonstrating correction for some curves by growth on the unfused concave side.

Distraction instrumentation may be used in certain cases. This mode of treatment, however, is associated with an increased risk of neurologic deficit. If correction of the congenital spinal deformity is contemplated, thorough investigation for intraspinal pathology (eg, MRI or contrast-enhanced CT scanning) must be done before operation. The presence of a diastematomyelia without neurologic deficit does not require treatment. If correction of the spinal deformity is contemplated, however, then the diastematomyelia must be addressed surgically. Hemivertebrae excision may be considered in cases of a

lumbosacral hemivertebrae with spinal decompensation (see Fig. 13-18).

Treatment of congenital kyphotic deformities is surgical. Patients with failure of formation causing either pure kyphosis or kyphoscoliosis are at high risk for spinal cord compression. Posterior hemivertebrae or failure of formation of a vertebral body should be treated by immediate surgical stabilization. These patients generally benefit from a combined anterior and posterior surgical spinal fusion (Fig. 13-19).

With failures of segmentation, a progressive kyphosis may ensue, although this rarely leads to neurologic deficit. A short, posterior fusion arrests spinal growth and halts progression of the deformity. If the deformity exceeds 50 degrees, anterior fusion must be done in conjunction with the posterior spinal fusion; otherwise progression may occur by bending of the fusion mass. Any neurologic deficit associated with congenital kyphosis or congenital kyphoscoliosis

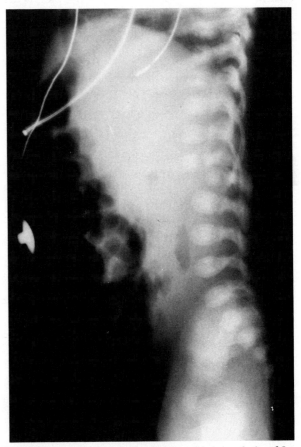

FIGURE 13-19. Six-week-old boy with hypoplasia of L1 with kyphosis. At 14 months of age, the patient underwent AP spinal fusion to prevent progression.

must be treated by spinal cord decompression and stabilization.

BACK PAIN IN CHILDREN

The child presenting with a chief complaint of back pain warrants careful evaluation because, although back pain is a common complaint in adults, back pain in children is uncommon.

The normal child may have occasional complaints of back pain after strenuous physical activity, prolonged sitting or standing, or repetitive heavy lifting. Back pain may also accompany a viral illness. Repetitive or chronic backache symptoms should be carefully investigated. There are many causes of backache in children (Table 13-4), and the cause can be established in about 85% of cases.

The child and family should be questioned to quantitate and characterize the pain. The pain should be characterized as to nature, intensity, location, and time of occurrence. Was the onset of the pain acute or insidious? Is it associated with any other illnesses? Is it activity related? Is it relieved by rest? Does it occur in the morning, the afternoon, or with repeated stress? Are there any associated bowel or bladder symptoms? What makes the pain better? What makes it worse? Is there associated night pain? Does aspirin relieve the pain? Are there associated radicular symptoms, leg pains, or paresthesia? Does the child have any complaints of a systemic illness, such as fever, weight loss, or general malaise? Is there a history of injury? Is the pain associated with repetitive trauma, such as gymnastic activities or other sports?

By taking a careful history, the physician should be able to narrow down the possible sources of the back pain. For example, if the patient is complaining

TABLE 13-4.
Causes of Back Pain in Children

Tumors
Spine
Spinal cord
Herniated nucleus pulposus
Spondylolysis
Spondylolisthesis
Scheuermann kyphosis
Postural kyphosis
Vertebral osteomyelitis
Diskitis
Overuse syndromes
Rheumatologic condition

of back pain usually at night with symptoms relieved by aspirin, an osteoid osteoma or osteoblastoma should be suspected. Pain during athletic events, such as gymnastics or blocking in a football lineman, are suggestive of spondylolysis or spondylolisthesis. Leg pain with or without associated back pain may be radicular pain associated with a herniated nucleus pulposus or may be secondary to hamstring tightness because of cauda equina irritation from a spondylolysis or spondylolisthesis. Back pain in children with or without neurologic deficits may also be a manifestation of intraspinal pathology.

Physical examination of the child presenting with the chief complaint of back pain should consist of a general overall evaluation, including examination of the head and neck, the upper and lower extremities, gait, and spine. A careful, detailed neurologic examination, including muscle, reflex, and sensory testing, is mandatory. The presence of normal or abnormal contours of the spine in either the coronal or sagittal plane should be noted. Skin lesions, such as nevi, sinuses, hair patches, or abnormal pigmentation over the lumbosacral area may indicate spinal dysraphism. The Adams forward-bend test should be performed, looking for evidence of scoliosis or an exaggerated kyphosis. Spinal motion should be assessed to be certain that the patient reverses the normal lumbar lordosis. Any loss of normal spinal motion or failure to reverse lumbar lordosis on forward flexion is suggestive of a pathologic condition and should be investigated.

The back should be palpated for any areas of tenderness over the spine or paraspinous region. The flank should be percussed, looking for areas of tenderness that may indicate a visceral abnormality. The abdomen should be palpated for masses. Limb lengths should be measured. Thighs and calves should be measured for any evidence of atrophy. Straight-leg raising tests are performed looking for signs of nerve root irritation or excessive hamstring tightness. The sacroiliac region, particularly the sacroiliac joints, should be examined for any signs of joint pathology. Signs of meningeal irritation should be sought.

In the child presenting with the chief complaint of back pain, a supine AP and lateral radiograph of the involved area of the spine is taken to assess bony detail. Standing PA and lateral radiographs can be ordered if the patient is being assessed for scoliosis or kyphosis associated with the pain. If spondylolisthesis or spondylolysis is suspected, a cone-down lateral view of the L3 to S1 region should be ordered. Oblique views may also be helpful.

If plain films are negative, special studies may be warranted. Bone scanning is useful in the face of a negative radiograph in diagnosing stress fractures, bone tumors, or infections of the spine. CT scanning may be helpful in documenting the anatomic details of lesions seen on plain films. For soft tissue lesions around the spine or for evaluating the spinal cord, MRI is the diagnostic procedure of choice.

Depending on the patient's clinical history, physical examination, and radiographic findings, certain laboratory studies may be helpful. A complete blood count and an erythrocyte sedimentation rate, although nonspecific, may be abnormal in infections, tumors, or rheumatologic conditions. If a collagen disease is suspected, HLA-B27 and rheumatoid factors may help in the diagnosis.

Some of the common etiologies of back pain in children are covered in the remainder of this section. Other causes, such as vertebral osteomyelitis, diskitis, and neoplastic lesions, are discussed elsewhere in the text.

Scheuermann Kyphosis

Scheuermann kyphosis is a structural sagittal plane deformity in the thoracic or the thoracolumbar spine. Patients have an increased kyphosis in the thoracic or thoracolumbar spine with associated diagnostic radiographic changes. Normal thoracic kyphosis is generally accepted to be between 20 and 45 degrees. The degree of kyphosis in the thoracic spine increases with age. Kyphosis should never be present at the thoracolumbar junction. Any kyphotic deformity present at this level is considered abnormal.

The incidence of Scheuermann kyphosis is thought to be between 0.4% and 8%, with a slight female predominance. The diagnosis is usually made during the adolescent growth spurt and is rarely made in patients younger than 10 years of age. An increased incidence of spondylolysis and spondylolisthesis is reported in patients with Scheuermann kyphosis as well a 20% to 30% incidence of an associated scoliosis in the region of the kyphosis.

The etiology of Scheuermann disease is unknown. Many theories have been advanced, including mechanical, metabolic, and endocrinologic. There is a definite hereditary component, but no mode of inheritance is known. Patients with Scheuermann kyphosis are generally taller than comparably aged patients, and their skeletal age is advanced over their chronologic age.

Histologic changes demonstrate that vertebral growth end-plate cartilage is abnormal, with a decreased collagen/proteoglycan ratio on electron microscopic examination. Enchondral ossification is profoundly altered in affected segments, and there are increased proteoglycan levels. The matrix of the end plates is abnormal, thus interfering with normal vertebral growth.

The two types of thoracic Scheuermann kyphosis are: kyphosis with the apex at the T7-T9 level and kyphosis with the apex in the lower thoracic spine at the thoracolumbar junction (T11-T12). There is generally an associated secondary increased lumbar lordosis. The so-called lumbar Scheuermann kyphosis has the apex at L1-L2. This condition is generally more common in boys and in young athletes. It is thought to have a traumatic etiology.

Clinically, most patients with thoracic Scheuermann kyphosis present with a history of deformity. The child is often brought in by the parent because of poor posture or is referred from a school screening program. The incidence of pain in the adolescent is low, although about 20% of patients present with a history of discomfort in the region of the kyphosis. In patients with lumbar Scheuermann kyphosis, the chief complaint is generally that of pain (80%). The pain is usually intermittent in nature. It is characterized as dull and aching and is generally activity related and relieved by rest.

On physical examination, patients with upper thoracic Scheuermann disease present with a kyphotic deformity. This is best demonstrated in the forward flexed position (Fig. 13-20). The flexibility of the kyphosis can be demonstrated by having the patient either hyperextend from a prone position or sit on a chair with the hands held behind the head and hyperextend. Lack of flexibility indicates the structural nature of the kyphotic deformity in contrast to patients with flexible postural kyphosis. These patients also have a hyperlordosis in the lumbar spine. In lower thoracic Scheuermann disease, the kyphosis is at the thoracolumbar junction. There may also be hypokyphosis above the thoracolumbar junction and hypolordosis in the lumbar spine.

Hamstring tightness may be present in these patients. Because of the high association of scoliosis with Scheuermann kyphosis, this too must assessed. The thoracic Scheuermann patient may have tenderness to palpation above or below the apex of the kyphosis. In the lumbar variety, tenderness to palpation is generally in the region of the curve apex.

Each patient should have a careful neurologic examination. Although rare, with extreme degrees of

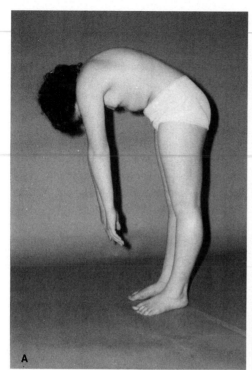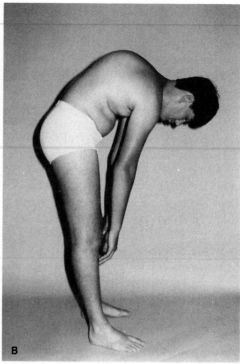

FIGURE 13-20. (A) Thirteen-year-old patient with normal sagittal plane spine contours on forward flexion. (B) Thirteen-year-old patient with Scheuermann kyphosis. Note the sharp angular thoracic spine kyphosis on forward flexion.

kyphosis, neurologic deficit can ensue. In addition, there is an association of epidural cyst, causing spastic paraparesis in patients with Scheuermann kyphosis.

A paucity of natural history data are available on Scheuermann kyphosis. Many authors think that, in the thoracic variety, if pain is present, it subsides with growth and that there are few adverse long-term sequelae of the condition. Others postulate that the incidence of pain with Scheuermann kyphosis increases throughout life, as may the deformity. The pain in adults with Scheuermann disease is generally described as the feeling of tiredness in the back. These patients may have pain in the hyperlordotic lumbar spine or at the apex of the kyphosis because of ankylosis.

The diagnosis of Scheuermann kyphosis is confirmed on a standing lateral radiograph of the spine. The radiograph should be taken with the arms parallel to the floor and resting on a support (Fig. 13-21). It is important to see the entire spine to measure the thoracic kyphosis, lumbar lordosis, and any secondary cervicothoracic curves that may accompany the kyphosis. The kyphosis is measured by determining the angle between the maximally tilted end vertebrae (similar to the Cobb method for measuring

scoliosis). A PA scoliosis film should be obtained to detect the presence and magnitude of any associated scoliosis.

The radiographic diagnosis of Scheuermann kyphosis is made by the presence of irregularities of the vertebral end plates, anterior vertebral body wedging, Schmorl nodes, and decreased intervertebral disk space height. In older patients, degenerative changes may be evident. The end-plate irregularity, Schmorl nodes, and disk space narrowing are often but not always seen. There is some discrepancy in the literature regarding the number of consecutive vertebrae that need be wedged to make the diagnosis of Scheuermann kyphosis. By one criterion (Sorenson criterion), there should be wedging in three or more adjacent vertebrae of more than 5 degrees. In other studies, the diagnosis is made by the presence of only one wedged vertebrae of more than 5 degrees. This compounds the problem of determining the natural history.

On the PA radiograph, any evidence of interpedicular widening should be noted because of the association of epidural cysts with Scheuermann kyphosis. Any scoliosis present should be assessed; curves rarely exceed 20 degrees. The flexibility of the

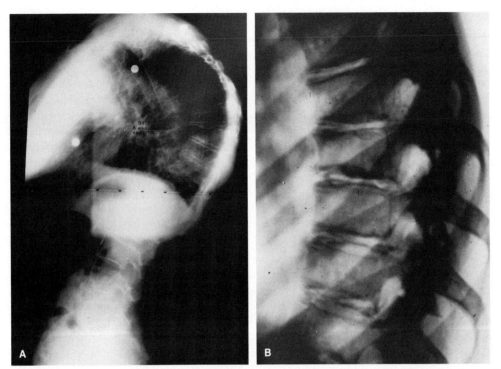

FIGURE 13-21. (A) Standing lateral radiograph of patient with Scheuermann disease (94 degrees). Note the marked vertebral wedging at the curve apex. (B) Coned-down views of spine in another patient with Scheuermann disease. Note the vertebral wedging, end-plate irregularity, and disk space narrowing.

kyphosis is best demonstrated in a supine hyperextension lateral view with a "bump" under the apex of the kyphosis.

In lumbar Scheuermann disease, irregularities of the vertebral end plates are usually present, as are Schmorl nodes. The intervertebral disk spaces are normal, and there is no evidence of vertebral wedging.

In a patient with an apparent exaggerated kyphosis, the differential diagnosis includes postural round back. In postural round back, there is a slight increase in the thoracic kyphosis. The kyphosis, however, is flexible, as demonstrated on the prone or sitting hyperextension tests. On the standing lateral radiograph, there are no structural changes as noted for Scheuermann kyphosis. The kyphosis in postural kyphosis patients is usually in the range of 45 to 60 degrees. On the supine hyperextension lateral view, the deformity is totally flexible. The question remains of whether a postural kyphosis left untreated may progress and get secondary bony changes resembling Scheuermann disease. Postural kyphosis, if flexible, should be treated by exercising.

Thoracic hyperkyphosis is also seen in patients with various types of skeletal dysplasia, such as spondyloepiphyseal dysplasia congenita and Morquio disease. These conditions can usually be diagnosed by the clinical examination and other radiographic features. Ankylosing spondylitis may present a similar picture, but 97% of these patients are HLA-B27–positive. Kyphosis may also be present in patients who had a laminectomy before skeletal maturity and in patients who had radiation to the spine for a regional tumor, such as Wilms tumor or neuroblastoma. Kyphosis may also been seen with eosinophilic granuloma. Type II congenital kyphosis (failure of segmentation) may be confused with Scheuermann disease. It may be necessary to use polytomography to identify the anterior failure of segmentation seen in this condition to differentiate it from Scheuermann kyphosis.

The treatment of Scheuermann kyphosis is controversial. Lumbar Scheuermann disease generally responds well to nonoperative measures, such as nonsteroidal antiinflammatory agents and temporary activity restriction. There are no adverse long-term sequelae from lumbar Scheuermann disease.

Some authors think that the natural history of thoracic Scheuermann kyphosis is benign and therefore needs no treatment. Others report increasing pain with progression of the deformity. It is uncertain whether treatment prevents any of the consequences that may occur without treatment. Treatment of Scheuermann kyphosis in the skeletally immature patient is recommended in the hope of preventing excessive deformity that may cause pain and cosmetic concerns. Exercises alone are not beneficial. Hyperextension body casts changed at monthly intervals to correct the curvature may be used in the skeletally immature patient with a rigid Scheuermann kyphosis (ie, less than 10 or 15 degrees of correction on hyperextension lateral radiograph). Once the correction has been obtained, it can then be maintained using a Milwaukee brace. In those patients with a somewhat flexible Scheuermann kyphosis, the Milwaukee brace is prescribed. In some centers, particularly in Europe, casting alone is used as a treatment for this condition. Treatment is generally continued until the patient reaches skeletal maturity. In immature patients, some of the anterior wedging associated with Scheuermann kyphosis can be corrected by treatment. Follow-up studies of patients treated for Scheuermann kyphosis demonstrate increase of the kyphosis over time even after brace treatment.

Surgery is rarely indicated in patients with Scheuermann kyphosis. In patients with curves greater than 75 degrees and with pain unresponsive to nonoperative measures, spinal fusion can be considered. Treatment of kyphosis of this magnitude requires anterior and posterior spinal fusion throughout the length of the kyphosis. Cord decompression is indicated for the rare patient who has neurologic deficits secondary to epidural cysts or increased kyphotic angulation.

Spondylolysis and Spondylolisthesis

Spondylolysis is a descriptive term referring to a defect in the pars interarticularis. The defect may be unilateral or bilateral and may be associated with spondylolisthesis. *Spondylolisthesis* refers to the anterior displacement (translation) of a vertebra with respect to the vertebra caudal to it. This translation may also be accompanied by an angular deformity (kyphosis). These two topics are considered together in that the most common cause of spondylolisthesis in children is spondylolysis.

Spondylolysis occurs most commonly at the L5-S1 level and less frequently at the L4-L5 region. Spondylolytic lesions may occur at other lumbar regions or at multiple levels. Spondylolytic lesions are found in about 5% of the general population. Spon-

dylolysis is an acquired condition. It has not been reported in infants and is rarely present before 5 years of age. There is an increased incidence of spondylolysis and spondylolisthesis up to the age of 20 years, after which the incidence remains stable.

Spondylolisthesis is classified into five types (Table 13-5). It is further classified by the degree of angular and translational displacement. The diagnosis and treatment of the condition depends on the type.

Spondylolysis is thought to be an acquired condition secondary to a stress fracture at the pars intraarticularis. Experimental studies showed that extension movements of the spine, particularly in combination with lateral flexion, increase the shear stress at the pars interarticularis. Clinical evidence for this theory includes the high association (four times more than normal) in female gymnasts, football linemen, and soldiers carrying back packs. This etiologic theory is also supported by a reported higher association in patients with Scheuermann kyphosis with secondary excessive lumbar lordosis. In contrast, spondylolysis has never been seen in patients who have never walked.

Evidence supports the concept the spondylolysis and spondylolisthesis may be inherited conditions. There is a high association of the condition in family members of affected patients. There are racial and gender differences, with the lowest incidence in black females and the highest incidence in white males. Most patients with type I spondylolisthesis have abnormalities at the lumbosacral junction with poor development of the superior aspect of the sacrum and superior sacral facets and with associated sacral spina bifida. Similar congenital changes have also been reported in about one third of patients with type II spondylolisthesis. Thus, these conditions may be genetic, acquired, or both.

TABLE 13-5.
Classification of Spondylolisthesis

Type	Description
I	Dysplastic
IIA	Fracture in pars interarticularis (stress fracture)
B	Elongated intact pars interarticularis
C	Acute fracture
III	Degenerative
IV	Traumatic (fracture in other than pars interarticularis)
V	Pathologic

(Adapted from Wiltse LL, Newman PH, MacNab I. Clin Orthop 1976;117:23–29)

The presenting complaints of patients with spondylolysis and spondylolisthesis are determined primarily by the age of the patient and, in spondylolisthesis, by the type. Although pain is the most common presenting complaint in the adult, it is relatively uncommon in children or the symptomatology is usually mild. Children most commonly present with gait abnormalities, postural deformity, and hamstring tightness. Back pain is usually localized to the lower-back region, with occasional radiation to the buttocks and the thighs. Occasional L5 radiculopathies are present, although this is not common in children.

The adult patient with type III degenerative spondylolisthesis generally is older than 40 years of age, and woman are more commonly affected than men. Pain in degenerative spondylolisthesis is often similar to the pain patterns in patients with a herniated nucleus pulposus (ie, the patient has pain radiating down the leg and complaints of sciatica). Patients may complain of pain similar to spinal stenosis and have claudication-type symptoms (ie, pain and cramping in the calves and back brought on by walking and relieved by sitting in a flexed spinal posture). In most cases of spondylolysis and spondylolisthesis, pain is precipitated by activity, especially flexion and extension on a repetitive basis, and relieved by rest or lowered activity levels.

Each patient must have a complete physical examination, including detailed neurologic examination. About 80% of children with spondylolysis and spondylolisthesis have evidence of hamstring tightness. The etiology for this is unknown but is thought to be instability in the area of the spondylolysis and spondylolisthesis resulting in cauda equina irritation. Hamstring tightness is responsible for the postural abnormalities often seen as the presenting complaint of the patients with spondylolisthesis. Restrictive flexion secondary to the hamstring tightness and the pelvic tilt gives the patient a stiff-legged gait with a short stride length. The pelvis rotates as the child takes a step, and often the children walks on tiptoes with the knees slightly flexed. The hamstring tightness may be so severe in some children that, in performing a straight-leg raising test in a supine position, the leg can only be lifted several inches off the table.

The physical findings referable to the back depend on the type and degree of the slip. Patients may present with mild tenderness to palpation in the area of the spondylolysis or spondylolisthesis. In severe grades of slip, a "step-off" may be palpated. There may be an apparent increase in lumbar lordosis with a backward tilting of the pelvis (Fig. 13-22). The pa-

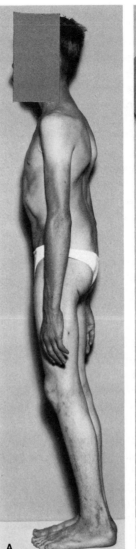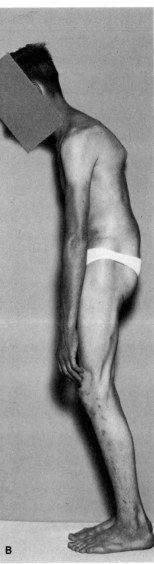

FIGURE 13-22. High-grade spondylolisthesis, physical findings. (**A**) Note the flattening of the buttock, anterior protrusion of the pelvis, visible lumbar slip-off, and apparent shortening of the trunk. (**B**) Displaying characteristic hamstring tightness, limiting his ability to touch his toes without flexing the knees. (Turner RH, Bianco AJ. Spondylolysis and spondylolisthesis in children and teenagers. J Bone Joint Surg 1971;53A:1298)

tient may present with protrusion of the lower abdomen, and in severe cases of spondylolisthesis, a deep transverse abdominal crease may be noted. A detailed neurologic examination, including deep tendon reflexes, sensory examination, and motor strength, should be performed on each patient with particular attention to any dysesthesia near the sacrum and rectum. A history of bowel or bladder dysfunction may be indicative of cauda equina syndrome.

About one third of patients with symptomatic spondylolisthesis have evidence of scoliosis. The scoliosis most commonly seen in association with symptomatic spondylolisthesis is generally not structural. It is more commonly seen in patients with high-degree slips. The curve is usually in the lumbar region and resolves with the resolution of the symptoms of the spondylolisthesis. Some patients have a characteristic idiopathic scoliosis that is unaffected by the spondylolisthesis or its treatment.

Spondylolisthesis in patients with isthmic spondylolysis may occur any time after the pars fractures. Most slippage occurs during the adolescent growth spurt. Rarely are significant increases in the degree of spondylolisthesis seen after skeletal maturity.

If spondylolysis or spondylolisthesis is clinically suspected, standing PA and standing lateral radiographs of the spine with a cone-down lateral view of L3 to the sacrum are indicated. In most cases, the pars interarticular defect can be seen on the spot lateral views. The defect is usually at the L5 to S1 level. Defects at the L4 level are more common in patients who have complete or partial sacralization of the L5 vertebra. If the defect is not visualized on the lateral film and the condition is suspected, an oblique view may be helpful. On this view, one can see what has been described as a Scotty dog with a broken neck or wearing a collar (Fig. 13-23). In about 20% of patients, the lytic defect is unilateral and may be accompanied by reactive sclerosis in the opposite pedicle, lamina, or both. This situation often presents a difficult diagnostic dilemma in that the sclerotic region can be confused with lesions such as osteoid osteoma and osteoblastoma. If the lesion is not visualized on plain radiograph, technetium bone scanning or Spect scan may be helpful in identifying the lesion. In an acute injury, a "hot" bone scan may allow for early detection. Bone scanning is also used to assess whether an established lesion has the potential to heal. If the lesion is "cold," there is an established nonunion, and hence immobilization would probably not result in healing of the stress fracture.

In type I spondylolisthesis, the entire posterior arch slips forward (Fig. 13-24). There is dysplasia of the superior articular facets of the sacrum and inferior articular facets of L5. Type I slips are generally limited to 25% to 30% slippage unless the pars becomes attenuated or fractures, allowing for severe degrees of slippage to occur.

In type II spondylolisthesis, the spinous process and posterior elements remain behind (Fig. 13-25).

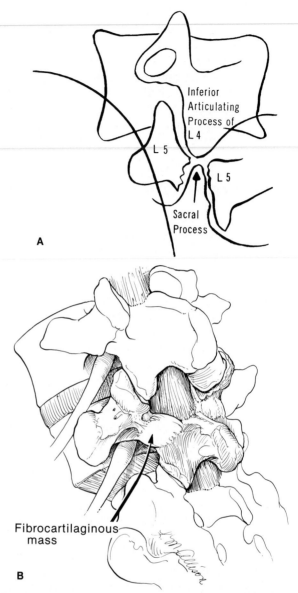

FIGURE 13-23. (A) Diagram of oblique radiograph of lumbosacral junction, showing cleft in isthmus of the fifth lumbar vertebra. The articular process of the sacrum projects upward and penetrates the cleft, meeting the inferior articular process of the fourth lumbar vertebra. (B) Pathology of spondylolisthesis showing the relation of the nerve root as it courses through the intervertebral foramen. The continuity of the pars interarticularis is bridged at the defect by a fibrous or fibrocartilaginous mass that rarely may encroach on the nerve root of L5.

Other changes should be noted, including the shape of the sacrum (ie, whether it is flattened or dome-shaped; Fig. 13-26) and the amount of wedging of L5 (Fig. 13-27). In the adult disk space, narrowing and degenerative changes at the intervertebral disk and posterior elements should be noted. Patients with

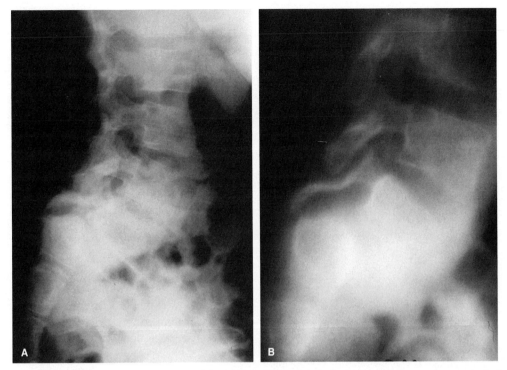

FIGURE 13-24. (A) Nine-year-old girl with type I spondylolisthesis. Note how pars interarticularis has become attenuated, allowing for severe slippage (translation and angulation). The entire posterior arch has slipped forward. (B) Polytome demonstrating the elongation of pars interarticularis.

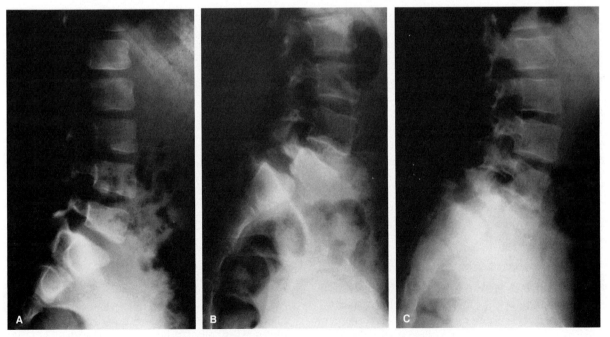

FIGURE 13-25. (A) Six-year-old female gymnast who complained of mild backache. Narrowing of pars interarticularis noted in radiograph. (B) At age 11, she had increasing pain. Radiograph demonstrates a lytic defect (type IIA) of the pars interarticularis and significant translation; surgery was recommended but refused. (C) Because of increasing pain, surgery was performed at age 12. The preoperative radiograph demonstrates increasing anterior translation and lumbosacral angulation (kyphosis).

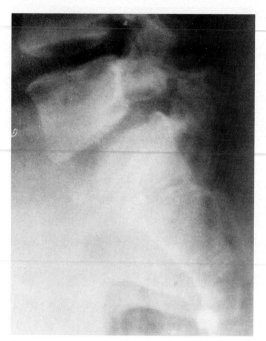

FIGURE 13-26. Spondylolisthesis. Note the attempt at formation of a supporting ledge at the anterior edge of the sacrum.

tients who do not have resolution of symptoms by nonoperative measures. Myelography is rarely indicated in the child or adolescent with spondylolisthesis unless the patient has signs or symptoms of nerve root compression or cauda equina syndrome. In the adult patient, other diagnostic tests, such as EMG, motor nerve condition studies, and psychological testing, may be considered.

Most children with spondylolysis can be treated successfully without surgery. If the diagnosis is made as an incidental finding, no activity restrictions are necessary. The patient should, however, be followed through skeletal maturity with standing spot lateral radiographs of the lumbosacral spine every 6 to 8 months to watch for the development of spondylolisthesis.

In a patient with spondylolysis with acute onset of symptoms, bone scanning is helpful to assess the lesion and to follow healing. In such patients, particularly athletes, there is some evidence to suggest that immobilization in a cast or brace allows for heal-

a more rounded S1 and a more wedge-shaped L5 have a greater risk of progression.

Spondylolisthesis is graded on a scale of 1 to 4 depending on the percentage of anterior translation of L5 on S1, with grade 1 being a 25% slip; grade 2, a 50% slip; grade 3, a 75% slip; and grade 4, a complete slip (Figs. 13-28 and 13-29). The term *spondyloptosis* is used to describe complete displacement of L5 in front of S1. It is important in assessing spondylolisthetic patients to have standing lateral radiographs of the lumbosacral junction because instability is not uncommon, particularly in childhood (Fig. 13-28). Several standard methods of measurements are used to quantitate spondylolisthesis; these include the percentage of translation, sagittal roll, and slip angle (Figs. 13-30 and 13-31). These measurements of angulation or lumbosacral kyphosis are important prognostic indicators.

Additional radiographic studies may be in order, especially in the adult patient with degenerative spondylolisthesis. These studies include flexion–extension lateral views to detect instability and CT scanning with or without myelographic enhancement to assess the integrity of the disk and to look for other potential sources of the discomfort. They are also useful to ascertain the specific pathology in spondylolisthesis associated with or causing spinal stenosis and to rule out intraspinal pathology in pa-

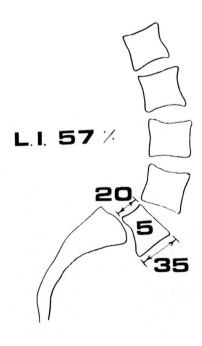

LUMBAR INDEX

FIGURE 13-27. The lumbar index represents the degree of trapezoidal deformation of the fifth lumbar vertebral body. Although a decreased lumbar index is secondary to increased slipping, when considered in conjunction with other factors, such as the adolescent growth spurt, a dome-shaped first sacral vertebra, and female gender, it indicates that the patient is at risk for progression of slipping. (Boxall D, Bradford DS, Winter RB, Moe JH. Management of severe spondylolisthesis in children and adolescents. J Bone Joint Surg 1979;61A:479)

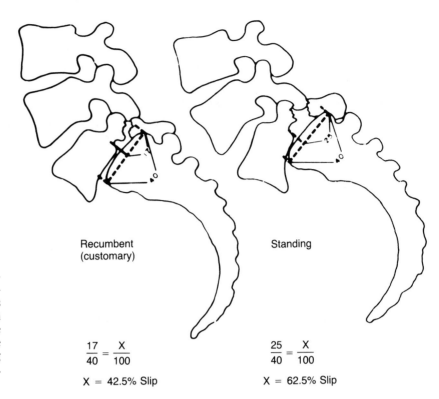

FIGURE 13-28. Spondylolisthesis, demonstrating the accuracy of the standing radiograph. The displacement is measured as a percentage of the width of the adjacent vertebral body. The standing and recumbent views are compared. (Lowe RW, et al. Standing roentgenograms in spondylolisthesis. Clin Orthop 1976;117:80)

Recumbent (customary)

$$\frac{17}{40} = \frac{X}{100}$$

X = 42.5% Slip

Standing

$$\frac{25}{40} = \frac{X}{100}$$

X = 62.5% Slip

ing of the lesion. There are some differences of opinion about whether the cast should extend from the nipple line to include one or both legs or if the same results may be achieved in a TLSO. If this treatment is attempted, the patient can be followed by serial radiographs and bone scans to assess healing.

Most patients with nonacute lesions can be successfully treated by activity restriction and exercises, including hamstring stretching. If symptoms are more severe, a short period of bed rest may be tried before immobilization in a TLSO. Exercises should be prescribed. Nonsteroidal antiinflammatory medications are a useful adjuvant to treatment.

If the patient does not respond to conservative management, other conditions, including neurologic conditions and tumors of the spine and spinal cord, must be ruled out before instituting surgical treatment. In patients whose symptoms do not respond to nonoperative treatment, lumbosacral intertransverse process fusion of L5 to S1 has a 90% chance of obtaining a solid fusion with relief of symptomatology, including resolution of hamstring tightness. In patients with isolated or multiple defects in the L1 to L4 region, surgical repair of the defect by one of many available techniques is often recommended to allow for sparing of lumbar motion segments.

In asymptomatic patients who have spondylolisthesis with less than a 25% slip, no treatment is indicated. Natural history indicates that the likelihood

of having future problems is essentially the same as that of the general population. With slips greater than 25%, there is an increased likelihood of the patient having lower-back symptoms compared with the general population. Certain clinical and radiographic risk factors have been determined to be associated with future pain, progressive deformity, and increasing degree of spondylolisthesis (Table 13-6).

In the skeletally immature patient with less than a 50% slip, nonoperative measures should be tried in attempt to control symptomatology. These measures are similar to those described previously for the treatment of spondylolysis. About two thirds of these patients have resolution of symptomatology with nonoperative treatment.

Indications for surgery in the skeletally immature patient are failure of relief of symptoms by nonoperative measures or a slip of greater than 50%. L4–sacrum intertransverse process fusion is recommended in those patients with a greater than 50% slip, and L5–sacrum fusion is recommended for those patients with a less than 50% slip. By this method, 90% of children can expect to have a solid fusion within in 1 year of surgery and gain resolution of any mild neurologic symptoms, including hamstring tightness, over the ensuing 12 to 18 months. Nonunions and curve progression despite a solid fusion, however, have been reported in children undergoing in situ fusion. Because of these problems, particularly

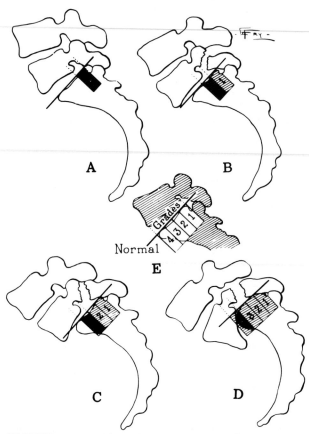

FIGURE 13-29. Meyerding grading system for spondylolisthesis, demonstrating the degrees of slipping of the fifth lumbar vertebra on the sacrum. (Meyerding HW. Spondylolisthesis. Surg Gynecol Obstet 1932;54:374)

with high-grade slips, many authors advocate fusion and closed reduction, followed by pantaloon casting for about 3 months to decrease the sagittal rotation and improve the cosmetic deformity. Although sagittal role or slip angle can be changed by closed methods, vertebral translation is generally unaltered or is changed little by these techniques. Decompression is rarely necessary in childhood spondylolisthesis and must be accompanied by a fusion to prevent further progression.

In the adult being treated for type I or type II spondylolisthesis, careful assessment must be done to rule out other associated conditions (eg, herniated nucleus pulposus) and to evaluate disk degeneration and nerve compression. In the adult, the symptomatology is generally confined to back pain. In situ fusion may be all that is necessary. If the patient has leg pain, however, decompression and fusion may be warranted. In the adult patient with spondylolisthesis with or without radiculopathy, it is incumbent on the surgeon to obtain a solid fusion. Many surgeons advocate internal fixation along with a spinal

fusion. Internal fixation is most commonly attained by means of pedicle screws, plates, or rods. In the adult, because the risk of further displacement is minimal, pantaloon cast immobilization as advocated in children is unnecessary.

In the adult with degenerative spondylolisthesis (type III), the source of the pain must be sought before recommending surgical treatment. These patients rarely develop spondylolisthesis greater than 25%. Radiographs show evidence of degenerative disk disease as well as degeneration of the facet joints. Some patients develop retrolisthesis, and others may develop intraspinal synovial cysts. A complete diagnostic evaluation must be done in these patients, including diskography to ascertain the source of the pain. Adult patients require a much more extensive work-up, including the possibility of EMG, motor nerve conduction studies, psychological testing, diskography, epidural steroid injections, or nerve root blocks, to ascertain the cause of pain and prognosticate the effectiveness of treatment. Most patients with degenerative spondylolisthesis can also be

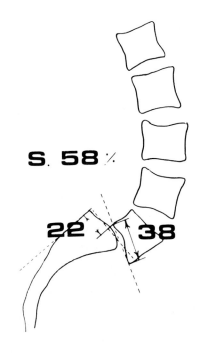

% SLIP

FIGURE 13-30. Percentage of slipping. A line is extended upward from the posterior surface of the first sacral vertebral body, and a second line is drawn downward from the posterior surface of the fifth lumbar vertebral body. The extent of slip is the distance between these two lines. This measurement is expressed as a percentage of the AP dimension of the fifth lumbar vertebral body. (Boxall D, Bradford DS, Winter RB, Moe JH. Management of severe spondylolisthesis in children and adolescents. J Bone Joint Surg 1979;61A:479)

treated nonoperatively. In those who fail conservative treatment, exhaustive diagnostic measures must be undertaken to determine the source of pain.

Herniated Nucleus Pulposus

Of all cases of herniated nucleus pulposus reported, less than 3% occur in children. An estimated 30% to 60% of cases reported have an associated history of trauma. There is a male predominance. Herniated nucleus pulposus in children is associated with additional vertebral disease, including sacralized L5, lumbarized S1 (either complete or incomplete), asymmetric articular facets, and spina bifida.

Symptoms of a herniated nucleus pulposus in the child may be minimal or they may be characteristic of the adult condition. In children, however, there is occasionally an associated scoliosis secondary to muscle spasm. The neurologic symptoms in children are less common and less severe. Herniated nucleus pulposus may also occur in association with a slipped vertebral apophysis or fracture of the ver-

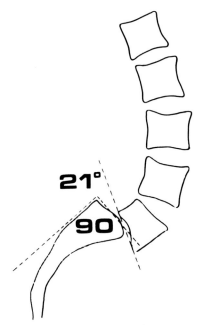

FIGURE 13-31. The slip angle measures the degree of forward tilting of the fifth lumbar vertebral body over the first sacral vertebral body, or the kyphosis at the level of slipping. The angle is formed by a line drawn perpendicular to the posterior aspect of the first sacral body and one drawn parallel to the inferior aspect of the fifth lumbar vertebral body. It represents the degree of instability and potential for progression, particularly when the slip angle is high and a significant increase is noted in the standing roentgenogram as compared with the supine roentgenogram. (Boxall D, Bradford DS, Winter RB, Moe JH. Management of severe spondylolisthesis in children adolescents. J Bone Joint Surg 1979;61A:479)

TABLE 13-6.
Risk Factors in Spondylolisthesis for Pain, Progression, and Deformity

CLINICAL RISK FACTORS

Younger age

Female patient

Recurrent symptoms

Hamstring tightness, if associated with gait abnormalities or postural deformity

RADIOGRAPHIC RISK FACTORS

Type I greater risk than type II

Greater than 50% slip

Increased risk with increased slip angle

L5–S1 instability with rounded sacral dome and vertical sacrum

(Adapted from Heinsinger RN. Spondylolysis and spondylolisthesis. J Bone Joint Surg 1990;71A:1098–1107)

tebral apophysis. The most common levels involved in children are L4 to L5 and L5 to S1. Treatment recommendations are the same as those in the adult.

BACK PAIN IN ADULTS

Back pain in the adult is one of the most common and costly medical problems. About 80% to 90% of the adult population suffers from back pain during their life. Most cases of back pain resolve spontaneously. Half of patients who complain of back pain are generally asymptomatic within 2 weeks, and 90% are asymptomatic after 3 months. It is estimated that 1 year after symptom onset, only 2% of all adults with back pain have persistent pain.

Back pain is the most common cause of disability for patients under 45 years of age. Although back pain is a common complaint, in 80% to 90% of cases, a pathologic etiology cannot be determined. Epidemiologic studies determined that risk factors related to the development of back pain include job dissatisfaction, repetitive lifting, low-frequency vibration, low educational level, smoking, and social problems.

In the adult patient who presents with backache, the history, careful physical examination of the musculoskeletal system, and complete neurologic examination generally allow the physician to make the diagnosis. Diagnostic tests are only used to confirm the suspected diagnosis. Most causes of back pain are self-limiting. Over half of patients with back pain recover within 7 days. Patients who have back pain-associated sciatica (pain down the distribution of the nerve roots contributing to the sciatic nerve) generally recover within 4 weeks.

Historically, the onset of the patient's pain should be assessed in terms of whether it is acute or chronic and whether it had an insidious onset or whether it can be related to a traumatic event. Risk factors should be sought. Pain should be characterized regarding location and whether it is confined to the back or the leg. It is important to determine the pattern of the pain. In patients with sciatica, the pain (and sometimes numbness or tingling) characteristically radiates down the distribution of one of the nerve roots that contributes to the sciatic nerve, characteristically L4, L5, or S1. If the pain does not radiate below the knee but is localized primarily to the back, buttock, hip, and distal thigh, it is likely to be referred pain rather than pain caused by compressive irritation of one of the nerve roots of the sciatic nerve.

The patient should be asked about the effect of position and activity on the pain. The patient should also be queried about muscle weakness or numbness and its location. Medications taken by the patient and the their effect on pain should be noted. The effect of previous treatments should also be assessed. A necessary line of questions includes whether or not there is workman's compensation or litigation involved. Job description and satisfaction should also be assessed. The patient must also be questioned about the symptoms impact activities of daily living. Swelling, erythema, and pain in other joints should be noted because they may be indicative of a generalized condition, such as metabolic bone disease or rheumatoid spondylitis. The patient should specifically be asked about urinary incontinence or retention or change in pattern of stream, which may indicate

bowel or bladder dysfunction. Complaints of non-anatomic sensory loss (eg, stocking-glove anesthesia or nonspecific motor loss throughout the entire lower extremities) should alert the physician to the possibility of a neuropathy or a nonorganic cause of the symptoms. Psychosocial factors can contribute to back pain or response to treatment in patients with chronic back pain. It is important to use additional studies, including psychological inventories such as the Minnesota Multiphasic Personality Inventory, to assess these patients.

In most cases, the pathologic condition causing the patient's symptoms can be ruled in or out by the history alone. Careful physical examination, however, must be done. The patient should be evaluated in a standing position to assess the presence or absence of the normal sagittal and coronal plane contours. The spine should be assessed in flexion, extension, and lateral bending. Restriction of motion or abnormality in any of these motions should be noted. The effect of various motions on the patient's back or leg pain should be noted. The spine should be examined in the prone position. The entire spine should be palpated, assessing both the soft tissues and bone elements for tenderness. The effect of palpation on the patient's symptomatology should also be noted. The sacroiliac joint should be examined, as should the hips. Pathology in these areas may be confused with pain of spinal origin. Each dermatomic region must be assessed for all sensory modalities (Fig. 13-32). Motor function in each muscle group must be graded. Reflexes should be tested and any asymmetry noted (Table 13-7). A positive Babinski sign may indicate an upper motor neuron lesion. As-

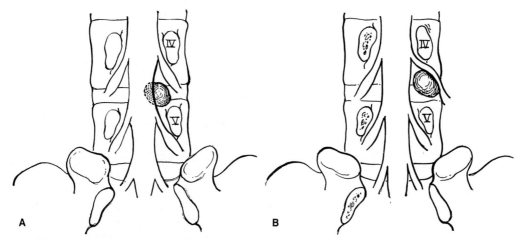

FIGURE 13-32. (A) The usual relation of the protruded disk at the fourth lumbar interspace. The fifth lumbar nerve root is compressed. (B) An uncommon relation of the protruded disk at the fourth lumbar interspace. The fourth lumbar nerve root is compressed.

TABLE 13-7.
Reflexes

DEEP TENDON REFLEXES
Biceps: C5
Brachioradialis: C5, C6
Triceps: C7, C8
Patella: L3, L4
Achilles: L5–S1

SUPERFICIAL REFLEXES
Upper abdominal: T5–T10
Lower abdominal: T10–T12
Cremasteric: L1, L2

SPHINCTERIC REFLEXES
Bladder: S3–S4
Anus: S3–S4

sessment of rectal tone and perianal sensation is imperative in any patient complaining of back pain. The straight-leg raising test should be performed both in the supine and prone (femoral stretch) positions. In the supine position, the test is performed by passively elevating the patient's leg with the knee extended and pelvis stable. The test is positive if this maneuver reproduces sciatic pain (radiating below the knee). If the patient only complains of back pain or tightness of the hamstring muscles behind the thigh, the test is considered negative.

The straight-leg raising test is one of the so-called tension signs indicative of neural irritability. This specific test should be done on both legs. If the patient's asymptomatic straight-leg raising test elicits sciatic pain down the contralateral leg, this called a positive contralateral straight-leg raising test and indicates nerve root irritation.

Another tension sign is the bow-string test; this is a straight-leg raise performed with the knee flexed. With the leg held in this position, the popliteal fossa is palpated. A positive bow-string test occurs if, during the compression of the tibial nerve in the popliteal fossa, the patient complains of radiating pain both proximally and distally or of paraesthesia in the distribution of any particular branch of the sciatic nerve.

The reverse straight-leg raising test (femoral stretch test) is performed with the patient in the prone position. The leg is extended from the hip, stretching the femoral nerve. Any pain along the distribution of the femoral nerve is considered a positive stretch test.

Pulses should be evaluated in the lower extremity. Patients with spinal stenosis have symptoms of claudication. The presence of palpable pulses in the extremities is helpful in ruling out a vascular cause of the claudication symptoms.

It is important during the physical examination to look for inconsistencies. The Wadell tests for nonorganic causes of lower-back pain are useful in evaluating patients with chronic backache (Table 13-8).

TABLE 13-8.
Nonorganic Physical Signs in Lower-Back Pain

Category	Test	Comment
Tenderness	Superficial palpation	Inordinate, widespread sensitivity to light touch of the superficial soft tissues over the lumbar spine is nonanatomic and suggests amplified symptoms.
	Nonanatomic testing	Tenderness is poorly localized.
Simulation (to assess patient cooperation and reliability)	Axial loading	Light pressure to the skull of standing patient should not significantly increase symptoms.
	Rotation	Physician should rotate the standing patient's pelvis and shoulders in the same plane; this does not move the lumbar spine and should not increase pain.
Distraction	Straight-leg raising	Physician asks the seated patient to straighten the knee. Patients with true sciatic tension arch backward and complain. These results should closely match those of the traditional, recumbent straight-leg raising test.
Regional		Diffuse motor weakness or bizarre sensory deficits suggest functional regional disturbance if they involve multiple muscle groups and cannot be explained by neuroanatomy principles.
Overreaction		Excessive and inappropriate grimacing, groaning, or collapse during a simple request is disproportionate.

(Adapted from Waddell G, McCulloch JA, Kummel E, Venner RM. Nonorganic physical signs in low back pain. Spine 1980;5:117–125)

The urgency with which the physician must proceed with further diagnostic work-up depends on whether the patient has a history or physical examination compatible with lumbar radiculopathy, keeping in mind the natural history. The remainder of the diagnostic tests and treatment alternatives depend on whether the patient has acute or chronic back pain and whether there is an associated radiculopathy.

Acute Back Pain With Lumbar Radiculopathy

The most common cause of lumbar radiculopathy in patients younger than 40 years of age is a herniated nucleus pulposus. The nucleus pulposus may bulge into the canal. Tears of the fibers of the annulus fibrosis may allow the disk to extrude through the annulus, or the disk may sequester through the annulus and lie free in the spinal canal or neural foramina. Nerve root compression may cause secondary in-

flammation of the nerve root, giving the patient subjective symptoms of pain, numbness, or tingling along the distribution of the particular nerve root. The most commonly affected nerve roots are L5 and S1. In the lumbar spine, the exiting nerve root is named for the vertebra about which it exits. Therefore, the L5 nerve root exits before the L5 to S1 disk space below the L5 pedicle. Thus, L5 to S1 disk herniation usually causes irritation of the S1 nerve root (Fig. 13-33). Herniations occur less frequently at higher levels. Pain associated with a herniated nucleus pulposus varies from mild pain along the distribution of the nerve to severe incapacitating pain.

Physical examination of the patient with a herniated nucleus pulposus generally reveals restricted range of motion with forward flexion increasing the pain. The patient may list to one side. Sensory and motor examination may show evidence of nerve root compression with decrease in sensation, muscle weakness, or both and diminished reflexes in the region of the affected nerve (see Table 13-7 and Fig. 13-32). Circumference of extremities should be measured to detect any evidence of atrophy. Acute nerve

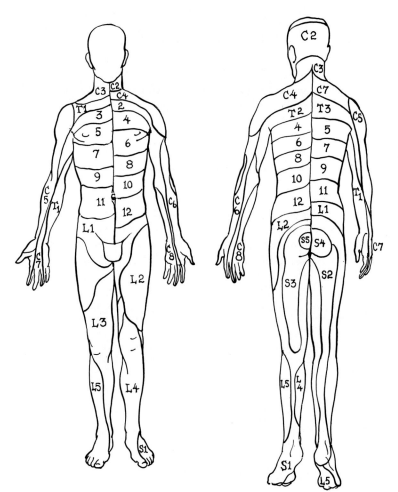

FIGURE 13-33. Distribution of spinal dermatomes. Considerable overlap occurs; consequently, involvement of a single spinal segment may not be evident.

root irritation is evidenced by positive tension signs and straight-leg raising, contralateral straight-leg raising, and bow-string stretch tests. A contralateral straight-leg raising test is the most specific sign of herniated nucleus pulposus.

The natural history of acute lumbar radiculopathy is that about half resolve within 4 weeks. Diagnostic studies thus are not indicated initially. The patient should be treated with a short period of bed rest (1 to 2 days), limitation or modification of activities, and in some cases, antiinflammatory drugs (aspirin or a nonsteroidal antiinflammatory agents). Epidural steroid injections may provide short-term relief for patients with a herniated nucleus pulposus. Treatment modalities advocated in the past (traction, spinal manipulation, corsets or braces, and physical therapy) have little scientific validity. As the adult symptoms resolve, it is important to get the patient on a rehabilitation program to prevent recurrent episodes of back pain and disability. Patients should be encouraged to increase their activity level and begin a conditioning and physical fitness program.

Because it is unusual for an acute herniated nucleus pulposus to cause bilateral sciatica, the presence of bilateral lower-extremity neurologic signs and symptoms should alert the physician to the possibility of a central disk herniation or, rarely, intraspinal pathology other than disk herniation. The presence of back pain, sciatica, and bowel or bladder dysfunction associated with motor weakness is referred to as *cauda equina syndrome* and is generally caused by extrinsic compression of the thecal sac in the area of the cauda equina. Cauda equina syndrome often requires immediate surgical intervention. Only patients with acute cauda equina syndrome should undergo immediate diagnostic evaluation. These patients should have immediate MRI, myelography, or both to determine the cause of the cauda equina syndrome before surgical intervention.

In patients with persistent symptomatology despite nonoperative treatment or progressive neurologic deficit, further diagnostic evaluation is often necessary. Plain lumbosacral radiographs rarely provide diagnostic information. With aging, normal degenerative changes occur in the lumbar spine that often confuse the diagnostic picture. Changes of spine degeneration are seen in as many of 70% of radiographs. These radiographic changes have little effect on management outcomes. Plain radiographs, however, may be taken to rule out other pathologic conditions, such as infection or tumor.

The ideal diagnostic confirmatory test for herniated nucleus pulposus is MRI. MRI is both sensitive and specific. CT scanning can act as an alternative if MRI is not available. Patients who have CT scans should have a myelogram to assess the thecal sac both proximal and distal to the suspected level so that abnormalities simulating radiculopathies are not missed. If radiographic studies correlate with the patient history and physical findings, treatment outcomes are generally favorable. If the patient's symptomatology persists despite nonoperative measures, then operative intervention can be considered. Discrepancies between the radiographic findings and the patient's clinical picture require further investigation.

In the face of a static neurologic deficit, there is no evidence to suggest that surgical intervention offers any improvement in weakness or sensory deficit over continued nonoperative treatment. In the short-term, however, most surgically treated patients with acute lumbar radiculopathy are pain free in a relatively shorter time. Limited surgical disk excision has a success rate of 90% in patients who have good correlation between history, physical examination, and diagnostic studies. Laminectomy is often the procedure of choice when surgery is indicated. If half or more of both or all of one facet joint is injured causing secondary instability, fusion across the segment may be necessary. In the absence of facet joint injury, fusion in conjunction with diskectomy is unnecessary.

Procedures such as chemonucleolysis, percutaneous diskectomy, and microsurgical diskectomy have been advocated to decrease hospitalization, minimize perineural scarring associated with laminectomy, and speed rehabilitation. Chemonucleolysis has the potential complications of anaphylactic shock and neurologic deficit secondary to acute transverse myelitis. It is contraindicated in patients who previously underwent operative treatment or have evidence of spinal stenosis. Transverse myelitis has been reported in patients undergoing chemonucleolysis using chymopapain and having concomitant diskography. Percutaneous diskectomy may not be used in patients with sequestered fragments or in the presence of spinal stenosis. With microdiskectomy, sequestered fragments can be missed, and the lateral recess may not be adequately decompressed.

Chronic Back Pain

Assessment of the patient with chronic lower-back pain with or without radicular pain is much more difficult than that of the patient with acute pain. Chronic back pain is usually defined as back pain present for at least 6 months and not responsive to nonoperative interventions. This is the most difficult group of patients facing the clinician. As with the patient with acute onset of back pain, the chronic pain must be characterized regarding onset location, radiation, pattern, effect of positions, associated weakness, bowel or bladder symptomatology, and effect of medications. Most important, however, a psychosocial history needs to be taken. How the pain affects the patient's lifestyle is important; any litigation or workman's compensation involved must be noted. Previous treatment modalities and their effects must be carefully documented because many patients with chronic lower-back pain previously had either surgical or nonoperative treatment. Each patient must have a complete and thorough physical examination, including neurologic examination. It is important to test the patient for nonorganic physical signs. Many patients previously were seen by multiple physicians. Psychosocial evaluation of these patients is often necessary.

The establishment of special centers devoted to the assessment and treatment of patients with chronic back disorders use the multidisciplinary approach. These clinics employ physicians, surgeons, psychologists, social workers, occupational therapists, vocational rehabilitation counselors, and others to evaluate these difficult and often complex patients.

In the evaluation of a patient with chronic back pain, plain films are not often helpful. Degenerative changes may be seen on plain radiographs in a high percentage of normal patients. This is secondary to the normal aging process. Spina bifida occulta, Schmorl nodes, vacuum dicks, mild scoliosis, transitional vertebrae (sacralization of L5 or lumbarization of S1, partially or completely) occur as frequently in asymptomatic patients as in patients with lower-back pain.

Plain radiographs may be helpful when the diagnosis of metabolic bone disease, tumor, fracture, or traumatic injury of the spine is suspected. As mentioned in the section on spondylolisthesis, degenerative spondylolisthesis may be evident on plain radiographs secondary to facet joint degeneration with subsequent subluxation. Subluxation may occur in a posterior direction (retrolisthesis). These conditions in some cases cause nerve root compression and radicular symptoms. Inflammatory disease may also be detected on plain radiographs. If the patient has any other joint complaints in association with spinal pain, radiographs of the sacroiliac joint may help to make the diagnosis of ankylosing spondylitis.

In the patient with chronic back pain, MRI is useful in determining the presence of recurrent disk herniation. MRI is especially helpful in patients who have had previous lumbar spine surgery and continue to have chronic back pain to differentiate recurrent disk herniation from dural scarring. Gadolinium-enhanced MRI increases diagnostic accuracy for identifying recurrent disk herniation. MRI has the ability to reveal early degenerative changes in the disk. The MRI is, however, overly sensitive in that about 40% of asymptomatic people older than 50 years of age have an abnormal signal on MRI. It is also difficult to visualize the lateral recesses with MRI.

Myelography, once the most common diagnostic test in the evaluation of a patient with back pain, has limited use because of the increased diagnostic sensitivity and specificity of MRI and CT scanning. Myelography complications include seizures, arachnoiditis, and induction of nausea and vomiting. It is also inadequate for evaluating pathology in the lateral recesses. Myelography with water-soluble dye is most commonly used in conjunction with CT scanning to evaluate the thecal sac proximally and distally to the suspected level.

CT scanning is useful in revealing the anatomic parameters of spinal stenosis and lateral recess stenosis as well as foraminal stenosis. CT scanning is also useful in patients suspected of having vertebral osteomyelitis, tumors of the spine, and unrecognized trauma. In patients with chronic back pain and radiculopathy, electromyography may be useful in documenting a radiculopathy and in differentiating a neuropathy from a myelopathy. Motor nerve conduction velocity and sensory nerve conduction velocity testing may also help in differentiating neuropathies. Electrodiagnostic studies help differentiate patients with peripheral neuropathy or generalized or demyelinating disorders from patients with compressive neuropathy.

The various diagnostic evaluations must be used in conjunction with the patient's history and physical findings to help the physician arrive at a diagnosis and appropriate plan of management. Few patients with chronic back pain require surgical intervention. The most common conditions requiring back surgery in the adult are recurrent disk herniation, spinal stenosis, and segmental lumbar instability. Patients with chronic back pain without evidence of any of the above conditions should be treated nonoperatively. Patients who do not improve with symptomatic treatment (ie, limited periods of rest, antiinflammatory agents, exercise and muscle strengthening programs) should be evaluated in a comprehensive back pain clinic. These patients generally need the multidisciplinary approach to provide for lifestyle modification and rehabilitation. Otherwise, this limited group of patients continues to be a financial, social, and economic burden on society.

Spinal Stenosis

Spinal stenosis is a generic term that refers to any narrowing of the nerve root canal or intervertebral foramen. Stenosis of the spinal canal can occur primarily, as in congenital spinal stenosis, or it can be a developmental condition, such as in achondroplasia. Most often, it occurs secondary to degenerative changes in the lumbar disk and facet joints, leading to compression of the dural sac by the ligamentum flavum disk or bony hypertrophy of the fact joints. Spinal stenosis can also occur after an infectious process or a traumatic injury to the spine. Men and women in the seventh and eighth decades of life are the group primarily affected by degenerative spinal stenosis.

The clinical presentation of spinal stenosis is variable. The most common symptom scenario is that of either unilateral or bilateral leg pain precipitated by walking and relieved by rest. Other patients complain of pain or paraesthesia in the buttocks, thighs, or groin or in various distributions near the lower extremity.

Physical findings are variable. Tension signs are often absent. Neurologic deficits may or may not be present. Most patients, however, have aggravations of symptomatology by extension of the lumbar spine with relief of symptoms by forward flexion. Because of the claudication-type symptoms, the main differential diagnostic disorder is vascular claudication. All peripheral pulses should be checked; vascular consultation may be needed. Plain radiographs generally reveal degenerative changes of the spine consistent with aging changes. Patients may show evidence of degenerative spondylolisthesis or retrolisthesis. The diagnosis of spinal stenosis can best be made by myelography followed by CT scanning.

Nonoperative management may be tried, including antiinflammatory agents and epidural steroid injections, but these methods are generally unsuccessful. The treatment of choice for spinal stenosis is often surgical decompression of the stenosed area. All bone and soft tissues compressing the thecal sac or roots should be removed, with care taken when possible to preserve the facet joints to avoid creating segmental instability and the need for a fusion. About 70% to 85% of patients have good results from this procedure.

Annotated Bibliography

Spinal Deformity

Bradford DS, Lonstein JE, Moe JH, Ogalvie JW, Winter RB. Moe's textbook of scoliosis and spinal deformities, ed 2. Philadelphia, WB Saunders, 1987.
This is the classic textbook of spinal deformity. This text covers all aspects of scoliosis and other spinal deformities. It has an extensive bibliography and is well illustrated.

Ceballos T, Ferrer-Torrelles M, Castillo F, Fernandez-Paredes E. Prognosis of infantile scoliosis. J Bone Joint Surg 1980;62A: 863.
This article reviews the authors' experience with infantile scoliosis.

Frigueiredo UM, James JIP. Juvenile idiopathic scoliosis. J Bone Joint Surg 1981;63B:61.
The article presents a review of 98 patients with juvenile idiopathic scoliosis. Curve patterns are analyzed, and the results of treatment by observation, bracing, and surgery are presented.

Lonstein JE, Carlson M. Prognostication in idiopathic scoliosis. J Bone Joint Surg 1984;66A:1061.
The authors studied the risk of progression in 727 patients with idiopathic scoliosis. The risk of progression versus skeletal maturity, as well as other risk factors in progression, are discussed.

Lonstein JE, Weinstein SL, Keller RB, Englar GL, Tolo VT. AAOS instructional course on adolescent idiopathic scoliosis. AAOS Instruct Course Lect 1989;38:105.
This lecture covers screening, diagnosis, prevalence, natural history, nonoperative treatment, and pre- and interoperative considerations in the surgical management of adolescent idiopathic scoliosis.

Lovallo JL, Banta JV, Renshaw TS. Adolescent idiopathic scoliosis treated by Harrington rod distraction and fusion. J Bone Joint Surg 1986;68A:1326.
In a 44-month follow-up of 133 surgically treated patients, the authors demonstrated that single Harrington distraction rod and fusion followed by 6 months in a postoperative cast is a safe and effective treatment for adolescent idiopathic scoliosis. There were no neurologic injuries.

Mehta MH, Morel G. The nonoperative treatment of infantile idiopathic scoliosis. In: Zorab PA, Siegler D, eds. Scoliosis. London, Academic Press, 1979;71.
This is a summary chapter on the approach to the patient with infantile idiopathic scoliosis and the results of nonoperative treatment.

Mielke CH, Lonstein JE, Denis F, Vandenbrink K, Winter RB. Surgical treatment of adolescent idiopathic scoliosis: a comparative analysis. J Bone Joint Surg 1989;71A:1170.
The authors reported a detailed review of 352 patients with single right or double thoracic curves undergoing posterior arthrodesis with one of four instrumentation systems. The authors demonstrated satisfactory outcome with each system and outlined the applicability of each depending on AP and sagittal plain deformity.

Tolo VT, Gillespie R. The characteristics of juvenile idiopathic scoliosis and results of its treatment. J Bone Joint Surg 1978;60B: 181.
This is a review article of 59 patients with juvenile idiopathic scoliosis. The prognostic value of the rib–vertebral angle is discussed.

Weinstein SL, Ponseti IV. Curve progression in idiopathic scoliosis: long term follow-up. J Bone Joint Surg 1983;65A:447.
The authors discuss the factors in curve progression after skeletal maturity in a group of 102 untreated patients followed for an average of 40 years.

Weinstein SL, Zavala DC, Ponseti IV. Idiopathic scoliosis: long term follow-up. Prognosis in untreated patients. J Bone Joint Surg 1981;63A:702.

The authors followed 194 patients with untreated adolescent idiopathic scoliosis for an average of 39.3 years. The authors studied the effects on pulmonary function, psychological effects, mortality, morbidity, and backache in this large, untreated population.

Winter RB, ed. Scoliosis. Orthop Clin North Am 1988;19:1.
This monograph covers all aspects of scoliosis of varying causes.

Winter RB, Lonstein JE, Drogt J, Noren CA. The effectiveness of bracing in the nonoperative treatment of idiopathic scoliosis. Spine 1986;11:790.
The authors reviewed 95 high-risk patients with thoracic curves treated with the Milwaukee brace. The average follow-up was 2.5 years out of the brace or until surgery. The brace was effective in halting progression in 84% of cases, much improved over natural history.

Congenital Spinal Deformity

McMaster M, David C. Hemivertebrae as a cause of scoliosis: a review of 104 patients. J Bone Joint Surg 1986;68B:588.
The authors reviewed the natural history of 154 hemivertebrae in 104 patients. The authors determined the various risk factors, including the type of hemivertebrae, location, age of the patient, and number of hemivertebrae as well as their relation to each other.

McMaster MJ, Ohtsuka K. The natural history of congenital scoliosis: a study of 251 patients. J Bone Joint Surg 1982;64A: 1128.
The authors reviewed the natural history of 251 patients with congenital scoliosis. Abnormalities are classified in regard to prognosis for each pattern and curve location.

Winter RB. Congenital spine deformity. New York, Thieme Stratton, 1983.
This book provides a comprehensive look at all aspects of congenital spinal deformities based on the author's extensive experience.

Winter RB, Moe JH, Lonstein JE. Surgical treatment of congenital kyphosis: a review of 94 patients 5 years or older with 2 years or more follow-up of 77 patients. Spine 1985;10:224.
The authors reported on a 7-year average follow-up of 94 patients with congenital kyphosis. The results of posterior fusion alone versus combined anterior and posterior fusion are presented.

Winter RB, Moe J, Lonstein JE. Posterior spinal arthrodesis for congenital scoliosis: analysis of 290 patients 5 to 19 years old. J Bone Joint Surg 1984;66A:1188.
This article reports on a 6-year average follow-up of 290 patients between 5 and 19 years of age who were treated by posterior spinal arthrodesis with or without Harrington instrumentation. The authors report that the most common problem was bending of the fusion mass.

Back Pain in Children

Bunnell WA. Back pain in children. Orthop Clin North Am 1982;13: 587.
In this review article, back pain in children is separated into four etiologic groups: mechanical, developmental, inflammatory, and neoplastic.

Emans JB. Diagnosing the cause of back pain in children and adolescents. J Musculoskeletal Medicine 1989;46.
In this review article on back pain in children and adolescents, the author provides a diagnostic approach.

Fredrickson BE, Baker D, McHolick WJ, et al. The natural history of spondylolysis and spondylolisthesis. J Bone Joint Surg 1984;66A:699.
This article describes a prospective study of 500 unselected first-grade children and their families, discussing the incidence, relation of listhesis to lysis, and cause of disease.

Freeman BL, Donati NL. Spinal arthrodesis for severe spondylolisthesis in children and adolescents. J Bone Joint Surg 1989;71A:594.
The authors report on a 12-year follow-up of 12 patients with grade III or IV (over 50%) spondylolisthesis. The article demonstrated that posterior in situ arthrodesis is effective, reliable, and safe for treatment of severe spondylolisthesis.

Harris IE, Weinstein SL. Long term follow-up of patients with grade III and VI spondylolisthesis: treatment with and without posterior fusion. J Bone Joint Surg 1987;69A:960.
This article compares an 18-year follow-up of 11 patients with grades III and IV spondylolisthesis treated nonoperatively with a 24-year follow-up of 21 surgically treated patients. The surgical group was less symptomatic and less restricted in their activities than the nonsurgical group. In situ fusion gave good functional long-term results in grades III and IV spondylolisthesis.

Hensinger RN. Current concepts reviews: spondylolysis and spondylolisthesis in children and adolescents. J Bone Joint Surg 1989;71A:1098.
This superb review article covers all aspects of the topic and has an extensive bibliography.

King HA. Evaluating the child with back pain. Pediatr Clin North Am 1986;33:1889.
This review article covers the history, physical examination, radiographic examination, and differential diagnosis of the child presenting with the chief complaint of back pain.

Lowe TG. Scheuermann's disease and postural round back. J Bone Joint Surg 1990;72A:940.
This is an excellent review article on the topic of Scheuermann's disease with a complete bibliography.

Murray PM, Weinstein SL, Spratt K. Natural history and long term follow-up of Scheuermann's kyphosis. J Bone Joint Surg 1993;75A:236.
The authors report on a 31-year follow-up of 81 patients with Scheuermann's kyphosis. Pulmonary function, pain, work attendance, and disability are evaluated.

Peek RD, Wiltse L, Reynolds JB, et al. Arthrodesis without decompression for grade III and IV isthmic spondylolisthesis in adults who have severe sciatica. J Bone Joint Surg 1989;81A: 62.
The authors report on in situ fusions in 8 patients who had back pain and sciatica caused by grade III or IV isthmic spondylolisthesis of the lumbar vertebrae and the sacrum. All patients achieved a solid fusion with excellent relief of back pain and sciatica at 5.5-year average follow-up.

Pizzutillo PD, Hummer CD. Nonoperative treatment for painful adolescent spondylolysis or spondylolisthesis. J Pediatr Orthop 1989;9:538.
The authors demonstrate symptomatic relief of pain in two-thirds of patients with spondylolysis and grade and I and II spondylolisthesis treated nonoperatively. Adolescents with symptomatic grade III and IV spondylolisthesis are appropriately treated surgically.

Sachs B, Bradford D, Winter R, et al. Scheuermann's kyphosis: follow-up of Milwaukee brace treatment. J Bone Joint Surg 1987;69A:50.
This article describes the long-term follow-up of 120 patients treated for Scheuermann's disease with a Milwaukee brace, with a minimum follow-up of 5 years after treatment. The authors demonstrate that the Milwaukee brace is an effective method of treating patients with Scheuermann's kyphosis.

Saraste H. Long term clinical and radiographical follow-up of spondylolysis and spondylolisthesis. J Pediatr Orthop 1987;7: 631.
The author reports on a long-term (mean, 29 years) clinical and radiographic follow-up of 255 patients with spondylolisthesis and spondylolysis. Half of these patients were treated for lower back symptoms.

Back Pain in Adults

Allan DV, Wadell G. An historical perspective on low back pain and disability. Acta Orthop Scand 1989;60(Suppl 234):1.
This is a superb monograph that reviews the history of lower-back pain and sciatica for the past 3500 years. The authors also discuss the problem of chronic disability screening.

Bolender NF, Schönström NSR, Spengler DM. Role of computed tomography and myelography in the diagnosis of a central spinal stenosis. J Bone Joint Surg 1985;66A:240.
The authors demonstrate that the AP diameter of the dural sac, as determined by a myelogram or from high-resolution CT scans, is the most reliable indicator of lumbar stenosis.

Eismont FJ, Currier B. Current concepts review: surgical management of the lumbar intervertebral disc disease. J Bone Joint Surg 1989;71A:1266.
This is an excellent review article on management of the lumbar spine intervertebral disk disease. The authors discuss treatment by various modalities and the status of imaging techniques.

Frymoyer JW. Back pain and sciatica. N Engl J Med 1988;318:291.
This review article covers all aspects of the surgical and nonsurgical treatment of adults with lumbar spine disorders.

Frymoyer JW, Newberg A, Pope MH, et al. Spine radiographs in patients with low back pain: an epidemiologic study in men. J Bone Joint Surg 1984;66A:1048.
The authors demonstrate that degenerative changes of the lumbar spine increase with age. They report that congenital and developmental changes and aging changes of the spine occur in frequencies that do not support the use of radiographs in back pain as a predictive tool for individual cases.

Kelsey JL, White AA III. Epidemiology and impact of low back pain. Spine 1980;5:133.
This article reports that back pain is the most common cause of disability for people under 45 years of age. A herniated disk is the most common problem in the age group of 30 to 39 years and is associated more with sedentary occupations than active occupations. Degenerative changes seen on spinal radiographs are more closely linked to the natural aging process.

Weber H. Lumbar disc herniation: a controlled prospective study with 10 years of observations. Spine 1983;8:131.
In this study, between 85% and 90% of surgically treated and nonsurgically treated patients with disk hernias were asymptomatic after 4 years. Only 2% of subjects in both groups were symptomatic after 10 years. After 1 year, the surgical group had less pain, but after 4 years there was no statistically significant difference in relief of symptoms between the two groups.

Weinstein JN, Wiesel SW. Lumbar spine. Philadelphia, WB Saunders, 1990.
This text, from the International Society for the Study of the Lumbar Spine, covers all aspects of adult lumbar spine disease in great detail and has a superb bibliography.

Turek's Orthopaedics: Principles and Their Application, Fifth Edition,
edited by Stuart L. Weinstein and Joseph A. Buckwalter.
J.B. Lippincott Company, Philadelphia, © 1994.

14

Stuart L. Weinstein

The Pediatric Hip

CONGENITAL HIP DYSPLASIA	DEVELOPMENTAL COXA VARA
AND DISLOCATION	SLIPPED CAPITAL FEMORAL
LEGG-CALVÉ-PERTHES DISEASE	EPIPHYSIS
TRANSIENT SYNOVITIS	

CONGENITAL HIP DYSPLASIA AND DISLOCATION

The diagnosis of congenital hip dysplasia and dislocation is difficult to make in a newborn. The diagnosis is based on the subtleties of the physical examination. The consequences of not making the diagnosis may be disastrous to the patient. A confusing area in the literature is the terminology used to discuss this condition. Various authors use the terms *instability, dysplasia, subluxation,* and *dislocation* interchangeably. We prefer to use the term *congenital hip dysplasia* (or congenital dysplasia of the hip, CDH) to refer to any hip in which the normal relation between the femoral head and the acetabulum is altered.

In normal embryonic development, the hip joint components, the femoral head and acetabulum, develop from the same primitive mesenchymal cells. In the seventh week of gestation, a cleft develops in these precartilaginous cells, defining the femoral head and acetabulum. By 11 weeks of gestation, the hip joint is fully formed. Although rare, this is theoretically the earliest point in development that a hip dislocation could occur. At birth, the femoral head is deeply seated in the acetabulum and held there by the surface tension of the synovial fluid. A normal infant's hip is extremely difficult to dislocate even after division of the hip joint capsule. In hips with dysplasia, however, this tight fit between the femoral head and the acetabulum is lost, and the head can be easily displaced from the acetabulum. The femoral head displacement is usually in a posterosuperior direction. Pathologic specimens of this condition show varying degrees of hip joint malformation from mild capsular laxity to severe acetabular, femoral head, and neck malformations. Therefore, *congenital hip dysplasia* probably appropriately refers to the many stages of this complex deformity.

We use the term CDH clinically for any hip that may be provoked to subluxate (partial contact between the femoral head and the acetabulum) or dislocate (no contact between the femoral head and acetabulum) or for any hip in which the

487

femoral head is either subluxated or dislocated in relation to the acetabulum but that can be reduced into the acetabulum. We prefer to use the term *congenital hip dislocation* when there is no contact between the femoral head and the acetabulum and the femoral head is not reducible. True dislocations in the newborn are rare and are usually associated with generalized conditions or anomalies such as arthrogryposis or myelodysplasia. These antenatal teratologic dislocations are at the extreme end of the CDH pathologic spectrum and account for only 2% of the cases seen in most series. The diagnosis and prognosis of these two separate conditions (dysplasia versus dislocation) are quite different.

The incidence of CDH varies considerably and is influenced by geographic and ethnic factors as well as the diagnostic criteria used, the acumen of the examiner, and the age of the patient at diagnosis. The results of newborn screening programs estimate that 1 in 100 newborns have some evidence of hip instability but that the true incidence of dislocation is between 1 and 1.5 per 1000 live births.

The cause of CDH remains unknown. Ethnic and genetic factors no doubt play a key role. The incidence of CDH has been reported to be as high as 25 to 50 cases per 1000 live births in Lapps and North American Indians and to be almost nonexistent among Chinese and blacks. Up to one third of patients may give a positive family history for CDH. The genetic effects of the condition may be manifest primarily by acetabular dysplasia, joint laxity, or a combination of both. The role of excessive femoral neck anteversion or acetabular anteversion in the development of CDH remains controversial. Intrauterine mechanical and neuromuscular mechanisms can profoundly affect the intrauterine development of the hip.

In white infants, there is an increased incidence of CDH in first-born children. It has been postulated that the prima gravida uterus and abdominal muscles are unstretched and subject the fetus to prolonged periods of abnormal positioning. This tends to force the fetus against the mothers spine, limiting motions of the hip, particularly hip abduction. This "crowding phenomenon" may also be manifested by the association of other abnormalities thought to be due to the intrauterine compression, such as torticollis (up to 20% of patients with torticollis may have associated CDH) and metatarsus adductus. CDH is also manifested in patients with oligohydramnios, another condition that causes limited fetal mobility. The left hip is more frequently involved; in the uterus, it is

the left side that is most often forced into the adducted position against the mother's sacrum.

Breech presentation is another strong associative feature. About 60% of children with CDH are first-born children. In first-born children, there is a high association of breech presentation. About 30% to 50% of patients with CDH are delivered in the breech presentation. About 60% of breech presentations are in first-born children, and most breech-born infants have leg-folding mechanism arrests. Children born frank breech (knees in the extended position) are at an even greater risk of developing hip instability. This is evidenced by the higher incidence of CDH in children born with congenital recurvatum or dislocation of the knee. Eighty percent of the cases of CDH occur in girls. A contributory factor is that twice as many girls are born breech as boys. The extrauterine environment may also have a profound effect on the development of CDH. Societies in which swaddling is used postnatally (hips kept extended and adducted), for example, in many native North American tribes, the incidence of CDH is considerably higher than expected.

Hip joint laxity, either genetically determined or secondary to maternal estrogens and those hormones necessary for pelvic relaxation at delivery, may have an effect on the development of CDH. These hormones have been thought to cause temporary laxity of the hip joint capsule in the newborn, particularly the newborn girl. Hip joint laxity, however, is seen often in newborn infants. This may allow for some instability in the absence of a positive Ortolani sign. CDH is extremely rare in conditions characterized by excessive laxity such as Down, Ehlers-Danlos, and Marfan syndromes.

Most CDH cases are detectable at birth; however, despite newborn screening programs, some cases are missed. The diagnostic test for CDH is caused by the femoral head gliding in and out of the acetabulum over a ridge of abnormal acetabular cartilage. This test was originally described by LeDamany. He referred to the sensation palpated as *signe de ressaut*. The Italian pediatrician, Ortolani, in 1936 described the pathogenesis of this diagnostic sign and referred to the sensation palpated as the *segno dello scotto*. This palpable sensation has been likened to the femoral head gliding in and out of the acetabulum over a ridge. This ridge of hypertrophied acetabular cartilage (Fig. 14-1) was called the *neolimbus* by Ortolani. Unfortunately, inadequate translation of both LaDamany's and Ortolani's work into English has resulted into the use of the term *click* to describe this

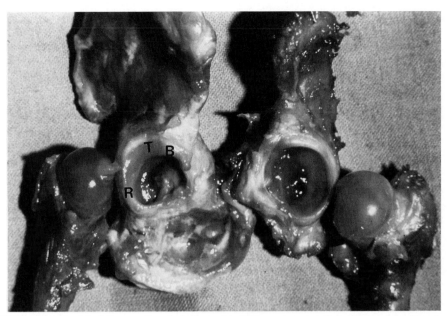

FIGURE 14-1. In this full-term female infant with fairly severe dysplasia of the right hip, the acetabulum and femoral head are smaller on the right than on the left. Extending along the posterosuperior margin of the articular surface of the right dysplastic acetabulum is a shallow trough (T). At the anterior end of this trough is a bulge (B), and extending posteriorly along the inferior and anterior margin of the trough down to the inferior margin of the acetabulum is a ridge (R) that separates the primary acetabulum inferiorly and anteriorly from the trough and the rest of the secondary acetabulum superiorly and posteriorly. (Ponseti IV. Morphology of the acetabulum in congenital dislocation of the hip: gross, histological, and roentgenographic studies. J Bone Joint Surg 1978;60A:586–599)

diagnostic sign. Experienced evaluators of hips in newborns realize that many high-pitched soft tissue clicks are often elicited in the hip examination of newborns that have no diagnostic significance. Unfortunately, this poor understanding of the pathology of the diagnostic sign in CDH has led to the misdiagnosis and overtreatment of infants. This diagnostic maneuver must be done gently. In the newborn period, such findings as asymmetry of the gluteal, thigh, or labial folds (asymmetric thigh and skin folds occur in a significant percentage of normal infants); limitation of abduction; or asymmetry of range of motion may make the physician suspect the presence of hip dysplasia, but the most reliable diagnostic sign is the Ortolani sign. The Ortolani test is performed with the infant in the supine position and the hips and knees flexed at 90 degrees. The middle finger is placed over the greater trochanter, while the thumb is placed on the lesser trochanter bilaterally. The hips are then slowly abducted with pressure over the greater trochanter. A palpable sensation indicates reduction of a dislocated or subluxated hip. Also with the legs in mid-abduction--adduction, posterior pressure can be applied to the lesser trochanters with the thumbs,

and a similar sensation can be palpated, indicating whether the hip is subluxating or dislocating. (The provocation portion of the diagnostic test is often referred to as the *Barlow maneuver.*) It is essential that this test be performed with the infant relaxed.

Some evidence suggests that a small number of cases of CDH may occur late. It is therefore extremely important to continually look for this condition after the newborn period when the disorder is manifested by the secondary adaptive signs. It is especially important to look for CDH in high-risk infants. The high-risk group of infants includes those who have a combination of any of the following risk factors: breech position, female, positive family history, lower limb deformity, torticollis, metatarsus adductus, significant persistent asymmetric thigh folds, excessive ligamentous laxity, any other significant musculoskeletal abnormality, and ethnic background associated with an increased incidence of CDH.

The longer after the newborn period, the greater is the likelihood of the patient exhibiting physical findings secondary to adaptive changes. With persistent subluxation or dislocation, the patient develops secondary contractures of the adductor muscles on the involved side. This leads to limited abduction (Fig. 14-2), the key late diagnostic finding in CDH. In addition, after the newborn period, the incidence of a positive Ortolani sign decreases markedly, particularly after 1 to 2 months of age. The disturbed relation between the proximal femur and the acetabulum may, in addition to limitation of abduction, lead to the presence of asymmetry of the gluteal, thigh, buttock, or labial folds. The patient may manifest apparent shortening of the femur (Allis sign) in comparison to the opposite side (Fig. 14-3) or "pistoning" or "telescoping" of the involved extremity, depending on the laxity of the hip joint capsule. In a child of walking age with unilateral CDH, the apparent limb length inequality may result in a limp secondary to the apparent shortening of the extremity. This also may lead to a secondary equinus deformity of the ankle. Clinically, bilateral dislocations are much more difficult to detect because the physical findings may be symmetric. Also in bilateral CDH, the child may walk with a waddling gait and hyperlordosis of the lumbar spine. Any gait abnormality in a child should not be dismissed without a careful clinical and radiographic evaluation of the hips.

The diagnosis of CDH in the newborn period is a clinical one. The femoral ossific nucleus is not present in the newborn, and a great portion of the pelvis of an infant is cartilaginous. Thus, normal relations are difficult to interpret radiographically, and all treatment decisions in the newborn nursery should be based on the clinical examination. Routine radiographs are generally unnecessary. A normal-appearing radiograph does not rule out the presence of CDH. Complete dislocations may be missed, and mild degrees of dysplasia are not easily detected.

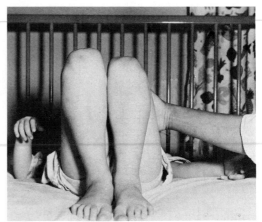

FIGURE 14-3. The Allis or Galeazzi sign. The knee is lower on the dislocated side.

Newer diagnostic tests, such as ultrasonography, may be helpful in screening children with suspected CDH. With increasing age and lack of the normal relation between the proximal femur and the acetabulum, the anatomic changes of this abnormal relation become increasingly evident. The femoral ossific nucleus, which normally appears between 4 and 7 months of age, may be delayed in its appearance and its general overall development stunted. The proximal femur is seen to lie laterally with varying degrees of proximal migration compared with the ilium. The Shenton line is disrupted. The acetabulum fails to develop, as manifested by an increase in the slope of the acetabular roof (Fig. 14-4). Most important is the accurate positioning of the child for the radio-

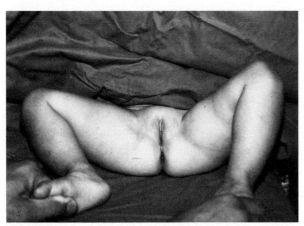

FIGURE 14-2. Eighteen-month-old girl with left congenital hip dysplasia. Note the limited abduction of left hip compared with the right.

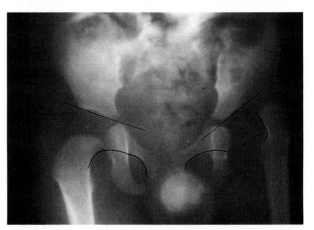

FIGURE 14-4. Eleven-month-old boy with left congenital hip dysplasia. Note the delayed appearance of left femoral ossific nucleus, disruption of the Shenton line with proximal migration of the femur, and lack of development of the acetabulum manifested by an increased slope of the acetabular roof.

graph. The lower extremities must be aligned and in neutral rotation.

In the newborn, the primary pathoanatomy consists of varying degrees of capsular laxity and the thickening of the acetabular cartilage in the superior, posterior, and inferior aspects of the acetabulum. This thickening in the cartilage was called *neolimbus* by Ortolani (see Fig. 14-1). It is the sensation of the femoral head gliding in and out of the acetabulum over this thickened ridge that produces the Ortolani sign. Without treatment, this ridge of hypertrophied acetabular cartilage may become more prominent, and within a few weeks or months after birth, the femoral head may remain dislocated into a secondary acetabulum. The child manifests the secondary adaptive physical findings mentioned previously. Pathologically, the anatomic obstacles to reduction change and become more difficult to overcome. The extraarticular and intraarticular pathologic changes may prevent concentric reduction. Extraarticular obstacles may include contraction of the adductor longus and the iliopsoas muscles as a consequence of the dislocation. The most common secondary change is varying degrees of anteromedial capsular constriction. The ligamentum teres may become thickened and hypertrophied or elongated, and in some cases, its sheer bulk precludes reduction. In the crawling or walking child, the constant pull of ligamentum teres on its attachment at the base of the acetabulum may cause hypertrophy of the transverse acetabular ligament, which secondarily decreases the diameter of the acetabulum. A true inverted labrum or limbus (hypertrophied labrum) may also be an obstacle reduction in the late diagnosed CDH. This, however, is a rare finding and is seen only in teratologic dislocations (2%) and in previously failed closed reductions, in which case it is an iatrogenic condition.

To understand the natural history of untreated CDH, it is important to appreciate that the normal concave shape of the acetabulum develops in response to the presence of a spherical femoral head. Experimental studies in animals as well as observations in humans with unreduced congenital hip dislocations show that the acetabulum does not develop its normal concave shape. Instead, with a complete dislocation, the triradiate cartilage grows normally, and hence the innominate bone reaches its normal length (Fig. 14-5); but the acetabular cartilage atrophies and degenerates, and the acetabulum appears flattened. The depth of the acetabulum increases normally as a result of continued interstitial growth within the acetabular cartilage, oppositional growth at the periphery of this cartilage, and periosteal new

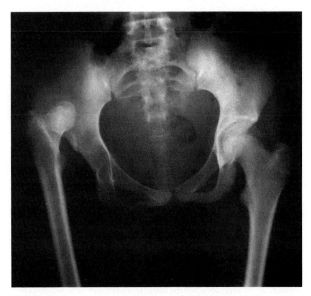

FIGURE 14-5. Untreated right congenital hip dysplasia in an adult. Note the lack of development of acetabular shape and depth. No secondary acetabulum exists. The left hip is normal.

bone growth at the edge of the acetabulum along the ilium. The depth of the acetabulum is further increased at puberty by the development of secondary centers of ossification in the three pelvic bones. For this normal growth and development to occur, a concentric relation must be maintained between the femoral head and the acetabulum throughout growth.

Most unstable hips at birth stabilize in a short time. A certain percentage of untreated hips, however, go on to subluxation (partial contact with the acetabulum) or dislocation (no contact between the femoral head and acetabulum), and some hips may remain located but retain dysplastic features. Unfortunately, the means to determine which of the unstable hips will attain spontaneous stability are not available, and hence all unstable hips in the newborn period must be treated to ensure the proper environment for hip joint development.

It is important to make the diagnosis early and institute treatment so that normal development may occur. If the hip remains completely dislocated, its natural history depends on two factors: the presence or absence of a false acetabulum and bilateralness.

In the absence of a false acetabulum, most patients with complete dislocations do well, maintaining a good range of motion and little functional disability. Completely dislocated hips with well-developed false acetabuli, however, are more likely to develop degenerative joint disease in the false acetabulum and have a poor clinical result (Fig. 14-6). Degenerative joint disease in the false acetabulum usually occurs in the fourth and fifth decades of life. In bilateral complete dislocations, lower-back pain may occur. This may be secondary to the hyperlordosis of the lumbar spine associated with the hip flexion adduction deformities caused by the dislocations.

In unilateral complete dislocations, the natural history is affected by the secondary problems of limb length inequality, ipsilateral knee deformity, pain (usually on the lateral side of the knee), secondary scoliosis, and gait disturbances. In these patients, the same factors concerning the development of secondary degenerative changes in any false acetabulum that may occur are also applicable.

After the neonatal period, *dysplasia* refers to inadequate development of the acetabulum, femoral head, or both. All subluxated hips are by definition dysplastic. Radiographically, however, the major difference between dysplasia and subluxation is the intactness of the Shenton line (Fig. 14-7). In subluxation, the Shenton line is disrupted, and the femoral head is superiorly or laterally displaced from the medial wall of the acetabulum. In dysplasia, the normal Shenton line relation is intact. Unfortunately, in the CDH natural history literature, these two radiographic and clinical entities are often not separated. In addition, the development of secondary degenerative arthritis in the dysplastic hip may convert it to a subluxated hip. Since the physical signs of hip dysplasia are usually lacking, cases are often diag-

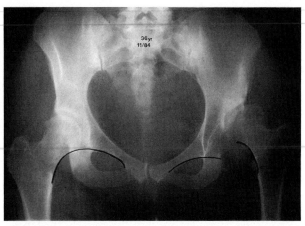

FIGURE 14-7. Radiographically, the major difference between dysplasia and subluxation is the intactness of the Shenton line. The right hip is dysplastic (Shenton line intact). The left hip is subluxated (Shenton line disrupted). All subluxated hips are, by definition, dysplastic. (Weinstein SL. Natural history of congenital hip dislocation [CDH] and hip dysplasia. Clin Orthop 1987;225:62–76)

nosed only incidentally on radiographs taken for other reasons or not until the patient develops symptoms.

The natural history of hip subluxation clearly indicates that this condition leads to the development of radiographic degenerative joint disease and clinical disability. The more severe the subluxation, the earlier is the symptom onset. Those patients with the most severe subluxations usually develop symptoms of degenerative joint disease during the second decade of life. The symptoms of degenerative joint disease and hip subluxation and dysplasia often predate radiographic changes of degenerative joint disease (decreased joint space, cyst formation, double acetabular floor, inferomedial femoral head osteophyte) by as much as 10 years. Often, the only radiographic feature present at symptom onset may be increased sclerosis in the weight-bearing area. In the absence of subluxation, the natural history of dysplasia cannot accurately be predicted, but there is a definite association of hip dysplasia with radiographic degenerative joint disease, especially in female patients.

Once the diagnosis of CDH is made, treatment should be initiated immediately. The use of triple diapers in the treatment of CDH in the newborn should be condemned. It is ineffective and gives the family a false sense of security. Pathologic changes seen in the newborn with CDH are reversible in 95% of cases with simple, appropriately applied treatment methods. The most widely used device in North America is the Pavlik harness (Fig. 14-8). The Pavlik harness prevents adduction and extension while al-

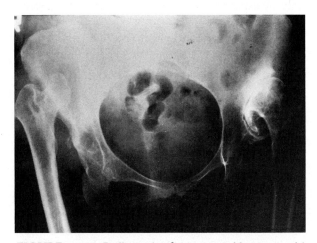

FIGURE 14-6. Radiograph of a 43-year-old woman with complete dislocation of both hips. She has no symptoms on the right but has disabling symptoms from the left hip. She has no false acetabulum on the right but has a well-developed false acetabulum on the left with secondary degenerative changes present. (Weinstein SL. Natural history of congenital hip dislocation [CDH] and hip dysplasia. Clin Orthop 1987;225:62–76)

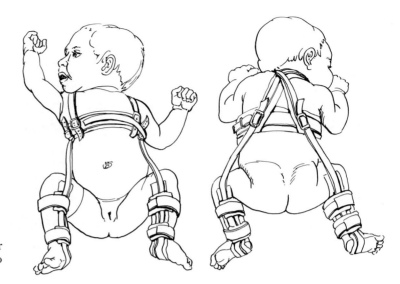

FIGURE 14-8. Pavlik harness. The posterior strap acts as a check rein against adduction to prevent redislocation.

lowing further flexion, abduction, and rotation. This position allows for gentle spontaneous reduction of dislocated hips. Stretching of tight adductors is also achieved with the Pavlik harness. The device is worn full-time until hip stability is achieved. Use of the Pavlik harness must be accompanied by extensive parent education by the physician. Patient noncompliance is the main cause of failure of this device. Appropriate application of the device is essential. Careful follow-up at weekly intervals is extremely important. Adjustments in the flexion and abduction straps of the Pavlik harness must be made to accommodate the hip stability assessed by physical examination of the patient. Clinical hip stability is usually obtained within 2 to 4 weeks of treatment by this method. Most physicians use the harness for a period of 6 to 12 weeks on a full-time basis. Initial radiographs or sonograms should be obtained in the harness to document adequate flexion and redirection of the femoral shaft toward the triradiate cartilage in the harness. Once clinical stability is obtained, a radiograph is not indicated until about 3 months of age to determine acetabular development. The Pavlik harness may be used in dysplasia and subluxation up to 6 months of age. Once the child begins to crawl, use of the Pavlik harness is extremely difficult, and the success rate with the harness decreases to less than 50%.

If hip stability is not achieved in the previously mentioned time frame, treatment with the Pavlik harness should be discontinued and alternative methods of treatment employed. The Pavlik harness is contraindicated in the patient who has CDH in association with conditions of muscle imbalance (eg, upper-level meningomyelocele), joint stiffness (eg, arthrogryposis), or excess ligamentous laxity, (eg,

Ehlers-Danlos syndrome). Applied correctly and used for the appropriate indications, the Pavlik harness may achieve 95% successful results in treatment of CDH. Inappropriately applied and poorly monitored use of the harness is associated with problems such as inferior hip dislocations from prolonged excess flexion of the hip in the harness. This hyperflexion may also be associated with femoral nerve palsies, which are usually transient. Brachial plexus palsies from pressure of the shoulder straps have also been reported. The parent must pay attention to skin care in the groin folds and the popliteal fossa area to prevent skin maceration and breakdown. The most devastating complication of the Pavlik harness is aseptic necrosis of the femoral head. Reported incidence of this complication ranges from 9% to 15%. This is generally produced by excess of tightening of the abduction strap. It has been well-documented that the hyperabduction position of the hip compromises the vascular supply to the proximal femur.

In a child with dysplasia or subluxation who is older than 6 months at age, a fixed-abduction orthosis (see Fig. 14-8) may be used to try and achieve hip stability and allow for growth and development of the hip joint. It can be used only if the hip is well reduced on a radiograph taken in the orthoses. The complications of fixed-abduction orthoses include skin problems and aseptic necrosis. It is important in positioning the fixed-abduction orthoses that the hip not be placed in extreme positions of abduction to avoid aseptic necrosis.

In the late diagnosed case or the case that fails treatment with a Pavlik harness and is not amenable to a fixed-abduction orthosis, the obstacles to reduction are different, treatment has greater risks, and the results are less predictable. The general goals of

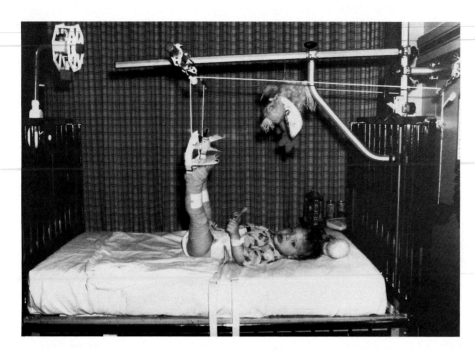

FIGURE 14-9. Preliminary traction. Bryant traction was used before attempted closed reduction to stretch soft tissue structures about the hip.

treatment in the late diagnosed case are to obtain and maintain a reduction, to allow for femoral head and acetabular development, and to avoid a development of aseptic necrosis.

In these cases or in those that have failed Pavlik harness treatment, closed reduction is indicated. Closed reduction is generally preceded by a 1- to 2-week period of traction (Fig. 14-9). The purpose of the traction is to allow gradual stretching of the soft tissue structures impeding reduction as well as of the neurovascular bundle. The primary purpose of traction is the avoidance of aseptic necrosis, the most devastating complication of the treatment of CDH. The traction can be applied in the hospital or at home. Generally, 1 to 2 weeks is sufficient. Skin traction is usually adequate, and skeletal traction is rarely necessary. The skin tapes should be applied above the knee to distribute the traction over a large area. Complications of traction include skin loss and ischemia of the lower extremities due to inappropriate application. Neurocirculatory checks must be done frequently and traction applied in a carefully supervised fashion. Home traction has become popular because of the decreased cost and convenience. Home traction should follow a 24-hour hospitalization to familiarize the parents with application of the traction and how to look for problems. It can only be used with cooperative, informed parents.

Closed reductions are usually performed in the operating room setting. Under general anesthesia, the hip is gently manipulated into the acetabulum. Ar-

throgography is extremely helpful in assessing the adequacy of reduction (Fig. 14-10). Because a large portion of the acetabulum is cartilaginous, the relations of the femoral head and acetabulum are nicely visualized on arthrography. The use of arthrography can help to assess any obstacles to reduction and also the quality of reduction. Reduction is then maintained by a well-molded cast (Fig. 14-11) for a variable

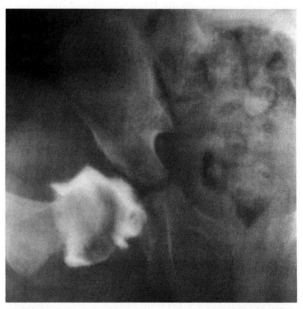

FIGURE 14-10. Attempted closed reduction under arthrographic control. Note pooling of dye medially. The hip cannot be reduced.

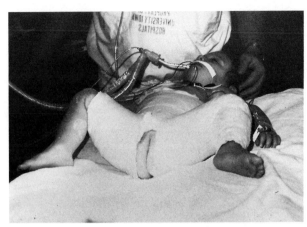

FIGURE 14-11. Reduction of left congenital hip dysplasia is maintained by a well-molded 1½ hip spica cast.

amount of time (range, 6 weeks to 4 months), depending on the child's age. The so-called human position of hyperflexion and limited abduction should be used in closed reductions. Extreme positions of abduction, as well as abduction and internal rotation, should be avoided because of their association with the development of aseptic necrosis. After removal of the cast, a fixed-abduction orthosis is applied and worn at night and during napping hours until acetabular development has returned to normal. The postoperative reduction can be confirmed by the use of single-cut tomography, computed tomographic (CT) scanning, or ultrasound.

Open reductions are indicated for failure to obtain a closed reduction, failure to maintain a closed reduction, or an unstable reduction. If an open reduction is necessary, it can be done through a variety of surgical approaches. During the open reduction, each obstacle to reduction must be addressed. The most common obstacle is the tight anteromedial joint capsule, which must be released. The transverse acetabular ligament often requires sectioning, and the ligamentum teres may need to be removed. A true inverted labrum or limbus should never be excised but only radially incised because excision of this tissue may interfere with the normal growth and development of the acetabulum.

After the age of 2 years, there is a high likelihood of a patient requiring an open reduction to obtain and maintain a reduction. By the age of 4 years, preliminary traction should not be used, but open reduction should be accompanied by a femoral shortening (removal of a section of the proximal femur) to decrease the incidence of aseptic necrosis. Between the ages of 2 and 4 years, the question of whether to use femoral shortening versus traction before open reduction remains unanswered.

The acetabulum has potential for growth for many years once a closed or open reduction has been obtained. If, however, the acetabulum does not make adequate progress toward normal development after a closed or open reduction, one of several types of innominate osteotomy should be performed to increase femoral head coverage (Fig. 14-12).

All children with CDH have associated femoral neck anteversion. In general, children reduced before they are 2 years of age rarely require derotation osteotomies to correct the anteversion. This usually corrects once the reduction is obtained. Aseptic necrosis is the most devastating complication associated with the treatment of CDH. Aseptic necrosis may be caused by many errors in treatment, as mentioned previously. In the newborn, excessive use of abduction or the abduction internal rotation position can cause aseptic necrosis. In the older child, aseptic necrosis may be caused by insufficient use of prereduction traction, failure to perform an adductor tenotomy, injuries to the blood vessels during surgery, failure to do femoral shortening, or persistence of closed techniques in the face of obstacles to reduction.

In adolescent patients with residual dysplasia, deformity may be present in the femoral head, acetabulum, or both. In these cases, normal anatomy and relation must be restored. In many cases, osteotomies are necessary on both the femoral and pelvic sides of the hip joint.

LEGG-CALVÉ-PERTHES DISEASE

Legg-Calvé-Perthes disease (LCPD) is a disorder of the hip in young children. The disease is characterized by varying degrees of necrosis of the femoral ossific nucleus. It is most common in the age range of 4 to 8 years, but has been reported in children as young as 2 years of age and also in the late teen-age years. It is more common in boys than girls by a ratio of 4:1, and the incidence of bilateralness is about 10% to 12%.

Epidemiologic studies of patients with Legg-Calvé-Perthes disease reveal an incidence of a positive family history of about 10%. There is a high association of abnormal birth presentation, such as breech or transverse lie, in affected patients. There are also racial and ethnic factors, with LCPD being more common in Japanese, Eskimos, and Central Europeans and uncommon in native Australians, Polynesians, American Indians, and blacks.

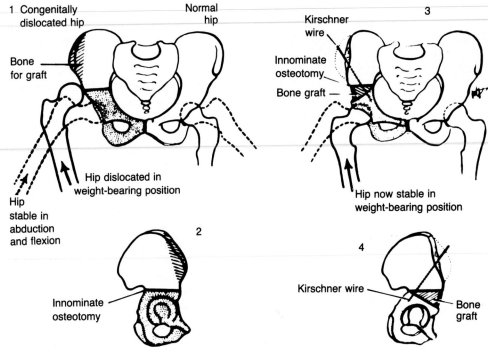

FIGURE 14-12. Technique of Salter innominate osteotomy. Diagram of principle involved. (Salter RB. Innominate osteotomy in the treatment of congenital dislocation and subluxation of the hip. J Bone Joint Surg 1961;43B:518)

Other epidemiologic factors include lower birth weights and delay in skeletal maturation as evidenced by retarded bone age. Affected children are shorter than nonaffected children. Anthropometric studies have confirmed this growth delay, with affected children being smaller in all dimensions except head circumference and with the distal portion of the extremities affected more than the proximal. The short stature of the patients affected with the disorder at a young age tends to correct during adolescence, while those affected at an older age tend to be small throughout life. An abnormality of growth hormone–dependent somatomedin in males with LCPD has recently been demonstrated.

An increased incidence of LCPD is seen in later-born children, particularly the third to the sixth child, and in lower socioeconomic groups.

LCPD is more common in certain geographic areas, particularly in urban rather than rural communities. Parental age of affected patients is higher than in the general population. Affected children have an increased association of genital urinary tract abnormalities, inguinal hernia, and minor congenital abnormalities.

The cause of LCPD remains unknown. LCPD has been thought to be an inflammatory disease, secondary to trauma or a developmental disorder. Toxic synovitis is thought by some authors to be a precursor to LCPD; however, a literature review of patients with toxic synovitis revealed that only about 3% subsequently develop LCPD. The most widely accepted etiologic theories are those involving interruption of the vascular supply to the femoral head. It has been well demonstrated in animal studies and confirmed by human pathologic material that LCPD is caused by repetitive episodes of infarction. Recent studies have postulated that the cause of the vascular embarrassment may be disturbed venous drainage, intraosseous venous hypertension, or increased blood viscosity leading to decreased blood flow.

Some evidence suggests that LCPD may be a generalized disorder of epiphyseal hyaline cartilage and thus should be called Legg-Calvé-Perthes syndrome. This may account for the delayed skeletal maturation and for the disease's manifestation in the hip because of the unusual and precarious blood supply of the proximal femur, which makes the femoral head especially vulnerable.

Skeletal surveys in patients with LCPD demonstrate irregularities of ossification in other epiph-

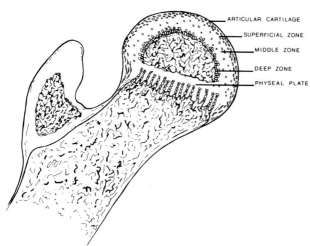

FIGURE 14-13. Anatomic regions of the proximal femur in a growing child. (Weinstein SL. Legg-Calvé-Perthes disease. In: Morrissy RT, ed. Lovell and Winter's pediatric orthopaedics, vol 2. 1990:854)

yses and abnormalities in the contralateral, so-called unaffected capital epiphysis compared with matched controls.

Histologic changes of the epiphyseal and physeal cartilage of patients with LCPD were described as early as 1913 by Perthes. The superficial zone of the cartilage covering the affected femoral head is normal but thickened (Fig. 14-13). In the middle layer of the epiphyseal cartilage, however, two types of abnormalities are seen: areas of extreme hypercellularity,

with the cells varying in size and shape and often arranged in clusters; and in other areas, a loose, fibrocartilaginous-like matrix. These abnormal areas in the epiphyseal cartilage have different histochemical and ultrastructural properties than normal cartilage or fibrocartilage. Areas of small secondary ossification centers are evident, with bony trabeculae of uneven thickness forming directly on the abnormal cartilage matrix.

The physeal plate in LCPD shows evidence of cleft formation with amorphous debris and extravasation of blood. In the metaphyseal region, enchondral ossification is normal in some areas; but in other areas, the proliferating cells are separated by a fibrillated cartilaginous matrix that does not calcify. The cells in these areas do not degenerate but continue to proliferate without enchondral ossification. This is evidenced by "tongues" of cartilage extending into the metaphysis as bone growth proceeds in adjoining areas (Fig. 14-14).

Catterall demonstrated thickening, abnormal staining, sporadic calcification, and diminished evidence of ossification in the deep zone of the articular cartilage of the unaffected hip. He also demonstrated the physeal plate in these unaffected hips to be thinner than normal, with irregular cell columns and cartilage masses remaining unossified in the primary spongiosa. Similar histologic changes have been seen in the acetabular cartilage and other epiphyses.

Thus, the epidemiologic, anthropometric, radio-

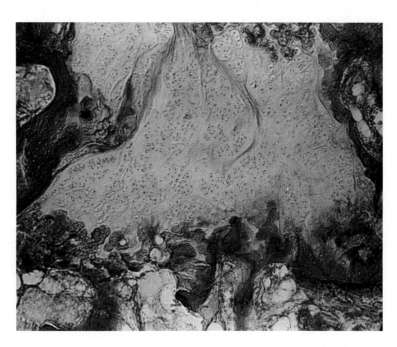

FIGURE 14-14. Photomicrograph (×80) showing a large area of cartilage in between the bone trabeculae of the femoral neck (case 1). (Ponseti IV. Legg-Perthes disease: observations on pathological changes in two cases. J Bone Joint Surg 1956;38A:739)

graphic, and histologic data lend support to the concept of the susceptible child. LCPD may thus represent a localized manifestation of the generalized transient disorder of the epiphyseal hyaline cartilage, clinically manifested in the proximal femur because of its unusual and precarious blood supply. The persistence of the abnormally soft cartilage through which blood vessels have to penetrate into the femoral head could cause repeated episodes of infarction and prolong the disease.

LCPD must not be thought of as simply aseptic necrosis similar to that seen in the adult or child after a femoral neck fracture or a traumatic dislocation of the hip. After a fracture at the femoral neck or a traumatic dislocation of the hip in a child, the vascular insult usually heals rapidly without going through the prolonged stages of fragmentation and repair that are seen in LCPD.

Patients with LCPD most commonly present with a history of the insidious onset of a limp. Most patients do not complain of much discomfort unless specifically questioned about this aspect. Pain when present is usually activity related and relieved by rest. Because of its mild nature, most patients do not present for medical attention until weeks or months after the clinical onset of disease. The pain that patients experience is generally localized to the groin or referred to the anteromedial thigh or knee region. Failure to recognize that thigh or knee pain in the child may be secondary to hip pathology may cause further delay in the diagnosis. Some children present with more acute symptom onset. As with most childhood musculoskeletal disorders, patients with LCPD usually present with limited hip motion, particularly abduction and medial rotation. Early in the course of the disease, the limited abduction is secondary to muscle spasm of the adductor muscles; however, with time, subsequent deformities may develop, and limitation of abduction may become permanent. Occasionally, long-standing adductor spasm leads to adductor contracture. The Trendelenburg test in patients with LCPD is often positive. These children most commonly have evidence of thigh, calf, and buttock atrophy from inactivity secondary to pain. This is further evidence of the long-standing nature of the condition before detection. Limb length should be measured; inequality is indicative of significant head collapse and a poor prognosis. Evaluation of the patient's overall height, weight, and bone age may be helpful in the differential diagnosis and may provide confirmatory evidence of the disorder. Laboratory studies are generally not helpful in LCPD, although they may be necessary to rule out other conditions.

The diagnosis is made and the condition followed by plain radiographs taken in the anteroposterior (AP) and frog-leg lateral positions. These radiographs are generally sufficient for the assessment of the patient and for subsequent follow-up evaluations. From the plain radiographs, the physician can determine the stage of the disease and the extent of epiphyseal involvement. Additional radiographic or imaging studies may be helpful in the initial assessment or follow-up of the condition.

Radionuclide bone scanning with technetium and pin-hole collimation may be helpful in the early stages of the disease when the diagnosis is in question, but this is rarely necessary. Some investigators consider scanning helpful in determining the extent of the epiphyseal involvement and hence prognosis.

Magnetic resonance imaging (MRI) is widely available in many medical centers. It appears to be sensitive in detecting infarction, but as of yet cannot accurately portray the stages of healing. Its role in the management of LCPD is yet to be defined.

There are four radiographic stages of LCPD. In the initial stage, the earliest radiographic signs of LCPD are failure of the ossific nucleus to grow compared with the unaffected hip and widening of the medial joint space caused by hypertrophy of the articular cartilage of the femoral head (Fig. 14-15). The physician may also see a relative increase in radiodensity of the femoral ossific nucleus in relation to the femoral neck. Radiolucencies may be present in the metaphysis with thinning and irregularity of the physeal plate (Figs. 14-16 and 14-17). A subchondral radiolucent zone (crescent sign) may also be present. This radiolucent zone generally corresponds to the extent of the necrotic portion of the ossific nucleus (Fig. 14-18).

The second radiographic stage is the fragmentation phase. In this phase, the physician sees resorption of the necrotic portion of the ossific nucleus (Fig. 14-19). This is followed by a reparative or reossification phase, in which the physician sees return to normal radiodensities of the ossific nucleus until the lesion is completely healed (see Fig. 14-19).

The femoral head and neck may become deformed as a result of the disease, the repair process, or premature physeal plate closure. The actual deformity that develops is profoundly influenced by the duration of the disease. This in turn is proportional to the extent of the epiphyseal involvement, the age of disease onset, the remodeling potential of

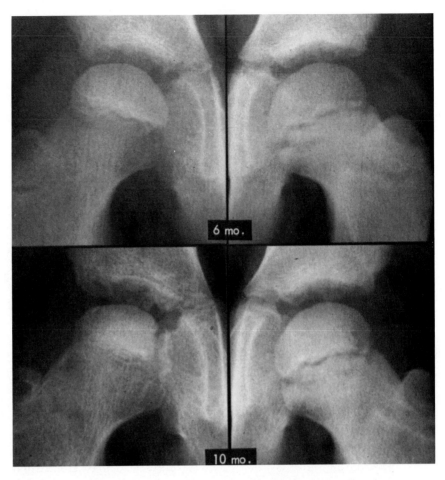

FIGURE 14-15. AP radiograph of the hip in a patient who developed Legg-Calvé-Perthes disease. On the initial film taken 6 months after onset of symptoms, the right ossific nucleus is smaller than the left, and the medial joint space is widened. Note also the retained density of the ossific nucleus compared with that of the normal hip and the relative osteopenia of the viable bone of the proximal femur and pelvis. Ten months after onset of symptoms, the evolution of the radiographic changes is seen. (Weinstein SL. Legg-Calvé-Perthes disease. AAOS Instr Course Lect Ser 1983;32:272)

the patient, and the stage of disease when treatment is initiated. An additional factor may be the type of treatment.

Prognostic factors must be gleaned from series of long-term follow-ups. In the 20- to 40-year post–symptom-onset follow-ups, most patients (70% to 90%) are active and free of pain. Most patients maintain a good range of motion despite the fact that few patients have normal-appearing radiographs. Clinical deterioration, increasing pain, decreasing range of motion, and loss of function are observed in only those patients with flattened irregular femoral heads at the time of primary healing and in those with evidence of premature physeal closure. The follow-up studies beyond 40 years, however, demonstrate marked reduction in function, with most patients developing degenerative joint disease by the sixth or seventh decade.

Reviews of long-term series of patients with LCPD identify certain clinical and radiographic features that have prognostic value. These interrelated factors include deformity of the femoral head and hip joint incongruence, age of disease onset, extent of epiphyseal involvement, growth disturbance secondary to premature physeal closure, protracted disease course, acetabular and femoral head remodeling potential, type of treatment, and stage during which treatment is initiated.

Partial or anterior head involvement leads to a more favorable prognosis than whole femoral head involvement. Catterall demonstrated the importance of the extent of epiphyseal involvement relating to prognosis and proposed four groups based on the presence or absence of seven radiographic signs in 97 untreated hips (Table 14-1; see Figs. 14-16 and 14-19). He reported that 90% of the good results in untreated patients were in groups 1 and 2, while 90% of the poor results were in groups 3 and 4.

Salter and Thompson recently proposed a simplified, two-group classification based on prognosis: group A had less than 50% femoral head involvement (Catterall groups 1 and 2); and group B had more than 50% femoral head involvement (Catterall

(text continues on page 504)

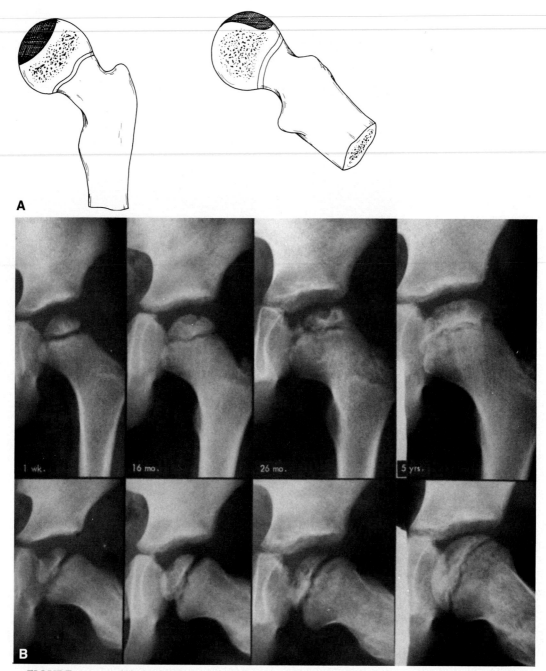

FIGURE 14-16. (A) Catterall group 1 disease: anterior head involvement, with no evidence of sequestrum or of a subchondral fracture line or metaphyseal abnormalities. (B) Catterall group 1 disease 1 week to 5 years after onset of symptoms. (Weinstein SL. Legg-Calvé-Perthes disease. In: Morrissy RT, ed. Lovell and Winter's pediatric orthopaedics, vol 2. 1990:863)

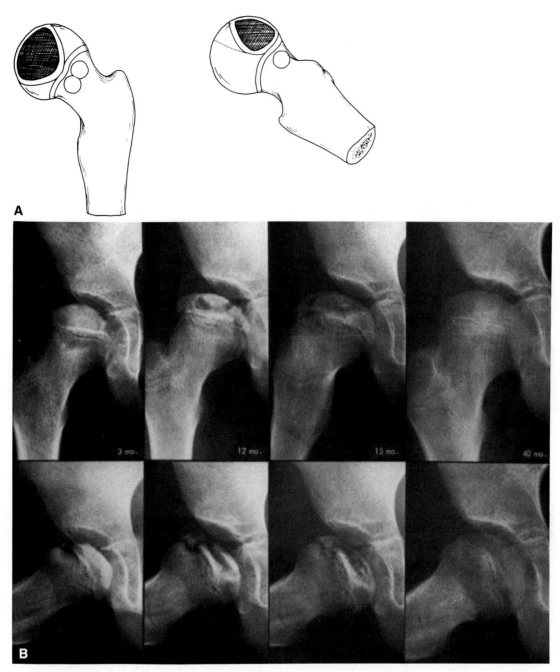

FIGURE 14-17. **(A)** Catterall group 2 disease: anterolateral involvement, sequestrum formation, and a clear junction between the involved and uninvolved areas. There are anterolateral metaphyseal lesions, and the subchondral fracture line is in the anterior half of the head. The lateral column is intact. **(B)** Catterall group 2 disease 3 to 40 months after onset of symptoms. Note the intact lateral pillar. (Weinstein SL. Legg-Calvé-Perthes disease. In: Morrissy RT, ed. Lovell and Winter's pediatric orthopaedics, vol 2. 1990:864)

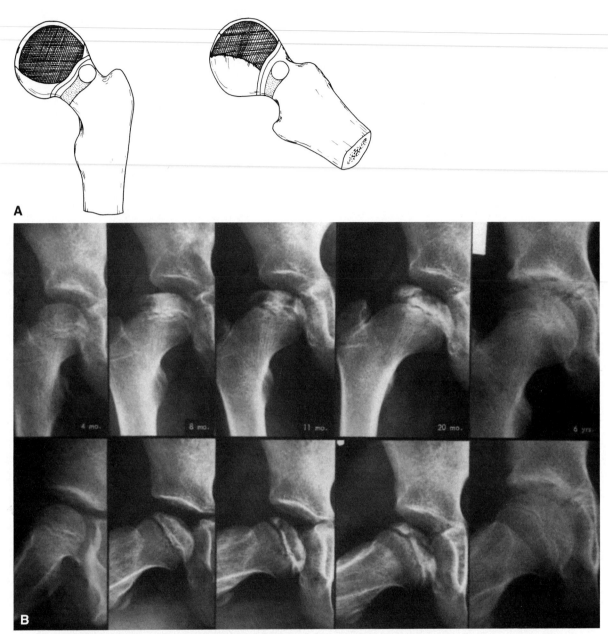

FIGURE 14-18. (A) Catterall group 3 disease: large sequestrum involving three quarters of the head. The junction between the involved and uninvolved portions is sclerotic. Metaphyseal lesions are diffuse, particularly anterolaterally, and the subchondral fracture line extends to the posterior half of the epiphysis. The lateral column is involved. (B) Catterall group 3 disease 4 months to 6 years after onset of symptoms. Note involvement of the lateral pillar as well as the subchondral radiolucent zone on the radiograph taken 8 months after onset of symptoms. (Weinstein SL. Legg-Calvé-Perthes disease. In: Morrissy RT, ed. Lovell and Winter's pediatric orthopaedics, vol 2. 1990:865)

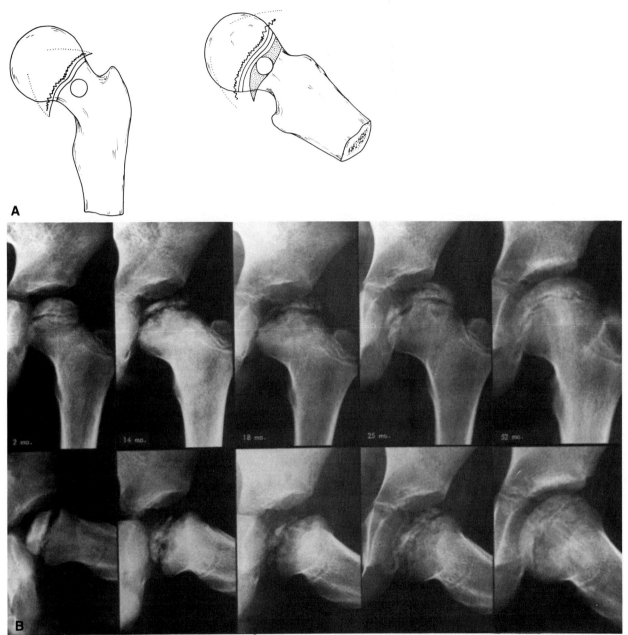

FIGURE 14-19. (A) Catterall group 4 disease: whole head involvement with either diffuse or central metaphyseal lesions and posterior remodeling of the epiphysis. (B) Catterall group 4 disease 2 to 52 months after onset of symptoms. Note the stage: 14 months—fragmentation; 18 months—early reossification; 25 months—late reossification; 52 months—healed. Note also the growth arrest line and evidence of reactivation of the growth plate along the femoral neck. (Weinstein SL. Legg-Calvé-Perthes disease. In: Morrissy RT, ed. Lovell and Winter's pediatric orthopaedics, vol 2. 1990:866)

TABLE 14-1.
Catterall Groups

Group	Characteristics	Prognosis
1	Anterior head involvement, no evidence of sequestrum or of a subchondral fracture line or metaphyseal abnormalities	Patients uniformly do well.
2	Anterolateral involvement, sequestrum formation and a clear junction between the involved and uninvolved areas. There are anterolateral metaphyseal lesions, and the subchondral fracture line is in the anterior half of the head.	Clinical results are generally good.
3	Large sequestrum involving three quarters of the head. The junction between the involved and uninvolved portions is sclerotic. Metaphyseal lesions are diffuse, particularly anterolaterally, and the subchondral fracture line extends to the posterior half of the epiphysis.	Healing is slower and less complete.
4	Whole head involvement with either diffuse or central metaphyseal lesions and posterior remodeling of the epiphysis	Patients have a poor long-term prognosis.

groups 3 and 4). The major determining factor between groups A and B is the presence or absence of a viable lateral pillar of the epiphysis. This intact lateral column (Catterall group 2, Salter-Thompson group A) may thus shield the epiphysis from collapse and subsequent deformity (see Figs. 14-17 and 14-18).

Catterall identified other radiographic signs of prognostic value (Fig. 14-20). These at-risk signs include the Gage sign (radiolucency in the lateral epiphysis and metaphysis) and calcification lateral to the epiphysis. These two signs indicate early ossification in the enlarged epiphysis and are therefore present only when the head is deformed but at a stage when the changes are reversible. Another at-risk sign is metaphyseal lesions. These radiolucencies may herald the potential for growth disturbance of the physeal plate. The final two at-risk signs are lateral subluxation and a horizontal growth plate. Lateral subluxation indicates a widened femoral head. The horizontal growth plate indicates a developing deformity that, if left untreated, leads to a fixed deformity, hinge abduction, and further deformity. These radiographic at-risk signs are manifested clinically by loss of motion and adduction contracture. Catterall reported no poor results in patients not manifesting two or more at risk signs.

The extent of epiphyseal involvement is related to the duration of the disease. In general, the greater the extent of epiphyseal involvement, the longer the duration and course of the disease. End results are worse with prolonged disease duration.

Age of disease onset is a significant factor in relation to outcome. The younger the patient at disease onset, the better is the prognosis. Eight years of age appears to be the watershed age in most long-term series. Age at healing, however, is probably a more important factor. Because of the overall skeletal maturation delay and the knowledge that this is usually compensated for during the adolescent growth spurt, patients affected at a younger age have an enhanced

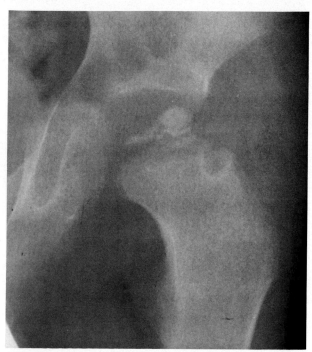

FIGURE 14-20. A 6-year, 5-month-old boy with Catterall group 4 disease and all the at-risk signs. (Weinstein SL. Legg-Calvé-Perthes disease. In: Morrissy RT, ed. Lovell and Winter's pediatric orthopaedics, vol 2. 1990:867)

potential for femoral head and acetabular remodeling. Femoral head at-risk signs are also less likely to occur in younger patients, particularly those younger than 5 years of age.

The development of the acetabulum depends on the geometric pattern within it during growth, and because the acetabulum continues to have significant development potential up to age 8 or 9 years of age, if a young patient does develop deformity, the immature acetabulum conforms to the altered femoral head shape. This leads to aspheric congruency, which may be compatible with normal function for many years.

The patient history, physical examination, and plain radiographs are usually sufficient to make a diagnosis of LCPD. Diagnosis early in the initial phase of the disease, however, must be differentiated from conditions such as transient synovitis (Table 14-2) and septic arthritis (primary or secondary to proximal femoral osteomyelitis). A complete blood count, including white blood cell differential, erythrocyte sedimentation rate, and hip joint aspiration, and analysis of the fluid may be necessary to rule out infection. All laboratory studies of LCPD are generally normal, although the erythrocyte sedimentation rate may be slightly elevated. In early cases, if all the laboratory studies are normal, and doubt as to the diagnosis persists, radionuclide scanning may be helpful.

In patients with bilateral hip involvement, generalized disorders, such as multiple epiphyseal dysplasia and hypothyroidism, must be considered. Patients with bilateral involvement, particularly those with atypical radiographic features, must have a careful family history obtained as well as a bone survey to rule out a metabolic or a genetic condition. In children younger than 4 years of age, Meyer dysplasia, a benign resolving condition, must be considered.

Most patients with LCPD (60%) do not need treatment. Treatment modalities have evolved from the earliest treatments of weight relief until the head was reossified to the present day containment methods. The essence of containment is that, to prevent deformities of the diseased epiphysis, the femoral head must be contained within the depths of the acetabulum to equalize the pressure on the head and subject it to the molding action of the acetabulum. Containment is an attempt to reduce the forces through the hip joint by establishing an actual or relative varus relation between the femoral head and the acetabulum. Considering all methods of containment, the physician must realize that the femoral head represents over three fourths of a sphere and the acetabulum only half of a sphere. Therefore, no method of containment can provide a totally contained femoral head within the acetabulum during all portions of the gait cycle.

The primary goals in the treatment of LCPD are to prevent deformity, alter growth disturbance, and prevent degenerative joint disease. To attain these goals, the patient must be assessed clinically and radiographically. Clinically, the patient is evaluated for at-risk signs of pain and loss of motion. AP and lateral radiographs are evaluated to determine the radiographic stage of the disease, the extent of epiphyseal involvement, and the presence of any at-risk signs. The optimal time for treatment is during the radiographic initial or fragmentation stage of the disease. Once the head is in the reossification stage, little further deformity occurs; thus, to influence deformity, treatment must initiated earlier. Some difficulties may be encountered in determining the extent of epiphyseal involvement, especially early in the disease process, and radionuclide scanning or MRI may be helpful.

Treatment is *not* indicated if the child demonstrates none of the clinical or radiographic at-risk signs, if the patients has Catterall group 1 disease (Salter-Thompson group A), or if the disease is already in the reossification stage. A child who demonstrates clinical or radiographic at-risk signs, regardless of the extent of epiphyseal involvement, should receive treatment. Even patients with Catterall group 2 disease who are at risk' may end up with a poor result without treatment.

TABLE 14-2.
Differential Diagnosis of Congenital Hip Dysplasia

Chondrolysis
Gaucher disease
Hemophilia
Hypothyroidism
Juvenile rheumatoid arthritis
Lymphoma
Mucopolysaccharridosis
Multiple epiphyseal dysplasia
Meyer dysplasia
Neoplasm
Old congenital hip dysplasia residuals
Osteomyelitis of proximal femur with secondary septic arthritis
Septic arthritis
Sickle cell disease
Spondyloepiphyseal dysplasia
Toxic synovitis
Traumatic aseptic necrosis

The first principle of treatment is restoration of motion. Motion enhances synovial nutrition and thus cartilage nutrition. Restoration of motion can be accomplished by putting the patient at rest with skin traction and progressive abduction to relieve the adductor spasm. Occasionally, surgical release of the contracted adductors may be necessary. Restoration of motion allows abduction of the hip, which reduces the force on the hip joint and allows positioning of the uncovered anterolateral aspect of the femoral head in the acetabulum (containment). Mobilization of the hip joint may also be obtained by use of progressive abduction casts. If containment treatment can be maintained, it appears to give superior results in severely involved patients (Catterall groups 3 and 4, or Salter-Thompson group B) compared with no treatment.

Arthrography is a useful adjunct in determining whether the head actually can be contained and, if so, in what position this is best accomplished. Arthrography demonstrates any flattening of the femoral head that may not be seen on plain film. More important, it may demonstrate the hinge abduction phenomenon, which is a contraindication to any type of containment treatment. Once the femoral head becomes deformed and is no longer containable within the acetabulum, the only motion that is allowed is in the flexion and extension plane, with abduction leading to hinging on the lateral edge of the acetabulum. This hinge abduction causes acetabular and secondary femoral head deformity (Fig. 14-21).

The three most commonly advocated methods of containment treatment are abduction bracing, femoral osteotomy, and innominate osteotomy. The most widely used abduction braces are modifications of the Atlanta-Scottish Rite orthosis (Fig. 14-22). These devices provide for containment solely by abduction of the hips without fixed internal rotation. Containment is provided for by the degree of abduction of the brace as well as the amount of hip flexion required to walk with the legs in abduction. Free motion is allowed in the knee and ankle. These

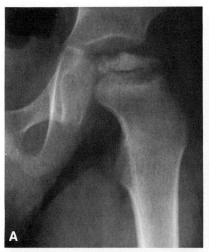
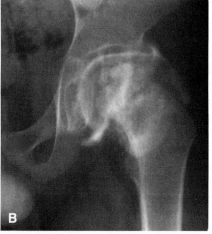
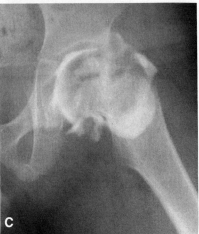

FIGURE 14-21. A 4-year, 9-month-old boy with Catterall group 4 disease and at-risk status. (A) Plain film. (B) Arthrogram in neutral abduction, adduction, and rotation. Note enlargement and flattening of the cartilaginous femoral head and how the lateral margin of the acetabulum is deformed by the femoral head. (C) Arthrogram in abduction and slight external rotation. Note how the femoral head hinges on the lateral edge of the acetabulum, further deforming the lateral acetabulum. Also note the slight pooling of dye medially. (Weinstein SL. Legg-Calvé-Perthes disease. In: Morrissy RT, ed. Lovell and Winter's pediatric orthopaedics, vol 2. 1990:872)

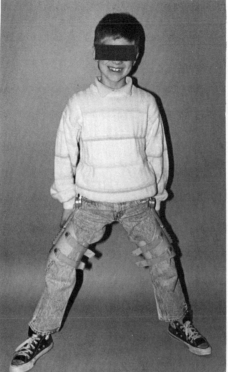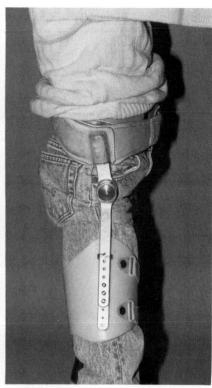

FIGURE 14-22. An abduction orthosis. (Weinstein SL. Legg-Calvé-Perthes disease. In: Morrissy RT, ed. Lovell and Winter's pediatric orthopaedics, vol 2. 1990:874)

devices are well tolerated by patients and less cumbersome than previously used braces. Early radiographic anatomic treatment results are comparable to previously used containment weight-bearing methods. The negative aspects of bracing include prolonged treatment times and the necessity of having a compliant patient. If an orthosis is used to treat LCPD, containment must be demonstrated in the brace on a radiograph in the weight-bearing position. The average time in a brace is 6 to 14 months, with the brace being discontinued once the head is in the reossification stage of the disease. Recent studies, however, question the efficacy of brace treatment in LCPD.

Surgical methods of providing and maintaining containment offer the advantage of early mobilization and avoidance of prolonged brace or cast treatment. Varus osteotomy with or without rotation offers the advantage of deep seating of the femoral head and positioning of the vulnerable anterolateral portion of the head away from the deforming influences of the acetabular margin (Fig. 14-23). It has been reported that this procedure improves disturbed venous drainage and relieves interosseous venous hypertension, thus accelerating the healing process. This, however, has not been conclusively confirmed. Prerequisites for the procedure include full range of mo-

tion, congruency between the head and the acetabulum, and the ability to seat the head in abduction and internal rotation. As with all containment treatment modalities, to have any effect, treatment must be instituted in the initial or fragmentation stage of the disease. The negative aspects of this treatment include the associated risks and costs of the surgical procedure in addition to a second surgical procedure necessary for any hardware removal. The affected limb is also shortened by the procedure. The varus angulation normally decreases with growth, but if there has been physeal plate damage by the disease, this remodeling potential may be lost, leaving the patient with a permanent varus deformity and limb shortening.

Innominate osteotomy provides for containment by redirection of the acetabular roof, providing better coverage for the anterolateral portion of the head. It places the head in relative flexion, abduction, and internal rotation with respect to the acetabulum in the weight-bearing position. Any shortening caused by the disease process is corrected. Prerequisites for innominate osteotomy include a full range of hip joint motion, joint congruency with the ability to seat the head in flexion, abduction, and internal rotation. The procedure must be done in the initial or fragmentation stage of the disease. The disadvantages of in-

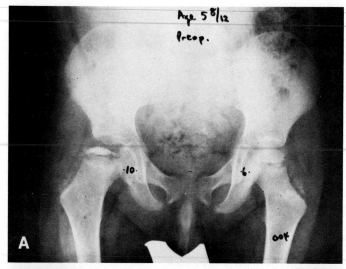

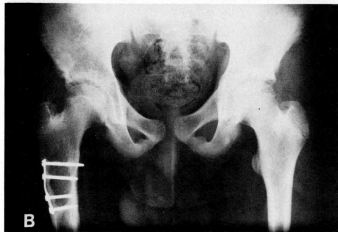

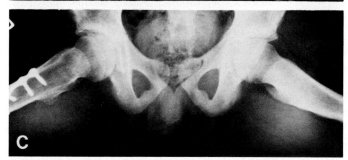

FIGURE 14-23. Varus/derotation osteotomy of Axer. This embodies the principle of containment of the diseased femoral head in the treatment of Legg-Calvé-Perthes disease, which is achieved by surgical means. Postoperatively, the child is permitted to walk with no restrictions, and the range of motion is full, so that the molding effect of the acetabulum on the femoral head is attained. (A) Severe involvement of femoral epiphysis in a boy 5 years and 8 months of age, 9 months after onset of limp and pain and in the left hip. (B and C) Ten years after varus/derotation osteotomy, excellent develolpment of the femoral head is seen. (Courtesy of Dr. A. Axer)

nominate osteotomy are the inherent risks of the surgical procedure, the fact that the operation is being performed on the normal side of the joint, and the suggestion that the procedure may increase the forces on the femoral head by lateralizing the acetabulum and increasing the lever arm of the abductors. Satisfactory anatomic results have been reported for all these containment methods in carefully selected patients.

Regardless of the method of containment treatment chosen, any episode indicative of loss of containment (ie, recurrent pain and loss of range of motion) must be treated aggressively by rest and traction or casting to restore lost motion.

For noncontainable hips, particularly those that demonstrate the hinge abduction phenomenon on arthrography, the physician must consider other alternatives. These salvage procedures include Chiari osteotomy, cheilectomy, abduction extension oste-otomy, and acetabular shelf procedures alone or in combination with femoral osteotomies. These procedures must be viewed as salvage procedures with the limited aims of pain relief, correction of limb length inequality, and improvement of movement and abductor weakness. Cheilectomy removes the anterolateral portion of the head that is impinging on the acetabulum in abduction. This procedure must only be done after the physis is closed; otherwise, a slipped capital femoral epiphysis (SCFE) may ensue. This procedure does not correct any residual short-ening or abductor weakness. The Chiari osteotomy improves the lateral coverage of the deformed fem-oral head but does not reduce the lateral impingement in abduction and may exacerbate any existing ab-ductor weakness. Its role in LCPD is yet to be defined. Abduction extension osteotomy of the femur is in-dicated when arthrography demonstrates joint con-gruency improved by the extended, adducted posi-tion. Preliminary results indicate improvement in limb length, decrease in limp, and improvement in function and range of motion.

Long-term series of patients with uniform treat-ment matched for age and degree of epiphyseal in-volvement are needed to determine the most effective treatment of LCPD. As our fundamental under-standing of LCPD increases, so too will our under-standing of how various treatment modalities influ-ence this complex growth disturbance.

TRANSIENT SYNOVITIS

Transient synovitis is the most common source of hip pain in the young child. This condition is often referred to in the literature by other terms, including *irritable hip, toxic synovitis, observation hip, coxitis serosa,* and *coxalgia fugax,* to name a few.

The cause of the condition is unknown. Because a high percentage of the children have a recent his-tory of an upper respiratory tract infection, a viral etiology has been suspected, as has an allergic re-action to an infectious agent. A history of trauma can sometimes be associated with symptom onset, but no causal relation has been established. Biopsy ma-terial from patients with transient synovitis dem-onstrates nonspecific inflammatory changes and sy-novial hypertrophy.

Transient synovitis is the most common cause of hip pain and limp in children under 10 years of age. Affected children range in age from 3 to 12 years,

with the average patient being between 5 and 6 years of age. Boys are affected two to three times as often as girls. Right and left hips are affected equally. Ninety-five percent of cases are unilateral.

Children with transient synovitis traditionally present with a history of hip pain or limp. The pain onset is acute in about half of cases, with symptoms being present for 1 to 3 days before presentation. In the other half of patients, the symptoms of limp or pain are more chronic in nature, often being present for weeks to months. The pain in most cases is mild, but in some children, it may be severe enough to awaken the child at night. In some cases, pain may not be admitted to by the patient. Pain when present is usually localized to the groin region but may be referred to the medial thigh or knee region. A careful medical history should be sought, looking for any history of antecedent infection, such as an upper re-spiratory infection, otitis media, strep throat, trauma, or other precipitating factors.

Physical examination is characterized by guarded rotation of the hip joint. Pain can usually be elicited at the extremes of motion, especially abduction and medial rotation. In some children, guarding may be evident by gently trying to roll the leg into internal rotation while the hip is extended. Patients may have evidence of thigh atrophy, depending on the duration of symptoms. There may also be tenderness to pal-pation in the groin. The gait of an affected child is usually antalgic. The child may walk with the hip in slight flexion, external rotation, and abduction.

The child may have a low-grade fever on pre-sentation. The sedimentation rate is usually normal but may be mildly elevated. The white blood cell count is generally normal with a normal differential.

Radiographs may demonstrate slightly widened joint space medially (Fig. 14-24). Bone density is nor-mal in all cases; if alteration in normal densities is present, another source of the hip pain should be sought. Loss of the hip capsular shadow outline has been reported in cases of toxic synovitis; this sign, however, is a radiologic artifact related to holding the hip in abduction and external rotation. Bone scanning may reveal normal or increased uptake in the proximal femoral epiphysis. Ultrasonography may demonstrate the presence of a mild effusion.

The differential diagnosis of this condition is im-portant in that certain of these conditions can have devastating consequences if not diagnosed. Septic arthritis must be ruled out. Children with septic ar-thritis generally present with pain, elevated temper-ature, elevated white blood cell count, and elevated

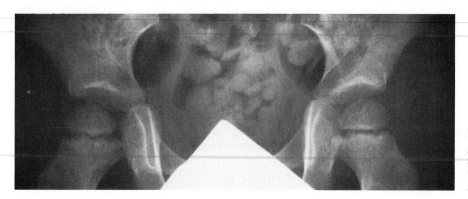

FIGURE 14-24. AP radiograph of a child with transient synovitis of the right hip. Note the slightly widened medial joint space in the right hip.

sedimentation rate. Septic arthritis of the hip may be accompanied by osteomyelitis of the proximal femur (see Chap. 4). Aspiration of the joint must be done when the diagnosis is uncertain. An arthrogram should be done at the same time as the aspiration to make sure that the hip joint has been entered. Rheumatic fever must also be excluded. The hip may be the first joint involved before the development of migratory polyarthralgia. These patients usually give a history of a β-hemolytic streptococcal infection 1 to 3 weeks before the onset of hip pain. Other major or minor manifestations of this disorder should be sought.

LCPD often presents in a similar manner. It occurs in the same age range as transient synovitis but has a slightly greater male predominance. Most LCPD patients have retardation of bone age. Bone scans in the early stages of LCPD may show decreased uptake in the femoral head. In the future, MRI scans may prove to be helpful to differentiate LCPD from transient synovitis. Many studies in the literature suggest that transient synovitis is a precursor to LCPD disease. The literature, however, suggests that in only 1% to 3% of cases of transient synovitis are associated with the later development of LPCD.

Juvenile rheumatoid arthritis, SCFE, and tumors, particularly osteoid osteoma of the proximal femur, must be included in the differential diagnosis of any child with hip pain. Osteoid osteoma usually is accompanied by a history of night pain relieved by aspirin. SCFE is usually seen in the obese adolescent during the growth spurt and has typical radiographic features.

Long-term follow-up studies of patients with transient synovitis reveal that many of the patients have secondary coxa magna and a widened femoral neck as a residual of the condition. The question of whether these patients will develop degenerative arthritis over the long-term remains to be answered.

Rest is the primary method of treatment for this condition. When the diagnosis is in question or the patient is particularly uncomfortable, hospitalization is often necessary. Light skin traction may be applied for comfort. Antiinflammatory agents may be used for a short time to relieve pain. As symptoms resolve, crutch-protected weight bearing may begin, with gradual resumption of full weight bearing as symptoms abate. Most patients have resolution of symptoms in 3 to 7 days, but in many patients, symptoms may persist for weeks to months. The condition is self-limiting; most children have only a single episode of hip pain, and recurrences are uncommon unless the child is returned to full activity before symptoms resolve.

DEVELOPMENTAL COXA VARA

The term *coxa vara* is a descriptive term referring to the angular relation between the femoral head or neck, or both, and the femoral shaft, which is less than the normal value for the patient's age. This abnormal relation may be congenital, developmental, or acquired. It is most important to distinguish between these three etiologic groups because each has its own natural history. This section deals only with developmental coxa vara.

Developmental coxa vara refers to defects localized to the cervical region of the proximal femur that are accompanied by a widened and vertically oriented physeal plate (Fig. 14-25). The shaft of the femur is normal. Clinical and radiographic features are not present at birth. Developmental coxa vara is an extremely rare condition equally affecting boys and girls. About 30% of the cases are bilateral. A familial tendency has been reported, but the exact mode of inheritance is unknown. The cause of developmental coxa vara is unknown, but many theories have been

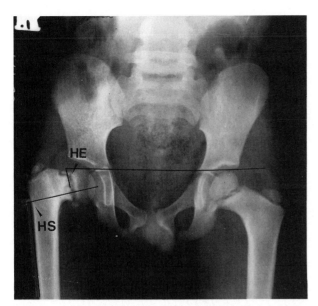

FIGURE 14-25. Coxa vara development. Note head–shaft angle (HS) and Hilgenreiner epiphyseal angle (HE).

postulated, including an embryonic vascular disturbance and regional dysplasia of the proximal femur.

Clinically, most patients present to the physician for a limb length inequality or abnormal gait. Although the gait abnormality may be evident when the child starts to walk, patients generally do not seek medical attention until the child is 3 to 7 years of age. The limp or waddling gait (in bilateral cases) is painless and usually progressive. Older children may complain of easy fatigability. Limb shortening is usually evident.

On physical examination, patients have short stature. Examination of the involved extremity reveals limited abduction and internal rotation, a positive Trendelenburg test, limb shortening, and trochanteric elevation. In bilateral cases, hyperlordosis of the lumbar spine is present, and the patient may have genu valgum. Limb length inequalities in developmental coxa vara rarely exceed 2 cm. In bilateral cases, the amount of shortening may be asymmetric.

The diagnosis can be made by an AP radiograph of the femurs and hips. The diagnosis is made by the presence of anatomic coxa vara, widened vertically oriented physeal plate, shortened neck, normal straight femoral shaft, and separate triangular ossification center on the inferior part of the femoral neck. This triangular ossification center may appear irregular and fragmented. A vertically oriented physeal plate borders the triangular fragment medially, while lateral to it is a vertical defect in the femoral neck. The femoral head is spherical and the acetabulum

generally normal, although mild dysplasia may be apparent in comparison to the opposite, normal side.

Various measurements have been made to quantify the relations in the proximal femur (see Fig. 14-25). These include the head–shaft angle, the neck–shaft angle, and the Hilgenreiner epiphyseal angle. The head–shaft angle has been found best to follow progression of deformity in that the neck–shaft angle remains fairly constant even in the face of progressive deformity. Most recently, the Hilgenreiner epiphyseal angle has been found to be a method of evaluation and prognostication for patients with developmental coxa vara.

Developmental coxa vara must be differentiated from congenital coxa vara and coxa vara acquired secondary to other conditions. Congenital coxa vara is detectable at birth and is accompanied by shortening of the proximal femur. Congenital coxa vara with a short femur is part of the spectrum of proximal femoral focal deficiency. The varus in this condition is generally in the subtrochanteric region or in the upper femur, and varying degrees of femoral shortening are seen. The head is abnormal in appearance, and acetabular dysplasia is generally present. The varus relation in this condition generally does not worsen with time and in general need not be addressed. Anatomic coxa vara can also be seen in patients with metabolic bone disease such as rickets, fibrous dysplasia, osteogenesis imperfecta, Ollier disease, SCFE, and sepsis. A radiographic appearance similar to developmental coxa vara is seen in patients with coxa vara secondary to metaphyseal chondrodysplasia and in patients with coxa vara and cleidocranial dysostosis. Coxa vara associated with cleidocranial dysostosis is usually present at birth, and patients have clavicular abnormalities, wormian bones, and abnormal dentition. In metaphyseal chondrodysplasia, there is generalized widening of the physeal plates. The hip radiographic abnormalities are bilateral and symmetric, and the femoral shafts are bowed. In bilateral cases of developmental coxa vara, the deformity may not be symmetric.

The goals of treatment in developmental coxa vara are to promote ossification of the defect and correct the varus deformity, allowing restoration of the mechanical advantage of the hip abductors to improve gait and to equalize limb lengths. In progressive coxa vara, the natural history suggests that there is increasing deformity (Fig. 14-26), decreasing function, and early degenerative joint disease. The general indications for surgical treatment include increasing coxa vara and a neck–shaft angle of less than 100 degrees. In mild, nonprogressive cases with

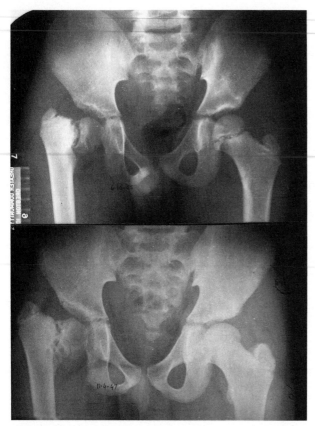

FIGURE 14-26. Coxa vara development. Note triangular fragment and worsening of condition over a 2-year period (*bottom*).

a neck–shaft angle of greater than 100 degrees and a Hilgenreiner epiphyseal angle of less than 45 degrees, resolution of the defect may occur, and observation of the patient with serial follow-up radiographs is indicated. In patients with a limp, progressive deformity, and a Hilgenreiner epiphyseal angle of greater than 60 degrees, intertrochanteric or subtrochanteric abduction osteotomy is the treatment of choice (Fig. 14-27). In these patients, the neck–shaft angle should be restored to decrease the shear stress across the vertical defect. With surgery, the defect generally heals, but growth plate arrest may be seen in a significant number of patients, leading to limb length inequality. Generally, patients older than 5 years of age at the time of surgery maintain their correction.

SLIPPED CAPITAL FEMORAL EPIPHYSIS

Slipped capital femoral epiphysis is a disorder in which there is a displacement of the capital femoral epiphysis from the metaphysis through the physeal plate (Fig. 14-28). The term *slipped capital femoral epiphysis* is actually a misnomer in that the head is held in the acetabulum by the ligamentum teres, and thus it is actually the neck that comes upward and outward while the head remains posterior and

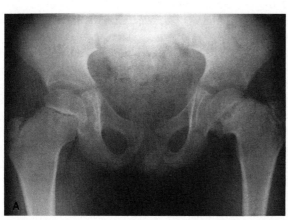

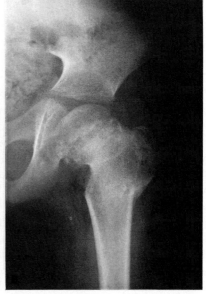

FIGURE 14-27. (**A**) Eight-year-old boy with coxa vara. (**B**) Eighteen months after abduction osteotomy.

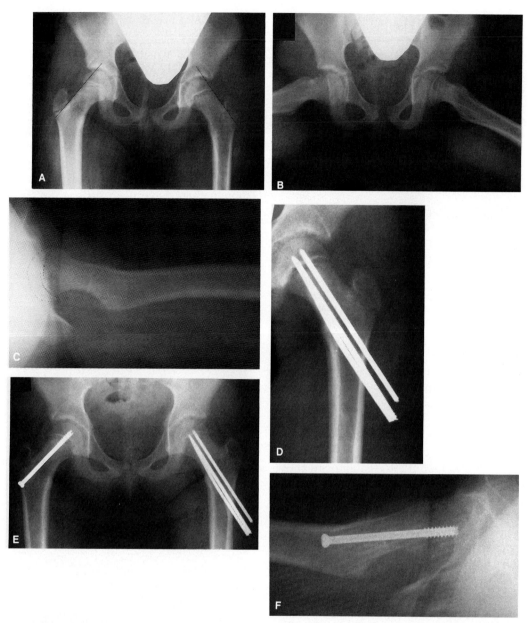

FIGURE 14-28. Ten-year-old girl with left hip pain for 3 months. (**A**) AP radiograph of pelvis. Note the Klein line. It should normally intersect at least 20% of the femoral head. (**B**) Lauenstein view demonstrates mild slip on left side. (**C**) True lateral view of left hip demonstrating mild slip. (**D**) The slip was treated with multiple threaded pins. (**E**) One year later, the patient complained of pain in the right groin and had a minimal slip. The right-sided slip was treated with a single screw (AP view). (**F**) Lateral view of postoperative pinning. Note central position of screw in epiphysis.

downward in the acetabulum (Fig. 14-29). In most cases, a varus relation exists between the head and neck, but occasionally the slip is into valgus, with the head displaced superiorly and posteriorly in relation to the neck.

The overall incidence of SCFE in the general population is about 2 cases per 100,000. The inci-

dence of SCFE is higher in blacks, particularly black girls. The disorder generally occurs in the age range of 10 to 14 years in girls (mean, 11.5 years) and 10 to 16 years in boys (mean, 13.5 years). Seventy percent of affected patients have delayed skeletal maturation. Skeletal age may lag behind chronologic age by as much as 20 months. There is a male predom-

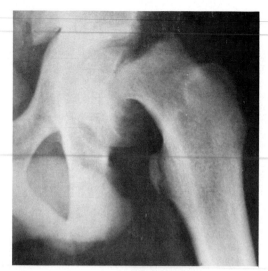

FIGURE 14-29. Complete slipped upper femoral epiphysis. Commonly termed *acute slipped epiphysis*, in reality, it is a form of fracture displacement that can also occur at other epiphyseal sites.

inance of 2.5:1. The left hip is twice as often affected as the right hip. Other epidemiologic factors may include seasonal variations and social class.

Affected patients have a tendency toward obesity. Almost half of affected patients are above the 95th percentile in weight for their age. Three fourths of affected boys and half of affected girls are above the 90th percentile in weight for their height. It has been disproved that tall thin people are predisposed to this condition.

The incidence of bilateralness of SCFE is generally accepted as being 25%. This figure may be low in that about half of bilateral slips are asymptomatic. This factor becomes important when considering the natural history of the disease.

Pathologically, the synovium from patients with SCFE generally exhibits changes characteristic of synovitis, with hypertrophy and hyperplasia of the synovial cells, villus formation, increased vascularity, and round cell infiltration. Light microscopic studies reveal that the physis is widened and irregular, sometimes reaching 12 mm in width (normal is 2.6 to 6 mm). Normally, the resting zone accounts for 60% to 70% of the width of the physis, whereas the hypertrophic zone accounts for only 15% to 30% of the width. In SCFE, the hypertrophic zone may constitute up to 80% of the physis width. Light microscopic studies also document that the actual slip takes place through the zone of hypertrophy, with occasional extension into the calcifying cartilage (Fig. 14-30). On the basis of histologic studies, it is apparent that the slip occurs through the weakest structural area of the plate, the hypertrophic zone.

The etiology of SCFE is unknown. All etiologic agents probably act either by altering the strength of the zone of hypertrophy or by affecting the shear stress to which the plate is exposed. Although trauma may be a contributing factor, it is certainly not the sole etiology; we know that the pathology of SCFE differs from that seen in physeal fractures.

Hormonal and endocrine abnormalities have long been implicated in the etiology of SCFE. Although there have been no specific endocrine abnormalities detected in patients with SCFE, there are numerous reports of SCFE associated with specific endocrine abnormalities, such as primary hypothyroidism, hypothyroidism secondary to panhypopituitarism, intracranial tumors, hypogonadism, treatment with chorionic gonadotropin, and treatment of hypothyroidism and growth hormone deficiency with growth hormone. SCFE has also been reported in

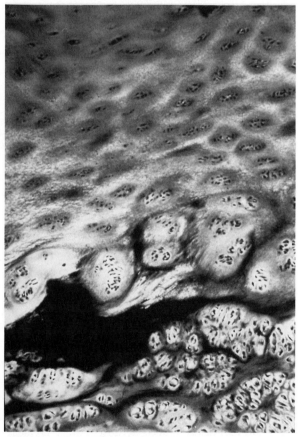

FIGURE 14-30. Physeal plate from a patient with slipped capital femoral epiphysis. Note slip (cleft) in zone of hypertrophy. Also note the abnormal architecture of the physeal plate. The zone of hypertrophy is increased in width, and the cells are in clusters and clumps.

patients undergoing radiation to the pelvis, patients with rickets, and patients with renal osteodystrophy.

Experimentally, the administration of growth hormone in castrated rats leads to increased thickness of the zone of hypertrophy and decreased shear strength. Estrogen, on the other hand, given to otherwise normal rats, leads to thinning of the growth plate and increased shear strength in similar experiments (Fig. 14-31).

Hormonal factors have been repudiated to contribute to the slippage because 78% of slips occur during the adolescent growth spurt, and in girls, slips occur before menarche. Hormonal theories have been used to account for many of the epidemiologic factors. For example, the age range of occurrence corresponds to the adolescent growth spurt for boys and girls. The gender prevalence of boys may be accounted for by boys having a longer and more rapid growth spurt. The high percentage of obesity (adiposogenital syndrome patients) has been attributed to an abnormal relation between growth hormone and sex hormone, giving a relative predominance to the growth effect. Thus, hormonal imbalance may lead to a structural weakening of the growth plate, leaving it more susceptible to slipping.

Other etiologic theories include SCFE being a localized manifestation of a generalized systemic disorder, secondary to a biochemical abnormality in cartilage collagen production or secondary to a mechanical disturbance caused by shear forces applied to a retroverted proximal femoral epiphysis. Genetic factors may contribute but have thus far not been identified. SCFE is probably a multifactorial disorder, with the slip representing the final manifestation of one of several predisposing factors.

On the basis of the patient's history, physical examination, and radiographs, SCFE can be classified into four categories—preslip, acute, acute on chronic, and chronic.

In the preslip phase, patients complain initially of weakness in the leg or limping on exertion; pain may occur in the groin, adductor region, or knee with prolonged standing or walking. On physical examination in this phase, the most consistent positive finding is lack of medial rotation of the hip in extension. When the affected leg is fixed, the thigh goes into abduction and external rotation, a sign pathopneumonic for SCFE. Radiographically, there is generalized bone atrophy and disuse osteopenia of the hemipelvis and upper femur only in those pa-

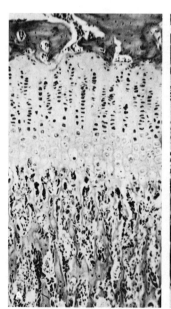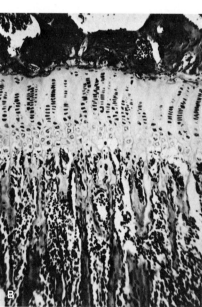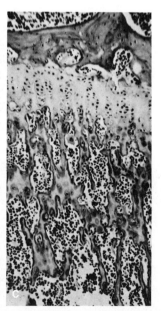

FIGURE 14-31. Effect of growth and sex hormone on the epiphyseal plate. (**A**) Growth hormone treated. The plate is thickened mainly by marked proliferation and accumulation of maturing chondrocytes. The layer of hypertrophied chondrocytes is fragile because it is deficient in matrix. (**B**) Untreated control. The layer of maturing chondrocytes is narrow and contributes little to the thickness of the plate. (**C**) Treated with sex hormones. The entire plate is narrow, the chondrocytes lack the orderly columnar arrangement, mature cartilage cells are rare, and bony trabeculae are numerous and thick. Epiphyseal separation is unlikely. (Harris WR. The endocrine basis for slipping of the upper femoral epiphysis. J Bone Joint Surg 1950;32B:5)

tients who limped or limited their activity. There is widening, irregularity, and blurring to the physeal plate (Fig. 14-32). The preslip may in actuality be a minimal slip that is not seen on standard radiograph but may possibly be seen on CT or MRI scans.

An acute slip is the "abrupt displacement through the proximal epiphyseal cartilage plate in which there was a preexisting epiphysiolysis." Acute slips account for about 10% of the slips in most large reported series (see Fig. 14-29). The clinical criterion of having the acute onset of symptoms for less than 2 weeks is generally accepted as the clinical definition of an acute slip. A review of the literature, however, reveals that 76% of patients with acute slips give a history of mild prodromal symptoms for 1 to 3 months before their acute episode, thus indicating that they probably had a preslip or mild slip preceding their acute symptom onset. These prodromal symptoms of mild weakness, limp, and intermittent groin, medial thigh, or knee pain are usually followed by some history of minor trauma or of direct trauma, with immediate increase in pain and inability to use the extremity. The pain is usually severe enough to prevent weight bearing. If the patient can walk, it is with difficulty and with a limp. SCFE in the patient with a history of mild prodromal symptoms may better be classified as an acute-on-chronic slip.

If the patient with an acute SCFE can walk, it is with an antalgic gait. These patients have an external rotation deformity, shortening, and marked limitation of motion. Any attempted motion is painful because of the marked spasm of the hip muscles. In general, the greater the amount of slip, the greater is the restriction of motion. The physical examination must be performed gently so as not to cause further dis-

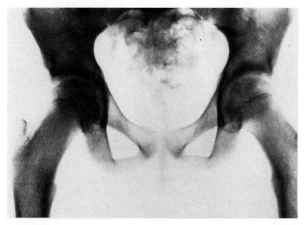

FIGURE 14-32. Before slip. Note widened, irregular, and blurry physeal plate on left hip. Left hemipelvis is relatively osteopenic.

placement. In the acute slip, because of pain, the physician may not be able to elicit the classic sign of SCFE (thigh abduction and external rotation as the thigh is flexed). There is generally thigh or calf atrophy present, except in those few patients without any prior symptoms.

Patients with chronic SCFE generally have a history of groin or medial thigh pain for months to years. A high percentage have knee or lower medial thigh pain as their initial symptom. They may give a history of exacerbations and remissions of the pain or limp. On physical examination, all these patients have limitation of motion (particularly medial rotation) and shortening, and most have thigh or calf atrophy.

Radiographs must be taken in two planes: AP and true lateral. Because of the unstable nature of the hip, the frog-leg lateral view may accentuate the deformity in the acute or acute-on-chronic slip.

The diagnosis of SCFE can be made on the AP radiograph by drawing a line along the superior basal margin of the neck. Normally, it should transect 20% or more of the epiphyses (see Fig. 14-28). Widening and irregularity of the physeal growth plate and decreased height of the epiphyses in the central acetabulum are also seen, and the medial junction of the epiphyses and the metaphyses fall outside the acetabulum. The lateral view is probably the best to detect the slip because the head is posterior in relation to the neck at first and thus may be missed on the AP view. In minimal slips, the displacement is initially posterior and may only be seen on the lateral radiograph.

In the acute slip, there is no radiographic evidence of healing or of remodeling, and the contour of the neck is sharply demarcated (see Fig. 14-29). In the acute-on-chronic SCFE or in the chronic SCFE, there may be evidence of healing and remodeling along the femoral neck.

Radiographically, slips may be classified by the maximal anatomic displacement either on the AP or lateral radiograph. One classification is as follows:

Preslip: normal relation of the epiphyses to the shaft, but the physis is widened and slightly irregular

Minimal slip: maximal displacement is less than one third the diameter of the neck

Moderate slip: greater than 1 cm of displacement but less than half the diameter of the neck

Severe slip: displacement greater than half the diameter of the neck

CT and MRI scans have been done to demonstrate predisposing factors such as retroversion or a widened physeal plate in the radiographically normal hip to try and predict a propensity to slip. The role of these modalities must await further investigation.

Review of the literature on natural history is at best controversial. There are few long-term studies of patients with SCFE, and included in these are few untreated patients.

In large series of patients with degenerative joint disease, the percentage of patients with known SCFE is small, averaging about 5%. The actual incidence may be higher because controversy exists about whether a higher percentage of patients with so-called primary degenerative arthritis had unrecognized slips or whether these radiographic features are merely secondary to primary degenerative joint disease.

The amount of deformity appears to be related to long-term prognosis, with degenerative joint disease and function being related to the severity of deformity. Those with moderate slips retain good function for many years, whereas those with severe slips have early degenerative joint disease and poor function. Poor results are occasionally seen even in minimal slips, usually as a result of a complication of treatment. The radiographic changes, however, do not always correlate with clinical symptoms over time.

Specific goals in the treatment of SCFE are to prevent further displacement of the epiphysis and to promote closure of the physeal plate. Treatment of SCFE should be considered an emergency. Once the diagnosis is made, the patient should not be allowed to bear weight. Treatment should be initiated immediately. Delay in treatment may result in further displacement of the femoral epiphysis with compromise of the remaining intact blood supply to the epiphysis. Further displacement also leads to increasing deformity and secondary increased risk of degenerative joint disease over time. Long-term goals of treatment include restoration of a functional range of motion, freedom from pain, and avoidance of aseptic necrosis and chondrolysis. Treatment considerations are based on the clinical classification (preslip, acute, acute on chronic, chronic) and the radiographic classification (mild, moderate, severe).

General principles of treatment of SCFE include reduction of acute slips and the acute component of acute-on-chronic slips followed by stabilization of the epiphysis. Chronic slips and the chronic component of acute-on-chronic slips should never be reduced but only stabilized. Any attempt at reduction of chronic components runs the risk of aseptic necrosis (the most common cause of a poor result) and long-term disability.

In acute slips, aseptic necrosis may occur with the sudden acute displacement of the epiphysis by interruption of blood supply to the capital femoral epiphysis. Reduction attempts of the slip must be gentle. Reduction can be obtained safely by the use of traction. Traction can be either by skin or skeletal methods. Because of the large size of these patients, skeletal traction is preferred. Traction is applied through a distal femoral pin placed just proximal to the distal femoral physeal plate. Longitudinal traction is applied as well as traction to the lateral extension of the traction pin so that an internal rotation moment to the traction can be applied. The acute component can usually be reduced within 24 hours.

Skin traction methods (Buck, Russell, split Russell, and so forth) also employ an internal rotation moment by the use of an internal rotation strap applied to the thigh. Manipulative reduction carries an increased risk of aseptic necrosis, especially by the overreduction of the displacement, and is therefore not recommended.

Stabilization of the acute slip can be accomplished by either epiphysis pinning or epiphysiodesis. The most widely used method of stabilization is pinning with multiple large threaded pins or bone screws (see Fig. 14-28). These techniques require the use of image intensification in the operating room. Radiographic control intraoperatively must include the ability to obtain images at 90 degrees to each other to minimize the risk of pin penetration, which is thought to be associated with chondrolysis. The fixation device must enter the epiphysis perpendicular to the physeal plate of the femoral head. The fixation device must cross the physis into the head but must be well short of the subchondral cortex. The pins or screws should be in the center of the epiphysis on the AP and lateral views of the hip (see Fig. 14-28). Pins should also avoid the superior quadrant of the femoral head to avoid the lateral epiphyseal vessels. Pins in this quadrant are associated with a higher incidence of aseptic necrosis.

Postoperatively, patients are kept to light weight bearing until they are pain free and have a comfortable range of motion. Rapid advance to full weight bearing may then begin.

All patients must be followed closely until the physeal plate closes. Loss of range of motion after treatment may be the first sign of chondrolysis. Pain in the other hip (groin, medial thigh, or knee) warrants careful investigation. Most bilateral slips are diagnosed within 1 year of the diagnosis of the initial slip. A bursitis occasionally develops over the extension of pins protruding beyond the femoral cortex.

This should be treated symptomatically until the physeal plate closes. Removal of pins or screws before physeal closure may allow for further epiphyseal displacement and complications. It is generally recommended that pins or screws be removed once the physeal plate is closed.

Although less widely used, epiphysiodesis, usually by open curettage of the physeal plate and bone grafting, is an alternative method of stabilization. Epiphysiodesis offers the advantages of providing added vascular channels between the metaphysis and the epiphysis, rapid fusion of the physeal plate (2 to 3 months), and avoidance of a second operation for hardware removal. The disadvantages of this technique are increased surgical time and blood loss and the need for postoperative casting for up to 3 months. Continued slipping may occur if the bone graft fails or the physis fails to close.

Chronic slips should not have attempts at reduction but should be treated by stabilization procedures primarily regardless of their degree of displacement. Long-term results of mild and moderate slips are generally good concerning function and range of motion. A certain amount of remodeling of the proximal femur can be expected.

Severe slips can also be treated by stabilization procedures primarily. Debate exists about whether these slips should be treated by realignment procedures in addition to stabilization to improve joint kinematics and hence long-term outcome. Long-term follow-up studies indicate that the greatest risk to the long-term outcome of patients with SCFE is the development of aseptic necrosis or chondrolysis, not malalignment. The use of realignment procedures (neck, intertrochanteric, or subtrochanteric osteotomy or manipulative reductions in chronic slips) is associated with significantly higher complication rates than either pinning in situ or epiphysiodesis alone. Realignment procedures should therefore be reserved for those situations in which restricted range of motion impairs function after plate physeal closure.

Aseptic necrosis is the most devastating complication of SCFE. It is most commonly associated, with acute slips with the abrupt displacement of the epiphysis disrupting retinacular vessels. In chronic slips, aseptic necrosis can occur as a result of treatment. As mentioned previously, attempts at reduction of chronic slips, overreduction of acute slips, improper pin placement, and femoral neck osteotomies are associated with this complication.

Chondrolysis or cartilage necrosis is often associated with SCFE. Chondrolysis is manifest clinically by loss of range of motion, pain, limp, and joint con-

tracture. Radiographically, the condition is manifest by loss of joint space, irregularity of the subchondral bone of the femoral head and the acetabulum, and disuse osteopenia. It can occur in untreated slips, but this is unusual (it can also occur as an isolated disorder). The cause of this condition remains unknown, but it is associated with prolonged immobilization, unrecognized pin penetration, severe slips, and a long duration of symptoms before treatment. Whether the condition represents an autoimmune phenomenon or other source of interference with cartilage nutrition remains to be proved. Treatment of chondrolysis is difficult. Symptomatic treatment should begin immediately and should include antiinflammatory agents and bed rest in skeletal traction to relieve pain and contractures. The role of continuous passive motion with or without a surgical capsulectomy is yet to be defined.

The key to the management of SCFE is prompt diagnosis and management by accepted techniques that have a high rate of success with minimal risk of complications.

Annotated Bibliography

Congenital Hip Dysplasia and Dislocation

Coleman SS. Congenital dysplasia and dislocation of the hip. St Louis, CV Mosby, 1978.
This is a superb monograph on CHD that deals with all aspects of this condition.

Hensinger RN. Congenital dislocation of the hip: treatment in infancy to walking age. Orthop Clin North Am 1987;18:597.
This review article on the fundamentals of diagnosis and management of CDH is primarily concerned with management in the first 12 to 18 months of life.

Mubarak SJ, Garfin S, Vance R, McKinnon B, Sutherland D. Pitfalls in the use of the Pavlik harness for treatment of congenital dysplasia, subluxation and dislocation of the hip. J Bone Joint Surg 1981;63A:1239.
The authors review 18 cases of failure of management of CDH with the Pavlik harness. They describe the pitfalls in the use of the most common device employed in the management of CDH. The appropriate protocol for use of the Pavlik harness is described.

Ponseti IV. Growth and development of the acetabulum in the normal child: anatomical, histological and roentgenographic studies. J Bone Joint Surg 1978;60A:575.
This classic article deals with normal acetabular development based on anatomic, histologic, and radiologic evaluation of the normal hip. Information in this article is essential to the management of CDH.

Ponseti IV. Morphology of the acetabulum in congenital dislocation of the hip: gross, histological and roentgenographic studies. J Bone Joint Surg 1978;60A:586.
The author describes acetabular development in CDH in contrast to previous studies of normal development. Alteration in ossification of acetabulum is described in late, reduced CDH by the development of accessory ossification centers. The pathology of the "neolimbus" is described.

Tachdjian MD. Congenital dislocation of the hip. New York, Churchill Livingstone, 1982.
This is a compilation of articles by experts in the field on all aspects of CDH. It is an excellent reference text with an extensive bibliography.

Weinstein SL. Natural history of congenital hip dislocation (CDH) and hip dysplasia. Clin Orthop 1987;225:62.
This is a review article on normal growth and development of the hip joint, epidemiology and causes of the condition, and natural history in the newborn and the untreated adult. It includes an extensive bibliography.

Legg-Calvé-Perthes Disease

Catterall A. The natural history of Perthes disease. J Bone Joint Surg 1971;53B:37.
This classic article describes the radiographic extent of epiphyseal involvement and prognosis based on natural history in a large group of untreated patients.

Catterall A. Legg-Calvé-Perthes disease: current problems in orthopaedics. New York, Churchill Livingstone, 1982.
This is a superb monograph on the subject by the leading authority. The author addresses all aspects of the disease. The monograph is beautifully illustrated and well referenced.

Martinez AG, Weinstein SL, Dietz FR. The weight-bearing abduction brace for the treatment of Legg-Perthes disease. J Bone Joint Surg 1992;74A:12.
This study reviewed 31 patients, with 34 hips, who had severe Legg-Perthes disease (5 hips with Catterall group 3 disease and 29 hips with Catterall group 4 disease). These patients were treated with weight-bearing abduction orthoses. The mean duration of follow-up was 7 years. The authors concluded that, although containment is the most widely accepted principle of treatment for patients who have Legg-Perthes disease, and the Atlanta-Scottish Rite orthosis is the most commonly used orthosis for this condition, there are few clinical data supporting the effectiveness of this device. On the basis of the results of their studies, the authors did not recommend the use of a weight-bearing abduction brace for the treatment of severely involved hips. These results were also confirmed by another study in the same issue of the journal from the Atlanta-Scottish Rite Hospital.

McAndrew MP, Weinstein SL. A long term follow-up of Legg Calvé Perthes disease. J Bone Joint Surg 1984;66A:860.
The authors describe a longitudinal 48-year average follow-up of a group of patients with Perthes disease. Marked deterioration of function was seen between 36 and 48 years of follow-up. By an average age of 56 years, 40% of patients had undergone arthroplasty, and an additional 10% had disabling osteoarthritis.

Salter RB. The present status of surgical treatment for Legg Perthes disease. J Bone Joint Surg 1984;66A:961.
The is an excellent review article on the pathology and pathogenesis of the disease and the principles of containment. The author outlines containment treatment methods and highlights indications and results of surgical containment. A discussion of late treatment to correct existing deformity is provided.

Salter RB, Thompson GH. The prognostic significance of the subchondral fracture and a two group classification of the femoral head involvement. J Bone Joint Surg 1984;66A:479.
The authors introduce a two-group classification based on the extent of epiphyseal involvement. Group A has less than 50% femoral head involvement; group B has greater than 50% femoral head involvement. The significance of subchondral fracture is presented.

Stulberg SD, Cooperman DR, Wallenstein R. The natural history of Legg Calvé Perthes disease. J Bone Joint Surg 1981;63A:1095.
This article describe a long-term follow-up study of a large number of patients from three hospitals. The authors describe five radio-graphic classes of deformity at maturity and discuss the long-term prognosis of each class.

Weinstein SL. Legg-Calvé-Perthes disease. In: Morrissy RM, ed. Lovell and Winter's pediatric orthopaedics. Philadelphia, JB Lippincott, 1990:851.
This textbook chapter covers all aspects of Legg-Calvé-Perthes disease in detail and has an extensive bibliography.

Transient Synovitis

De Valderrama JAF. The "observation hip" syndrome and its late sequela. J Bone Joint Surg 1965;45B:462.
This article describes a follow-up study of 23 patients with an average 21-year follow-up (range, 15 to 30 years). Twelve patients had evidence of coxa magna, osteoarthritis, and widening of the femoral neck. The author discusses possible mechanisms for causation of coxa magna.

Haveisen DC, Weiner DS, Weiner SD. The characterization of treatment synovitis of the hip in children. J Pediatr Orthop 1986;6:11.
This is an excellent, well-referenced review of the topic and includes a 30-year retrospective review of 497 cases. The authors report a detailed radiographic and clinical follow-up of 147 cases.

Nachemson A, Scheller S. A clinical and radiological follow-up study of transient synovitis of the hip. Acta Orthop Scand 1969;40:479.
The study described is a 20- or 22-year follow-up of 73 cases of transient synovitis. Of the original pool, 6% (102 patients) subsequently developed Perthes disease. There was a statistically significant difference in the incidence of coxa magna, cysts, and radiodensity in the femoral heads of affected patients, but these were of no clinical significance. The paper documents the benign natural history of this condition.

Sharwood PF. The irritable hip syndrome in children: a long term follow-up. Acta Orthop Scand 1981;52:633.
The author reviews 101 children with irritable hip syndrome who were followed an average of 8.2 years (range, 5 to 15 years). Most patients had prompt resolution of symptoms (within 16 days). Only one subsequent case of Perthes disease and one of coxa magna were seen, both in patients who had prolonged symptoms and radiologic abnormalities on presentation.

Wingstrand H, Egund N, Carlin NO, Forsberg L, Gustafson T, Sunden G. Intracapsular pressure in transient synovitis of the hip. Acta Orthop Scand 1985;56:204.
The authors evaluated 14 patients with sonography, scintigraphy, and intracapsular pressure recording and aspiration. They found an effusion in all cases and increased intracapsular pressure with the hip in extension. The authors recommended treatment with rest with the hip joint in about 45-degree flexion to reduce intracapsular pressure and decrease the risk of ischemia to the femoral head from vascular tamponade.

Developmental Coxa Vara

Amstutz HC. Developmental (infantile) coxa vara: a distinct entity—report of 2 patients with a previously normal roentgenograms. Clin Orthop 1970;72:242.
The author distinguishes between developmental coxa vara and proximal femoral focal deficiency. Two patients are reported who had normal hip radiographs obtained incidentally during the first year of life and later developed developmental coxa vara. The author further refines a classification previously presented.

Amstutz HC, Wilson PD Jr. Dysgenesis of the proximal femur (coxa vara) and its surgical management. J Bone Joint Surg 1962;44A:1.
This classic article includes classification of coxa vara into the categories of congenital and acquired. The authors discuss in detail

the general characteristics and treatment of patients with congenital short femur with coxa vara, congenital bowed femur with coxa vara, and congenital coxa vara.

Schmidt TL, Kalamchi A. The fate of the capital femoral physis and acetabular development in developmental coxa vara. J Pediatr Orthop 1982;2:534.
A retrospective review of 22 hips in 15 children with developmental coxa vara. The authors found that acetabular depth did not improve if the neck–shaft angle was not corrected to at least 140 degrees. Premature physeal plate closure was a frequent sequelae (89%) of valgus osteotomy, leading to relatively greater trochanteric overgrowth and the development of limb length inequality.

Weinstein JN, Kuo KN, Millar EA. Congenital coxa vara: A retrospective review. J Pediatr Orthop 1984;4:70.
This article describes a retrospective long-term review of 22 cases of congenital coxa vara. This study presents the Hilgenreiner epiphyseal angle and the natural history and surgical indications based on this angle.

Slipped Capital Femoral Epiphysis

Canale ST. Problems and complications of slipped capital femoral epiphysis. AAOS Instruct Course Lect Ser 1989;38::281.

Crawford AH. The role of osteotomy in the treatment of slipped capital femoral epiphysis. AAOS Instruct Course Lect Ser 1989;38::273.

Morrissy RT. Principles of in situ fixation in chronic slipped capital femoral epiphysis: instructional course on slipped capital femoral epiphysis. AAOS Instruct Course Lect Ser 1989;38:257.

Weiner DS. Bone graft epiphysiodesis in the treatment of slipped capital femoral epiphysis. AAOS Instruct Course Lect Ser 1989;38::263.
These are excellent, well-referenced review articles on the management and complications of management of SCFE.

Carney BT, Weinstein SL, Noble J. Long term follow up of slipped capital femoral epiphysis. J Bone Joint Surg 1991;73A:667.
This article describes a long-term follow-up study of 155 hips in 124 patients, with a mean follow-up of 41 years after onset of symptoms. The authors determined that the natural history of the malunited slip is mild deterioration related to the severity of the slip and complications. Techniques of realignment are associated with a risk of appreciable complications and adversely affect the natural history of the disease. Regardless of the severity of the slip, pinning in situ provides the best long-term function and delay of degenerative arthritis, with a low risk of complications.

Walters R, Simon SR. Joint destruction: A sequel of unrecognized pin penetration in patients with slipped capital femoral epiphysis. In: The hip: proceedings of the Eighth Open Scientific Meeting of the Hip Society. St Louis, CV Mosby, 1980:145.
Evidence is presented implicating unrecognized pin penetration as a cause of chondrolysis after pinning of a slip. The authors demonstrated the blind spot afforded by right-angle radiographs that allows for pin penetration to occur yet be unrecognized radiographically.

Weinstein SL. Background on slipped capital femoral epiphysis. AAOS Instruct Course Lect Ser 1984;33:310.
This review article covers the epidemiology, causes, pathology, clinical features, and natural history of SCFE and includes an extensive bibliography.

Turek's Orthopaedics: Principles and Their Application, Fifth Edition,
edited by Stuart L. Weinstein and Joseph A. Buckwalter.
J.B. Lippincott Company, Philadelphia, © 1994.

15

Mark A. Mehlhoff

The Adult Hip

EMBRYOLOGY
VASCULAR SUPPLY
SURGICAL APPROACHES
　Anterior Approach
　Anterolateral and Direct Lateral
　　Approaches
　Posterior Approach
BIOMECHANICS
EXAMINATION OF THE
　PATIENT WITH HIP PAIN
　History
　Physical Examination
　Radiographic Evaluation

DISEASES OF THE HIP
　Osteoarthritis
　Rheumatoid Arthritis
　Avascular Necrosis
　Paget Disease
TREATMENT OF HIP DISEASES
　Osteotomy
　Hip Arthrodesis
　Total-Hip Arthroplasty
　Revision Total-Hip Arthroplasty

The deep stable ball-and-socket configuration of the hip joint allows considerable range of motion. The adult proximal femur is composed of the greater and lesser trochanters, the femoral neck, and a nearly spherical femoral head that articulates with a horseshoe-shaped acetabulum. The acetabulum has deepened articular anterior, posterior, and superior walls that surround the nonarticular acetabular fossa that contain the ligamentum teres, branches of the obturator artery, and fat. The fibrocartilaginous acetabular labrum encircles the outer edge of the femoral head, attaching at the periphery of the acetabulum and inferiorly attaching to the transverse acetabular ligament at the base of the acetabular fossa. The joint capsule envelops the hip joint, attaching to the bony pelvis on the acetabular side and on the femoral side, attaching anteriorly along the intertrochanteric line and posteriorly 1.5 cm proximal to the intertrochanteric line. The anterior joint capsule thickens to form the iliofemoral ligament or the ligament of Bigelow. Slightly hyperextending the hip moves the force of body weight posterior to the hip joint, tightening the ligament of Bigelow, stabilizing the hip joint, and allowing the gluteus maximus to relax its antigravity function.

EMBRYOLOGY

The elements of the hip differentiate in situ from the lower limb bud mesenchyme at the level of the lumbar and first sacral segments. The overlying ectoderm develops a well-defined bridge-like structure called the *apical ectodermal ridge*. Under the influence of the apical ectodermal ridge, the underlying mesoderm is stimulated to elaborate limb elements in a proximal distal sequence. The ridge and underlying mesoderm are mutually dependent on one another to initiate and maintain normal limb development. The normal sequence of limb bud formation and hip joint development can be divided into five general phases as described by O'Rahilly and Gardner (Fig. 15-1):

1. Condensation of the mesenchyme occurs by cellular aggregation to form a *blastema* (a growing mass of mesenchymal tissue before definitive tissues can be distinguished).
2. Chondrification begins in the region of the future bone and divides the blastema.
3. Formation of interzones occurs as the areas between the centers of the chondrification remain as densely cellular avascular regions se-

creting extracellular material that maintains and widens the homogenous interzone.

4. Formation of synovial mesenchyme occurs as the synovium differentiates at the periphery of the interzone and later is responsible for the development of the synovial lining, the joint capsule, the intracapsular ligaments and tendons, and menisci.
5. Cavitation begins in the central part of the interzones with small multiple cavities that eventually coalesce to form the joint cavity. At about the same time, a synovial membrane develops that undergoes vascular invasion with accompanying macrophages and other cell types.

This process occurs about 4.5 to 7 weeks after fertilization, and, when concluded, a joint cavity line by synovium and hyaline cartilage has been formed. Because of this sequence of differentiation, the development of congenital hip dislocation must occur after the hip joint has formed.

At birth, the acetabulum has formed from the ilium, ischium, and pubis as they join at the triradiate cartilage. The proximal femur consists of the femoral head and neck and the greater and lesser trochanters. Secondary ossification centers form in the femoral head and greater trochanter. The triradiate cartilage fuses in boys on average at 15 years of age and in girls on average at 13 years of age. The femoral head growth plate fuses on average at 17 years of age in boys and at 14 years of age in girls. The greater trochanteric physis fuses on average at 16 years of age in boys and at 14 years of age in girls.

VASCULAR SUPPLY

The medial and lateral femoral circumflex arteries arising from the profunda femoris or less frequently from the femoral artery are the primary arteries supplying the developing proximal femur with occasional contributions from the artery of the ligamentum teres. The circumflex femoral arteries travel to the femoral neck to form an extracapsular ring surrounding the base of the neck. The medial, lateral, and posterior parts of the ring are a continuation of the medial femoral circumflex, while the lateral femoral circumflex supplies only the anterior portion of the ring. Only occasionally do the two portions of the ring form a complete anastomosis (Fig. 15-2). Branches from the extracapsular arterial ring, known as *ascending cervical* or *retinacular vessels*, then penetrate the capsule on the anterior, posterior, medial, and lateral femoral neck surfaces and ascend beneath the synovium, sending branches to the metaphysis and epiphysis and forming a subsynovial anastomotic

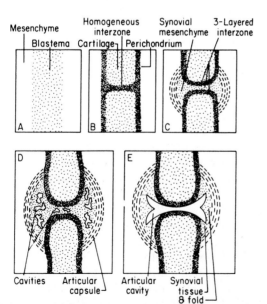

FIGURE 15-1. Diagram of the development of a synovial joint. (**A**) Joints develop from the blastema, not the surrounding mesenchyme. (**B**) Chondrification has occurred. The interzone remains avascular and highly cellular. (**C**) The synovial mesenchyme develops from the periphery of the interzone and becomes vascularized. Following shortly after differentiation of synovial membrane is cavitation, which may begin centrally in the interzone or peripherally (**D**) and merge to form the joint cavity (**E**). (O'Rahilly R, Gardner E. In: Sokoloff L, ed. The joints and synovial fluid, Vol 1. New York, Academic Press 1978)

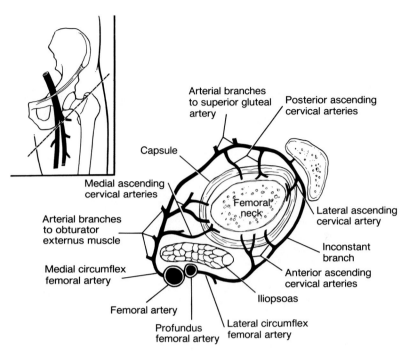

FIGURE 15-2. Cross section of the proximal part of the left femur at the base of the neck, showing the extracapsular arterial ring. Broken lines indicate inconstant connections between anterior and lateral ascending cervical arteries. The lateral ascending cervical artery branches after traversing the capsule. In young children, this artery can be compressed in the narrow space between the femoral neck and greater trochanter as the artery passes through the capsule. (Trueta J. The normal vascular anatomy of the human femoral head during growth. J Bone Joint Surg 1957;39B:358–394)

ring on the surface of the femoral neck at the margin of the articular cartilage.

Before the appearance of the secondary ossification centers, vertical intraosseous metaphyseal vessels help supply the capital femoral epiphysis. As epiphyseal ossification begins, however, the epiphyseal growth plate becomes a barrier to the blood flow between the epiphysis and the metaphysis. The intraosseous blood supply to the epiphysis then occurs from the lateral epiphyseal vessels, which arise from the lateral ascending cervical arteries and advance horizontally within the bone toward the center of the capital femoral epiphysis. The lateral ascending cervical vessels originate from the medial femoral circumflex artery, and therefore this vessel is responsible for most of the capital femoral epiphysis vascular supply. In addition, medial epiphyseal vessels occasionally arising from the ligamentum teres artery penetrate the head, supplying varying amounts of the epiphysis. In general, however, these vessels do not play a major role in contributing to the epiphyseal blood supply, especially in the infant and growing child. After 7 years of age, the medial epiphyseal vessels may become more prominent and supply a larger area of the capital femoral epiphysis.

The vascular patterns established during growth persist throughout life. In adults, the lateral epiphyseal arteries enter the head superiorly and posterosuperiorly, following closely the lines of the old epiphyseal plate running downward and medially. The medial epiphyseal arteries originating from the ligamentum teres run laterally until they meet and

anastomose with the lateral epiphyseal vessels. The metaphysis is supplied by superior and inferior metaphyseal arteries, which arise from the ascending cervical arteries and form the encircling subsynovial anastomotic ring at the margin of the articular cartilage (circulus articuli vasculosus). Once inside the bone, the epiphyseal and metaphyseal vessels anastomose freely with one another and with intramedullary vessels (Fig. 15-3).

SURGICAL APPROACHES

The surgical exposure of the hip joint can be achieved through a variety of approaches. When considering approaches for adult reconstructive problems and procedures, there are three basic approaches (Fig. 15-4).

Anterior Approach

The anterior approach, also known as the Smith-Petersen approach, uses two muscular and internervous planes. Superficially, the dissection is carried out between the sartorius (femoral nerve) and the tensor fascia femoris (superior gluteal nerve) muscles. The deep dissection lies between the rectus femoris (femoral nerve) and the gluteus medius (superior gluteal nerve) muscles. The skin incision runs proximally along the anterior half of the iliac crest, turning distally at the anterosuperior iliac spine, running distally about 10 cm on the anterolateral thigh at the

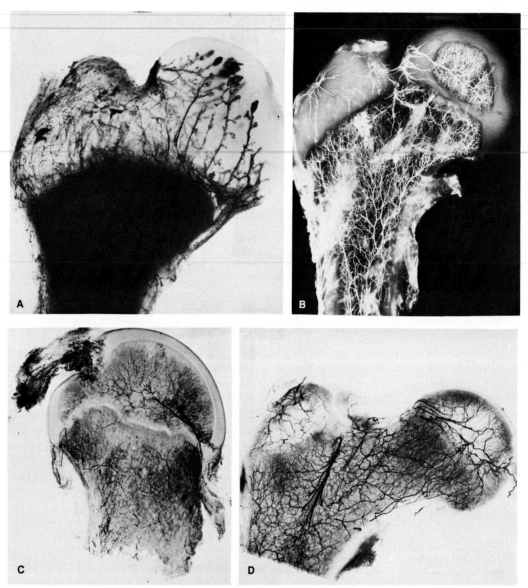

FIGURE 15-3. The vascular pattern of the femoral head during growth. (A) At birth: Main supply from lateral epiphyseal and metaphyseal vessels. (B) After 4 months: Exclusive supply from lateral epiphyseal vessels. Cartilaginous growth plate is a barrier to metaphyseal vessels. (C) After 7 years of age: Vessels from the ligamentum teres penetrate and join the lateral epiphyseal vessels. Cartilaginous growth plate is still a barrier. Metaphysis is vascular and becomes more so as epiphyseal fusion approaches. (D) Adulthood: Epiphyseal plate barrier has disappeared. Anastomoses have formed between lateral epiphyseal, medial epiphyseal, superior metaphyseal, and inferior metaphyseal vessels. (Trueta J. The normal vascular anatomy of the human femoral head during growth. J Bone Joint Surg 1957;39B:358)

medial edge of the tensor fascia femoris muscles. Palpation helps define the interval between the sartorius and the tensor fascia femoris. This interval is then developed, taking care to identify and protect the lateral femoral cutaneous nerve. The interval between the muscle is developed, retracting the sartorius medially and the tensor fascia femoris laterally, exposing the underlying gluteus medius muscle and

the ascending branch of the lateral femoral circumflex artery, which is then ligated. The plane between the rectus femoris and the gluteus medius is identified next, and the reflected head attachments of the rectus femoris to the anteroinferior iliac spine, bony pelvis, and hip capsule are divided. The interval deep to the gluteus minimus and between the hip capsule and the iliopsoas as it crosses toward the lesser trochanter

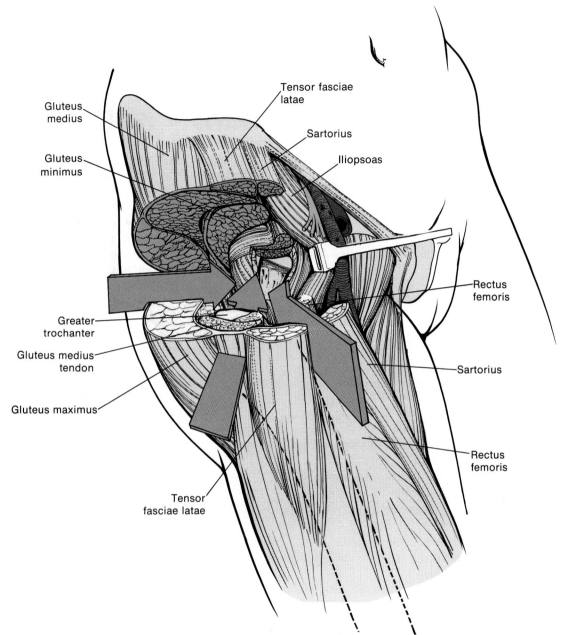

Gluteus medius

Gluteus minimus

Tensor fasciae latae

Sartorius

Iliopsoas

Rectus femoris

Greater trochanter

Gluteus medius tendon

Gluteus maximus

Sartorius

Rectus femoris

Tensor fasciae latae

FIGURE 15-4. The intermuscular intervals used in the anterior, anterolateral, and posterior approaches to the hip. (Hoppenfeld S, de Boer P. Surgical exposures in orthopaedics: the anatomic approach. Philadelphia, JB Lippincott, 1984)

is developed next. Deep retractors are placed on the hip capsule, both medially and laterally, giving exposure of the hip joint. The exposure can be expanded by subperiosteal dissection of the hip abductors off of the ilium; by osteotomy of the anteroinferior iliac spine, allowing further retraction of the rectus femoris; or by developing the dissection distally along the femur anterior to the tensor fascia femoris and then splitting the tensor fascia lata.

Anterolateral and Direct Lateral Approaches

A variety of approaches are best called anterolateral or direct lateral approaches. This type of approach was first described by Watson-Jones and has subsequently been modified. In general, the approaches differ in their management of the greater trochanter and of the deep structures about the hip, but they all use the same superficial interval between the gluteus medius (superior gluteal nerve) and the tensor fascia femoris (superior gluteal nerve) muscles. The approach is not an internervous approach because both these muscles are innervated by the superior gluteal nerve; however, dissection generally stops short of damaging the main branch of the superior gluteal nerve as it passes to the tensor fascia femoris muscle near its insertion on the iliac crest.

The skin incision can be made in a variety of ways but in general is centered over the greater trochanter, extending distally along the lateral femur and extending proximally either gently anteriorly toward the anterosuperior iliac spine or gently posteriorly toward the posterosuperior iliac spine. The deep fascia is incised posterior to the tensor fascia femoris muscle, and the interval between it and the gluteus medius muscle is then developed.

The various approaches differ in the manner in which the deep dissection is carried out. An anterolateral approach leaves the greater trochanter and attached abductor musculature intact, and dissection is carried out anterior to the greater trochanter. This exposure can be facilitated by partial release of the anterior portions of gluteus medius and gluteus minimus as they insert on the greater trochanter. As in the anterior approach, the interval between the hip capsule and the rectus femoris and iliopsoas is identified. This generally is accomplished by resection of the insertion of the reflected head of the rectus femoris muscle and blunt dissection of any capsular attachments of the muscle, then placing retractors in the interval, retracting the rectus femoris and iliopsoas medially. Laterally, a retractor is placed deep to the gluteus minimus on the superior surface of the hip capsule.

The direct lateral approach uses the same superficial dissection between the gluteus medius and tensor fascia femoris. An intracapsular osteotomy of the greater trochanter, with the gluteus medius and minimus and short external rotators attached, gains exposure of the hip joint by taking the osteotomized fragment of bone and muscular attachments superiorly.

A modification of this approach uses the functional thick tendinous periosteal continuity between the vastus lateralis and the gluteus medius muscle. The same superficial interval is developed; however, deeply the anterior one third of the gluteus medius is divided from bone in continuity with the anterior one third of the vastus lateralis muscle. The insertion of the gluteus minimus muscle is resected, and the capsule is then exposed. The entire flap is retracted anteriorly to expose the femoral neck.

Posterior Approach

The posterior approach does not use an intramuscular plane but rather splits the fibers of the gluteus maximus muscle (inferior gluteal nerve) to gain exposure of the posterior aspect of the gluteus medius and the greater trochanter. The skin incision is centered over the greater trochanter, extending distally along the lateral shaft of the femur and proximally extending slightly posteriorly in line with the fibers of the gluteus maximum muscle along the posterior edge of the underlying gluteus medius muscle. The deep fascia is distally incised longitudinally along the tensor fascia lata, and proximally the fascia and gluteus maximum muscle are split. The greater trochanteric bursa is incised, exposing the posterior aspect of the gluteus medius and the short external rotator muscles. The medial femoral circumflex vessel is identified and ligated as it courses beneath the quadratus femoris muscle on the posterior surface of the base of the femoral neck. The short external rotator muscles are detached from their insertion on the femur and the greater trochanter; the posterior aspect of the hip capsule is thus exposed, and capsulotomy and dislocation of the femoral head can be accomplished.

BIOMECHANICS

Diarthrodial joints have opposing surfaces covered with hyaline cartilage, which allows for a nearly frictionless surface. Important biomechanical and physiologic questions arise in determining how this cartilage reacts to the applied forces that result from joint function. These questions can in part be answered by examining some biomechanical concepts.

Stress is defined as internal force per unit area as the result of an external load. The internal stress applied to articular cartilage depends on the magnitude of the applied load (joint reaction force) and the surface area of cartilage over which the load is applied. Therefore, the congruency of the total surface area of the hip joint and the magnitude of that area become important parameters that affect cartilage function. Cartilage is able to attenuate internal stress as a result of applied loads because of its viscoelastic properties. When a load is applied to cartilage, there is an initial deformation as a result of that load, but with time, additional deformation results because of *creep* (deformation or change in strain of material over time as a result of the constant load). With removal of the load, there is an initial rapid recovery to normal shape and volume followed by a slower, sustained recovery of volume. These properties depend on hyaline cartilage's ability to maintain its structure as a superhydrated matrix of proteoglycans and collagen.

The proximal femur has unique anatomic relations that create mechanical advantages for hip function. With growth, the femoral neck shaft angle decreases from a more valgus position to an average of 125 degrees. This moves the greater trochanter laterally and increases the abductor lever arm, thus increasing the mechanical advantage of the abductor muscles. In the coronal plane, the femoral neck is anteverted or placed anterior to the dicondylar plane of the knee. This anteversion angle averages 8 to 15 degrees in adults, lengthening the lever arm of the gluteus maximus and increasing its efficiency.

The compressive forces that act across the hip joint in stance are a summation of the force of the body weight and the muscle forces around the hip. These forces are represented in Figure 15-5, with A, the abductor muscle force, and K, the partial body weight (body weight minus the weight of the supporting leg). The direction of A is defined by the direction of the pull of the abductor muscles, and the direction of K is vertical. In single-legged stance, the partial body weight acts medially to the hip joint through a center of gravity slightly anterior to the L3-4 interspace and slightly to the contralateral side of the midline. This force creates a moment around the hip that causes the pelvis to rotate downward and the hip to adduct. The abductors create a force lateral to the hip joint, counteracting that force maintaining the pelvis level. In a static equilibrium, these two vectors establish a third resultant compressive vector joint reaction force that acts through the center of rotation of the femoral head to the point of intersection of the vectors representing abductor muscle force and partial body weight. The resultant vector (R) establishes an angle that averages 16 degrees from the vertical and perpendicular to the weight-bearing surface of the hip joint. The magnitude of this compressive vector can be determined by either vector addition of abductor muscle force and partial body weight or by assuming a static equilibrium and determining the moments created by forces K and A around the hip. Distance *a* is about three times distance *b*; thus, to maintain static equi-

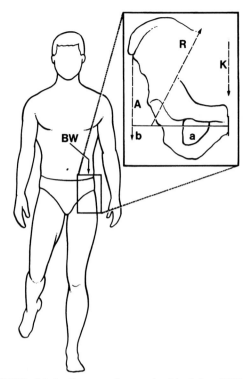

FIGURE 15-5. *Forces* acting at the hip joint. BW, body weight; A, abductor muscle force; K, partial body weight (BW − weight of leg); R, joint reaction force (distance a is about three times distance b); EF, sum of all hip forces; EM, sum of all hip movements. In a static equilibrium, the sum of all forces around the hip must equal zero: EF = 0, or A + K − R = O; that is A + K = R. Additionally, the sum of all moments must equal zero (moment equals force times distance from center of rotation): EM = O, or Ab − Ka = O (the direction of A and K are opposite, so one is given a minus or negative value). Thus, Ab = Ka; A = K $\frac{a}{b}$; (3a = b); A = 3K, or R = 4K. Summary: The abductor muscle force is about three times the partial body weight, and the joint reaction force is about four times the partial body weight.

librium, the abductor muscle force must be three times the partial body weight. Because in a static equilibrium the sum of all forces is zero, the abductor muscle force plus the partial body weight must equal the joint reaction force. Thus, the total compressive force, or the joint reaction force, is about four times the partial body weight.

The activities of daily living create joint reaction forces across the hip, ranging from 2.5 to 6 times body weight. Activities as simple as getting off and on a bedpan can create forces several times body weight. Forces during gait can be reduced by using a cane in the opposite hand. The cane works through a long lever arm, and small loads applied to the cane can significantly reduce the joint reaction force. Similarly, the changes in the bony architecture of the proximal femur can significantly alter the joint reaction force. Coxa valga deformities shorten the abductor lever arm and thus decrease the mechanical advantage of the abductors, causing the force required to significantly increase and thus also increasing the joint reaction force. When the abductor musculature is unable to balance the moment created by the body weight, the pelvis drops during gait. This is compensated for by walking with an abductor lurch (Trendelenburg), with the body weight shifted over the center of the hip, reducing the lever arm and the moment over which body weight acts and allowing the abductor muscles to generate less force to maintain a level pelvis.

EXAMINATION OF THE PATIENT WITH HIP PAIN

History

The most common reason for medical or surgical intervention in diseases of the hip is disabling pain. Therefore, it is important to qualify and quantify the amount of pain the patient is having. Pain from the hip joint generally localizes to the groin, buttock, or proximal thigh, and it is important to differentiate from pain originating in the back, sacroiliac joint, knees, or visceral organs. A certain degree of subjectivity exists for the patient, the examiner, or both; nevertheless, an attempt to quantify the pain should be made. A determination of the patient's ability to work, level of activity, walking capacity, functional abilities (eg, use of stairs, ability to put on shoes and socks), and whether walking aids (cane, crutch) are needed should be recorded. Most importantly, the physician must determine the impact the pain is having on the patient's occupation, recreational lifestyle, activities of daily living, and overall quality of life. When these parameters are determined along with information regarding the patient's age, general medical condition, physical examination, and radiographic and serologic analyses, the physician may proceed with a rational plan for treatment.

If a determination is made that surgery is the most appropriate treatment, a general history and examination regarding the patient's overall medical condition, especially with regard to previous dental, genitourinary, gastrointestinal, cardiovascular, pulmonary, neurologic, and infectious disease history, is mandatory. History of thrombophlebitis, pulmonary embolus, and deep vein thrombosis must also be reviewed.

Physical Examination

A detailed physical examination is essential in the assessment of hip function and disease. The examination should include an assessment of overall hip and lower extremity function as well as a detailed general examination. An observation of the patient's gait should be recorded with the determination of limp and stride length, limb alignment, muscle strength, and overall body mechanics. An assessment of the degree of pain, muscle strength, range of motion, and length of the limbs should be directly measured. In single stance, a positive Trendelenburg sign is an expression of unfavorable geometry of the hip or weakness of the abductors, or both. In contrast, a Trendelenburg lurch or abductor lurch, which may or may not be associated with a positive Trendelenburg sign, represents an attempt by the patient to reduce pain by shifting the body weight closer to the center of the hip (Fig. 15-6). This must also be differentiated from a limp secondary to a shortened extremity. Contractures about the hip can also alter gait patterns. Abductor muscle strength is assessed by the Trendelenburg test and by side-lying hip abduction. Both active and passive range of motion should be recorded as well as the presence and magnitude of any contractures around the hip. Overall lower extremity limb alignment should be recorded both in stance and during gait. Limb length should be recorded, and if the patient uses shoe lifts, the patient should ambulate both with and without the lift. Likewise, if a patient uses an assistive device to ambulate, the patient should, if possible, walk both with and without the device. The groin, buttock, thigh, and greater trochanter should be palpated for areas of tenderness or masses. Range of motion should be recorded in both knees, ankles, and feet. The contralateral hip and spine should be thoroughly evaluated. An assessment of lower extremity vascular supply should also be carried out.

Upper extremity function should be examined, especially if the patient has multiple joint disease or if the use of ambulatory devices after a surgical procedure will be required. Additionally, a functional assessment of the patient's ability to put on shoes and socks and climb stairs should be recorded. An overall assessment of the patient's general medical condition is mandatory. Currently, reports are at-

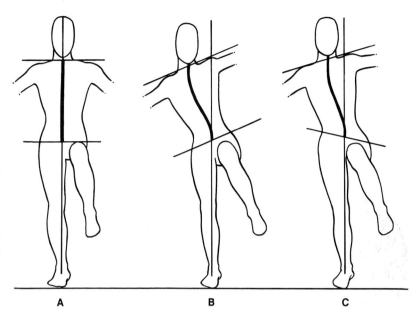

FIGURE 15-6. Trendelenburg sign and Trendelenburg lurch (Duchenne sign). (**A**) Negative Trendelenburg sign and lurch. (**B**) Negative Trendelenburg sign and positive Trendelenburg lurch. (**C**) Positive Trendelenburg sign and lurch. (Johnston RC, Fitzgerald RH Jr, Harris WH, Poss R, Muller ME, Sledge CB. Clinical and radiographic evaluation of total hip replacement. J Bone Joint Surg 1990;72A: 161–168)

A   B   C

tempting to standardize the terminology for reporting the results of the clinical and radiographic evaluation of patients undergoing total-hip replacement.

Radiographic Evaluation

The radiographic evaluation of the hip joint should include anteroposterior (AP) views of both the affected hip and the pelvis. Shoot-through lateral or Lowenstein lateral radiographs should also be obtained. Depending on the disease process being evaluated, computed tomographic (CT) scanning, magnetic resonance imaging (MRI) scanning, tomographic evaluation, or radionucleotide imaging may be warranted. These studies are discussed individually in the subsequent sections on the various disease entities as they affect the hip.

DISEASES OF THE HIP

Osteoarthritis

Any discussion regarding the evaluation and treatment of osteoarthritis of any joint should begin with an appreciation of articular cartilage. Articular cartilage is a uniquely arranged suprahydrated structure of collagen (80% to 90% type II collagen) and proteoglycans. The proteoglycans exist aggregated on long filaments of hyaluronic acid, stabilized by low-molecular-weight glycoproteins. They exist linked within a collagen framework, maintaining an electronegative domain that allows cartilage to withstand shear and compression. Despite the relatively acellular character of articular cartilage, it is not inert, and in conjunction with underlying subchondral bone, cartilage functions to maintain itself to withstand tremendous forces while supplying a nearly friction-free surface for joint function. When the ability of cartilage to maintain its structural and physiologic integrity is overcome, the subsequent morphologic, biochemical, inflammatory, and immunologic changes that result produce the disease state osteoarthritis. The actual etiology of osteoarthritis is unknown but may be secondary to changes in the joint biomechanics, changes in physiologic properties of cartilage, changes in subchondral and trabecular bone physiology, or combinations thereof. Speculation exists about the role of inflammatory and immunologic processes in the development of osteoarthritis. The body of evidence best supports the hypothesis that a primary insult to cartilage results in the release of factors that may accelerate the destruction of cartilage and mediate changes leading to progressive softening, ulceration, and focal degeneration of articular cartilage, with neoformation of peripheral osteophytes at the joint margins. Whether osteoarthritis is a primary disease of cartilage, an inability of cartilage to respond to deleterious changes in its environment, or results from morphologic changes in the underlying subchondral bone remains unknown. The pathogenesis of osteoarthritis proceeds when the magnitude of unit load exceeds the physiologic limit of cartilage repair and function.

Osteoarthritis can be divided into two types—primary and secondary. *Primary osteoarthritis* results from a defect in cartilage's ability to maintain itself. *Secondary osteoarthritis* results when the cartilage's ability for homeostasis has been altered by inflammatory, metabolic, structural, or biomechanical factors. Common causes of secondary arthritis are listed in the Table 15-1.

Epidemiology

Osteoarthritis of the hip develops in 5% of the population older than 55 years, and it is estimated that about half of these patients eventually require hip surgery. The incidence of osteoarthritis of the hip in men and women is about the same; however, women are more likely to develop the disease at a younger age, probably secondary to the higher incidence of congenital hip dysplasia in women. Men, on the other hand, have an increased incidence of childhood hip diseases that occur later in life (Perthes and slipped capital femoral epiphysis) and subsequently may develop osteoarthritis secondary to these abnormalities at an older age. Other childhood hip diseases that are associated with the development of osteoarthritis as an adult include multiple epiphyseal dysplasia, Morquio disease, spondyloepiphyseal dysplasia, the osteochondral dysplasias, and avascular necrosis (AVN) from systemic diseases such as sickle cell anemia. Thus, congenital and childhood hip disorders can alter normal hip development, resulting in hip dysplasia, joint incongruities, joint stress concentrations, and altered hip biomechanics, which may predispose to cartilage degeneration and the development of osteoarthritis of the hip later in life (Fig. 15-7).

Climate, geography, and race do not significantly impact on the incidence of osteoarthritis of the hip, with the exception that a decreased incidence is found in some Asian races (Hong Kong Chinese), Indians, and South African blacks. It is speculated that this may be secondary to a decreased incidence of congenital childhood hip disease in these ethnic groups.

TABLE 15-1.
Common Causes of Arthritis

PRIMARY
Idiopathic

SECONDARY
Inflammatory
  Rheumatoid arthritis
  Septic arthritis
  Spondyloarthropathies
Endocrine
  Acromegaly
  Hyperparathyroidism
Traumatic
Developmental defects
  Congenital hip dysplasia
  Legg-Calvé-Perthes disease
  Slipped capital femoral epiphysis
  Inherited childhood dysplasia (ie, multiple epiphyseal
    dysplasia)
Metabolic
  Ochronosis
  Hemachromatosis
  Wilson disease
  Chondrocalcinosis
  Gout
  Paget disease
Neuropathic disorders
Avascular necrosis
Hemophilia

Etiology

Although the etiology of primary osteoarthritis of the hip is unknown, several etiologic factors are associated with the development of osteoarthritis.

Increased age is the strongest risk factor associated with the development of osteoarthritis, with several epidemiologic studies indicating an increasing incidence of osteoarthritis with age. Aging is associated with changes in cartilage properties to withstand fatigue forces, changes in joint congruity, and changes in peripheral nerve function, all or some of which may make cartilage more susceptible to the development of osteoarthritis.

Although obesity has been clearly shown to be associated with an increased incidence of osteoarthritis of the knee, there is no evidence that obesity predisposes the hip joint to the development of this disease.

There are conflicting reports on the effect of increased forces on the normal hip joint and their relation to the development of osteoarthritis. For example, football players, farmers, retired athletes, and miners were observed to have an increased incidence of osteoarthritis of the hip, whereas other studies involving marathon runners and female physical education instructors failed to show any correlation.

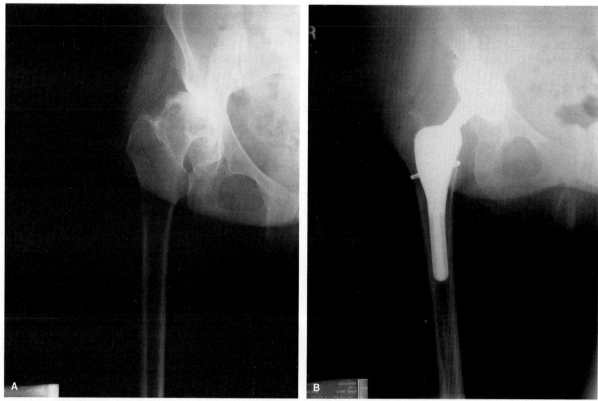

FIGURE 15-7. (A) AP radiograph of a 50-year-old woman who developed degenerative arthritis of the right hip secondary to congenital dislocation of the hip, which was treated conservatively as a child with abduction bracing. (B) Radiograph illustrating the postoperative result using a custom femoral component and placing the acetabular component in a slightly upward and inward position, resting the component on existing acetabular bone stock. The 3-year follow-up was excellent.

In general, there is little evidence to support the concept of a primary defect in cartilage as the etiologic factor for the development of osteoarthritis. Several conditions, however, may directly or indirectly alter the cartilaginous matrix and influence the development of secondary osteoarthritis. Hemosiderin in hemochromatosis, copper in Wilson disease, hemogentisic acid in ochronotic arthropathy, monosodium urate crystals in gouty arthritis, and calcium pyrophosphate dihydrate deposition disease are conditions that may have an effect on the development of osteoarthritis.

Trauma may result in direct injury to cartilage, or an unreduced or poorly reduced intraarticular fracture may leave incongruous joint surfaces, altering joint and cartilage function. This may lead to stress concentrations, cartilage failure, and posttraumatic arthritis. Primary inflammatory conditions that affect the hip joint also may result in secondary arthritis. Examples include rheumatoid arthritis, bacterial infections, and tuberculous infections in which the primary disease process alters cartilage homeo-

stasis and precedes the secondary changes of osteoarthritis.

Finally, there are reports of acetabular labral tears and intraarticular acetabular labrum as etiologic factors in the development of osteoarthritis of the hip.

These factors, combined with the incidence of adult hip sequela secondary to childhood hip disease as well as other factors, lead some authors to question the etiologic significance of primary osteoarthritis of the hip. The hypothesis put forth is that a significantly higher percentage of osteoarthritis of the hip may be secondary osteoarthritis with an identifiable underlying cause. (See Table 15-1 for a list of causes of secondary osteoarthritis.)

Pathology

The gross pathology of cartilage degeneration in osteoarthritis of the hip is highly variable. Early in the disease, the cartilage may undergo softening and thinning and obtain a yellowish to brown discoloration. Progression of the disease results in fibrillation,

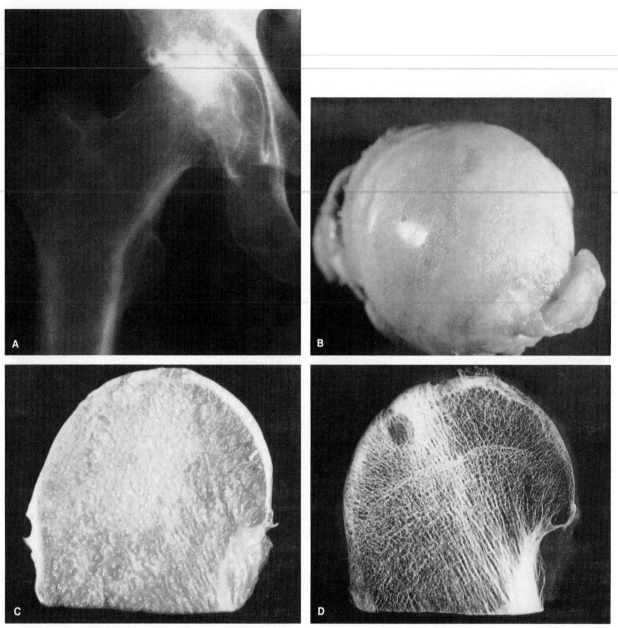

FIGURE 15-8. (A) Radiograph of the hip joint in a patient complaining of pain and limitation of motion in that joint. Note the diminished joint space in the superior aspect of the joint, together with sclerosis evident on both the acetabular and femoral sides of the joint. In this patient, there is no significant migrating of the joint, either medially or laterally, and this finding may be considered characteristic of the early stage of osteoarthritis of the hip joint. (B) Gross photograph of the femoral head removed from the patient shown in A. Note the absence of the articular cartilage on the superior and lateral aspect of the femoral head and the polished appearance of the exposed bone (eburnation). The remaining surrounding cartilage has a somewhat yellow color, and its surface is roughened. (C) A slice through the femoral head shown in B reveals the absence of the articular cartilage over the superolateral surface. However, the sphericity of the joint is fairly well maintained, and there is no significant osteophyte formation. This finding is in keeping with the lack of significant migration seen in the radiograph. (In later stages of the disease when migration has occurred, osteophyte formation is prominent.) (D) Radiograph of the specimen shown in C. Note the sclerosis of the bone underlying the superolateral surface of the femoral head. Within this sclerotic bone, a cyst can be seen. (The specimen radiograph often reveals gross anatomic features more clearly than the specimen itself.) (E) A histologic preparation of the specimen shown in B through D. The sclerosis of the bone in the eburnated portion of the femoral head and the fibrous-filled area of bone lysis are evident. (F) A section through the articular cartilage at the margin of the eburnated area shows thinning and irregularity of the surface of the cartilage without obvious chondrocyte proliferation. (Bullough PG, Vigorifa VJ. Atlas of orthopaedic pathology with clinical and radiographic correlations. University Park Press, 1984:7.10)

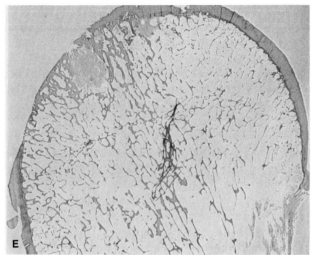
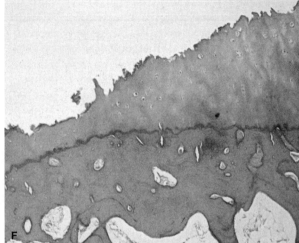

FIGURE 15-8. (*Continued*)

fissuring, and ulceration of articular cartilage. Eventually, the cartilage may become completely absent, leaving bare eburnated bone. Bits and tufts of fibrous tissue or fibrocartilage appear within the eburnated sclerotic surfaces. The femoral neck enlarges, and osteophytes form at the joint margins. Large osteophytes are especially common on the medial acetabular floor, near the acetabular fossa, and at the acetabular periphery and the medial femoral neck. The osteophytes have a central core of bone capped with hyaline and fibrocartilage. The subchondral bone adjacent to the areas of diseased cartilage may become dense and sclerotic. These changes may be present on both the femoral and acetabular surfaces and are most common at the areas of highest load transfer across the joint. Osteoarthritic cysts form within the femoral head and the acetabulum and generally occur near the joint surfaces. They are surrounded by a layer of sclerotic bone and contain a hemogenic, clear or cloudy, gelatinous fluid. The appearance of the synovium is also highly variable. It can appear normal or may have thickened areas with villi and infolding. Histologically, it may also appear normal or may have areas of hypervascularity, hemorrhage, fibrosis, or inflammatory infiltrates. Special staining techniques may even reveal immune complexes. The capsule thickens and has areas of fibrosis that may lead to joint contractures about the hip.

Histologically, the cartilage changes seen depend on the stage of the disease. Early changes of the cartilage surface include fibrillation of uncalcified cartilage (a structural abnormality of cartilage characterized by splitting and fraying of the tissue). In the mild form, fibrillation is confined to the superficial areas of the cartilage, but in the more severe forms, it extends deeper and can be associated with thinning of the cartilage surface secondary to the loss of tissue. When the full depth of cartilage is lost and the underlying bone exposed, an ulcerated lesion exists. The cartilage may also show a relatively smooth thinning without the vertical splitting and severe fibrillation. Horizontal cleft formation may also be seen in the areas between the calcified and uncalcified zones of cartilage and may predispose to full-thickness loss of cartilage superficial to the cleft. Changes in cartilage cellularity accompany the morphologic changes seen. Initially, there may be a mild, diffuse hypercellularity; in the later stages, the chondrocytes may be found clustered together in brood capsules or clones. The tide mark may also show areas of irregularity, duplication, and neovascularization. These changes may initially be focal but with later stages of the disease are progressive and become generalized. Eventually, the cartilage surface is destroyed, leaving bare eburnated subchondral bone. Areas of fibrous or fibrocartilaginous tissue, as well as areas of new bone formation and variable areas of osteonecrosis, may be present within these eburnated surfaces (Fig. 15-8).

JOINT SPACE NARROWING. Early in the disease, the loss of cartilage is accompanied radiographically by the progressive loss of joint space but with the preservation of subchondral contours. As the disease progresses, the subchondral bone plate over both sides of the joint may hypertrophy and appear sclerotic. With further disease, there is loss of subchondral bone plate contour and eventually progressive bone loss leading to femoral head migration. In the final stages of disease, after bone loss and migration have stabilized, there may be reappearance of small amounts of joint space. It has been postulated that this reappearance of small amounts of joint space in the end stages of osteoarthritis of the hip may be secondary to attempts at repair and resurfacing of the eburnated bone surface with fibrous tissue and fibrocartilage.

OSTEOPHYTES. Osteophyte formation in osteoarthritis of the hip is common and, as opposed to the osteophytes formation found in otherwise normal senescent hips, tends to be larger and more progressive. Figure 15-9 summarizes the distribution of osteophytes as described by Bombelli. One investigator found no prognostic significance in the presence and location of osteophytes.

CYSTS. Cysts are common in osteoarthritis of the hip. They tend to be small and located near the subarticular areas of the acetabulum and femoral head within the areas of highest stress transfer. In general, loss of cartilage with exposure of subchondral bone is required before the appearance of cystic changes. Several authors noted that acetabular cysts appear sooner and more frequently than femoral head cysts and suggest that the initial bone changes of osteoarthritis may occur in the acetabulum.

Radiographic Evaluation

The radiographic evaluation of osteoarthritis of the hip must differentiate between true osteoarthritic change and the normal changes that occur with aging. The hallmark of osteoarthritis is progressive thinning of cartilage that eventually exposes subchondral bone and is associated with structural changes in bone. Radiographically, this is manifested as joint space narrowing. Joint space narrowing, however, may also be a normal finding of senescence. Both processes may also be accompanied by osteophyte formation. Their differences lie in the extent of involvement. Aging is characterized by mild cartilage fibrillation, smaller amounts of cartilage narrowing, smaller osteophyte formation, and maintenance of joint function. Osteoarthritis, on the other hand, is characterized by progressive narrowing of the joint space, full-thickness cartilage loss, exposure and eburnation of subchondral bone, large osteophyte formation, cyst formation, and the progressive loss of joint function (see Fig. 15-9).

Therefore, joint space narrowing and the formation of osteophytes does not, in and of itself, confirm the diagnosis of osteoarthritis of the hip. Guidelines in determining the presence of osteoarthritis include: local or generalized loss of joint space (less than 3 mm in patients older than 70 years of age or

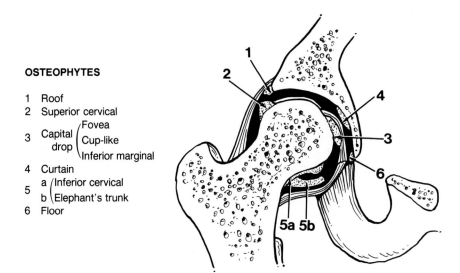

OSTEOPHYTES

1 Roof
2 Superior cervical
3 Capital drop { Fovea / Cup-like / Inferior marginal
4 Curtain
5 a { Inferior cervical / b Elephant's trunk
6 Floor

FIGURE 15-9. In a completely developed osteoarthritic hip, there are three principal osteophytes on the femoral head: the superior cervical (2), starting as the superior marginal osteophyte; the inferior cervical (5a), starting as the inferior marginal osteophyte; and the capital drop (3). There are three on the acetabulum: the roof osteophyte (1), the curtain osteophyte (4), and the floor osteophyte (6). The capital drop is made by the fusion of the fovea osteophyte, the inferior marginal osteophyte, and the cup-like osteophyte. The inferior cervical osteophyte may assume the shape of an elephant's trunk (5b). (Bombelli R. The role of osteotomy as a consequent therapy. In: Osteoarthritis of the hip: classification and pathogenesis. Berlin, Heidelberg, New York, Springer-Verlag, 1983)

less than 4 mm in patients younger than 70 years of age), the presence of an acetabular cyst, an increase in subchondral sclerosis, and a loss of parallelism of the subchondral plate in the weight-bearing segment. The presence of cysts and osteophytes should be recorded. Various predisposing conditions (ie, Perthes disease or congenital dislocation of the hip) complicate the radiographic picture and may cause earlier degenerative changes to appear and consequently require the radiographic changes to be interpreted and recorded accordingly. Other parameters that require evaluation are the presence and degree of acetabular dysplasia as measured by the center edge angle of Wiberg (an angle that defines the acetabular coverage of the femoral head); the presence, direction, and extent of femoral head migration; and the quantitative assessment of overall acetabular and femoral bone stock.

Treatment

Symptoms do not necessarily parallel the degree of degenerative change. Severe degenerative joint disease may exist with relatively little or no pain and with good function despite limited motion and deformity. On the other hand, severe pain and loss of function may occur early in the course of the disease. The need for treatment of osteoarthritis of the hip is determined by the severity of pain and the degree to which such symptoms interfere with the activities of daily living.

Conservative treatment should focus on attempts to protect the joint, reduce symptoms, and restore and maintain joint function. The simple measures of reducing stressful activities, resting, and using ambulatory aids may reduce the stress on the hip joint and relieve symptoms. Heat, massage, gentle range-of-motion exercise, and muscle strengthening exercises can restore and help maintain range of motion and reduce muscle spasm and pain. Nonsteroidal antiinflammatory medications can help reduce inflammatory symptoms and can add an analgesic effect. These measures many times are successful in alleviating symptoms to the point that surgical treatment can be avoided or delayed. When these measures fail to reduce symptoms and maintain hip function, or when the local pathologic processes make increasing degeneration of the hip joint and bone loss inevitable, surgical intervention should be considered.

The goals of all surgical procedures around the hip for osteoarthritis are to relieve pain and improve function with a minimum of bone destruction. The various surgical alternatives include fusion, femoral or pelvic osteotomy, resection arthroplasty, hemiarthroplasty, cup arthroplasty, and total-hip arthroplasty. The choice of the most appropriate surgical procedure depends on a number of variables. The decision-making process should include consideration of patient age and expectations, weight, occupation, life-style and activity level, level of symptoms, involvement of other joints, history of previous infection, history of previous hip surgery, and overall medical condition and an overall assessment of what is possible with the patient's existing bony anatomy. The benefits, risks, and complications of any surgical procedure must be discussed in detail, and it is imperative that the patient have realistic expectations regarding the outcome of any proposed surgical procedure. A detailed discussion of the various surgical alternatives is presented later in this chapter.

Rheumatoid Arthritis

Rheumatoid arthritis is a chronic, systemic, inflammatory disorder with a predilection for articular cartilage. The hip joint is less frequently afflicted in the adult form of rheumatoid arthritis than other joints; however, its involvement may result in disabling symptoms and significant diminishment of function. Likewise, juvenile rheumatoid arthritis also more frequently involves larger, more rapidly growing joints, including the knees, wrists, elbows, and ankles and less commonly affects the hip joints. It has been estimated that about 1% of the United States adult population has rheumatoid arthritis. Therefore, it is reasonable to estimate that between 4 and 6 million cases of rheumatoid arthritis are found in the United States. The disease affects women more frequently, with a female/male ratio of between 2:1 and 4:1. The disease affects all ages but generally increases in incidence with advancing age. In women, the peak incidence is between the fourth and sixth decades.

Etiology

Extensive research continues to be done, but the exact etiology of rheumatoid arthritis remains obscure. Regardless of its cause, it may be described as an inflammatory process that somehow is triggered and centers in the joints with articular cartilage. The inflammation manifests as a stimulus for synovium to hypertrophy and become increasingly hyperplastic and hypervascular with increasing cellularity. This hypertrophic synovial tissue invades and degrades articular cartilage. The actual destruction of articular cartilage is done in large part by *rheumatoid pannus,* a fibrovascular granulation tissue that protrudes from the inflamed synovium into articular cartilage. It contains fibroblasts, small vessels, and multiple inflammatory cells that are responsible for the destruction of articular cartilage and its underlying bone.

Pathology

Pathology within the hip joint generally involves varying degrees of articular cartilage loss secondary to the inflammatory process. This usually involves the entire femoral head, resulting in concentric loss of cartilage and subsequent concentric joint space narrowing. There may also be varying amounts of bone loss and even femoral head collapse. Varying degrees of cyst formation occur, and in about 5% of patients, significant protrusio acetabuli develops.

Radiographic Evaluation

Radiography of the hip joint shows varying degrees of osteopenia and loss of joint space. The loss of joint space, in contrast to that seen in osteoarthritis, is generally concentric, and varying degrees of protrusio acetabuli may be present. Osteophyte formation is rare, and subchondral sclerosis is not a prominent feature. Cysts may develop within both the femoral head and the acetabulum. These changes may culminate in varying degrees of femoral head collapse, and in severely advanced cases, autofusion may occur with severe limitation of range of motion (Fig. 15-10).

Treatment

Conservative measures as they apply to the management of osteoarthritis also apply to hip diseases secondary to rheumatoid arthritis. The use of ambulatory devices, physical therapy, and nonsteroidal antiinflammatory medications can help to reduce inflammatory symptoms, decrease pain, and increase function. Additionally, in rheumatoid arthritis, a variety of medical approaches and treatments may be administered in a systemic attempt to reduce the overall inflammatory response within the body. This may include a variety of remitting agents and steroids not within the scope of this discussion.

With regard to surgical management, a number of options require discussion.

HIP ARTHRODESIS. Hip arthrodesis has a limited role in the treatment of rheumatoid arthritis of the hip because often the disease is bilateral. The

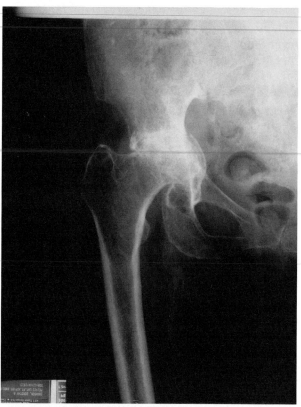

FIGURE 15-10. Right AP hip radiograph of a 76-year-old woman with a history of long-standing rheumatoid arthritis. The radiograph is an example of severe acetabuli protrusio with fracture of the medial wall and near autofusion of the hip joint secondary to the degenerative and inflammatory changes.

involvement of adjacent joints makes the role of the hip arthrodesis extremely limited.

HEMIARTHROPLASTY. Hemiarthroplasty also has a limited role in the treatment of hip disease secondary to rheumatoid arthritis. The focus of the inflammatory response is articular cartilage, and a hemiarthroplasty does not replace or remove the cartilage on the acetabular side of the joint, thereby leaving a focus for ongoing inflammatory disease and making the use of hemiarthroplasty limited.

SYNOVECTOMY. Both favorable and discouraging results using synovectomy in rheumatoid arthritis of the hip have been reported. One of the main concerns with regard to trying to perform an adequate synovectomy of the hip joint is that of causing AVN within the femoral head.

OSTEOTOMY. Osteotomy likewise has an extremely limited role in the treatment of rheumatoid arthritis of the hip joint. It does not remove the articular cartilage, which is the stimulus for the inflammatory process. Additionally, the articular involvement tends to be concentric and does not allow the ability to rotate less involved areas of articular cartilage into the superior weight-bearing area. Therefore, osteotomy has little if any role in the treatment of rheumatoid arthritis of the hip.

TOTAL-HIP ARTHROPLASTY. Total-hip arthroplasty remains the mainstay in the treatment of end-stage rheumatoid arthritis of the hip. The technique and results of total-hip arthroplasty are discussed later in this chapter.

TOTAL-JOINT REPLACEMENT IN JUVENILE RHEUMATOID ARTHRITIS. Juvenile rheumatoid arthritis may involve the hip joints to such a degree as to cause crippling disability. Total-hip replacement can provide dramatic improvement in both function and life-style in patients so afflicted. Total-hip replacement in juvenile rheumatoid arthritis may present an array of technical complexity because of the small size of the patient and deficiencies in the femoral and acetabular bone stock. These problems may require customized or miniature components. Additionally, although the early result of cemented total-hip arthroplasty may be good, these patients are young, and the total-hip replacement must withstand many years of function. One study indicated that this was offset somewhat by low functional demand in these patients because of other joint involvement. Another study reported on an average 4.8-year follow-up of cemented total-hip replacement in juvenile rheumatoid arthritis in patients with an average age of 46 years. There was an 18% loosening rate in this group of patients. The advent of cementless techniques, especially the role of cementless, customized techniques, may play a part in the future in improving these results.

Avascular Necrosis

Avascular necrosis is the death or necrosis of bone secondary to the loss of its vascular supply. The most common cause of AVN is trauma. Displaced subcapital and high transcervical femoral neck fractures can disrupt the vascular supply to the femoral head and are associated with a high incidence of AVN. The traumatic variety generally occurs in an older patient population, is unilateral, and is generally associated with a healing fracture or a nonunion. When present, the process generally involves the entire femoral head and is associated with an internal fixation device and

a prolonged period of either partial or no weight bearing. These factors combine to make early diagnosis difficult, and AVN is generally diagnosed after the collapse of the femoral head, failure of internal fixation, or development of gross nonunion. If symptoms are sufficient to warrant treatment, the surgery of choice is either endoprosthesis or total-hip arthroplasty, depending in part on the presence of acetabular involvement and the age and activity level of the patient.

Nontraumatic or idiopathic AVN occurs in younger people and is bilateral more than half of the time. Its exact etiology is unclear. There may be a causal relation between fat embolism and osteonecrosis. It has been postulated that these fat emboli may accumulate in intraosseous arterioles, causing a vascular occlusion. The source of these fat emboli has been postulated to be the fatty liver of alcohol-associated liver disease or of those taking high-dose steroids, or the coalescence of endogenous plasma lipoproteins resulting in continuous or intermittent fat embolism. Clinical and experimental studies have shown that prolonged steroid treatment is associated with fat emboli in subchondral arterioles, fat cell hypertrophy, and a gradual increase in femoral head intramedullary pressure. Bilateral hip involvement occurs in up to 80% of cases of steroid-induced osteonecrosis.

A second hypothesis suggests that bone functions as a starling resister, likening osteonecrosis to a compartment syndrome within bone. The starling resister concept requires that blood flow depends on external pressure. The femoral head acts as a closed osseous compartment in which increased intravenous pressures cause a venous outflow obstruction and secondary ischemia. This outflow obstruction may be secondary to fat cell hypertrophy causing increased pressure in the closed osseous compartment and resulting in venous congestion and decreased outflow. In a study by Warner and colleagues, however, in which high-dose steroids were administered to rabbits, no significant elevation of intramedullary pressure or venous outflow resistance was found, suggesting the possibility of a direct cytotoxic effect of steroids on osteocytes.

Therefore, the etiology of idiopathic AVN may be multifactorial and includes arterial insufficiency, venous occlusion, intravascular or extravascular sinusoidal occlusion, and direct cytotoxic effects. In contrast to the elderly patient with posttraumatic AVN in whom surgery generally is reconstructive, the patient with idiopathic AVN is generally younger, and the goal is to preserve, not to replace, the femoral head. A primary goal, therefore, must be early diagnosis.

Diagnosis

HISTORY. Many patients are completely asymptomatic in the early stages of AVN. When symptoms do develop, they are generally associated with a *crescent sign* (a radiolucent crescent below and parallel to the articular surface), subchondral collapse, or gross flattening of the articular surgery. These findings are all thought to be secondary to fracture of bone (subchondral plate), and they usually manifest as pain, limp, and decreased painful range of motion. Some patients may develop symptoms before any radiographic change, and these may be secondary to increased intraosseous pressure or microfracture.

The most common cause of AVN is trauma secondary to either fracture or dislocation. Nontraumatic AVN, however, has been shown to be associated with a number of conditions. The most common of these are the use of systemic corticosteroids, excessive alcohol use, and sickle cell disease. Ficat and Arlet divided these relations into definite and probable (Table 15-2). Determination of these factors is important in obtaining a thorough patient history.

PHYSICAL EXAMINATION. Findings on physical examination are generally nonspecific. The patient may have decreased or painful range of motion, a limp, or muscle weakness. Limb shortening may be present if gross femoral head collapse has occurred. As always, a general examination is mandatory to rule out findings suggestive of a more generalized arthritic or systemic disorder.

LABORATORY FINDINGS. Laboratory findings are generally within normal limits. They are useful in ruling out other systemic disorders. In black patients, a test for sickle cell disease should be performed.

IMAGING TECHNIQUES. A variety of techniques are available for the diagnosis of AVN, including plain radiographs, tomograms, CT scan, technetium bone scan, single-photon emission computed tomography, and MRI. Radiographs of the hip must include both AP and lateral projections; the lateral radiograph is most sensitive in detecting early flattening or the crescent sign within the femoral head. Every case of bone necrosis passes through a preradiographic phase, and therefore, early in the course of the disease, the radiographs are normal. When radiographic changes do appear, they are due to the reaction of living bone to the ischemia. Varying amounts of osteopenia may occur initially in association with cystic or sclerotic changes within the femoral head. The development of the crescent sign is secondary to subchondral bony collapse and manifests as a radiolucent crescent below and parallel to the articular surface or subchondral bone. These changes are thought to be secondary to subchondral resorption of dead bone with revascularization and new bone formation. Investigators have postulated that the progression of disease results from this mixture of osteoblastic new bone formation and osteoclastic resorption, with the latter predominantly in the subchondral area. This results in weakening of the subchondral bony plate and leads to microfracture and collapse. Finally, varying degrees of femoral head collapse lead to flattening and obvious loss of femoral head congruency, joint space narrowing, acetabular involvement, and frank degenerative change. Tomograms are useful in outlining the extent and location of infarct and in determining the status of the articular surface and subchondral bony plate.

TECHNETIUM BONE SCAN. Technetium bone scanning is useful in helping to diagnosis AVN. The initial phases of the avascular process during which the ischemic necrosis takes place are generally clinically silent, and the patient is asymptomatic. Therefore, decreased uptake is generally not found. Rather, patients are often in the reparative phase of osteonecrosis, and the scans usually demonstrate the increased activity of new bone formation. Occasionally, there can be both increased and decreased areas of

TABLE 15-2.
Etiologic Associations in Avascular Necrosis

DEFINITE
Major trauma
Caisson disease
Sickle cell disease
Postirradiation
Major arterial disease
Gaucher disease

PROBABLE
Minor trauma
Steroid associated
Hyperuricemia
Venous occlusion
Lipodystrophies (including alcoholism)
Connective tissue disease
Osteoporosis or osteomalacia

(Ficat RP, Arlet J. In: Hungerford DS, ed. Ischaemia and necrosis of bone. Baltimore, Williams & Wilkins, 1980)

isotope activity within the femoral head. Few conditions produce decreased activity, and therefore, diminished radioisotope activity within the femoral head is virtually diagnostic of AVN.

COMPUTED TOMOGRAPHY. CT scans, like tomograms, can be useful in specifically identifying the extent and location of the infarct and in helping to determine articular surface involvement. They may also identify changes in the femoral head sooner than plain radiographs.

MAGNETIC RESONANCE IMAGING. MRI is being used with increasing frequency and has been found to have greater sensitivity and accuracy in the diagnosis of AVN than both technetium bone scanning and CT scanning. MRI scanning depends on the hydrogen ion content within tissue. Bone marrow generally has a strong signal secondary to its hydrogen-rich fat content. MRI scanning, therefore, is able to detect early signal reduction in AVN as decreases in hydrogen ion content occur with the osteonecrosis, revascularization, and new bone formation (Fig. 15-11).

OTHER DIAGNOSTIC TECHNIQUES. Investigators described the use of direct intraosseous pressure measurements and intraosseous venography in the diagnosis of AVN and reported that these studies are sensitive in the detection of early AVN. Others,

however, were unable to reproduce these results and found these methods to be no more useful than technetium bone scanning. Additionally, these methods suffer from the concomitant increased risks of invasive techniques. With the increasing accuracy of MRI, their usefulness is diminishing. Occasionally, biopsy may be required to confirm the diagnosis.

Staging

The staging of AVN is important because it helps guide and serve as a basis for treatment.

Staging systems for AVN developed out of the recognition that radiographic, pathologic, and clinical findings occur in a generally accepted sequence of events that describes the evolution of femoral head change. There are two commonly used radiographic staging systems. Ficat and Arlet classified AVN into five stages (Table 15-3):

Stage 0: This stage refers to a hip that is both clinically and radiographically normal. This is a preclinical condition whose only pathologic finding is that of increased intraosseous pressure.

Stage 1: This is the earliest point in the disease at which clinical manifestations are appreciated. These findings generally include pain and a limited range of motion of the hip. The pain generally is in the groin, is occasionally

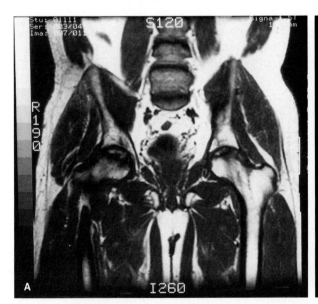
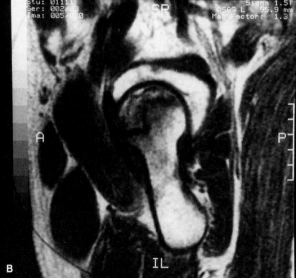

FIGURE 15-11. (A) MRI scan of a 39-year-old black man who developed a bilateral avascular necrosis of the hips. The MRI study illustrates the area of the infarct bilaterally that involves the superior weight-bearing area of the femoral head. (B) The significance of its size is illustrated on the transverse section, with nearly the entire anterior aspect of the femoral head being involved with necrotic revascularizing bone.

TABLE 15-3.
Staging of Avascular Necrosis

Stage	Description	Radiographic Findings
0	Fat embolism Intraosseous vascular occlusion Inflammatory Focal intravascular coagulation	Normal
1	Osteonecrosis	Normal to patchy, small areas of increased density
2	Revascularization	Round head, sclerotic area adjacent to articular surface
3	Collapse and deformity	Crescent sign and collapse, flattening, sequestrum formation
4	Degenerative change	Joint incongruity, joint line narrowing, general findings of degenerative change

(Lange TA. Staging of aseptic necrosis. In: Bassett FH, ed. Instructional course lectures, vol 37. Park Ridge, IL, American Academy of Orthopaedic Surgeons, 1988:33)

associated with radiation to the thigh, and is seen in about half of cases. Examination of the hip may reveal limited motion, especially medial internal rotation and abduction. Standard AP and lateral radiographs are usually normal. There may be subtle changes in blurring of the trabecular pattern or patchy osteoporosis in comparison to the opposite side, but these changes generally are not significant. Therefore, this stage also is for the most part a preradiographic stage.

Stage 2: In this stage, the clinical findings of pain and decreased range of motion persist, and the initial radiographic findings appear. The radiographs show changes in the trabecular pattern of the femoral head as well as possible findings of osteoporosis, sclerosis, or cystic formation. Stage 2 disease has also been divided into substages 2A and 2B in an attempt to identify the transition phase to stage 3. In stage 2A, there is no flattening of the femoral head, and the femoral head maintains a normal joint line and normal articular surface contour. Additionally, stage 2A may be qualified as predominantly sclerotic or predominantly cystic, depending on the overall appearance of the femoral head. Stage 2B disease represents the transition phase, is heralded by the appearance of the crescent sign, and is the predecessor to early flattening of the femoral head, which also may initially be present in stage 2B disease.

Stage 3: Stage 3 is characterized by the pathognomonic appearance of a sequestrum within the femoral head. The normal contour of the femoral head is now broken, and flattening is present. Varying degrees of femoral collapse may be present, but the joint space is pre-

served. Clinical findings include increasing pain and loss of motion as well as progressive functional incapacity and limp.

Stage 4: This is the final stage of AVN and is characterized by progressive loss of articular cartilage, narrowing joint space, and involvement of the acetabulum. There may be worsening flattening or collapse of the femoral head. The clinical findings are that of advanced osteoarthritis.

The Ficat system is essentially descriptive and does not grade or evaluate the extent of the disease process.

Steinberg and colleagues presented a grading system that quantitates the extent and type of femoral head involvement. Table 15-4 summarizes the Steinberg grading system.

Treatment

The goal of all treatment is to arrest the progression of the disease and to prevent late collapse of the femoral head and the development of progressive degenerative arthritis. The type of treatment is in part dependent on the stage at which the disease is diagnosed. The goal of all treatment, especially in younger patients, is to try to preserve or salvage the normal femoral head and prevent degenerative change.

Nonoperative treatment has been shown to be ineffective in the treatment of AVN. In a group of patients treated nonoperatively with both normal weight bearing and restricted weight bearing, regardless of the weight bearing status, the overall progression rate of disease was 92%. Of those hips

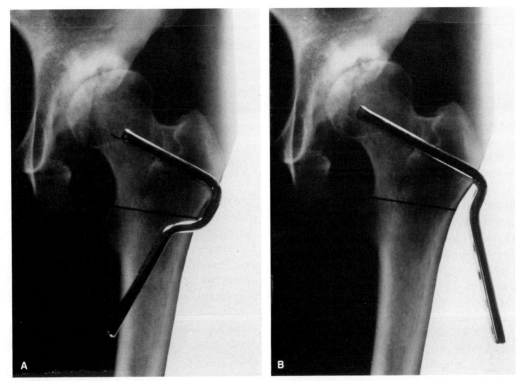

FIGURE 15-15. Depending on whether varus (A) or valgus (B) correction is desired, the suitable angled blade plate is chosen.

Varus Osteotomy

The classic radiographic candidate for varus osteotomy is the patient whose hip has a spherical femoral head, moderate or absent acetabular dysplasia (a center edge angle of at least 15 to 20 degrees), signs of lateral overloading of the sourcil (the acetabular subchondral bone plate), and a valgus neck–shaft angle of more than 135 degrees. If radiographs in abduction demonstrate improved congruency of the hip, then varus osteotomy may be indicated. By performing varus osteotomy with medial shaft displacement, the abductors, psoas, and adductors are relatively relaxed, thus unloading the hip joint, and the weight-bearing surface is increased. Medial shaft displacement of 10 to 15 mm is desirable not only to decrease the force of the abductors but also to keep the ipsilateral knee centered over the femoral head. Appropriately selected candidates achieved long-term, good to excellent results in over 90% of cases. Varus osteotomy carries with it, however, the certainty of 1 cm of shortening, the presence of a Trendelenburg gait for about 1 year, and a prominent greater trochanter. Patients must be aware of the longer convalescent period intrinsic to this operation.

Valgus Osteotomy

When the femoral head is no longer spherical, the goals of decreasing unit load and improving congruency may be achieved by a valgus osteotomy. Osteophytes that form in predictable locations on the femoral head and acetabulum are exploited to achieve the desired results. The capital drop and inferior cervical osteophytes of the femoral neck are brought into contact with the floor osteophytes of the acetabulum by adduction of the hip. With these osteophytes serving as a fulcrum, the superior and lateral joint space is widened. An assessment of the magnitude of correction can be obtained by examination under fluoroscopy, tracings, or radiographs obtained in various degrees of hip adduction. Sufficient valgus correction should be done so that lateral traction on the superior capsule results in the stimulation of formation of the roof osteophytes. Pain relief is achieved by: (1) unloading the hip joint (abductor and psoas relaxation), (2) changing the bone-on-bone contact from the painful innervated superior femoral head and acetabulum to the noninnervated medial osteophyte, (3) decreasing the lever arm body weight by shifting it medially to the new center of rotation of the femoral head, the osteophytes, and

(4) improving the congruity of the joint and thus increasing the weight-bearing surface. Further long-term improvement may come from the formation of the roof osteophyte, which further increases the weight-bearing surface and cartilage healing.

Extension

In addition to the angular correction in the coronal plane, correction in the sagittal plane can increase the effectiveness of osteotomy. Biplane correction is desirable for two reasons. First, in acetabular dysplasia, the femoral head is uncovered not only laterally (the frontal plane) but anteriorly (the sagittal plane). Better coverage is achieved by correction in both planes. Second, fixed flexion contractures can be eliminated by extension correction to a degree at least equal to the magnitude of the flexion contracture. By doing so, the functional arc of motion is returned to within the anatomic arc, and an important source of pain and impingement is removed. The use of the term *extension* is often confusing. Extension refers to the angular correction of the femur in the sagittal plane after osteotomy. Thus, with extension, the apex of the angle is directed anteriorly. To achieve this correction, the femur is flexed to the desired degree, the osteotomy is performed, and then the distal fragment is brought parallel to the floor, thus achieving the extension correction. Thus, the proximal fragment is flexed, but the final angular correction of the femur is said to be extended.

Rotation

Patients with dysplastic hips usually have a constellation of anatomic variation on the pelvic and femoral sides of the joint. The acetabulum is deficient both laterally and anteriorly; the femoral neck is in excessive valgus (greater than 135 degrees); anteversion is increased. The true degree of femoral anteversion (and hence the true neck–shaft valgus) can be determined by fluoroscopic or other methods. It is likely that a neck–shaft angle of 150 degrees seen on AP radiograph is in reality a combination of a 140- to 145-degree neck–shaft angle and a 25-degree femoral anteversion. Preoperative planning for a varus extension osteotomy should allow for 10 to 15 degrees of rotation (leave 15 degrees of residual internal rotation to allow for normal gait) and varus correction of 10 to 20 degrees.

Limb Alignment and Limb Length

The planning of the intertrochanteric osteotomy must include an assessment of leg lengths and the effects of osteotomy on the mechanical axis of the limb. Of particular interest is the effect of hip alignment on the ipsilateral knee. When varus osteotomy is performed, a medial shaft displacement is required, so that mechanical axis of the extremity remains through the center of the knee. Similarly, in valgus osteotomy, lateral shaft displacement is required.

Hip Arthrodesis

The increasing success of total-hip arthroplasty has expanded its indications to increasingly younger patient populations. However, the procedure of choice for adolescent and young adult patients with unilateral, noninflammatory, end-stage hip disease not amenable to osteotomy remains hip arthrodesis. Successful hip arthrodesis allows durable, pain-free function at nearly normal levels of physical activity, including manual labor. In a time of increasing patient demand and a near panacean attitude regarding the outcome of total-hip arthroplasty, we need only remember the increasing frequency and complexity of revision total-hip arthroplasty to remind us of the potential outcome when prosthetic devices are placed in patients whose functional demands exceed the mechanical and physiologic limitations of the prosthetic device. Only when patients have been fully informed of both the advantages and disadvantages of total-hip arthroplasty and hip arthrodesis, as well as realistic functional limitations regarding activity with these two procedures, can an informed and appropriate treatment decision be reached.

Indications and Contraindications

A freely mobile and disease-free spine, ipsilateral knee joint, and contralateral hip joint are prerequisites for successful hip arthrodesis. The most common indication for hip arthrodesis is arthritis of the hip joint in young, active patients. Causes may include arthritis secondary to sepsis or osteomyelitis, failed osteotomy, failed cup arthroplasty, posttraumatic arthritis, or arthritis secondary to congenital or childhood hip diseases such as slipped capital femoral epiphysis, Legg-Calvé-Perthes disease, or congenital hip dislocation. AVN may also be an indication for hip arthrodesis; however, one must bear in mind the frequency with which AVN is bilateral and the difficulty that exists in trying to achieve fusion when dealing with avascular bone.

Contraindications to hip arthrodesis include significant loss of motion or advanced degenerative changes in the ipsilateral knee, contralateral hip, or lumbar spine. Bilateral hip arthrodesis is contraindicated, but fusion on one side with total-hip replacement on the contralateral side is a procedure that may deserve consideration. Active infection also is a contraindication to this procedure.

It is imperative that the patient be made aware of the functional limitations that will exist on the patient's occupation and life-style as a result of having a fused hip. These limitations must be contrasted with a frank discussion regarding the potential long-term complications of total-hip arthroplasty in young, active patients. When this is accomplished, the patient can become an active participant in the decision-making process.

A variety of operative techniques exist for achieving hip arthrodesis. Hip arthrodeses are increasingly being converted to total-hip arthroplasties once patients reach a suitable age; therefore, one of the important issues in deciding operative technique for achieving hip fusion is the management of the abductor musculature. If future conversion to total-hip arthroplasty is a consideration, efforts to maintain the abductor muscles may prove beneficial. Investigators reported satisfactory results in 31 of 33 patients who underwent such a conversion, with unlimited walking ability being achieved in 28 patients.

Methods that preserve the abductor musculature include the use of Barr bolts. In this technique, the hip is dislocated, and the femoral head and acetabulum are denuded of cartilage down to bleeding bony surfaces. Fixation is then achieved using bolts that cross the greater trochanter, the femoral neck, and then the ilium, where nuts are placed on the inner pelvis. This transarticular bolting does not require pelvic, femoral, or trochanteric osteotomy and preserves abductor musculature. Postoperatively, a hip spica cast is necessary.

Alternatively, cobra plate fixation has been used to rigidly fix the hip fusion construct. This requires both pelvic and trochanteric osteotomy. The distal fragment of the pelvis is displaced medially, and after appropriate preparation of the femoral head, the femoral head and femur are firmly secured beneath the iliac wing with a laterally placed cobra plate. This type of fixation does not require supplementary cast fixation, but it is significantly more traumatic to the abductor musculature.

The optimal position for hip arthrodesis is neutral to slight adduction (about 5 degrees), 35 to 40 degrees of hip flexion, and neutral to 5 degrees of external rotation.

Results

A review was conducted of the long-term results of hip arthrodesis in young patients. The average age at the time of fusion was 14 years, and the average duration of arthrodesis was 38 years. Overall, 78% of patients were satisfied with the results of their arthrodesis, and many were employed in strenuous occupations. Some level of low-back discomfort was seen in 57% of patients, and some knee discomfort occurred in 45% of patients. Overall, 13% of patients had conversion to a total-hip arthroplasty for these problems. Arthroplasty was valuable in relieving the low-back discomfort but not in relieving knee discomfort.

Another long-term follow-up of hip arthrodesis found that most patients could function at a higher level for many years and were able to work in most occupations. Back and knee pain were common after long follow-up, but these symptoms were usually not incapacitating.

Total-Hip Arthroplasty

Total-hip arthroplasty has been an extremely successful procedure for adult patients with hip disease. This remains, however, a nonbiologic solution, carrying with it the risk of complications and the questions of long-term implant survivability, implant wear, biocompatibility, and host bone response. The options in total-hip arthroplasty include cemented and cementless (bioingrowth) techniques.

Indications

The ideal candidate for total-hip arthroplasty is an elderly patient with hip disease that causes a level of pain and disability unresponsive to conservative measures, significantly impairing the patient's quality of life and warranting the risk of the surgical procedure. Patients younger than 60 years of age, those involved in strenuous activities, and patients with histories of previous hip infection are generally considered poor candidates for total-hip arthroplasty, and aggressive conservative treatment, fusion, or osteotomy should be considered. Many patients younger than 60 years of age with disabling hip symptoms, however, are unresponsive to conservative treatment and have disease and bony anatomy that preclude surgical options other than total-hip replacement. Their quality of life may be so encumbered as to warrant the risk of this procedure. Reports of high failure rates of cemented total-hip arthroplasty in young, active patients have been the impetus for the surge of cementless techniques for total-hip replacement. It may well be appropriate to proceed with cementless total-hip replacement in these patients, but only with the full knowledge that the long-term questions of implant longevity, implant biocompatibility, long-term polyethylene wear, and long-term response of bone to the presence of a cementless implant remain at this time unanswered.

Cemented Total-Hip Arthroplasty

Much of the orthopaedic literature regarding cemented total-hip arthroplasty is conflicting and controversial. Problems in comparison between variations in basic clinical and radiographic evaluations and the lack of standardized definitions for failure and success contribute to these controversies. Many reports have varying patient populations, use varying prosthetic implants, and include large numbers of patients lost to follow-up, making the observed failure rates difficult to interpret. Additionally, many reports represent the results of surgeons early in their experience with cemented total-hip replacement. In an attempt to account for some of these problems, survivorship analysis has been used to try to predict longitudinally the incidence of failure of a prosthesis. Unfortunately, standardized criteria to define component failure are poorly established, with most reports using revision surgery as the criterion for component failure and not including other clinical and radiographic parameters that may help identify failure in a patient who did not undergo arthroplasty. Therefore, when making comparisons within the orthopaedic literature, it is important to define the patient population, the type of prosthesis used, and the criteria used to determine success or failure. Finally, the cause of failure must be differentiated among the femoral, the acetabular, and both components; among implant, polyethylene, and polymethyl methacrylate (PMMA) failure; and among mechanical loosening, infection, dislocation, and fracture.

Intermediate and long-term follow-up of the original Mueller prosthesis indicates a significant percentage of failure and revision. Using component migration as a criteria for radiographic failure, one author found an overall incidence of aseptic loosening of 29% for the acetabular and 40% for the femoral component at an average 10-year follow-up. Long-term follow-up reports of the original Charnley prosthesis, on the other hand, have more encouraging results. Unfortunately, critical analysis of these reports reveal that they suffer from many of the shortcomings previously outlined. Nevertheless, the results indicate relatively good results with cemented Charnley-type total-hip arthroplasty using what would be considered poor cement techniques by today's standards. The results presented in Table 15-6 indicate that there is about a 90% success rate with cemented Charnley total-hip arthroplasty in an elderly patient population at 10-year follow-up. The data, however, also reveal an increased percentage of radiographic component loosening, suggesting a higher impending failure rate. The wide range of reported values is probably best explained by differences in clinical and radiographic interpretation. Nevertheless, it appears that, of surviving prostheses, between an additional 5% and 30% of femoral and acetabular components have worrisome radiographic findings at 10-year follow-up.

In a group of patients undergoing revision for aseptic loosening, plain radiographs predicted only 36% of actual loose acetabular components. The clinical significance of these findings is unclear, with some authors finding little correlation and others finding significant clinical correlation, especially on the acetabular side. Even though many radiographic loose components may clinically provide satisfactory function, however, it is clear that the rate of clinical failure progressively increases in the presence of loose components. Most data indicate that femoral component loosening is nonlinear and decreases with time, while acetabular component loosening increases linearly with time (Fig. 15-16).

Young, active patients are especially susceptible to failure of cemented devices. About a 20% revision rate in cemented total-hip arthroplasty occurred in young patients at 5-year follow-up. Based on radiographic review, significantly higher percentages of impending failures occurred, especially on the acetabular side. Poor results were also reported when using cemented, metal-backed acetabular components in patients younger than 30 years of age, with 9 of 10 patients developing loosening at average 11-year follow-up. High failure rates were associated with young age, previous diagnosis of AVN, previously failed hemiarthroplasty, previously failed cup arthroplasty, heavy activity, and increased weight.

TABLE 15-6.
Results of Cemented Total Hip Arthroplasty

Study	Hips		Diagnosis				Follow-up (y)	Mean Age (y)	Radiographic Failures	Clinical Failures (Revised)
	At Operation	At Follow-Up	OA	RA	AVN	Other				
Eftekhar, 1971	256	128	76	31	0	13	7–8	66	No femoral loosening observed	5% (1.4% acetabular loosening; 3.6% infection)
Charnley, 1972	338	210	70	26	0	4	4–7	60s	?	4.8% (1% acetabular loosening; 3.8% infection)
Charnley & Cupic, 1973	185	106	66	27	0	7	9–10	65	?	9.6% (2% acetabular loosening; 1% femoral loosening; 6.6% infection)
Charnley, 1977	396	138	68*	31	0	1	13.2	?	112 reviewed had 25% grade III & IV acetabular changes†	5% (1.5% mechanical failure; 3.5% infection)
Stauffer, 1982	333	231	56	7.5	3	33.5	10	63.6	36.8% (29.9% femoral; 11.3% acetabular)‡	8.2%
Johnston, 1983	326	178	?	?	?	?	10	?	16.9% (9% femoral; 7.6% acetabular)§	1.5% (aseptic loosening)
Older, 1986	215	153	93	0.5	0.5	6	11	67	15% loose acetabulum (grades III & IV)†	6% (2% aseptic loosening)
Brady, 1986	352	170	58	5	14	23	10	60.8	?	8.8%
Jinnah, 1986	149	39	43.4	15.4	11.9	19.3	10	63	Possible loosening: 25.3% acetabular; 22.8% femoral∥	10.8% using survivorship analysis; 12.4% observed failure rate
Dall, 1986	470	98	76	4	4	16	12	61.4	6.1%	14.3% (9.2% acetabular failure; 4.1% femoral failure)
McCoy, 1988	100	40	50	22.5	5	17	15	60	50% had radiolucencies or cement failure	9.2% using survivorship analysis
Hozack, 1990	1139	1041	—	—	—	—	10	65	25% acetabular; 9.6% femoral	3.5%
Johnston, 1993	330	322	74	5	1	20	20	60	22% acetabular; 7% femoral	13% acetabular; 6% femoral

OA, osteoarthritis; RA, rheumatoid arthritis; AVN, avascular necrosis.

* 14.6% had previous surgery.

† Grade III: severe demarcation (circumferential lucency); grade IV: migration.

‡ Femoral failure: (1) any prosthesis–cement lucency, (2) complete bone–cement lucency, (3) migration. Acetabular failure: (1) lucency > 1 mm around entire acetabulum, (2) migration.

§ Femoral failure: (1) lucency > 2 mm in any zone, (2) cement failure, (3) migration. Acetabular failure: (1) lucency around 80%–100% of component with some portion > 2 mm, (2) migration.

∥ Possible femoral loosening: (1) any prosthesis–cement lucency, (2) 50% of bone–cement lucency with a minimal width > 1 mm. Possible acetabular loosening: complete cement–bone lucency with a maximal width > 2 mm.

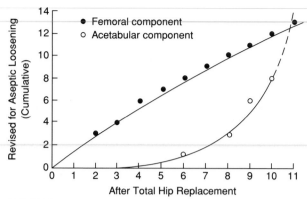

FIGURE 15-16. Cumulative revisions required for loosening of the femoral and the acetabular components over time. (Sutherland CJ, Wilde AH, Borden LS, Marks KE. A ten year follow-up of one hundred consecutive Muller curved-stem total hip replacement arthroplasties. J Bone Joint Surg 1982;64A:970)

The increased failure rates in young patients and the high percentage of worrisome radiographic changes, especially as seen on both the femoral and acetabular side of total-hip arthroplasty, prompted the development of improved cement technique and component design. These improvements include better preparation of the bony surfaces to receive cement, plugging the femoral canal, improved cement introduction techniques (cement gun), improved component designs, and preparation techniques that improve the mechanical properties of cement, thus increasing its fatigue life (vacuum-mixing centrifugation and canal pressurization). Figure 15-17 represents a radiographic example of improved cemented techniques on the femoral side.

Using these improved cementing techniques, the reported radiographic and clinical results for the femoral component have been dramatically improved. Using contemporary cementing techniques, one author reported a 1.1% incidence of definitely loose femoral components (evidence of migration, appearance of cement mantle crack, or stem fracture); a 0% incidence of probably loose femoral components (continuous radiolucent line at the bone–cement interface not present on the immediate postoperative radiograph); and a 4% incidence of possibly loose femoral components (development of 50% or more radiolucent lines at the bone–cement interface) at average 3.3-year follow-up. In a later review of hybrid total-hip arthroplasty (cementless acetabular and cemented femoral components), the same author reported a 0% incidence of femoral loosening at 3.5-year follow-up. Another investigator reported a 2%

femoral loosening rate at 5-year follow-up, and in a review comparing a matched group of early cement technique and a later group of cemented femoral components using contemporary techniques, still another investigator found a 21% incidence of definitely loose femoral components in the early group compared with 0% definitely or probably loose and only 4% possibly loose femoral components in a later group. These authors also found that the rate of loosening was in part technique dependent, with femoral component loosening correlating with excessive malpositioning (greater than 5 degrees of varus or valgus) of components and inadequate cement mantle, especially in zone 4 at the tip of the femoral prosthesis. Interestingly, a minimal 20-year review of total-hip arthroplasty performed by a single surgeon adhering to the design and surgical concepts of the original Charnley prosthesis produced remarkable results, especially on the femoral side. With excellent clinical follow-up (98%) using combined radiographic loosening or revision arthroplasty as an endpoint for failure, only 7% of femoral components and 22% of acetabular components had loosened, with 85% of patients retaining their original prosthesis. Similar findings regarding a large group with the Charnley prosthesis also were confirmed, with a 92% survivorship of the prosthesis at 10 years.

The issues of collared versus collarless, cobalt-chromium versus titanium, and anatomic versus straight femoral components are ongoing and undecided. It appears, however, that improved cementing techniques have improved the results of cemented femoral components. It also appears reasonable to extrapolate the previously reported finding that femoral component loosening is nonlinear, decreasing with time, to contemporarily cemented femoral components, suggesting that a lower early failure rate will also result in a lower late failure rate.

The reports on cemented acetabular components are more conflicting. Several authors reported excellent long-term results with cemented acetabular components in select groups of elderly patients. One author, however, reported a 25% incidence of radiographic loosening of cemented acetabular components at 10- to 14-year follow-up, and another reported a loosening rate of 29% at 10-year follow-up. Loosening of cemented acetabular components may be associated with significant bone stock deficiency, making revision surgery technically more difficult and the results less predictable. In comparison with the femur, the acetabular bony geometry makes it less

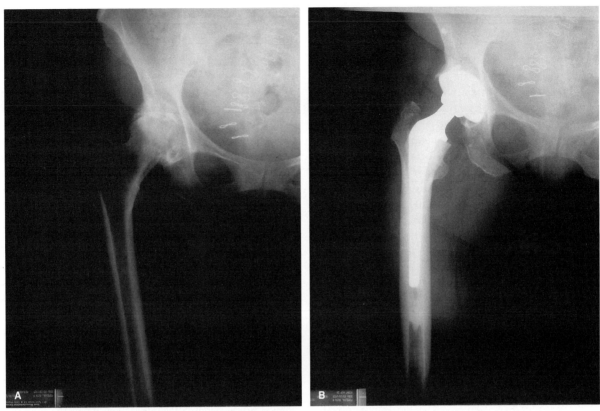

FIGURE 15-17. Preoperative (A) and postoperative (B) radiographs in a 67-year-old woman with osteoarthritis of the right hip joint. The patient underwent a hybrid total hip arthroplasty with uncemented acetabular component and cemented femoral component. The femoral side illustrates cement technique that can be achieved with plugging of the femoral canal, vacuum mixing of methyl methacrylate, and pressurization injection techniques into the proximal femur.

amenable to significant improvements in cement techniques. Preventing the lamination of blood with cement and preserving the subchondral bone plate are important in improving cemented acetabular results, and many surgeons have adopted these principles. Additionally, finite element analysis suggests that metal backing of a polyethylene acetabular component stiffens the component and allows for a more uniform distribution of stress. This redistribution of stress reduces the magnitude of peak stresses within the surrounding PMMA, trabecular bone, and subchondral bone. Additionally, the use of a metal shell makes the component modular, which allows exchange of polyethylene liners. These advantages must be weighed, however, against the knowledge that metal backing of an acetabular component reduces the available space for polyethylene, thereby decreasing the potential thickness of the polyethylene acetabular liner. This problem is increased in cemented applications, in which appropriately thick

mantles further decrease the diameter of any acetabular implant. Decreased polyethylene thickness is associated with accelerated wear rates and increased polyethylene debris; investigations suggested this may be associated with significant osteolytic changes. Therefore, questions regarding metal backing, all polyethylene cups, femoral head implant size, and minimal cement mantle and polyethylene thickness remain controversial.

Despite these improvements, a 6% aseptic loosening rate of cemented metal-backed acetabular components was reported in a group of relatively young patients (average age 41 years) at average follow-up of 6.5 years. In a study on the same group of patients at an average 11.3-year follow-up, the revision rate for aseptic acetabular loosening increased to 12.5%. Overall, 41% of patients had either loosened components or showed radiographic evidence of loosening. In patients older than 30 years of age, 14% showed radiographic evidence of loosening, but none had been revised. A 7.5% aseptic loosening rate was reported in a group of relatively young patients (average age, 44 years) at average follow-up of 7.6 years. Therefore, despite the addition of metal backing to the acetabular component, as well as improvements in bone and cement preparation, failure rates of cemented acetabular components, especially in younger patients, remain unacceptably high. Additionally, a study in which the only variable was the presence or absence of metal backing in a cemented acetabular component revealed that metal backing actually led to a significantly higher failure rate for radiolucency, loosening, and revision. At 5.2-year follow-up, only 2% of all polyethylene cemented components required revision, giving a somewhat contrary viewpoint regarding the efficacy of metal backing. In summary, the previously reported worrisome linear failure rate of cemented acetabular components suggests an increased failure rate of even contemporarily cemented acetabular designs (metal and nonmetal backed), leading to the increasing use of cementless acetabular techniques.

Cementless Total-Hip Arthroplasty

Most investigators in the United States have adopted the principle of microporosity when applying cementless techniques to total-hip arthroplasty. This principle involves applying a porous coating to an implant that theoretically allows actual bone ingrowth into the open pore structure as the basis to achieve lasting fixation. Investigative work in this area has included the search for optimal metal alloys, ingrowth surfaces, and implant designs. All designs, however, must have an optimal pore size and achieve initial rigid fixation and intimate bony apposition to achieve bone ingrowth.

A number of animal studies documented the ability of bone to grow into porous surfaces. This work defined the ideal pore characteristics of the surface to allow for bone ingrowth. It has been determined that a minimal pore size of 100 μm is necessary for bone ingrowth and that a pore size in the range of 200 to 450 μm is required for haversian remodeling to occur, allowing the optimal mechanical strength for bone prosthesis fixation.

The most commonly used metal super alloys are cobalt-chromium (Co-Cr-Mo) and titanium (Ti-6AL-4V) alloys. Both alloys have demonstrated excellent biocompatibility. Porous materials are used as a surface layer bonded to these solid alloy components to form a composite prosthetic device. The most widely used ingrowth surfaces are cobalt-chromium–beaded surfaces, titanium beaded or wire mesh surfaces, or titanium alloy plasma-sprayed surfaces. Cobalt-chromium beads are applied to the underlying component by gravity sintering, which requires high temperatures to fuse the porous material onto the underlying substrate. Because of the high temperatures required, changes can occur in the microstructure of the substrate that may adversely affect its fatigue strength. Titanium alloy is also susceptible to degradation of fatigue properties by sintering heat; therefore, titanium beads or wire mesh (fiber metal) are generally applied by diffusion bonding, which incorporates both heat and pressure to fuse the porous material to the substrate, allowing for relatively lower temperatures and fewer microstructural alterations. Both materials, however, are of concern because the coating process affects the fatigue characteristics of femoral components. Because of the generally much larger size of ingrowth femoral components that is necessary to achieve intimate bony contact and rigid fixation, however, fatigue failure has not been a significant clinical problem. Cobalt-chrome and titanium also are different in their relative stiffness. The modulus of elasticity of cobalt-chrome is two times greater than that of titanium. Because the stiffness of a component varies as the fourth power of its radius, however, most ingrowth components are of sufficient size to be an order of magnitude stiffer than cortical bone, thus raising the question of the significance of the difference in the modulus of elasticity of a component as it affects the stress transfer and long-term bony remodeling around an implant.

A third method of achieving a porous surface, titanium plasma spraying, uses a presurgical gas mixture to spray a molten mixture of titanium onto the implant. The substrate does not undergo intensive direct heating, which would result in weakening of the metal. The characteristics of the porous surface are controlled through variations in particle size and pressure. When compared with bead or meshed surfaces, the resulting porosity is generally more limited, but this has not proved to be a problem clinically.

A variety of cementless designs have been used. The early experience with these designs leaves us with some uncertainty as to the relative importance of a number of design variables. Controversy exists regarding the use of cobalt-chrome versus titanium, straight versus anatomic femoral stems, collared versus collarless femoral stems, ingrowth surfaces, and other questions about the size, shape, and geometry of prostheses. As the debate continues, a general conclusion that can be drawn from previous work is that clinical results improve with the degree of fit achieved at surgery. It also was shown that distal fixation using fully porous-coated femoral stems may produce deleterious proximal bone resorption secondary to undesirable stress transfers.

Animal research demonstrated that relative displacements between the implant and surrounding host bone in excess of 30 μm inhibit bone formation within porous-coated implant surfaces. Rather, a well-organized fibrous tissue connective layer develops. A canine cementless acetabulum study showed that initial bone prosthesis apposition gaps in excess of 0.5 mm resulted in significantly less bone ingrowth. These findings raise questions about what actually is necessary to achieve a successful ingrowth prosthesis. It appears that successful biologic fixation is probably a combination of some limited bony ingrowth with additional extensive fibrous tissue ingrowth. Human retrieval analysis studies of total-hip arthroplasties are limited. A review demonstrated that bone ingrowth does occur into both beaded and fiber metal surfaces but that large areas of fibrous tissue generally also occur. One author described bony ingrowth into the distal aspects of fully coated prostheses where the prosthesis contacted the endosteal cortical surface.

Additional concerns regarding ion release from the significantly increased surface areas of ingrowth components have led some to investigate other implant surfaces. One author reported histologic analysis that occurred around stable press-fit Moore-type (smooth-surface) implants. This author found a relatively benign fibrous-type membrane with a fibrocartilaginous response in areas under compressive load. Another group investigated implant designs using press-fit techniques without ingrowth surfaces. Other surfaces under investigation also include hydroxyapatite coatings, with initial encouraging results.

The structure of synthetic hydroxyapatites is similar to that of naturally occurring hydroxyapatites found in bone. Studies of titanium alloy implants that are plasma sprayed with a 50-μm layer of hydroxyapatite found the hydroxyapatite to be mechanically stable. Animal and clinical studies in this area showed accelerated and enhanced apposition of bone to the implants without an intervening layer of fibrous tissue. D'Antonio reported a minimal 2-year follow-up of 92 proximally coated titanium femoral implants with excellent clinical and radiographic results. No local or systemic toxicity to hydroxyapatite was found, yet concern remains for this type of implant because the material was shown to be slowly resorbed by biologic tissues, and the long-term mechanical stability of the coating remains unanswered.

A study reported on two cases of loosened, cementless cobalt-chromium femoral components, which resulted in local metallosis with elevated serum levels of cobalt and an aggressive inflammatory reaction characterized by multinucleated foreign body–type giant cells. The authors compared this to metallic debris released in a similar manner observed with metal on metal-type replacements. High local levels of metal can develop and are associated with the possible problems of sensitivity, inflammation response, and systemic toxicity. Researchers described two-fold increases in serum titanium levels in patients with loose titanium femoral components.

Of more serious concern is the speculation that elevated levels of metallic debris may be carcinogenic. A direct association of metal implants and malignant change have been extremely difficult to establish in humans, but there have been several reports of tumors developing in patients with total-hip arthroplasties. Figure 15-18 is an example of a cementless device.

CLINICAL REPORTS. Reports reviewing the clinical results of cementless total-hip arthroplasties have been limited. These reports must be compared with the cemented results that can be obtained using contemporarily designed components and cement techniques, remembering that patient selection criteria may be different for cementless techniques. Researches reported on the 2-year results in 307 patients and the 5-year results in 89 patients in whom a modified cobalt-chrome Austin-Moore–type femoral prosthesis (the anatomic medullary locking prosthesis) was used. The overall clinical results were excellent, and no correlation was found between clinical results and the patient's age, gender, or underlying disease. Radiographically, 85% of the components were thought to have bone ingrowth, and this ingrowth was primarily cortical in nature, arising from regions where the implant was in contact with the endosteal bone. Clinical and radiographic results improved significantly when a press fit of the prosthesis was obtained in the isthmus of the femur. Therefore, significantly improved results were obtained with this prosthesis when larger-diameter components were used. The axial rigidity of an implant, however, increases directly with the square of the stem diameter, and structural rigidity increases as the fourth power of the stem diameter. Thus, small increases in stem diameter greatly increase its rigidity. Since in a com-

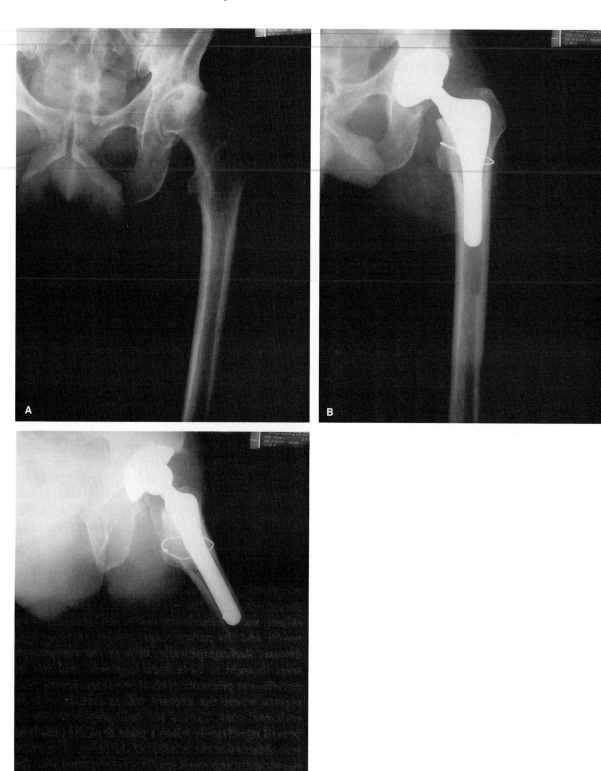

FIGURE 15-18. (A) AP radiograph of a 56-year-old man with osteoarthritis of his left hip joint. The custom cementless femoral component shows excellent fit and fill characteristics on both the AP (B) and lateral (C) radiographs.

posite structure, load is preferentially carried by the more rigid material, the less rigid surrounding bone is relieved of stress to a greater degree with a larger stem. Therefore, to optimize fixation by bone ingrowth using this design, large implants are necessary to contact the diaphyseal cortical bone, which in turn increases the likelihood of stress relief of the proximal femur. To date, this has not been reported as a significant problem, but the potential for long-term problems due to proximal femoral bone loss cannot be discounted. Moderate or severe resorptive bony problem changes were seen in 12% of the patients. Nearly all these cases occurred in patients with larger-diameter implants that achieved isthmus press fit and had radiographic evidence of bone ingrowth.

At 5-year follow-up of patients with cementless porous-coated anatomic prostheses, clinical results were thought to be excellent. Using revision or radiographic evidence of migration as endpoints for failure, there was a 93% survivorship at 5 years. Between 16% and 23% of patients, however, reported mild thigh pain at each of the yearly follow-up visits. The most disturbing finding was that of late subsidence occurring in 3% of femurs and 4% of acetabula.

The 2-year follow-up of 118 porous-coated anatomic total-hip arthroplasties from a multicenter study also was reported. The patient's clinical performance was considered comparable to cemented total-hip arthroplasty and was in large part dependent on surgical technique, especially on the femoral side. Maximal filling of the proximal femur using larger femoral components resulted in increased radiographic evidence of bone ingrowth, stable fixation of the implant, and improved clinical results. Proximal femoral bony remodeling changes were observed, especially when good proximal femoral component press fit was achieved.

A series of patients younger than 45 years old at the time of total-hip arthroplasty was reviewed at an average 4.5-year follow-up. Generally good results were found, with only about a 7% failure rate. Twenty-three percent of the patients had some degree of thigh pain, with 5% being overly troublesome. In this study, no correlation between age, Charnley functional classification, previous hip operations, obesity, occupation, level of activity, or preoperative diagnosis and clinical outcome was established.

The 5-year clinical results were reported on 69 patients with a cementless, long, curved titanium femoral component (biologic ingrowth anatomic system). The rationale behind a longer component is to achieve multiple-point contact inside a curved medullary canal, providing the torsional stability essential for bone ingrowth. The overall clinical results were excellent. Three percent of patients required femoral revision, but none was from aseptic loosening.

Another study reported on an average 6.5-year follow-up of cementless titanium fiber-metal–coated total-hip arthroplasty. This was a relatively young group of patients, with average age of 49 years. The acetabular results were excellent, with no loosening or revisions; however, there was a 9% rate of femoral loosening, with a 5% revision rate and an 8% rate of distal endosteal cortical revision. The clinical success of the femoral implants was found to be related to the extent of both metaphyseal and diaphyseal femoral implant fit and fill, with closer approximation of implant to corticoendosteal surface, achieving an improved result.

These reports and others suggest that the early results of cementless hemispherical ingrowth acetabular components are excellent both clinically and radiographically. (These early reports also suggest an improved result over that of earlier published series.) A retrieval study of porous-coated ingrowth acetabular components has ingrowth of bone occupying a mean of 32% of available surface area, with dense, well-organized fibrous tissue occupying the nonossified areas. It has been postulated that these fibrous tissue–bone interfaces inhibit the deposition of particulate debris but that bone ingrowth provides a better barrier for this process. When compared with results of contemporary cemented femoral implants, however, results with cementless femoral implants indicate increased failure rates and increased thigh pain. These findings, however, are generally in younger, more active patient populations, which may bias the results.

As the numbers and length of follow-up for primary total hip arthroplasty increase, the incidence of revision is becoming increasingly more frequent and the surgery more complex. There are a number of indications for revision, including infection, implant breakage, dislocation, femoral fracture, and significant implant-related osteolysis. The single most common indication for revision is aseptic loosening of one or both components, which may be associated with pain and progressive loss of bone stock. The pain generally is intermittent and associated with increased activity, and tends to be progressive. The complexity and complication rate of revision surgery are of sufficient magnitude that symptoms should significantly limit the patient's function before revision is indicated. In some situations, however, patients may have few symptoms, but revision arthroplasty may still be indicated because progressive loss of bone stock is occurring.

The exact mechanisms by which this well-documented clinical phenomenon occurs are unknown but probably are related to the particulate debris generated from total hip arthroplasty and its ability to induce a foreign body granulomatous response. This debris falls into three categories: polyethylene debris from the acetabular component, PMMA debris associated with cemented implants, and metal debris. The host's response to these materials is the invasion of inflammatory cells and the formation of granulomas. In addition, particulate debris can cause a third body wear phenomenon between articulating surfaces, increasing the amount of debris present. Furthermore, metal debris may have a direct cytotoxic cellular affect.

The bone–cement interface membrane from radiographically loose prostheses has been studied, and the findings support the postulate that this membrane is capable of secreting prostaglandin E_2 and collagenase, which may in part be responsible for the bone lysis seen in some patients. Motion and particulate PMMA have been implicated in converting a relatively benign soft tissue membrane into one capable of active bone osteolysis. The membranes taken from focal points of bone osteolysis surrounding clinically well-fixed prostheses have been characterized and contain histiocytes and foreign-body giant cells demonstrating high osteoclastic activity and were associated with particulate PMMA. Evidence suggests that the stimulus to the induction or formation of these problems may be secondary to the body's response to particulate PMMA or polyethylene debris. Therefore, relatively asymptomatic but radiographically loose components mandate frequent follow-up to determine any ongoing loss of bone stock that may be occurring, since it would be advantageous to revise a component while existing bone stock remains optimal for revision fixation. Even in the absence of significant symptoms, the ongoing loss of bone is an indication for revision.

Similar findings have been reported in mechanically stable prostheses associated with areas of periprosthetic bone loss. Linear relationships between the amount of polyethylene wear debris, the number of macrophages (most macrophages had intracellular particles of polyetyhlene), and the degree of bone resorption have been observed. Areas of osteolysis along the shaft of otherwise well-fixed femoral components suggest that the joint fluid may actually penetrate extensively along the implant. Recent evidence also suggests that a similar phenomenon may occur around well-fixed, mechanically stable acetabular components. Figure 15-19 demonstrates the osteolytic phenomenon around loose components.

Revision total-hip replacement presents the surgeon with increasing degrees of difficulty that tax ingenuity and surgical skills and that call for an array of prosthetic sizes, grafting materials, and surgical instrumentation. As in primary total-hip arthroplasty, both cemented and cementless techniques may be appropriate at different times in approaching the problem of a failed total-hip arthroplasty. The overall clinical results, however, are frequently compromised by significantly increased complication rates and rates of aseptic loosening. This is particularly true in patients who are younger, active, and overweight and in those with inadequate bone stock, infection, fracture nonunion, or history of multiple previous failures. Review of multiple studies revealed that the complications during revision of cemented total-hip arthroplasty are frequent: deep infection, 1% to 5%; dislocation, 2% to 15%; intraoperative fracture, 1% to 9%; postoperative fracture, 2% to 7%; nerve palsies, 1% to 5%; wound hematomas, 3% to 15%; trochanteric nonunion, 3% to 20%; and nonfatal pulmonary emboli, 2% to 3%. Additionally, roentgenographic and clinical loosening has been reported in 2.5% to 62%, with most studies having relatively short follow-up. These studies collectively also reveal a rerevision rate of 7.5% to 20.8%. Nevertheless, patients with cemented revisions have reported improvements in pain level, function, and overall satisfaction. This is documented by several surgical reports indicating good or excellent results in 50% to 60% of patients undergoing cemented revision. At times, largely depending on the quality of the existing bone stock, the results of cemented revision total-hip arthroplasty can approach the results obtained in primary replacement.

The revision of failed total-hip arthroplasty presents the surgeon with a variety of both acetabular and femoral bone stock deficiencies. Each of these deficiencies must be individualized at the time of reconstructive surgery, but there are general patterns of bone stock loss that allow the categorization of various defects. This enables surgeons to identify, plan, reconstruct, and report their approaches to the various problems and the results that are attainable.

On the acetabular side, the American Academy of Orthopaedic Surgeons has established a classification system of acetabular defects: type I, segmental or noncontained defects (significant rim defects); type II, cavitary contained defects; type III, combinations of types I and II; type IV, pelvic discontinuities; and type V, arthrodesis.

The Committee on the Hip has recently intro-

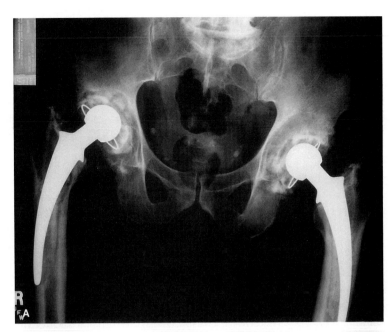

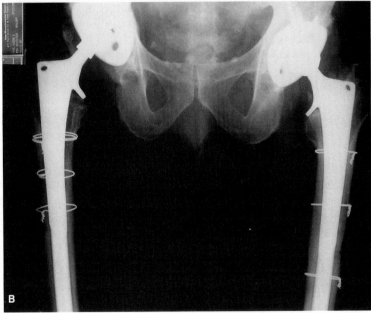

FIGURE 15-19. (A) Radiograph of a 66-year-old white man who developed bilateral femoral and acetabular loosening of cemented total hip arthroplasties placed 8 years previously. The right hip shows gross loosening of the acetabular component with significant osteolysis and loss of acetabular bone stock. There has also been significant distal and varus subsidence of the right femoral component, with endosteal scalloping of bone in the proximomedial one third of the femur and significant lateral cortical erosion of the distal one third of the femoral component. Similar but not as dramatic findings are found on the left hip. (B) Postoperative radiograph shows reconstruction with cementless acetabular and femoral techniques. The acetabula are reconstructed using large, cementless acetabular devices, maximizing component host bone contact and using auxiliary screw fixation. The femoral components are cementless devices of sufficient length to bypass the embarrassed lateral cortex of both femurs by at least two canal diameters. Attempts to restore appropriate leg lengths have been made by placing varying neck lengths.

duced a comprehensive classification system that has two basic classes of femoral abnormalities—segmental and cavitary. *Segmental defects* are defined as any loss of supporting cortical shell, and *cavitary defects* are defined as the loss of cancellous or endosteal cortical bone without violation of the outer cortical shell. Segmental deficiencies can be further divided as partial, complete, or intercalary. Ectasia is a form of cavitary defect in which the femoral medullary canal is expanded. Additional categories include combined, malalignment, femoral stenosis, and femoral discontinuity.

Clinical Reports

A 29% mechanical failure rate at 8.1 years of follow-up was reported in 99 of 110 cemented revision total-hip arthroplasties. Of the remaining patients, 63% had good or excellent results and 7% had fair results. The presence of progressive radiolucent lines was thought to be an ominous sign. The authors believed that the initial quality of a well-fixed, uncomplicated cemented revision compared favorably with a primary total-hip arthroplasty but concluded that the durability of that result is substantially less certain. At average 3.6-year follow-up of 139 cemented hip revisions, overall mechanical failure occurred in 16% of hips, and most were due to aseptic loosening. Additionally, 33% of the patients had either fair or poor results. There was a 13% rate of femoral perforation, 3.4% incidence of deep infection, 8.2% rate of postoperative dislocation, and 6.2% incidence of trochanteric complications with trochanteric osteotomy. Femoral component loosening correlated with varus positioning, inadequate cement technique, and younger age. Loosening of either the acetabular or femoral component correlated with poor bone quality and failure to restore normal hip center position. In a large series of patients undergoing revision between 1968 and 1978 with an average of 4.5 years of follow-up, 90% of the patients who had undergone cemented revision believed that their condition had improved. However, radiographic analysis revealed probable loosening in 20% of acetabular and 44% of femoral components. Overall, 27% of patients clinically were thought to have had poor results. The clinical results were poorer in patients who underwent revision secondary to recurrent dislocation or acetabular loosening. Overall, 45% of patients showed probable radiographic loosening, and 21% had clinically symptomatic loosening. An interesting conclusion from this study was that when revising a failed femoral component, one should revise the acetabular component only if it is definitely loose. In a group of patients who had undergone numerous revisions for multiple failed cemented total-hip arthroplasties, at 3-year follow-up, about 50% had satisfactory results after a second or third revision, with the remainder having poor clinical results, evidence of radiographic loosening, or both. Failure rates were 24% after a second revision at a mean of 3.4 years and 15% after a third revision. There was a significantly increased rate of acetabular loosening if the original revision had been performed for acetabular loosening as opposed to other conditions (eg, malposition). There also was a trend toward repeated failure of cemented acetabular components in patients with congenital dislocation of the hip who had undergone previous multiple cemented revisions for aseptic loosening. Poor bone stock was also associated with increased revision rates. Based on the data, the authors recommended that the stem of a femoral component bypass any femoral cortical defect by at least two stem diameters and that one consider bone grafting for these defects. However, they were unable to verify that cemented long-stem femoral components improved fixation and prevented or delayed eventual loosening. Overall complications were frequent. The survivorship analysis at average 9-year follow-up of cemented revision total-hip arthroplasty in a group of older patients (average age, 71 years) was reported with special emphasis on autograft acetabular augmentation or reconstruction for bone defects and overall surgical technique. Survivorship data revealed a cumulative survival rate of 85% at 14 years. However, 6.7% of patients required a second revision, and an additional 13.3% were considered candidates for revision. Significantly larger percentages of patients had radiographic criteria suggestive of loosening that had not yet required revision.

It is apparent from the review of published reports that the results of cemented revision total-hip arthroplasty do not approach what we would expect from using contemporary cemented techniques. However, most current reports are from patients who have not benefited from advances in cemented technique. It seems reasonable to extrapolate that these improvements should also improve the results of cemented revision total-hip arthroplasty provided a suitable bony environment is present to accept the presence of PMMA. Therefore, in elderly, sedentary individuals in whom femoral bone stock remains good, the continued cautious use of cemented femoral revision techniques seems warranted (Fig. 15-20). Additionally, in those femoral reconstructions with significant loss of bone, particulate allograft femoral reconstructions (Ling technique) are showing promising early results, with significant clinical improvements of pain and function as well as what appears to be reestablishment of lost femoral bone stock. In comparison with the femur, the bony geometry and current methods of cement introduction make the acetabulum less amenable to significant improvement in cement technique, especially in the presence of sclerotic bony surfaces and the frequent loss of bone stock that accompanies a failed cemented acetabular component. This conclusion seems to be supported by the reports in which the incidence of complications of cemented acetabular revisions was high. These problems have led to the widespread use of cementless acetabular components in revision total-hip arthroplasty and the increasing use of cemented allograft reconstructions. Initial clinical and radiographic experience of cementless methods has been excellent, supporting their increasing use in revision of failed cemented acetabular components. Also, various investigators have explored the use of particulate acetabular allograft reconstructions many times in combination with structural allograft or structure reinforcement using protrusio rings, wire mesh, or plates to achieve containment of the particulate allograft. These techniques can be especially useful in examples of massive acetabular bone destruction in which the bony foundation is first reestablished using the above-mentioned techniques and then all polyethylene cups are cemented into these reconstructions. Analogous reconstructions using large-bulk structural acetabular components have also been reported.

As stated in the previous section, the incidence of failure in cemented revision total-hip arthroplasty remains unacceptably high, particularly on the acetabular side. This is especially true in cases in which the patients are young, active, overweight, or in which there has been significant loss of bone stock. For these reasons, the use of cementless techniques in performing revision total-hip arthroplasty has become increasingly popular.

On the acetabular side, various approaches are available for the revision of failed acetabular components, including: fixed ingrown cups, bipolar prostheses, and cemented acetabular cups. Each of these approaches can be combined with the use of autograft or allograft in either particulate or structural form. They may also be combined with various metallic reinforcements. The quality of existing acetabular bone stock—including the location, size, and type of acetabular defect—and the patient's age, weight, medical condition, and functional requirements help to determine the appropriate reconstruction method. In general, fixed hemispherical bone-ingrowth–type devices that do not require structural or nonstructural graft for inherent stability when host bone contact can be maximized are the preferred initial choices in revision surgery. Inherent three-dimensional stability is mandatory in the use of fixed hemispheric cups. The stability can be achieved through a variety of press-fit techniques, including acetabular components that have attached peripheral fins, pegs, or raised edges for rotational stability or, in certain situations, the use of screws placed through the component to achieve stability. Underreaming of the acetabulum with impaction of slightly oversized components is another method of achieving stability. The role of allograft in reconstructing bone loss is crucial for restoring lost bone stock, but its role as a structural supporting material for the prosthesis must be minimized if possible. The size and location of acetabular defects may mandate the use of acetabular allograft for reconstruction to achieve component stability. Questions about the minimal contact area of prosthesis to host bone versus allograft or autograft bone remain unanswered. It is likely that varying

degrees of host–prosthesis contact are required, depending on the type and location of the acetabular defect. Finally, certain defects may be best approached through combinations of bone graft, stabilization plates, protrusio rings, custom implants, and standard implants used with or without cement (Fig. 15-21).

With the use of nonstructural particulate graft, one can accept as little as 30% host bone contact and expect a satisfactory short-term result. Additionally, with the use of segmental but nonstructural grafts, as little as 40% host bone contact is required, provided the host bone extends to at least the lateral summit of the hemisphere of the socket in the coronal plan. Although the acceptable area of host bone versus allograft bone for prosthesis contact has not been quantified, it has been stated that one could expect a good, short-term result provided cavitary defects are filled, the rim is reconstructed, and the component can achieve adequate stability based on host bone, not relying on segmental allograft for stability.

In situations in which the use of structural cement or allografting is necessary for prosthesis support, increasing evidence suggests that graft failure may be secondary to graft nonunion and possible fatigue fracture with subsequent nonunion. In these situations, acetabular components that allow the use of screws through the dome to firmly fix the acetabular component to as much host bone as possible have been recommended, as has interfragmentary screw compression of the allograft to host bone augmented by a buttress support plating to further enhance the stability. Cementing the component into the structural allograft bed has been suggested when the component rests largely on the allograft. This is in part because one cannot expect any significant stabilizing biologic interface between the component and the dead allograft surface. However, the use of large segmental acetabular allografts has been reported in a structural role into which uncemented acetabular components have been placed. Additionally, these components have not been augmented by any additional fixation such as screws. In this concept, the prosthesis–allograft construct in essence is allowed to "float" within the host bone, such that if collapse of the allograft occurs, the component theoretically seeks and migrates to a stable position. The use of cementless acetabular components in large segmental allografts has been reported with good short-term results. The average 3.5-year follow-up of acetabular allograft reconstruction during acetabular revision using non–metal-backed cemented components has been reported. The results are dif-

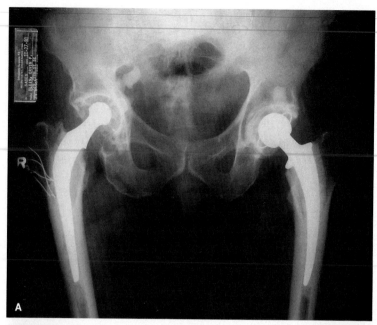

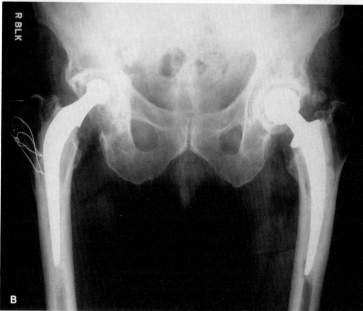

FIGURE 15-20. Radiographs of an 82-year-old man who underwent cementless acetabular and cemented femoral revision of a loose left total hip arthroplasty. (A) One-year postoperative result of this patient's original total hips. He has a cemented Charnley device placed on the right side and a cemented Mueller device placed on the left side. (B) Eleven-year-old follow-up of the same hips. The right side is functioning nicely, with no evidence of loosening on either the acetabular or femoral side. The left hip, on the other hand, has clear evidence of loosening of the femoral component, with distal and varus migration of the device and endosteal scalloping of the medial femoral bone stock along the distal one third of the component. AP (C) and lateral (D) views of the left hip at 11-year follow-up reveal circumferential radiolucencies at the acetabular component. At the time of surgery, both the acetabular and femoral components were grossly loose. (E) Postoperative revision using a cementless acetabular device and a cemented femoral component.

ficult to interpret, since no description was given of the size of the graft, nor was the percentage of host versus allograft component contact reported. Nevertheless, only one failure or graft collapse was reported. Additionally, three-dimensional CT radioisotopic bone scanning revealed uniform uptake of the isotope consistent with revascularization of the grafts. The radiographic and clinical results suggested that allograft and host bone remodeled in response to stress and that allograft incorporated into host bone.

The short-term results, however, must be tempered by the report that at an average of 7 years of follow-up, there was a 20% radiographic resorption of autogenous femoral head allografts used in a acetabular reconstruction for congenital dislocation of the hip. These were cemented, non–metal-backed components and were all done for primary total arthroplasty. The grafts were used in a supporting structure role, and the authors thought the reason for their collapse was in part the loss of posterior support for the acetabular component. This report

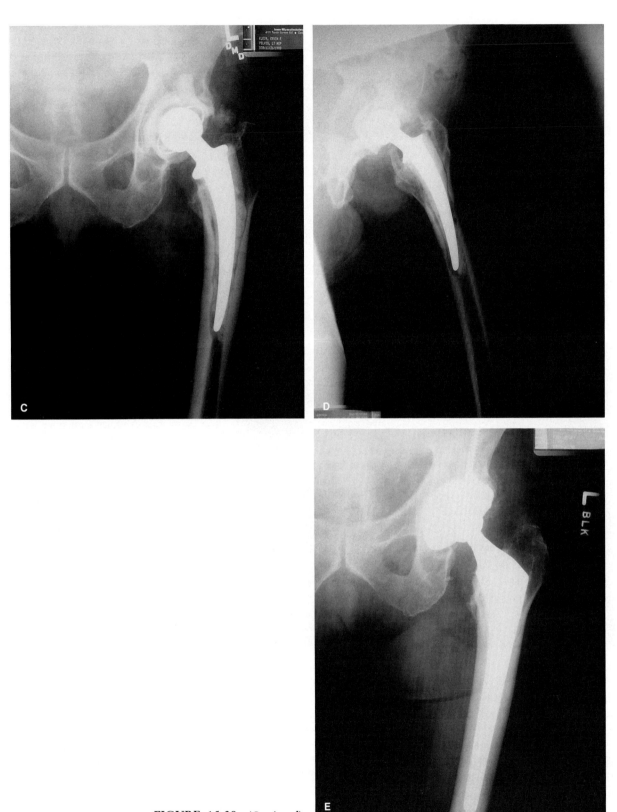

FIGURE 15-20. (*Continued*)

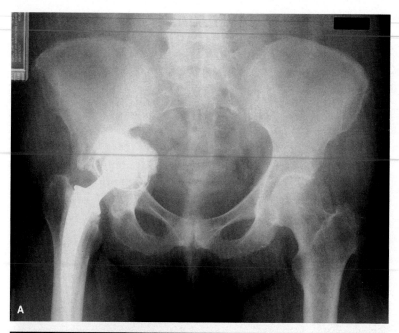

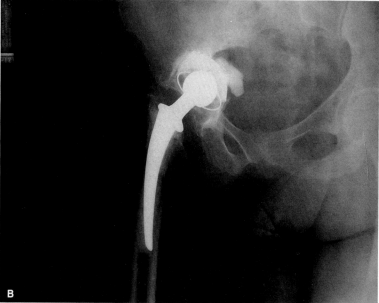

FIGURE 15-21. (A) Radiograph of a 72-year-old woman who had a previous acetabular revision for aseptic loosening using a large bolus of methyl methacrylate to accommodate for the original acetabular bony destruction. There has been medial and superior migration of the acetabulum. (**B** and **C**) Oblique right hip radiographs further illustrate the loosening of this acetabular component, with severe medial migration breaching the medial acetabular wall. (**D**) Immediate postoperative radiograph reconstructs the deficiency with a massive medial allograft and cementless acetabular component of sufficient size to make use of peripheral host bone contact. (**E**) One-year follow-up of the same hip shows remodeling of the medial graft with maintenance of good position of the acetabular component.

raises questions about the long-term viability of either allograft or autograft reconstruction when used in a supporting role.

In an ongoing follow-up of a group of patients in whom bulk, weight-bearing, femoral head allografts were used to augment severe acetabular deficiencies, at mean 10-year follow-up, all grafts united, but nearly half of these reconstructions resulted in failure of acetabular fixation. Biologic union of the allograft was believed to have resulted in revascularization, which led to a deterioration of its struc-

tural, load-bearing properties, ending in acetabular loosening and failure of the reconstruction.

Repeated cemented revisions of failed cemented acetabular components have a high percentage of failure; therefore, the choice of cementless revision is appealing. The use of hemispherical ingrowth cups with the appropriate use of either morselized or segmental allografting while maximizing the host bone–prosthesis interface contact to achieve fixation provides the most promising solution for the future. Finally, there continues to be a debate regarding hip

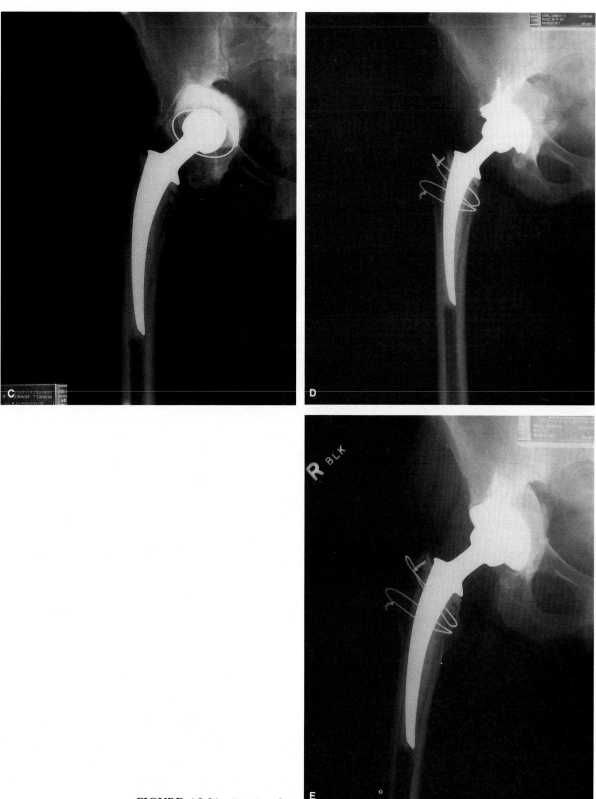

FIGURE 15-21. (*Continued*)

center position during acetabular reconstruction revision with massive amounts of bone loss. The debate centers on the positioning of the center of the hip. The question that remains unanswered is whether to try to place the center of the hip in the anatomic position or to move the hip joint to a position in the pelvis that provides the most stable supporting host bone.

In a group of 37 hips in which the acetabular component had been placed a minimum of 35 mm above the interteardrop line, 16% of the components were loose at 10 years, but only one component required revision. The authors emphasized the importance of medial placement of the cup when using the high hip center technique.

These questions currently are unanswered, but relatively small displacements of the hip center to obtain good apposition to host bone are probably acceptable and preferable to placing the components on structural allograft. However, as one moves more superiorly in the ilium, the amount of bone stock available for acetabular fixation markedly decreases as the iliac wing is reached and relatively larger displacements of hip center may contribute to increasing failure rates. Other solutions involve maximizing the anteroposterior dimension of the acetabulum and using large or jumbo cups, either alone or with relatively smaller quantities of autograft or allograft in attempts to maximize implant–host contact while minimizing superior displacement of the hip center. In a series of cementless revision acetabular components with 80% of hips treated with bone grafting, generally a mixture of local autogenous and freeze-dried allograft, there was a 5% revision rate for infection or instability and none for aseptic loosening. The concept of maximizing host bone coverage was emphasized. Additionally, it has been postulated that the length of time the total hip reconstruction can be expected to function increases if the stresses on the components are reduced. Therefore, according to their mathematical model, the single most important factor in minimizing the load of a hip prosthesis is the placement of the hip center in its anatomic position. In addition to this, although the causes of dislocation are multifactorial, the position of the hip center in a nonanatomic position increases the risk of dislocation.

The use of bipolar components in acetabular revision surgery may occasionally be indicated. Several investigators have reported migration with the use of either morselized or segmental allograft reconstruction when using bipolar components. A migration rate of 52% using particulate graft has been reported, 11% of these being progressive. Other studies have also shown significant rates of migration, including superior and medial migration. The extent of socket migration and deficient acetabuli appears to be related to the location of the graft, the relative size of the socket, the quality of the supporting native bone, and the ability of host bone to heal the added bone graft. When the largest possible bipolar component was used with minimal grafting, results were acceptable, but rates were significantly poorer when bipolar components were combined with massive allografting.

The high migration rate of bipolar components when used in conjunction with particulate allograft suggests that the most stable environment for particulate allograft incorporation is one in which there is no motion of the acetabular component (eg, fixed acetabular cup). However, information conflicts, since several reports have indicated that bipolar components in select situations can give relatively good results if their use is limited to acetabuli that have intact peripheral rims and only cavitary medial bone loss. Acceptable levels of pain relief and functional gain have been reported in 47 patients. The authors of this study, however, point out that the technique is indicated only in completely contained defects with intact peripheral rims in which the contained defect primarily is central and not superior. In these situations, by careful packing and placing of the particular graft as well as appropriate sizing of the bipolar component to obtain complete rim contact, good results were reported. Several basic principles were recommended to minimize migration when reconstructing deficient acetabuli with bipolar components: (1) reconstruct central contained acetabular defects; (2) maximize contact with the patient's rim of native bone; (3) use sufficient amounts of graft well prepared and tightly packed; and (4) minimize joint reactive forces by modifying the activity level during the early postoperative period of graft maturation. If these principles can be adhered to, the inherent stability of a bipolar component may make it a useful reconstructive technique in situations in which recurrent dislocation or weakened abductor musculature is a concern.

Finally, in select situations in patients in whom functional demands are low, longevity is short, and appropriate acetabular bone stock remains, the selected use of cemented reconstructions may be appropriate.

Reports reviewing cementless revision of loosened femoral components have also been limited and suffer from the problems of short follow-up and lack of clinical and radiographic completeness as well as a lack of a standardized classification system for femoral bone stock deficiency. Nevertheless, the early results of cementless femoral component revision are encouraging. A number of reviews have reported clinical success rates of 73% to 90% at follow-up of 2 to 6 years. Additionally, attempts have been made to correlate clinical results with classification systems that describe the extent of femoral bone stock deficiency encountered during cementless revision arthroplasty. Loosening of cemented femoral components can result in femoral bone stock loss. This bone loss has been categorized in a number of ways but in general relates to the quality of remaining bone stock as it is affected by segmental bone loss, cavitary and cortical defects, cortical thinning, femoral canal expansion, and condition of the greater trochanter and attached abductor musculature, as well as overall femoral bone density. The goals of femoral reconstruction include leg length equalization, restoration of hip biomechanics, maintenance of the abductor mechanism, restoration of femoral integrity, and rigid, lasting prosthetic fixation. In general, as the quality of remaining femoral bone stock diminishes, the technical complexity of revision surgery increases and the clinical outcome becomes less predictable. Additionally, the role and usefulness of cemented revision techniques significantly declines. This is in part secondary to the sclerotic endosteal bone surfaces that accompany loosened cemented components, thereby leaving a poor surface on which to obtain a microinterlock with PMMA. Additionally, loss of bone stock may in part be secondary to the physiologic response to loose particulate PMMA debris that can result from loosened femoral compo-

nents. The use of a cementless femoral component may allow some recovery of bone, whereas a cemented revision component is less likely to allow for this. However, the role of cemented revision in elderly, less active patients who still have good-quality bone stock remaining and in whom in a microinterlock of PMMA bone cement with bone can be obtained must be emphasized. In these select patients, the use of cemented revision is valid. However, in patients in whom significant destruction has occurred or in whom bone surfaces have become extremely sclerotic, the role of cemented revision significantly diminishes.

The extent and location of femoral bone loss in revision surgery require an array of femoral components from which to select the appropriate component size and shape to match existing femoral geometry. This generally requires the meticulous removal of all cement and soft tissue membrane. Remaining femoral bone stock is then assessed to determine whether three-dimensional implant stability can be achieved by carefully machining the endosteal bone surfaces to accept a femoral component. If so, revision may be accomplished in this fashion, taking care to reestablish soft tissue tension and limb length. Occasionally, particulate allograft may be used as a filler within the medullary canal as a means of bone grafting cavitary defects.

If faced with large, structural segmental defects, the choices are either to use large, custom-type implants that replace the lost bone with metal and generally mandate cemented application because of the inability to achieve uncemented fixation in remaining host bone or to use an allograft–femoral prosthesis

(text continues on page 571)

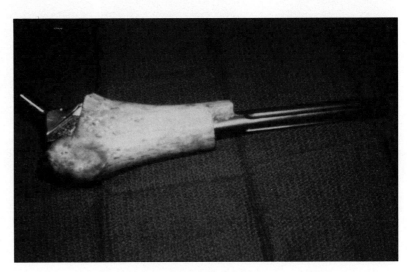

FIGURE 15-22. One technique for the use of a proximal femoral structural allograft. In this technique, a femoral device is cemented into a circumferential proximal femoral allograft. A step-cut is used at the host bone–allograft junction. This composite is then impacted into the remainder of the proximal host femur, with bending stability coming from the intramedullary portion of the femoral component as it rests in the distal host bone and with torsional stability coming from the step-cut articulation between the host bone and the allograft. The femoral component is cemented into the allograft and placed without cement into the host bone, thus allowing compression at the host bone–allograft junction without fear of interposed methyl methacrylate.

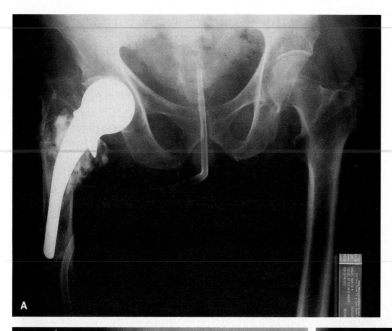

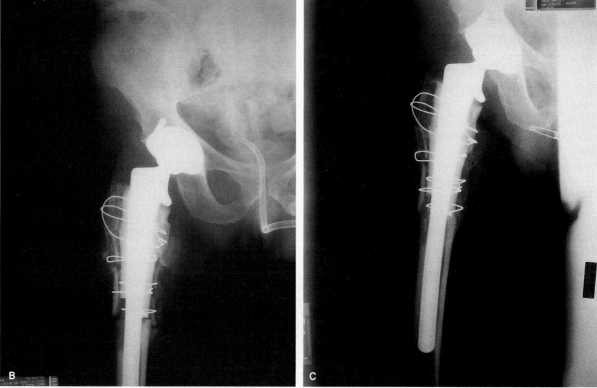

FIGURE 15-23. (A) Ten-year follow-up of a 68-year-old man who had a cemented endoprosthesis placed for a previous femoral neck fracture. The patient subsequently developed severe osteolysis and bony destruction of the proximal one third of his femur. (B) Immediate postoperative result using a composite circumferential femoral allograft as was shown in Figure 15-21. The remaining host bone from the proximal femur is circumferentially circlaged around the allograft construct. (C) Two-year follow-up of this patient shows bony union between the allograft and the host bone along the medial step-cut as well as incorporation of the circlaged femoral host bone around the proximal one third of the femur.

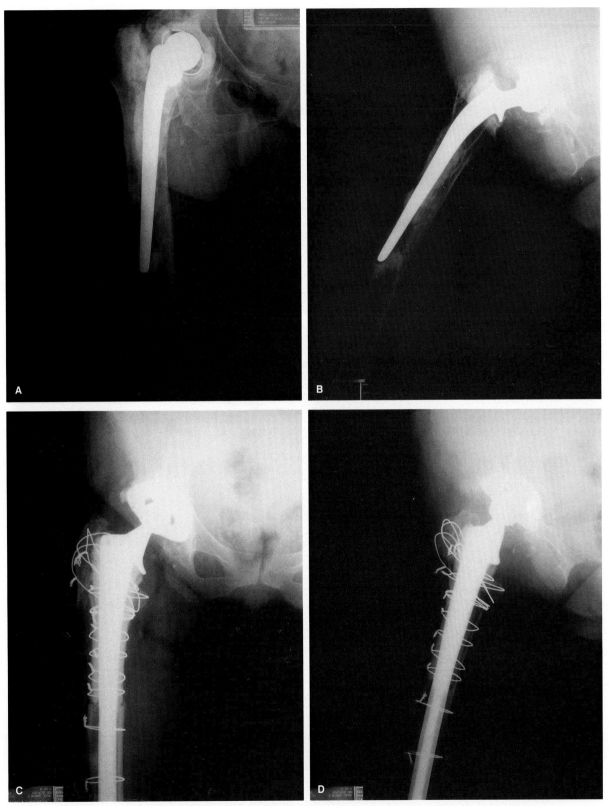

FIGURE 15-24. Radiographs of a patient who developed severe osteolysis and destruction of prox-imofemoral bone stock. The proximal femur was reconstructed using a structural proximofemoral allograft composite, as illustrated in Figure 15-21. The remnant of the greater trochanter was circum-ferentially circlaged to the allograft.

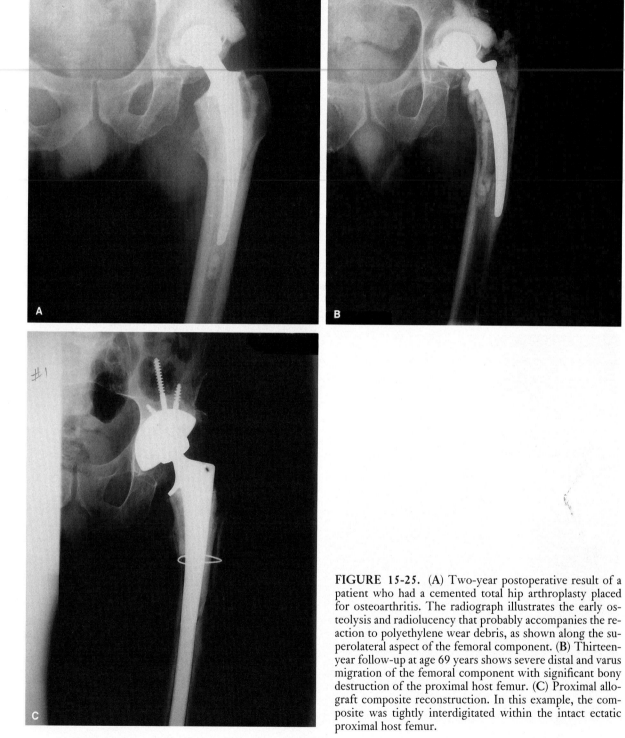

FIGURE 15-25. (A) Two-year postoperative result of a patient who had a cemented total hip arthroplasty placed for osteoarthritis. The radiograph illustrates the early osteolysis and radiolucency that probably accompanies the reaction to polyethylene wear debris, as shown along the superolateral aspect of the femoral component. (B) Thirteen-year follow-up at age 69 years shows severe distal and varus migration of the femoral component with significant bony destruction of the proximal host femur. (C) Proximal allograft composite reconstruction. In this example, the composite was tightly interdigitated within the intact ectatic proximal host femur.

composite in either a cemented or cementless application. The advantages of an allograft composite are that it replaces lost bone stock and allows bony union to remaining host bone further enhancing stability. Osseous allografts are nonviable at the time of implantation but serve as a structural material that undergoes subsequent revascularization, osseous remodeling, and bone healing. The revascularization is slow and variable in location. These allografts may be either circumferential replacing varying lengths or segments of proximal femur or they may be onlay-type grafts attached to the host femur by means of circlage fixation, replacing varying incomplete segments of proximal femur (Fig. 15-22). Additionally, struts of cortical allograft may be useful in reinforcing host bone or host–allograft bone composites by circumferentially circlaging them to the femur in a "barrel stave" fashion. The role of bone cement in these complex revision cases remains controversial. Cement probably is useful when attaching the femoral component to a segmental femoral allograft as

the bone cement interface in an allograft probably will not revascularize and therefore should remain stable. Bone cement may be used in the host bone if necessary to obtain rigid fixation. However, it may hamper host–allograft bone union by not allowing compressive forces at the osteotomy site or by directly interposing cement between the host and the allograft, thereby preventing bone healing. Therefore, if possible, one should avoid the use of cement in host bone. Stability may be enhanced through the use of a step-cut osteotomy, and union may be facilitated using autogenous bone graft at the host–allograft junction. Examples of allograft techniques are shown in Figures 15-22 through 15-26.

A small series of massive segmental proximal femoral allografting with an average of 3 years of follow-up has been reported as having excellent results. A series of proximal femoral allograft reconstructions with mean 4-year follow-up femoral or femoral head allograft reconstructions in deficient proximal femurs has also been reported. Seventy-

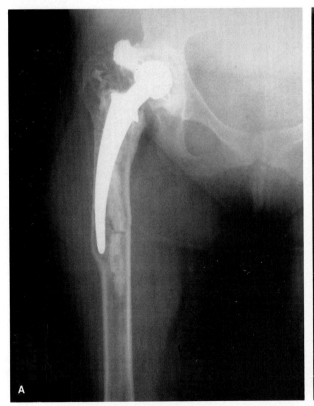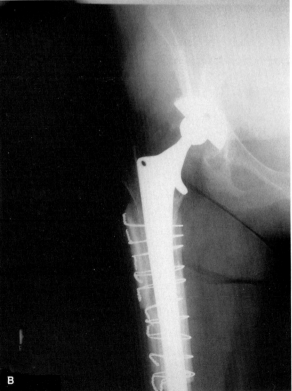

FIGURE 15-26. Radiographs showing a loose cemented acetabular and femoral component with a significant distal varus subsidence of the femoral component. Additionally, there is significant ectasia of the lateral cortical femoral bone with an undisplaced femoral fracture at the level of the distal one third of the component. This was reconstructed using a cementless acetabular device and a large cementless femoral device augmented with peripheral allograft strut bone grafting to augment the deficient lateral femoral cortex and to stabilize the fracture.

five percent of femoral head reconstructions failed; entire proximal femurs fared better, with 82% attaining host–allograft union, but 64% of components subsided. Subsidence was thought to be secondary to the use of cementless femoral components unable to achieve any biologic fixation in dead allograft, and the authors recommended cementing into the allograft.

Bone allografts have been used to augment bone stock deficiencies in patients undergoing two-stage reconstruction and reimplantation after failed total-hip replacement secondary to infection. Rates of success were good, and the result provided a better functional outcome than the alternative of resection arthroplasty or attempted fusion.

Finally, a technique has been reported on in which the proximal femoral canal is plugged and then densely packed with particulate allograft. Into this allograft bed, a tamped cavity is formed to accommodate a cemented femoral component, essentially establishing a cemented particulate allograft composite contained within the remaining proximal femoral bone stock. Excellent early clinical results have been reported as well as what appears to be the radiographic reconstitution of proximal femoral bone stock.

Annotated Bibliography

Berry DJ, Chandler HP, Reilly DT. The use of bone allografts in two-stage reconstruction after failure of hip replacements due to infection. J Bone Joint Surg 1991;73A:1460.
A classification system for femoral abnormalities for both primary and revision total-hip arthroplasty is presented.

Bradway JK, Bernard F. The natural history of the silent hip in bilateral atraumatic osteonecrosis. J Arthroplasty 1993;8:383.
Fifteen hips were identified that fit the strict selection criteria of no history of symptoms, normal AP radiograph, and negative ^{99m}Tc bone scan (if available) at the time of contralateral total-hip arthroplasty. At a mean of 23 months later, all 15 silent hips developed collapse secondary to AVN, indicating that when vascular necrosis develops in a hip joint, a high percentage of patients quickly progress to collapse and secondary symptoms.

D'Antonio JA, Capello WN, Borden LS, et al. Classification and management of acetabular abnormalities in total hip arthroplasty. Clin Orthop 1989;243:1260.
A classification system for acetabular abnormalities for both primary and revision total-hip arthroplasty is presented.

Johnston RC, Fitzgerald RH Jr, Harris WH, et al. Clinical and radiographic evaluation of total hip replacement. J Bone Joint Surg 1990;72A:161.
The authors outline a consensus reporting methods for total-hip arthroplasty, including clinical and radiographic parameters for both cemented and cementless replacements. Clinical parameters measured include pain, ability to work, level of activity, walking capacity, patient satisfaction, and results of physical examination. Radiographic parameters include position of the implant, presence of migration, changes in the cement mantle, presence of radiolu-

cencies, and measurements of bone remodeling. Detailed evaluation schemes are presented.

Murtell JM, Pierson RN, Jacobs JJ, Rosenberg AG, Maley M, Galante JO. Primary total hip reconstruction with a titanium fiber–coated prosthesis inserted without cement. J Bone Joint Surg 1993;75A:554.
Results of a prospective study of 121 cementless Harris-Galante total-hip arthroplasties are reported, with an average follow-up of 67 months. Nine percent of femoral components were considered loose, and 8% of femurs had distal cortical osteolysis. Overall survivorship analysis revealed a 97% chance of survival.

Padgett DE, Kull L, Rosenberry A, Summer D, Galante JO. Revision of the acetabular component without cement after total hip arthroplasty. J Bone Joint Surg 1993;75A:663.
The results of 129 of 138 cementless acetabular revisions are reported, with an average follow-up of 44 months. There was a 5% revision rate for either infections or dislocation. There were no reported cases of aseptic loosening. The technique of maximization of host-bone coverage and of packing of all defects with cancellous autogenous graft, allograft, or both was successful for all classes of acetabular deficiencies.

Pellicci PM, Wilson PD, Sledge CB, et al. Long-term results of revision total hip replacement. J Bone Joint Surg 1985;67A:513.
The results of 99 of 110 cemented revision arthroplasties are reported, with an average follow-up of 8.1 years. Twenty-nine percent of these revisions had failed. Most had shown progressive radiolucencies with time.

Poss R. The role of osteotomy in the treatment of osteoarthritis of the hip: current concepts review. J Bone Joint Surg 1984;66A:144.
The evolution of modern osteotomy approaches is reviewed. Questions of patient selection, operative procedure, and analysis of reported results are also reviewed.

Scher MA, Jakim I. Intertrochanteric osteotomy and autogenous bone grafting for avascular necrosis of the femoral head. J Bone Joint Surg 1993;75A:1119.
The authors report results of a prospective study of 45 hips with Ficat stage 3 disease that underwent valgus flexion intertrochanteric osteotomy, curettage of necrotic bone, and autogenous grafting. Cumulative survival was 87% at 5 years, with a mean postoperative Harris hip score of 90 ± 7 points.

Schulte KR, Callaghan JJ, Kelley SS, Johnston RC. The outcome of Charnley total hip arthroplasty with cement after a minimum 20-year follow-up. J Bone Joint Surg 1993;75A:961.
The results of 330 cemented Charnley total-hip arthroplasties are reviewed. Of the 322 hips for which the outcome was known, 90% had retained the original implant until the patient died or until the most recent examination. Of the 98 hips of patients who lived for at least 20 years, 85% had retained the original prosthesis.

Sponseller PD, McBeath AA, Perpich M. Hip arthrodesis in young patients. J Bone Joint Surg 1984;66A:853.
Fifty-three patients under 35 years old at the time of hip arthrodesis are retrospectively reviewed at an average follow-up of 38 years. Seventy-eight percent were satisfied with the arthrodesis, but significant percentages reported low back and knee discomfort.

Warner JP, Phillip JH, Brodsky GL, Thornhill TS. Studies of nontraumatic osteonecrosis: the role of decompression in the treatment of nontraumatic osteonecrosis of the femoral head. Clin Orthop 1987;225:104.
This study reports the 5-year results of core decompression in nontraumatic (predominantly steroid-associated) osteonecrosis of the femoral head. A lack of correlation between pressure manometrics, venography, and clinical outcome was observed. Recommendations for core decompression in Ficat stage 0, I, and IIA (sclerotic predominant) disease are outlined.

Turek's Orthopaedics: Principles and Their Application, Fifth Edition,
edited by Stuart L. Weinstein and Joseph A. Buckwalter.
J.B. Lippincott Company, Philadelphia, © 1994.

16

Peter D. Pizzutillo

The Pediatric Leg and Knee

Although trauma of the leg and knee in children is of major concern, a host of other problems due to congenital anomalies, infections, developmental deformities, and intrauterine problems have a major impact on both the growth and development of the child's leg and knee. Traumatic insults may be subdivided into macrotrauma and microtrauma. Macrotrauma that involves the bone may affect the physis and lead to leg length discrepancy and angular deformity. The application of repetitive subliminal forces on the growing limb may have other expressions, which are further elucidated in this chapter.

CONGENITAL SUBLUXATION AND DISLOCATION OF THE KNEE

Hyperextension of the knee in newborn infants may be caused by aberrations in intrauterine positions, such as the frank breech position, which slowly stretches the hamstrings and soft tissues of the posterior aspect of the knee. The term *genu recurvatum* refers to a mild degree of hyperextension of the knee and is usually noted in normal children who have had breech presentation. Infants with genu recurvatum display knees that may actively hyperextend to 20 degrees and yet demonstrate normal passive flexion. These infants are capable of actively flexing their knees, and no treatment is usually necessary because knee anatomy and stability are normal. Special attention must be directed to the hip joint because a significantly higher incidence of hip instability is associated with the breech position.

Congenital subluxation of the knee indicates a more severe degree of deformity and instability of the knee. More than half of these infants have associated congenital dislocation of the hip. The range of motion of the knee may reveal up to 45 degrees of hyperextension of the knee with no passive flexion (Fig. 16-1). Bilateral knee involvement is the rule. Treatment should be initiated immediately after birth and usually requires serial splinting or casting of the knees into flexion with daily adjustments until 90 degrees of flexion is attained. A brace, such as the Pavlik harness, may then be used to allow motion of the knee in flexion and simultaneously prevent knee extension. The Pavlik harness simultaneously treats coexisting hip instability. The radiographic appearance of the hyperextended knee reveals normal centers of secondary ossification at the distal femur. Lateral radiographs of the hyperextended knee demonstrate normal orientation between the proximal tibia and distal femur (Fig. 16-2), while the lateral view of congenital subluxation of the knee demon-

strates anterior subluxation of the proximal tibia on the femur. After 4 to 6 weeks of treatment, patients with congenital subluxation of the knee demonstrate complete flexion of the knee without a tendency for recurrent hyperextension. The growth and development of the knee in this group of patients has been demonstrated to be normal without recurrence of deformity or instability.

Congenital dislocation of the knee is a severe clinical problem seen in association with other conditions such as Larsen syndrome or myelomeningocele. Long-standing dissociation of the knee joint in utero results in stretching of the posterior capsule of the knee with anterior displacement of the hamstring muscles. The hamstrings no longer act as flexors of the knee but rather as extensors and thus foster persistent deformity. Shortly after birth, splinting and casting is required to improve femorotibial alignment and to obtain flexion of the knee. Surgical correction is frequently necessary to reduce the dislocation of the knee because the rectus femoris is short and fibrotic. Lengthening of the rectus femoris usually results in 90 degrees of flexion of the knee, allowing good function; however, normal growth and development of the knee is not the rule. If left untreated, congenital dislocation of the knee produces severe rotational deformities of the knee with significant anterolateral displacement of the tibia on the femur and progressive alteration in the congruency of the distal femur and proximal tibia (Fig. 16-3). Bracing of the untreated knee is virtually impossible, and

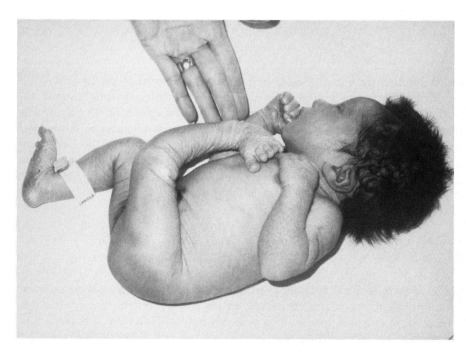

FIGURE 16-1. Newborn infant illustrates hyperextension of the knee consistent with congenital subluxation of the knee.

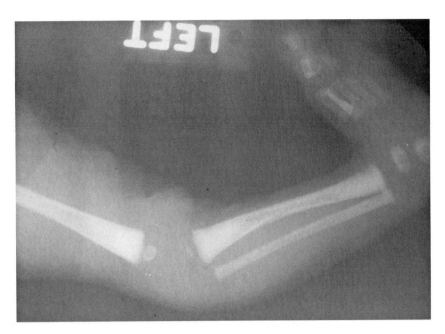

FIGURE 16-2. Lateral radiograph of the knee demonstrates normal orientation of proximal tibia to distal femur in hyperextension of the knee.

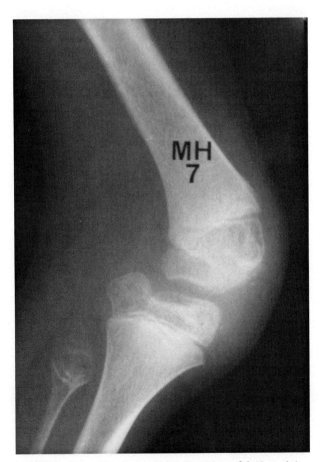

FIGURE 16-3. Severe rotational distortion of the knee joint with secondary changes to the distal femur and proximal tibial epiphysis.

many children are limited in their ability to stand, transfer, and ambulate. Although normal range of motion of the knee is not usually obtained by early surgical intervention, sufficient flexion of the knee is maintained to permit activities of daily living.

TIBIA VARA (BLOUNT DISEASE)

Normal growth and development of the lower extremities exhibits physiologic varus or bowing of the lower limbs until 2 to 3 years of age, at which time physiologic genu valgum (knock knees) usually develops in conjunction with spontaneous resolution of internal tibial torsion (Fig. 16-4). Physiologic bowing is accentuated by persistence of severe degrees of internal tibial torsion. When a toddler presents with evidence of severe bowing of the lower extremities with genu varum, it is necessary to rule out rickets, metaphyseal dysostosis, and tibia vara (Blount disease).

Tibia vara is frequently seen in obese children and in early walkers (eg, 7 months of age) and has a higher incidence in Jamaican children. Infantile Blount disease is detected before 3 years of age and is usually bilateral. These children are brought by their parents with complaint of bowing of the lower extremities (Fig. 16-5).

Physical examination of children with tibia vara reveals full flexion and extension of the knees with

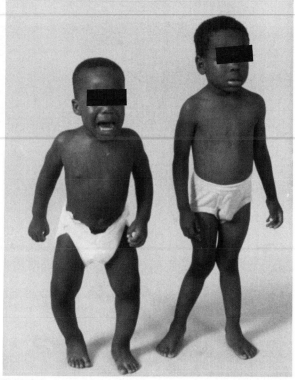

FIGURE 16-4. Normal genu varum evolves to a physiologic genu valgum by 3 years of age in normal growth and development.

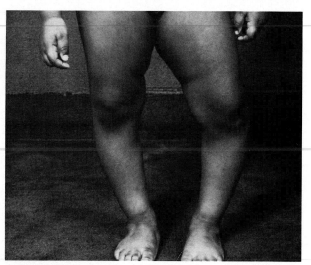

FIGURE 16-5. Rotational deformity of the proximal tibia, especially when unilateral, suggests tibia vara.

occasional observation of mild laxity of the lateral side of the knee. The degree of laxity of the knee correlates directly with the duration of deformity and the age of the child. The treatment of infantile Blount disease is controversial. A Blount brace that uses a lateral pad system with medially directed forces to correct bowing or a long-leg brace with a locked knee and three-point system to correct the bow have been used, but results are difficult to evaluate because spontaneous resolution of deformity has been reported. Langenskiold classified tibia vara into seven stages. Spontaneous improvement and successful bracing are noted in the first three stages; however, once stage 4 deformity has occurred, surgical correction is required. Progressive varus deformity increases compressive forces on the medial physis of the knee, inhibits medial tibial physeal growth, and stresses the lateral ligaments of the knee.

Radiographic evaluation of the knee in infantile tibia vara reveals early changes involving "thumb printing" of the medial aspect of the proximal tibial epiphysis that may gradually progress to a depression of the metaphysis (Fig. 16-6). Concomitant changes occur at the knee joint with overgrowth of the medial

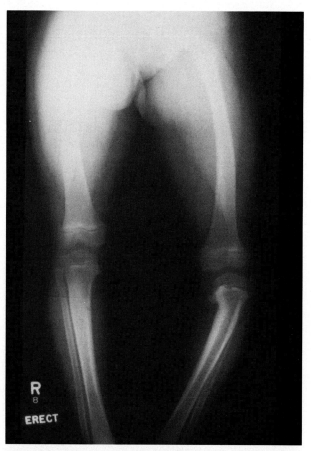

FIGURE 16-6. This radiograph demonstrates mild epiphyseal involvement of the proximal right tibia with significant depression of the epiphysis, physis, and proximal metaphysis of the left proximal tibia consistent with tibia vara.

femoral condyle and at the ankle joint with alterations of the axis of the ankle into internal rotation.

Blank reported that obese children with 30 degrees of varus at the knee are biomechanically susceptible to inhibition of growth of the proximal tibial physis. Surgical correction of tibia vara requires osteotomy of the proximal tibia in the metaphyseal area. The tibial tubercle must not be violated to avoid early closure of the anterior proximal tibial physis with secondary deformity. Overcorrection of the proximal tibial osteotomy into valgus is needed to discourage recurrence of varus deformity. Repeat osteotomy may be required in young children, and their parents should be forewarned of this possibility. Ligamentous laxity noted at the lateral aspect of the knee in children with tibia vara may be addressed by bracing after surgical realignment. Although laxity of the knee joint is an irreversible problem in the adult, ligamentous laxity in infantile tibia vara may be corrected by appropriate surgical realignment of the lower leg and bracing of the knee.

Adolescent Blount disease occurs in the second decade of life, is seen in patients who are above the 95th percentile for height and weight, and is usually unilateral. The radiographic appearance of adolescent Blount disease differs from the infantile form and exhibits diminished height of the medial half of the proximal tibial epiphysis (Fig. 16-7). Only in advanced stages do radiographic changes develop at the medial physis and metaphysis, with histologic evidence of disorganized physeal cells and bony bridging between epiphysis and metaphysis. Significant deformity may develop with secondary laxity of the ligaments requiring surgical realignment of the proximal tibia with closure of the remainder of the proximal tibial physis. When there is marked overgrowth of the medial femoral condyle with resultant valgus alignment of the knee joint, it is extremely important to first realign the distal femur by distal femoral osteotomy and then correct the proximal tibial deformity.

CONGENITAL PSEUDARTHROSIS OF THE TIBIA

Congenital pseudarthrosis of the tibia is a rare condition with an incidence of 1 in 190,000 live births. Bilateral involvement is rare. The etiology of congenital pseudarthrosis of the tibia is unknown and appears to be the end expression of several different pathologic conditions. The most common associated condition is neurofibromatosis. There are scattered

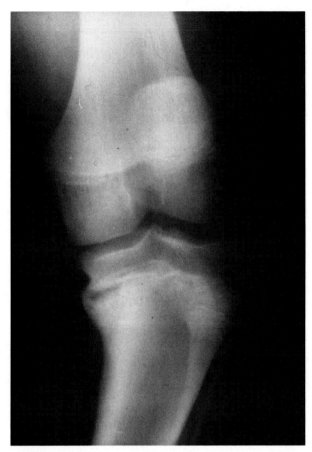

FIGURE 16-7. Radiograph documents diminished height of the medial half of the proximal tibial physis consistent with adolescent Blount disease.

reports of congenital pseudarthrosis of the tibia that is hereditary (see Chap. 7).

Fracture and frank pseudarthrosis are rarely present at birth. There are three forms of congenital pseudarthrosis of the tibia: dysplastic, cystic, and late. The dysplastic congenital pseudarthrosis of the tibia is typified by anterolateral bow of the tibia, sclerosis of the diaphysis, and complete or incomplete obliteration of the medullary canal. The dysplastic form requires protection by bracing because fracture is likely to occur once ambulation is initiated. Fracture of the dysplastic type usually results in nonunion and has a frequent association with neurofibromatosis. The cystic form of congenital pseudarthrosis of the tibia reveals cyst-like changes in the distal tibia that result in anterolateral deformation of the tibia with weight bearing. Protection is required to prevent fracture. The late form of congenital pseudarthrosis of the tibia occurs in the previously normal lower leg that develops pseudarthrosis after fracture secondary to minimal trauma and is not associated with neurofibromatosis.

The management of established congenital pseudarthrosis of the tibia is controversial but relies on stabilization of the nonunion of the tibia, bone grafting, and transposition of vascularized fibular grafts. The Ilizarov technique of bone transfer of a segment from the proximal tibia with compression of the pseudarthrosis has had successful early results, but long-term prognosis is not yet established.

POSTEROMEDIAL BOW OF THE TIBIA

Posteromedial bow of the tibia is thought to occur as a result of intrauterine position. In addition to a visible and palpable bowing of the tibia and fibula, clinical evaluation reveals excessive dorsiflexion of the foot and ankle. Involvement is unilateral, with the involved limb shorter than the opposite normal lower leg. Progressive improvement in the posteromedial bow is the rule without increased risk of fracture. Foot and ankle function is normal, and leg length discrepancy is the primary concern. Leg length discrepancy may be addressed primarily through shoe lifts or epiphysiodesis of the opposite tibia. Brace treatment to protect the tibia from fracture or to stimulate improved alignment is unnecessary, as is osteotomy of the tibia and fibula. When leg length discrepancy exceeds 5 cm, leg lengthening of the involved tibia and fibula may be done without risk of pseudarthrosis.

DISCOID MENISCUS

The discoid meniscus typically involves the lateral meniscus with occasional involvement of the medial meniscus. The etiology of this problem is yet unknown, although Kaplan described aberrant attachment of the ligament of Wrisberg from the posterior horn of the lateral meniscus to the lateral aspect of the medial femoral condyle. Kaplan theorized that this attachment translates the meniscus laterally and medially with each flexion and extension of the knee, and he thus postulated an "irritative etiology for the hypertrophy seen in this meniscus."

Children with a discoid meniscus present with a loud popping sound and painless lateral translation of their knee with each arc of flexion and extension. The presentation of this problem typically occurs in

the first decade of life and may be of significant concern to parents. The affected children demonstrate no other physical problems. Examination of the knee is otherwise unremarkable, with no clinical deformity.

The radiographic appearance of the knee may demonstrate widening of half the joint space compared with its opposite side. Arthrography of the knee or magnetic resonance imaging (MRI) more specifically demonstrates a flat, quadrangular-shaped meniscus instead of the normally well-defined triangular meniscus (Fig. 16-8).

Older children may present with intermittent popping of the knee or true locking, which is unusual. If knee pain develops, evaluation is necessary to rule out complex tears or degeneration that may occur within the substance of the discoid meniscus. Treatment recommendations for painful meniscal tears or degeneration involve partial resection and contouring of the meniscus to maintain a stable peripheral attachment.

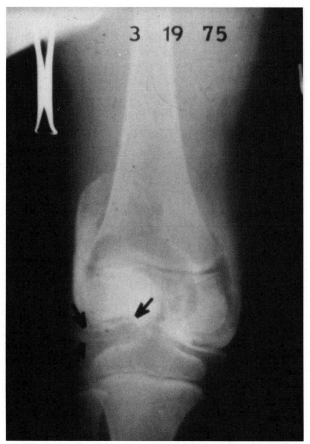

FIGURE 16-8. Arthrography of the knee demonstrates a quadrangularly shaped meniscus seen in discoid meniscus.

POPLITEAL CYST

The presence of a popliteal cyst in a child does not suggest knee pathology as it does in the adult. The cyst is noted in the area of the medial head of the gastrocnemius and semimembranosus insertion. It is typically discovered by a parent and is rarely symptomatic. The popliteal cyst is soft, nontender, and transilluminated. It is most commonly unilateral. Aspiration of the cyst reveals clear, yellow gelatinous fluid. Routine radiographs of the knee are normal, with soft tissue swelling noted and no osseous changes or soft tissue calcification. The natural history of popliteal cysts in children is one of spontaneous resolution with rare indication for operative intervention. Differential diagnosis of popliteal cysts includes fibromas, lipoma, vascular anomalies, inflammatory conditions such as juvenile rheumatoid arthritis, and malignant tumors. If the suspicion of a malignant lesion exists, aggressive evaluation through ultrasonography, computed tomographic scan, MRI, and if necessary, aspiration and open biopsy is warranted.

OSGOOD-SCHLATTER DISEASE

Osgood-Schlatter disease is a common problem that is typically seen in athletic boys at an average age of 14 years. Patients present with a painful bump at the anterior tibial tubercle. The etiology of Osgood-Schlatter disease is repetitive microtrauma with stress injury occurring within the cartilaginous substance of the anterior tibial tubercle. The traumatic etiology of this problem has been established from histologic evaluation of the tibial tubercle as well as from the clinical observation that Osgood-Schlatter disease occurs with an incidence of 21% in athletic children as opposed to 4.5% in sedentary children. Symptoms may span the spectrum from pain solely with direct contact of the tibial tubercle to pain during physical activities, such as running and jumping, to chronic pain associated with activities of daily living.

Clinical examination reveals full flexion and extension of the knee without evidence of effusion or instability. The anterior tibial tubercle is prominent and painful to direct palpation or percussion (Fig. 16-9). Frequently, there is significant weakness and atrophy of the thigh muscles and contracture of the hamstrings. Radiographic evaluation of the knee is normal except for soft tissue swelling anterior to the tibial tubercle. Fragmentation of the ossification cen-

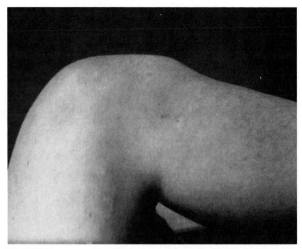

FIGURE 16-9. Physical examination of the child with Osgood-Schlatter disease reveals prominence of the anterior tibial tubercle, which is usually painful to direct palpation.

ter of the tibial tubercle is not diagnostic and may be seen in the knees of asymptomatic children.

Treatment depends on the stage of involvement. In children who have pain merely with contact and are able to be athletically active without symptoms, no intervention is required except for provision of knee pads during sports. In patients who have pain during sports activity in the absence of direct knee contact or who have pain with activities of daily living, rest from offending activities and temporary substitution of nonoffensive activities is recommended. Icing of the knee aids in diminishing the inflammatory phase and complements a physical therapy program of strengthening and stretching. The use of antiinflammatory medication and immobilization in casts has not substantially influenced the duration of treatment.

OSTEOCHONDRITIS DISSECANS OF THE KNEE

Osteochondritis dissecans was first noted by Pare in 1558, and the term *osteochondritis dissecans* was applied to this condition by Koenig in 1887. The etiology of this problem has been suggested as embolic phenomena as well as avascular necrosis; however, no end arterial system has ever been demonstrated at the distal end of the femur. Smillie suggested that repetitive trauma imposed by the tibial spine on the medial femoral condyle could result in osteochondritis dissecans, and research by others has supported this thesis. The lateral aspect of the medial femoral condyle is most frequently involved. Radiographic appearance reveals a defect at the margin of the condyle involving an osseous fragment surrounded by a lucent defect (Fig. 16-10). The lesion may be missed on routine anteroposterior (AP) radiographs and is more reliably visualized on AP tunnel view of the knee. Lesions may occur on either the medial or lateral condyle of the knee. A lesion noted at the posterior aspect of either femoral condyle or a lesion noted simultaneously at both the medial and lateral condyles represents a physiologic defect in ossification rather than a pathologic entity. Ossification defects spontaneously resolve with resultant normal radiographic appearance.

Patients may present with pain on activity or with pain, recurrent effusion, and giving way and locking of the knee. The latter complex suggests disruption of the articular cartilage overlying the osteochondral defect with mechanical loosening of the fragment. MRI or arthroscopy aids in determining the integrity of the articular cartilage. In patients with an intact articular surface and open distal femoral physis, immobilization of the knee frequently results in healing of the osteochondritis dissecans without surgical intervention. Immobilization is not effective in the mature knee.

When the articular surface of the condyle is disrupted, it is important to stabilize the fragment and to encourage revascularization by drilling the base of the lesion or by bone grafting of large osteochondral defects. This results in healing of the fragment in 80% of patients. In patients with a chronic lesion,

the bony component is minimal and surrounded by cartilage. Attempts to internally fix this lesion are fruitless, and prudent treatment involves excision of the fragment followed by a rehabilitation program. When a large portion of the weight-bearing surface of the medial compartment of the knee is involved, degenerative arthritis of the knee with narrowing and sclerosis of the joint can be expected to occur at an early age.

CONGENITAL DISLOCATION OF THE PATELLA

Patients with congenital dislocation of the patella exhibit complete lateral displacement of the patella from the distal femoral groove (Fig. 16-11). Although fixed dislocation of the patella is common, patients may demonstrate recurrent dislocations of the patella with each flexion and extension of the knee. Typically, the patella is hypoplastic, and the distal femur demonstrates a shallow intercondylar groove with a hypoplastic lateral femoral condyle.

Fixed congenital dislocation of the patella occurs in association with a variety of syndromes, and recurrent dislocation of the patella occurs in Down and Ehler-Danlos syndromes.

Patients with fixed congenital dislocation of the knee are able to ambulate without discomfort or instability and infrequently require surgical intervention. Recurrent dislocation of the patella that is painful or associated with frequent falling requires soft

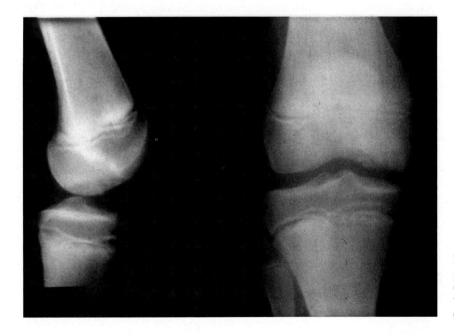

FIGURE 16-10. Radiograph depicting defects of the medial femoral condyle on both AP and lateral views indicative of osteochondritis dissecans.

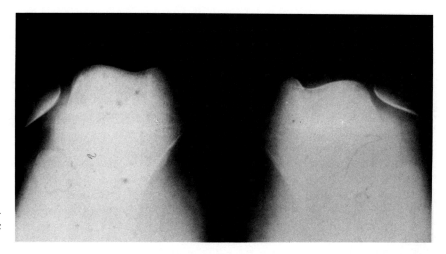

FIGURE 16-11. Lateral dislocation of both patellas with hypoplastic lateral femoral condyle.

tissue reconstruction involving lateral retinacular release, medial plication, and occasionally, realignment of the distal attachment of the patellar tendon.

PATELLAR LESIONS

Bipartite patella is characterized radiographically by an incompletely ossified portion of the patella. Involvement of the superolateral corner of the patella occurs in 75% of cases. Although bipartite patella is usually discovered as an incidental radiographic finding, it may become painful with overuse. Physical examination demonstrates local tenderness with palpation at the bipartite segment of the patella. Intervention of a surgical nature is rarely required because symptoms resolve with rest.

Patellar cysts are usually noted as incidental radiographic findings but may present in patients with knee pain. Typically, cysts are bilateral, well-circumscribed lesions of the patella. Biopsy of patellar cysts reveals nothing more than a cyst with synovial fluid. Surgical intervention is not indicated.

Sinding-Larsen-Johansson syndrome refers to lesions at either the proximal or distal poles of the patella that are the result of repetitive microtrauma. Healthy, athletic boys are commonly affected. Radiographic evaluation of the knee may be normal or may demonstrate an ill-defined border at the involved pole of the patella. Uptake on bone scan is intense at the involved site. Treatment consists of rest from running and jumping activities with resolution of the pain in 2 to 4 weeks. Healing of the lesion may be demonstrated radiographically by increased ossification at the pole of the patella with increased longitudinal length of the patella. Surgical intervention is not indicated.

TRAUMA

Tears of the extensor mechanism of the knee are rare in children but do occur and may result in complete disruption of the extensor mechanism requiring surgical reattachment to the patella. These may be associated with collagen disorders or may occur in otherwise healthy children. After healing and a comprehensive rehabilitation program, normal range of motion and function of the knee is expected.

Traumatic dislocation of the knee joint in children is rare and carries the same ominous prognosis as dislocation of the knee in the adult.

Fractures of the knee include avulsion of the tibial eminence and physeal fractures of the proximal tibia and distal femur. Avulsion of the tibial eminence may be reduced by complete extension of the knee. If radiographs of the knee in full extension demonstrate anatomic reduction of the fracture, immobilization of the knee in this position is expected to result in excellent return of function. Inability to fully extend the injured knee is a clinical indication that reduction is not anatomic; open reduction with internal fixation is then indicated.

Fracture of the proximal tibial physis requires a tremendous amount of energy and carries the same poor prognosis as dislocations of the knee with potential compromise of the popliteal vessels and nerves (Fig. 16-12). This injury is an orthopaedic and vascular emergency requiring rapid evaluation and intervention.

Fracture of the distal femoral physis may mimic injury of the medial collateral ligament and may require stress radiographs for definitive diagnosis. Physical examination reveals a swollen knee with palpable tenderness near the distal femoral physis.

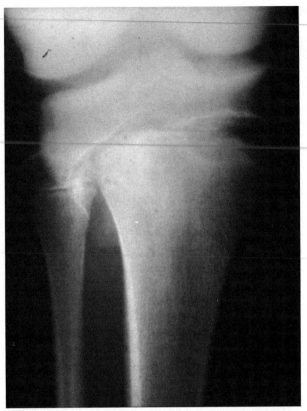

FIGURE 16-12. Fracture of the proximal tibia physis is a devastating injury with frequent compromise of popliteal vessels and nerves.

Minimally displaced fractures of the distal femoral epiphysis may be treated by immobilization in a long-leg cast, while those fractures that are completely displaced from the metaphysis of the femur require closed reduction with the use of internal fixation and hip spica casting. Premature closure of the distal femoral physis is common owing to the significant energy required to produce this fracture. Complete cessation of growth of the distal femoral physis may occur with resultant leg length discrepancy; partial closure of the physis results in progressive angular deformity of the knee.

LIGAMENTOUS INJURY

Although there has been a growing interest in reconstruction of the anterior cruciate deficient knee, the indications for reconstruction, as well as its efficacy in the immature knee, is yet to be demonstrated. The natural history of the anterior cruciate deficient knee in the child and adolescent is unknown; thus, intraarticular ligament reconstructions that violate the

growth plates of the knee must be considered investigational. The child and young adolescent who present with anterior cruciate deficiency with loss of secondary restraints and significant instability may be treated with an extensive physical therapy program and bracing to defer reconstruction of the knee to a later age.

ANTERIOR KNEE PAIN

Anterior knee pain in the child and adolescent is a symptom complex similar to that of adults with the diagnosis of chondromalacia patella.

Patients typically complain about vague anterior knee pain and swelling that is associated with activities such as prolonged walking, running, or jumping. Pain is made worse by prolonged sitting, stair climbing, squatting, and inclement weather, and there exists a sense that the involved knee will give way. Patients with anterior knee pain demonstrate full range of motion of the knee and no instability. There may be low-grade synovitis, and significant muscle weakness of the lower extremity is frequently present. A comprehensive rehabilitation program is the treatment of choice without the need for bracing, arthroscopic evaluation, or other interventional modalities.

RECURRENT SUBLUXATION AND DISLOCATION OF THE PATELLA

Recurrent dislocation of the patella is uncommon. It is usually the result of posttraumatic dislocation and failure of restitution of medial restraining structures of the knee. Children with ligamentous laxity, such as Ehlers-Danlos syndrome, are also subjected to recurrent subluxation of the patella. Patients with posttraumatic dislocations of the patella, as well as those with excessive ligamentous laxity, may demonstrate recurrent subluxation.

Recurrent subluxation and dislocation of the knee most commonly occur laterally. The patient presents with a complaint of sudden knee pain and with a sensation of instability or giving way of the knee. In the case of frank dislocation, the patient may actually fall. With recurrent subluxation and dislocation, the vicious cycle of pain and reflex weakness of the dynamic stabilizers of the knee result in activity-related pain, swelling, and instability. Physical examination reveals a hypermobile patella with lateral displacement of the patella and may reveal contracture of lateral retinaculum with only minimal medial displacement of the lateral edge of the patella from the lateral femoral condyle. Patella alta and abnormalities of the Q angle are occasionally noted. Multiple radiographic studies of the patellofemoral junction have been unreliable in analysis of this problem. Routine radiographs of the knee are required, however, to rule out fractures involving the lateral femoral condyle or the patella. Treatment of lateral subluxation of the patella requires an intensive physical therapy program and may require lateral retinacular release. Dislocation of the patella is not usually successfully treated by nonsurgical techniques and requires specific analysis of contributing factors before surgical treatment. In most adolescent patients, proximal realignment of the extensor mechanism with lateral retinacular release and medial retinacular plication results in restoration of normal patellofemoral mechanics. The Hauser procedure, with bony transposition of the patellar tendon insertion medially, is contraindicated in the immature knee because of damage to the anterior aspect of the proximal tibial physis with secondary deformity of the proximal tibia and distal migration of the patellar. After operation, an intensive physical therapy program is required.

JUMPER'S KNEE

Jumper's knee is a term that has been applied to the pathology that occurs at the junction of the quadriceps tendon and the superior pole of the patella or,

more commonly, to the junction of the distal pole of the patella and the patellar tendon. Pain is typically described as a dull ache that initially occurs after sports activity and eventually evolves to pain that is present during activities of daily living and precludes participation in sports. Physical examination of the knee reveals full extension of the knee, but flexion is limited when compared with the opposite, uninvolved side. There is no evidence of joint line tenderness or effusion; however, when the knee is examined in rested extension, there is marked tenderness to palpation of the patellar tendon adjacent to the distal pole of the patella. Early diagnosis results in the most successful treatment programs; and although considered a self-resolving problem in the past, Jumper's knee is now known to be a treacherous problem that can have permanent and irreversible effects. Histologic studies have demonstrated a partial tear of the patellar tendon fibers with fibrous proliferation and myxomatous degeneration of the tendon associated with an inflammatory response that occasionally results in softening of the distal pole of the patella.

Conservative treatment involves rest from running and jumping activities, occasionally requiring crutches and avoidance of weight bearing. Antiinflammatory medication, ice, stretching of the rectus femoris contracture, and a gradual strengthening program have been successful. Marked atrophy and weakness of the quadriceps is universal. Local steroid injections should be avoided because of the risk of

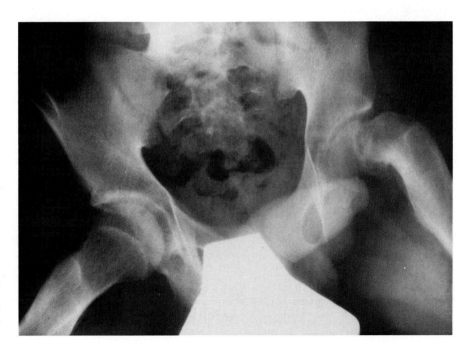

FIGURE 16-13. Hip disease, such as slipped capital femoral epiphysis, frequently presents as knee or medial thigh pain in the growing child.

spontaneous rupture of the patellar tendon. When conservative treatment fails, surgical treatment is indicated. Surgical treatment involves excision of the necrotic segment of the patellar tendon and occasionally transection of the distal pole of the patella.

MISCELLANEOUS

It is extremely important in dealing with a growing child who complains of knee pain to rule out hip disease, such as Perthes disease or slipped capital femoral epiphysis, which may present as knee pain (Fig. 16-13).

Neoplasms may also present with musculoskeletal complaints and frequently involve the knee. Leukemia is still the most common malignancy in childhood and may directly present as knee pain. Osteoid osteoma and osteoblastoma do occur in children and may require a bone scan for earlier identification.

Monoarticular juvenile rheumatoid arthritis most commonly presents with a swollen, tender, painful knee. Infection of the knee in children and adolescents is unusual and is more common in the adult.

Neuromuscular diseases may present with knee pain. These include dystonia, with alterations in gait, as well as Duchenne muscular dystrophy, which again may present with knee pain and alterations in gait.

Annotated Bibliography

Boyd HB. Pathology and natural history of congenital pseudarthrosis of the tibia. Clin Orthop 1982;16:5.
This is a classic article describing Boyd's classification of congenital pseudarthrosis of the tibia. It clearly characterizes the types of deformities that are seen and also has prognostic value.

Dinham JM. Popliteal cysts in children: the case against surgery. J Bone Joint Surg 1975;57B:69.
This article convincingly demonstrates that the natural history of popliteal cysts in children is that of spontaneous resolution. Twenty-one of 50 cysts that were treated surgically demonstrated recurrent formation of cysts in less than 1 year.

Green WT, Banks HH. Osteochondritis dissecans in children. J Bone Joint Surg 1953;35A:26.
This classic report is as true today as it was when it was first published. It characterizes osteochondritis dissecans in children. It also substantiates the value of nonoperative treatment in healing of this lesion.

Kaplan EB. Discoid lateral meniscus of the knee joint: nature, mechanism, and operative treatment. J Bone Joint Surg 1957;39A:77.
This is an elegant study of the problem by Dr. Kaplan. It identifies the aberrant ligamentous attachment of the ligament of Wrisberg to the discoid meniscus and gives an excellent description of the anatomic and pathologic anatomy.

Kling TF Jr, Hensinger RN. Angular and torsional deformities of the lower limbs in children. Clin Orthop 1983;176:136.
This is an excellent review of the commonly encountered angular and torsional problems in early childhood and discusses presentation, differential diagnosis, and recommended treatment.

Kujala UM, Kvist M, Heinonen O. Osgood-Schlatter disease in adolescent athlete: retrospective study of incidence and duration. Am J Sports Med 1985;13:236.
This study confirms the effect of increased activity in the adolescent with Osgood-Schlatter disease. A questionnaire and evaluation demonstrated that 21% of adolescents involved in sports, as opposed to 4.5% of those who were not active, were affected by Osgood-Schlatter disease.

Langenskiold A. Tibia vara: a critical review. Clin Orthop 1989;246:195.
The presentation, treatment, and radiographic classification of tibia vara, or Blount disease, are discussed.

Medlar RC, Lyne ED. Sinding-Larsen Johansson disease: its etiology and natural history. J Bone Joint Surg 1978;60A:1113.
The clinical characteristics, presentation, and suspected etiology are presented in this study of adolescent patients. It concludes by noting that this disease has a self-limiting course that requires some dramatic treatment.

Nogi J, MacEwen GD. Congenital dislocation of the knee. J Pediatr Orthop 1982;2:509.
This article describes congenital dislocation of the knee and its associated abnormalities and expected outcomes.

Ogden JA, Southwick WO. Osgood-Schlatter disease and tibial tuberosity development. Clin Orthop 1976;116:180.
The authors compare the normal growth and development of the tibial tuberosity with radiographic appearance of 53 patients with Osgood-Schlatter disease and note that this problem is an overuse disorder due to the inability of the secondary ossification centers to withstand the strong tensile forces.

Pappas AM. Congenital posteromedial bowing of the tibia and fibula. J Pediatr Orthop 1984;4:525.
The growth and development of 33 patients with congenital posteromedial bowing of the tibia and fibula are documented with the demonstration of progressive improvement and leg length discrepancy.

Riseborough EJ, Barrett IR, Shapiro F. Growth disturbances following distal femoral physeal fracture-separations. J Bone Joint Surg 1983;65A:885.
This article demonstrates the high incidence of early growth plate disorders associated with this injury.

Roberts JM. Fractures and dislocation of the knee. In: Rockwood CA Jr, Wilkins KE, King RE, eds. Fractures in children, vol 3. Philadelphia, JB Lippincott, 1984:891.
This article clearly describes the pathophysiology of this fracture and indicates that closed reduction can be obtained in almost all cases.

Salenius P, Vankka E. The development of the tibiofemoral angle in children. J Bone Joint Surg 1975;57A:259.
This study demonstrates the normal progression of children born with genu varum to genu valgum after 2 to 3 years of age.

Shelton WR, Canale ST. Fractures of the tibia through the proximal tibial epiphyseal cartilage. J Bone Joint Surg 1979;61A:167.
This report documents the serious complications associated with this injury involving compartment syndrome and nerve and arterial damage.

Stanislavjevic S, Zemenick G, Miller D. Congenital, irreducible, permanent lateral dislocation of the patella. Clin Orthop 1976;116:190.
In addition to the authors' recommended treatment of proximal realignment of the dislocated patella, a comprehensive review of the literature is presented.

Turek's Orthopaedics: Principles and Their Application, Fifth Edition,
edited by Stuart L. Weinstein and Joseph A. Buckwalter.
J.B. Lippincott Company, Philadelphia, © 1994.

17

Russell E. Windsor

The Adult Knee

SOFT TISSUE DISORDERS
    Popliteal Cysts
    Bursitis and Tendinitis
    Quadriceps Tendon Rupture and
        Patellar Tendon Rupture
PATELLOFEMORAL DISORDERS
    Lateral Patellar Compression
        Syndrome
    Patellar Subluxation and
        Dislocation
    Chondromalacia Patellae and
        Patellofemoral Arthritis
LIGAMENT INJURIES
    Location

    Tests
    Classification
    Radiologic Evaluation
    Treatment
MENISCAL INJURIES
OSTEONECROSIS
ARTHRITIS OF THE KNEE
FRACTURES OF THE PATELLA
FRACTURES OF THE FEMORAL
    CONDYLES
FRACTURES OF THE TIBIAL
    PLATEAU
INFECTION

SOFT TISSUE DISORDERS

Popliteal Cysts

Distention of the semimembranosus bursa gives rise to a popliteal or Baker cyst. In children, a popliteal cyst occurs as a primary condition. It usually appears in the back of the knee as a painless swelling. Although its cause is unknown, the cyst is possibly due to friction of the flexed knee against a school chair or bench. It may be bilateral and usually resolves spontaneously. In adults, the occurrence of a popliteal cyst is nearly always secondary to pathologic changes in the knee joint, such as patellofemoral arthrosis, meniscal tears, or any form of synovitis. It presents as an aching pain in the back of the knee, and aspiration of synovial fluid confirms the diagnosis. Occasionally, the cyst becomes so large that it ruptures, spilling synovial fluid into the surrounding tissues, and causes a syndrome that mimics acute thrombophlebitis. Popliteal cysts usually resolve spontaneously and only rarely need excision.

Bursitis and Tendinitis

Numerous bursae around the knee may become infected or inflamed (Fig. 17-1). The prepatellar bursa lies anterior to the patella and is subcutaneous. It becomes chronically inflamed from prolonged kneeling and usually produces no effusion. Treatment consists of aspiration of the serosanguineous fluid with injection of a cortisone derivative. Rarely, excision is necessary. Other bursae that may become inflamed are the semimembranosus, pes anserinus, and infrapatellar bursae. Inflammation is usually due to overuse and is treated by heat, exercise, and antiinflammatory medications.

Tendinitis can affect any of the tendons that insert around the knee, that is, the pes anserinus, semimembranosus, biceps femoris, quadriceps extensor mechanism, and popliteal tendons and the iliotibial band (Fig. 17-2). Most patients can be treated with rest, exercise modification, locally applied heat, and occasional use of antiinflammatory medications.

Traction apophysitis of the patella (Sinding-Larsen disease) affects the region overlying the tibial tubercle insertion of the patellar ligament. It may occur proximally at the lower pole of the patella (jumper's knee). These conditions usually are seen in basketball or volleyball athletes who put excessive strain on the patellar ligament. The iliotibial band syndrome is due to chronic rubbing of a tight iliotibial band over the prominent lateral femoral condyle. Bicyclists and long-distance runners often develop this syndrome. These conditions can also be treated by rest, exercise modification, locally applied heat, or antiinflammatory medications.

Quadriceps Tendon Rupture and Patellar Tendon Rupture

Significant force generated across the knee extensor mechanism may result in rupture of the quadriceps tendon insertion on the proximal pole of the patella or the patellar ligament from the distal pole of the patella. Excessive eccentric loading of the extensor mechanism during a maximal contraction results in its disruption. In elderly patients, the ruptures occur in the tendinous region, where there is a tenuous blood supply. In younger patients, tears occur in the quadriceps muscle. Ruptures also occur in patients with a history of diabetes mellitus, chronic renal failure, hyperthyroidism, gout, and multiple cortisone injections. Magnetic resonance imaging (MRI) is a valuable tool in diagnosing acute ruptures. However, the physical examination confirms the diagnosis: the patient cannot actively extend the knee against resistance, and a palpable defect is usually present. The treatment of choice for rupture of the quadriceps tendon or of the patellar tendon is surgical repair.

PATELLOFEMORAL DISORDERS

The patella is effectively anchored to the knee by four structures in a cruciform arrangement: the pa-

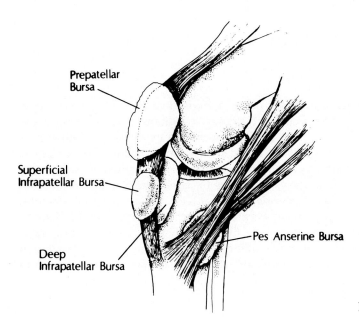

FIGURE 17-1. The bursae of the knee.

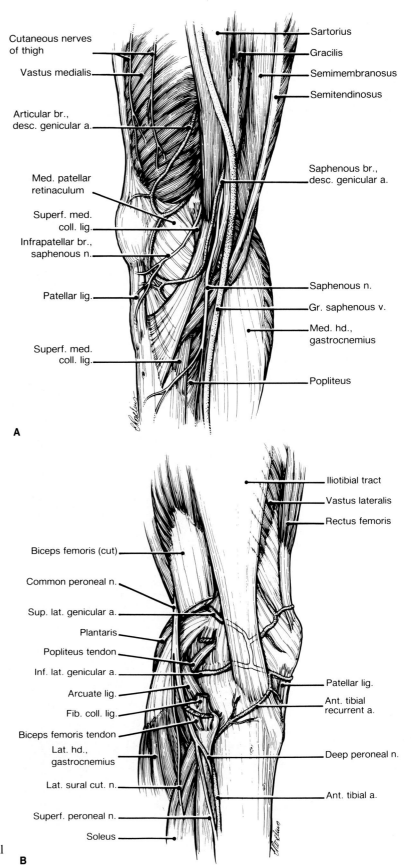

FIGURE 17-2. The medial (A) and lateral (B) aspects of the knee joint.

tellar tendon, the lateral retinaculum, the medial retinaculum, and the quadriceps tendon (Fig. 17-3). There are several congenital anomalies of the patella, including bipartite patella, congenital absence of the patella (patellar aplasia), a small patella (patellar hypoplasia), and a large patella (patella magna). The patellofemoral joint is biomechanically complex, but the most important function of the patella is to improve the efficiency of the quadriceps by increasing the lever arm of the extensor mechanism. The thickness of the patella displaces the patellar tendon away from the femorotibial contact point throughout knee range of motion, thereby increasing the moment arm of the patellar tendon. It has been shown that 3.3 times the body weight is generated across the patellofemoral joint at 60 degrees of knee flexion during stair climbing, and up to 7.8 times the body weight at 130 degrees during deep knee bends. Patellofemoral contact pressures are uniformly spread over all contact areas, but peak pressures are highest between 60 and 90 degrees of flexion.

The symptoms of patellar dysfunction include anterior knee pain, giving way, locking, and swelling. Occasionally, pain may be referred to the joint lines, mimicking the symptoms associated with meniscal tears.

Lateral Patellar Compression Syndrome

The lateral patellar compression syndrome is characterized by pain. Pain is characteristically dull, poorly localized, and increased by activities that overload the patellofemoral joint. Symptoms may follow a trauma. A sense of the knee buckling may occur, which makes this syndrome difficult to differentiate from patients with true patellar instability. True episodes of patellar instability, however, followed by considerable swelling that persists a few days, are lacking. An apprehension test (whereby the patient becomes apprehensive when the physician attempts to move the patella medially and laterally

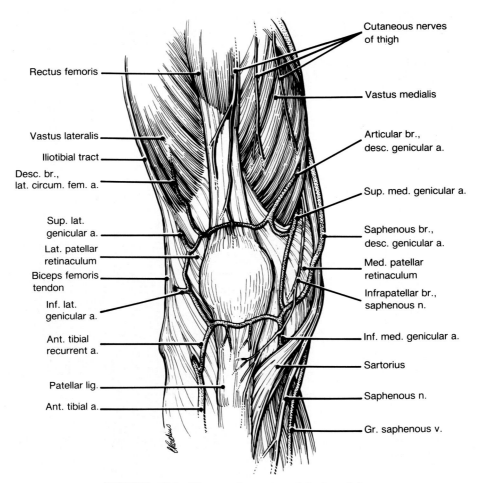

FIGURE 17-3. The anterior aspect of the knee joint.

with the knee extended, simulating the feeling of instability) is negative, and only minor tracking abnormalities of the patella are present.

On physical examination, squinting of the patellae is easily appreciated. There may be a mild varus relation between the tibia and the femur. The intramedullary axes of the femur and tibia are usually parallel and connected by an oblique patellar tendon, which slopes downward and laterally (bayonet deformity). A half-squat usually provokes pain. A quadriceps angle of greater than 20 degrees is abnormal. This angle is formed by a line drawn through the center of the long axis of the thigh across the midportion of the patella and a line drawn along the patellar tendon. The lateral retinaculum is considered tight if the patella is unable to be moved medially more than one fourth of its width. Pain on compression of the patella against the femoral sulcus is usually present. Patellofemoral radiographs in the form of axial views in different degrees of extension show the patella not to be laterally displaced (Fig. 17-4). The pain is thought to result from excessive lateral loading of the patellar ridge. Excessive lateral ligamentous tension may also contribute to the syndrome.

Treatment consists of rest, restriction of activity, quadriceps training, antiinflammatory medication, rehabilitation program, and taping. Occasionally, surgical treatment is necessary and includes lateral retinacular release done by open arthrotomy or arthroscopic means. An overall compilation of the data in the literature showed 73% satisfactory results in 879 procedures reported.

Patellar Subluxation and Dislocation

Patellar subluxation and dislocation can be grouped together as patellar instability. *Subluxation* is an alteration of normal patellar tracking, but with the patella still within the femoral sulcus. *Dislocation* occurs when the patella is completely displaced out of the sulcus. The following clinical situations can be encountered: acute dislocation, chronic subluxation, and recurrent, habitual, and permanent dislocation of the patella.

Acute Dislocation of the Patella

The term *acute dislocation of the patella* is applied after the first episode of dislocation. The dislocation occurs after a twisting movement of the knee that causes the patient to fall to the ground. The patella is observed lying on the lateral side of the knee. As

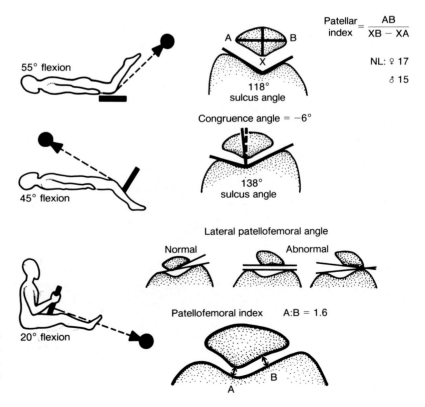

FIGURE 17-4. Schematic representations of the different radiographic evaluations of the patella: the Hughston (55 degrees), Merchant (45 degrees), and Laurin (20 degrees) patella views.

the knee is straightened, the patella relocates in the sulcus with a rapid onset of swelling. It is unusual to observe the patella still in the dislocated position in the emergency department. Knee aspiration generally demonstrates a hemarthrosis. The knee is grossly swollen with medial retinacular tenderness. The differential diagnosis includes anterior cruciate ligament injury and rupture of the quadriceps or patellar tendon. Radiographically, lateral placement of the patella on an axial, skyline (Merchant) view may be evident (Fig. 17-5). Oblique and notch radiographic views may be necessary to exclude the presence of an osteochondral fracture of the medial patellar facet. Initial treatment includes immobilization in extension for 4 weeks followed by quadriceps strengthening. The rate of recurrent dislocation is 33%. Surgical repair of the medial retinaculum with proximal quadriceps muscle realignment is indicated for recurrence and for acute dislocation with associated osteochondral fracture.

Chronic Subluxation of the Patella

Patients with chronic subluxation of the patella have patellar pain and axial radiographic views that reveal a lateral displacement of the patella. These knees represent an intermediate grade of dysplasia between lateral patellar compression syndrome and recurrent dislocation of the patella. Patients may experience patellar instability. Treatment is initially nonoperative, but if this fails, a lateral retinacular release or major realignment procedure may be considered.

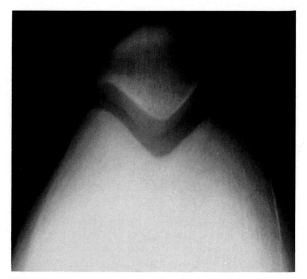

FIGURE 17-5. A 45-degree (Merchant) axial view of the patellofemoral joint.

Recurrent Dislocation of the Patella

Recurrent dislocation of the patella occurs after an acute dislocation and may occur as a result of trivial injuries. The patient may demonstrate quadriceps atrophy and hypoplasia of the vastus medialis obliquus. The quadriceps angle may be increased. The patient demonstrates significant apprehension when the patella is displaced laterally with the knee flexed 20 to 30 degrees. A flattened sulcus may be observed, and patella alta with hyperextension deformity of the knee may also contribute to chronic dislocation. Conservative treatment consists of quadriceps strengthening and the use of a patellar cut-out brace. Surgical treatment consists of lateral retinacular release or a proximal realignment. Occasionally, in severely dysplastic knees, both proximal and distal realignments are necessary. Distal realignments usually consist of changing the location of the distal insertion of the patellar tendon at the tibial tubercle. Successful stabilization of the knee occurs in 85% of cases. However, some degree of pain may persist.

Chronic Dislocation of the Patella

In knees with chronic dislocation of the patella, the patella dislocates laterally each time the knee is flexed and returns toward the midline with extension of the knee (habitual dislocation). In the most severe cases, the patella is permanently dislocated laterally (permanent dislocation). This disorder is usually first detected in children in the first decade. It may be associated with contracture of the quadriceps or chronic injections into the thigh, which may cause quadriceps fibrosis and contracture. Surgical treatment is directed toward realigning the patella and lengthening the contracted quadriceps.

Chondromalacia Patellae and Patellofemoral Arthritis

Chondromalacia patellae and patellofemoral arthritis are secondary to damaged or softened articular cartilage of the patellofemoral joint. The term *chondromalacia* should be used only to describe the changes that occur in the articular cartilage. Observable age-related changes in chondromalacia occur commonly after the second decade and in almost all knees after the fourth decade. Outerbridge classified chondromalacia in four different grades:

Grade I—softening and swelling

Grade II—fragmentation and fissuring in a 0.5-inch or smaller area

Grade III—fragmentation and fissuring in a 0.5-inch or larger area

Grade IV—cartilage erosion down to bone

Most chondromalacia is idiopathic in nature. It may, however, result from lateral patellar compression syndrome, patellar instability, trauma, previous anterior cruciate ligament surgery, prolonged immobilization for fracture treatment, or synovial conditions affecting the articular cartilage surface. Pain is associated with increased patellar pressure and basal degeneration of the cartilage. Chondromalacia should be limited to disorders that involve only the articular cartilage. If the disease has progressed to involve changes of the bone (osteophyte formation, subchondral sclerosis, and cysts) and of the synovium (synovitis), it should be classified as patellofemoral arthritis.

Patellofemoral arthritis involves predominantly the lateral joint line in most cases. Narrowing of the joint line, with osteophytes on the lateral patellar border and trochlea, subchondral sclerosis of the lateral facet, and possibly cyst formation, may be present on axial radiographs. Most often, patellofemoral arthrosis appears to arise de novo in a structurally normal joint for which no obvious cause can be assigned. There is a frequently associated femorotibial arthrosis. Nonoperative treatment consists of isometric quadriceps exercises, knee braces, and anti-inflammatory medications. Surgical treatment involves procedures that relieve stress on the patellofemoral joint and that directly address the pathology of the articular cartilage. Patellar cartilage shaving can be done open or arthroscopically and yields the best results (83% satisfactory) in the earlier stages of chondromalacia. Subchondral bone drilling with cortical abrasion yields more unpredictable results (60% satisfactory), as does lateral retinacular release. Elevation of the tibial tubercle (Fig.17-6), patellar resurfacing, and patellectomy show limited success (70% satisfactory) and are formidable procedures with high complication rates.

LIGAMENT INJURIES

Location

Medial Structures

The medial collateral ligament (superficial and deep portions) and the posterior capsular ligament, termed the *posterior oblique ligament*, are augmented by the dynamic stabilizing effect of the capsular arm of the semimembranosus tendon and its aponeurosis, the oblique popliteal ligament. The medial head of the gastrocnemius provides dynamic support to the medial compartment. The posterior oblique ligament is firmly attached to and contiguous with the medial meniscus. This ligament is the main deterrent to external rotation of the knee.

Lateral Structures

The lateral collateral ligament is the major static support to varus stress, while the iliotibial tract provides both dynamic and static support. The posterolateral capsule is composed of the lateral collateral ligament, the arcuate ligament, and the aponeurosis of the popliteus muscle. These structures form the arcuate complex, whose function is augmented by the dynamic effects of the biceps femoris, popliteus muscle, and the lateral head of the gastrocnemius muscle.

Anterior Cruciate Ligament

The anterior cruciate ligament is the primary structure controlling anterior displacement in the unloaded knee. The ligament is composed of anteromedial and posterolateral bundles. Some authors found that the fiber bundles were not isometric but that the anteromedial bundle lengthens and the pos-

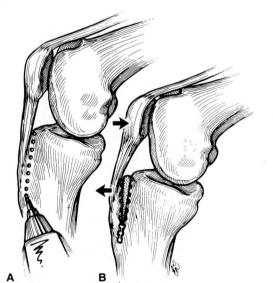

FIGURE 17-6. The Maquet tibial tubercle elevation. The procedure is designed to decrease the patellofemoral contact pressures for the treatment of severe chondromalacia and arthritis of the patella.

terolateral bundle shortens during flexion. Tibial rotation is better resisted by a combination of capsular structures, collateral ligaments, joint surface, and meniscal geometry, while the cruciates play only a secondary role. The medial collateral ligament provides significant resistance to the anterior drawer test only after the anterior cruciate is disrupted and when both ligaments are lost. Injuries to the medial structures further compromise anterior stability when they accompany anterior cruciate ligament injuries.

Posterior Cruciate Ligament

The posterior cruciate ligament is believed to be the most important of the knee ligaments because of its cross-sectional area, tensile strength, and location in the central axis of the knee joint since it provides 95% of the total resistance to posterior displacement of the tibia. The posterior cruciate ligament prevents posterior translation at all angles of flexion. Absence of the posterior cruciate ligament has no effect on primary varus or external rotation of the tibia so long as the lateral collateral ligament and capsular structures are intact. The anterior portion, which forms the bulk of the ligament, tightens in flexion, whereas the smaller posterior portion tightens in extension. Lying anterior to the posterior cruciate ligament, connecting the posterior horn of the lateral meniscus to the medial femoral condyle, is the ligament of Humphrey. The ligament of Wrisberg passes posterior to the posterior cruciate ligament to attach to the posterior cruciate ligament.

Tests

Valgus Stress Test

The valgus stress test should be performed on the normal extremity first for later comparison. The involved knee is flexed to 30 degrees, and a gentle valgus stress is applied to the knee with one hand placed on the lateral aspect of the thigh and the other hand grasping the foot and ankle. It tests for medial ligamentous laxity.

Varus Stress Test

The varus stress test is similar to the valgus stress test and is carried out with the knee both in full extension and in 30 degrees of flexion. The integrity of the lateral ligamentous structures is tested by this maneuver. Flexing the knee 30 degrees removes the lateral stabilizing effect of the iliotibial band so that the lateral collateral ligament can be isolated for examination.

Anterior Drawer Test

The anterior drawer test evaluates the integrity of the anterior cruciate ligament (Fig. 17-7). The hip is flexed to 45 degrees with the knee flexed to 80 or 90 degrees. The examiner stabilizes the foot with his or her buttocks. The hand is placed around the proximal tibia, and the tibia is displaced anteriorly in a to-and-fro manner after the hamstrings are adequately relaxed.

Lachman Test

The Lachman test also assesses anterior knee laxity and stiffness with the knee in about 20 degrees of flexion and applying an anterior drawer to the proximal calf (Fig. 17-8). Endpoint stiffness is assessed. A soft endpoint signifies a torn anterior cruciate ligament, whereas a firm endpoint demonstrates an intact structure.

Pivot Shift Test

The pivot shift test demonstrates anterior subluxation and reduction of the tibia with knee flexion and extension from 10 to 40 degrees as a result of anterior cruciate ligament disruption (Fig. 17-9).

Posterior Drawer Test

The posterior drawer test demonstrates the integrity of the posterior cruciate ligament. The knee

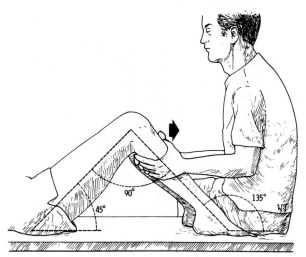

FIGURE 17-7. The anterior drawer test is performed with the patient supine and the affected knee bent 90 degrees. An anterior force is applied by the examiner.

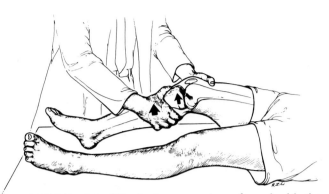

FIGURE 17-8. The Lachman test is performed with the knee flexed between 15 and 30 degrees. An anterior force is applied by the examiner.

is flexed to 90 degrees, and posterior force is exerted on the tibia in an attempt to subluxate it posteriorly in relation to the femur (Fig. 17-10). A sag may be demonstrated anteriorly in comparison with the other intact knee. The examiner should be aware of the position of the tibia before starting the test.

Posterior Pivot Shift Test

The posterior pivot shift test is used to diagnose injuries to the posterolateral ligament complex. The clinician supports the limb with a hand under the heel, with the knee in full extension and neutral rotation (Fig. 17-11). A valgus stress is applied, and the knee is flexed. In a positive test, at about 20 to 30 degrees of flexion, the tibia externally rotates, and the lateral tibial plateau subluxates posteriorly and remains in this position during further flexion. When the knee is extended, the tibia reduces.

Classification

Sprain

A *sprain* is an injury to a joint ligament that stretches or tears ligamentous fibers but does not completely disrupt the ligament. A *first-degree sprain* is a tear of a minimal number of fibers of a ligament with localized tenderness and no instability. A *second-degree sprain* tears more ligamentous fibers with slight to moderate abnormal motion. In a *third-degree sprain*, there is a complete tear of the ligament with disruption of fibers and demonstrable instability. Third-degree sprains are further subdivided as follows:

Grade I—less than 0.5-cm opening of the joint surfaces
Grade II—0.5- to 1-cm opening of the joint surfaces
Grade III—rupture larger than 1 cm

Instability

Instability is divided into *straight* and *rotatory*. There are four types of straight instability:

Medial—caused by a tear of the medial ligaments combined with a tear of the posterior cruciate ligament. In full extension, the knee joint opens on the medial side with a valgus stress test with the knee in a fully extended position. This instability indicates disruption of the medial collateral ligament, the medial capsular ligament, the anterior cruciate ligament, the posterior oblique ligament, and the medial portion of the posterior capsule.
Lateral—results from a tear of lateral structures

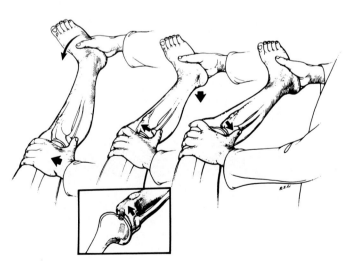

FIGURE 17-9. The pivot shift test of Galway and MacIntosh is performed with the knee in full extension. A valgus and internal rotation stress is applied.

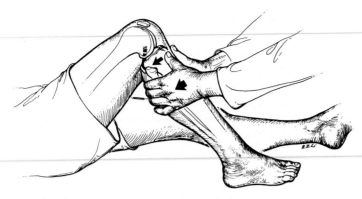

FIGURE 17-10. The posterior drawer test is done with the knee flexed 90 degrees. A posteriorly directed force is applied to the tibia.

and the posterior cruciate ligament. The knee opens on the lateral side with a varus stress test with the knee in the fully extended position. It indicates disruption of the lateral capsular ligament, the lateral collateral ligament, and commonly, the posterior cruciate ligament.

Posterior—develops after disruption of the posterior cruciate ligament, the arcuate ligament complex, and the posterior oblique ligament complex.

Anterior—caused by disruption of the anterior cruciate ligament, the lateral capsular ligament, and the medial capsular ligament.

There are four types of rotatory instability:

Anteromedial—manifested in tibial abduction, adduction, external tibial rotation, and anterior tibial translation and causes the medial tibial plateau to translate or subluxate anteriorly in relation to the femur. This implies disruption of the medial capsular ligament, medial collateral ligament, posterior oblique ligament, and anterior cruciate ligament. An intact me-

dial meniscus may provide added stability in this instability.

Anterolateral—shown by excessive internal rotation of the tibia on the femur with the knee at 90 degrees of flexion. This implies disruption of the lateral capsular ligament, the arcuate complex, and the anterior cruciate ligament.

Posterolateral—when the lateral tibial plateau rotates posteriorly in relation to the femur with lateral opening of the joint. This implies disruption of the popliteus tendon, the arcuate complex, and the lateral capsular ligament, and at times injury to the posterior cruciate ligament. This results in an external rotatory subluxation in which the tibia rotates around an axis in the intact posterior cruciate ligament.

Posteromedial—manifested by medial tibial plateau rotation posteriorly in reference to the femur with medial opening of the joint. This implies a disruption of the medial collateral ligament, the medial capsular ligament, the posterior oblique ligament, the anterior cruciate ligament, and the medial portion of the posterior capsule.

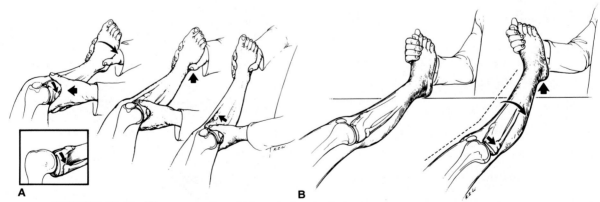

FIGURE 17-11. The reverse pivot shift test is done in flexion. An external rotation and valgus stress are applied.

Radiologic Evaluation

Standard anteroposterior and lateral views are required, with Merchant (axial) and tunnel views providing additional information if knee motion is sufficient to allow these radiographs to be taken. Injury to ligaments is not demonstrated on these views, but they show avulsion injuries to the ligament bone insertions, loose bodies, and other osteochondral fragments. A Segond fracture, an avulsion of the middle third of the lateral capsule from the tibial plateau, can be seen and has come to be known as the *lateral capsular sign*, indicating injury to the anterior cruciate ligament. Arthrography and MRI are useful tests in diagnosing acute and chronic ligamentous injuries (Fig. 17-12). MRI also shows the integrity of the menisci, which becomes important in the discussion of operative and nonoperative treatment of anterior cruciate ligament injuries.

Treatment

Isolated tears of the medial collateral ligament with intact cruciate ligaments can be treated nonsurgically. The mechanism of injury is a blow to the lateral aspect of the leg with the foot firmly planted. When valgus and rotation are coupled, tears may first occur in the medial collateral ligament and progress to involve the posterior oblique ligament and possibly the anterior cruciate ligament. Medial opening in full extension indicates concomitant injury to the cruciate

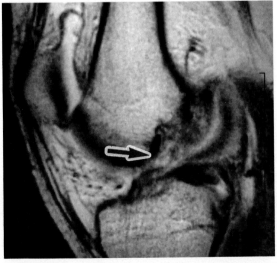

FIGURE 17-12. MRI of the knee showing absence of the normal low-intensity signal of the anterior cruciate ligament, indicating a tear or disruption of the ligament.

ligaments. Conservative treatment with early mobilization is the treatment of choice in isolated tears of the medial collateral ligament and results in more complete and rapid recovery. The ligament must be protected from harmful stress during the regeneration and maturation phases of healing. Controlled functional stress is helpful in stimulating and directing the repair response.

Treatment of anterior cruciate ligament injuries is controversial and includes both operative and nonoperative treatment options, which are applied to the patient on an individual basis based on the patient's age and activity level. The mechanism of anterior cruciate ligament tears is based on a valgus and rotatory twist on the knee with the foot firmly planted on the ground. Hyperextension injuries also can rupture the anterior cruciate ligament. Past reports demonstrated that successful rehabilitation of an anterior cruciate ligament injury can be obtained by nonoperative means in older patients with limited activities. Many recent studies, however, showed that only a small percentage (15% to 33%) of patients reach their preinjury activities. Thus, these patients stop certain activities or have pain or instability during rigorous sports. There is also a 40% chance that subsequent injury to the menisci will occur after a giving-way episode resulting from chronic anterior cruciate ligament insufficiency. Repeated injuries eventually result in further deterioration of knee function and the development of osteoarthritis. Bony changes are proliferative rather than degenerative with osteophyte formation close to the joint cartilage. Osteophytes are seen as early as 26 days postoperatively and are formed through chondroid metamorphosis of fibrous tissue and subsequent enchondral ossification. Therefore, surgical intervention has become more commonly indicated for anterior cruciate ligament injuries in older as well as younger athletic patients who wish to maintain their preinjury levels of performance.

Two methods of surgically reconstructing the anterior cruciate ligament are commonly used. Since the ligament does not heal by itself owing to the synovial fluid environment and its limited arterial blood supply, substitute structures are used to restore stability to the knee. The gracilis and semimembranosus tendons are used together, which avoids disruption of the extensor mechanism. These structures can be positioned by arthroscopic means, preventing excessive intraarticular scarring and minimizing potential complications to the extensor mechanism (Fig. 17-13). This material is ideal for acute reconstruction of the anterior cruciate ligament. Use of the central

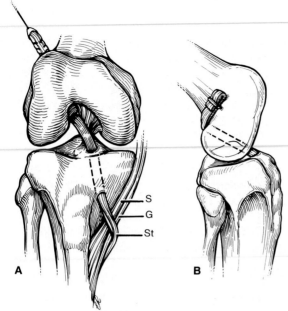

FIGURE 17-13. Anterior cruciate ligament reconstruction using the transfer of the semitendinosis tendon secured proximally with a staple. The gracilis tendon may also be used along with the semitendinosis tendons to add strength to the overall surgical construct.

one third of the patellar ligament and its bony attachments to the patella and tibial tubercle is the most common method for reconstructing the anterior cruciate ligament by arthroscopic means. More serious, multiligament injuries may not be conducive to ar-

throscopically assisted reconstruction, but the patellar ligament substitute represents the strongest natural material for restoring ligamentous integrity to the knee. The ligament measures 9 to 12 mm wide and is placed in an isometric position to allow equal tension placed on it in flexion and extension (Fig. 17-14). The rehabilitation program commences on the first postoperative day and continues for about 6 to 12 months. The length of rehabilitation depends on the ultimate activity level the patient wishes to regain.

The treatment of combined medial collateral and anterior cruciate ligament disruption involves stapling the medial collateral ligament to the tibia or femur in type III tears. In chronic insufficiency, it may be necessary to reconstruct the medial collateral ligament with the semitendinosus tendon and to use the middle third of the patellar ligament to substitute for the deficient anterior cruciate ligament. If the graft is inappropriately placed, limitation of motion occurs. If the graft is placed too far anteriorly in the tibia, knee extension is limited. If the graft is placed too far anteriorly in the femur, knee flexion decreases.

Treatment of posterior cruciate ligament injuries depends on the associated ligamentous injuries that may be present. Injuries to the posterior cruciate ligament may occur by several different mechanisms. A direct blow to the flexed knee is the most common mechanism for isolated posterior cruciate ligament injury. The force is usually applied to the proximal tibia with the knee flexed and imparts a forceful posterior drawer to a horizontally oriented posterior

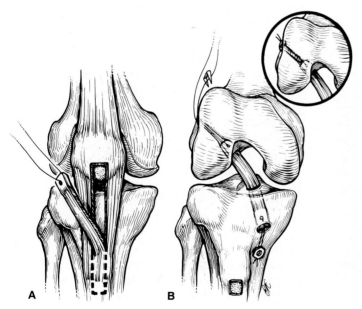

FIGURE 17-14. Anterior cruciate ligament reconstruction using the bone–patellar tendon–bone preparation. The middle third of the patellar tendon is used.

cruciate ligament, causing it to fail. Forced hyperextension and severe varus or valgus stress may cause disruption of the posterior cruciate ligament in combination with collateral ligament injury or knee dislocation. Injury to the posterolateral corner of the knee is frequent and results from a posteriorly directed blow to the anteromedial knee with the knee in extension.

Treatment of an isolated posterior cruciate ligament injury is controversial. The literature contains many reports of successful outcomes without surgery. It is not yet been proved that surgical reconstruction prevents later onset of degenerative arthritis in posterior cruciate–deficient knees. Characteristically, knees with an isolated deficiency of the posterior cruciate ligament are not unstable, and patients return to near full function. Combined ligament injuries, however, can present instability symptoms and have a poorer outcome if not surgically corrected. Treatment of an isolated posterior cruciate ligament injury is, in general, nonoperative. A vigorous quadriceps strengthening program is begun as soon as the patient's symptoms allow. Hamstring exercises are initially avoided. Some authors follow these patients yearly with bone scans to determine onset of arthritic bony changes. Surgical reconstruction is recommended when these changes are observed.

Avulsion injuries to the posterior cruciate ligament (usually the tibial bone insertion) should be surgically reattached because excellent functional results are obtained without the complications of more involved reconstructive techniques. If posterior translation of the tibia at 90 degrees of flexion is less than 10 mm, nonoperative treatment may suffice.

Direct surgical repair of the posterior cruciate ligament has met with limited success; generally, tissue autografts are needed, with the middle third of the patellar ligament used most commonly. Some surgeons use patellar ligament allografts, but the data are too sparse to recommend common use of this substitute. The patellar ligament autograft can be positioned using arthroscopic techniques (Fig. 17-15). If there is a combined injury to the posterolateral structures, open surgical augmentation should be performed. A strip of iliotibial band substitutes for an injured popliteus tendon, and the biceps femoris tendon satisfactorily works for a ruptured lateral collateral ligament. In knees with injury to the lateral collateral ligament in addition to the posterior cruciate ligament, the patient may demonstrate a varus alignment with a lateral thrust during gait. High tibial osteotomy is necessary in addition to the ligament

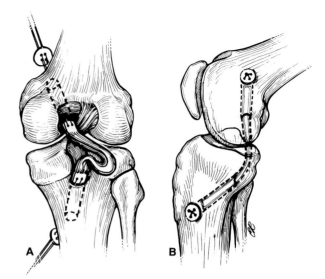

FIGURE 17-15. The Clancy technique of posterior cruciate reconstruction uses the same bone–patellar tendon–bone preparation that is seen in the anterior cruciate ligament reconstructions. However, the placement of bone tunnels is different.

reconstruction to remove stress from the lateral tibial plateau and to decrease the early onset of lateral compartment osteoarthritis.

The treatment of combined anterior and posterior cruciate ligament injuries is surgical. If both injuries are present, a history of knee dislocation should be suspected, and evaluation of the arterial circulation should take prime importance before further treatment commences. It is difficult to reconstruct the knee keeping the ligament substitutes in relatively isometric (anatomic) positions. It is possible, however, to reconstruct both ligaments with open or arthroscopic techniques. The arthroscopic method causes less scarring than the open method by arthrotomy since dissection of the surrounding soft tissue structures is minimized. The semitendinosus and gracilis tendons are used for the anterior cruciate ligament, and the middle third of the patellar ligament substitutes for the posterior cruciate ligament. An alternative method is to use Achilles or patellar tendon allograft to reconstruct either or both ligaments.

Treatment of isolated lateral collateral ligament injuries is usually nonoperative. It should be reconstructed if there is a large lateral thrust during gait. The anterior two thirds of the biceps femoris tendon is the standard anatomic substitute for the lateral collateral ligament. It is brought from its insertion on the fibular head and is placed in an isometric position on the lateral femoral condyle.

MENISCAL INJURIES

The menisci are C-shaped wedges of fibrocartilage interposed between the femoral and tibial condyles. They are extensions of the tibia and serve to deepen the articular surfaces of the tibial plateau to better accommodate the condyles of the femur (Fig. 17-16). The peripheral border of each meniscus is thick, convex, and attached to the inside capsule of the joint. The opposite border tapers to a thin, narrow, free edge. The proximal surfaces are concave and contact the femoral condyles, whereas the distal surfaces are flat and lie on top of the tibia. The medial meniscus is somewhat semicircular in form, while the lateral meniscus is more circular in shape and covers a larger percentage of the articular surface of the tibial condyle than the medial meniscus.

One function of the menisci is weight bearing. Biomechanical studies showed that at least half of the compressive load of the knee joint is transmitted through the meniscus in extension, while about 85% of the load is transmitted in 90 degrees of flexion. Complete and partial meniscectomies result in a significant increase in the load per unit area across the joint. Another proposed function of the menisci is knee joint stability. Although meniscectomy alone may not significantly increase joint instability, meniscectomy in association with anterior cruciate ligament insufficiency significantly increases the anterior laxity of the knee. The menisci also increase the congruity between the condyles of the femur and tibia and contribute significantly to overall joint conformity. The anterior and posterior translation of the menisci during flexion and extension protects the articular surfaces from injury. The menisci also have been shown to serve a proprioceptive role in the knee.

The vascular anatomy of the menisci is of prime importance in the healing of these structures after injury. The vascular supply to the medial and lateral menisci of the knee originates predominantly in both the medial and lateral genicular arteries (both inferior and superior branches). Branches from these vessels give rise to a perimeniscal capillary plexus within the synovial and capsular tissues of the knee. The peripheral penetration of the menisci by this vascular network is 10% to 30% of the width of the medial meniscus and 10% to 25% of the width of the lateral meniscus. After injury in the vascular zone, a fibrin clot forms that is rich in inflammatory cells. Vessels from the perimeniscal capillary plexus proliferate through this fibrin "scaffold," accompanied by the proliferation of undifferentiated mesenchymal cells. The lesion is filled with a cellular, fibrovascular granulation tissue that "glues" the wound edges together and appears to be continuous with the adjacent normal meniscal fibrocartilage. The initial strength of this tissue is minimal, but increased collagen synthesis within the granulation tissue slowly results in a fibrous scar.

Knowledge of healing of peripheral meniscal tears has given rise to the rationale for meniscal surgical repair. There are different techniques of repair by open arthrotomy and by arthroscopy, but most make use of a fibrin clot that is placed surgically into the tear before tightening the sutures to provide a fibrin scaffold to facilitate healing by scar. Meniscal tears that extend beyond the vascular zone do not heal regardless of technique, and partial meniscec-

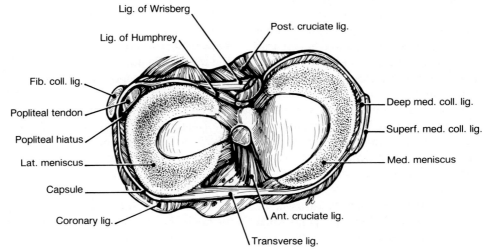

FIGURE 17-16. Depiction of the menisci of the knee with the associated intermeniscal ligaments.

tomy is the procedure of choice. Although meniscectomy was once performed by open arthrotomy, the procedure is almost universally done today by arthroscopic means. Injuries that involve menisci and the anterior cruciate ligament, however, should be surgically repaired whenever possible.

The diagnosis of meniscal injuries is usually suspected from the history and physical examination. The patient commonly presents with an injury giving pain directly over one of the joint lines. The Steinman, Appley, and MacMurray tests reproduce the pain along the joint line. The MacMurray test actually reproduces the locking that occurs with a bucket-handle–type tear as the knee is twisted back and forth during flexion and extension. These tests, however, can be negative in a large number of clinically significant meniscal injuries. Often, the knee may present with joint line discomfort only at the maximal degree of knee flexion. The patient may feel occasional locking but most of the time just experiences pain at the joint line when stressful weight-bearing activities are performed.

The diagnosis of a meniscal tear is confirmed by arthrogram or MRI techniques. Nonoperative treatment consisting of antiinflammatory medications and careful exercise may allow the menisci to heal. These treatment methods should last 6 to 8 weeks to allow for the possibility of meniscal healing to occur. If the patient still complains of symptoms after 6 weeks, arthroscopic subtotal meniscectomy should be undertaken.

OSTEONECROSIS

Osteonecrosis indicates death of a segment of the weight-bearing portion of the femoral condyle or tibial plateau with associated subchondral fracture and collapse. In the typical case, the patient, who is usually older than 60 years of age, presents with a precise and dramatic description of severe pain with sudden onset, well localized to the medial side of the knee. Often, the patient recalls exactly the activity he or she was doing at the onset of symptoms. During the acute phase, the knee appears locked because of pain, effusion, and muscle contracture. Although it is most common in the medial femoral condyle, osteonecrosis may also occur in the lateral femoral condyle and tibial plateau. The tibial lesions occur on the medial side. Radiographs may be normal, but bone scintigraphy is markedly abnormal. MRI also shows this lesion during the acute phase before it is clearly shown on plain radiographs. After 2 or 3

months, radiographs typically show flattening and radiolucency of the subchondral bone of the medial femoral condyle with a sclerotic line of demarcation around the lesion. Degenerative changes may also be present at this time if a large weight-bearing area of the femoral condyle is involved.

The condition may present in a similar manner to a spontaneous tear of the medial meniscus and should be differentiated from it in a patient who is older than 60 years of age. Most cases are idiopathic in nature. Vascular and traumatic theories also have been proposed, with the vascular theory being the most widely accepted. Fat embolism has been suggested as a possible mechanism. Bone microcirculation is contained within an expandable compartment, and an increase in bone marrow pressure can cause bone ischemia. Elevated bone marrow pressure is found in patients on steroid therapy, but it is also found in osteoarthritis of the knee.

Osteonecrosis presents radiographically in five stages. In stage 1, the radiographs are normal, but bone scintigraphy is abnormal. Slight flattening of the condyle is seen in stage 2. An area of radiolucency with a distal sclerosis and a faint halo of bony reaction is found in stage 3. Stage 4 shows a calcified plate with radiolucency surrounded by a definite sclerotic halo. Stage 5 represents narrowing of the joint space with subchondral sclerosis and osteophyte formation typical of osteoarthritis.

The differential diagnosis includes osteochondritis dissecans, osteoarthritis, meniscal tears, and pes anserinus bursitis. The area of the lesion is important in predicting which knee will develop osteoarthritis. Knees with lesions smaller than 5 cm² have a better clinical and radiographic prognosis.

Treatment of osteonecrosis consists mostly of conservative therapy in which the patient uses a cane to relieve joint reaction force on the weight-bearing limb. If the disease progresses, a few cases can be treated by arthrotomy or arthroscopy and drilling of the lesion with or without removal of the loose fragment. Core decompression has been tried with limited success. High tibial osteotomy, hemiarthroplasty, and total-knee replacement are reserved for knees in which advanced osteoarthritis has developed. Care should be taken to resect the entire osteonecrotic area during total-knee replacement.

ARTHRITIS OF THE KNEE

Arthritis of the knee results from a wearing away of the articular cartilage of the joint. Arthritis may be idiopathic, or it can result from trauma, rheumatoid synovitis, pigmented villonodular synovitis, and seronegative arthropathies such as gout, chondrocalcinosis, osteonecrosis, and idiopathic disorders. Osteoarthritis is predominantly a mechanical deterioration that may be associated with malalignment of the knee. Familial, genetic predisposition may exist, however, and osteoarthritis may result from and be associated with significant synovitis. Rheumatoid arthritis is associated with significant synovitis, with 80% of patients having a positive rheumatoid factor, indicating an autoimmune basis for cartilage destruction.

The knee is the most commonly affected joint with osteoarthritis. Posttraumatic etiologies include torn menisci with previous complete meniscectomy, fractures, patellar instability, and loose bodies caused by chondromalacia or synovial chondromatosis. Mechanical varus or valgus malalignment with obesity may cause abnormal loading of the knee over time and produce premature degeneration of the joint cartilage. Infection causes joint cartilage destruction owing to the proteolytic enzymes released by the leukocytes that enter the knee to combat infection where the enzymes are nonselective in their destructive capabilities.

Clinically, the patient with arthritis presents initially with stiffness and pain. Characteristically, the patient has stiffness on initiation of gait (gelling), which gets better as the knee "warms up." There may be an antalgic or painful gait in which the stance phase of the walking cycle is shortened. A knee with varus malalignment may demonstrate a lateral thrust due to instability of the lateral collateral ligament. A patient with valgus malalignment may show a medial thrust due to an incompetent medial collateral ligament. The knee may show swelling caused by an effusion and synovitis. Locking may also occur as the bare bony surfaces grate against each other, causing severe pain. Osteophytes may also be palpable on clinical examination.

Radiographically, weight-bearing views should be obtained to give the appearance of the knee while it is under stress. A weight-bearing view in full extension shows most of the clinical destruction of the joint. Only the posterior condyles may be involved, however, in which case a weight-bearing view with the knee flexed 40 degrees shows joint space narrowing, indicating significant cartilage destruction.

Osteoarthritis is characterized by joint space narrowing, osteophytes, cortical sclerosis on the weight-bearing bony surfaces, and subchondral cysts. Usually, the medial or lateral joint with mechanical malalignment is seen on the radiograph with or without patellofemoral involvement. Rheumatoid arthritis, on the other hand, demonstrates a more symmetric joint destruction appearance on the standing radiographs without osteophytes.

Treatment of the arthritic knee should initially consist of a period of rest and avoidance of weight bearing if the knee is painful. Occasionally, a splint or elastic bandage is needed to allow the synovitis to calm down. Moist heat may be applied to decrease stiffness. Ice should be used if the knee becomes acutely swollen and painful. Nonsteroidal antiinflammatory medications may be prescribed to decrease the synovitis. Prudent use of intraarticular cortisone injections may be used; however, the use of cortisone injections at frequent intervals (eg, every month) has been shown to accelerate arthritic deterioration. After the acute pain and synovitis has calmed, gentle exercises and stretching of the joint may begin. Exercises often slow the onset of permanent stiffness and flexion contractures.

Surgical intervention is indicated if the patient has persistent pain that is not relieved by rest, antiinflammatory medications, and cortisone injections.

Joint débridement is the first surgical method of treatment. A radical resection of the synovium and removal of osteophytes with shaving of degenerated cartilage down to subchondral bone through an open arthrotomy was used in the past. However, arthroscopic débridement is now the procedure of choice. It can be redone in the future if the patient feels successful long-term pain relief was obtained. Débridement is less predictable if there is mechanical deformity of the joint. Knees with loose bodies and cartilage tears were shown to do well with arthroscopic intervention.

Advanced arthritis poses a more formidable problem for the surgeon. The surgical decision is based primarily on the age and activity of the patient, the mechanical deformity, and the type of arthritis. For isolated patellofemoral arthritis, there are three options: patellectomy, tibial tubercle elevation, or patellofemoral joint replacement.

Patellectomy removes the patella but yields a permanent weakness of 30% when compared with the uninvolved normal knee and is generally reserved for severe posttraumatic injuries to the patella in young patients. Tibial tubercle advancement decreases contact pressure on the patellofemoral joint, which in turn may decrease arthritic pain. Patellofemoral arthroplasty involves replacing the articular surfaces of the patella or patellofemoral joint with implants. All three of these procedures achieve limited success in completely removing pain and are successful only 65% to 70% of the time.

Knee arthrodesis is reserved for the young, heavy, active person who has premature severe destruction of the knee due to arthritis (Fig. 17-17). Most of the time, however, the patient refuses arthrodesis owing to the postoperative appearance and the inability to bend the knee after the procedure. The procedure provides permanent pain relief and allows the patient to return to durable, active work.

Medial joint osteoarthritis in a patient younger than 60 years of age can be treated by upper tibial osteotomy. This procedure alters the mechanical axis of the knee by the removal of a triangular wedge of bone based laterally from the proximal aspect of the tibia above the tibial tubercle (Fig. 17-18). Success remains durable in patients who have a postoperative alignment of at least 8 degrees of valgus and who are not obese. The correction is done on the tibial side since most of the bone destruction is tibial. Women tolerate the postoperative valgus alignment less well than men and represent a relative contraindication for the procedure. The procedure is not indicated in grossly obese patients, unstable knees, or

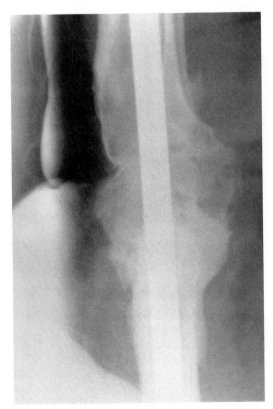

FIGURE 17-17. Knee arthrodesis using an intramedullary rod.

knees with less than 75 degrees of motion, greater than a 15-degree flexion contracture, and instability. Deformities of up to 10 degrees of varus can be treated in this manner. There are numerous techniques of fixation of the fragments after osteotomy, including staples, plates, and cylinder casts. The procedure allows the patient to remain active and delays the time when total-knee replacement becomes necessary. The procedure permits participation in rigorous sports.

Hemiarthroplasty is reserved for patients older than 60 years of age who have isolated medial or lateral joint osteoarthritis. The indications are the same as those for upper tibial osteotomy but in an older age group. The success of the operation is controversial, with some centers claiming great functional improvement and durability, while others show shorter times of pain relief and premature mechanical failure. The procedure is not indicated if other joint compartments demonstrate advanced destructive arthritic damage. In these cases, total-knee replacement is the procedure of choice.

For the young, active patient with a valgus arthritic deformity, supracondylar femoral osteotomy is the treatment of choice (Fig. 17-19). Arthritic knees with valgus malalignment typically have bone destruction located on the lateral femoral condyle. Hence, correction of the deformity should be on the femoral side. A medial varus femoral osteotomy is performed, with the widest base of the wedge located medially. The osteotomy fragments are fixed in place with supracondylar blade plates. This procedure yields satisfactory results in 80% of the cases and enables a young patient with advanced arthritis to return to an active life-style.

In older patients with advanced osteoarthritis, total-knee replacement is the preferred treatment (Fig. 17-20). The indications for joint replacement have been stretched for younger patients with tricompartmental (medial and lateral tibiofemoral and patellofemoral) disease owing to the predictable pain relief and durability of the implants over time. Joint replacement for the young, active patient, however, ensures the need for future revision surgery, thus the operation should be delayed as long as possible for these patients. Age is not a factor in recommending total-knee replacement for rheumatoid arthritic patients because the disease generally affects the patient's overall activity level significantly so that wear and loosening of the implants are of less concern.

Total-knee replacement has been shown to provide predictable pain relief and yields satisfactory results in 90% of properly selected patients with

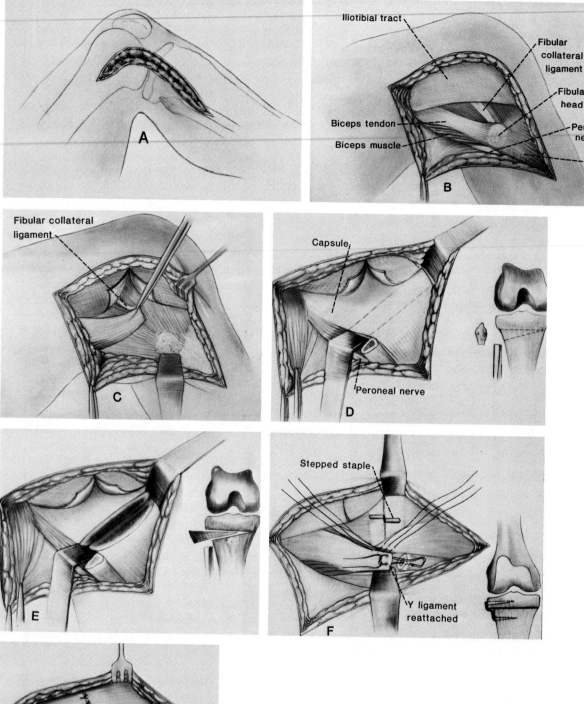

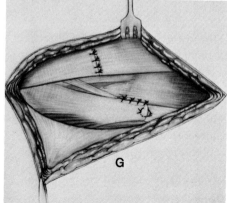

FIGURE 17-18. Proximal tibial osteotomy is performed by removal of a laterally based wedge of bone from the proximal tibia, which in turn creates a valgus alignment to restore the normal mechanical axis to the leg. The tibiofibular joint must be released or the proximal fibular head should be resected to allow closure of the osteotomy.

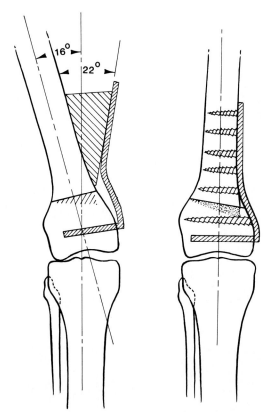

FIGURE 17-19. Supracondylar femoral osteotomy is performed by removing a medially based wedge of bone to restore the mechanical axis of the leg.

rheumatoid or osteoarthritis. Initial designs consisted of linked metal hinges that were implanted with acrylic cement. These designs demonstrated premature failure and a high infection rate. Knee replacement designs can be categorized as hinged or unhinged designs. Hinged designs are constrained and are linked, whereas unhinged designs contact each other without being mechanically connected. The unhinged designs rely on the stability of the collateral and cruciate ligaments and articular architecture of the implants. Hinged designs have become largely obsolete owing to their high failure rate and infection risk.

In 1974, the total condylar prosthesis was designed, which is an unlinked replacement with a cupped tibial surface. It originally provided 90 degrees of motion, which permitted patients to walk without pain. This prosthesis yields 94% survivorship over 12 years (Fig. 17-21). The benefits of this prosthesis are: predictable pain relief, durability, decreased infection rate compared with hinged designs, bone preservation, and good function. Its success became so great that an entire family of prosthetic

designs became known as total condylar–type prostheses. These prostheses can be further subdivided into groups that preserve the posterior cruciate ligament and those that sacrifice or substitute for it (Fig. 17-22). The original total condylar prosthesis sacrificed the posterior cruciate ligament and provided only 90 degrees of motion. This motion was insufficient to allow the patient to get out of an automobile easily, climb or descend stairs, or tie shoes. In 1978, the total condylar design was further modified to substitute for the posterior cruciate ligament and to provide up to 120 degrees of motion. This prosthesis has also demonstrated excellent survivorship of 96% over 10 years. Implants that preserve the posterior cruciate ligament have shown similar survivorship.

Restoration of the mechanical joint axis is important to prevent premature failure of the prosthesis (Fig. 17-23). Implants that were placed in excessive varus demonstrated premature loosening and settling of the implant in tibial bone. Ideal alignment is 3 to 8 degrees of valgus. Knees with severe preoperative

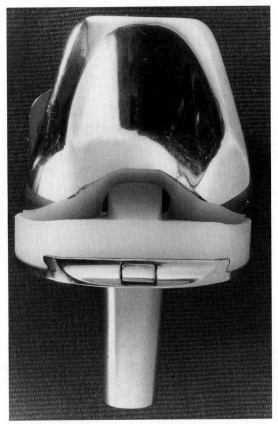

FIGURE 17-20. The posteriorly stabilized condylar total-knee prosthesis. The design allows for up to 130 degrees of flexion.

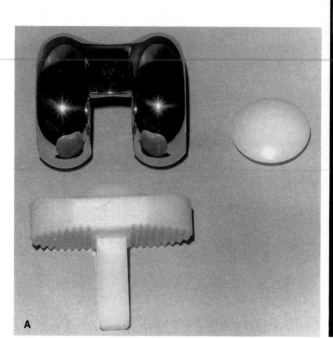
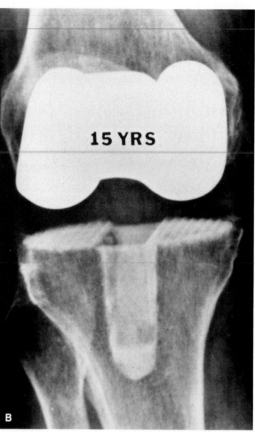

FIGURE 17-21. (A) The original total-condylar prosthesis, which has shown up to 20 years of durability. (B) This prosthesis has provided pain relief without evidence of mechanical failure for 15 years.

malalignment need release of the soft tissues and ligaments to restore alignment to normal. Knees with severe varus deformity need subperiosteal release of the medial collateral ligament from the proximal portion of the tibia. This is required because the medial collateral ligament becomes contracted as the varus alignment becomes more severe. In valgus knees, the iliotibial band, popliteus tendon, and lateral collateral ligament frequently need to be released from the femur. Flexion contractures are corrected by removal of osteophytes from the posterior femoral condyles and release of the posterior joint capsule; occasionally, more distal femoral bone needs removal. The knee should be stable in flexion, and extension and hyperextension (recurvatum) of the joint should be avoided. The tibial component should be placed in the bone with the tray perpendicular to the long axis of the tibial shaft. This position ensures long-term survival of the implant. The femoral component is placed in 3 to 8 degrees of valgus, de-

pending on the patients height and preoperative alignment.

The complications of total-knee replacement include: loosening, wear, infection, peroneal nerve palsy in knees with valgus deformity and flexion contracture, dislocation, settling into the cancellous bone, stress fracture of the patella, and osteolysis due to metal and polyethylene wear debris. Loosening, wear, dislocation, and settling can be corrected by revision total-knee replacement. Infection is particularly difficult to treat owing to the implants acting as foreign bodies in the knee, making antibiotic treatment and drainage alone unpredictable and doomed to failure. The infection can be suppressed by antibiotics alone in medically infirm patients. In healthy patients, however, definitive treatment of the infection is achieved by removal of the prostheses and acrylic cement with complete débridement of all infected tissue, a 6-week course of intravenous antibiotics maintaining a minimal bacteriocidal con-

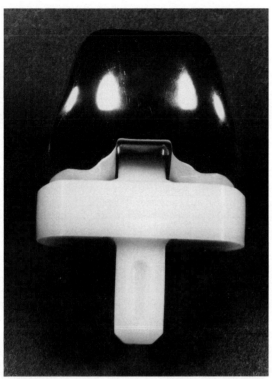

FIGURE 17-22. The first design of the posteriorly stabilized condylar prosthesis. The Cam mechanism in the middle of the prosthesis substitutes for the posterior cruciate ligament.

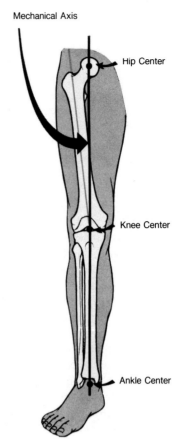

FIGURE 17-23. The normal mechanical axis of the leg.

centration of 1:8, followed by reimplantation of a new knee replacement. Definitive cure of the infection can be obtained in 98% of cases using this treatment protocol. If the patient's bone is too much destroyed or if the knee is at too great a risk of infection owing to an immunosuppressed medical state, arthrodesis is the treatment of choice. Occasionally, in the medically infirm patient, the knee may be allowed to stiffen without a new knee replacement being implanted.

FRACTURES OF THE PATELLA

Fractures of the patella occur as a result of direct trauma to the anterior aspect of the knee. A powerful force generated by the quadriceps muscle, however, may generate enough energy to fracture one of the poles of the patella (Fig. 17-24). Forces across the patellofemoral joint increase with flexion. A fall from a height may generate a combination of excessive force across the patella and significant quadriceps contraction to cause bone failure.

Horizontal transverse fractures generally result from excessive quadriceps force. A direct blow across the patella of moderate force may also yield a clean, transverse fracture. Fractures may be divided into displaced or undisplaced. Undisplaced fractures heal

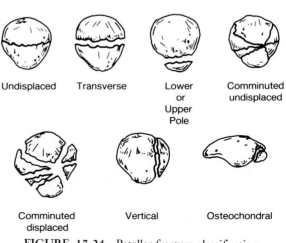

FIGURE 17-24. Patellar fracture classification.

well by immobilizing the knee in a cylinder cast for 6 weeks, followed by active assisted flexion and range-of-motion exercises. In patients with little pain, a knee immobilizer may be used instead of a cast, with early motion beginning almost immediately. Apical transverse fractures at the proximal or distal poles of the patella can also be treated in this manner. On physical examination, the patient usually has significant pain on direct palpation of the patellar region. Pain may prevent the patient from actively extending the knee. The lateral radiographs of the knee show minimal displacement of the fracture fragments.

Displaced fractures of the patella must be surgically corrected. The physical examination often elicits significant anterior knee pain on direct palpation. The patient is totally unable to extend actively the knee against resistance. There is often a palpable defect that can be appreciated right over the patella. A transverse patellar fracture is best treated by tension band wiring with open reduction and internal fixation (Fig. 17-25). The tension band–wiring technique is the most widely accepted way to manage the fracture, although some surgeons use cancellous screws if the fracture fragments are large enough to contain them (Fig. 17-26). Displaced apical fractures are best managed by excision of the small fragment and direct suturing of the quadriceps or patellar tendon to the remaining large bone fragment.

Stellate, comminuted fractures of the patella usually result from severe trauma to the patella and pose difficult fixation problems. The bone fragments are often so small that metallic fixation screws or wires cannot adequately hold them. If there is a single large fragment located proximally or distally, a partial patellectomy is performed, with the remaining bone attached to the extensor mechanism. If all the fragments are small, a total patellectomy should be performed.

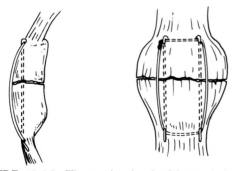

FIGURE 17-25. The tension band wiring technique for patellar fracture reduction.

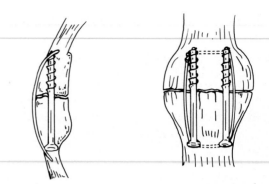

FIGURE 17-26. Cancellous screws may also be used in the tension band wiring technique if the bone fragments are large enough to hold the screws. Otherwise, nonthreaded pins are used.

The patient should be made aware that although healing of bone may be achieved with patellar fractures, crepitus and pain may still remain to some degree. Traumatic chondromalacia generally is due to the severe compressive load that was placed across the patellar cartilage to generate a fracture. Patellar arthritis may also result, depending on the severity of the fracture.

FRACTURES OF THE FEMORAL CONDYLES

Fractures of the distal part of the femur are defined as fractures involving the distal 9 to 15 cm of the bone, measured proximally from the articular surface of the condyles. They may involve the diaphyseal bone as well as the metaphyseal region. There may also be fractures that display intraarticular extension. These fractures remain difficult problems; namely, reduction and fixation of many fragments in osteoporotic bone, restoration of perfect limb alignment, and equalization of the leg lengths. Treatment is also controversial.

The fractures in the supracondylar and condylar regions of the femur usually occur from significant trauma. There is inherent mechanical weakness in the intercondylar regions so that intraarticular extension of the fracture into this region frequently occurs. The metaphyseal region in older patients may be osteoporotic, making the possibility of severe crushing of the bone fragments likely.

Two deforming forces add difficulty to the treatment of these fractures: the amount of initial trauma and unbalanced muscle pull on the fragments. The distal fragment may be flexed by the gastrocnemius muscles. The heads of the gastrocnemius muscles may rotate and spread the condylar fragments in intercondylar fractures. Valgus or varus deformity can be produced by the adductors. In T-, Y-, or V-shaped fractures of the supracondylar and intercondylar region, the proximal fragment may be driven into the distal fragment, wedging the condyles apart.

Architectural malunion of the femoral condyles may result in limitation of flexion, and surgical dissection through the quadriceps muscle may also contribute to knee stiffness even though proper reduction of the fragments is performed. Other circulatory dangers exist. The popliteal artery resides close to the osteoarticular region of the knee joint, and the artery is held relatively immobile in the adductor canal superiorly and in the soleus canal anteriorly. Thus, injury to the artery should be ruled out by arteriography.

Most fractures occur as a result of high-velocity motor vehicle accidents. The second most frequent cause is a fall on the flexed knee. Falls from a height also are responsible for a limited number of fractures. There are major differences between the fractures sustained by young patients and those caused in the elderly population. Fractures that occur in young patients require higher energy, which leads to more soft tissue damage. They are often more comminuted or open and may often have an intraarticular extension. Fractures in the elderly involve osteoporotic soft bone. The fracture energy is much lower, leading to less soft tissue damage and less frequent intraarticular extension.

A variety of classifications of distal femur fractures can help the surgeon decide on appropriate treatment. The simplest classification is by Neer and colleagues. In group I, the fragments are minimally displaced. Group IIA is represented by medial displacement of the condyles, whereas group IIB reflects lateral displacement of the femoral condyles. Group III fractures are comminuted and involve the shaft as well. This classification is popular in the United States. The AO-ASIF classification has become the most widely accepted classification system, however, although it is more detailed than previous ones (Fig. 17-27). The AO-ASIF classification is broken down into three large groups with subgroups:

Extraarticular
Type A1—partial supracondylar
Type A2—simple supracondylar

> *Type A2a*—with lateral displacement of the condyles

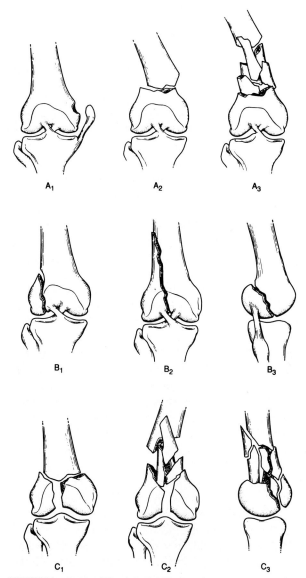

FIGURE 17-27. The AO/ASIF classification of supracondylar femur fractures.

> *Type A2b*—with medial displacement of the condyles

Type A3—comminuted supracondylar

Intraarticular
Type B1—sagittal marginal split of part of a condyle
Type B2—sagittal vertical split (entire condyle)
Type B3—coronal fracture of one condyle

Intraarticular and Extraarticular
Type C1—simple intercondylar
Type C2—intercondylar fracture plus additional supracondylar comminution
Type C3—supraintercondylar plus additional intraarticular comminution

The incidence of open fractures varies from 8% to 38%. Arterial injury is unusual, and if the popliteal artery is lacerated or crushed, surgical intervention must commence within 6 hours of trauma. Peroneal nerve injuries are rare.

Nonoperative, conservative treatment may be applied to undisplaced, minimally displaced, stable, or impacted supracondylar fractures. Plaster casts or splints can be placed to hold the fragments in position until healing occurs 6 to 12 weeks later. Occasionally, closed manipulation of the fracture and casting is possible. The advantage of the treatment is a short hospitalization period. However, there is the risk of joint stiffness. Skeletal traction through the tibial tuberosity or femoral condyles may also be used for a week, followed by closed reduction and spica cast immobilization.

Traction is the most widely known conservative method. It has been used in the forms of skin traction, a single tibial skeletal pin, and double (tibial and femoral) skeletal pins. This treatment requires frequent manipulation of the fracture fragments and radiographic documentation of the reduction to assess adequacy of treatment. Functional cast braces have been used successfully for supracondylar fractures and also for supraintercondylar fractures. Cast braces provide immobilization of the fracture but also allow early mobilization of the joint to prevent stiffness.

Early studies indicated that distal femoral fractures were best treated by closed methods. At that time, open treatment was frequently followed by major complications, such as infection, slow recovery of motion, and malrotation as well as residual varus and recurvatum deformities. Currently, closed treatment should be reserved for relatively well-aligned and undisplaced fractures, using reduction by traction and early conversion to cast braces. Surgical correction is reserved for displaced fractures and those that involve the articular surface. Open fractures must be treated by open irrigation, with fixation of the fracture by either internal plates or external pins. Numerous fixation devices have been created to adequately fix these fractures: the angled blade plate, condylar buttress plate, condylar compression screw plate, intramedullary devices such as the Rush rods, Zickel supracondylar nails, Ender nails coupled to cancellous screws, interlocking intramedullary nails, and the sewn retrograde intramedullary rod (Fig. 17-28). The intramedullary devices require less surgical dissection, allow earlier weight bearing, and are load sharing. They are only useful for extraarticular or nondisplaced fractures, some length is necessary for their use, and occasionally they require external support with a brace. Bone grafting with cancellous bone taken from the iliac crest is generally required for most open-reduction and internal-fixation procedures.

After surgical correction, partial weight bearing is allowed until evidence of fracture healing is seen radiographically. Radiographs should be made at regular monthly intervals to assess healing and maintenance of the reduction. Complications include: limitation of motion, malunion, nonunion, implant failure, sepsis, and traumatic osteoarthritis. The incidence of infection varies from 0% to 28%, depending on the severity of the treated injuries. Nonunion after closed treatment ranges from 0% to 22% and after open treatment varies from 14% to 19% in the older series and 0% to 6% in the most recent series. Malunion occurs in about half of cases treated nonoperatively, and its incidence is substantially decreased by open methods.

FRACTURES OF THE TIBIAL PLATEAU

Proximal tibial plateau fractures involve the articular cartilage, the epiphysis, and the metaphysis. Tibial plateau fractures occur in one of the most important load-bearing joints since the tibial plateau during stance acts as a platform on which the femur and the remainder of the body rest. Treatment is controversial, with equal numbers of specialists advocating operative and nonoperative intervention. The treatment goal is to obtain a stable, well-aligned, mobile joint with minimal articular cartilage irregularities. In cases of severe trauma in which parts of the joint may be exposed, the surrounding soft tissue must also be sufficient if open reduction and internal fixation are needed. If these conditions are met, future degenerative arthritis may be prevented.

The mechanism of injury is multifactorial and depends on the weight-bearing status of the limb during impact, the quality of the bone, and energy of the deforming force. The forces that produce the fractures of the tibial plateaus are valgus, compression, or both. The "nutcracker theory" is based on the medial collateral ligament acting as a rigid hinge during a valgus (abduction) stress. The femoral condyle is then driven into the lateral tibial plateau. Most condylar fractures are produced by the prominent anterior part of the lateral femoral condyle in exten-

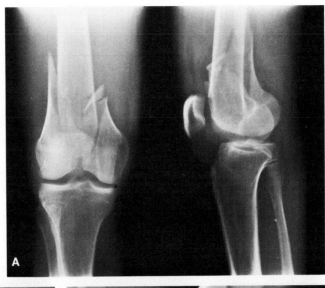

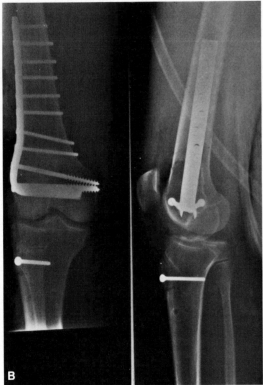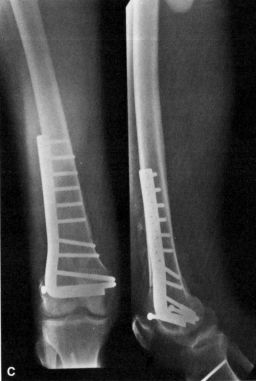

FIGURE 17-28. (A) A closed C_2 supracondylar femur fracture. (B) Fixation was achieved with a 95-degree angled blade plate. (C) The fracture healed with normal alignment.

sion. The mechanisms that produce lateral, medial, and bicondylar fractures are similar. The force is directed primarily distally but may proceed in a medial or lateral direction, splitting off one or both of the condyles. In fractures of the lateral tibial plateau, the medial collateral ligament may still be torn, creating an unstable mediolateral relation between tibia and femur.

As with femoral condyle fractures, there are many classifications of tibial condyle fractures present in the literature. The Rasmussen and the Hohl classifications are the most frequently used and are the most detailed. The AO-ASIF classification is too simplistic to derive meaningful data and reporting of results, although it is widely used by European surgeons. The Rasmussen classification follows:

Lateral Plateau Fracture
Split
Split compression
Compression

 Anterior
 Posterior
 Central
 Total

Medial Plateau Fracture
Split
Split compression
Compression

Bicondylar Fracture
Split
Split compression

The Hohl classification (Fig. 17-29) is as follows:

Type I—minimally displaced
Type II—local compression

Type III—split compression
Type IV—total condylar
Type V—split
Type VI—rim avulsion or compression
Type VII—bicondylar

A precise classification is useful for analyzing and studying the results of various treatment modalities and for comparing them.

The clinical evaluation involves a physical examination of the knee as well as other body areas that also may have been injured. An effusion is often present. Tenderness is felt over the tibial plateau. Evacuation of the hemarthrosis can be done to facilitate the examination. Fat globules may be seen in the aspirate. Ligament and stability testing should be done when the patient is more comfortable. The angular instability is predominantly caused by the bone depression and displacement, but it may also be ligamentous. Testing should be done in full extension and in slight flexion of 20 degrees if the patient is comfortable enough to allow manipulation of the knee. The stability should be compared with the opposite normal side. The extremity should be examined

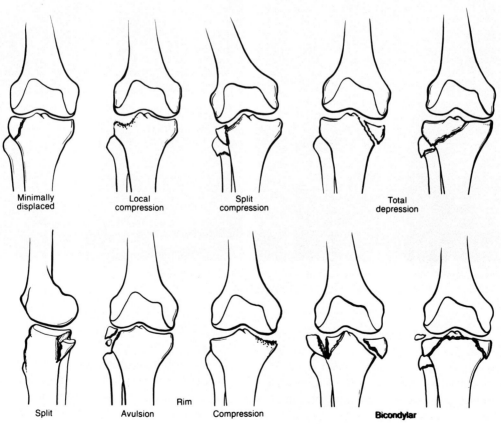

FIGURE 17-29. The Hohl classification of tibial plateau fractures.

for neurovascular complications. Peroneal nerve and popliteal artery injuries are rare but usually occur with large fractures associated with knee dislocation.

The radiographic evaluation consists of plain radiography. Varus and valgus stress films are recommended to show the association of ligament injuries. Fracture anatomy is most accurately delineated by tomography. The classification of the fracture types, so important to the therapeutic decision, can be undertaken only knowing precisely the location, the extent, and the displacement of the fracture or depressed fragments.

Until 30 years ago, most fractures were treated nonoperatively by traction or cast immobilization. With the arrival of more sophisticated internal fixation techniques, surgical intervention has become more common. The goal of surgical treatment is restoration of the anatomic congruency of the tibial articular surface in addition to the ligament stability and maintenance of the mechanical alignment. There are still situations in which nonoperative treatment is indicated, however. Traction, casts, and cast braces

are used and yield acceptable functional results, although the anatomic correction is less than ideal.

Displacement of the articular surfaces determines the need for surgical correction (Fig. 17-30). Some authors only accept less than a 1-mm displacement, whereas other authors accept as much as 10 mm. Most investigators accept 5 mm of fragment displacement before considering open reduction. In fractures with severe displacement and crushed bone defects, surgical intervention is necessary to restore stability and joint congruency. Since articular cartilage derives its nutrition from the joint fluid and not the underlying bone, the cartilage must be brought to its anatomic position and supported with new bone taken from the iliac crest. Large bone defects remain, and the trabecular bone does not "spring back" into place after deformation. The only material that can fill the defect is autologous bone graft.

Different techniques are used for management of tibial plateau fractures. Arthroscopy with arthroscopically assisted placement of cancellous bone screws percutaneously was described and is best

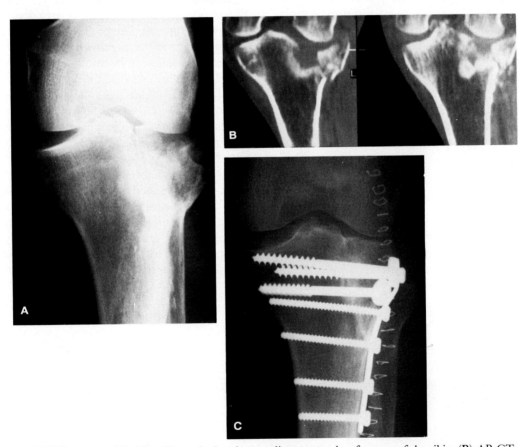

FIGURE 17-30. (A) AP radiograph showing a split-compression fracture of the tibia. (B) AP CT scan showing the depressed articular surface of the tibia. (C) A postoperative radiograph showing reduction and fixation of the fracture with a buttress plate. Iliac crest bone graft should be used.

suited for relatively mildly displaced fragments without significant comminution or crushing of bone (Fig. 17-31). Arthroscopy evacuates the hematoma and allows visualization of the articular surfaces. It also allows evaluation of the menisci, which can tear in as many as half of cases. If there is disruption of the collateral ligaments, open reduction and internal fixation are necessary along with ligament repair. Therefore, percutaneous pin fixation with arthroscopy is only well suited for relatively nondisplaced fractures or fractures over which the skin coverage is tenuous.

Open reduction and internal fixation are the treatment of choice for displaced split, split-compression, and bicondylar fractures. Usually, an extensile exposure is required through which the meniscus and its attachments are retracted superiorly to allow clear vision of the tibial articular surface. The fragments are temporarily fixed with small-diameter, nonthreaded pins to provide adequate fracture control while placing on the desired fixation device (blade plate, buttress plate, and screws). Depressed fragments with overlying articular cartilage must be elevated to the level of the normal tibial articular surface. The space left after the elevation of the fragments is filled with bone obtained from the iliac crest.

Postoperative care stresses early mobilization, but full weight bearing is not allowed for 6 to 8 weeks and for as long as 12 weeks, depending on bone quality. Although it is less likely to develop in well-reduced fractures, osteoarthritis may still occur prematurely.

INFECTION

Infection of the knee represents an orthopaedic emergency. Organisms may be introduced by direct inoculation (needle aspiration, arthroscopy, open arthrotomy) or by a hematogenous route (gonorrhea, Lyme disease, juvenile sepsis resulting from trauma). The knee usually presents with an acute onset of pain, effusion, and synovitis with or without fever or chills. Juvenile hematogenous sepsis usually is accompanied by fever, but a high index of suspicion by the orthopaedic surgeon should be present. Aspiration of purulent material usually confirms the diagnosis. Plain radiographs show the intraarticular fluid accumulation, and bone scintigraphy is positive after a longer time has passed (about 4 days). However, the surgeon should not wait until radiographic changes are seen before securing the diagnosis because it comes late in the infective process, and delay in treatment causes destruction of the articular cartilage by the proteolytic enzymes secreted by the polymorphonuclear leukocytes and macrophages. The key to success is early diagnosis. The treatment should commence at the earliest possible moment after obtaining an aspiration of the joint fluid for culture and sensitivity studies and immediate Gram stain. The rheumatology literature supports treatment of joint infection by serial aspirations and antibiotic therapy. The serial aspirations serve to drain the joint of infective material. The goal of treatment is to drain the joint so that the organism is removed. Leukocytosis in the joint can be minimized so that the proteolytic enzymes secreted by these cells do not destroy the articular cartilage. The microbial organisms themselves do not create significant cartilage destruction; it is the proteolytic enzymes discharged from macrophages and polymorphonuclear leukocytes that cause the destruction.

The orthopaedic literature supports formal incision and drainage instead of repeated aspirations since aspiration alone does not provide adequate drainage of multiloculated infections with abscess formation. The procedure can be done by arthroscopic means or by formal arthrotomy. Débridement of childhood sepsis should be done by arthrotomy

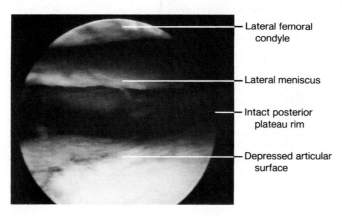

— Lateral femoral condyle

— Lateral meniscus

— Intact posterior plateau rim

— Depressed articular surface

FIGURE 17-31. Arthroscopic view of a depressed tibial plateau fracture. Occasionally, reduction can be accomplished by arthroscopic means through elevation and percutaneous screw fixation.

since the infection arises from the circulation adjacent to the growth plate, an area not readily attainable by arthroscopy. A 3- to 6-week course of intravenous antibiotics is necessary, and duration is based on the virulence of the organism.

Gonococcal infection of the knee, however, may be treated by antibiotics alone owing to the exquisite sensitivity of the organism to intravenous penicillin. Tuberculosis may also occur in the knee and can be treated by standard intravenous antibiotic therapy. Lyme disease also is treated solely by antibiotics.

A particularly difficult knee infection to treat is that which occurs in a knee with a total-knee prosthetic replacement. Chronic infection may be shown radiographically by radiolucency at the bone–cement interface of the prosthesis (Fig. 17-32). If infection is diagnosed within 3 weeks of onset, successful incision and drainage with retention of the components is successful 27% of the time. However, the most successful and accepted way to definitively treat the infection is by a two-stage procedure. In the first stage, a complete débridement and drainage, including re-

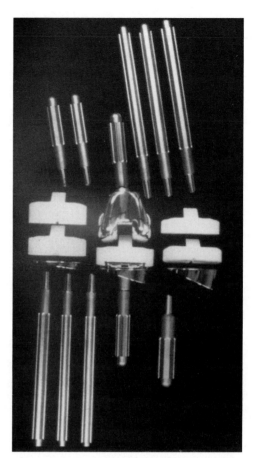

FIGURE 17-33. Example of a total-knee replacement system with modular metal wedges and intramedullary stems. The "core" prosthesis is a posteriorly stabilized design.

moval of the total-joint prosthesis and acrylic cement, is performed. A 6-week course of antibiotic therapy with minimal bactericidal concentration of 1:8 follows the first stage. At the conclusion of antibiotic therapy, a new knee replacement is inserted as the second stage. The procedure is successful in eradicating the original infection in 98% of cases, but the use of modular and custom-designed implants may be necessary to augment any bone loss that may have developed during the active course of the infection (Fig. 17-33).

Annotated Bibliography

Aglietti P, Insall J, Deschamps G, et al. The results of treatment of idiopathic osteonecrosis of the knee. J Bone Joint Surg 1983;65B:588.
This article characterizes the clinical course of osteonecrosis based on radiographic area of involvement.

Ahlback S, Bauer GCH, Bohme WH. Spontaneous osteonecrosis of the knee. Arthritis Rheum 1968;11:705.
The is the first description of osteonecrosis affecting the knee.

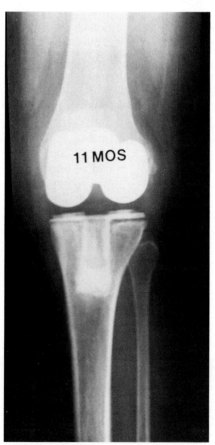

FIGURE 17-32. AP radiograph of an infected total-knee replacement showing a radiolucency at the cement–bone interface beneath the medial plateau of the tibial component.

Arnoczky SP, Warren RF. Microvasculature of the meniscus and its response to injury: an experimental study in the dog. Am J Sports Med 1983;11:131.
This essential article forms the basis of meniscal repair.

Arnoczky SP, Warren RF, Spivak JM. Meniscal repair using an exogenous fibrin clot: an experimental study in dogs. J Bone Joint Surg 1988;70A:1209.
Further data are provided that support the success of meniscal repair.

Clancy WG Jr, Shelbourne KD, Zoellner GB, et al. Treatment of knee joint instability secondary to rupture of the posterior cruciate ligament. J Bone Joint Surg 1983;65A:310.
This is the best report on open reconstruction of the posterior cruciate ligament using the middle third of the patellar ligament. The procedure is now frequently done arthroscopically.

Fulkerson J, Becker GJ, Meaney JA, et al. Anteromedial tibial tubercle transfer without bone graft. Am J Sports Med 1990;18:490.
This article describes Fulkerson's technique for bringing the tibial tubercle anteromedially for treatment of chondromalacia patella and patellar arthritis.

Hungerford DS. Disorders of the patellofemoral joint. Baltimore, Williams & Wilkins, 1990.
This textbook is the standard reference for patellofemoral disorders.

Insall JN, Joseph DM, Msika C. High tibial osteotomy for varus gonarthrosis: a long-term follow-up study. J Bone Joint Surg 1984;66A:1041.
The authors provide a follow-up of valgus upper tibial osteotomy.

Insall JN, Windsor RE, Scott WN, Kelly MA, Aglietti P, eds. Surgery of the knee, ed 2. New York, Churchill Livingstone, 1993.
One of the standard textbooks on knee surgery, this edition was updated to include expanded treatment for all disorders of the knee.

Lotke PA. Osteonecrosis of the knee: current concepts review. J Bone Joint Surg 1988;70A:470.
This review updates current theories on this condition.

Mooney V, Nickel VL, Harvey JP, et al. Cast–brace treatment for fractures of the distal part of the femur. J Bone Joint Surg 1970;52A:1563.
This was the first published report on the use of cast braces for the treatment of distal femoral fractures.

Neer CS, Grantham SA, Shelton M. Supracondylar fractures of the adult femur: a study of 110 cases. J Bone Joint Surg 1967;49:591.
This report presents a classification of supracondylar femur fractures with results of conservative and surgical treatment.

Noyes F, Mooar P, Matthews D, Butler D. The symptomatic anterior-deficient knee: part I. J Bone Joint Surg 1983;65A:154.
This study presents the natural history of anterior cruciate–deficient knees.

Outerbridge RE. The etiology of chondromalacia patellae. J Bone Joint Surg 1961;46B:752.
This article first describes the lesions and classification of chondromalacia.

Scaglione NE, Warren RF, Wickiewicz TL, et al. Primary repair with semitendinosus tendon augmentation of anterior cruciate ligament injuries. Am J Sports Med 1990;18:64.
This article describes primary repair of the anterior cruciate with augmentation, which serves as a basis for present treatment with the hamstring tendons alone without primary repair.

Siliski JM, Mahring M, Hofer P. Supracondylar-intercondylar fractures of the femur: treatment by internal fixation. J Bone Joint Surg 1989;71:95.
This study specifically analyzes the clinical results of rigid internal fixation of the fractures.

Stern SH, Insall JN. Posterior stabilized prosthesis: results after follow-up of nine to twelve years. J Bone Joint Surg 1992;74A:980.
The article demonstrates the success of this implant after it was modified to allow more knee flexion and to substitute for the posterior cruciate ligament.

Stewart MJ, Sisk TD, Wallace SL. Fractures of the distal third of the femur: a comparison of methods of treatment. J Bone Joint Surg 1966;48:784.
This old but important study compared the different treatment methods available at that time for the treatment of distal femur fractures, with most of the treatments being nonsurgical.

Vince KG, Insall JN, Kelly MA. The total condylar prosthesis: 10 to 12-year results of a cemented knee replacement. J Bone Joint Surg 1989;71B:793.
The authors present a long-term evaluation of the original total condylar prosthesis design that sacrificed the posterior cruciate ligament.

Turek's Orthopaedics: Principles and Their Application, Fifth Edition,
edited by Stuart L. Weinstein and Joseph A. Buckwalter.
J.B. Lippincott Company, Philadelphia, © 1994.

18

Stuart L. Weinstein

The Pediatric Foot

PES PLANUS	**SEVER DISEASE**
TARSAL COALITION	**METATARSUS ADDUCTUS**
CONGENITAL VERTICAL TALUS	**CLUBFOOT**
CALCANEAL VALGUS	**IDIOPATHIC TOE-WALKING**
KÖHLER DISEASE	**TORSIONAL PROBLEMS**
FREIBERG INFARCTION	

Anatomically, the foot can be divided into three sections: the forefoot, midfoot, and hindfoot. The forefoot consists of the metatarsals and phalanges. The cuneiform, cuboid, and navicular bones comprise the midfoot, and the hindfoot consists of the calcaneus and talus. The three foot segments are linked together by strong ligaments; because of this linkage, all foot movements occur concurrently. Supination and pronation are combination movements in the individual foot joints: *supination* refers to the sole pointing inward, and *pronation* refers to sole turning outward (Fig. 18-1). Varus (inversion) and valgus (eversion) are motions of a foot segment on a theoretic longitudinal axis (Fig. 18-2). When the foot is supinated, the heel goes into varus. When the foot is pronated, the heel goes into valgus (Fig. 18-3). Adduction and abduction are motions of the foot segment on a theoretic vertical axis (Fig. 18-4).

PES PLANUS

Pes planus is a term describing any condition of the foot in which the longitudinal arch is lowered. It is important to distinguish between physiologic pes planus and pes planus secondary to pathologic conditions.

Physiologic pes planus (hypermobile flatfoot, flexible flatfoot) is characterized by varying degrees of loss of the longitudinal arch of the foot on weight bearing. The foot assumes an apparent pronated posture with abduction of the forefoot and varying degrees of heel valgus (Fig. 18-5). The important distinguishing characteristic between physiologic and pathologic pes planus is flexibility. In the physiologic type, the foot remains flexible.

Ninety percent of normal children younger than 2 years have varying degrees

615

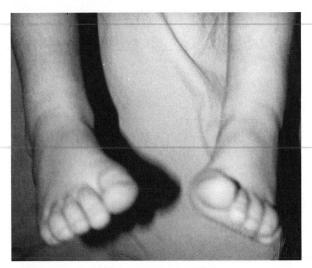

FIGURE 18-1. Foot supination (sole turning inward).

of pes planus. This is due to the normal joint hypermobility in this age group and the normal infant fat pad along the medial aspect of the foot (Fig. 18-6). In addition, the normal wide-based stance assumed by newly standing or walking children causes the weight-bearing line to fall medial to first or second ray, resulting in the hypermobile foot assuming a pes planus posture.

Between 3 and 5 years of age, the normal longitudinal arch develops in most patients. It is estimated that by age 10 years, only 4% of the population have persistent pes planus.

The normal longitudinal arch of the foot is determined by maintenance of the normal relations between the bones of the foot. These relations are maintained by the supporting ligamentous and capsular structures and can be affected by functional stresses applied to the foot in weight bearing and by muscle contraction. The foot musculature does not maintain the longitudinal arch. Its purpose is to maintain balance, adjust the foot to uneven ground, and propel the body. Biomechanically, when the foot is supinated, the articulations of the midfoot are "locked," and the foot is a rigid structure. When the foot is pronated, however, greater mobility is allowed at the midfoot joints, and maximal motion can occur at the talonavicular and calcaneocuboid joints. The position of heel valgus and forefoot abduction with lowering of the longitudinal arch is often referred to as a *pronated foot,* while in actuality, the forefoot is supinated to varying degrees in relation to the hind foot. Thus, in true physiologic pes planus, as the calcaneus assumes a valgus position, the lateral aspect of the forefoot is in contact only with the ground if the forefoot supinates to some degree in relation to the hind foot.

The normal weight-bearing pattern includes ground contact with the lateral border of the foot and with the first and fifth metatarsals. In pes planus, as the calcaneus assumes a more valgus position, the talar head loses some of its support and assumes a more vertically oriented position, with subsequent

(text continues on page 620)

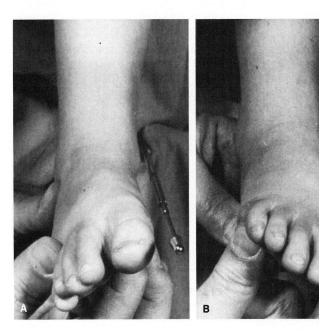

FIGURE 18-2. Forefoot varus (inversion; **A**) and forefoot valgus (eversion; **B**) are motions of a foot segment on a theoretical longitudinal axis.

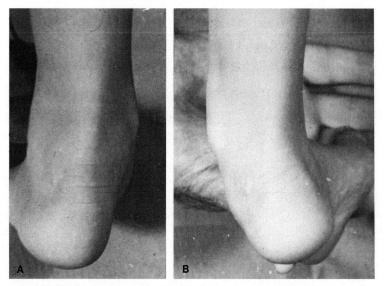

FIGURE 18-3. (A) Heel valgus (eversion) when foot is pronated. (B) Heel varus (inversion) when foot is supinated.

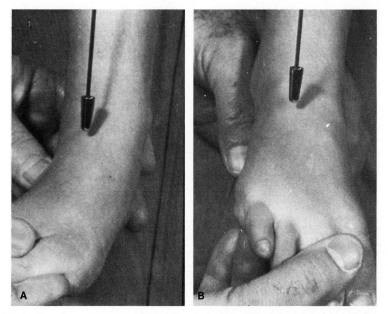

FIGURE 18-4. Forefoot adduction (**A**) and forefoot abduction (**B**) are motions of a foot segment on a theoretic vertical axis.

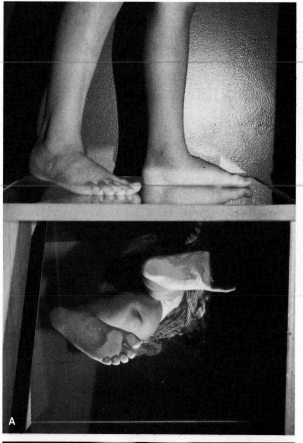

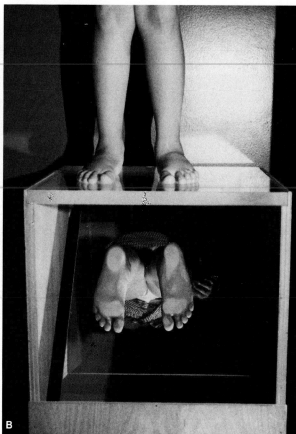

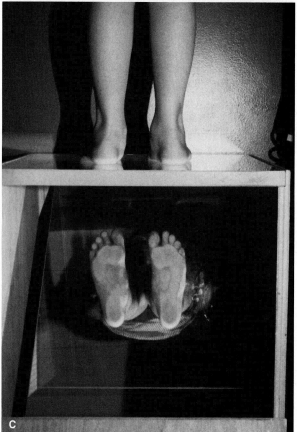

FIGURE 18-5. (A and B) Physiologic pes planus. Note loss of longitudinal arch and apparent pronated posture with abduction of the forefoot. (C) Physiologic pes planus. Note heel valgus position with loss of longitudinal arch. (D) Physiologic pes planus. With the leg dangling over the examination table in the non–weight-bearing position, the foot assumes a normal appearance to the arch. (E) Physiologic pes planus tiptoe test. When the patient stands on tiptoes, normal appearance of the arch is apparent.

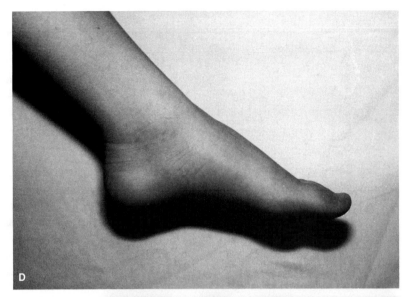

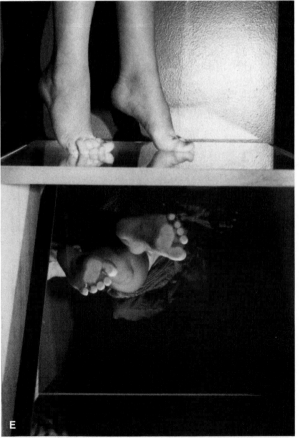

FIGURE 18-5. *(Continued)*

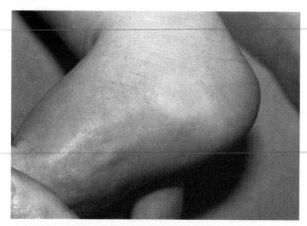

FIGURE 18-6. Four-month-old infant with physiologic pes planus. Note prominence of the medial fat pad contributing to the appearance of pes planus (fat pad is blanched by finger pressure to emphasize its location).

loss of the normal arch (Fig. 18-7). Body weight shifts medially, altering the normal weight-bearing pattern and causing increasing ground contact with the medial aspect of the foot. With time, the Achilles tendon may shorten and act as an everter of the foot, accentuating the deformity.

Many theories have been advanced over the years about the cause of physiologic pes planus, most centering around abnormal bone configuration, muscle imbalance, or ligamentous laxity. The etiology of persistent physiologic pes planus, however, remains unknown. Many patients have a positive family history of a similar condition or evidence of generalized ligamentous laxity. Physiologic pes planus may also be associated with obesity. A positive family history should be sought for conditions associated with joint laxity, such as Marfan and Ehlers-Danlos

syndromes. Physiologic pes planus is occasionally seen as a residual of the calcaneal valgus foot deformity (discussed later). It is important to obtain a family history of treatment of similar conditions because this may have significant bearing on the patient education necessary in prescribing treatment modalities to the family.

Most children with physiologic pes planus are asymptomatic. They are brought in by their parents because of the assumption that flatfeet are abnormal and harmful to their child if not treated. Occasionally, some children may complain of symptoms that are referable to foot strain after prolonged activity and generally relieved by rest. Associated leg aches are not uncommon in patients who present with symptomatic pes planus, but because these are present in a large portion of normal people, a cause-and-effect relation is difficult to establish.

Each patient should be thoroughly examined for excessive joint laxity manifested by the ability to hyperextend the metacarpal phalangeal joints, appose the thumb to the forearm, and hyperextend the elbows and knees. The foot has normal to slightly increased subtalar motion. In weight bearing, varying degrees of loss of the longitudinal medial arch are noted. The heel is in valgus and the forefoot in abduction (see Fig. 18-5). With loss of the longitudinal arch on weight bearing, the center of gravity is shifted medially to the second metatarsal or medially to the first metatarsal. The patient may have a toe-in gait in an attempt to shift the weight-bearing axis laterally.

Foot flexibility may be demonstrated in two ways: by examining the feet in the resting position and by the tip-toe test. The patient should be examined with legs dangling over the examination table

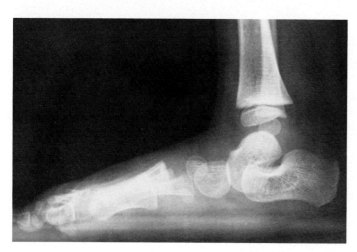

FIGURE 18-7. Physiologic pes planus, standing lateral radiograph. The longitudinal arch is depressed; the talus points directly downward instead of forward in line with the navicular and metatarsals.

(see Fig. 18-5). In this position, the physiologic pes planus foot assumes a normal contour to the longitudinal arch. In the tip-toe test, the patient's feet are observed when the patient walks on tip toes (see Fig. 18-5). In this position, the normal arch is restored, with the heel going to a neutral or slightly varus position. Muscle strength of the foot should be normal.

It is important to rule out hypermobile flatfoot associated with a short Achilles tendon by history and physical examination (Fig. 18-8). This condition, which is often familial, is evidenced by contracture of the gastrocnemius in association with the same clinical features as described previously. This condition is usually symptomatic and associated with long-term disability. These patients can usually correct the deformity by involuntary muscular effort, as demonstrated by the patient restoring the arch by standing on tip toes. In addition, in the non–weight-bearing position, the normal arch is generally present. Contracture of the Achilles tendon is best assessed with the knee in extension and the talonavicular joint locked in inversion so that dorsiflexion is measured only at the ankle. The radiographic features of this condition are characteristic (Fig. 18-9). These patients may also show evidence of hypermobility at the midtarsal joints, which allows the heel to touch the floor despite a contracted Achilles tendon. Without treatment, this condition may cause severe disabling pain.

In the child presenting with a complaint of flatfeet, pathologic causes of pes planus must be ruled out. These include congenital vertical talus, oblique talus, tarsal coalition, tumor, foreign body reaction, and Köhler disease of the navicular and accessory navicular. Accessory navicular bones are seen in about 12% of the population and are a normal variant. Two patterns are evident. In one pattern, the accessory navicular is a sesamoid bone within the posterior tibial tendon (Fig. 18-10). It is anatomically separate from the navicular and usually does not cause symptoms. In the second form, the accessory navicular is in close association with the navicular as an ossification center, causing a change in shape of the navicular. This type may be associated with pain, particularly during adolescence (Fig. 18-11). Accessory navicular is not a cause of hypermobile flatfoot, but because both conditions are common, they may be present together. Accessory naviculars may be treated symptomatically, but excision may be required if conservative measures fail.

The foot with a vertical talus assumes a convex plantar surface that is rigid and has characteristic radiographic findings (Figs. 18-12 to 18-14). Neuromuscular causes of pes planus, such as cerebral palsy and muscular dystrophy, can be diagnosed by their typical diagnostic characteristics. The most severe form of physiologic pes planus is referred to as an *oblique talus* because of its radiologic appearance. It has features similar to vertical talus on the standing lateral view, but normal alignment is restored on plantar flexion lateral radiographs. Tarsal coalitions have rigidity of subtalar motion, may be associated with peroneal spastic flatfoot, and are diagnosed radiographically (Figs. 18-15 through 18-18). Other causes of pes planus include the so-called skewfoot or Z foot (see metatarsus adductus) and surgically overcorrected clubfeet.

Radiographs are generally not indicated in the asymptomatic child with a physiologic pes planus. In severe cases, standing anteroposterior (AP) and lateral radiographs should be obtained. On the normal standing AP radiograph, the talocalcaneal angle should be between 15 and 35 degrees (Fig. 18-19). Diversion of the AP talocalcaneal angle to greater than 35 degrees is evidence of heel valgus. The midtalar line passing medial to the first metatarsal with the navicular displaced laterally is evidence of forefoot abduction. On the standing lateral radiograph, the normal lateral talocalcaneal angle is between 25 and 50 degrees. The talus first metatarsal angle should be about 0 degrees. On the lateral view, the exact location of loss of longitudinal arch can be determined. This sag may occur at the talonavicular joint, first naviculocuneiform joint, and first metatarsocuneiform joint, or combinations thereof. On the standing lateral radiograph, the talus is more vertically oriented, with the metatarsals and the calcaneus

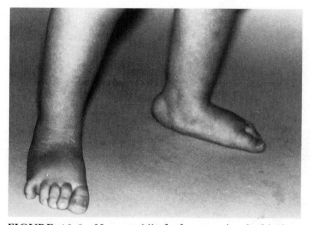

FIGURE 18-8. Hypermobile flatfoot associated with short Achilles tendon. Typical appearance is similar to that of physiologic pes planus.

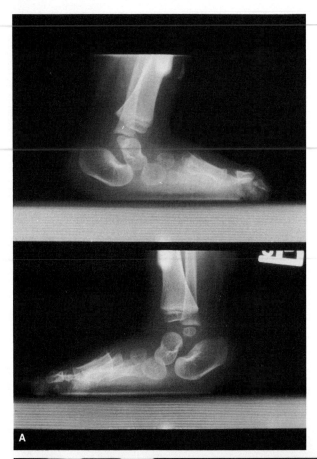

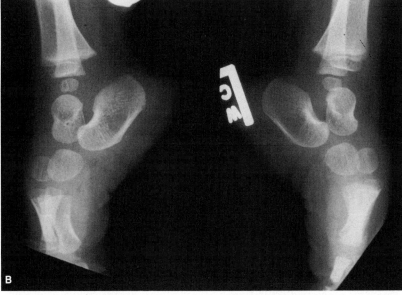

FIGURE 18-9. Hypermobile flatfoot associated with short Achilles tendon. (A) Standing lateral radiographs reveal talus in plantar flexion, calcaneus in equinus indicative of contracted Achilles tendon. (B) Forced plantar flexion lateral radiograph. The forefoot is colinear with the longitudinal axis of the talus, indicative of passive correctability of this deformity. The patient's condition resolved with Achilles tendon lengthening.

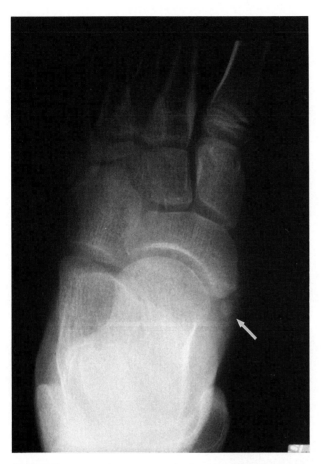

FIGURE 18-10. Accessory navicular. Note the appearance of sesamoid bone within the posterior tibial tendon.

in a more horizontal position than normal because of flattening of the arch (see Fig. 18-7).

If the patient presents with a painful flatfoot, oblique views and Harris views (radiograph taken from behind the foot with the x-ray beam at a 45-degree angle) may be helpful in defining a tarsal coalition or a pathologic process. If tumor, infection, or a stress fracture is suspected, bone scanning may be helpful. Computed tomography (CT) is indicated if talocalcaneotarsal coalition is suspected (see Fig. 18-18). The diagnosis of physiologic pes planus is one of exclusion.

The natural history of physiologic pes planus is unfortunately clouded by medical and nonmedical mythology. To most parents and many physicians and paramedical personnel, flatfeet are considered a significant health problem. Unfortunately, good natural history data on this condition are lacking.

Treatments offered in the past have been based on the assumption that patients will have problems in the future if the condition is not treated. In normal children, aged 1 to 3 years, whose parents bring them in for concerns over flatfeet, reassurance and explanation of the cause of pes planus are essential. The parents should be informed about the presence of the normal fat pad, the normal hyperlaxity of infancy, the often familial nature of the condition. They should also be reassured that, in most children, an arch will develop by 5 years of age. The parents should be informed of the benign natural history of

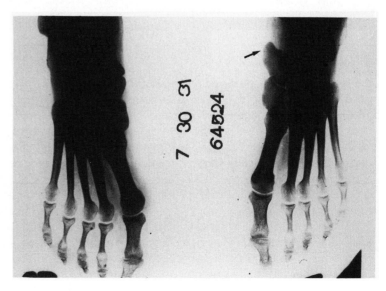

FIGURE 18-11. Accessory navicular. This type of accessory navicular has fused to the primary navicular, altering its shape and leading to prominence of the tuberosity.

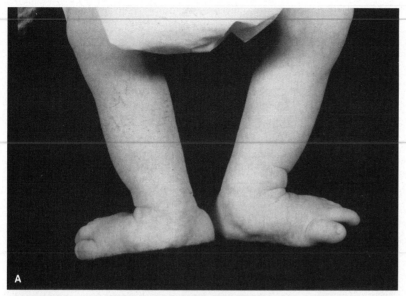

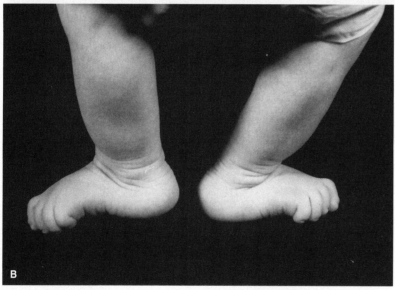

FIGURE 18-12. Congenital vertical talus. Newborn with sacral agenesis and bilateral congenital vertical talus. The heels are in valgus and the forefoot is abducted. The foot has the characteristic rocker-bottom deformity.

the condition. Appropriate literature should be supplied to the family so they can reassure themselves and other family members who may expect some treatment because of what they have heard from others, what they have read, or treatment they underwent as children. Many parents are under the false assumption that so-called corrective shoes are responsible for the natural development of the longitudinal arch.

The same conservative recommendations apply to all other children with the diagnosis of physiologic pes planus. The educational aspects of the natural history of the condition cannot be overemphasized.

The parents should be instructed that treatment modalities offered in the past were offered without any scientific basis. A recent prospective randomized study of patients with flexible flatfeet treated by corrective shoes and inserts revealed that all patients improved moderately after 3 years of treatment, and no greater improvement was seen in patients who were treated vigorously, even those treated with custom-made inserts. All treatments in the past, including exercises, varying shoe modifications, and inserts, have been proved to be ineffective.

In a child with a painful flexible flatfoot, the diagnosis must be reassessed and sources of painful

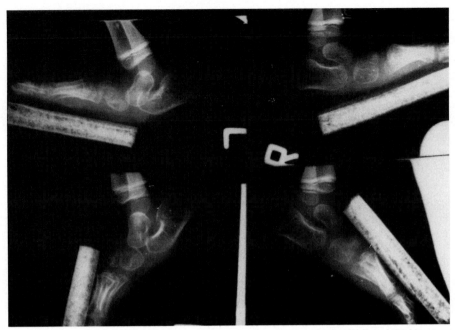

FIGURE 18-13. Congenital vertical talus of left foot. (Hypermobile flatfoot with contracted Achilles tendon on the right foot.) In the simulated weight-bearing views (*upper left and upper right*), both feet have the evidence of a rocker-bottom deformity with dorsiflexion occurring at the midfoot, the hind foot is in equinus, and the forefoot is in dorsiflexion. The talus is more severely plantar flexed on the left than the right. Both calcanea are in equinus, and on the left foot there is disruption of the calcaneal cuboid joint. On the plantar flexion views (*bottom*), note on the right side the longitudinal axis of the talus is colinear with the forefoot; but on the left (side with congenital vertical talus), the longitudinal axis of the talus is not colinear with the longitudinal axis of the metatarsals, indicative of the rigid nature of the deformity.

flatfeet eliminated. Prophylactic treatment of any type is unwarranted. Treatment for flexible flatfeet is only indicated if the patient presents with pain, usually in the foot or calf, or if the patient has severe excessive shoe wear. The discomfort in the foot and the associated leg aches, which occur in about 15% to 30% of normal people, should be treated symptomatically with acetaminophen, local heat, and massage. If fatigue symptoms or discomfort with increasing activity persists, shoe modifications can be considered. It is important to emphasize that these modifications are not corrective. High-top tennis shoes with a good longitudinal arch can usually be recommended. If symptoms persist, other noncorrective adaptive measures may be tried, such as a medial heel wedge, a long shoe counter, or a navicular pad.

For the more severe symptomatic physiologic pes planus that fails to respond to conservative measures, a more formal shoe orthotic, such as a University of California Biomechanics Lab insert or custom-made insert, may distribute body weight more evenly across

the sole of the foot and take the pressure off the prominent talar head. These modalities, however, are expensive, must be changed frequently with foot growth, and have no scientific basis for their use. The use of shoe modification inserts tends to label the child as having a problem. The use of these devices to appease parents or grandparents should be discouraged.

In young patients with hypermobile flatfoot and a short tendo Achilles, heel cord stretching exercises should be instituted. If symptoms develop or the contracture persists, tendo Achilles lengthening can be considered. The only operative indications in true physiologic pes planus flatfoot are severe malalignment problems causing excessive abnormal shoe wear or pain. Achilles tendon stretching or casting may be of some benefit. Surgical options for these indications are rarely indicated. In in the past, these included soft tissue procedures alone; arthrodeses of the various tarsal joints; osteotomies; and combined osteotomies, arthrodeses, and soft tissue procedures, all

(text continues on page 628)

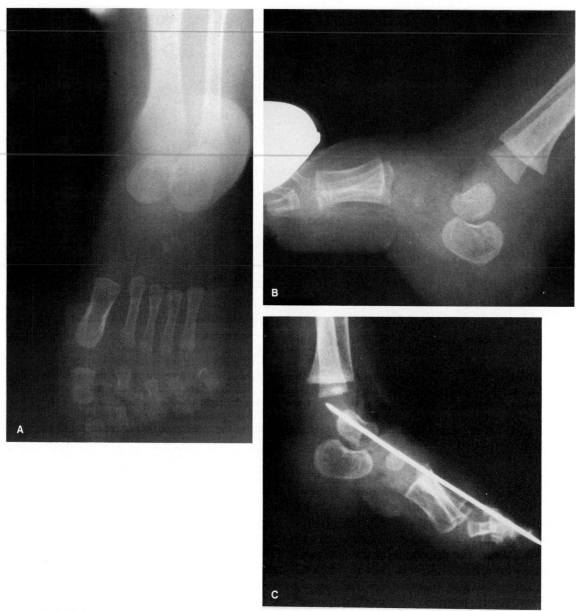

FIGURE 18-14. Congenital vertical talus. (**A**) Standing AP view demonstrates increased angle between talus and calcaneus indicative of the hindfoot valgus. (**B**) Lateral view of plantar flexion indicates failure of realignment of the metatarsals with the long axis of the talus. (**C**) Postsurgical realignment of forefoot, midfoot, and hindfoot. (**D** and **E**) Standing PA and lateral radiographs 6 years after operation demonstrating restoration of normal anatomic relations.

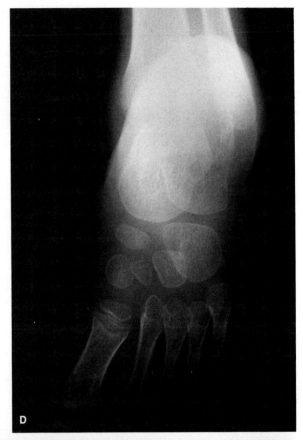

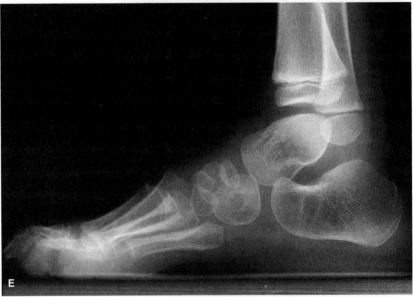

FIGURE 18-14. *(Continued)*

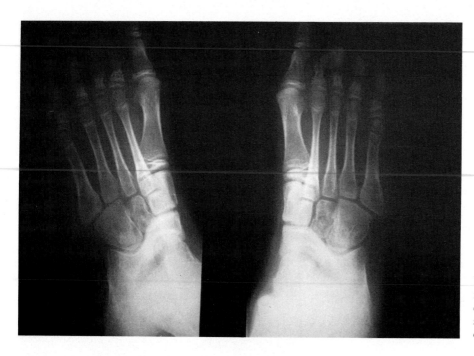

FIGURE 18-15. Calcaneal navicular coalition. Forty-five-degree oblique view demonstrates calcaneal navicular coalitions.

with the goal of restoring the normal longitudinal arch, relieving pain, and preserving as much motion as possible. Results of these procedures have been poor.

TARSAL COALITION

The term *tarsal coalition* refers to the union of two or more tarsal bones by fibrous, cartilaginous, or bony tissue. This entity is often called *peroneal spastic flatfoot* because of the high association with contracture of the peroneal tendons. The most common sites of coalition are between the calcaneus and the navicular and between the talus and calcaneus. The most com-

mon talocalcaneal coalition is between the sustentaculum and the talus, with rare coalitions involving the anterior or posterior facet. Other tarsal coalitions are much less common. The coalitions may be complete or partial. When the coalitions are fibrous, they are called *syndesmosis*. When the coalitions are cartilaginous, they are referred to as *synchondroses*. Bony unions are referred to as *synostosis*. Tarsal coalition

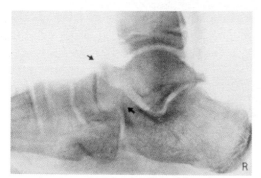

FIGURE 18-16. Calcaneal navicular coalition. In a patient with calcaneal navicular bar, standing lateral radiograph demonstrates prominence of the anterior process of the calcaneus and a spur at the superior talonavicular articulation.

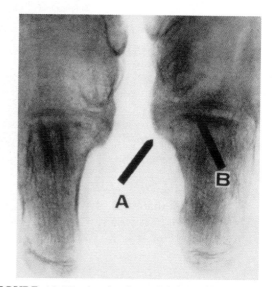

FIGURE 18-17. A talocalcaneal bridge. Harris views of both feet. Note the prominence of the sustentaculum (*arrow A*); talocalcaneal articulation is obliterated in the medial portion (*arrow B*).

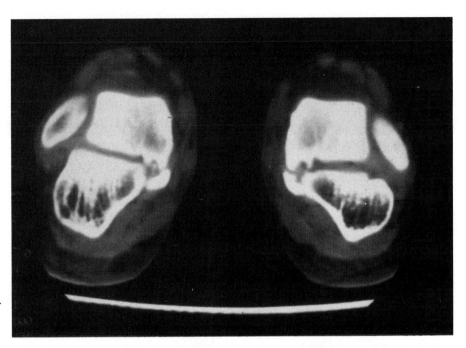

FIGURE 18-18. Talocalcaneal coalition. Frontal section of a CT scan demonstrates tarsal coalition at middle facet joint.

represents the most common nonneuromuscular cause of pathologic pes planus.

The true incidence of tarsal coalition is unknown. It is estimated, however, that less than 1% to 2% of the population is affected. Although tarsal coalitions may be multiple, rarely is there more than one coalition per foot. Bilateralness, however, is common.

Demonstration of coalitions in fetal specimens lends support to the theory of failure of segmentation as the etiology of tarsal coalitions (Fig. 18-20). This incomplete segmentation of the mesenchymal anlage of the tarsal bones gives rise to the fibrous or cartilaginous coalition, which may ossify later in life. Bilateralness has been reported in up to 70% of calcaneonavicular coalitions and in 20% to 50% of talocalcaneal coalitions. Tarsal coalitions are thought to be an inherited condition, with the most widely accepted pattern being autosomal dominant inheritance with variable penetrance.

Because the true incidence of tarsal coalitions in the population is unknown, the natural history is uncertain. It is apparent that many patients with tarsal coalitions have no symptoms, and many patients with coalitions treated symptomatically can go well into adult life without persistent pain or disability. Symptoms most commonly develop when the coalition begins to ossify. Ossification of the coalition restricts subtalar motion. This alteration in subtalar mechanics leads to increased stress at adjacent joints, particularly the ankle and talonavicular joints. If a coalition re-

mains fibrous (syndesmosis), symptoms may never develop because of the mobility allowed through the syndesmosis. With increasing ossification of a cartilaginous (synchondrosis) coalition, decreased mobility ensues, increasing the likelihood of the patient developing clinical symptoms. The altered subtalar joint mechanics over time may lead to degenerative joint disease in adjacent joints, causing persistent pain and disability. The limited subtalar motion also causes increased laxity in adjacent joints, particularly the ankle joint, leading to increased incidence of sprains and secondary joint alterations.

The typical patient with tarsal coalition presents during the second decade of life with pain or decreased subtalar motion. Occasionally, the patient complains of a limp, discomfort in the calf region, or nonspecific foot pain. The pain is often localized to the anterior, medial, or lateral aspect of the subtalar joint or to the talonavicular region. The onset of pain is usually insidious or associated with a traumatic event such as a nonresolving ankle sprain. Pain is usually made worse by activities like running and jumping or prolonged standing; it is usually relieved by rest. The symptom onset depends on the nature of the coalition (fibrous, cartilaginous, or bony) and the specific joint involved. Children with the rare talonavicular coalition may present between 2 and 4 years of age. Typically, patients with calcaneonavicular coalitions present between 8 and 12 years of age, and those with talocalcaneal coalitions between

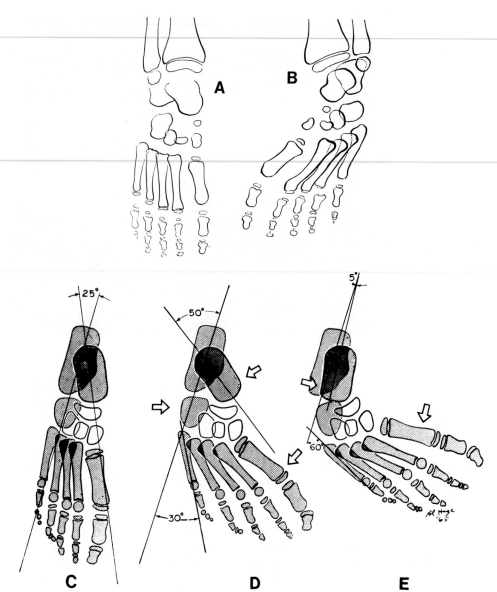

FIGURE 18-19. Congenital metatarsus varus. (A) The talus, the scaphoid, the first cuneiform, and the first metatarsal form a straight line. The anterior ends of the talus and the calcaneus are separated. (B) The first metatarsal is carried medially and is in line only with the inner cuneiform and the scaphoid, the latter lying lateral to the talar head. The talus and the calcaneus are in the flatfoot position, the anterior ends lying in a divergent relationship. The inversion of the forefoot causes the cuneiforms to overlap and the lateral aspect of the metatarsals to be visualized. The metatarsals normally are bowed dorsalward, and in this view they are wrongly identified as deformed. (C) Diagram of roentgenogram of a normal foot; (D) a foot with metatarsus adductus; and (E) a clubfoot. Arrows indicate directions and sites of molding during corrective manipulation and plaster-cast application. (Ponseti IV, Becker JH. Congenital metatarsus adductus. J Bone Joint Surg 1966;48A:702)

12 and 14 years of age. In any child presenting with a painful rigid foot, tarsal coalition must be ruled out.

Physical examination in patients with tarsal coalition generally reveals decreased hindfoot or midfoot motion, or both. Most commonly, the heel is in valgus and the forefoot in abduction (Fig. 18-21). The patient may walk with an antalgic gait, and if symptoms are long-standing and the pain is significant, disuse atrophy may be noted on calf measurements. In about half of cases, contractures of the peroneal muscles is present. This is evidenced by

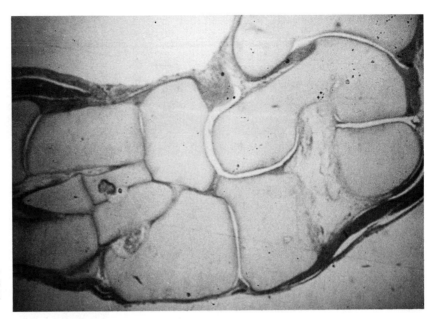

FIGURE 18-20. Tarsal coalition. Fetal specimen demonstrating fibrous tarsal coalition between calcaneus and navicular.

prominence of the peroneal tendons in the lateral aspect of the ankle and foot (Fig. 18-22). Attempt at inversion of the deformity causes pain and discomfort along the peroneal region (Fig. 18-23). The peroneal tendons are contracted secondary to prolonged positioning of the foot in valgus. True muscle spasms of the peroneal tendons are rare. Increased ankle ligamentous laxity is most commonly seen in patients with long-standing symptoms, particularly those with

talocalcaneal coalitions. There may also be varying degrees of loss of the longitudinal arch. Pathologic conditions affecting the subtalar joint, including tumors, rheumatoid arthritis, and traumatic injuries, may mimic the physical findings of tarsal coalition.

When tarsal coalitions are suspected, standing AP, lateral, and 45-degree medial oblique radiographs should be obtained (see Fig. 18-15). The diagnosis of a calcaneonavicular coalition can usually

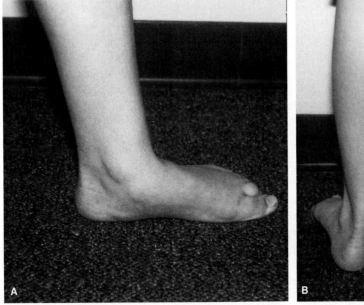
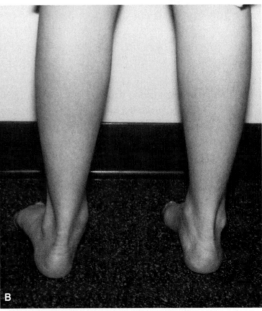

FIGURE 18-21. Tarsal coalition. Note the position of the involved left foot with the forefoot in abduction (A) and heel in valgus (B). Also note the loss of the longitudinal arch.

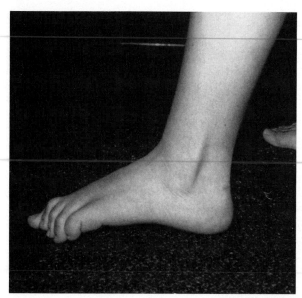

FIGURE 18-22. Tarsal coalition. Note prominence of the perineal tendons on the lateral aspect of the ankle because of prolonged positioning of the hindfoot in valgus and forefoot in abduction.

be made on these standard radiographs. The 45-degree medial oblique radiograph usually demonstrates this coalition. If the coalition is fibrous or cartilaginous, however, it may not be obvious on plain radiographs. Other findings that indicate a possible calcaneonavicular coalition include elongation at the anterior portion of the calcaneus to a point of close proximity to the navicular and irregular, sclerotic margins of the two bones in close approximation (see Fig. 18-16).

Before the development of CT scanning, talocalcaneal coalitions were often difficult to diagnosis. In suspected talocalcaneal coalitions, Harris views taken from behind the foot at an angle 45 degrees from the horizontal demonstrate the posterior and medial facets of the subtalar joint. Normally, these are parallel, but coalitions may be diagnosed by the loss of the parallel orientation between the two facets, presence of fusion, or irregular or sclerotic surfaces (see Fig. 18-17). Other types of tomography also have been used to demonstrate talocalcaneal coalitions; however, CT is the diagnostic method of choice for demonstrating these coalitions. Coronal sections should be obtained to document the coalition (see Fig. 18-18). These sections not only document the presence of the coalition but also clearly define its extent. CT scans are most helpful in planning surgical management of this condition.

In patients with talocalcaneal coalitions, abnor-

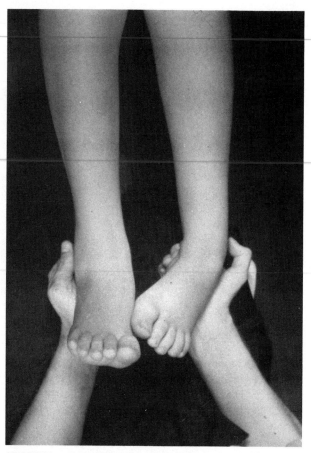

FIGURE 18-23. Tarsal coalition. There is inability to supinate the involved right foot secondary to tarsal coalition with restricted subtalar motion.

mal subtalar mechanics may be evident radiographically by secondary adaptive changes. These include dorsal beaking or lipping at the head or neck of the talus (see Fig. 18-16). This is secondary to stretching of the talonavicular ligaments because of the navicular impinging on the head of the talus. The lateral aspect of the talus may appear broadened, with the undersurface of the talar neck having a concave appearance. There may be apparent narrowing of the posterior talocalcaneal joint space and inability to determine the definition of the middle talocalcaneal articulation.

Radiographs of the ankle joint may demonstrate an apparent ball-and-socket ankle; this is manifest by convexity of the dome of the talus on both the AP and lateral views. In patients presenting with repeated ankle sprains and radiographic evidence of a ball-and-socket ankle, tarsal coalition should be sought. In these cases, the radiographic changes at the ankle joint are secondary to long-standing ankle instability and adaptive changes of the tibial talar articulation.

Initial management of calcaneonavicular coalitions should be nonoperative because the natural history indicates that many patients have no symptoms and the literature review of various treatment programs indicates some success with nonoperative treatment. Nonoperative treatment measures are based on immobilizing the subtalar joint. Shoe orthotics, ankle–foot orthoses, nonsteroidal antiinflammatory agents, and activity restriction may be tried as a first line of treatment. If these fail, a period of cast immobilization with a short-leg walking cast for 3 to 6 weeks should be tried. If symptoms recur or are not alleviated by conservative measures, surgical excision is indicated. The most commonly used surgical technique is wide excision of the bar and interposition of either extensor digitorum brevis tendons or fat. Patients are immobilized in a cast for about 7 to 10 days, followed by range of motion exercise and protected weight bearing. Full weight bearing is allowed in 4 to 6 weeks. The main indication for surgery is pain relief, not restoration of joint motion, although with calcaneonavicular bar excisions, restoration and maintenance of joint motion can be expected if the patient does not have secondary degenerative joint disease changes. If symptoms persist and secondary degenerative joint disease is present in the adjacent joints, triple arthrodesis remains the only option for relief of the patient's symptoms. Success rates of surgery in calcaneonavicular coalitions are best in young patients with cartilaginous bars and no evidence of degenerative joint disease at the talonavicular joint. Talar beaking is not a contraindication for surgery because it does not necessarily represent degenerative changes.

The treatment of talocalcaneal coalitions is somewhat more difficult. Usual treatment should center around nonoperative measures as indicated previously for calcaneonavicular coalitions. If these nonoperative measures fail to provide lasting relief of the patient's symptoms, resection of the coalition with interposition of fat or bone wax should be considered. Specific criteria for resectability of these coalitions are lacking. Long-term series with large numbers of patients are unavailable. Contraindications to resection, however, are an extensive coalition and degenerative joint disease at the adjacent joints. In these circumstances, subtalar fusion or triple arthrodesis should be considered. The most common cause of failure in surgical management of tarsal coalitions is incomplete resection.

CONGENITAL VERTICAL TALUS

Congenital vertical talus is a rare deformity of the foot. It is characterized by a rigid flatfoot deformity, with the plantar aspect of the foot having a convex contour. The heel is in valgus, and the forefoot is abducted (see Fig. 18-12). This entity has also been called *congenital convex pes planus, congenital convex pes valgus,* and *congenital flatfoot with talonavicular dislocation.* All these terms are descriptive either of the clinical or radiographic appearance of the foot.

Congenital vertical talus rarely exists alone. It is usually associated with other congenital abnormalities, musculoskeletal defects, or disorders of the central nervous system. There is a high incidence of congenital vertical talus in children with myelomeningocele (10% having congenital vertical talus), congenital hip dysplasia, and several trisomies (13 to 15, 18). This entity is more common in boys than girls, and there appears to be a familial tendency. It may be bilateral, but if unilateral, it may be associated with a pathologic condition of the opposite foot, including clubfoot, metatarsus adductus, or calcaneal valgus deformity.

Clinically, the condition can be diagnosed at birth. The involved foot is usually smaller than the opposite side with decreased circumference of the calf. In the newborn, the dorsal aspect of the foot may be in close approximation to the distal aspect of the tibia, similar to the foot position in the calcaneal valgus deformity. Unlike calcaneal valgus, however, this position is rigid, and the foot cannot be flexed in a plantar direction. The sole of the foot has a convex appearance, the rocker-bottom deformity. The hindfoot is in the equinovalgus position with the Achilles tendon contracted. The forefoot is in the abducted dorsiflexed position. The head of the talus is easily palpable on the plantar medial aspect of the foot at the apex of the foot convexity. The deformity is rigid; it cannot be manipulated into the normal position. The head of the talus is covered dorsolaterally by the displaced navicular. Attempts at manipulation fail to reduce the talonavicular joint. The clinical appearance may mimic a hypermobile flatfoot or calcaneal valgus deformity. In both these conditions, however, normal relations, particularly the talonavicular relation, can be restored by plantar flexion.

AP and simulated standing or standing lateral radiographs should be obtained. Standing or simulated standing lateral radiographs reveal the calcaneus to be in equinus and talus to be vertically oriented parallel to the long axis of the tibia (see Fig.

18-13). Because of the extreme plantar flexion of the talus, only the posterior aspect of dome articulates with the distal aspect of the tibia. In children younger than 3 to 5 years of age, the navicular is not ossified, and hence the talonavicular dislocation can only be inferred by noting that the forefoot is displaced dorsally in relation to the talus. Occasionally, a concave depression may be noted on the talar neck induced by the dorsolateral subluxation of the navicular. Once the navicular is ossified, the talonavicular dislocation is easily demonstrated. Radiographs may also demonstrate disruption of the calcaneocuboid joint with dorsolateral displacement of the cuboid. The diagnosis can be confirmed radiographically by a forced plantar flexion lateral view.

In congenital vertical talus, the normal bony relations are not restored on the plantar flexion lateral view. The long axis of the talus is plantar to the cuboid, as opposed to dorsal, and the long axis of the metatarsals cannot be brought into colinear alignment with the long axis of the talus (see Fig. 18-13).

Pathoanatomic studies of a few specimens of congenital vertical talus confirm the anatomic distortions evident by the clinical and radiographic presentation. The specimens reported are similar in their clinical features, all demonstrating hindfoot valgus, equinus deformity, and the dorsolateral subluxation of the navicular on the talus. The talus itself may be hypoplastic with a facet joint on the dorsal neck at the point of articulation with the navicular. The sustentaculum talus is hypoplastic and the anterior facet joint absent. The peroneal and posterior tibialis tendons are displaced dorsally, resulting in muscle imbalance. The etiology of this condition is unknown.

The natural history of congenital vertical talus depends not only on the foot deformity but also on any associated musculoskeletal or central nervous system disorder. In general, without treatment the ambulatory patient develops significant callosities over the head of the talus. This results in pain and skin breakdown over the talar head. The gait of these children is awkward, and shoeing may be a significant problem.

The treatment of congenital vertical talus depends on whether associated conditions are present. In the isolated deformity, surgical correction is almost always necessary. The foot should be manipulated to try to stretch the dorsolateral soft tissues. The manipulations are followed by casting with a long-leg cast changed at weekly intervals. The purpose of the manipulation and casting is to stretch the dorsolateral constricted soft tissues to minimize surgical complications, particularly skin necrosis. Manipulation and casting should be begun immediately at birth and continued for 6 to 10 weeks. Surgical correction is then performed either as a single or multistage procedure. The surgical correction involves lengthening the contracted dorsolateral structures, reducing the talonavicular or calcaneocuboid (or both) joint subluxations, and correcting of the equinus deformity through a posterior capsulotomy of the ankle and subtalar joint and Achilles tendon lengthening. Reinforcement of the soft tissue structures on the plantar aspect of the navicular by use of the posterior tibial tendon is generally indicated (see Fig. 18-14). In older children (over 2.5 years of age), surgical correction is often accompanied by an extraarticular subtalar arthrodesis at the time of surgical correction or as an adjunctive procedure at a later time. Surgical corrections are aimed at restoring normal bony alignment and muscle balance. Complication rates of surgery are high and include aseptic necrosis of the talus, loss of reduction, and stiffness, particularly of the subtalar joint. Success rates are better in children treated surgically when younger than 1 year of age. Tendon transfers may be needed at a later date to restore muscle balance. In the adolescent or adult with untreated or recurrent congenital vertical talus, triple arthrodesis may be the only way to restore normal bony alignment.

CALCANEAL VALGUS

Calcaneal valgus (pes calcaneal valgus, talipes calcaneal valgus, congenital talipes calcaneal valgus) is one of the most common foot deformities seen at birth. The entire foot is held in the dorsiflexed everted position, and in its most severe form, the foot lies adjacent to the anterior border of the tibia (Fig. 18-24). Calcaneal valgus is thought to be secondary to intrauterine molding. It is most common in firstborn children and in children of young mothers. It has a female predominance of 1:0.6 and is estimated to occur in 1 of every 1000 live births.

Clinically, the foot is held in dorsiflexion near the tibia with the forefoot in varying degrees of abduction and the heel in varying degrees of valgus. The peroneal tendons may be subluxated anterior to the lateral malleolus. The soft tissues on the dorsal and lateral aspect of the foot are contracted and restrict plantar flexion and inversion. There may be a transverse crease just distal to the ankle joint on the dorsal aspect of the foot. The foot can generally be manipulated to neutral or just short of the neutral position and, occasionally in mild cases, just beyond

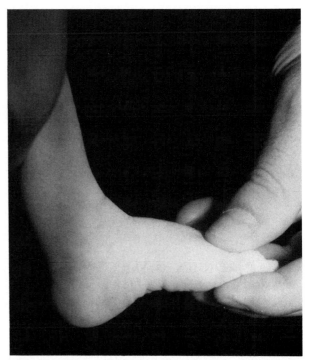

FIGURE 18-25. Calcaneal valgus deformity. The foot can easily be manipulated to or just short of the neutral position.

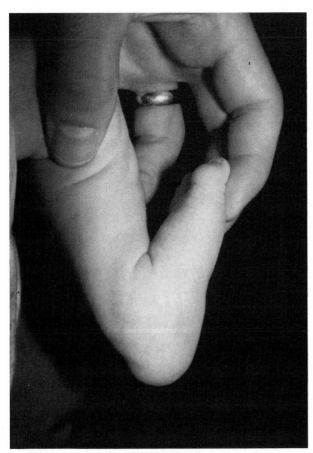

FIGURE 18-24. Calcaneal valgus deformity. There is close approximation of the dorsum of the foot to the anterior aspect of the distal tibia.

this position (Fig. 18-25). The deformity may be accompanied by a mild abduction of the forefoot in varying degrees of heel valgus. There is an occasional association of this deformity with external rotation contractures in the hip and with other conditions thought to be secondary to intrauterine molding deformities (eg, congenital hip dysplasia and torticollis).

It is important to rule out neuromuscular causes of calcaneal valgus deformity, such as myelomeningocele and arthrogryposis, as well as congenital vertical talus. In congenital vertical talus, the Achilles tendon is contracted, the hindfoot is in equinus, and there is a rocker-bottom deformity. Half the cases of vertical talus are associated with a neuromuscular deformity. All cases of posteromedial bowing of the tibia are associated with a calcaneal valgus deformity of the foot.

Radiographs are not necessary to make the diagnosis of pes calcaneal valgus. The foot can be palpated to show normal alignment with no subluxation at the talonavicular joint. Radiographs are only nec-

essary when the diagnosis is in question. It is important to stimulate the foot to make certain that the plantar flexors are present.

The natural history of pes calcaneal valgus is one of spontaneous correction. Persistence of some of the deformity may lead to a flexible flatfoot. Casting is rarely necessary. Treatment should be directed at instructing the parents in stretching exercises. The foot should be gently manipulated into plantar flexion and inversion. In general, the deformity is corrected by 2 to 4 months of age. If it is persistent, however, manipulation and casting can be considered.

KÖHLER DISEASE

Köhler disease is an osteochondrosis that affects the tarsal navicular. It is a self-limited condition characterized by pain or swelling in the area of the tarsal navicular in association with certain radiographic features. It occurs in the age range of 4 to 7 years, with 80% of cases occurring in boys. One fourth to one third of cases are bilateral.

The cause of Köhler disease is unknown, but it is thought to be related to repetitive trauma and interruption of blood supply to the tarsal navicular. The tarsal navicular is the last bone of the foot to ossify. The appearance of the ossification center varies and is gender related. In girls, the tarsal navicular ossifies between 18 months and 2 years of age. In boys, the ossification occurs between 2.5 and 3 years of age. The normal ossification center has a smooth contour and uniform density. In otherwise normal children who have delay in appearance of the ossification center of the navicular, however, it may appear flat or fragmented with multiple ossification centers of increased density and irregular contour. Several ossification centers may eventually coalesce to form the navicular. Postmortem studies of the navicular in children reveal that the blood supply is tenuous, being supplied by only a single vessel until age 6 years.

Köhler disease is more common in patients (male or female) in whom ossification is delayed. The pathogenesis may be secondary to traumatic interruption of the vasculature to the tarsal navicular at a crucial stage in ossification.

Clinically, children present to the physician with complaints of pain and tenderness to palpation over the tarsal navicular. Localized swelling is occasionally evident. There may be palpable thickening of the soft tissues around the tarsal navicular. Many affected children walk with an antalgic gait and bear weight on the lateral aspect of the foot to avoid pressure over the medial aspect and the tarsal navicular. Active and passive range of motion are normal.

Radiographically, the navicular shows evidence of flattening, sclerosis, and irregular ossification (Fig. 18-26). On the standing lateral view, the navicular has a decreased AP diameter with evidence of varying amounts of flattening. Multiple centers of ossification may be present. As mentioned previously, these radiographic features may be a normal variation in as many as one third of children, particularly those who have late-onset ossification. Therefore, the diagnosis of Köhler disease is made only with the combination of the clinical signs and symptoms and the radiographic features.

Children with clinical Köhler disease may have similar radiographic changes in the opposite navicular and be totally asymptomatic. In the normal child, the radiographic appearance is assumed to be secondary to coalescence of multiple ossification centers, while in the child with Köhler disease, the radiographic features represent the changes of avascular necrosis, with invasion by granulation tissue, resorption of necrotic trabeculae, and deposition of new bone.

The natural history of Köhler disease is relatively benign. No long-term disabilities have been reported

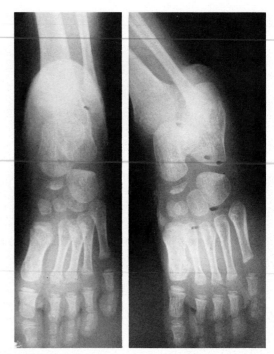

FIGURE 18-26. Köhler disease or osteochondrosis of the tarsal navicular.

in patients who have Köhler disease despite lack of treatment. In most cases, the navicular assumes a relatively normal appearance within 1 to 3 years after symptom onset.

Treatment of the condition is designed to relieve symptoms and not to hasten the reparative process. Treatment for Köhler disease is nonsurgical and depends on the magnitude of symptoms. In patients with mild symptoms, restriction of activities may be all that is necessary. In children with more severe symptoms, a longitudinal arch support can be considered to more evenly distribute the patient's body weight in weight bearing. These measures, in conjunction with avoidance of strenuous activities such as jumping and running, usually relieve symptoms. In patients with more severe symptoms, immobilization in a short-leg cast for 3 to 4 weeks usually provides good relief of symptoms. The patient may need to use crutches with touch weight bearing for a short time but then may bear full weight on the cast as long as symptoms do not recur. Cast treatment should be continued until the patient is asymptomatic. In severe cases, the use of a short-leg walking cast improves the natural history of symptoms dramatically but has no effect on the radiographic course of the disease. Without treatment, most patients have intermittent symptoms for 1 to 3 years that is activity-related and relieved by rest.

FREIBERG INFARCTION

Freiberg infarction is another type of osteochondrosis. Specifically, it is an aseptic necrosis of the metatarsal head. Three fourths of cases occur in girls, and the second metatarsal head is the most commonly involved, although the disease may affect the third or fourth metatarsal head. Freiberg disease rarely occurs before the age of 13 or 14 years.

The etiology of Freiberg infarction is unknown, but it is thought to be similar to that of osteochondritis dissecans of the knee. The second metatarsal is the longest and the most rigid metatarsal. It is subjected to the greatest amount of stress in walking. Freiberg infarction is sometimes seen with an accompanying stress fracture of the metatarsal.

Clinically, patients present with pain and tenderness around the second metatarsophalangeal joint. They may complain of stiffness and have a limp secondary to the pain. On physical examination, the discomfort is well localized. There may be palpable swelling at the second metatarsophalangeal joint. Pain may be elicited on passive range of motion. Motion may be limited and painful. The history may be one of exacerbations and remissions, with pain aggravated by activity and relieved by rest.

Radiographically, the second metatarsal head may have a flattened, enlarged appearance with areas of increased sclerosis and fragmentation. The affected metatarsophalangeal joint may be narrowed, and in long-standing disease, secondary degenerative changes may be evident (Fig. 18-27).

The natural history of Freiberg infarction is variable. In many cases, the condition is self-limited, with revascularization of the affected metatarsal head. The disease process may leave the metatarsal head deformed. Many patients have no pain or discomfort and good range of motion. In some cases, however, the disease course involves exacerbations and remissions. Significant deformity may ensue, and secondary degenerative changes may occur at the metatarsophalangeal joint.

The goal of treatment is to obtain healing of the aseptic necrosis. Initial treatment should be symptomatic. Symptomatic treatment includes decreasing activities and using metatarsal pads inserted in the shoe or metatarsal bars on the sole of the shoe. These latter two measures are designed to allow for weight-bearing on the metatarsal neck as opposed to the metatarsal head to decrease the stresses applied to the metatarsal head. In patients who have more acute symptoms, a short-leg walking cast with or without crutches may provide relief. If the joint is free of

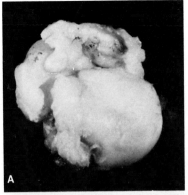

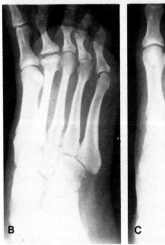

FIGURE 18-27. Freiberg infarction (osteochondrosis of the metatarsal head). (**A**) Frontal view of the resected metatarsal head. The articular cartilage is irregular with areas of loss of articular surface. There are multiple indentations about the head. The capsule about the periphery is thickened, and secondary osteoarthritic spurs are present. A cleft at the margin suggests formation of a loose body by separation. (**B** and **C**) Radiographs of the second metatarsal head before resection showing sclerosis, irregularity, widening, and spurring with flattening.

degenerative changes and symptoms persist, removal of the necrotic fragment alone may provide symptomatic relief. A foot orthosis designed to provide pressure relief over the second metatarsal head may be used on a long-term basis once the acute symptoms have subsided or after surgical removal of the necrotic segment. Mild symptoms may be treated by an orthosis alone.

In patients with long-standing symptoms who fail nonoperative treatment, surgical treatment may be offered. This may include removal of the loose fragment and resection of the base of the proximal phalanx. Alternatively, resection of the metatarsophalangeal joint may be required, with syndactylization of the second and third toe to avoid significant shortening that may follow resection of the metatarsophalangeal joint. This usually provides good relief of symptoms.

SEVER DISEASE

Sever disease, or calcaneal apophysitis, is one of the most common overuse syndromes seen in growing children. It most commonly occurs in the age range of 6 to 12 years and is thought to be due to repeated microtrauma. Most affected children are extremely active. This condition may thus represent chronic strain at the insertion of the tendo Achilles.

Affected children present with activity-related pain over the posterior aspect of the calcaneus. Physical examination reveals tenderness to compression over the calcaneal apophysis. Symptoms may cause discomfort with passive ankle dorsiflexion. The condition must be differentiated from other sources of heel pain in young children (Table 18-1).

In normal children, the calcaneal apophysis appears at an average of 5.6 years of age in girls (range, 3 to 8.5 years) and 7.9 years of age in boys (range, 6 to 10 years). In many normal children, the calcaneal apophysis may appear fragmented and then coalesce from two to three separate ossification centers. This normal ossification variant, in combination with symptomatology, is considered diagnostic of Sever disease (Fig. 18-28). If patients have bilateral symptoms, radiographs are often not necessary. In unilateral cases, however, radiographs of both feet should be obtained to rule out other causes of heel pain, such as retrocalcaneal bursitis, stress fractures, infection, rheumatologic conditions, and neoplastic lesions.

Sever disease is a self-limiting condition. In cases of severe symptoms, activity restriction may be necessary. If this alone does not relieve symptoms or if symptoms are acute, a short-leg walking cast may be applied for 3 to 4 weeks. This usually is adequate to curtail symptoms. Longer periods of casting or activity restriction of up to 1 to 3 months may be necessary in some cases. No long-term disability or deformity has been reported from Sever disease.

METATARSUS ADDUCTUS

A wide variety of terms are used to describe this clinical entity, including *metatarsus adductus, metatarsus varus, skewfoot, serpentine foot, pes adductus, metatar*

TABLE 18-1.
Sources of Heel Pain in Childhood

OVERUSE/OVERGROWTH/TRAUMATIC
Calcaneal apophysitis
Contusion/strain
Stress fracture of calcaneus
Fracture of calcaneus

DEVELOPMENTAL
Tarsal coalition

INFLAMMATORY
Tendinitis (Achilles, patellar, flexor hallux longus)
Plantar fasciitis
Retrocalcaneal bursitis
Periostitis
Os trigonum inflammation

INFECTIOUS
Soft tissue infection
Abscess
Calcaneal osteomyelitis

RHEUMATOLOGIC
Juvenile rheumatoid arthritis
Reiter syndrome
Miscellaneous

TUMORS
BENIGN
Osteoid osteoma
Osteochondroma
Chondroblastoma
Bone cyst (solitary or aneurysmal)
MALIGNANT (RARE)
Leukemia
Metastatic

NEUROLOGIC
Tarsal tunnel syndrome

(Micheli LJ, Ireland ML. Prevention and management of calcaneal apophysitis in children: an overuse syndrome. J Pediatr Orthop 1987;7:34–38)

sus adductovarus, hooked forefoot, metatarsus internus, and *congenital metatarsus varus*. These terms unfortunately are used inconsistently throughout the medical literature. The two most widely used terms are metatarsus adductus and metatarsus varus, which describe slightly different forefoot variations but are synonymous. In this condition, the forefoot is generally adducted and occasionally inverted (varus) at the tarsometatarsal joint, and the hindfoot is generally neutral to valgus (Fig. 18-29; see Fig. 18-19).

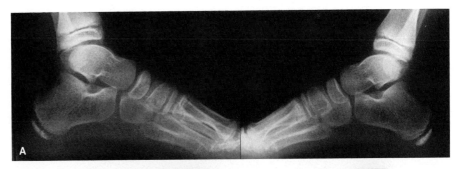

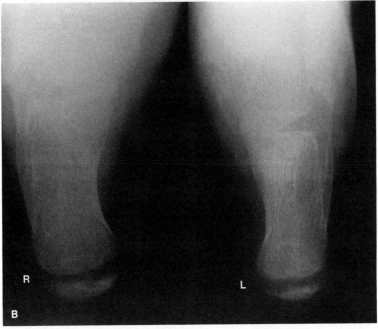

FIGURE 18-28. Severe disease of the calcaneal apophysis. (A) Standing lateral radiograph. (B) Calcaneal views. Note sclerotic fragmented appearance of the right symptomatic calcaneus as opposed to the sclerotic semifragmented appearance of the asymptomatic left side. (Ponseti IV, Becker JH. Congenital metatarsus adductus. J Bone Joint Surg 1966; 48A:702)

Metatarsus adductus is present at birth but often is overlooked by the family until the child is between 3 months and 1 year of age.

Metatarsus adductus is the most common congenital foot deformity. Its incidence is 1 in 1000 live births. It has a female predominance of 4:3 and a 5% incidence of the condition in first-degree relatives. There is no known pattern of inheritance, but the risk of a second sibling being affected is 1 in 20. Two thirds of patients have involvement of both feet. There is a strong association between metatarsus adductus and congenital hip dysplasia and dislocation.

The cause of metatarsus adductus is unknown. It is thought to be secondary to intrauterine molding because 59% of patients are firstborn children. Other etiologic theories include peroneal muscle weakness with overactive anterior tibialis and posterior tibialis; abnormal insertion of the tibialis posterior tendons on the first cuneiform rather than their usual site on the navicular; and posture habits caused by prone sleeping with the buttocks elevated, hips and knees in complete flexion, feet adducted and tucked beneath the buttocks, and sitting on the adducted feet. Persistent soft tissue contractures may lead to secondary tarsal changes, making the deformity rigid with time.

Clinically, the deformity is present at birth but usually not noticed by the parents until the child begins to crawl or walk. Occasionally, patients present to a physician in the toddler years when the parents complain of the child in-toeing or having difficulty with wearing shoes. On physical examination, all the metatarsals are adducted and the forefoot is occasionally in varus (see Fig. 18-29). The heel is in neutral to slight valgus. The great toe is often widely separated from the second toe, and the base of the fifth metatarsal and the cuboid are prominent on the lateral aspect of the foot. The medial border of the foot is concave, and the lateral border is convex. Medial tibial torsion often accompanies metatarsus

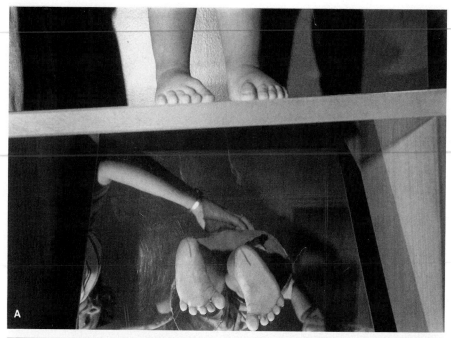

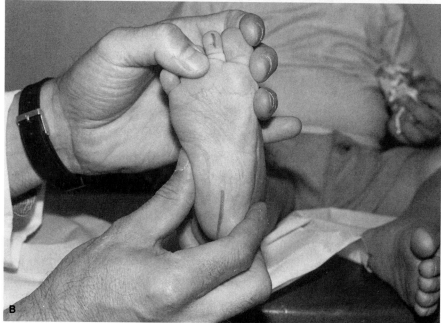

FIGURE 18-29. (A) Thirteen-month-old boy with bilateral metatarsus adductus. The left foot is abducted and the right forefoot is adducted and in slight varus. The heel bisector is at the fourth toe on the left foot and between the third and fourth toes on the right foot. (B) Note passive correctability of deformity. Forefoot can be passively abducted beyond the heel bisector.

adductus. The Achilles tendon is not tight, and the foot can be fully dorsiflexed at the ankle joint. The deformity is often accentuated by overactivity in the abductor hallucis and the short toe flexors.

The deformity is often classified subjectively as mild, moderate, or severe, depending on whether the forefoot can be passively corrected to neutral or to an overcorrected position. Severe deformities are rigid and not passively correctable. The ratio of supple to rigid deformity is about 10:1. The term *serpentine*

foot is often used for a rigid adducted forefoot with an accompanying heel valgus.

The heel bisector should pass through the second toe. In a mild deformity, the bisector passes through the third toe; in a moderate deformity, it passes between the third and fourth toes or just the fourth toe; and in a severe deformity, the heel bisector passes between the fourth and fifth toes. The deformity is said to be flexible or passively correctable if the forefoot (second toe) can be passively abducted beyond the heel bisector (see Fig. 18-29). Many patients exhibit dynamic hallux varus, whereby the great toe deviates medially during stance phase but the metatarsals are normally aligned.

Radiographs are not required to make the diagnosis of metatarsus adductus. Radiographs can, however, document deformity and are used by some to classify the deformity. Radiographs, if taken, should be in the standing position or with the foot resting in a simulated standing position on the radiograph cassette. Radiographs demonstrate sharp medial angulation of the tarsometatarsal joints, with the first metatarsal being more severely adducted than the fifth (see Fig. 18-19). Normally, a line drawn through the longitudinal axis of the first metatarsal is parallel or diverges laterally from a line drawn through the longitudinal axis of the talus. In metatarsus adductus, the first metatarsal line falls medial to the talar line. In the weight-bearing or simulated weight-bearing film, the calcaneal line should bisect the cuboid and the base of the fourth metatarsal. In metatarsus adductus, the calcaneal line passes through the lateral portion of the cuboid and through the base of the fifth metatarsal. Heel valgus is evidenced by a greater than 35-degree AP talocalcaneal angle and by medial and forward displacement of the head of the talus in relation to the anterior portion of the calcaneus. The navicular (generally not seen on radiographs in this age group) is neutral or displaced laterally on the talar head (see Fig. 18-19).

The natural history of metatarsus adductus is generally benign. It is estimated that 85% to 90% of cases resolve spontaneously without treatment. In childhood, persistent metatarsus adductus leads to an in-toeing gait and occasional complaints of stumbling or tripping. Adults with uncorrected metatarsus adductus rarely complain of pain but may have hallux valgus and bunions. Shoe wear may be a problem in patients with uncorrected metatarsus adductus. Patients may complain of pain in the lateral foot and in the tarsometatarsal joints. Shoes may irritate this area. It is thus important in infancy to select patients who require treatment.

Treatment decisions for metatarsus adductus are based on the passive correctability of the deformity. In patients in whom the deformity corrects by stimulation of the lateral border of the foot or in those in whom the heel is stabilized, the deformity can be passively corrected or overcorrected, and only observation is necessary. Most cases correct spontaneously. In most large series, if the foot remained passively correctable, the deformity had corrected spontaneously by the age of 3 years. Parents should not be encouraged to do manipulations. Manipulations by parents are generally poorly done and may accentuate heel valgus and only minimally correct forefoot adduction. There is no scientific validity for the use of straight-last or reverse-last shoes in the treatment of metatarsus adductus. Denis Browne splints should not be used because they may accentuate heel valgus.

In patients with rigid, severe, nonpassively correctable metatarsus adductus, manipulation and casting are indicated. Two main components of the deformity, adduction of the metatarsals and varying degrees of valgus of the heel, must be corrected simultaneously. Improper manipulation and casting treatment of metatarsus adductus lead to a pronation deformity of the foot. A flatfoot with residuals of metatarsus adductus and severe heel valgus is a significantly worse problem than the original deformity.

The hindfoot deformity is corrected by supinating the calcaneus underneath the talus. With the calcaneus supinated, the cuneiform, navicular, and cuboid bones are inverted, bringing the bases of the metatarsals in proper alignment with the talus and calcaneus (see Fig. 18-19). The metatarsals are then abducted, with counterpressure applied over the cuboid bone. It is important not to pronate the forefoot because a cavus deformity will result. The manipulations of the foot are sustained for several minutes, and this is followed by the application of a thinly padded, well-molded, toe-to-groin plaster cast changed at biweekly intervals until the foot is in the slightly overcorrected position. Complete correction usually requires 3 to 4 long-leg plaster applications. The casting treatment is complete when the lateral aspect of the foot is no longer convex, the heel is in neutral to slight valgus position, and the forefoot has been completely corrected past neutral. Successful treatment of metatarsus adductus by manipulations and casting in patients older than 8 months of age is not likely, and surgical correction may be necessary.

Surgical correction for metatarsus adductus is indicated only in patients with significant cosmetic or shoe-wearing problems. In patients younger than 2 years of age with rigid metatarsus adductus, first metatarsal cuneiform capsulotomy and release of the abductor hallucis, followed by casting, is usually successful. In older children, corrective bone surgery may be necessary.

CLUBFOOT

Talipes equinovarus is the term most commonly used for clubfeet. *Talipes* is a generic term for any foot deformity that centers around the talus. *Equinus* im-

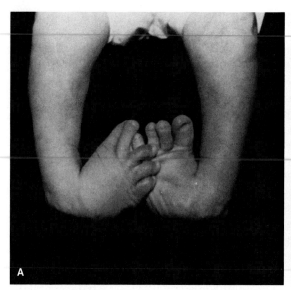
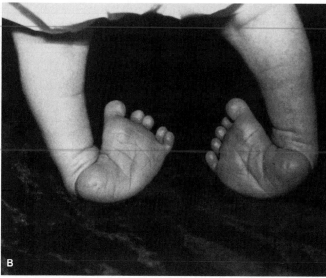

FIGURE 18-30. Severe clubfoot deformity. The heel is in severe varus, and the forefoot is adducted and inverted. The cavus deformity results from the slightly pronated position of the forefoot in relation to the hind foot.

plies that the foot is flexed in the plantar direction. The term *talipes equinocavovarus* is sometimes used to denote the varying amounts of cavus of the forefoot evident in patients with clubfeet. In the clubfoot, the heel is in varus, and the first metatarsal is in severe plantar flexion, while the fifth metatarsal is normally aligned with the cuboid and calcaneus (Figs. 18-30 and 18-31; see Fig. 18-19). Cavus is caused by eversion of the forefoot in relation to the hindfoot.

Clubfoot is a complex foot deformity that is readily apparent at birth. All clubfeet are not of the same severity, although all have the basic components of adduction and inversion of the forefoot and midfoot, heel varus, and fixed equinus. The soft tissue changes vary from mild to severe. Clubfoot should best be thought of as a spectrum of deformities. Clubfoot may occur as an isolated disorder or in combination with various syndromes and other associated anomalies, such as arthrogryposis, sacral agenesis, amniotic bands, Larsen syndrome, diastrophic dwarfism, Freeman-Sheldon syndrome, and myelodysplasia.

The incidence of idiopathic clubfoot is estimated to be 1 to 2 per 1000 live births. It has a male predominance of 2:1 and an incidence of bilateralness estimated to be about 50%. There is an increased incidence in certain racial and ethnic groups, such as Polynesians, Maoris, and South African blacks, with a much higher incidence if the patient has a positive family history for clubfoot.

The etiology of congenital clubfoot in otherwise normal patients remains unknown. Many theories

have been advanced, including intrauterine molding defect, blastemic defect of the tarsal cartilage, primary nerve lesion with secondary muscle dysfunction, vascular abnormalities, arrested embryonic development, abnormal tendon insertions, and primary fibrotic contracture. The most widely accepted theory

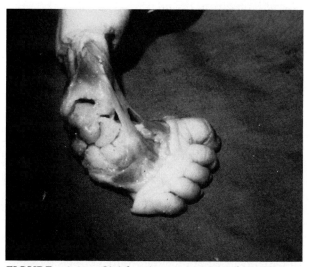

FIGURE 18-31. Clubfoot in a 3-day-old infant. The navicular is medially displaced and articulates only with the medial aspect of the head of the talus. The cuneiforms are seen to the right of the navicular, and the cuboid is underneath it. The calcaneocuboid joint is directed posteromedially. The anterior two thirds of the os calcis is seen underneath the talus. The tendons of the anterior tibialis extensor hallucis longus and the extensor digitorum longus are medially displaced. (Ponseti IV, Campos J. Observations on pathogenesis and treatment of congenital clubfoot. Corr 1972;84:50–60)

is that of polygenic inheritance modified by environmental factors.

Clinically, the deformity is readily apparent at birth. The child presents with the foot in severe supination with a fixed equinus deformity, heel varus, forefoot and midfoot adduction, and varying amounts of cavus. The involved foot is generally smaller than the opposite side with varying amounts of calf atrophy.

The head of the talus is prominent and easily palpable on the dorsolateral aspect of the foot. Depending on the severity of the cavus deformity, there may be a deep skin crease across the plantar medial aspect of the midfoot. The foot cannot be passively manipulated into the neutral position.

Radiographs are often useful in documenting the deformity. The calcaneus, talus, and cuboid are usually ossified at birth. The navicular does not ossify until about 3 years of age. The normal values of bony relations on standing AP and lateral views of the foot are somewhat variable and age dependent (Fig. 18-32).

Radiographs are useful in documenting the deformity (photographs are also useful for this purpose), for follow-up, in assessing the results of nonoperative treatment, and in planning for operative correction of the deformity if necessary. It is best to obtain the initial radiographs in the maximally corrected position. This position varies depending on the flexibility of the individual clubfoot.

In the clubfoot deformity, the talus and calcaneus exhibit parallelism on both the AP and lateral radiographs, indicating hindfoot varus and equinus (see Fig. 18-31). The talus first metatarsal angle is negative, indicating adduction of the forefoot. Because of the inversion of the forefoot, the metatarsals appear overlapped. The cuboid is medially displaced on the AP view, indicating the adduction at the midfoot; and on the lateral view, the first metatarsal is in plantar flexion to a greater degree than the fifth metatarsal, indicating cavus deformity.

Pathoanatomically, many specimens of clubfeet have been described, all showing varying degrees of similar abnormalities (see Fig. 18-31). In the clubfoot, the talar body is in plantar flexion with the neck angulated medially. The navicular articulates with the medial aspect of the talar neck, and the navicular tuberosity is in close approximation with the medial malleolus. The calcaneus is directly underneath the talus, and the cuboid is medially displaced beneath the navicular. The midfoot is thus adducted and inverted in relation to the talus. The dorsal tendons are medially displaced, and the head of the talus is prominent laterally.

Anatomically, the involved talus is generally smaller than the noninvolved side, with the neck in varying degrees of medial deviation. The navicular is wedged shaped laterally, with a prominent tuberosity. The calcaneus is small, often with an absent anterior facet. The posterior facet shows varying degrees of hypoplasia and may be linked directly to the middle facet. In unilateral deformities, the foot is always smaller than the noninvolved side, and the calf has varying degrees of atrophy. The tuberosity of the navicular is held in close approximation to the talar neck, the sustentaculum ,and the medial mal-

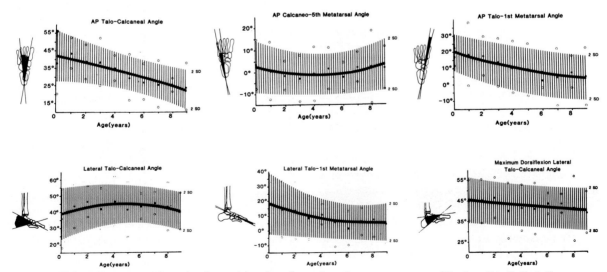

FIGURE 18-32. Normal radiographic values for various foot measurements. (Vanderwilde R, Staheli LT, Chew DE, Malagon V. Measurements on radiographs of the foot in normal infants and children. J Bone Joint Surg 1988;70A:407–415)

leolus by the shortened, thickened tibionavicular ligament, calcaneonavicular ligament, and sheath of the posterior tibial tendon.

Clubfoot deformity, regardless of etiology or associated clinical problems, results in a severe handicap unless corrected. The surface area for weight bearing is the lateral aspect of the foot; without treatment, even an otherwise normal patient develops pressure sores and sinuses by the fourth or fifth decade of life (Fig. 18-33).

The criteria for successful treatment of a clubfoot deformity vary in the orthopaedic literature. Some judge success only by radiographic criteria, others by function, and others by certain clinical criteria. Thus, the literature on treatment is difficult to compare.

The goal of treatment in clubfoot deformity is to obtain and maintain the foot in plantar-grade position. Treatment should be initiated immediately on diagnosis, preferably within the first week of life. Treatment for the newborn with clubfoot is by manipulation and then casting to maintain the correction obtained through manipulation. Corrections begun at a later age may be more difficult owing to ligamentous contracture and joint deformity. Toe-to-groin plaster casts are used to maintain the corrections obtained through manipulation. The equinus deformity is the last deformity corrected to prevent development of a rocker-bottom foot. Casts are changed at weekly intervals, and most deformities are corrected in 2 to 3 months. Successful treatment rates by casting regimens alone vary in the literature from 15% to 90%. Night splinting is often used for prolonged periods (several years) to maintain correction.

Depending on the initial severity, clubfeet have a natural tendency to recur. The more severe and rigid the initial deformity, the greater the risk of recurrence. Recurrences may be treated by serial manipulations and casting followed by occasional tendon transfers to correct for any muscle imbalance.

Deformities that fail to respond to manipulation and casting or that recur may require extensive posterior, medial, and lateral soft tissue releases. The releases are best done at a young age but can be done satisfactorily in children until 5 years of age.

In children older than 3 years of age, lateral column shortening procedures (decancellation of the cuboid or wedge resection of the cuboid in excision of the anterior end of the calcaneus) are often performed in conjunction with posteromedial releases. This is because the greater length of the lateral foot column compared with the medial foot column is thought to be secondary to the medial soft tissue contractures.

The major complications of the extensive posterior, medial, subtalar, and lateral releases performed for residual, resistant, or recurrent clubfoot include skin sloughing on posteromedial aspect of the foot, overcorrection of the deformity, residual forefoot adductus, and incomplete correction of the deformity.

Triple arthrodesis may be necessary for recurrent or persistent clubfoot deformity in older children. These procedures are best offered to the patient at 10 to 12 years of age, when foot growth is complete.

IDIOPATHIC TOE-WALKING

This entity is also called *habitual toe-walking, hereditary tendo Achilles contracture,* or *congenital short tendo calcaneus*. Parents notice that the child is walking on the toes either all or most of the time. Idiopathic toe-walking is thought to be an inherited condition because up to 70% of patients have a positive family history. The condition is bilateral and predominantly affects boys (3:1). About 20% of these children have evidence of a learning disability, and an occasional child carries the diagnosis of hyperkinesia with minimal brain dysfunction.

When a child begins to stand and walk, toe-walking is a normal gait variation. Generally, within the first 6 months after walking, the gait may progress from the toe–toe gait or an occasional toe–toe gait to a toe–heel gait and eventually to a heel–toe gait. The mature heel–toe gait pattern is generally established by the time a child is 3 years of age. Careful history of gait development should be obtained in each pa-

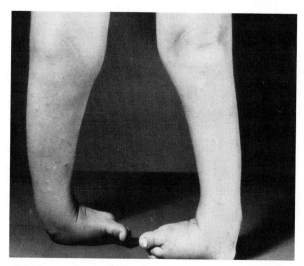

FIGURE 18-33. Four-year-old girl with bilateral untreated clubfeet.

tient who presents with a chief complaint of toe-walking. Patients with the diagnosis of idiopathic toe-walking have nearly always walked on their toes.

Physical examination includes range of motion of the upper and lower extremities as well as a careful neurologic examination and observation of the patient's gait. Variable amounts of contracture and restriction of ankle dorsiflexion are noted. The amount of contracture or restriction of motion may not be symmetric. These patients have normal sensory examinations and no evidence of muscle weakness. Deep tendon reflexes should be intact without evidence of hyperactivity. The spine should be evaluated for evidence of hair patches, dimpling, hyperpigmentation, or nevi, which are suggestive of spinal dysraphism. There should be minimal or no contracture of the hamstrings, and the patient should have good control of the upper extremities.

The child's gait should be carefully evaluated. Many patients with idiopathic toe-walking can walk on their heels and have a heel–toe gait periodically, but the observed gait pattern usually is toe–toe. Idiopathic toe-walkers with heel cord contractures can generally get their heels down in standing only through knee hyperextension (Fig. 18-34).

Idiopathic toe-walking is the diagnosis of exclusion. All conditions that may be associated with an equinus deformity and contracture of the tendo Achilles must be ruled out. Cerebral palsy can be ruled out by the absence of increased deep tendon reflexes, hypertonicity, hamstring contractures, and the lack of posturing abnormalities of the upper extremity during gait. Gait analysis may be of help in differentiating the idiopathic toe-walker from the cerebral palsy patient. Other conditions, such as spinal dysraphism, muscular dystrophy, tethered spinal cord, or other central nervous system dysfunctions, must be ruled out. Electromyographs, motor nerve conduction studies, spine films, CT scan of the brain, or magnetic resonance imaging (MRI) may be necessary. Muscle biopsy to rule out muscular dystrophy is also warranted on occasion. Any child with a unilateral deformity, particularly of recent onset, should have an etiologic source sought. A neurologic consultation is often in order.

The typical patient with idiopathic toe-walking has no abnormal findings other than those referable to the equinus deformity with varying degrees of contracture of the Achilles tendon. They have normal sensation, no pain, and no muscle dysfunction.

Treatment of the condition varies according to the age of the patient and the degree of contracture of the Achilles tendon. In patients who are younger

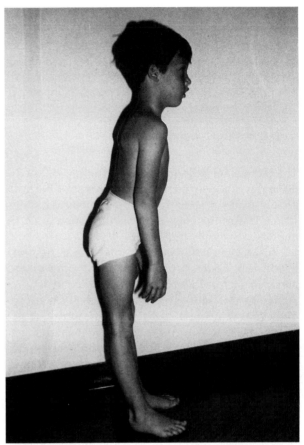

FIGURE 18-34. Three-year-old male idiopathic toe-walker. The heels can be brought to the floor by knee hyperextension.

than 3 to 4 years of age and have no or minimal contracture of the Achilles tendon, passive range of motion and stretching exercises are indicated. The child's progress should be monitored carefully. If ankle dorsiflexion to at least 10 degrees cannot be restored by this method in 3 to 4 months, serial casts should be applied. If, however, the ankle can be passively dorsiflexed to neutral or beyond, but the child habitually toe-walks, use of a hinged or nonhinged ankle foot orthosis is an option to prevent plantar flexion. These can be used for a period of weeks to months, depending on the clinical situation. The patient should be continually reevaluated and progress reassessed. In most cases, serial casting in dorsiflexion for 4 to 6 weeks is usually sufficient to resolve the problem. Many patients require postcasting ankle–foot orthoses, passive range of motion, and careful follow-up to ensure that the condition does not recur. In most cases, these noninvasive procedures provide resolution of the problem. For the child who fails to respond to serial casting or is otherwise not a candidate for this procedure, Achilles tendon lengthening provides uniformly good results. Surgical Achilles tendon lengthening is followed by 3 weeks in a non–weight-bearing short-leg cast, then 3 weeks in a weight-bearing short-leg cast. Recurrences after this procedure are rare.

TORSIONAL PROBLEMS

The parents' or grandparents' perception of an abnormal position of the legs of an infant or the way a child walks frequently results in medical consultation. Unfortunately, these concerns often result in unnecessary, costly treatment.

In the newborn, the proximal femur (femoral head, neck, and trochanter) is usually anteverted about 40 degrees in relation to the transcondylar axis of the distal femur. The intermalleolar axis of the distal tibia in relation to the interplateau axis of the proximal tibia is in about 3 degrees of lateral rotation. During the first year of life, femoral anteversion decreases by about 8 degrees and thereafter decreases by about 1 degree per year until the adult configuration of about 10 to 15 degrees of anteversion is reached at maturity. Tibial version also increases throughout life until the adult lateral version of 15 to 20 degrees is reached at maturity. Version of more than two standard deviations beyond the mean is referred to as *torsion*.

Any child who is brought in for evaluation because the parents perceive an abnormality should be carefully checked to see whether the child is merely in the normal stages of development or has a torsional problem. The most common torsional problems are femoral antetorsion and medial tibial torsion. The normal values for version vary according to the age of the patient (Fig. 18-35) The cause of the torsional problems is unknown but may be due to persistent version or genetic factors. Postnatal sitting and sleeping postures have been implicated as mechanisms that either cause torsional abnormalities or contribute to their lack of resolution, but no conclusive proof exists. Excessive ligament laxity on a genetic basis has been thought by some investigators to contribute to persistent femoral antetorsion in that many children with femoral antetorsion have accompanying physiologic pes planus, genu recurvatum, and excessive lumbar lordosis. The latter two may actually be compensatory measures for femoral antetorsion.

Any child brought in by parents for complaints of in-toeing should have a careful history and phys-

ical examination. The history should include the age at which the parents first noted the deformity, how they think it effects the child's function, and any perceived disability because of the deformity. Sleeping and sitting postures should be assessed and a complete history of normal growth and development obtained. The age at onset of walking should be evaluated. Any delay in development of walking beyond 18 months of age may be suggestive of a neuromuscular abnormality such as cerebral palsy. A family history of similar problems should be sought.

Careful physical examination must include a complete neurologic examination and a torsional profile of the patient. The most common abnormalities seen are those of femoral antetorsion, medial tibial torsion, and metatarsus adductus. Other conditions, such as an overactive abductor hallucis, clubfoot deformity, or dynamic in-toeing because of muscle imbalance, must be ruled out.

The parents may complain that the child's problem is worse at the end of the day or when tired, which may indicate failure of compensatory mechanisms. The problem may be of great concern to parents, who often scold the child for walking in a way that is more comfortable because of the child's rotational profile.

The child should be observed walking and running in an unobstructed area. The position of the patella and the feet should be noted. The physician should assess the foot progression angle. The foot progression angle is the axis of the foot as the child walks along an imaginary line of progression. This can be estimated or special paper (footprint paper) can be used to assess the foot progression angle. Negative foot progression angles designate in-toeing; positive foot progression angles designating out-toeing. The normal foot progression angle is usually positive.

Hip rotation should be assessed with the hip in extension in the prone position. The knee is flexed to 90 degrees, and rotation is assessed medially and laterally in relation to the gluteal cleft. The pelvis should be stabilized, and no force should be exerted on the limb. Internal and external rotation are assessed and compared with normal, age-matched values (Figs. 18-36 and 18-37).

Tibial rotation is next assessed by use of either the thigh–foot or transmalleolar axis (Fig. 18-38). In most cases, the thigh–foot axis is sufficient. Tibial rotation can be assessed in several ways. With the patient in the prone position and the knees flexed to 90 degrees, the thigh–foot axis can easily be assessed and compared with normal, age-matched values. If

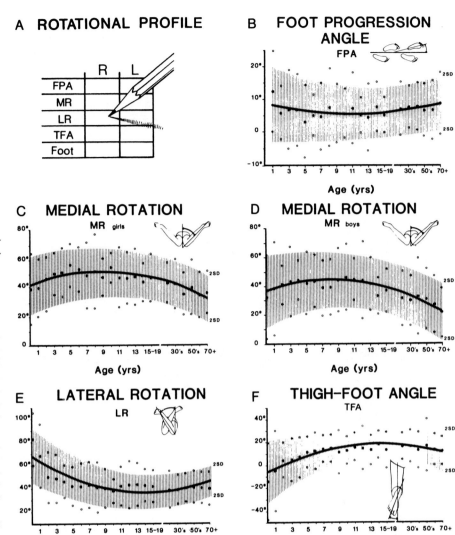

FIGURE 18-35. The rotational profile. (**A**) The method of recording and the degree of measurement for each element of the profile are depicted. This simple chart includes the vital information necessary to establish the diagnosis and to document deformity. (**B** through **F**) Normal values with the profile based on 1000 normal limbs are shown. In each figure, the age is listed on the abscissa on a logarithmic scale, and the degrees are shown on the ordinate scale. The mean values are shown in the solid line with a ±2 standard deviation normal range shown in the shaded areas. A gender difference was found from medial rotation, so values are shown independently. (Staheli LT. The lower limb. In: Morrissy RT, ed. Lovell and Winter's pediatric orthopedics, ed 3. Philadelphia, JB Lippincott, 1990:742)

the patient has a foot deformity, the transmalleolar axis should be used. The transmalleolar axis is assessed by placing the thumb and index finger on the medial and lateral malleoli, respectively, to define the intermalleolar axis; a perpendicular axis is then defined, and the angles between the perpendicular and intermalleolar axis and the long axis of the thigh are assessed. A simpler assessment of the intermalleolar axis is done with the patient sitting with the legs hanging free over the table and the knees at 90 degrees. The thumb and index finger can be placed on the medial and lateral malleoli, respectively, and the intermalleolar axis can be assessed in relation to the tibial tubercle, determining the degree of tibial rotation.

The patient's feet should be examined for evidence of metatarsus adductus and residual deformity secondary to previous clubfoot treatment. The cause of the patient's in-toeing gait may be one or more abnormalities in the lower extremity. Occasionally, a rotational profile of the parent may reveal a torsional problem that explains the torsional problem in the child or lack of resolution of the problem in the older child.

Radiographs or special studies are rarely necessary in children with torsional problems. In the infant, congenital hip dysplasia must be ruled out, and if clinical examination warrants, radiographs may be necessary. Determination of version is best done by CT or MRI with cuts through the axis of the femoral neck and the femoral condyles. Torsion of the tibia is easily measured clinically, and hence radiographs or special studies are rarely necessary.

The natural history of torsional problems is one

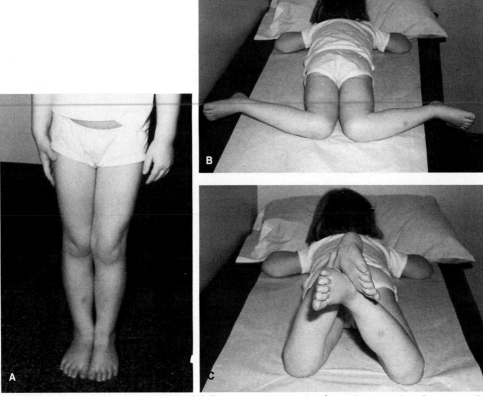

FIGURE 18-36. Femoral antetorsion. (**A**) Four-year-old girl with femoral antetorsion. In the standing view, the patella points inward. In the prone position, excessive femoral antetorsion indicated by internal rotation to about 90 degrees (**B**) and by restricted external rotation (**C**).

of gradual resolution, and hence treatment of these conditions is rarely necessary. Treatment by devices such as corrective shoes, twister cables, and alteration of sleeping or sitting habits have never been shown to affect the natural history of these conditions and should therefore be avoided. Education of the family regarding the natural history of these conditions is important. The family should be reassured that most torsional problems resolve spontaneously in the course of normal growth. The parents should also be reassured that if there is a positive family history of torsional problems, complete resolution may not occur, but in most cases, no functional disability ensues.

Infants and children before walking age may be brought in by parents for complaints of the feet pointing out. Careful examination of the hips should be done to rule out congenital hip dysplasia. External rotation contractures are normal in the infant and gradually resolve with time. Treatment is never indicated.

In the child who has not reached walking age who comes in with the parents complaining of one foot turning out, a careful hip examination should be performed to rule out any associated congenital hip dysplasia. In general, the out-turned foot is the more normal foot because this condition usually coexists with metatarsus adductus or medial tibial torsion on the opposite side. The natural history should be explained to the parents and observation recommended.

In the prewalking years, the most common cause of in-turning of the lower extremities is metatarsus adductus. Congenital hip dysplasia must, however, be ruled out.

In the walking child between 1 and 3 years of age, the most common cause of in-toeing is medial tibial torsion. This may or may not be accompanied by metatarsus adductus. Reassurance and observation is the treatment of choice.

In the older child, particularly after 3 years of

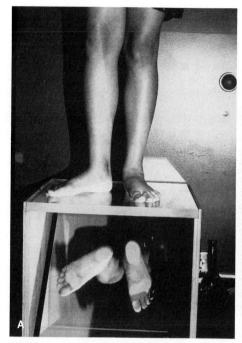
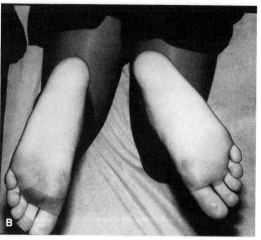

FIGURE 18-37. Lateral tibial torsion. (A) Twelve-year-old girl with lateral tibial torsion. (B) Unilateral abnormality in the thigh–foot axis is seen.

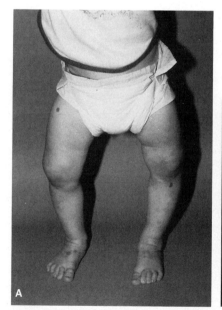
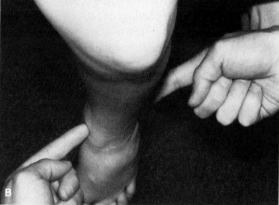

FIGURE 18-38. Medial tibial torsion. (A) Eighteen-month-old boy with medial tibial torsion and physiologic bowing. (B) Tibial rotation is assessed by visualizing relation of intermalleolar axis in reference to the tibial tubercle with patient sitting with leg over the edge of the examination table.

age, medial femoral torsion is a common cause of an in-toeing gait. Natural history studies indicate that medial femoral torsion is not associated with degenerative joint disease over the long-term, and hence observation is the only treatment warranted. Radiographs or special studies are not indicated unless there is asymmetry.

Surgical treatment for medial tibial torsion or medial femoral torsion is rarely indicated. Surgical correction can be considered in cases of medial tibial torsion if the child is older than 8 years of age (when spontaneous correction is no longer possible), if the discrepancy is more than three to four standard deviations from the mean, and if the deformity is causing the child significant functional or cosmetic problems. Supramalleolar osteotomy is usually the treatment of choice when surgical correction is contemplated.

Lateral tibial torsion is not an uncommon problem and usually does not resolve with age. Lateral tibial torsion can be considered for correction if it is greater than 30 degrees and causes significant functional or cosmetic deformity to the child (see Fig. 18-37).

Medial femoral torsion can be considered for correction if the child is older than 8 years of age and has more than three standard deviations from the mean of torsional deformity (medial rotation greater than 85 degrees, lateral rotation less than 10 degrees, or anteversion greater than 50 degrees). Consideration can be given for correction either at the intertrochanteric level or the supracondylar region; most surgeons prefer the intertrochanteric region. In teenagers, closed intramedullary rotational osteotomy can be considered.

In a certain number of children with severe femoral antetorsion, lateral tibial torsion compensates for the deformity. Surgical treatment should be avoided because the rotational osteotomies would need to be performed in the femur and the tibia, and subsequent patellofemoral malalignment problems could ensue.

Annotated Bibliography

Physiologic Pes Planus

Grogan DP, Gasser SI, Ogden JA. The painful accessory navicular: a clinical and histopathologic study. Foot Ankle 1989;10:164.
The authors present a review of 22 skeletally immature patients with 39 accessory navicular bones seen during a 4-year period. Twenty-five of the feet were treated surgically after failure of conservative treatment. Symptoms were relieved in all surgically treated patients. Detailed histologic studies of the excised specimens are presented. The changes were consistent with the theory that chronic chondroosseous tensile failure could occur and that this condition is responsible for the clinical findings.

Harris RI, Beath T. Hypermobile flat feet with short tendoachilles. J Bone Joint Surg 1948;30A:116.
This is a classic study of flatfeet in 3600 Canadian army recruits. The authors found that flexible flatfoot produces disability only when it occurs in combination with a contracted tendo Achilles.

Penneau K, Lutter LD, Winter RD. Pes planus: radiographic changes with foot orthoses and shoes. Foot Ankle 1982;2:299.
This article reports on a radiographic study of 10 children with flexible flatfeet. Radiographs were taken barefoot, with a Thomas heel, with an over-the-counter insert, and with two specially molded plastic foot orthoses. The study showed no difference between the barefoot radiographs and those in which an appliance was used.

Staheli LT, Chew DE, Corbett M. The longitudinal arch: a survey of eight hundred and eighty-two feet in normal children and adults. J Bone Joint Surg 1987;69A:426.
This article reports on a study of 441 normal subjects (1 to 80 years old) that was conducted to determine the configuration of the longitudinal arch. The authors found that flatfeet are usual in infants, common in children, and within the normal range of observations in adults.

Tachdjian MO. The child's foot. Philadelphia, WB Saunders, 1985:556.
This chapter provides an excellent review of flexible flatfoot, covering all aspects including surgical considerations. It includes an extensive bibliography.

Wenger DR, Mauldin D, Speck G, et al. Corrective shoes and inserts as treatment for flexible flat foot in infants and children. J Bone Joint Surg 1989;71A:800.
This article reports on a randomized prospective study of 98 patients treated by various "accepted" methods for flexible flatfoot. The authors demonstrated that flexible flatfoot improved naturally over the 3 years of the study and that the degree of improvement was not affected by wearing of a corrective shoe or a shoe with an insert.

Tarsal Coalition

Gonzalez T, Kumar SJ. Calcaneal navicular coalition treated by resection and interposition of the extensor digitorum brevis muscle. J Bone Joint Surg 1990;72A:71.
The authors present a 2- to 20-year follow-up of 75 calcaneal navicular coalitions treated by resection and interposition of the extensor digitorum brevis muscle. Good or excellent long-term results were reported in 77% of the cases. The best results were reported in patients between 11 and 15 years of age who had a cartilaginous coalition. Talar beaking was not a contraindication to surgery.

Herzenberg JE, Goldner GL, Martinez S, Silverman PM. Computerized tomography of talocalcaneal tarsal coalition: a clinical and anatomic study. Foot Ankle 1986;6:273.
The authors compared CT scanning with plain radiography and plain tomography in the clinical anatomic study. CT was demonstrated to be superior in identifying the anatomy of the subtalar joint. Coalitions were demonstrated by the authors in the evaluation of 22 patients with peroneal spastic flatfoot.

Leonard MA. The inheritance of tarsal coalition and its relationship to spastic flat foot. J Bone Joint Surg 1974;56B:522.
The author evaluated 31 index patients with tarsal coalitions and peroneal spastic flatfoot and 90 of their first-degree relatives. Thirty-nine percent of the first-degree relatives were found to have some type of tarsal coalition, but none was ever symptomatic. The study demonstrates that tarsal coalitions are inherited probably as an autosomal dominant disorder and that tarsal coalition is probably not a rare phenomenon.

Mosier KM, Asher M. Tarsal coalitions and peroneal spastic flat foot: a review. J Bone Joint Surg 1984;66A:976.
The authors present a superb review of the history, etiology, hereditary evidence, incidence, clinical presentations, pathomechanics, radiologic diagnosis, differential diagnosis, and treatment of tarsal coalitions. This article was published before the use of CT scanning in diagnosis and also before several long-term reviews of treatment. The background information and bibliography on tarsal coalition are superb.

Olney BW, Asher MA. Excision of symptomatic coalition of the middle facet of the talocalcaneal joint. J Bone Joint Surg 1987;69A:539.
The authors report excision of the middle facet of the talocalcaneal joint and autogenous fat grafting in nine patients with 10 symptomatic coalitions. Eight of 10 feet had satisfactory results.

Percy EC, Mann DL. Tarsal coalition: a review of the literature and presentation of 13 cases. Foot Ankle 1988;9:40.
This article adds 13 cases to the world literature. The introductory material surveying the world literature is excellent.

Swiontkowski MF, Scranton PE, Hansen S. Tarsal coalitions: long-term results of surgical treatment. J Pediatr Orthop 1983;3:287.
The authors reviewed 40 patients who underwent 57 operations for tarsal coalition. Poor results were correlated with inadequate resection or advanced degenerative joint disease. Talar beaking does not necessarily represent early degenerative joint disease but does represent talonavicular ligament traction spurs, which are not necessarily associated with articular degeneration but are caused by increased stress across the talonavicular joint. This beaking is not a contraindication to bar resection.

Congenital Vertical Talus

Coleman SS, Stelling FH, Jarrett J. Pathomechanics and treatment of congenital vertical talus. Clin Orthop Relat Res 1970;70:62.
The authors present a classification of congenital vertical talus, discuss the pathophysiology, and present a surgical method of management.

Ogata K, Shoenecker PL, Sheridan J. Congenital vertical talus and its familial occurrence: an analysis of 36 patients. Clin Orthop Relat Res 1979;139:128.
The authors report the follow-up of 36 patients with 57 feet with congenital vertical talus. A high incidence of associated congenital hip dislocation, arthrogryposis, congenital hypoplasia of the tibia, and central nervous system abnormalities was noted. Half of the patients with a primary isolated form of congenital vertical talus had a positive family history of foot deformities in first-degree relatives. A method of surgical correction is presented.

Oppenheim W, Smith C, Christie W. Congenital vertical talus. Foot Ankle 1985;5:198.
The authors present a series of 15 congenital vertical tali in 12 patients. They found that the best result was obtained with early subtalar arthrodesis (Grice operation) and plantar K-wire fixations. Attempts to augment push-off power with tendon transfers were unrewarding. Casting alone revealed the worst results. Half of patients had associated abnormalities.

Calcaneal Valgus

Larsen B, Reimann I, Becker-Andersen H. Congenital calcaneal valgus. Acta Orthop Scand 1974;45:145.
In this article, 125 cases of congenital calcaneal valgus are presented. Forty-nine percent were treated with manipulation and taping; 51% were treated with observation alone. The authors demonstrate no significant difference in the outcome between the two groups. The follow-up was between 3 and 11 years, and most feet were normal. Pronation of the feet was often seen when the patients began to walk, and many had slight residual valgus compared with the other side.

Witzenstein H. The significance of congenital pes calcaneal valgus in the origin of pes planovalgus in childhood. Acta Orthop Scand 1960;30:64.
The authors reviewed 2735 consecutive newborns and followed the patients for 2 years. One-hundred and forty-seven of the patients had more than 20 degrees of heel valgus; 333 had 10 to 15 degrees; 759 had 0 to 5 degrees; and 1496 had 0 degrees. When seen at 2 years of age, 43% of the 147 patients with at least 20 degrees of valgus had flatfeet. Twenty-three percent of the group with normal valgus had flatfeet. The authors conclude that severe calcaneal valgus is associated with a flatfoot deformity in later life.

Wynne-Davies R. Family studies and the cause of congenital clubfoot: talipes equinovarus, talipes calcaneal valgus, and metatarsus varus. J Bone Joint Surg 1964;46B:445.
This article deals with family history, associated abnormalities, and causes of clubfoot, metatarsus varus, and calcaneal valgus deformity. This is an excellent review article on the epidemiology and etiology of these three foot conditions.

Köhler Disease

Ippolito E, Ricciardi Polini PT, Falez F. Köhler's disease of the tarsal navicular: long-term follow-up of 12 cases. J Pediatr Orthop 1984;4:416.
The authors report an average 33-year follow-up of 12 patients with Köhler disease of the tarsal navicula. Complete restoration of normal navicular anatomy averaged 8 months. Treatment did not affect the radiographic course of the disease. All patients reconstituted normal navicular shape, were asymptomatic, and had no evidence of degenerative joint disease.

Karp MG. Köhler's disease of the tarsal scaphoid: an end result study. J Bone Joint Surg 1937;19:84.
The author reports 45 cases of Köhler disease of the tarsal navicular (39 boys, 6 girls). Treatment had no effect on the radiographic course of the disease. The radiographs of 50 normal children (25 boys, 25 girls) were evaluated for scaphoid development with radiographs taken every 6 months from age 9 months to 4 years. In over half the female patients, a well-developed ossific nucleus of the scaphoid was apparent at 2 years of age; it was apparent by 3.5 years of age in all the patients. More than one third of the male patients were older than 3.5 years of age before the scaphoid appeared. The average age of appearance of the ossific nucleus for girls is 18 months to 2 years and for boys, 2.5 to 3 years of age. The authors also discussed ossification patterns of the scaphoid in relation to time of appearance. The radiographic appearance is unrelated to the duration of symptoms or to treatment. Normal delayed development of the appearance of the ossific nucleus to the scaphoid may simulate a radiographic picture similar to that seen in Köhler disease.

Waugh W. The ossification and vascularization of the tarsal navicular and the relation to Köhler's disease. J Bone Joint Surg 1958;40B:765.
This article reports on an excellent study of the vascular supply to the tarsal navicular and a radiographic study of 52 normal children's feet. Radiographs were taken at 6-month intervals between the ages of 2 and 5 years to assess normal ossification patterns in the navicular. On the basis of the vascular injection studies and the clinical follow-up, the author proposes that Köhler disease of the navicular is caused by compression of the bony nucleus at a critical phase during the growth of a navicular whose appearance is delayed.

Williams GA, Cowell HR. Köhler's disease of the tarsal navicular. Clin Orthop Relat Res 1981;158:53.
The authors reviewed 20 patients with Köhler disease of the tarsal navicular with an average follow-up of 9.5 years. All patients were

asymptomatic and had reconstituted the navicular to the normal radiographic appearance. Short-leg casting significantly affected the morbidity in patients, reducing the symptomatic period from 15 months (untreated patients) to less than 3 months.

Freiberg Infarction

Freiberg AH. The so called infarction of the second metatarsal bone. J Bone Joint Surg 1926;8:257.
The author, who described the etiology of the condition in 1913, discusses Köhler's opinion that the etiology of the condition is probably not traumatic. This is a classic paper.

Smillie IS. Freiberg's infarction (Köehler's second disease). J Bone Joint Surg 1955;39B:580.
In this review of 41 cases, female patients predominated. The author proposes a traumatic etiology (ie, stress fracture) for the disease. Treatment options at various disease stages are discussed.

Sever Disease

Micheli LJ, Ireland ML. Prevention and management of calcaneal apophysitis in children: an overuse syndrome. J Pediatr Orthop 1987;7:34.
The authors present an excellent historical review and extensive discussion on the differential diagnosis of heel pain in the child and adolescent. The authors present a large series (85 children, 137 heels) of calcaneal apophysitis (Sever disease) treated by a physical therapy program of lower-extremity stretching, particularly the Achilles tendon, ankle dorsiflexion strengthening, and orthotics. All patients were able to return to their sport of choice 2 months after the diagnosis. The authors proposed that the cause of the condition is an overuse syndrome.

Metatarsus Adductus

Berg EE. A reappraisal of metatarsus adductus and skewfoot. J Bone Joint Surg 1986;68A:1185.
The author describes a radiographic classification in 84 patients with 124 feet with a minimal follow-up of 2 years. The study was devised to determine prospectively whether radiographic evaluation can provide better prognostic information than the usual clinical criteria. The author proposes a four-group classification based on the anteroposterior radiographs: simple metatarsus adductus, complex metatarsus adductus, simple skewfoot, and complex skewfoot. The author reports that all patients with complex skewfoot had flatfoot at follow-up and that there was a strong association with the use of Denis Browne splints and flatfoot deformity at follow-up. Ninety-seven percent of untreated feet responded favorably. The period of cast treatment for patients with complex skewfoot deformity was required twice as long as for those with simple metatarsus adductus, and all had flatfoot at follow-up. This article includes an extensive bibliography.

Bleck EE. Metatarsus adductus: classification relationship to outcomes of treatment. J Pediatr Orthop 1983;3:2.
This was a retrospective study of the results of treatment of 160 children (265 feet) classified by flexibility according to the extent of passive abduction of the forefoot against the stabilized hindfoot with reference to the heel bisector. Results of treatment were statistically significantly better when treatment was begun between the ages of 1 day and 8 months. The only significant predictor of a good outcome was the age of the patient. The recurrence rate was 12%. Severity and flexibility did not appear to affect the treatment outcome. This is an excellent review of the subject with an extensive bibliography.

Ponseti IV, Becker JR. J Bone Joint Surg 1966;48A:702.
The authors report on 379 patients. Three hundred and thirty-five required no treatment. All were passively correctable. All dem-

onstrated slight progression of metatarsus adductus with resolution by 3 years of age. All had complete correction of the forefoot, some having mild flatfoot with minimal metatarsus adductus that was not handicapping. Forty-four patients (11.6%) were not passively correctable and required active treatment. The authors describe the method of casting as well as a follow-up of 57 patients treated by this method. This is a superb article that outlines and demonstrates the method of cast correction of metatarsus adductus.

Clubfoot

Ippolito E, Ponseti IV. Congenital clubfoot of the human fetus: a histologic study. J Bone Joint Surg 1980;62A:8.
The authors present a superb review of the pathologic anatomy of clubfoot, comparing 5 clubfeet with 3 normal control feet in subjects of the same ages. The authors propose a retracting fibrosis as the primary etiologic factor of clubfoot deformity.

Laaveg SJ, Ponseti IV. Long term results of treatment of congenital clubfoot. J Bone Joint Surg 1990;62A:23.
The authors present a mean 19-year follow-up of 104 clubfeet treated by a standardized approach. Ninety percent of patients were satisfied with both the appearance and function of the foot, with the average functional score being 88.5 points out of 100 possible points.

Tachdjian MO. The child's foot. Philadelphia, WB Saunders, 1985: 139.
The author presents an exhaustive review of congenital talipes equinovarus with an extensive bibliography.

Turco VJ. Resistant congenital clubfoot: one stage posteromedial release with internal fixation. J Bone Joint Surg 1979;61A:805.
The author reports modifications of his original technique (most widely used technique with surgical treatment of clubfoot) and end results in 149 feet. The author reports that the best results and fewest complications occurred in patients operated on between 1 and 2 years of age.

VanderWilde R, Staheli LT, Chew DE, Malagon V. Measurements on radiographs of the foot in normal infants and children. J Bone Joint Surg 1988;70A:407.
The authors present a radiographic review of feet of 74 normal infants and children ranging in age from 6 to 127 months. The authors present their results and compare these to results gleaned from the literature in other studies of normal feet.

Wynne-Davies R. Genetic and environmental factors in the etiology of talipes equinovarus. Clin Orthop Relat Res 1972;84:9.
This review article on the epidemiologic and etiologic theories on idiopathic clubfoot should be read in conjunction with this author's article listed under Calcaneal Valgus.

Idiopathic Toe-Walking

Griffin PT, Wheelhouse WW, Shiavi R, Bass W. Habitual toe walkers: clinical and electromyographic gait analysis. J Bone Joint Surg 1977;59A:97.
The authors report a clinical and electromyographic study of six children who are habitual toe-walkers compared to six otherwise normal children walking on their toes. The abnormalities noted on dynamic electromyograms reverted to normal in the habitual toe-walkers after plaster cast treatment.

Hall JE, Salter RB, Bhalla SK. Congenital short tendocalcaneous. J Bone Joint Surg 1967;49B:695.
This is the first description in the literature of idiopathic toe-walking, which the authors term congenital short tendocalcaneous. The authors reported on 20 patients with an average follow-up of 3 years (range, 1.5 to 7 years), all treated by Achilles tendon lengthening. All children were otherwise normal. The surgical outcome was good in every patient.

Kalen V, Adler N, Bleck EE. Electromyography of idiopathic toe walking. J Pediatr Orthop 1986;6:31.

The authors report dynamic electromyograms in 18 patients with idiopathic toe-walking as compared with normal children walking on their toes and cerebral palsy children with equinus deformities. Significant differences in phasic time were demonstrated between cerebral palsy and idiopathic toe-walking patients versus controls, but no significant differences were noted between idiopathic toe-walkers and the cerebral palsy patients. Because of these gait abnormalities, the authors conclude that idiopathic toe-walking may be due to an unknown nervous system deficiency.

Torsional Problems

Bleck EE. Developmental orthopaedics. III. Toddlers' developmental medicine. Childhood Neurol 1982;24:533.

This excellent review article covers not only torsional abnormalities but also angular deformities of the lower extremity. It includes excellent references.

Hubbard DD, Staheli LT, Chew DE, et al. Medial femoral torsion in osteoarthritis. J Pediatr Orthop 1988;8:540.

The authors measured anteversion in 44 hips in 32 patients with idiopathic osteoarthritis of the hip and compared this with mea-surements in 98 normal adult hips. The differences in the two groups were not significant. The authors did not find medial femoral torsion associated with osteoarthritis of the hip.

Kitaoka HB, Weiner DS, Cook AJ, et al. Relationship between femoral anteversion and osteoarthritis of the hip. J Pediatr Orthop 1989;9:396.

In a CT scanning study, the authors demonstrated no difference in anteversion between osteoarthritis subjects and controls with reference to anteversion. They concluded that rotational femoral osteotomies to prevent osteoarthritis are not warranted.

Staheli LT. Torsion-treatment indications. Clin Orthop Related Res 1989;242:61.

The author briefly discusses rotational problems in infants and children and presents the indications and methods of surgical treatment in the rare cases that require operative intervention.

Staheli LT, Corbett M, Wyss C. Lower extremity rotational problems in children: normal values to guide in management. J Bone Joint Surg 1985;67A;39.

The authors present the rotational profile and the normal values for progression angle, medial rotation, lateral rotation, and thigh-foot angle. This is a classic reference article for torsional deformities of the lower extremity.

Turek's Orthopaedics: Principles and Their Application, Fifth Edition,
edited by Stuart L. Weinstein and Joseph A. Buckwalter.
J.B. Lippincott Company, Philadelphia, © 1994.

19

Roger A. Mann

The Adult Ankle and Foot

Problems of the ankle and foot are a common source of pain and disability in adults. Unfortunately, many of the problems involving the forefoot are brought about by improper shoe wear. As a general rule, most of these problems can be accurately diagnosed by obtaining a careful history and carrying out a detailed physical examination. Radiographic studies of the foot in a weight-bearing position are useful in helping to define the anatomic abnormalities. At times, supplemental examinations including a bone scan, computed tomographic scan, or on rare occasions, magnetic resonance imaging may be indicated to help in making the diagnosis. As a general rule, most problems involve the forefoot and consist of deformities of the great toe or lesser toes. Various types of soft tissue problems, such as tendinitis or fasciitis, are common. Postural problems of the foot, arthroses of the foot and ankle, and foot problems in diabetic patients are less commonly observed. As a general rule, most foot problems respond well to conservative management. This usually consists of getting the patient into a more comfortable shoe, which is one with a wide toe and soft flexible sole. At times, an orthotic device may be indicated. Surgical intervention also may be indicated to correct a foot problem, but it should be used only if all conservative measures have been exhausted.

DISORDERS OF THE FIRST METATARSOPHALANGEAL JOINT

The first metatarsophalangeal joint provides almost half of the weight bearing of the forefoot and helps stabilize the longitudinal arch through the attachment of the plantar aponeurosis into its base. During walking, weight is rapidly transferred from the heel to the metatarsal head region. As a step is taken, the

toes are pushed into dorsiflexion, and the plantar aponeurosis, which arises from the tubercle of the calcaneus and passes to insert into the base of the proximal phalanx, is pulled over the metatarsal head. This dorsiflexion movement with the attached plantar aponeurosis depresses the metatarsal heads. This action of depression of the metatarsal heads provides stability to the longitudinal arch (Fig. 19-1). As various disorders of the first metatarsophalangeal joint

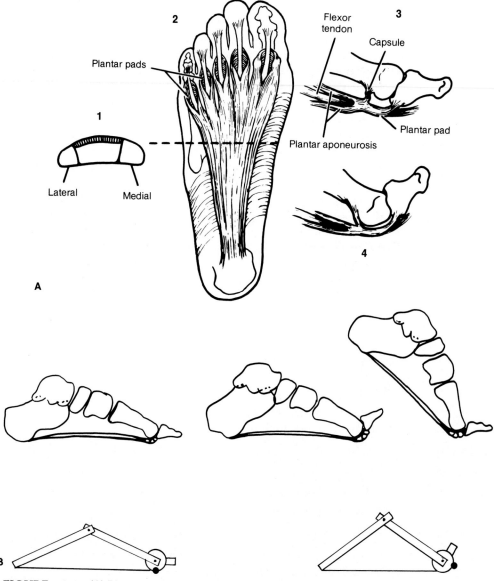

FIGURE 19-1. (A) Plantar aponeurosis. (1) Cross section. (2) Division of plantar aponeurosis around flexor tendons. (3) Components of the plantar pad and its insertion into the base of the proximal phalanx. (4) Toe in extension with the plantar pad drawn over the metatarsal head. (B) The windlass mechanism functions by the passive dorsiflexion of the metatarsophalangeal joints in the last half of the stance phase, which tightens the plantar aponeurosis and mechanically causes the longitudinal arch to rise. This is probably the main stabilizer of the longitudinal arch of the foot. (A from Mann R, Inman VT. Structure and function. In: Du Vries HL. Surgery of the foot, ed 2. St Louis, CV Mosby, 1965)

develop, all or part of the weight-bearing mechanism of the plantar aponeurosis can be disrupted. As a result, weight is transferred to the lesser metatarsals, and a painful callous may develop. It is therefore essential that any surgical procedure on the first metatarsophalangeal joint consider the basic biomechanics of the joint so that disruption of this normal function does not occur.

Hallux Valgus

A hallux valgus deformity results from lateral deviation of the proximal phalanx on the first metatarsal head (Fig. 19-2). As this deformity occurs, several secondary deformities are brought about. These include contracture of the soft tissues on the lateral side of the metatarsophalangeal joint, elongation of the capsular structures on the medial side of the metatarsophalangeal joint, and migration of the first metatarsal head off the sesamoid bones, which are

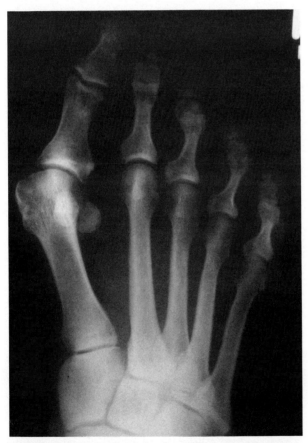

FIGURE 19-2. Radiograph of a hallux valgus deformity. Note the lateral deviation of the proximal phalanx on the metatarsal head, the medial deviation of the metatarsal head, and subluxation of the sesamoids.

anchored in place by the transverse metatarsal ligament and the adductor hallucis muscle. A medial eminence of varying degrees, commonly known as a *bunion*, results from the deformity of the first metatarsophalangeal joint. In addition, because of the deformity of the first metatarsophalangeal joint, the weight-bearing function of the great toe can be diminished, and a transfer lesion may occur in the form of a callous beneath the second metatarsal head. At times, due to pressure of the great toe against the second toe, the second metatarsophalangeal joint becomes subluxated or dislocated, and the toe then may ride up onto the dorsal aspect of the great toe.

Other conditions may be associated with a hallux valgus deformity or may be etiologic factors. These include contracture of the Achilles tendon, severe pronation of the foot (flatfoot), hypermobility of the first metatarsocuneiform joint, hyperelasticity of tissues, and shape of the metatarsophalangeal joint.

The clinical evaluation of a patient with a hallux valgus deformity begins with soliciting the patient's chief complaint. This is important because, although the patient may have a significant deformity of the first metatarsophalangeal joint producing a rather large, obvious bunion, the main complaint may be the dislocated second toe that is sitting on top of the great toe, or possibly the large callus beneath the second metatarsal head as a result of a transfer lesion due to instability of the first metatarsophalangeal joint. It is important to ascertain the level of activity of the patient because this helps in the decision-making process regarding what type of correction may be indicated. Most important, the patient's expectations must be carefully elicited and discussed. People can be particular about their feet. For example, the patient with a wide, thick foot with a mild deformity may believe that if this deformity were surgically corrected, they could then place their foot into any type of shoe they wish, and this is not always possible. Therefore, the wishes of the patient must be clearly understood so that the physician and patient both understand the likely outcome of treatment.

The physical examination of the patient with a hallux valgus deformity begins with the patient standing so that the physician can observe the posture of the foot. The physician should determine whether the heel touches the ground, the nature of the arch, and the overall configuration of the forefoot and the lesser toes. The patient is then seated and the range of motion of the ankle, subtalar, transverse tarsal, and metatarsophalangeal joints is observed. The examination of the first metatarsophalangeal joint is extremely important so that the physician can determine how much motion is present at the joint. Significantly decreased motion may affect the type of surgical procedure chosen. The mobility of the first metatarsocuneiform joint is observed by grasping the first metatarsal head and pushing it dorsally and in a plantar direction. In this manner, the physician gains an impression about how much mobility is present at the joint. In about 3% to 5% of patients, some increased mobility of the metatarsocuneiform joint exists, which influences the clinical decision-making. The neurovascular status of the foot should be carefully evaluated; if there is any question about the circulatory status of the foot, a Doppler study should be carried out.

Weight-bearing radiographs are obtained to ascertain the degree of the deformity. The following information should be obtained from the weight-bearing radiograph:

- The degree of hallux valgus, which is measured by a line that bisects the proximal phalanx and first metatarsal. This normally should be about 15 degrees or less (Fig. 19-3A).
- The intermetatarsal angle, which is determined by drawing a line through the first and second metatarsals. This angle should be 9 degrees or less (see Fig. 19-3A).
- The degree of distal metatarsal articular angle, which is the angle formed by the articular surface in relation to the long axis of the metatarsal. This angle is normally between 0 to 10 degrees of lateral deviation (see Fig. 19-3B).
- The degree of arthrosis present at the first metatarsophalangeal joint
- The shape of the metatarsal head. As a general rule, a person with a flat metatarsal head rarely has a hallux valgus deformity, whereas a person with a rounded metatarsal head has a greater tendency toward hallux valgus formation.
- The shape of the metatarsocuneiform joint should be carefully observed, and a severe medial angulation of the joint should make the physician conscious of a possible hypermobile metatarsocuneiform joint (see Fig. 19-3C).
- Is the metatarsophalangeal joint congruent or incongruent? A metatarsophalangeal joint is congruent when there is no lateral subluxation of the proximal phalanx on the metatarsal head. If there is lateral subluxation of the proximal phalanx on the metatarsal head, then the joint is considered incongruent. This determination is important because if the joint is congruent, a surgical procedure must be selected to correct the bunion without moving the proximal phalanx around on the metatarsal

head. On the other hand, if the joint is incongruent (subluxated), the proximal phalanx can be moved around on the metatarsal head to correct the deformity (see Fig. 19-3D).

Treatment of patients with a hallux valgus deformity includes informing them about the nature of the problem and then placing them into shoes that accommodate the deformity. At time, this is difficult because the shoes that are necessary to accommodate a hallux valgus deformity are often not fashionable. The basic principle is to get the stress off the metatarsal head area over the bunion, and this often produces relief of the bunion pain. If the patient has an accompanying callus beneath the second metatarsal head, a soft metatarsal support can be placed into the shoe to relieve the stress on the involved area. If the patient has a significant dislocation of the second metatarsophalangeal joint so that the great toe has slid underneath the second toe, holding it in the air, then probably an extradepth shoe, which has a thick toe box to accommodate a widened forefoot, can be used. As a general rule, the shoe should be a lace-type as opposed to a loafer so that the laces can be let out to accommodate the deformity. It is not possible for a person with a significant hallux valgus deformity to wear a tight-fitting high-heeled shoe comfortably.

If conservative measures fail, then the physician may consider surgical correction. At times, however, complete correction cannot be achieved by surgery, and this may be distressing for the patient. In younger patients, some motion may be lost at the metatarsophalangeal joint, and if the patient is involved in athletic endeavors in which good motion is needed, then surgery may be delayed until the patient's physical demands on the foot are diminished. This is not to say that a satisfactory result cannot be achieved in these patients, but most bunion operations provide about 85% to 90% patient satisfaction, which leaves 10% to 15% of the patients not satisfied. It is important that the patient be made aware of the risks of surgery when contemplating an operative procedure on the first metatarsophalangeal joint.

In the selection of an operative procedure, the first question that needs to be asked is whether the patient has a congruent or incongruent joint. As mentioned previously, if the joint is incongruent, then there is lateral subluxation of the proximal phalanx on the metatarsal head, and as a result, the correction is achieved by rolling the proximal phalanx around on the metatarsal head to realign it. If, however, there is no lateral subluxation of the proximal phalanx on

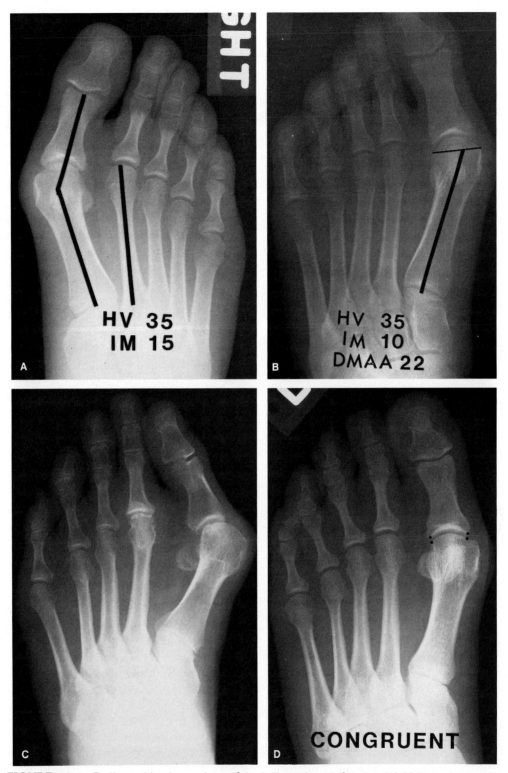

FIGURE 19-3. Radiographic observations of the hallux valgus deformity. **(A)** Hallux valgus angle: normal (less than 15 degrees). Intermetatarsal angle: normal (less than 9 degrees). **(B)** Distal metatarsal articular angle (DMAA): normal (less than 10 degrees lateral deviation). **(C)** Marked obliquity of the metatarsocuneiform joint should alert clinician to possible instability of this joint. **(D)** A congruent joint is one in which there is no lateral subluxation of the proximal phalanx on the articular surface of the metatarsal head. **(E)** The incongruent or subluxated joint has lateral deviation of the proximal phalanx on the metatarsal head.

the metatarsal head, and the deformity is as a result of a large medial eminence and lateral deviation of the distal metatarsal articular angle, then a surgical procedure that realigns the metatarsal head needs to be undertaken rather than one that realigns the proximal phalanx on the metatarsal head. For the patient who has a congruent joint and a hallux valgus deformity, there are three basic procedures that can be used: the chevron procedure; the Akin procedure along with excision of the medial eminence; and a distal soft tissue procedure, in which the soft tissues around the metatarsophalangeal joint are realigned and the medial eminence excised.

When there is an incongruent joint with lateral subluxation of the proximal phalanx on the metatarsal head, the procedures that usually result in satisfactory correction are the chevron procedure (provided the hallux valgus deformity is less than about 30 degrees, the intermetatarsal angle less than 14 degrees, and the patient younger than than 50 years of age), a distal soft tissue realignment procedure, usually with a proximal metatarsal osteotomy, or a Mitchell procedure. If the hallux valgus deformity becomes advanced, with a hallux valgus angle of greater than 40 degrees and an intermetatarsal angle greater than 20 degrees, the Mitchell procedure is no longer useful, and the distal soft tissue procedure, along with a proximal metatarsal osteotomy, or an arthrodesis of the first metatarsophalangeal joint usually produces a satisfactory result. If significant degenerative arthritis is present at the metatarsophalangeal joint, probably an arthrodesis of the joint or occasionally a double-stem implant can be used.

In the occasional patient who has hypermobility of the first metatarsocuneiform joint associated with a hallux valgus deformity, an arthrodesis of the first metatarsocuneiform articulation to provide stability to the joint along with correction of the intermetatarsal angle and a distal soft tissue realignment procedure are indicated.

It becomes obvious from the previous discussion that no one single operative procedure is most efficacious for all bunions. The distal soft tissue realignment with the addition of the proximal metatarsal osteotomy probably gives the most flexibility and is useful for the largest range of deformities; however, when significant arthrosis is present or there is a distal metatarsal articular angle of greater than 15 degrees, this procedure does not produce a satisfactory clinical result in all cases.

The following sections briefly describe each of the operative techniques presented previously. This is not meant to be a detailed surgical description but rather a presentation of the general principles of each operative procedure.

Chevron Procedure

The chevron procedure consists of a distal metatarsal osteotomy that is carried out through a medial approach to the metatarsal head. The distal metatarsal is exposed, with care taken not to excessively strip the soft tissues; the medial eminence is excised; and a chevron-shaped osteotomy with an angle of about 60 degrees is created with the apex starting about 7 to 10 mm proximal to the articular surface. The osteotomy site is then displaced laterally and impacted on the metatarsal shaft. If necessary, a pin may be used for stabilization. The small bony prominence that has been created by the lateral displacement of the metatarsal head is removed and the medial capsular tissue reapproximated. The patient is usually mobilized in a postoperative shoe and firm gauze and tape dressing for 6 to 8 weeks. This procedure usually provides satisfactory correction of a mild hallux valgus deformity with a hallux valgus angle of about 30 degrees and an intermetatarsal angle of less than 14 degrees. There may be some mild joint stiffness after the procedure, and occasionally the metatarsal shaft is shortened by 2 to 4 mm. The most devastating complication is that of avascular necrosis of the metatarsal head, which occurs in about 0.5% to 1% of cases. Although avascular necrosis occurs (which is probably due to excessive stripping, particularly on the lateral side of the metatarsal head where the blood supply is greatest), the result still may be satisfactory (Fig. 19-4).

Akin Procedure

The Akin procedure consists of an osteotomy of the proximal phalanx in which a medially based wedge of bone is removed to realign the proximal phalanx. It is most useful if a hallux valgus procedure has failed to correct completely the hallux valgus deformity and the great toe is still resting against the second toe. It may also be used in patients who have a congruent joint with a large medial eminence. In these patients, the medial eminence is removed by extending the incision proximally along the proximal phalanx, opening the joint capsule, excising the eminence, and then plicating the capsule. The osteotomy site in the proximal phalanx can be stabilized with an internal suture or possibly a pin. After operation, the patient is kept in a wooden shoe until the osteotomy site heals, which is about 6 to 8 weeks. This procedure is useful, but only within the strict limi-

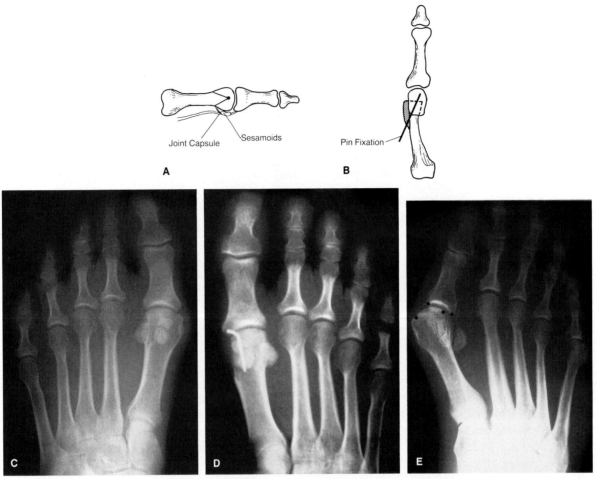

Joint Capsule   Sesamoids

A

Pin Fixation

B

C   **D**   **E**

FIGURE 19-4. Chevron procedure. (A) The apex of the Chevron osteotomy starts in the center of the metatarsal head and is brought proximally. (B) The osteotomy site is displaced laterally 20% to 30% of the width of the shaft. Preoperative (C) and postoperative (D) radiographs demonstrating the Chevron osteotomy. (Mann RA, Coughlin MJ. The video textbook of foot and ankle surgery. St Louis, Medical Video Productions, 1991)

tations mentioned previously. This procedure cannot correct an incongruent joint. The main complication of the procedure is that the proximal phalanx may become unstable and subluxate laterally, resulting in a significant recurrence of the deformity (Fig. 19-5).

Distal Soft Tissue Realignment

The distal soft tissue realignment procedure involves releasing the soft tissue contracture on the lateral side of the metatarsophalangeal joint, which consists of the adductor hallucis, transverse metatarsal ligament, and lateral joint capsule. The medial eminence is excised and the elongated capsular tissue on the medial side plicated. This procedure is indicated occasionally in the patient with a congruent joint but usually in the patient with an incongruent

joint with a hallux valgus angle of less than 30 degrees and an intermetatarsal angle of less than 12 to 14 degrees. The main complications associated with this procedure are recurrence of the deformity or inadequate correction due to the presence of a fixed intermetatarsal angle, which requires a basal metatarsal osteotomy to correct it. In my experience, a basal osteotomy needs to be added to this procedure between 80% and 90% of the time (Fig. 19-6).

Distal Soft Tissue Realignment and Basal Metatarsal Osteotomy

The distal soft tissue realignment is carried out as described previously. The basal osteotomy is a crescentic osteotomy that permits the correction of the intermetatarsal angle. The crescentic osteotomy

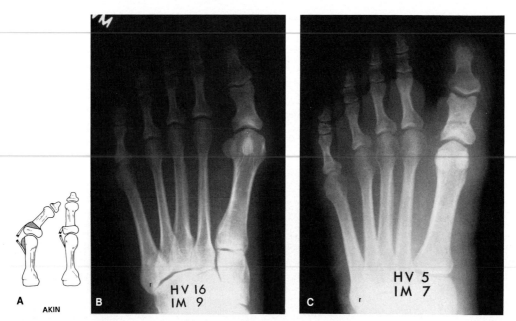

FIGURE 19-5. Akin procedure. (A) The medial eminence is excised, and a medially based wedge of bone is removed from the proximal phalanx. Preoperative (B) and postoperative (C) radiographs demonstrating an Akin procedure.

is simple to perform with a curved osteotomy blade and provides a stable osteotomy site with little or no shortening of the metatarsal. I prefer this osteotomy to either an opening or closing wedge osteotomy because the opening wedge is basically unstable and the closing wedge may produce shortening or dorsiflexion of the distal metatarsal. The main complication of this procedure is that of a hallux varus deformity in which the great toe deviates medially due to overcorrection of the metatarsal shaft laterally or overplication of the medial soft tissue structures (Fig. 19-7).

Arthrodesis of the Metatarsophalangeal Joint

Arthrodesis of the metatarsophalangeal joint is an excellent procedure for patients who have a severe deformity or significant arthroses of the metatarsophalangeal joint and as a salvage procedure for a failed bunion operation. The arthrodesis is done so that it produces about 15 degrees of valgus and 10 to 15 degrees of dorsiflexion in relation to the plantar aspect of the foot, which is 25 to 30 degrees in relation to the first metatarsal shaft, which is inclined in a plantar direction about 20 degrees. After arthrodesis, the patient can be ambulated in a postoperative wooden shoe until the arthrodesis site is solid, which is usually about 10 to 12 weeks after surgery. The main complications of arthrodesis are malalignment

of the arthrodesis site and nonunion, although that is uncommon. If sufficient valgus and dorsiflexion is not placed into the arthrodesis at the time of surgery, excessive wear on the interphalangeal joint occurs, and this is a potential problem (Fig. 19-8).

Silastic Prosthesis

The use of a Silastic prosthesis to replace the first metatarsophalangeal joint, in my estimation, is rarely indicated because stability of the joint is lost, which sometimes results in a transfer lesion to the adjacent metatarsal head. The active movement of the metatarsophalangeal joint is usually significantly decreased owing to an inability to reinsert the intrinsic muscles once the prosthesis has been placed. At times, there is a reaction to the prosthetic materials and a silicon synovitis results. The life expectancy of a prosthesis is rarely more than 5 years. Therefore, it should not be used in any patient who is young and expects to place a great deal of stress on the metatarsophalangeal joint.

Hallux Rigidus

Hallux rigidus is degenerative arthritis of the first metatarsophalangeal joint. As the pathologic process advances, a large ridge of bone develops on the dorsal

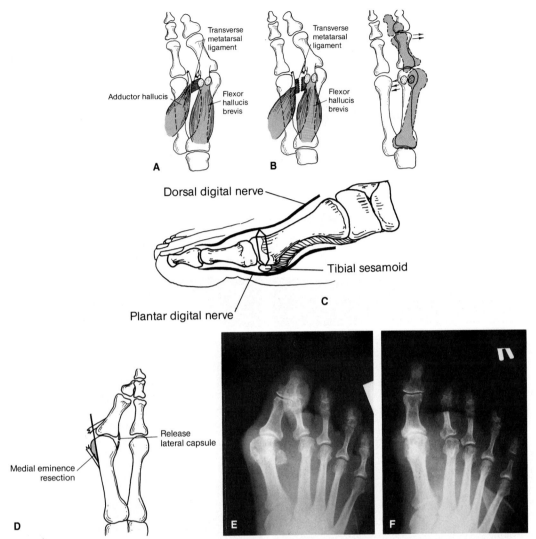

FIGURE 19-6. The distal soft tissue procedure. **(A)** The adductor tendon is released from its insertion into the base of the proximal phalanx and fibular sesamoid. **(B)** The transverse metatarsal ligament is transected and the lateral joint capsule released. **(C)** Through a longitudinal medial incision, a portion of the medial joint capsule is excised. **(D)** The medial eminence is excised in line with the medial aspect of the metatarsal shaft. **(E)** Preoperative radiograph. **(F)** Postoperative radiograph with satisfactory realignment of the metatarsophalangeal joint. (Mann RA, Coughlin MJ. The video textbook of foot and ankle surgery. St Louis, Medical Video Productions, 1991)

aspect of the metatarsal head, resulting in an impingement to the proximal phalanx. During normal gait, dorsiflexion occurs at the metatarsophalangeal joint, and if there is an obstruction to the dorsiflexion, then a significant impairment in gait may occur. This is particularly bothersome in patients who engage in athletics. The proliferative bone around the metatarsal head can also result in significant increased bulk of the joint, which makes shoe wearing difficult.

The patient's main complaint with hallux rigidus is that of pain with dorsiflexion of the metatarsophalangeal joint. This is aggravated by increased activities, particularly running and other athletic endeavors. The patient may also complain of the fact that, owing to the increased bulk of the joint, shoe wearing is difficult.

The physical examination frequently demonstrates an abrasion or ulceration over the osteophyte on the dorsal or dorsomedial aspect of the metatarsal head. The joint itself is enlarged, there is synovial

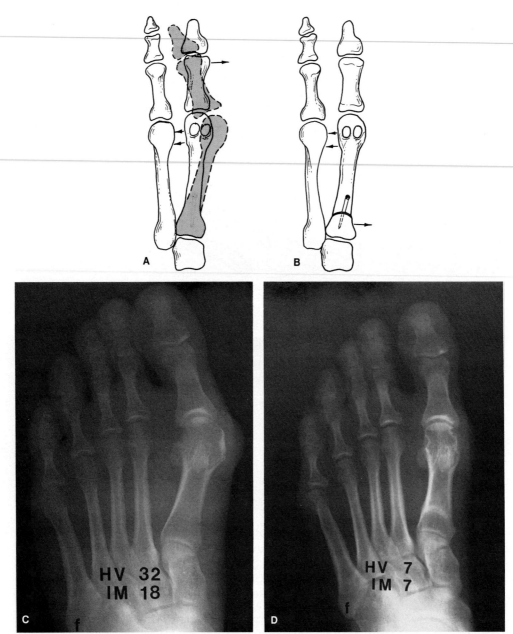

FIGURE 19-7. Distal soft tissue procedure with proximal crescentic metatarsal osteotomy. (**A**) To determine whether an osteotomy is necessary after the soft tissue release has been carried out, the first metatarsal head is pushed laterally. If there is any tendency for the metatarsal head to spring open, an osteotomy should be considered. We add an osteotomy to the distal soft tissue procedure about 85% of the time. (**B**) The osteotomy site is reduced by freeing the soft tissues about the osteotomy and displacing the proximal fragment medially while pushing the metatarsal head laterally. Preoperative (**C**) and postoperative (**D**) radiographs demonstrating correction of a moderate hallux valgus deformity with a distal soft tissue procedure and basal metatarsal osteotomy. (Mann RA, Coughlin MJ. The video textbook of foot and ankle surgery. St Louis, Medical Video Productions, 1991)

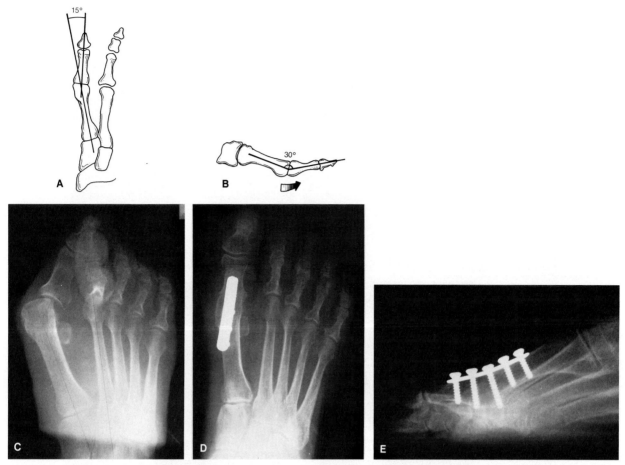

FIGURE 19-8. Arthrodesis of the metatarsophalangeal joint. Proper alignment of the arthrodesed joint is 15 degrees of valgus (**A**) and 30 degrees of dorsiflexion (**B**) in relation to the first metatarsal shaft, which translates to about 10 to 15 degrees of dorsiflexion in relation to the ground. Preoperative (**C**) and postoperative (**D** and **E**) radiographs of an arthrodesis of the first metatarsophalangeal joint using plate fixation. (Mann RA, Coughlin MJ. The video textbook of foot and ankle surgery. St Louis, Medical Video Productions, 1991)

thickening, and there is significant tenderness around the joint, particularly along the lateral aspect of the metatarsophalangeal joint and over the dorsal ridge (Fig. 19-9). There is usually significant restriction of dorsiflexion, and occasionally the proximal phalanx is held in a position of slight plantar flexion if the deformity is severe. Forced dorsiflexion of the joint causes pain.

The radiographs of the patient with hallux rigidus are characteristic, demonstrating degenerative arthritis of the metatarsophalangeal joint on the anteroposterior (AP) view. Besides the narrowing of the joint, significant osteophyte formation is often present along the lateral aspect of the joint. Medially, there rarely is significant osteophyte formation. On the lateral view, there is a dorsal osteophyte of vary-

ing degrees. Occasionally, there is an osteophyte on the dorsal aspect of the proximal phalanx as well.

Management of patients with hallux rigidus involves diminishing their level of activity if possible, placing them into a shoe that has adequate room for the metatarsophalangeal joint, and stiffening the shoe by inserting either an orthotic device or a piece of spring steel in the sole to decrease dorsiflexion at the metatarsophalangeal joint. Occasionally, nonsteroidal antiinflammatory medications can be beneficial.

If conservative management fails, then surgical intervention may be indicated if the neurovascular status of the foot is satisfactory.

The operative procedure of choice for this problem is a cheilectomy, which is a procedure in which the dorsal 20% to 30% of the metatarsal head is re-

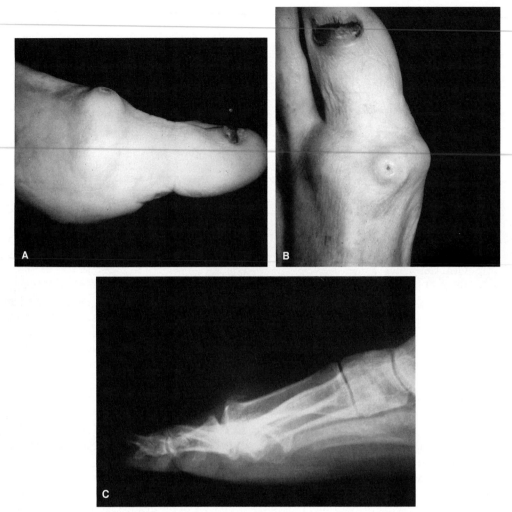

FIGURE 19-9. (A and B) First metatarsophalangeal joint in a patient with hallux rigidus. Note the increased bulk of the joint and marked osteophyte formation. (C) Lateral radiograph of a patient with hallux rigidus, with a large dorsal osteophyte that mechanically blocks dorsiflexion of the proximal phalanx.

moved along with the osteophytes along the lateral side of the metatarsal head. The principle of this procedure is to relieve the dorsal impingement of the proximal phalanx as dorsiflexion occurs, which usually relieves most of the pain. The procedure, however, only reestablishes about half of normal dorsiflexion, but this is usually sufficient to permit the patient to ambulate comfortably and resume most activities. Other methods of treatment include arthrodesis of the metatarsophalangeal joint, which provides a painless joint, although I believe this procedure should be held in abeyance and used if the cheilectomy fails. Occasionally, in an older person whose ambulatory capacity is limited, a Keller procedure can be used. In this procedure, the proximal one third of the proximal phalanx is excised along with the dorsal osteophyte. The problem with this procedure is that it detaches the intrinsic muscles from the base of the phalanx, and as a result, the toe may drift into dorsiflexion or possibly varus or valgus. It is, however, useful in the older patient with marginal circulation. The use of a prosthetic replacement of the metatarsophalangeal joint is rarely indicated in patients with hallux rigidus.

LESSER-TOE DEFORMITIES

Lesser-toe deformities are afflictions of the toes other than the great toe. They include mallet toe, hammertoe, and clawtoe deformities. Hard and soft corns also occur on the lesser toes.

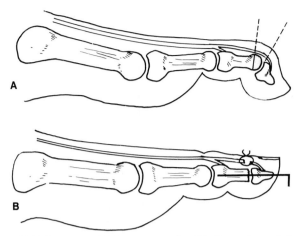

FIGURE 19-10. Mallet toe repair. (A) Resection of the condyles of the middle phalanx. (B) Intramedullary Kirschner wire fixation. (Mann RA, Coughlin MJ. The video textbook of foot and ankle surgery. St Louis, Medical Video Productions, 1991)

Mallet Toe

A mallet toe consists of a fixed flexion deformity of the distal interphalangeal joint, usually involving the second toe but possibly involving the third or fourth toes as well (Fig. 19-10). The patient's chief complaint is usually that of pain on the tip of the toe secondary to pressure from the ground or pain over the distal interphalangeal joint region secondary to pressure against the shoe.

The conservative management of the problem consists of adequate padding beneath the toe to lift the tip of the toe off the ground. This can be achieved by using small felt pads or wrapping the toe with lamb's wool. A shoe with an adequate shoe box is necessary to provide enough room for the toe and the material padding it. If conservative management fails, operative treatment can be undertaken.

The operative treatment of a mallet toe consists of removing the distal portion of the middle phalanx, which decompresses the distal interphalangeal joint. If the deformity is extremely fixed, then a release of the flexor digitorum longus tendon may also be carried out.

Hammertoe

A hammertoe deformity involves the proximal interphalangeal joint in which a flexion deformity, which may be either fixed or flexible, is present. The fixed deformity is one in which the proximal inter-

phalangeal joint cannot be straightened, and a flexible deformity is one in which the proximal interphalangeal joint can be brought back into anatomic alignment (Fig. 19-11). The patient's chief complaint is that of pain, usually over the tip of the toe and over the proximal interphalangeal joint. The patient may develop callus formation beneath the tip of the toe or over the proximal interphalangeal joint region. The conservative management is to adequately pad the area with lamb's wool or felt and to change the patient's shoe wear to accommodate the padding around the toe. If conservative management fails, then operative treatment can be carried out.

The operative treatment of a hammertoe consists of excising the distal portion of the proximal phalanx and then holding the toe in correct alignment for about 6 weeks, until a satisfactory fibrous union has occurred. Arthrodesis of the proximal interphalangeal joint can be attempted, although the fusion rate is low (about 50%). For this reason, usually a fibrous union is the procedure of choice.

Clawtoe

A clawtoe deformity consists of a combination of the aforementioned mallet toe and hammertoe deformities along with dorsiflexion at the metatarsophalangeal joint. This deformity may involve a single metatarsophalangeal joint or multiple metatarsophalangeal joints. The deformities can be either fixed

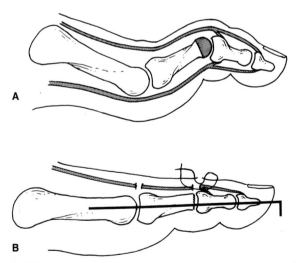

FIGURE 19-11. Fixed hammertoe repair. (A) Resection of the condyles of the proximal phalanx. (B) Intramedullary Kirschner wire fixation. (Mann RA, Coughlin MJ. The video textbook of foot and ankle surgery. St Louis, Medical Video Productions, 1991)

or flexible (Fig. 19-12). The etiology is usually idiopathic, although it may be associated with neurologic disorders. The patient's chief complaint is that of pain over the proximal interphalangeal joint region where the toes strike the top of the shoe, and if the deformity is severe enough at the metatarsophalangeal joint, where the patient develops callus formation beneath the metatarsal heads secondary to depression of the metatarsal heads by the dorsiflexion of the proximal phalanges.

The conservative management consists of fitting the patient into a shoe that has an adequate toe box to accommodate the dorsiflexion of the toes, adding soft insole material to the shoe, and using a soft metatarsal support, which is placed in the shoe just proximal to the metatarsal head region. In this manner, the pressure on the metatarsal heads is relieved. Obviously, with increased padding beneath the foot, the toe box area of the shoe must be of adequate size to accommodate both the shoe and the metatarsal supports.

Operative management of the clawtoe deformity can be undertaken if the conservative measures fail to achieve relief of the problem. If the patient has a fixed deformity, then release of the contracted structures on the dorsal aspect of the metatarsophalangeal joint, which consists of both extensor tendons, the joint capsule, and the collateral ligaments, is undertaken to straighten the contracture at the metatarsophalangeal joint. If a fixed hammertoe deformity is present, then a condylectomy with excision of the distal portion of the proximal phalanx is undertaken. A Girdlestone flexor tendon transfer, in which the flexor digitorum longus tendon is transposed to the dorsal aspect of the proximal phalanx, is carried out to provide increased plantar flexion pull at the metatarsophalangeal joint region. In these cases, pin fixation is often used to maintain satisfactory alignment of the corrected hammertoe and metatarsophalangeal joint until the soft tissues have had a chance to heal. This form of immobilization is used for about 4 to 6 weeks, depending on the severity of the deformity. If the deformity is a dynamic one and does not involve any fixed deformity, then a Girdlestone flexor tendon transfer alone may produce a satisfactory clinical result.

Hard Corn and Soft Corn

A corn is a keratotic lesion that develops on the skin in response to pressure against the skin by an external force (a shoe). As a general rule, a small bony prominence, termed an *exostosis*, lies beneath the skin, and the shoe covering the foot chafes against this area. Corns are divided into hard and soft corns, depending on their location. A hard corn occurs between the skin and the shoe, whereas a soft corn occurs between one toe and an adjacent toe. In both cases, however, the etiology is due to an underlying exostosis.

The patient's main complaint is that of buildup of hypertrophic skin over the exostosis. In time, this may become rather large and painful.

The conservative management is to trim the lesion and place a soft support around it to alleviate the pressure on the involved area. Usually, a broader, softer shoe helps to accommodate this problem.

If conservative management fails, then a surgical procedure may be undertaken that removes the offending prominence.

METATARSALGIA

Metatarsalgia is a generalized term for pain beneath the metatarsal head region. During normal walking, maximal pressure is applied to the metatarsal region for 50% to 60% of the stance time. As a result, any type of abnormality in this area may cause the patient significant disability. Metatarsalgia can be due to a bony problem, systemic disorders, dermatologic conditions, soft tissue problems, dysfunction of the metatarsophalangeal joint, or iatrogenic problems. In

CLAW TOE

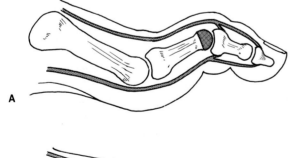

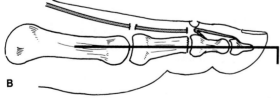

FIGURE 19-12. Fixed claw toe repair. (A) Excision of the condyles of the proximal phalanx, metatarsophalangeal joint capsular release, and extensor tenotomy. (B) Intramedullary Kirschner wire fixation stabilizes the toe. (Mann RA, Coughlin MJ. The video textbook of foot and ankle surgery. St Louis, Medical Video Productions, 1991)

many patients, metatarsalgia can be treated conservatively by obtaining a shoe of adequate size and then adequately padding the metatarsal area to relieve the areas of maximal pain. At times, however, this conservative management fails, and operative intervention is indicated.

Metatarsalgia due to a bony problem usually results in a callus beneath one or more metatarsal heads. This may be due to a prominent fibular condyle, a long metatarsal, a so-called Morton foot in which the first metatarsal is short, a hypermobile first ray in which the first metatarsocuneiform joint is of insufficient stability to provide adequate weight bearing, or after trauma in which a metatarsal may be pushed into a plantar or dorsal angulation. In most of these cases, a callus develops beneath the prominent metatarsal head, which is usually the source of the patient's pain. In these cases, adequate padding is placed around the area to alleviate the pressure on the involved metatarsal head. If this fails, then a surgical procedure may be indicated either to relieve the prominence or to elevate or shorten the metatarsal.

Metatarsalgia due to a systemic disorder is usually associated with rheumatoid arthritis, psoriatic arthritis, or gout. In these conditions, proliferative synovial tissue develops around the metatarsophalangeal joint, which results in an enlargement of the joint as well as a significant inflammatory response by the body. Under these circumstances, placing pressure on the metatarsal head region causes the patient significant discomfort and may make walking extremely difficult. Gout is usually localized to the first metatarsophalangeal joint, whereas rheumatoid and psoriatic arthritis involve multiple metatarsophalangeal joints.

Conservative management of this problem involves placing the patient into an adequate shoe, often an extra-depth shoe with a soft metatarsal support to relieve the pressure on the metatarsal heads. Gout can often be handled therapeutically, although in some cases with large tophaceous deposits, alteration in shoe wear is necessary.

If the conservative management of rheumatoid and psoriatic arthritis fails, then a forefoot reconstructive procedure is carried out, along with arthrodesis of the first metatarsophalangeal joint, to produce a foot with a soft metatarsal pad area and a stable first metatarsal joint.

Metatarsalgia due to dermatologic problems can often be a significant problem for the patient. The dermatologic problems most frequently encountered consist of a plantar wart, a seed corn, or hyperkeratotic skin. A wart is a vascular lesion secondary to a virus. It usually does not occur under a metatarsal head but rather off the weight-bearing surface. If the wart is large enough, however, it can produce disability. A wart is differentiated from a callus by carefully trimming the hyperkeratotic skin off the wart and observing small punctate bleeders secondary to the fine end arteries, which are present in a wart and not in a keratotic lesion. A wart can be treated either by dermal burning with liquid nitrogen; by using Cantharone, which after multiple applications usually relieves the wart; or occasionally by curettage. Burning the bottom of the foot with electrocautery or surgically excising the wart are not recommended unless other options fail because they result in a scar on the plantar aspect of the foot. A permanent scar on the plantar aspect of the foot may be symptomatic and difficult to treat.

A seed corn is a small invagination of skin that results in a small keratotic lesion, which at times can be painful. These usually can be managed by trimming the lesion; or if this fails, curettage may alleviate it. Hyperkeratotic skin is observed in some patients and is probably due to a biochemical abnormality that is poorly understood. In these patients, surgical intervention is not indicated; rather, frequent trimming of the hyperkeratotic skin usually is adequate treatment and often can be taught to the patient.

Metatarsalgia due to soft tissue problems includes atrophy of the plantar fat pad, a synovial cyst arising from the metatarsophalangeal joint, an interdigital neuroma, soft tissue tumors such as a lipoma, permanent changes secondary to a crush injury, or a plantar scar secondary to trauma. Atrophy of the plantar fat pad occurs most frequently in older people and can present a significant problem for the patient. Because of loss of adequate padding beneath the metatarsal heads, some callus formation often results, and the metatarsal heads are sensitive to weight bearing. Unfortunately, there is no way to remedy this situation other than to place the patient in a soft-soled shoe with adequate support in the metatarsal area to alleviate the discomfort.

Occasionally, a synovial cyst arises from the metatarsophalangeal joint and presents on the plantar aspect of the foot. These patients usually experience a squishy feeling and state that they feel as if they are walking on a small marble that moves around. These cysts can often be identified clinically, and if they do not respond to adequate padding, excision often has a satisfactory clinical result.

An interdigital neuroma produces a well-localized area of burning pain on the plantar aspect of the foot, which often radiates out toward the tips of the toes. It most frequently involves the third interspace, although it occasionally involves the second interspace. The etiology of an interdigital neuroma is not precisely known, although the nerve often becomes thickened secondary to increased hyalinization of the tissues surrounding it and the bursal structures above and below the transverse metatarsal ligament usually enlarge. The pain associated with an interdigital neuroma can be reproduced by squeezing the interspace in a dorsal plantar direction and, when pressure is applied to the interspace, squeezing the foot in a mediolateral direction. Conservative management consists of fitting the patient in a wide, soft shoe that also provides metatarsal support. If this fails, excision of the neuroma can be carried out through a dorsal approach to the web space, sectioning the transverse metatarsal ligament and resecting the nerve proximal to the metatarsal head region. This results in a satisfactory response in about 80% of patients.

A soft tissue tumor such as a lipoma can also produce metatarsalgia due to its physical prominence. If this fails to respond to conservative management, such as adequate padding and shoe wear, surgical excision may be carried out. Occasionally, after a crush injury, significant soft tissue damage is done to the foot, which results in fibrous and generalized tenderness around the soft tissue structures. These patients often complain of neuritic-type symptoms such as tingling and burning in the foot and sometimes have atrophy of the soft tissues as well. As a general rule, conservative management is indicated, although some patients do not respond well and are left with a foot that is chronically painful. A plantar scar secondary to an accidental laceration of the plantar aspect of the foot can produce significant discomfort and disability. The scar may become hypertrophic or painful if a nerve becomes entrapped in the scar. Under these circumstances, conservative management to adequately pad and protect the area should be attempted initially, but if this fails, either revision of the scar or excision of the nerve tissue that is entrapped, or both, may be of benefit. The prognosis in some of these cases is poor.

Metatarsalgia may be due to dysfunction of the metatarsophalangeal joint, which includes nonspecific synovitis, plantar plate degeneration, Freiberg infarction, or dysfunction secondary to subluxation or dislocation of the metatarsophalangeal joint.

Nonspecific synovitis is a condition in which the patient develops synovial proliferation around the second metatarsophalangeal joint. This usually starts spontaneously, and patients often feel as if they are walking on a painful lump on the bottom of the foot. The physical examination demonstrates generalized synovial thickening around the metatarsophalangeal joint. This is sometimes associated with a hammertoe. This condition often responds to conservative management consisting of adequate shoes and padding and nonsteroidal antiinflammatory medications. Occasionally, injection of corticosteroid into the joint relieves the condition. If the condition persists, synovectomy of the metatarsophalangeal joint should be considered. At times, this condition results in a patient developing a subluxation of the metatarsophalangeal joint frequently associated with a fixed hammertoe deformity.

Degeneration of the plantar plate occurs occasionally and is due to cystic changes in the dense plantar plate, which helps to stabilize the metatarsophalangeal joint. It is associated with pain beneath the metatarsal head and often a progressive cocking-up of the metatarsophalangeal joint. Usually, patients do not develop the generalized synovial reaction noted in patients with nonspecific synovitis. The problem can usually be handled conservatively, although occasionally arthroplasty of the metatarsophalangeal joint is indicated.

Freiberg infarction is an avascular necrosis of unknown etiology that occurs in the metatarsal head. This results in collapse of the metatarsophalangeal joint (Fig. 19-13). This process is often associated with generalized discomfort around the joint, and the joint may develop a significant synovial reaction or enlargement due to collapse of the bony structures. This condition can often be managed conservatively with adequate shoes and padding, although nonsteroidal antiinflammatory medications are useful during the acute phases. If the problem significantly limits the patient, arthroplasty may be indicated to remove some of the proliferative bone about the joint.

Subluxations and dislocations of the metatarsophalangeal joint are due to multiple causes, including degeneration of the plantar plate, which permits the extensor tendons to pull the proximal phalanx up into dorsiflexion; chronic pressure of the great toe against the second toe, which may result in a dislocated second metatarsophalangeal joint; nonspecific synovitis; or an undetermined etiology. When a severe subluxation or dislocation occurs, the proximal phalanx pushes the metatarsal head into a plantar position (Fig. 19-14). As a result, pain and often a large callus develop beneath the metatarsal head. The patient often complains of pain over the dorsal aspect of the toe as well because this strikes the top of the shoe. Under these circumstances, conservative man-

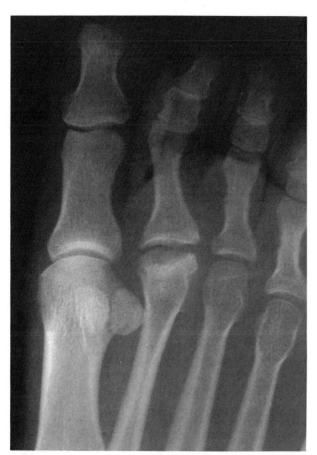

FIGURE 19-13. Radiograph of Freiberg infraction involving the second metatarsal head. This is an avascular necrosis of undetermined cause producing collapse of the metatarsal head.

conservative, with wide, soft shoes and an adequate support, but if this fails, revision of the scar may be indicated. The results of this type of surgery, however, often are not gratifying. Occasionally, after metatarsal surgery to alleviate pressure on one metatarsal, a condition known as a *transfer lesion* may occur. This results in pressure beneath the adjacent metatarsal head due to lack of weight bearing on the previously operated metatarsal. Under these circumstances, the transfer lesion may be as symptomatic as the original problem. Conservative management consists of wide, soft shoes and adequate padding. If this fails, occasionally a metatarsal osteotomy may relieve this condition.

As is apparent from this discussion, metatarsalgia can be a significant problem for the patient. Treatment basically consists of fitting the patient in a shoe that is of adequate size to allow the foot to spread out, relieving pressure against the foot in mediolateral and dorsal plantar directions. Soft metatarsal supports placed proximal to the painful area often permit the patient to live with the problem. Surgery is infrequently indicated in patients with metatarsalgia.

agement consists of a shoe with an adequate toe box to alleviate the pressure on the toe and metatarsal head along with adequate padding to relieve the pressure beneath the metatarsal head. If conservative measures fail, then some an operative procedure to reduce the metatarsophalangeal joint may be indicated. These procedures are often successful in alleviating this condition.

Metatarsalgia due to iatrogenic causes usually is a result of surgery on the metatarsal bones or is secondary to scars on the plantar aspect of the foot after surgery. As a general rule, scars on the plantar aspect of the foot should be avoided in dealing with maladies of the forefoot. Unfortunately, plantar scars, if misplaced beneath the metatarsal head, become chronically painful. Also, if the scar becomes hypertrophic, pain can result. Frequently, a plantar approach to the foot results in a certain degree of atrophy of the plantar fat pad, and this may produce the metatarsalgia. The management of this problem is

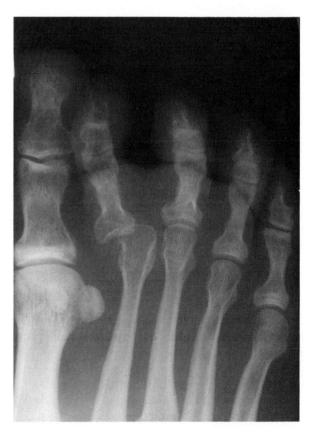

FIGURE 19-14. Subluxation of the second metatarsophalangeal joint in a dorsomedial direction.

POSTURAL PROBLEMS

The term *postural problems* refers to deformities in the overall shape of the foot. These include excessively low or high arches, which may be congenital or acquired. A low-arched foot is termed a *flatfoot*, and a high-arched foot is called a *cavus foot*. An abnormally high or low arch does not necessarily represent a clinical problem for the patient, particularly if it is congenital in nature. However, patients who have acquired deformities due to trauma, tendon degeneration, or arthritis often have symptoms.

Flatfoot (Pes Planus)

A general classification of flatfoot follows.

Congenital
Hypermobile flatfoot

Asymptomatic flexible flatfoot
Symptomatic flexible flatfoot
Flatfoot associated with accessory navicula
Flatfoot associated with a generalized dysplasia, such as Ehlers-Danlos or Marfan syndrome

Rigid flatfoot

Peroneal spastic flatfoot (tarsal coalition)
Congenital abnormality (eg, vertical talus)

Acquired
Traumatic

Subtalar joint dysfunction secondary to fracture or dislocation
Rupture of the posterior tibial tendon

Generalized arthritic conditions

Rheumatoid arthritis
Psoriatic arthritis

Neuromuscular imbalance

Cerebral palsy
Stroke
Polio

Diabetes
Charcot foot

The physical findings associated with a flatfoot generally are those of a lowered longitudinal arch. Secondary changes are noted when the patient stands, namely, an increased degree of valgus of the hindfoot and abduction of the forefoot. The clinical examination of the hypermobile foot frequently demonstrates marked instability of the talonavicular joint and at times a tight Achilles tendon. When testing for Achilles tendon tightness, it is imperative that the head of the talus be covered by the navicular and the foot brought up into dorsiflexion; otherwise, a false degree of dorsiflexion is observed.

The radiographic findings in the evaluation of a patient with pes planus should be obtained in a weight-bearing position. In the lateral radiograph, a line drawn through the long axis of the talus should nearly bisect the navicular and first metatarsal shaft (Fig. 19-15). *Mild flatfoot* is indicated by a sag in this line of up to 15 degrees; a sag from 15 to 40 degrees indicates *moderate flatfoot;* and a sag greater than 40 degrees indicates *severe flatfoot*. In the AP radiograph, a line drawn through the long axis of the talus and calcaneus should measure about 15 degrees. An increase in this angle indicates varying degrees of flatfoot. Observation of the talonavicular joint demonstrates lateral subluxation of the navicular off the head of the talus (see Fig. 19-15).

Conservative treatment of flatfoot involves fitting the patient with a firm shoe that has an extended medial counter to help support the talonavicular joint, a medial heel wedge to help tilt the heel into a neutral position, and a well-molded, semiflexible arch support to further support the longitudinal arch of the foot. These treatment modalities suffice in most patients with symptomatic hypermobile flatfoot of congenital etiology. Stabilization of the foot with arthrodesis of the joints of the hindfoot may be necessary in significantly symptomatic patients. The surgeon must always be cautious, however, when carrying out a stabilization procedure of the hindfoot because an excessively flexible foot is being replaced with a rigid foot, and this does not always ensure that the patient will become asymptomatic.

In specific cases, however, a painful rigid flatfoot due to a tarsal coalition is present. In these cases, arthrodesis results in a foot that is significantly more functional (Fig. 19-16). Patients with acquired flatfoot sometimes require surgical intervention to repair the abnormality. If the deformity is due to an injury that resulted in degenerative changes of the joints, then realignment and stabilization often result in a significantly more functional foot, although rarely a normal foot. Whenever arthrodesis is carried out around the foot, the main principle of the procedure is to produce a plantigrade foot, or one that can be placed flat on the ground. This foot posture enables the most function and least abnormal stress. Occasionally, a tendon transfer, rather than arthrodesis, can be used in patients with dysfunction of the posterior tibial tendon.

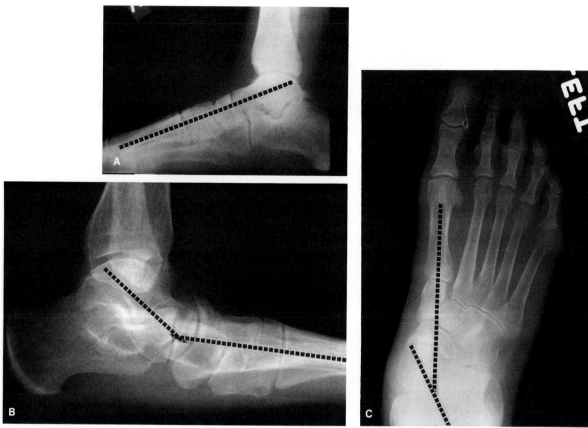

FIGURE 19-15. Radiographs of the flatfoot deformity. (A) Normal lateral radiograph demonstrating the relation between the long axis of the talus and first metatarsal. (B) In the flatfoot deformity, there is a sagging of the talonavicular joint. (C) In the AP view, there should be a straight line relation between the long axis of the talus and first metatarsal. In flatfoot, this line is disrupted, and there is medial deviation of the head of the talus.

Cavus Foot

A cavus, or high-arched, foot is the opposite of a flatfoot deformity. The foot is often stiff, and there may be an associated neuromuscular disorder. A general classification of the etiology of pes cavus follows.

Neuromuscular
Muscle disease
    Muscular dystrophy
Afflictions of the peripheral nerves
    Charcot-Marie-Tooth disease
    Intraspinal tumor
    Polyneuritis
Anterior horn cell disease of the spinal cord
    Poliomyelitis
    Spinal dysraphism
    Spinal cord tumor
    Syringomyelia

Long tract and central disease
    Freidreich ataxia
    Cerebral palsy

Congenital
Idiopathic cavus foot
Residual of a clubfoot
Arthrogryposis

Traumatic
Compartment syndrome—old
Contracture secondary to severe burn
Malunion of a fracture

On physical examination, the patient with a cavus deformity demonstrates a high arch while standing, which is associated with a varus deformity of the heel, adduction of the forefoot, and often clawing of the toes. The foot frequently is rigid with restricted motion in all the joints, fixed dorsiflexion contracture

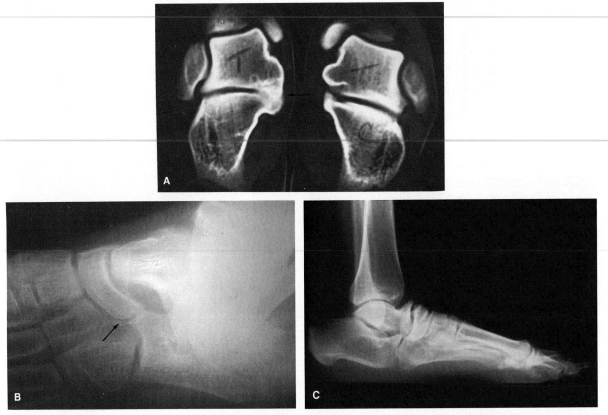

FIGURE 19-16. Tarsal coalitions. (A) Talocalcaneal middle facet coalition (*arrow*). (B) Calcaneonavicular coalition. (C) Changes secondary to a tarsal coalition consist of beaking and irregularity of the talonavicular joint, abnormal appearance of the subtalar joint, and lack of dorsiflexion pitch to the calcaneus.

of the metatarsophalangeal joints, and fixed hammering of the proximal interphalangeal joints.

The weight-bearing radiographs of the foot demonstrate an increased pitch to the calcaneus in relation to the floor of greater than 40 degrees, an elevated longitudinal arch, and frequently plantar flexion of metatarsals giving rise to a forefoot equinus (Fig. 19-17).

The patient with a cavus foot must be carefully evaluated for any neurologic problems as the possible etiology of the deformity, especially if the deformity is progressive.

The clinical treatment of the cavus foot is usually to provide a shoe with adequate support and cushioning to help absorb some of the impact of ground contact. If a neurologic disorder exists, a polypropylene ankle–foot orthosis (AFO) may be necessary to provide stability. Surgical treatment of the cavus foot depends on the precise etiology of the problem. The main goals of surgery are to produce a planti-

grade foot and, if possible, to lower the longitudinal arch. The type of surgical procedure indicated depend on the specific bony abnormality present and the location of the maximal deformity.

If, after careful evaluation, surgery is required on the rear foot to reduce the degree of cavus and varus, a Dwyer calcaneal osteotomy is carried out. This procedure permits the heel to be brought from a varus configuration into valgus and occasionally to slide proximally to reduce the pitch of the calcaneus. In addition, release of the plantar fascia and a first metatarsal osteotomy may provide a plantigrade foot without having to resort to a fusion-type procedure (Fig. 19-18). If muscle weakness is present, then a tendon transfer may be indicated to help stabilize the foot. Occasionally, a triple arthrodesis is needed to realign the foot, and under these circumstances, I recommend using a Siffert beak–type triple arthrodesis, which lowers the longitudinal arch while correcting the deformity (Fig. 19-19).

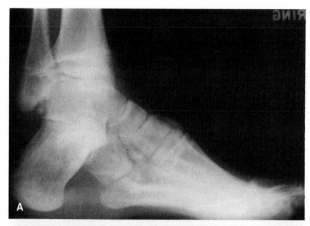

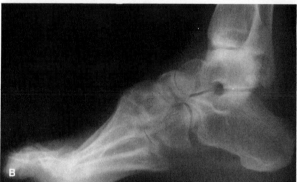

FIGURE 19-17. Radiographs of the cavus foot. (**A**) Marked dorsiflexion pitch of the calcaneus. Normal calcaneal pitch is 20 to 40 degrees. (**B**) Forefoot equinus resulting in a cavus foot. Note the almost normal-appearing pitch to the calcaneus. (Mann RA, Coughlin MJ. The video textbook of foot and ankle surgery. St Louis, Medical Video Productions, 1991)

THE DIABETIC FOOT

The diabetic foot presents a difficult problem in management. Many diabetics develop a peripheral neuropathy, making the foot insensitive to the stresses placed on the skin and underlying skeletal structures. As a result of the diminished sensation, ulceration of the skin of varying degrees may occur, along with skeletal changes, resulting in a Charcot foot. Because of lack of sensation and impaired tissue nutrition, the clinical condition is often advanced before the orthopaedist has the opportunity to see the patient. The most important factor in the management of the diabetic patient is education of the patient and family about the potential problems and need for constant surveillance and early recognition and treatment. When treatment is initiated, it must be a multispecialty approach with the help of the patient's internist and input from vascular, general, and plastic surgeons.

The most frequent problem faced by the diabetic is breakdown of the skin of the foot, usually over a bony prominence. The natural history of the problem has been classified to enable the clinician to systematically approach the problem.

Grade 0: Skin intact (may have bony deformities)
Grade 1: Localized superficial ulcer
Grade 2: Deep ulcer to tendon, bone, ligament, joint
Grade 3: Deep abscess, osteomyelitis
Grade 4: Gangrene of the toes or forefoot
Grade 5: Gangrene of the whole foot

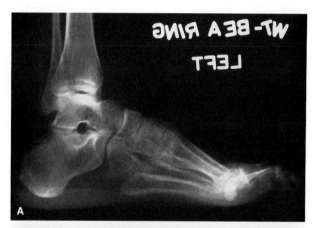

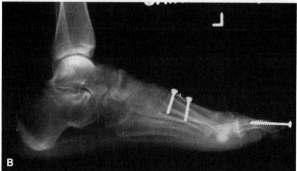

FIGURE 19-18. Operative correction of a cavus foot. (**A**) Preoperative deformity demonstrating the increased dorsiflexion pitch of the calcaneus and mild equinus of the forefoot. (**B**) Postoperative radiograph after a calcaneal osteotomy permitting dorsiflexion of the proximal fragment, dorsiflexion osteotomy of the first metatarsal, release of the plantar fascia, and fusion of the interphalangeal joint of the great toe. The longitudinal arch has been lengthened as a result of this procedure. (Mann RA, Coughlin MJ. The video textbook of foot and ankle surgery. St Louis, Medical Video Productions, 1991)

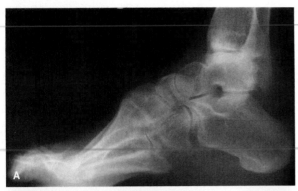

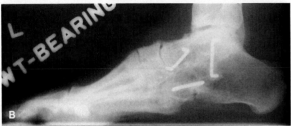

FIGURE 19-19. Results of the surgical treatment of a cavus foot using the Siffert triple arthrodesis. (A) Preoperative radiograph. (B) Postoperative radiograph demonstrating the flattening and stabilization of the longitudinal arch. (Mann RA, Coughlin MJ. The video textbook of foot and ankle surgery. St Louis, Medical Video Productions, 1991)

In reviewing the various grades of difficulties encountered by the diabetic patient, it becomes obvious that a more aggressive approach needs to be taken as the problem becomes more severe. If only a minor abrasion is present, the patient should be placed into shoes of adequate size, which often entails an extra-depth shoe with a Plastizote liner. This shoe provides the diabetic foot with an environment that should not place undue stress on the skin or over any bony prominences that are present. The soft Plastizote liner can be made to conform to the plantar aspect of the foot, alleviating pressure underneath metatarsal heads if necessary.

As the breakdown increases and other factors are introduced, such as involvement of tendons, joints, and bones, infection becomes a significant problem. The basic principle of treatment is first to gain control over the infected area by the initiation of appropriate antibiotics, surgical débridement, and readjustment of antibiotics, depending on the cultures obtained at the time of surgery. Adequate soft tissue débridement and bony resection must be carried out to permit healing.

The overall ability of the diabetic to heal a foot lesion is related to what is known as an *ischemic index.* This index involves use of Doppler ultrasound, whereby the blood pressure of the brachial artery is compared with that of the posterior tibial and dorsalis pedis, and even the toe. The ischemic index is derived by dividing the pressure in the lower extremity by the brachial artery pressure, and if a pulsatile flow is present with an ischemic index of over 0.45, healing can be expected in about 90% of cases. If inadequate blood supply is present, then a vascular surgeon should be consulted to evaluate the vascular tree of the lower extremity for the possibility of a localized block that could be remedied, thereby providing increased circulation to the foot and possibly healing.

At times, amputations of digits, forefoot (transmetatarsal amputation), or hindfoot (Syme amputation) is necessary. Limb length should be preserved if possible, but selection of the amputation site depends on the correlation of the ischemic index and the condition of the underlying skeletal structure.

Charcot changes of the foot, which are the direct result of the chronic sensory neuropathy, present an extremely difficult problem for both the patient and clinician. Charcot changes usually occur in the midfoot, although other joints can be involved, from the ankle to the metatarsophalangeal joints. Typically, patients experience a trivial trauma, continued to walk on the extremity because they have little or no sensation, and over time note significant swelling of the foot and ankle associated with possible deformity. A patient with a Charcot foot can sustain a complete tarsometatarsal dislocation and can continue to walk on the foot with little or no discomfort. If the diabetic patient presents with swelling of undetermined etiology through the midfoot, the physician should presume that an early Charcot foot may be developing and that the extremity needs to be placed at rest. This includes casting until such time that the swelling and increased warmth in the foot have subsided, after which the foot should be braced in a polypropylene AFO to keep stress off the involved area and distribute the pressure throughout the entire foot (Fig. 19-20). Early detection and treatment of the Charcot foot often prevents significant deformity.

In the patient who presents with a total collapse of the foot as a result of Charcot changes, bracing is extremely difficult owing to the bony prominences and the severe deformity of the foot. At times, it is necessary to resect bony prominences to prevent chronic skin breakdown.

The toenails of the diabetic patient also must be carefully managed to ensure that a simple ingrown

management fails, then stabilization of the involved joint may be considered.

Ankle Joint

The ankle joint is rarely afflicted with primary arthrosis, but after an ankle fracture or other various traumas to the ankle joint, degenerative arthritis can occur. The patient complains of pain that is well localized to the ankle joint, and this can often lead to a significant degree of disability. After a fracture of the ankle joint, a varus or valgus deformity may result in improper placement of the foot on the ground. The management of the patient with osteoarthritis of the ankle joint is often helped by use of a polypropylene AFO that maintains the ankle joint in a fixed position, relieving the stress across the joint (see Fig. 19-20). A rocker-bottom shoe sole permits the patient to roll over the foot, thereby relieving the stress on the ankle joint. If the pain and disability persist, then arthrodesis of the ankle joint can be considered.

When arthrodesis of the ankle joint is carried out, the ankle should be put into neutral position in terms of extension and flexion and into about 5 degrees of valgus (Fig. 19-21). The rotation of the foot in relation to the knee joint should be the same as on the uninvolved side. This usually is external rotation, although there is some individual variation. After a successful ankle arthrodesis, patients still maintain some dorsiflexion and plantar flexion motion of the foot, which is mediated through the talonavicular and subtalar joints. Arthrodesis usually results in restoration of function, although most patients cannot participate in running or jumping activities.

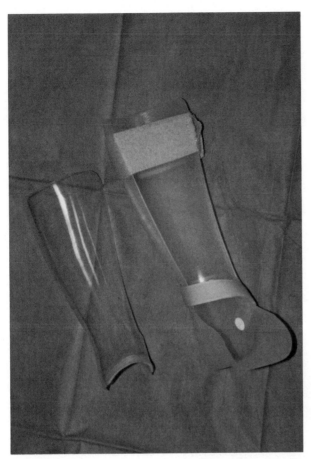

FIGURE 19-20. An ankle–foot orthosis may be used with and without an anterior shell to help contain the foot and ankle.

toenail does not develop into a more significant problem.

ARTHROSIS OF THE FOOT AND ANKLE

Arthrosis of the foot and ankle may be primary or secondary. Although primary arthrosis of the ankle and subtalar joint is uncommon, it does occur in the talonavicular, tarsometatarsal, and first metatarsophalangeal joints. Why some joints are affected by primary arthroses and others are usually affected after trauma remains an enigma. Because the foot and ankle are weight-bearing structures, joint afflictions may severely limit a person's ability to remain functional. As a general rule, the diagnosis of arthrosis is not difficult to make, and in most cases conservative management can benefit the patient. If conservative

Subtalar Joint

The subtalar joint rarely develops primary osteoarthritis but frequently develops changes after an interarticular calcaneal fracture. These changes result in loss of motion of the subtalar joint and sometimes in a lateral impingement against the fibula. Conservative treatment includes use of a polypropylene AFO, but in this case, the trim line of the brace can be made to permit 50% ankle joint motion, which gives the patient a smoother gait while providing support to the subtalar joint. If conservative measures

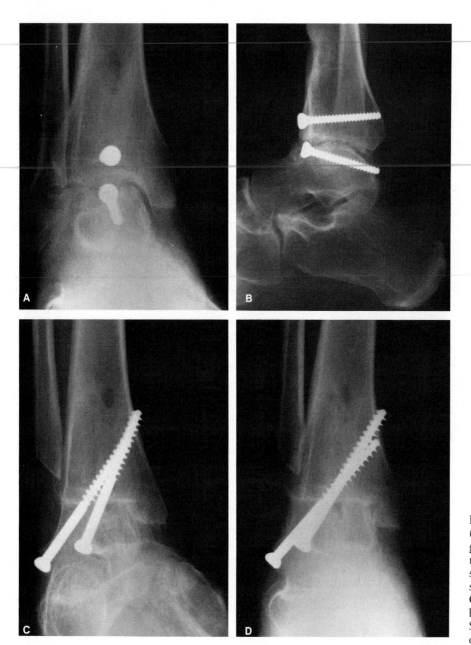

FIGURE 19-21. Ankle fusion. (A and B) Preoperative radiographs. (C and D) Postoperative radiographs demonstrating a satisfactory ankle fusion using screw fixation. (Mann RA, Coughlin MJ. The video textbook of foot and ankle surgery. St Louis, Medical Video Productions, 1991)

fail, then arthrodesis of the subtalar joint often produces a satisfactory clinical result.

When arthrodesis of the subtalar joint is carried out, the subtalar joint is placed into about 5 degrees of valgus. If a lateral impingement exists beneath the fibula, this should be excised at the time of the fusion. An isolated subtalar arthrodesis is also indicated in the patient who has a congenital talocalcaneal bar without other secondary changes around the foot.

After a successful subtalar arthrodesis, patients may resume most activities (Fig. 19-22).

Talonavicular Joint

The talonavicular joint may develop primary arthrosis, or arthrosis may follow trauma to this area. After trauma, a significant deformity of the talona-

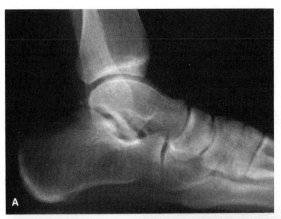

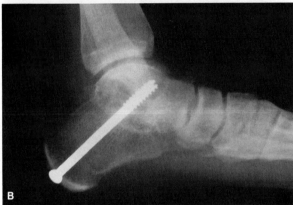

FIGURE 19-22. Subtalar joint arthrodesis. (A) Preoperative radiograph of arthrosis of the posterior facet of the subtalar joint. (B) Postoperative radiographs demonstrating satisfactory arthrodesis using screw fixation.

vicular joint may occur, and the head of the talus tends to drop in a plantar and medial direction. This results in a secondary deformity of the foot in which the calcaneus drifts into valgus and the forefoot into abduction, causing an acquired flatfoot deformity. The problem can be handled conservatively using a polypropylene AFO with the trim line cut to permit ankle joint motion. These patients sometimes have trouble with the orthosis, however, owing to the prominence of the navicular along the plantar medial aspect of the foot.

If conservative measures fail, an isolated arthrodesis of the talonavicular joint produces a satisfactory result in patients older than 50 years of age, but this usually should be combined with a fusion of the calcaneocuboid joint. This is also true in patients who are younger and very active. Fusion of the talonavicular joint results in significant limitation

of the subtalar joint motion because, for normal subtalar joint motion to occur, rotation of the navicular over the head of the talus must occur. After arthrodesis, because this motion is blocked, subtalar joint motion is blocked. After talonavicular fusion, however, patients remain functional.

Subtalar Joint and Talonavicular Joint Arthritis

Degenerative changes due to trauma can occur in several of the joints of the hindfoot, including both the talonavicular and subtalar joints. Occasionally, the calcaneocuboid joint is involved as well.

Under these circumstances, there may be a problem with malalignment of the foot as well as painful arthrosis. The use of a polypropylene AFO may provide adequate stability to the foot and diminish the discomfort. If conservative management fails, then a triple arthrodesis may be indicated.

A triple arthrodesis involves fusion of the subtalar (talocalcaneal), talonavicular, and calcaneocuboid joints. When a triple arthrodesis is carried out, only ankle joint motion is present, and all inversion and eversion function of the foot is lost. When carrying out such an arthrodesis, the subtalar joint needs to be placed into about 5 degrees of valgus, the talonavicular joint in a neutral position, and the forefoot rotated into a neutral position. This creates a plantigrade foot, so that when the foot comes into contact with the ground, there is no abnormal varus or valgus configuration to either the heel or forefoot (Fig. 19-23). If the triple arthrodesis is carried out incorrectly, abnormal weight bearing may result. After a successful triple arthrodesis, patients are functional, although there is some added stress to the ankle joint, which can be a problem in some cases. As a general rule, these patients can carry out most functions of daily living, although sports and running are difficult. These patients are encouraged to swim, ride a bicycle, hike, and engage in low-impact activities.

Tarsometatarsal Arthrosis

Arthrosis of the tarsometatarsal articulation can be primary, or it can be secondary to a Lisfranc fracture dislocation. In both cases, patients note progressive pain and sometimes a progressive abduction defor-

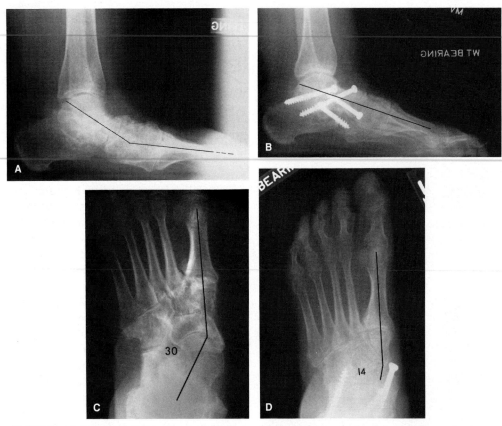

FIGURE 19-23. The triple arthrodesis consists of fusion of the subtalar, talonavicular and calcaneocuboid joints. Preoperative (**A**) and postoperative (**B**) lateral radiographs demonstrating reestablishment of the longitudinal arch. (**C** and **D**) AP view demonstrating correction of the abduction deformity of the forefoot. (Mann RA, Coughlin MJ. The video textbook of foot and ankle surgery. St Louis, Medical Video Productions, 1991)

mity of the forefoot, which results in flattening of the longitudinal arch. A prominence often develops, particularly near the first metatarsocuneiform articulation on the plantar medial aspect of the foot. A polypropylene AFO with a trim line cut to permit ankle joint motion and a full length foot piece often helps provide support. If a large plantar medial prominence is present, however, wearing a brace may be difficult. If conservative management is unsuccessful, arthrodesis to realign the tarsometatarsal articulations can be undertaken.

Arthrodesis of the tarsometatarsal articulation should be carried out to realign the foot and place it back into as normal a position as possible. If marked forefoot abduction is present as well as dorsiflexion at the tarsometatarsal articulation, an attempt should be made to correct this. Technically, this procedure is difficult because realignment of the foot at times

is difficult to achieve. After a successful arthrodesis, the patient has a plantigrade foot and stability of the involved joints. Some patients, however, complain of persistent stiffness in the foot after the fusion, and although they are highly functional, they are encouraged not to engage in high-impact sports.

Arthrosis of the First Metatarsophalangeal Joint

Primary arthrosis of the first metatarsophalangeal joint, frequently called *hallux rigidus*, is a common problem. These patients develop a large dorsal ridge on the metatarsal head, which results in an impingement of the proximal phalanx to dorsiflexion, limitation of motion, and pain. These patients can be fitted with a stiff-soled shoe with an adequate toe box to relieve stress on the soft tissues and underlying bony tissues and to limit joint motion. If conservative management fails, then usually a cheilectomy can be carried out (described previously). If this fails or the arthritic change is sufficiently severe, an arthrodesis can be carried out. Arthrodesis should placed the hallux into 15 degrees of valgus and about 30 degrees of dorsiflexion in relation to the first metatarsal, which is 10 to 15 degrees in relation to the ground (Fig. 19-24).

Rheumatoid Arthritis

Patients with rheumatoid arthritis may have involvement of the foot. In about 11% of patients who develop rheumatoid arthritis, it begins in the foot.

Because the foot is a weight-bearing structure, the resultant deformity may significantly limit the patient's ability to ambulate and obtain shoe wear. The rheumatoid process in the foot is the same as noted elsewhere in the body, manifested by marked proliferation of synovial tissue within the joints and subsequent invasion of the articular cartilage with destruction of the joint. As a result, significant foot deformities may occur. As a general rule, the forefoot is more frequently involved than the hindfoot or ankle joint.

The changes in the joints begin with a synovitis-type picture, and over time, the deformities may progress to subluxations and dislocations. This process, particularly in the forefoot, can be helped if synovectomies of the metatarsophalangeal joints are carried

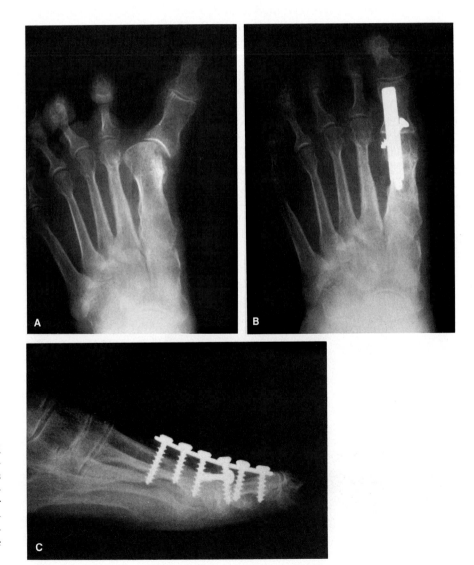

FIGURE 19-24. Arthrodesis of the first metatarsophalangeal joint. (A) Preoperative radiograph of a severe hallux varus deformity. (B and C) Postoperative radiographs taken after arthrodesis of the first metatarsophalangeal joint using an intrafragmentary screw and plate fixation.

out at an early stage, before significant capsular destruction has occurred. Unfortunately, the patient is not usually seen by the orthopaedic surgeon early in the disease process, and it is not until the toes are significantly deformed that the patient is referred to the orthopaedic surgeon.

The pathologic anatomy that is noted in the rheumatoid forefoot is that of a marked hallux valgus deformity associated with dislocations and lateral deviation of the lesser metatarsophalangeal joints. The plantar fat pad is drawn distally, and the metatarsal heads are held in a fixed position in the plantar aspect of the foot. This results in callus formation beneath the metatarsal heads, which may be severe and may even result in ulcerations. This situation sometimes is compounded by the formation of rheumatoid cysts, which further aggravate the problem. The toes develop severe hammering and become rigid. Patients with rheumatoid arthritis of the foot often end up walking on the metatarsal heads, and their toes do not participate in weight bearing.

Conservative treatment of the rheumatoid foot consists of fitting the patient with an extra-depth shoe that has a large toe box with enough room for the patient's forefoot deformities and for an orthotic device to help relieve the stress on the metatarsal heads (Fig. 19-25). If this type of conservative management is not successful, then surgical intervention is often of benefit to the patient.

Surgical treatment consists of arthrodesis of the first metatarsophalangeal joint to correct the deformity and create stability of the medial aspect of the

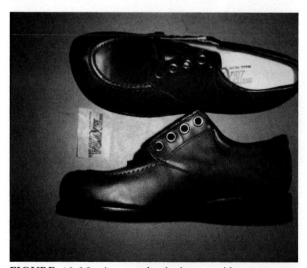

FIGURE 19-25. An extradepth shoe provides extra room in the toe box as well as extra width to accommodate a deformed foot.

foot. The lesser metatarsophalangeal joints are treated by resecting the metatarsal heads, which decompresses the metatarsophalangeal joint, permitting the fat pad to be drawn back down onto the plantar aspect of the foot and creating a soft cushion for the foot that relieves the metatarsalgia. The lesser-toe deformities are corrected by manual osteoclasis and pinning, which corrects the fixed deformities. After this procedure, patients often have increased ambulatory capacity and can wear store-bought shoes (Fig. 19-26).

Rheumatoid arthritis often involves the talonavicular joint, which may subluxate, resulting in a significant valgus deformity of the hindfoot with plantar flexion of the talus. This can result in a prominence on the plantar medial aspect of the foot, which may lead to ulceration. Attempts to treat subluxation of the talonavicular joint conservatively are difficult because of the stress being applied across the area. In addition, an orthotic device usually is not well tolerated because of the marked prominence of the talar head. As a general rule, early arthrodesis of the talonavicular joint, when it is affected, often leads to resolution of the patient's pain and helps to prevent the significant deformity that may follow.

The ankle joint may also be affected in the rheumatoid patient, but not as frequently as other joints. As with other joints that are affected with rheumatoid arthritis, the magnitude of the deformity can become extremely severe. Early on, the treatment may consist of nonsteroidal antiinflammatory medications, and if the symptoms progress, synovectomy of the ankle joint may be indicated. The use of a polypropylene AFO to keep some of the stress off the ankle joint, along with a mild rocker-bottom shoe, also may be of benefit. If these conservative measures fail or the deformity becomes too severe, arthrodesis of the ankle usually offers satisfactory resolution of the problem. If, however, other hindfoot joints are involved, such as the subtalar or talonavicular joint, the patient may not have complete relief after ankle fusion, and an AFO may be required.

MISCELLANEOUS

Heel Pain

Pain in the heel pad area may vary from an annoyance to a significantly disabling problem. Heel pain has multiple etiologies, and it is imperative that a careful history and physical examination be carried out to pinpoint, as precisely as possible, the etiology

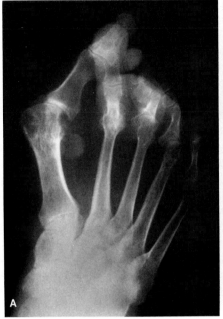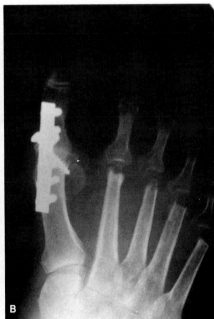

FIGURE 19-26. A rheumatoid foot. (A) Preoperative radiograph of typical rheumatoid changes with a severe hallux valgus deformity and subluxation and dislocation of the lesser metatarsophalangeal joints. (B) Reconstruction using an arthrodesis of the first metatarsophalangeal joint and arthroplasties of the lesser metatarsophalangeal joints.

of the pain. In this way, specific treatment can be formulated to relieve the condition. Heel pain can result from a disorder of the Achilles tendon or the soft tissues near the heel. It can be caused by a neurologic disorder, or it can be secondary to an abnormal bony prominence.

Heel pain associated with the Achilles tendon can be tendinitis of the distal portion of the tendon associated with pain on palpation and occasionally crepitus. If the pain is located at the insertion of the Achilles tendon into the calcaneus, it may be due to some degeneration of the Achilles tendon. In this case, there is thickening of the tendon near its insertion, which at times may become large. This can be associated with increased warmth over the area as well. Calcification at the insertion of the Achilles tendon may indicate some degeneration and on rare occasions is a source of pain. At times, pressure from a prominence on the posterosuperior aspect of the calcaneus, known as a *Haglund deformity,* can be the cause of the pain. In the patient with a Haglund deformity, a lateral radiograph of the calcaneus reveals a large posterosuperior prominence on the calcaneus that is responsible for the problem.

Soft tissue causes of heel pain include atrophy of the heel pad. This is most frequently seen in older patients who develop thinning of the fat pad, which decreases the cushion on the heel. The diagnosis is made by palpation of the heel pad and the observation of lack of adequate fatty tissue. Plantar fasciitis

may also cause heel pain and is usually located near the tubercle of the calcaneus or just distal to it. Palpation along the plantar fascia reveals the origin of the problem. At times, the fasciitis involves the origin of the abductor hallucis muscle, and in these cases, the pain is located along the plantar medial aspect of the heel and is aggravated by palpation of the origin of the muscle.

Neurologic causes of heel pain include tarsal tunnel syndrome, which is an entrapment of the posterior tibial nerve with involvement of the medial calcaneal nerve. This may be diagnosed by percussion over the posterior tibial nerve or its terminal branches, which would demonstrate a Tinel sign with radiation toward the heel. Lumbar disc disease at the L5 to S1 level also may be the source of heel pain. In these cases, the patient typically manifests some evidence of nerve root irritation, with back, buttocks, or leg pain, possibly associated with sensory motor or reflex changes. Heel pain also may be due to a nerve entrapment in which the nerve to the abductor digiti quinti muscle is stretched over the plantar fascia as it passes over it to cross the foot. In these cases, pain is often noted along the plantar medial aspect of the foot, just below the abductor hallucis muscle.

Bone-related causes of heel pain include a calcaneal spur on the plantar aspect of the foot. This is thought by some to be a common source of heel pain, but I believe in most cases it represents a fasciitis at the origin of plantar fascia as opposed to pain over the calcaneal spur. A calcaneal spur is present in more than half of people older than 50 years of age, and thus should probably not be considered an abnormality. Occasionally, a stress fracture may involve a calcaneal spur on the plantar aspect of the calcaneus as a cause of heel pain. This sometimes can be demonstrated radiographically and other times requires a bone scan. A bony ridge along the medial or lateral aspect of the insertion of the Achilles tendon may also be a source of heel pain. This bony ridge results in a mechanical problem, which results in chafing against the counter of the shoe.

The cause of heel pain can be multifactorial, but it is imperative that the clinician accurately diagnose it and direct the treatment accordingly. In general, treatment consists of nonsteroidal antiinflammatory medications, relief of stress over the involved bony prominence, use of a soft orthotic device in the shoe to relieve the heel, cast immobilization, or some combination of these. As a general rule, surgery is not necessary for heel pain. There certainly are exceptions to this, but the physician should be as conservative as possible in the management of heel pain.

Toenails

The two most frequent problems observed with toenails are ingrown toenails and a fungus infection known as *onychophytosis*. On rare occasions, a subungual exostosis may be a cause of toenail pain.

The ingrown toenail may be due to an intrinsic abnormality of the nail in which the nail is formed in an abnormal manner, resulting in the two edges of the nail pinching together. The other cause of an ingrown toenail is hypertrophy of the ungual labia, in which the skin grows up around the edge of the nail. In both these situations, the nail begins to grow into the skin, which results in an inflammatory reaction. If this is left untreated, a significant infection can result. The basis of treatment consists of removing the offending nail from the skin to allow the soft tissue inflammation to subside. Once this occurs, with proper nail care, the condition may resolve. Conservative management consists of permitting the nail to grow out over the skin, and if this occurs, the problem may resolve. If, however, the nail continues to grow into the skin, then surgical intervention should be considered.

The Winograd procedure generally resolves the problem. In this procedure, the medial or lateral margin of the nail is excised along with the nail bed. The only difficulty is that a nail horn forms in about 5% to 10% of cases, which may require further treatment. If the nail itself is deformed, the entire nail may be ablated and the nail bed removed. Simple avulsion of the nail, as a general rule, is not indicated because when the nail grows back, it generally becomes ingrown again. Treatment of the margin of the nail results in a much higher cure rate than excision of the entire nail.

Onychophytosis usually is managed conservatively by débridement of the nail. On occasion, the nail can become ingrown, but this is not common. If the problem is too severe, excision of the nail and nail bed, or a terminal Syme amputation, can be carried out. Simple avulsion of a nail with a fungal infection does not result in resolution of the problem.

Subungual exostosis can be painful and can result in a distorted-appearing nail. If the exostosis becomes too uncomfortable, the nail can be excised, although there is a propensity for the exostosis to recur if the base is not carefully curetted.

Annotated Bibliography

Mann RA. Surgery of the foot. St Louis, CV Mosby, 1986:1.
This general review article describes the biomechanics of the foot and ankle.

Disorders of the First Metatarsophalangeal Joint

Coughlin MJ. Arthrodesis of the first metatarsophalangeal joint with mini fragment plate fixation. Orthopaedics 1990;13:1037.
This article discusses the history of arthrodesis and the indications, surgical technique, results, and complications of this procedure.

Leventen EO. The chevron procedure: etiology and treatment of hallux valgus. Orthopaedics 1990;13:973.
This article discusses the indications, surgical technique, results of the chevron procedure.

Mann RA. Decision making in bunion surgery. AAOS Instruct Course Lect 1990;39:1.
This article discusses the basic concepts used and presents an algorithm that is helpful in the decision-making process in hallux valgus surgery.

Mann RA. Hallux rigidus. AAOS Instruct Course Lect 1990;39:15.
This review article discusses the etiology, physical findings, radiographic findings, and treatment of hallux rigidus using various techniques. It emphasizes cheilectomy and arthrodesis as the main surgical procedures.

Mann RA, Coughlin MJ. The great toe. In: The video textbook of foot and ankle surgery. St Louis, Medical Video Productions, 1991:145.
This book chapter presents a concise overview of hallux valgus surgery, including the indications, surgical technique, and complications of various surgical procedures.

Mann RA, Coughlin MJ. Hallux valgus: etiology, anatomy, treatment and surgical considerations. Clin Orthop 1981;157:31.
This article discusses treatment of the hallux valgus deformity using the distal soft tissue procedure. It points out the technical aspects of the procedure, results, and complications.

Mann RA, Rudicel S, Graves S. Hallux valgus repair utilizing a distal soft tissue procedure and proximal metatarsal osteotomy: a long term result. J Bone Joint Surg 1992;124:74A.
This is a detailed analysis of the surgical technique, postoperative results, and complications of a review of 109 operative procedures in 75 patients.

Plattner PF, Van Manen JW. Results of Akin type proximal osteotomy for correction of hallux valgus deformity. Orthopaedics 1990;13:989.
This article discusses results of the Akin procedure on a series of patients. It points out the indications and complications of this procedure.

Shereff MJ, Bejjani FJ, Kummer FJ. Kinematics of the first metatarsophalangeal joint. J Bone Joint Surg 1986;68A:392.
This article describes the motion of the first metatarsophalangeal joint in terms of its kinematics.

Lesser-Toe Deformities

Mann RA, Coughlin JM. Lesser toe deformities. In: The video textbook of foot and ankle surgery. St Louis, Medical Video Productions, 1991:37.
This concise book chapter reviews the various lesser-toe deformities. It discusses the definition, evaluation, surgical treatment, and complications of these various deformities.

Metatarsalgia

Mann RA. Intractable plantar keratosis. AAOS Instruct Course Lect 1984;33:287.
This article reviews the various types of callus formation on the plantar aspect of the foot. It outlines the conservative and operative management of these problems.

Mann RA, Reynolds JC. Interdigital neuroma: a clinical analysis. Foot Ankle 1983;3:238.
This article discusses the history, physical findings, and surgical procedure for treatment of the interdigital neuroma. It then analyzes the results of this procedure.

Postural Problems

Mann RA, Coughlin MJ. Postural problems of the foot. In: The video textbook of foot and ankle surgery. St Louis, Medical Video Productions, 1991:17.
This book chapter presents an overview of the various types of acquired flatfoot deformities. It points out the physical findings, methods of treatment, and technical aspects of surgery. The chapter further discusses the treatment of the cavus foot.

The Diabetic Foot

Wagner FW. The diabetic foot and amputations of the foot. In: Mann RA, ed. Surgery of the foot, ed 5. St Louis, CV Mosby, 1986:421.
This book chapter presents the problem of the diabetic foot along with a logical approach to treatment. It presents a series of algorithms that enables the clinician to better understand the various modalities of treatment of the diabetic foot.

Arthrosis of the Foot and Ankle

Mann RA, Coughlin MJ. Rheumatoid arthritis and arthrodesis about the foot. In: The video textbook of foot and ankle surgery. St Louis, Medical Video Productions, 1991:105.
This chapter describes the surgical treatment of the rheumatoid forefoot, presenting the various types of surgical procedures and postoperative care. It further discusses arthrodesis about the foot, which includes subtalar, talonavicular, and tarsometatarsal arthrodeses. It presents a discussion on triple arthrodesis and double arthrodesis.

Miscellaneous

Baxter DE, Pfeffer GB, Thigpen M. Chronic heel pain: treatment rationale. Orthop Clin North Am 1989;20:563.
This article discusses the various types of heel pain, methods of diagnosis, and conservative and operative management.

Index

Page numbers followed by *f* indicated illustrations; *t* following a page number indicates tabular material.